Proceedings of the XV Symposium Neuroradiologicum

Mutsumasa Takahashi · Yukunori Korogi · Ivan Moseley (Eds.)

Proceedings of the XV Symposium Neuroradiologicum

Kumamoto, 25 September – 1 October 1994

With 589 Figures (1118 Separate Illustrations) and 154 Tables

Springer

Professor Mutsumasa Takahashi
Chairmann, Department of Radiology
Kumamoto University School of Medicine
1-1-1 Honjo
Kumamoto 860
Japan

Yukunori Korogi
Assistant Professor
Department of Radiology
Kumamoto University School of Medicine
1-1-1 Honjo
Kumamoto 860
Japan

Dr Ivan Moseley
Director, Lysholm Department of Radiology
National Hospital for Neurology and Neurosurgery
Queen Square
London WC1N 3BG
United Kingdom

This book appears as a supplement to the journal **Neuroradiology** Volume 37/1995

ISBN 978-3-642-79436-0 ISBN 978-3-642-79434-6 (eBook)
DOI 10.1007/978-3-642-79434-6

Typesetting: Elsner & Behrens GmbH, Oftersheim

SPIN: 10474405 21/3130 – 5 4 3 2 1 0 – Printing on acid free paper

Foreword

Since the introduction of computed tomography in 1972, there have been considerable technical developments in neuroradiology, and the practice and content of our profession have changed markedly. Magnetic resonance imaging continues to expand in many areas of neuroradiology, replacing to a major degree the classical procedures such as angiography, computed tomography, functional radionuclide imaging and even some of the interventional neuroradiological techniques. The latter, on the other hand, are expanding in turn and have already become a major part of our speciality.

The XV Symposium Neuroradiologicum was held in Kumamoto, Japan, from 25 September to 1 October 1994, so that workers from around the world could report on and discuss the developments in neuroradiology since the previous Symposium in London in 1990. The 370 proffered papers accepted for presentation included almost 150 oral communications and about 220 posters. On this occasion an emphasis was placed not only on scientific communications, but also on educational programmes.

This volume contains the 266 papers accepted for publication from among the profferend papers, plus three special "New Horizons" lectures. The editors and publishers have made every effort to ensure that the proceedings have appeared as promptly as possible, while the contents are still of most value to the neuroscience community.

Our special gratitude is expressed to Professor Koichi Yamaguchi and Drs Tadayuki Maehara and Tadatoshi Tsuchigame for their support in publishing this volume. Thanks are also due to Nell Graville, Louisa H. Millar, Hannah Moseley, Jessie North and Chrissie Young for their editorial assistance.

Professor Mutsumasa Takahashi
President, XV Symphosium Neuroradiologicum
Kumamoto, September 1994

Contents

New Horizons Special Lecture I

New techniques/functional MRI

MRA

Vascular

Neoplasms

Degenerative

Inflammation

White matter, trauma, epilepsy

Paediatrics

Spine

Sella

Orbit

Head and neck

New Horizons Special Lecture II

New Horizons Special Lecture III

Intervention: aneurysms

Intervention: angioplasty

Intervention: fistulae

Intervention: AVMs

Spinal fistulae

Gamma knife

Contrast media

CT technique

Nuclear medicine

List of Authors

New Horizons Special Lecture I

Neuroradiology: its present science – its future challenges

D. C. Harwood-Nash

The Hospital for Sick Children, Toronto, Canada

Abstract. Neuroradiology is at the forefront of medicine, exciting and often turbulent, and at times most challenging. Not only has its advance been extraordinary, but the present and potential expansion of diagnostic and therapeutic capabilities of neuroradiology is taking us into areas never before conceived of. Genetics, neurophysiology, neurochemistry, computed 3D – guided surgery, endovascular therapy and magnetic source imaging are only a few of the noteworthy arenas – indeed, true new horizons. Concomitant has been the maturation and growth of neuroradiological societies worldwide and the birth of many new ones. These are attended by an increasing awareness of and concern with matters political, societal, financial and educational. The increasing need to speak with one voice, the voice of all neuroradiology, may even transcend individual national or even continental concerns. Communications, standards, journals, continuing education, research and specific professional qualifications need to be strengthened. The evolution and birth of the new World Federation of Neuroradiological Societies at this symposium, and its incorporating of future symposia with new directions, will provide a foundation matrix to accommodate the above matters successfully. This will ensure the continuing growth and strength of neuroradiology world-wide well into the next century.

Key words: Neuroradiology – Advances – World Federation – Societies, international

There is a tide in the affairs of men,
Which taken with the flood,
Leads on to fortune ...
We must take the current when it serves,
Or lose our ventures.

Shakespeare, *Julius Caesar* IV, iii

As we enter the second half of the last decade of this century, the extraordinary and revolutionary development and advance of neuroradiology are apparent. With such success of its present science, come the inevitable probabilities of future challenges. This XV Symposium Neuroradiologicum provides a most suitable forum and a most propitious time to reflect on the present, and to evolve a qualified consideration of our future, a future of neuroradiology as a whole and within its many parts and associations. This is for me not only a great privilege, but my personal view and perspective, anticipations and indeed fears. Couched in words of intense pride for our history, its legacy and its consequences, are one man's expectations, possibly delphic, yet hopefully pragmatic for what is to come in neuroradiology, its new horizons. It is a personal credo. Many other valid ideals and expectations surely exist, and many colleagues are certainly far more sophisticated technically and scientifically than I.

Present science

Neuroradiology is a vital, clinical and academic pursuit. It has had a remarkable period of growth from a relatively recent birth within medicine to its present maturity, one of extreme rapidity and success. This growth is not only in clinical stature, but in the sophistication of modern technical advances applied to the central nervous system (CNS), in research and computer techniques. MRI had their major, indeed revolutionary, impact upon the CNS, to be associated similarly with surgical angiography, and now the emerging functional imaging of the brain.

It is undoubtedly with some wistfulness that senior neuroradiologists look back upon the simpler but effective physical efforts and creativity required in the past for CNS imaging by air and contrast pneumencephalography and ventriculography, direct puncture and brachial retrograde angiography, and oil and air contrast myelography. Such efforts, albeit with some morbidity, demonstrating surface and vascular anatomy of the CNS, demanded an exquisite knowledge of this anatomy – knowledge that today regrettably seems to be falling short, a deficiency probably due to the technical ease of demonstration of an image per se and the detection often direct and dramatic of intraparenchymal abnormalities, a detection not available in previous years when they relied on the secondary effects on surface, ventricular and vascular and skeletal anatomy.

A number of outstanding pioneers of neuroradiology documented the growth of our specialty from those earlier days [1, 2], then through the decades [3–5] and often presented at a previous Symposium Neuroradiologicum [2, 6], dealing with both North America [3, 5] and Europe [7]. From pneumencephalography and ventriculography evolved CT, MRI and now 3D renditions of exquisite elegance. Direct angiography begat selective, then superselective, Seldinger technique catheter angiography with coils, glue, emboli, stents and again associated 3D and MR vasculography. From angiographic vascular

Correspondence to: D. C. Harwood-Nash, 555 University Avenue, Toronto, Ontario M5G 1X8, Canada

flow, and CSF flow by air or contrast, now come Doppler ultrasound and MR flow vasculography, often still not as comprehensive as the old and more invasive techniques. The ubiquitous "functional imaging" now embraces spectroscopy, PET and SPECT, regional O_2 utilization on MRI, and echoplanar MR techniques with the exciting potential of diffusion (cerebral ischemia and myelination) and perfusion imaging (cerebral blood flow and cortical activity). Intraparenchymal CSF flow still remains a mystery, as do the exact sequelae to intraventricular obstructive hydrocephalus and its resultant fluid disturbance within the brain substance or indeed its many pathways of absorption. Attendant emerging techniques for investigating brain activity, especially useful in charting cortical or deep anatomical activity, normally and in epilepsy, are magnetic source imaging and an increased tissue characterization using magnetic transfer imaging, as examples of significant advances. Sophisticated multihead gamma cameras and SPECT provide very precise and affordable functional images of the brain. Spectroscopy and PET are still undergoing lengthy evaluation studies towards their potential impact on neuroradiology as a whole, especially relative to neoplasm specificity and cortical mapping, and metabolic brain diseases as examples. The gamma knife and the operative "wand", in concert with sophisticated 3D imaging, are and should be involving the neuroradiologist at the forefront of these techniques. New intraoperative open MR equipment is now in clinical trials. New contrast agents are being directed at a cellular level.

Increasing sophistication of MR equipment and the rapidity by which new sequences and techniques emerge and change are seen week by week. Thus the catchword "functional imaging" is now embracing the CNS with a whirlwind of enthusiasm, technical sophistication and indeed challenges, truly if anything a tide in the affairs of medicine which neuroradiology must take at its flood in order to lead to scientific and clinical fortune. Neuroradiology is not just a technical art, it is a clinical science. Direct involvement in these advances, with expertise and knowledge and the dedication of the necessary time, is a major mandate for neuroradiology in the future.

Future challenges

The sea that is medicine is a wide, turbulent and often threatening are a fraught with political and economical shoals, yet with many fruits, surprises, calm waters, favorable winds and currents. How does one not only just keep up with the tides, but improve and sail better than others, and man one's clinical and academic ships with the best and most qualified possible? Not only must this be in clinical science and research but also in the very body politic of neuroradiology.

Clinical and scientific neuroradiology

The veritable avalanche of new techniques such as holography and other energy source imaging techniques on the horizon (microwave, heat, endogeneous magnetic fields, etc.) and the increasing sophistication of digital and filmless imaging, new vascular occlusion methods and the emerging direct endovascular scopes are, among others, significant new challenges. Physicists, machines, and computer consoles may perform the work. The neuroradiologist is in danger of being relegated, after the fact often, to reportage. Yet no man or woman can be everything to everyone. Areas of defined expertise and interest, often the finely focused, may soon occupy the majority of one's efforts and knowledge day to day. Future formal clinical neuroscience imaging divisions will need more and more people each doing a smaller spectrum of tasks, yet fully occupied but exquisitely trained and expert. Widespread freestanding neuroscience imaging departments may indeed become appropriate. Can there or will there be a place for the "general" neuroradiologists? Yes indeed, with increased clinical expertise commensurate with increased technical sophistication, but in more narrowed and basic diagnosic spectrum.

Innovations in contrast-tagged directed antibodies which are able to be imaged; new fluid flow techniques within the brain substance and cord; genetic disease being better defined and quantified; increased understanding of CNS metabolic disturbances, indeed new ones being identified with their cellular CNS sequelae, are all rapidly evolving. These are often outstripping our knowledge and capabilities of diagnosis even with good imaging. Specificity must soon parallel sensitivity. Is in vivo cellular imaging – virtual microscopy – near at hand? Probably.

Energy, innovation, realism and preparedness are probably the catchwords of the next decade for neuroradiologists and our colleagues. The general neuroradiologists in community clinical practices will undoubtedly still be essential but will have to become better informed and sophisticated. The academic center neuroradiologists, head and neck radiologists and interventional angiographers will have to become more finely focused practitioners, will have to know a lot more about less – by necessity, by circumstance and by demand. An increasing involvement upfront within all these areas of advancement and especially research in the neurosciences and related services is essential and becoming increasingly so [4].

No more can neuroradiology be questioned "What is your substance, whereof are you made, what millions of strange shadows on you tend" (Shakespeare, *Sonnet 53*). Not only are neuroradiologists, surgical cerebral angiographers, head and neck radiologists becoming prime management physicians as well as diagnostic imagers, but there is an important concomitant recent and growing development of subspecial interests, talents and clinical direction in pediatric neuroradiology and spine imaging. Such partners and offsprings now play a significant and identified part not only in neuroradiological but also in major general radiological meetings and educational organizations. *They must be kept within the body of neuroradiology.* An extraordinary successful, fully integrated, combined European meeting of neuroradiology, head and neck radiology and interventional angiography took place in Zürich in 1991, to be followed in North

America by a conjoint meeting of similar persuasions in 1993.

What of our sister persuasions of neurosurgery and neurology? Both are powerful and historically mature. Both, together with those clinicians and surgeons dealing with abnormalities of head and neck, eye, cancer and bone refer patients to neuroradiology for diagnosis and/or management. The question, however, must be put – if a diagnostic procedure is affordable and technically "button pressing" easy; if the knowledge of anatomy and pathology by those performing it good as it is in the above specialists; if one is the prime responsible physician – is it necessary to send the patient to anyone else? These questions are current in many countries and continents, in some more than in others. The rationale for neuroradiologists, head and neck radiologists, and surgical cerebral angiographers to be the prime practitioners of imaging techniques and their related procedures together with it essential requirements, provides a four-part response.

1. It is often not only the diagnostic technique that suffices, but judgment of imaging priorities and appropriateness is essential; a knowledge of and familiarity with all possible single or composite imaging techniques is mandatory. It is only neuroradiology and its associates with, however, optimum knowledge of anatomy and pathology that can accommodate this large spectrum day by day, a spectrum increasing in scope and sophistication week by week.
2. It necessitates a comprehensive, prolonged, specific and sophisticated period of training in all imaging modalities to achieve this. This experience must be performed with and taught by full-time practitioners, neuroradiologists and their associated persuasions.
3. A comprehensive and complete knowledge of anatomy, pathology, the metabolic, genetic, the clinical and surgical principles of the CNS and its diseases at all ages, together with those of associated spine and head and neck, is essential. An in-depth knowledge of the many variations of "normal" artifacts and the nuances of anatomical and pathological abnormalities that are so commonly shown on diagnostic imaging techniques present and emerging is essential and can only be obtained by comprehensive training. It is the cumulative knowledge and its wide spectrum that are paramount. It is the integration of "functional" with anatomical imaging that is essential. It is in neuroradiology and its associated persuasions that this must be accomplished.
4. Research within imaging and angiographic techniques relative to the investigation of anatomy and its disordered pathology must be based on sound scientific, technical and clinical bases. This can be only achieved by the leadership of neuroradiologists in coordination with physics, engineering, physiology, pathology, genetics, neurosurgery and neurology in particular. The imaging essessment of genetic and metabolic diseases, the anatomical bases of epilepsy, CSF flow, all embracing functional image is a major focus for the future. The planning and performance of intraoperative imaging must be a combined endeavour. Advances in molecular biology within disease processes of the CNS must have the relative imaging modalities (PET, MRI, spectroscopy) incorporated into neuroimaging. Such leadership and coordination is best initiated by neuroradiology and its associates.

It is thus apparent that, if these are true – and I believe them to be so – and if they are to continue to strengthen and expand, there is an essential need within neuroradiology and its associated persuasions of head and neck radiology and surgical CNS angiography worldwide for a vehicle whereby our professional societies can form a cohesive and constructive collegium. It is also apparent therefore that for neuroradiology best to invest this extraordinary history and legacy of expansion, excellence and innovation, it must continue to be the best, the best in training and education, in diagnostic and interventional techniques, in safety, in accuracy, in clinical and applied research.

This excellence must evolve at the residency and fellowship level, advance through academic, clinical and research centers, and then embrace national, continental and international societies.

International neuroradiology for the 21st century

To meet these many challenges worldwide; to maintain, indeed enhance, neuroradiology's high profile in the neurosciences; to adapt to the changing requirements of education, especially those of the new young breed of neuroradiologists; to assist the many and varying goals of individual national or international neuroradiological and allied societies, the World Federation of Neuroradiological Societies (WFNRS) [8] has been formally, constitutionally and legally inaugurated at this XV Symposium Neuroradiologicum in Kumamoto, Japan, September 1994.

The basic objective of the WFNRS is providing such a collegium, yet preserving the independence and mosaic of priorities of member societies, is the advancement of neuroradiology in all its aspects and the representation of neuroradiology throughout the world in matters of common interest by: establishing and maintaining *cooperation* between neuroradiological organizations and those of its allied persuasions worldwide; directing and enhancing the *prominent position* of neuroradiology within the radiological community through the appointment of leaders in neuroradiology worldwide as officers and committee members of the Federation; exchanging and *disseminating* knowledge and ideas in the field of neuroradiology; developing the best possible *standards* of neuroradiological facilities and practice; recommending and encouraging optimum standards of *education, training, and research* in neuroradiology and its allied sciences; providing appropriate neuroradiological *training and education* in allied countries requesting aid; facilitating *personal associations* between neuroradiologists throughout the world; and supporting scientific *symposia* and annual *scientific meetings* of member neuroradiological organizations in such a way that neuroradiology will keep its organizational and medical integrity intact. Neuroradiology must thus maintain and defend its integrity from influences which may arise within radiology in general or from without, from other neuroscience specialties. This collective international strength and wisdom is not only now mandatory, but provides a template and firm foundation for our younger members who, in the near future, will be our leaders. Such a coordinated and ordered organization must be able readily to react as future circumstances demand, must be innovative, not only to adapt but also to chart the future. Our present collective strength is remarkable in its potential.

The WFNRS also has a unique opportunity, based on the wealth of expertise and innovation in neuroradiology teaching throughout many countries through its members societies, and by embracing the Symposium Neuroradiologicum with its new formal foundation and future as the Federation's academic arm, to provide further leadership and new models for world education. A sensitivity toward the economics of travel and congress organization, and the present and potential rise in numbers of neuroradiologists and demands for neuroradiology worldwide, especially outside Europe and North America, is essential. From within the Symposium Neuroradiologicum, the major neuroradiological societies in North America, Europe and elsewhere, and our affiliated persuasions coordinated by the WFNRS, must soon evolve a new foundation of education suitable for increasing and varying needs. The demands and changing philosophies of the new breed of neuroradiologists must be accommodated, especially in rapidly developing countries. With what priorities and form should future symposia take, being the academic arm of the WFNRS? Is a periodic all-inclusive megameeting appropriate, one of such an excellence and scope as to be the only meeting worldwide that year? What are the position and future goals of the major societies in this context? Is the development of outreach programs for training and education appropriate to some member societies a priority?

What part should electronic techniques and transmission of communication and education take? As we near the 21st century, the stimulation and support of increased research, the attraction of the best trainee candidates, education, together with economic, political and professional challenges are priority concerns. The WFNRS will provide a vehicle for comprehensive and successful management, communication and enhancement of these principles and for approaching these questions, and thus provide effective collective wisdom and leadership.

The present science of neuroradiology is captivatingly exciting. The future challenges from all quarters are formidable but can, as before, be met and more. All of neuroradiology, head and neck radiology, and interventional neuroangiography, together with the Symposium Neuroradiologicum, assisted by the WFNRS, now have a unique opportunity to chart together an appropriate and successful course.

'Wouldst thou' – so the helmsman answered –
'Learn the secret of the sea?
Only those who brave its dangers
Comprehend its mystery!'

Longfellow, *The secret of the sea*

References

1. Bull JWD (1961) History of neuroradiology. Br J Radiol 34:69–84
2. Fischgold H, Bull JWD (1967) A short history of neuroradiology. In: Proceedings of the VIII Symposium Neuroradiologicum, Paris
3. Taveras JM (1980) The development of neuroradiology in the United States. AJNR 1:1–2
4. Taveras JM (1990) Neuroradiology: past, present, future. Radiology 175:593–601
5. Gutierrez C (1981) The birth and growth of neuroradiology in the USA. Neuroradiology 21:227–237
6. Greitz T (1987) The Symposium Neuroradiologicum. Acta Radiol 28:1
7. Cabanis EA (Ed) (1989) Contribution à l'histoire de la neuroradiologie européenne. Editions Pradel, Paris
8. Harwood-Nash DC (1991) The World Federation of Neuroradiological Societies: a proposal. AJNR 12:845–847

New techniques/ functional MRI

Diffusion-weighted MRI and perfusion echo-planar imaging in a rat stroke model

W. Reith [1], B. Elger [2], M. Forsting [1], S. Heiland [1], J. Seega [2], J. Weber [1], K. Sartor [1]

[1] Department of Neuroradiology, University of Heidelberg Medical School, D-69120 Heidelberg, Germany
[2] Biophysics, Knoll AG, D-67061 Ludwigshafen, Germany

Abstract. Two new MR techniques, diffusion-weighted imaging and perfusion imaging, are capable of displaying ischaemic areas within minutes after the onset of ischaemia. Ischaemia was induced in eight rats using the suture occlusion model. Reperfusion was achieved by withdrawal of the suture thread 1 h after permanent occlusion of the middle cerebral artery. Diffusion-weighted and perfusion images were acquired 30 min after vessel occlusion and 30 and 90 min after reperfusion. Infarction was confirmed and correlated to histology 24 h later. Both MRI techniques clearly demonstrated the ischaemic area within 30 min of vessel occlusion. After withdrawal of the suture, diffusion-weighted imaging showed a reduction in size of the ischaemic area. A delay in perfusion indicated the incompleteness of reperfusion and the persistance of an ischaemic area. The routine use of diffusion-weighted and perfusion MRI should allow rapid determination at the degree of ischaemia, including how much tissue can be salvaged and thus guide and optimise therapy.

Key words: Focal ischaemia – Reperfusion – Diffusion-weighted MRI – Perfusion imaging

New and more aggressive therapies for acute stroke require imaging methods capable of demonstrating the full extent of cerebral ischaemia as early as possible and of monitoring therapeutic strategies. One treatment strategy is the restoration of cerebral blood flow. Ischaemic brain injury may recover if blood flow is restored after a short period of ischaemia. Diffusion-weighted magnetic resonance imaging (DWI) is well established as a noninvasive method for early detection of cerebral ischaemia [1]. This technique also seems to be useful for monitoring the temporal and spatial evolution of early ischaemia at a time when T1- and T2-weighted images still appear normal. Combined with a model of experimental cerebral ischaemia, imaging methods such as DWI and perfusion imaging would be ideal for radiologists to monitor treatment effects [2].

Materials and methods

Focal cerebral ischaemia was induced in eight male Wistar rats using an endovascular occlusion technique of the middle cerebral artery

Correspondence to: W. Reith, Department of Neuroradiology, Kopfklinikum, University of Heidelberg Medical School, Im Neuenheimer Feld 400, D-69120 Heidelberg, Germany

Supported in part by the Deutsche Forschungsgemeinschaft (Ku 294/18-1), Germany

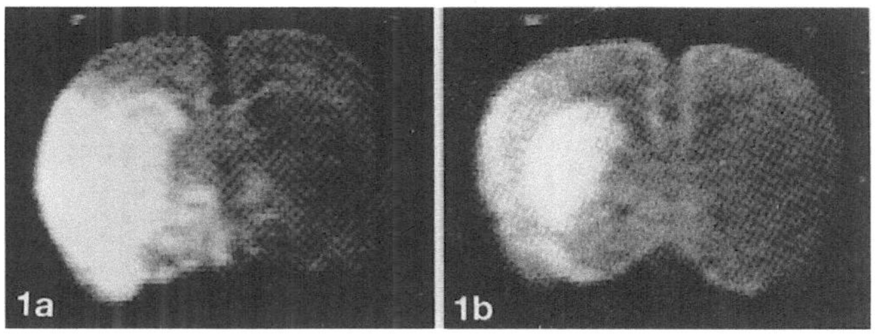

Fig. 1. Representative diffusion-weighted MRI (DWI) 30 min after middle cerebral artery (MCA) occlusion **(a)** and 30 min after reperfusion **(b)**. Before withdrawal of the nylon suture the hyperintense area involves both the caudoputamen and the adjacent neocortex on DWI. After withdrawal of the occluder, cortical hyperintensity reverts to nearly normal grey matter values.

(MCA) by inserting a nylon suture thread into the vessel [3]. Reperfusion was achieved by withdrawal of the suture after 1 h of occlusion. Thirty minutes after MCA occlusion coronal multislice DWI (TR 2000 ms, TE 45 ms, half-sine-shaped diffusion-sensitive gradient pulses with δ 10 ms and Δ 45 ms) were performed on a 2.0 T experimental MR scanner. Dynamic contrast-enhanced MRI studies, using echo-planar imaging (EPI) were performed after each DWI at a coronal slice (slice thickness 2 mm) through the optic chiasm. EPI scans were acquired at 1 s intervals over 48 s with bolus injection of 0.03 mmol/kg superparamagnetic iron oxide particles after the third image. The same MR protocol was used 30 and 90 min after reperfusion. Twenty-four hours after reperfusion the infarct area was determined by DWI, T2-weighted images (TR 2000 ms, TE 90 ms) and vital staining using the 2, 3, 5 triphenyl-tetrazolium-chloride (TTC) method.

Results

Both imaging techniques clearly detected the ischaemic area 30 min after MCA occlusion and furthermore showed a reduction of this area after reperfusion. By 30 min after MCA occlusion a hyperintense area was visible in both the lateral caudoputamen and adjacent neocortex (Fig. 1a), the area supplied by the MCA. DWI obtained 30 min after withdrawal of the occluder revealed a smaller hyperintense area, now only visible in the lateral caudoputamen (Fig. 1b). The hyperintensity in the adjacent neocortex reverted to nearly normal values for grey matter. TTC staining after 24 h showed the infarct to involve only the caudoputamen. DWI 30 min after MCA occlusion, 30 min and 90 min after reperfusion, and 24 h after reperfusion showed a marked reduction in lesion size after reperfusion (Fig. 2). Lesion size on DWI during reperfusion was less than during ischaemia and was reduced to 55% of the original area 24 h after reperfusion.

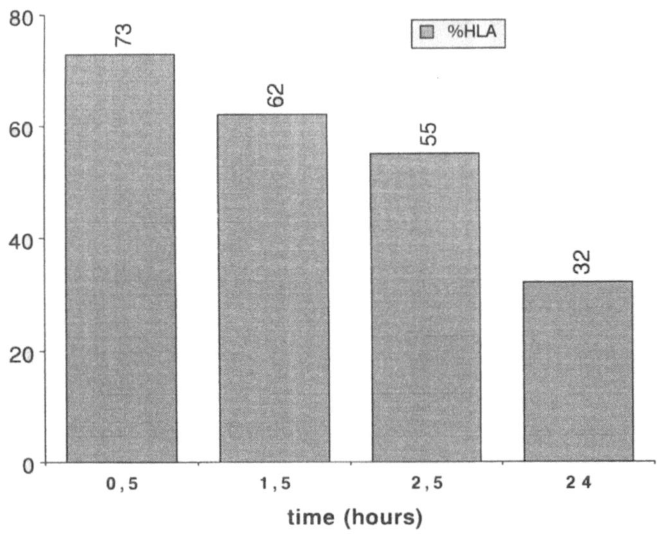

Fig. 2. Reduction of lesion size on DWI [percentage of hemisphere lesion area (%HLA)] 30 min after MCA occlusion, 30 min and 90 min after reperfusion and 24 h after reperfusion. The ischaemic area decreases significantly (55% reduction of %HLA)

Perfusion imaging revealed a perfusion deficit in the territory of the occluded MCA. Time intensity curves obtained in user-defined regions of interest in the ischaemic and nonischaemic hemispheres showed a decrease in signal intensity after bolus injection of iron oxide particles in the nonischaemic hemisphere, whereas in the nonperfused ischaemic region no signal alteration occurred. Time intensity curves of the same animal 30 min after reperfusion showed a delay, indicating that reperfusion was incomplete.

Discussion

DWI and perfusion EPI using superparamagnetic contrast agents are both capable of detecting cerebral ischaemia earlier than conventional MRI techniques. Perfusion studies qualitatively document hypoperfusion and reperfusion during and after temporary MCA occlusion. A delay in perfusion after reperfusion indicates incompleteness of reperfusion and persistence of ischaemia. DWI and perfusion imaging offer rapid, nonivasive, and quantitative ways to monitor the extent and degree of ischaemia. Because they can be employed very early after the onset of focal cerebral ischaemia, these techniques may be useful in assessing and adjusting cerebroprotective therapy while the ischaemic insult is still evolving. Furthermore, combined with an adequate model of focal cerebral ischaemia, these techniques can be used to monitor, in vivo, various aspects of therapy in acture stroke. Radiologists can use this tool to combine methodological and clinical research.

References

1. Minematsu K, Fisher M, Li L, Sotak CH (1993) Diffusion and perfusion magnetic resonance imaging studies to evaluate a noncompetitive *N*-methyl-D-aspartate antagonist and reperfusion in experimental stroke. Stroke 24:2074–2081
2. Rosen BR, Belliveau JW, Vevea JM, Brady TJ (1990) Perfusion imaging with NMR contrast agents. Magn Reson Med 14:1304–1311
3. Longa ZE, Weinstein PR, Carlson S, Cummins R (1989) Reversible middle cerebral artery occlusion without craniectomy in rats. Stroke 20:84–91

Comparison of conventional T2-weighted and diffusion-weighted MRI in identification of cystics lesion in the cerebrospinal fluid space

G. Y. Ko, D. E. Goo, H. K. Lee, D. C. Suh

Department of Diagnostic Radiology, Asan Medical Centre, University of Ulsan College of Medicine, Seoul, Korea

Abstract. We carried out 17 examinations to compare the utility of T2 (T2WIs) and diffusion-weighted (DWI) images for identification of cystic lesions in the cerebrospinal fluid space. Images were obtained at 1.0 T with T2-sequence (TR/TE = 2500/140 ms) and followed by the same scan parameters with additional diffusion-gradient pulses (4 mT/m; b value 250 s/mm^2). After visual comparison of 17 images, signals of the lesion, cistern, ventricle and parenchyma were measured for statistical analysis in 10 of them. In the visual comparison, all lesions were isointense to adjacent CSF on T2WI, but in 15 out of 17 the contrast was much improved on DWI. The difference in signal intensities between the lesions and the CSF was statistically significant on DWI ($P < 0.02$), but insignificant on T2-weighted images ($P > 0.10$). DWI can be more useful than T2WI in identification of cystic lesions in the CSF.

Key words: Brain – Magnetic resonance imaging – Diffusion study – Cysts

Correspondence to: G. Y. Ko, Department of Radiology, Asan Medical Center, University of Ulsan, 388-1 Poongnap-dong, Songpa-gu, Seoul 138-040, Korea

The application of strong diffusion-sensitizing gradients during spin-echo pulse sequences has been shown to be a

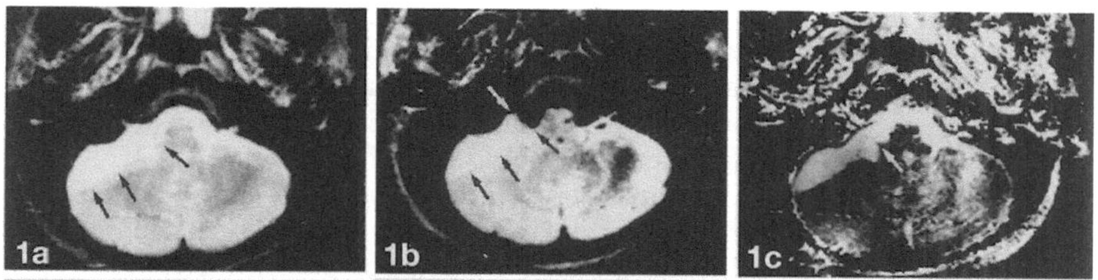

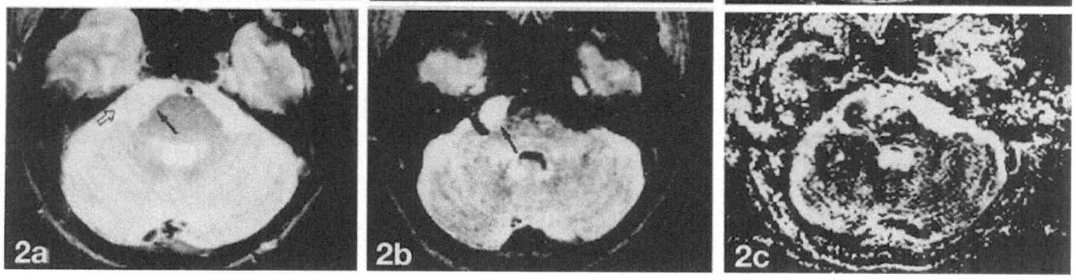

Fig. 1 a–c. An arachnoid cyst in the right cerebellopontine cistern (**a** T2WI, **b** DWI, **c** ADC image). The **a** right cerebellopontine cistern was widened, but the extent of the lesion was not apparent *(arrows)*. **b, c** The lesion's demarcation was obvious *(arrows)*. The signal from the lesion was higher than that of adjacent CSF on DWI and vice versa on an ADC image

Fig. 2 a–c. An epidermoid cyst in the right cerebellopontine cistern. **a** A suspicious mass *(arrow)* and mass effect on the right trigeminal nerve *(arrow)*. Lesion, cistern and ventricle were isointense. **b** The lesion demarcation and the contrast were much improved. **c** The signal intensity of the lesion was heterogeneously isointense to normal brain parenchyma *(arrow)*

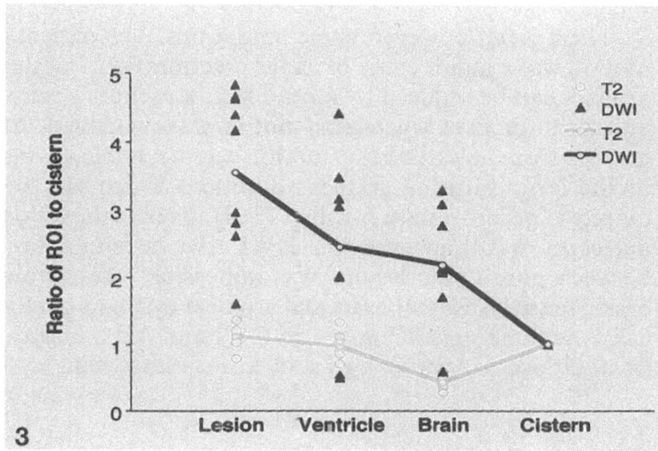

Fig. 3. The signal ratio curves of the lesions, ventricles and brain parenchyma to cisterns. The difference in signal intensity between the lesions and the CSF was markedly increased on DWI

method in which differences in molecular self-diffusion can be observed [1, 2]. The resultant diffusion-weighted images (DWI) were extremely sensitive to changes in the microscopic motions of water protons, and the contrast was proportional to the diffusion coefficient of tissues. Many preliminary studies of this technique have been reported showing utility of DWI in clinical applications [1–5]. The purpose of our study was to demonstrate the clinical utility of DWI in the identification of cystic lesions in the cerebrospinal fluid (CSF) space.

Materials and methods

We studied 17 lesions in 16 patients. These included 8 arachnoid cysts, 3 cisternal neurocysticercal cysts, two intraventricular cysts, one epidermoid cyst, one pineal cyst and two tumour-related cysts (a haemangioblastoma and a neurilemmoma). Ten lesions were surgically confirmed, and the rest were diagnosed by their typical MRI and laboratory findings.

Images were obtained at 1.0 T with a T2-weighted sequence (TR/TE = 2500/140 ms), followed by the same scan parameters with additional diffusion-gradient pulses (4 mT/m; b value = 250 s/mm^2) along the phase- and frequency-encoding axes. The study was performed without cardiac gating and the patient's head was immobilized by a sponge head rest with elastic bandage.

After visual comparison of the contrast between the lesion, the adjacent CSF space and parenchyma by two neuroradiologists, the signal intensities of the lesion, ventricle, cistern and parenchyma were measured in 10 cases. The difference in measured signal intensities was stastically analysed by a non-paired *t*-test.

Results

In the visual comparison, there was no difference between two reviewers. The 17 lesions were isointense to adjacent CSF on T2WI, but in 15, the contrast was much improved on DWI. In these, the lesions had higher signals than the CSF and parenchyma on DWI. Also, all lesions, except an epidermoid cyst, had higher signals than parenchyma but lower signals than CSF on apparent diffusion coefficient (ADC) images (Fig. 1). However, an epidermoid cyst was isointense to parenchyma on an ADC image (Fig. 2). An intraventricular cyst was isointense to CSF on DWI, but hypointense to ventricular CSF on ADC images, and so the demarcation was slightly improved. This finding corresponds with the CT ventriculography.

The average signal intensities of the lesions, ventricles, cisterns and parenchyma were 852 (standard deviation, 162) 772 (140), 722 (129), 317 (54) on T2WI, and 430 (99),

220 (97), 126 (76), and 246 (65) on DWI. The signal ratios of the lesions, ventricles and parenchyma to cisterns were 1.18, 1.07, 0.44 on T2WI and 3.41, 1.75, and 1.95 on DWI (Fig. 3). The difference in signal intensities between the lesions and CSF were statistically significant on DWI ($P < 0.02$), but insignificant on T2WI ($P > 0.10$).

Discussion

Tsuruda et al. have shown that DWI are highly sensitive to any motion, and bulk CSF flow contributes to accentuating image contrast between the cystic lesion and CSF [1]. In our study, DWI were able to show the lesion clearly in CSF (88-5), but also to determine if the lesion was cystic or solid by comparing the signals of the lesion and parenchyma. In fact, the signal of the epidermoid cyst, which was solid, was isointense to parenchyma on an ADC image.

There were, however, some limitations. The patient's motion was a major cause of image deterioration, but this artefact can be reduced by a head rest, a vacuum device, and sedation. Even when gross motion was controlled, the artefact from pulsatile brain motion was inevitable, owing to the long diffusion-gradient duration, which was required in order to raise b values [2, 3]. Even if the lesion detection was improved on DWI, the differentiation between pure cystic lesions was impossible. Arachnoid cysts, neurocysticercal cysts and a pineal cyst had practically the same signal changes on DWI and ADC images. In addition, a tumour cyst and a intraventricular cyst showed similar signal intensity on DWI and ADC images, but were not clearly differentiated from the adjacent CSF space. This finding was probably due to the stasis of CSF flow by obstruction, and if this phenomenon occurred, the lesion detection could be difficult.

In spite of these limitations, DWI showed good results for the detection of the lesion in the CSF space. Improved delineation was accentuated by pulsatile CSF flow. Therefore, invasive techniques such as cisternograhy or ventriculography can be avoided for evaluation of the CSF space. In conclusion, the DWI were valuable in the definition of the lesions that exist in the CSF space.

References

1. Tsuruda JS, Chew WM, Moseley ME, Norman D (1990) Diffusion-weighted MR imaging of the brain; value of differentiating between extraaxial cyst and epidermoid tumors. AJR 155:1059–1065
2. Bihan DL, Breton E, Lallemand D, Aubin ML, Vignaud J, Laval-Jeantet M (1988) Separation of diffusion and perfusion in intravoxel incoherent motion MR imaging. Radiology 168:497–505
3. King MD, Bruggen NV, Busza AL, Houseman J, Williams SR, Gadian DG (1992) Perfusion and diffusion MR imaging. Magn Res Med 24:288–301
4. Bihan DL, Turner R, Douek P, Patronas N (1992) Diffusion MR imaging: clinical applications. AJR 159:591–599
5. Henkelman RM (1990) Diffusion-weighted MR imaging: a useful adjunct to clinical diagnosis or a scientific curiosity? AJNR 11:932–934

Kinetic studies with echo-planar imaging

G. Krol, R. de la Paz, B. O'Malley

Memorial Sloan-Kettering and Cancer Center, New York, N.Y. 1002, USA

Abstract. With acquisition times in the millisecond range, echo-planar imaging is an ideal tool for scanning the actual motion or eliminating its detrimental effects. The technique appears to be sensitive to cerebrospinal fluid (CSF) flow and may be beneficial in the study of abnormal CSF circulation or obstruction of the pathways. The disadvantages of this technique include relatively long preparation time, offsetting the advantage of the intended total examination time reduction. The images are predominantly T2-weighted and the spatial resolution is rather low. At present, the Instascan is considered to be an experimental tool. The installation requires major hardware modifications and the modality has yet to be proven to cost effective.

Key words: Echo-planar imaging – Kinetic studies

Correspondence to: G. Krol

The major disadvantage of conventional MRI sequences is the long acquisition time. Even with fast sequences such as fast spin-echo (FSE), at least 2.5 min is needed to generate images of acceptable quality. Recently introduced Instascan echo-planar imaging allows very rapid, even real time image data acquisition.

Echo-planar images are acquired much more rapidly than conventional spin-echo images. The key difference acquisition is that conventional imaging requires a complete TR cycle for each of the phase-encoding steps to cover K-space, whereas the single-shot echo-planar imaging technique acquires the entire map of K-space in a single echo following a single radiofrequency excitation.

Materials and methods

We tested the Instascan in the assessment of kinetic motion in three healthy volunteers and one patient with a diagnosis of intracranial

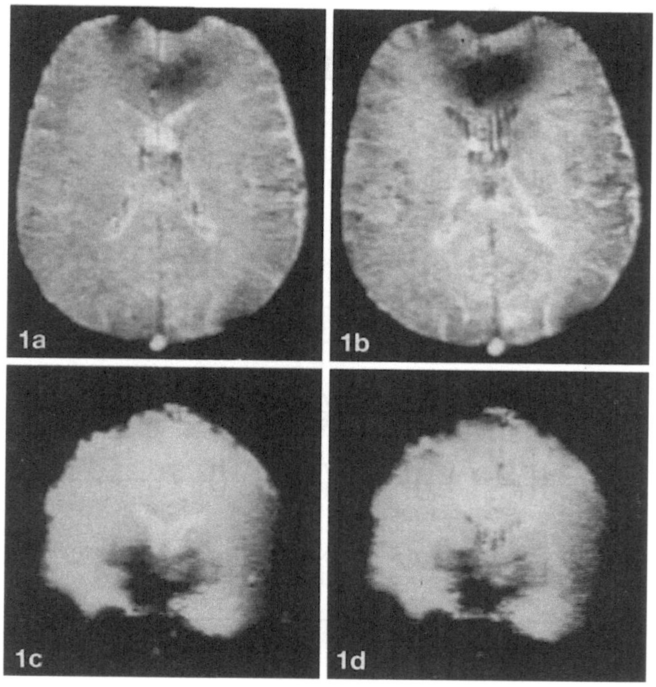

Fig. 1 a–d. Axial image of the head obtained during quiet breathing. **a** there is gradual overall loss of intensity through the sequence from the first to the last image, probably due to phase dispersion. There is an additional signal loss within the ventricles due to motion of CSF. This is more pronounced during a Valsalva maneuver. **b** A similar effect is noted on coronal images **(c, d)**

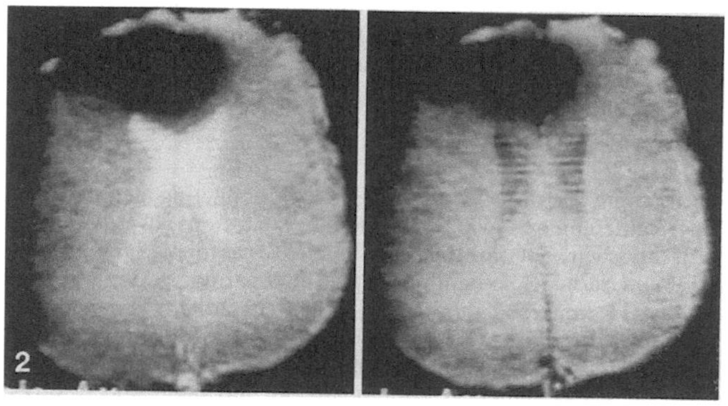

Fig. 2. Single axial acquisition, Valsalva maneuver applied in the middle of the sequence. The pattern of signal loss in this patient with low pressure hydrocephalus is increased compared to a normal volunteer

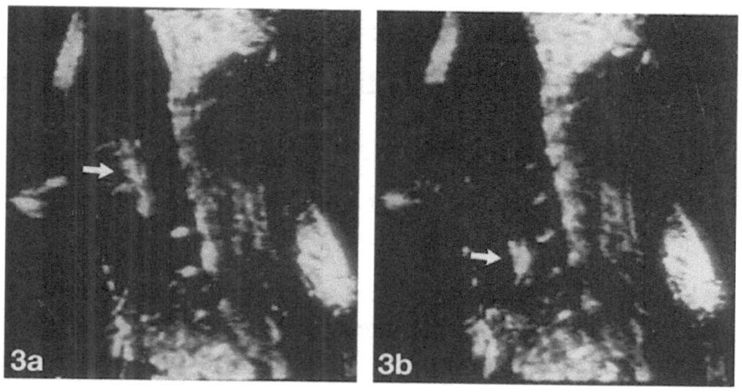

Fig. 3. Pharyngeal motion imaged immediately after swallowing one large bolus of water (progression of bolus is marked by *arrows)*

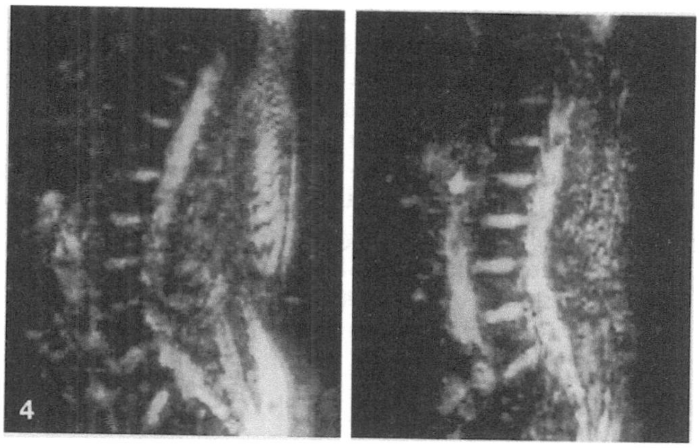

Fig. 4. Flexion and extension of the lumbar spine

hypotension. A single-shot gradient-echo sequence was used to assess cerebrospinal fluid (CSF) motion within the ventricular system of the brain (Fig. 1, 2), motion of the pharynx and larynx during swallowing (Fig. 3), movements of temporomandibular joints, flexion and extension of the spine (Fig. 4) and knee. A level of interest was chosen from a spin-echo localizing image. Slice thickness was 10 mm, TR 150, TE 67 ms and flip angle 60°. A combination of 256 × 128 matrix with 40 × 20 cm field of view provided symmetrical pixels of 1.5 × 1.5 mm. Twenty Instascan images were acquired in 8 s. For the display, the speed was adjusted to 10–20 frames per s.

Discussion

With acquisition times in the range of milliseconds, Instascan is an ideal modality for imaging tissues in motion. There are many exciting clinical implications, for example, measurements of blood flow, functional studies of the cerebral cortex, cardiac action, etc. Some of the obvious benefits of EPI in pediatrics and in imaging uncooperative patients are the reduction or elimination of sedation or anesthesia.

Cystic brain masses: use of variable-bandwidth steady-state free-precession MRI

R. D. Tien, A. K. Osumi, G. J. Felsberg, J. MacFall, M. Bernstein, E. R. Heinz

Department of Radiology (Neuroradiology), Duke University Medical Center Durham, North Carolina, USA

Abstract. Our objective was to evaluate variable-bandwidth steady-state free-precession (VBSSFP) MRI in characterization of epidermoid tumors and arachnoid cysts. Axial conventional spin-echo and VBSSFP MR images were obtained in 12 patients with epidermoid tumors and 23 with arachnoid cysts and examined for ability to characterize these two lesions and to delineate lesion margin. On conventional spin-echo MRI, characterization of epidermoid tumor and arachnoid cyst was occasionally difficult, because of atypical cases. On VBSSFP MRI, lesion characterization was improved by recognition of two distinct patterns of internal texture and margins of the lesions could be separated from surrounding cerebrospinal fluid. The 25 operated cases confirmed the imaging impression. VBSSFP MRI complements conventional spin-echo imaging to help characterize epidermoid tumors and arachnoid cysts. The improved characterization of these cystic masses with VBSSFP MRI can help radiologists and surgeons establish more accurate preoperative diagnoses and more appropriate treatment plans.

Key words: Brain neoplasms – Cyst – Magnetic resonance, pulse sequences – Magnetic resonance, technology

In clinical practice, the separation of arachnoid cyst from epidermoid tumor is frequently a dilemma. Both lesions may follow cerebrospinal fluid (CSF) signal on all conventional spin echo MR sequences [1]; differentiation is also hampered by the presence of repeated hemorrhages and septations within arachnoid cysts which may mimic the inhomogeneity of epidermoid tumors [2]. Epidermoid tumors, although frequently lobulated, may also show a smooth external surface similar to arachnoid cysts [3].

Steady-state free-precession (SSFP) MRI has been described as useful in characterizing complex cystic masses of the brain; however, artifacts due to the motion sensitivity of the sequence may limit application and interpretation [4]. More recently, variable-bandwidth steady-state free-precession (VBSSFP) has been shown to provide similar lesion characterization as SSFP images but with decreased pulsatility artifacts [5].

Materials and methods

MRI was carried out on 35 patients with cystic mass lesions of the brain suspected of being epidermoid tumor or arachnoid cyst. All studies were performed with a 1.5-T superconducting magnet. Axial T1-weighted images [600/20/2 (TR/TE/excitations)] were obtained with and without contrast medium (0.1 mmol/kg gadolinium-DTPA). Gradient-moment nulling without cardiac gating was used on long TR images (2800/30, 80/1). In all 35 patients, axial volume VBSSFP MR images were obtained by using the following parameters: 25-30/40-56/2 (TR/TE/Nex), 256 × 192 matrix, 20-cm field of view, 2-mm slice thickness without gap, 90° flip angle, and 32 slices, with a scan time under 5 min (Fig. 1). The lesions were surgically confirmed in the 25 cases with definite symptomatology.

Correspondence to: R. D. Tien, Department of Radiology, Duke University Medical Center, Box 3808, Durham, North Carolina, USA

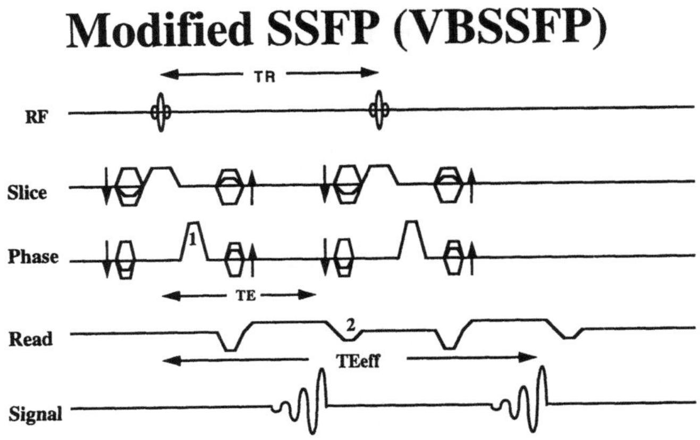

Fig. 1. Pulse diagram of axial variable-bandwidth steady-state free-precession (VBSSFP) sequence used in this study. The effective echo time (*TEeff*) is longer than the repetition time (*TR*) as each signal is the result of two successive excitations. Rephasing gradients are applied to maintain the steady state. As opposed to SSFP, the free induction decay in VBSSFP is dephased by a smaller crusher gradient (1) on the inplane axis, the readout dephase gradient (2) is smaller due to partial echo collection and the read gradient is smaller due to narrowed bandwidth. Using fractional echo-acquisition and small crusher gradients results in significantly reduced pulsatility and motion artifacts due to vascular and CSF motion; narrowing the bandwidth in this sequence compensates for loss in signal by fractional echo acquisition

Results

On the basis of the VBSSFP images, two discrete patterns of lesion appearance were seen. The first pattern (type 1) was characterized by lesion homogeneity; lesion signal was slightly hypointense to CSF centrally with a thin peripheral margin of hyperintensity (isointensity to CSF). This pattern was seen exclusively in all patients with arachnoid cysts (Fig. 2). In cases of large arachnoid cysts, additionally, a wavy pattern of hypointensity (to CSF) was seen centrally (Fig. 3). The second pattern (type 2) was characterized by lesion inhomogeneity; the lesion signal was more markedly hypointense to CSF. No peripheral margin of hyperintensity was seen and this pattern was

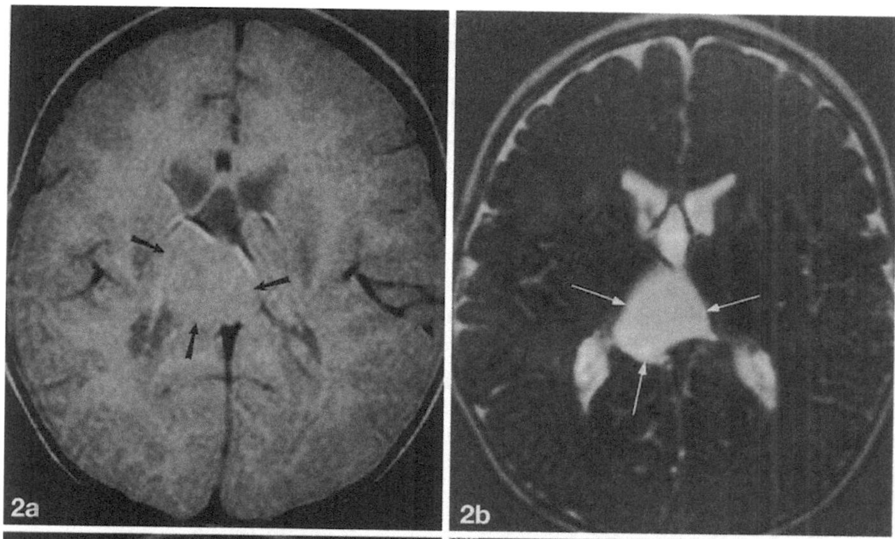

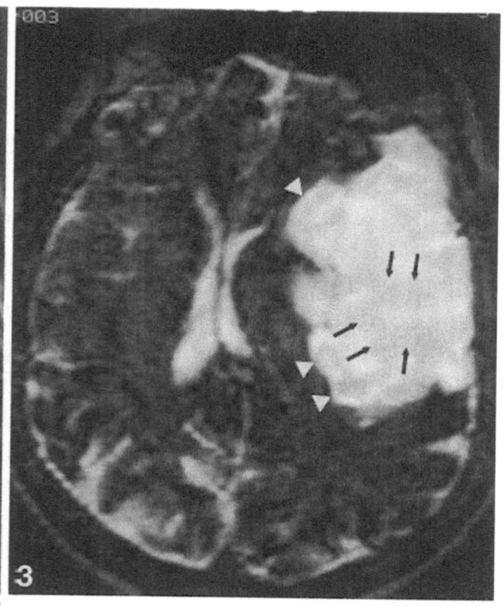

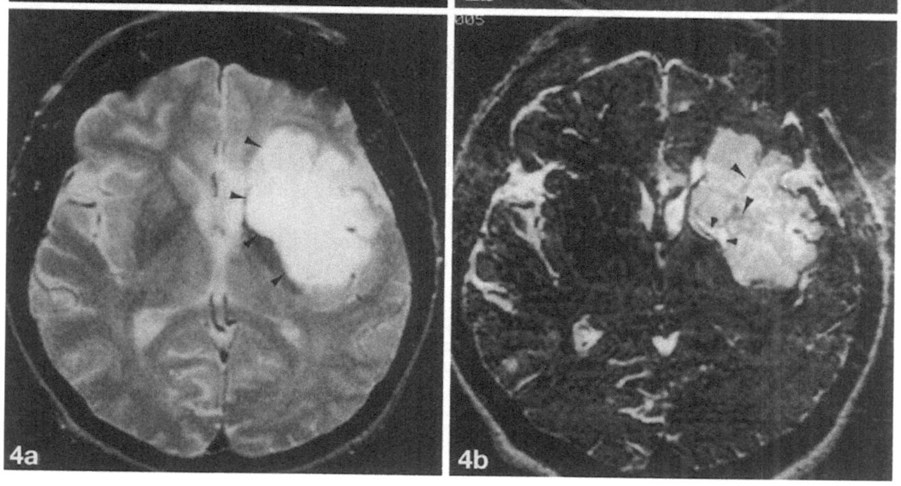

Fig. 2. Intraventricular arachnoid cyst in a 4-month-old boy. **a** T1-weighted image shows well-defined lesion in posterior third ventricle. Lesion is minimally heterogeneous and slightly hyperintense to ventricular CSF. No enhancement was seen after contrast medium. A proton-density image shows hyperintensity of the cyst (*arrows*) compared to ventricular CSF. T2-weighted image showed lesion homogeneity and minimal hyperintensity to ventricular CSF. **b** VBSSFP MRI shows type 1 pattern with homogeneous central hypointensity to ventricular CSF with marginal hyperintensity (*arrows*). Although the hyperintensity on proton-density spin-echo MRI was mildly atypical for an arachnoid cyst, the VBSSFP findings were typical and an arachnoid cyst was confirmed at surgery

Fig. 3. Large sylvian arachnoid cyst in a 51-year-old man. VBSSFP image shows type 1 pattern with lesion homogeneity and peripheral hyperintensity (*white arrowhead*). Note wavy pattern (*black arrows*) throughout cyst secondary to pulsation artifact. Arachnoid cyst was confirmed at surgery

Fig. 4a, b. Large sylvian epidermoid cyst in a 60-year-old woman. **a** T1-weighted image showed large, heterogeneous, lobulated lesion in left sylvian fissure slightly hyperintense to ventricular CSF. T2-weighted MR image shows lesion homogeneity and intensity similar to ventricular CSF. Smooth medial border (*arrowheads*) is slightly atypical for epidermoid tumor. **b** VBSSFP image shows type 2 pattern with lesional inhomogeneity and hypointensity to ventricular CSF. Linear regions of more pronounced hypointensity can be identified within the lesion (*large arrowheads*) consistent with lamellation. Note improved delineation of the tumor from the surrounding CSF (*small arrowheads*)

seen exclusively in epidermoid tumors (Fig. 4). Lace-like, more pronounced hypointense lamellations could be identified within the lesion. Depiction of the border between the lesion and the adjacent brain parenchyma or CSF in the ventricles, sulci, and cisterns was improved with VBSSFP when compared to conventional spin echo images; VBSSFP images consistently demonstrated one of the two patterns described above, in all cases allowing improved characterization of the lesions. All cases that went to surgery confirmed the preoperative diagnosis. However, on the basis of conventional spin echo, there were 9 patients with VBSSFP type 1 lesions and 2 patients with type 2 lesions who could not be confidently diagnosed preoperatively. The margins of all type 2 lesions could not be separated from surrounding CSF or post-operative encephalomalacia on conventional spin-echo imaging also.

Discussion

Specialized MRI pulse sequences have been used to further assist in differentiation of arachnoid cysts from epidermoid tumors. Recently, use of an SSFP MRI pulse sequence that exploits the T2 differences in cystic lesions has been reported and has been found to be of use in improving characterization of complex cystic masses [4]. However, there is still a moderate degree of motion sensitivity which can occasionally obscure accurate characterization of the internal architecture and the margins of lesions. The recent development of a modified SSFP MRI sequence (VBSSFP) has enabled generation of images with a definite decrease in pulsation-induced artifact without sacrificing extreme T2 weighting. It has been previously shown that use of VBSSFP results in images with significantly less pulsatility and motion artifact when compared to routine SSFP [5].

Using VBSSFP we were able to accurately characterize all lesions into two separate and distinct patterns. Type 1 pattern was seen in all cases of arachnoid cysts and larger arachnoid cysts showed, additionally, a distinct wavy pattern in which alternating regions of hypointensity and hyperintensity could be identified. Loss of signal within the arachnoid cyst on the VBSSFP images is likely due to pulsation-induced signal loss while the fluid along the periphery of the cyst is not subject to the same degree of motion and is therefore hyperintense. The wavy pattern demonstrated in larger arachnoid cysts reflects accentuated fluid motion within the cyst. Type 2 pattern was seen in all cases of epidermoid tumor. More pronounced linear regions of hypointensity could be identified within the lesion, suggesting a lamellated matrix. This corresponds to macroscopic pathologic observations in which progressive exfoliation of cholesterol crystals and keratinous material lined by squamous cell tissue, form lamellations within the cyst [6]. Accurate definiton of the border of the epidermoid tumor, or VBSSFP, was possible due to the high contrast differences between the lesion, the surrounding hyperintense CSF, and the markedly hypointense brain parenchyma.

In conclusion, although conventional spin-echo MRI may distinguish epidermoid tumor from arachnoid cyst in most cases, difficulty may arise in atypical cases or in the postoperative setting. Our results show that VBSSFP images are very helpful in further characterization of arachnoid cyst and epidermoid tumor and in delineation of the margins of these masses, adding confidence to imaging with conventional spin-echo MRI. The improved characterization of these cystic masses with VBSSFP MRI can help radiologists and surgeons establish more confident and accurate preoperative diagnoses and more appropriate treatment plans.

References

1. Osborn AG (1994) Diagnostic neuroradiology. Mosby, St. Louis, pp 633–635
2. Quint DJ (1992) Retroclival arachnoid cysts. AJNR 13:1503–1504
3. Goldberg HI (1991) Extraaxial brain tumors. In: Atlas SW (ed) Magnetic resonance imaging of the brain and spine. Raven Press, New York, p 365
4. Tien RD, MacFall J, Heinz R (1992) Evaluation of complex cystic masses of the brain: value of steady-state free-precession MR imaging. AJR 159:1049–1055
5. Tien RD, Bernstein M, MacFall J (1993) Pulsatile motion artifact reduction in 3D steady-state free-precession-echo brain imaging. Magn Reson Imaging 11:175–181
6. Russell DS, Rubinstein LJ (1989) Pathology of tumours of the nervous system, 5th edn. Williams and Wilkins, Baltimore, p 695

Restricted arterial expansion as a universal causative factor in communicating hydrocephalus

D. Greitz[1], J. Hannerz[2], B. M. Bellander[3], T. Hindmarsh[1]

[1] The Karolinska MR-Research Centre, Karolinska Hospital, Stockholm, Sweden
[2] Department of Neurology, Karolinska Hospital, Stockholm, Sweden
[3] Department of Neurosurgery, Karolinska Hospital, Stockholm, Sweden

Abstract. The cerebrospinal fluid (CSF) flow in the aqueduct and below the foramen magnum and the blood flow in the superior sagittal sinus (SSS) were examined in ten patients with communicating hydrocephalus and six controls, using cardiac-gated MR-phase images. The cervical CSF pulsations were found to be significantly decreased in communicating hydrocephalus reflecting a decreased expansion of the intracranial arteries, in accordance with a previous study. The stroke volume and the rise and delay times for the systolic peak in the SSS were also decreased, as was the pulsatility index for diastole. The reduced expansion of the arteries is regarded as the main causative factor in communicating hydrocephalus. According to the theory, any process that restricts this expansion, such as arterial disease and obstruction of the paravascular spaces, may cause communicating hydrocephalus. It is suggested that the same mechanism explains hydrocephalus accompanying obstruction of the subarachnoid space near the craniocervical junction as seen with cervical spinal stenosis and Chiari malformations.

Key words: Hydrocephalus – Arterial expansion – Cerebrospinal fluid, flow dynamics – Superior sagittal sinus, flow dynamics – Magnetic resonance imaging

Correspondence to: D. Greitz

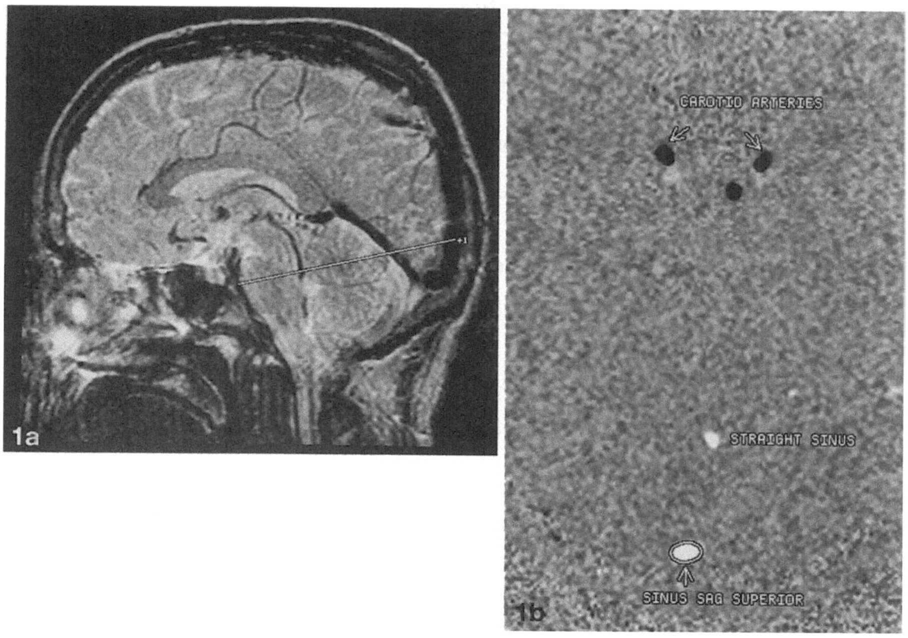

Fig. 1. Blood flow was studied in the distal parts of straight (SR) and superior sagittal sinuses (SSS) in a plane indicated by the *dotted line* **(a)**. The phase image **(b)** was used to estimate the flow perpendicular to the slice. Regions of interest were drawn to include the cross-sectional area of the vessel as shown in the SSS

Table 1. Clinical features of patients with communicating hydrocephalus

Patient	Dementia	Ataxia	Incontinence	Other symptoms
1	+	+	+	
2	+	+	+	
3	+	+	+	
4	+	+	+	
5	+	+	+	
6	+	+	+	
7	+			
8		+		
9	–	–	–	Dizziness
10	–	–	–	Headache, personality disturbance

In an MRI study of healthy volunteers [1] an analysis of intracranial hydrodynamics was made by applying the Monro-Kellie doctrine, which states that the sum of the intracranial volume of brain tissue, cerebrospinal fluid (CSF) and blood is constant at every moment. The main conclusions were that the cervical CSF flow reflects the expansion of the arteries and the flow in the aqueduct reflects the expansion of the brain. A pilot study of communicating hydrocephalus [2] has shown that the cervical CSF flow is decreased as compared to controls. This should imply a decreased expansion of the intracranial arteries. However, an almost significant increase of the aqueduct flow was also found. This was thought to be due to increased expansion of the brain in hydrocephalus causing large ventricular pulsations and an increased transmantle pressure gradient as well as ventricular dilatation. The present investigation was undertaken to test the validity of our previous findings.

Patients and methods

We examined ten patients with hydrocephalus (age 35–80 years, mean 64 years; Table 1) and six controls (age 39–73 years, mean 52 years). There were two patients without the classical symptoms of normal pressure hydrocephalus. The patients were examined on a 1.5 T MR imager using a standard head protocol. A retrospective cardiac gated cine phase sequence was used to measure the blood flow in the superior sagittal sinus (SSS) and in the straight sinus (SR). This sequence offered 24 images, covering the entire cardiac cycle. The slice thickness was 4 mm, with an in-plane resolution of 0.8 × 0.8 mm. The same sequence with a lower velocity encoding was used to measure the CSF flow in the aqueduct and below the foramen magnum at the level of C2.

In order to explore the alterations in the haemodynamics on the venous side, the flows were studied in the distal parts of the SR and SSS (Fig. 1a). Regions of interest were drawn to include the cross-sectional area of the vessel (Fig. 1b). Flow was calculated as mean velocity multiplied by the cross-sectional area. Pulsatile stroke volume, represented as the hatched area in Fig. 2a, was defined as the difference between the integrated total flow minus the lowest diastolic flow. Pulsatility was determined as described by Gosling and King [3]. The maximum vertical excursion of the flow profile divided by its mean height was used as the pulsatility index (Fig. 2b). The rise and delay times of the systolic peak were determined (Fig. 2c). An unpaired two-tailed *t*-test was used for statistical analysis.

Results

A highly significant decrease in cervical CSF flow was demonstrated in the hydrocephalic patients (Table 2) in accordance with the previous study. A tendency towards increased aqueduct flow was found, but this difference was not statisticaly significant. The stroke volume in the SSS (Fig. 2b) was reduced in the hydrocephalic patients (Table 3). The pulsatility index for systole was higher in the hydrocephalic group, but this finding was not significant (Table 4). The index for diastole, however, was

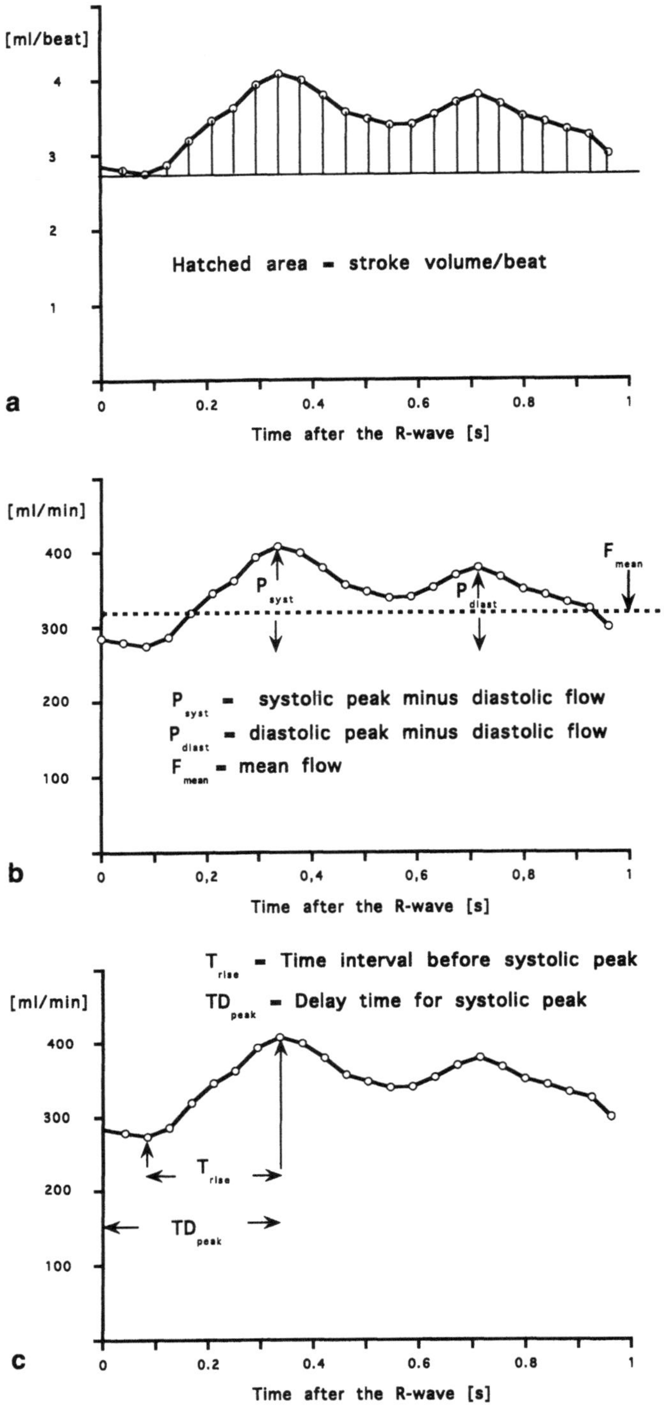

Fig. 2. a The stroke volume in the SSS (*hatched area*) defined as the total integrated flow minus the lowest diastolic flow. **b** The maximal excursion of the flow profile divided by its mean height was used as the pulsatility index. This index was used both for systole (P_{syst}/F_{mean}) and diastole (P_{diast}/F_{mean}). **c** The rise time and delay time for the systolic peak are indicated on the flow profile

significantly decreased. A shortening of the rise time and delay time for the systolic peak was found in the hydrocephalic group (Table 5). The blood flow in the SR and SSS did not differ between the two groups. However, when the two asymptomatic patients were excluded, the flow proved to be reduced in hydrocephalus (Table 6).

Table 2. CSF stroke volume ml/cardiac cycle

	Aqueduct	Foramen magnum
Normals	0.071	0.66
Hydrocephalus	0.091 (NS)	0.34 (P=0.0006)

Table 3. Pulsatile stroke volume in the superior sagittal sinus ml/beat ± SEM

Normals	0.93 ± 0.12
Hydrocephalus	0.67 ± 0.07 (P=0.05)

Table 4. Pulsatility index (PI) (peak flow minus diastolic flow divided by mean flow)

	PI systolic peak	PI diastolic peak
Normalsy	0.37	0.27
Hydrocephalus	0.47 (NS)	0.19 (P=0.03)

Table 5. Rise time (T_{rise}) and delay time (TD_{peak}) for the systolic peak of the SSS, ms ± SEM

	T_{rise}	TD_{peak}
Normals	294 ± 46	414 ± 49
Hydrocephalus	198 ± 12 (P=0.03)	295 ± 9 (P=0.009)

Table 6. Superior sagittal sinus (SSS) and straight sinus (SR) blood flow (ml/min) in the normal controls and the eight patients with classical symptoms of normal pressure hydrocephalus

	SSS	SR	SSS + SR
Normals	311	123	434
Hydrocephalus	233 (P=0.02)	92 (P=0.009)	325 (P=0.009)

Discussion

Our results confirm the earlier observations that the expansion of the intracranial arteries is reduced in communicating hydrocephalus. The decrease in the delay and rise times for the systolic peak in the SSS (Fig. 3) is believed to indicate a reduced compliance, causing increased pulsations intracranially. Increased pulsations have been demonstrated in animal experiments to cause hydrocephalus [4] and an up to six-fold increase in CSF pulse pressure has been found in patients with communicating hydrocephalus [5], although the mean CSF pressure is normal.

Our results may also offer an explanation for the reduced blood flow in communicating hydrocephalus. The venous counter pressure is thought to be essential for maintaining the normal cerebral blood flow. It is a well established fact in experimental hydrodynamics [6], that in certain circumstances, an increased outflow resistance, causing decreased perfusion pressure, may produce a paradoxically increased flow in collapsible vessels and vice versa. The decreased cervical CSF pulsations do not mean only a decreased filling of the spinal canal, but also a decreased refilling of the cranial cavity. This means reduced CSF pressure and reduced venous pressure during diastole in hydrocephalus. The reduced pulsatility in diastole corresponds to a decreased diastolic blood flow in the SSS. The decreased stroke volume in the SSS may also be caused by a reduced counter pressure.

This investigation supports the notion that reduced arterial expansion is the main aetiological factor in communicating hydrocephalus explaining both ventricular dilatation and the reduced cerebral blood flow. Accordingly any process which restricts arterial expansion – be it located in the vessel wall or in the paravascular spaces – may cause hydrocephalus. From this, it follows that the same mechanism may operate to cause hydrocephalus when there is an obstruction of the subarachnoid space at the level of the craniocervical junction, i. e. with cervical spinal stenosis (Fig. 4) or Chiari I and II malformations.

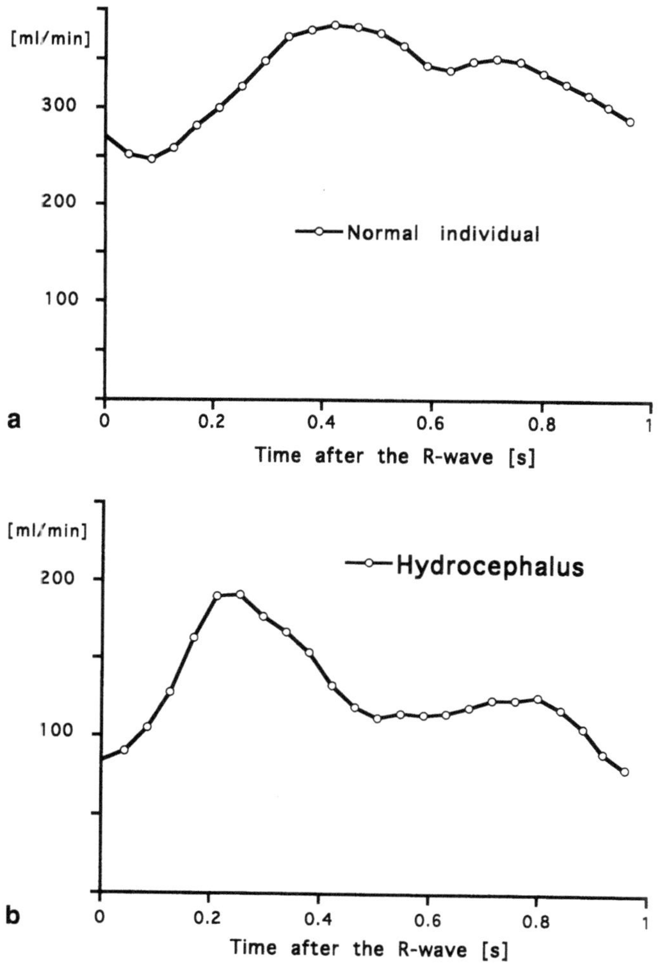

Fig. 3. Flow profile in the SSS of a normal volunteer **(a)** and a patient with hydrocephalus **(b)**. Note short rise and delay time for the systolic peak and the small diastolic peak in hydrocephalus

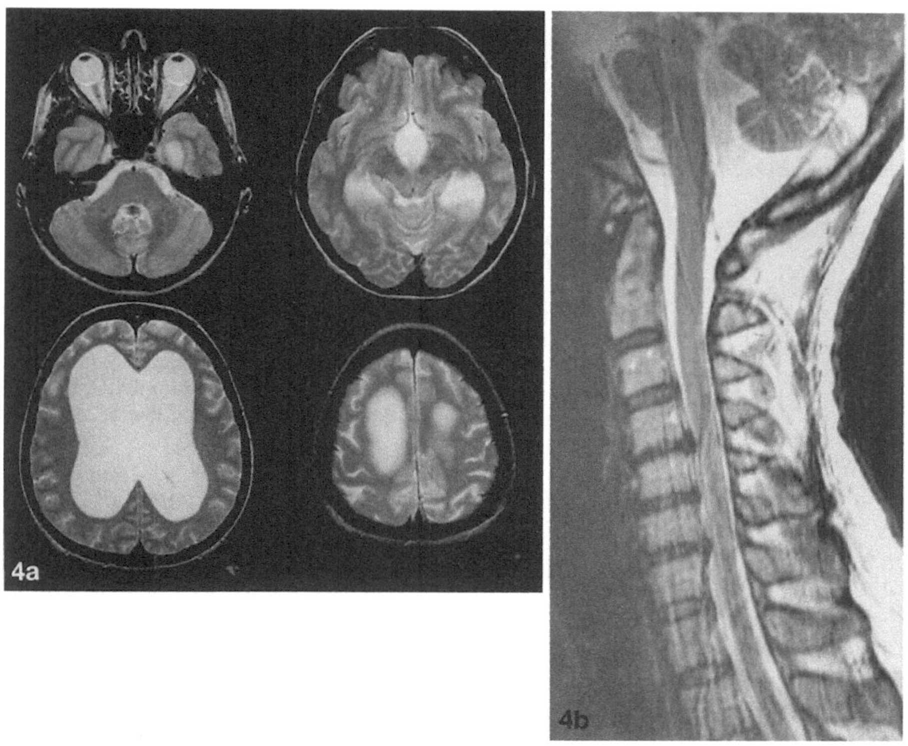

Fig. 4a, b. Patient 9. A 53-year-old, previously healthy woman presenting with dizziness and pain in the upper limbs. Marked hydrocephalus **(a)** and pronounced cervical spinal stenosis **(b)** were found. The cervical CSF pulsation was reduced (0.4 ml/beat). The cervical stenosis would restrict the CSF flow from the cranial cavity and decrease the intracranial compliance, causing decreased arterial expansion and hydrocephalus

References

1. Greitz D, Wirestam R, Franck A, Nordell B, Thomsen C, Ståhlberg F (1992) Pulsatile brain movement and associated hydrodynamics studied by magnetic resonance phase imaging. The Monro-Kellie doctrine revisited. Neuroradiology 34:370–380
2. Greitz D, Hannerz J, Rähn T, Bolander H, Ericsson A (1994) MR imaging of cerebrospinal fluid dynamics in health and disease. On the vascular pathogenesis of communicating hydrocephalus and benign intracranial hypertension. Acta Radiol 35:204–211
3. Gosling R, King D (1974) Arterial assessment of Doppler shift ultrasound. Proc R Soc Med 67:447–449
4. Di Rocco et al. (1978) Communicating hydrocephalus induced by mechanically increased amplitude of the intraventricular CSF pressure. Experimental studies. Exp Neurol 59:40
5. Ekstedt J, Friden H (1984) CSF hydrodynamics of the study of adult hydrocephalus syndrome. In: Shapiro K, Marmarou A, Portnoy H (eds) Hydrocephalus. Raven Press, New York, pp 363–382
6. Pedley TJ (1980) Flow in collapsible tubes. In Batchelor GK, Miles JW (eds) The fluid mechanics of large blood vessels. Cambridge University Press, Cambridge, pp 301–308

Brain plasticity in patients with central tumours: functional MRI and intraoperative electrophysiological mapping

T. Yousry [1], D. Schmidt [1], U. Schmid [2], A. Jassoy [1], D. Heiss [1], W. Eisner [2], M. Reiser [1]

[1] Department of Radiology, Ludwig Maximilians University, Munich, Germany
[2] Department of Neurosurgery, Ludwig Maximilians University, Munich, Germany

Abstract. Cortical representation of motor function anatomically is not static but shows a certain degree of plasticity. We wanted to detect the effect of a mass lesion in the central region on the motor hand area using functional magnetic resonance imaging (fMRI) and intraoperative motor mapping. We examined six patients and eight volunteers. The paradigm for fMRI and mapping was the opening and closure of the fist. In all volunteers and two patients the motor hand area was spotlike, and it was broader in three patients. In comparison to the relatively small representation areas found in healthy volunteers, tumours that lie in the vicinity of the motor hand area can induce its anatomical enlargement and displacement, most probably reflecting the brain's functional plasticity.

Key words: Tumour – Motor – Cortex – Magnetic resonance imaging

Functional MRI (fMRI) is based on the concept that a local increase in brain perfusion coupled with an unchanged oxygen consumption leads to a decreased concentration of deoxyhaemoglobin, thereby increasing the signal intensity. It was deduced that a local change in signal intensity located in the parenchyma and correlating in time with the onset and end of an specific task should correspond to the cortical representation of this activation. We have previously proven this assumption, by correlating fMRI with intraoperative mapping [1].

Somatomotor representation can be regarded as a flexible system, able to adapt to activity and behavioural changes. This capability is the basis for the potential of functional recovery after injury [2]. From intraoperative mapping we [3], and others [4], have found that a slow growing lesion can lead to a shift in the localization of functional representation. We wanted to assess the capability of fMRI to detect these changes.

Correspondence to: T. Yousry

Patients and methods

We examined eight volunteers and six patients (four gliomas, two cavernomas). The tumours were located in the central region, in or close to the precentral gyrus.

Imaging was performed on a 1.5 T imager. In order to evaluate the anatomical localization of the lesion, we performed a 3D FLASH sequence (RF spoiled, TR/TE 15/6 ms, FA 20°, FOV 200 mm). For MRI a 2D FLASH sequence (TR/TE 46.75/30 ms, FA 40°, FOV 200 mm, matrix 128×256 was performed. Twenty-seven measurements were obtained for each slice, 11 before, 6 during and 10 after an specific task: repetitive opening and closure of the fist.

For data analysis, we subtracted six summed pretask images from six summed task images. All bright areas were analysed. Those projecting into the parenchyma and showing a signal intensity change corresponding to the beginning and end of the task were further assessed. Based on their anatomical shape, they were divided into two categories: spotlike or broad. Intraoperative direct cortical stimulation [5] was performed on six of the patients immediately prior to tumour removal. Similarly, as outlined for fMRI, the motor hand area was defined and characterized as spotlike or broad.

Results

On fMRI, in all eight volunteers the motor hand area was spotlike. It was broad in four patients and spotlike in two. In one patient no motor hand area could be detected by fMRI.

Based on intraoperative mapping by direct electrical stimulation of the central area, the motor hand area was spotlike in one patient, and broad in four.

When comparing the findings of fMRI and intraoperative mapping, they correlated in four patients (three broad, one spotlike). In one patient the area was broad in fMRI and spotlike in intraoperative mapping.

Discussion

There is a debate concerning the anatomical substrate of the hyperintense area detected by fMRI, whether it corresponds to larger veins ("macrovasculature") or venules ("microvasculature") [6, 7]. The spotlike shape in all the volunteers and in two patients is compatible with both assumptions, whereas the broad area that projected into the cerebral parenchyma could only be explained by the presence of small veins. Usually, as known from stimulation experiments in primates [8, 9], the cortical representation of the motor hand area is apparently quite small, so probably only the result of the localized increased perfusion (always occurring) can be detected.

We and others have shown previously that a variety of peripheral neuronal [10], medullary [2] or cortical [2] pathologies can induce changes – namely enlargement – of cortical representation of motor function. The data of the present study that were collected with fMRI and intraoperative stimulation mapping suggest that the presence of a slow growing tumour can induce a redistribution in the cortical representation of motor hand function. The anatomical substrate of such reorganization that is based on neuronal plasticity [2, 10] may be reflected in the broader shape of the vascular phenomena visualized with fMRI. The close correlation with the intraoperative mapping shows that these changes are real.

Acknowledgements. Technical support by Jens Frahm, Max Planck Institute, Göttingen, is greatly appreciated. Financial support came from the Friedrich-Baur-Foundation Munich (to T. Y. and U. D. S.), the Weigand Foundation Munich and the Münchner Medizinische Wochenschrift (to T. Y.), and the Swiss National Science Foundation (grant no. 32-9001.86 to U. D. S.).

References

1. Yousry T, Schmid UD, Jassoy A, Schmidt D (1993) Validation of functional MRI by intraoperative direct cortical stimulation. Neuroradiology 35:S46
2. Levy WJ, Amassian VE, Schmid UD, Jungreis C (1991) Mapping of motor cortex gyral sites noninvasively by transcranial magnetic stimulation in normal subjects and patients. Electroencephalogr Clin Neurophysiol [Suppl] 43:51–75
3. Ebeling U, Schmid UD, Ying Z, Reulen HJ (1992) Safe surgery of lesions near the motor cortex using intra-operative mapping techniques: a report on 50 patients. Acta Neurochir (Wien) 119:23–28
4. Haglund MM, Berger MS, Shamseldin M, Lettich E, Ojemann GA (1994) Cortical localization of temporal lobe language sites in patients with gliomas. Neurosurgery 34:567–576
5. Schmid U, Ebeling U, Reulen H (1989) Electrophysiological localization of the human sensorimotor cortex. J Neurosurg 70:817–818
6. Menon RS, Ogawa S, Tank DW, Ugurbil K (1993) Tesla gradient recalled echo characteristics of photic stimulation-induced signal changes in the human primary visual cortex. Magn Reson Med 30:380–386
7. Lai S, Hopkins AL, Haacke EM, Li D, Wasserman BA, Buckley P, Friedman L, Meltzer H, Heders P, Friedland R (1993) Identification of vascular structures as a major source of signal contrast in high resolution 2D and 3D functional activation imaging of the motor cortex at 1.5 T: preliminary results. Magn Reson Med 30:387–392
8. Lemon RN (1988) The output map of the primate motor cortex. Trends Neurosci 11:501–506
9. Humphrey DR (1988) Representation of movements and muscles within the primate precentral motor cortex: historical and current perspecives. Fed Proc 45:2587–2699
10. Brasil-Neto JP, McShane LM, Fuhr P, Hallett M, Cohen LG (1992) Topographic mapping of the human motor cortex with magnetic stimulation: factors affecting accuracy and reproducibility. Electroencephalogr Clin Neurophysiol 85:9–16

Functional mapping of sensorimotor cortex with combined use of magnetoencephalography, functional MRI, and motor-evoked potentials

T. Morioka [1], A. Mizushima [2], T. Yamamoto [3], S. Tobimatsu [4], S. Matsumoto [2], K. Hasuo [2], S. Nishio [1], K. Fujii [1], M. Fukui [1]

[1] Department of Neurosurgery, Neurological Institute, Faculty of Medicine, Kyushu University, Fukuoka, Japan
[2] Department of Radiology, Faculty of Medicine, Kyushu University, Fukuoka, Japan
[3] Department of Otolaryngology, Faculty of Medicine, Kyushu University, Fukuoka, Japan
[4] Department of Clinical Neurophysiology, Neurological Institute, Faculty of Medicine, Kyushu University, Fukuoka, Japan

Abstract. In an attempt to localize a structural lesion precisely to the central sulcus, magnetoencephalography (MEG), functional magnetic resonance imaging (fMRI), and motor-evoked potentials (MEP) were carried out on three patients. The sensory cortex was identified with magnetic source imaging (MSI) of somatosensory-evoked magnetic fields using MEG and MRI. The motor area of the hand region was identified using fMRI, during a hand-squeezing task. In addition, transcranial magnetic stimulation localized the hand motor area on the scalp, which was mapped onto the MRI. There was good agreement between MSI, fMRI and MEP as to the gross location of the sensorimotor cortex and its relationship to the lesion. However, the precise localization of the motor cortex on fMRI could not be obtained due to inflow effect. The scalp mark over the motor cortex detected with MEP could not localize the entire motor strip. Thus, MSI, at present, proved to be the most reliable method for localizing peri-Rolandic lesions.

Key words: Functional magnetic resonance imaging – Magnetic source imaging – Magnetoencephalography – Motor-evoked potentials

Precise determination of the anatomical relationship between a peri-Rolandic lesion and the sensorimotor cortex is important in deciding upon an appropriate surgical strategy. Magnetic source imaging (MSI) by the combined use of the magnetoencephalography (MEG) and neuroradiological imaging provides complementary information for the identification of the somatosensory cortex. Current research extends MRI methods to provide information about biological function, with the motor cortex being visualized by motor task in addition to the concomitant anatomical information (functional MRI; fMRI). Furthermore, transcranial magnetic stimulation has been used to explore the functional anatomy of the motor cortex by measuring the motor-evoked potentials (MEP) following stimulation at multiple scalp sites. We compared these three mapping techniques of the sensorimotor cortex in three patients with peri-Rolandic lesion. A preliminary result has been reported elsewhere [1].

Correspondence to: T. Morioka, Department of Neurosurgery, Neurological Institute Faculty of Medicine, Kyushu University 60, 3-1-1 Maidashi, Higashi-ku, Fukuoka 812, Japan

Materials and methods

Three patients with peri-Rolandic lesions [intracerebral cyst, arteriovenous malformation (AVM) and parasagittal meningioma] were studied. Our sensory mapping technique with MEG and motor mapping techniques with MRI and MEP have been described previously [1, 2].

Results

There was good agreement between MSI, fMRI and MEP as to the gross location of the sensorimotor cortex and its relationship to the lesion in all cases. However, inflow effect on fMRI obscured precise localization of the motor cortex in one case. In a patient with long-T2 peritumoural oedema, fMRI failed to reveal activated hyperintense signals associated with hand-grasping. In two cases, the scalp mark over the motor cortex detected with MEP could not localize the entire motor strip. We describe an illustrative case.

A 32-year-old housewife was admitted with a history of generalized seizures. Angiography revealed an AVM in the left frontal lobe (Fig. 1A). She underwent a localizing procedure with MSI for the hand sensory area. MSI indicated that the current dipoles in response to somatosensory stimuli of contralateral index and thumb fingers were located posterior to the large sulcus, which was deduced to be the central sulcus (Fig. 1C). Thus, the AVM nidus was interpreted to be within the premotor area. On three-dimensional MSI, the spatial relationship between the sensory strip and the AVM nidus was visualized more precisely, and there were central and precentral sulci between the two (Fig. 1B). On fMRI, an activated hyperintense region was surmised to be the hand motor area (Fig. 1D), and this corresponded grossly to the precentral gyrus determined by MSI. The most hyperintense area was, however, a large cortical vein running on the central sulcus, which obscured the precise localization of the motor cortex. By MEP, the scalp mark over the hand motor area was consistent with the findings of fMRI (Fig. 1E), although the point on the scalp did not reflect the entire motor strip.

At the time of surgery, cortical recording of somatosensory-evoked potentials following median nerve stimulation was performed. The central sulcus was identified by the reversed polarity of the primary sensory N20 potential (Fig. 1F, G). The lesion was found to be within the premotor area, being consistent with preoperative functional mapping. The AVM nidus was totally removed without any neurological deficit.

Discussion

We have confirmed the accuracy of sensory mapping with MSI [1, 2]. However, it has not been applicable in assessment of the motor cortex. MRI has been successfully applied to image the human motor cortex functionally,

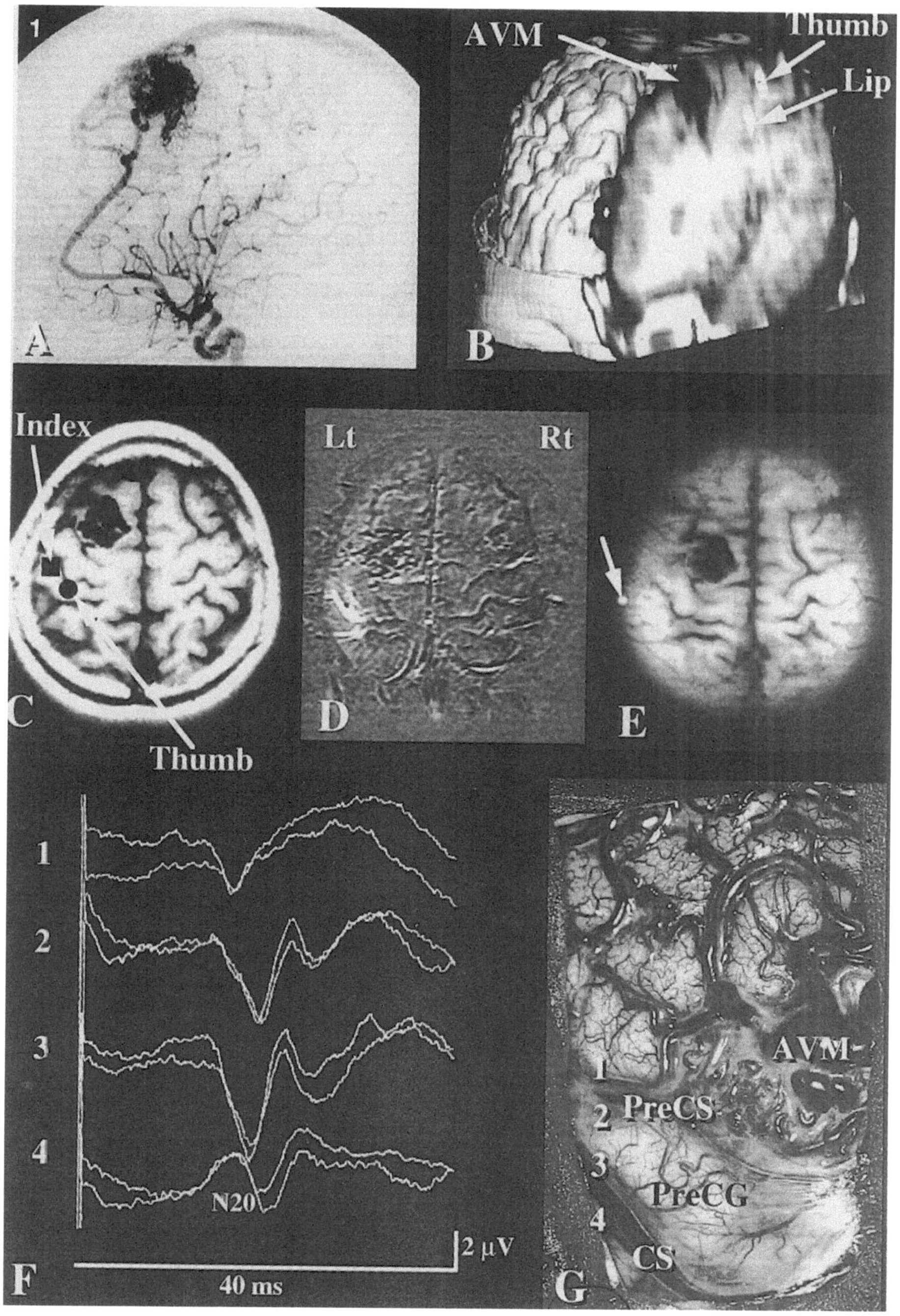

Fig. 1. A Lateral view of left carotid angiogram shows an arteriovenous malformation (AVM) in the left frontal lobe. **B** Three-dimensional magnetic source imaging (MSI) indicates the spatial relationship between the sensory strip (the current dipoles in response to sensory stimuli of contralateral thumb finger and lip) and AVM nidus. There are central and precentral sulci between these two. **C** An axial view of MSI indicates that the current dipoles in response to sensory stimuli of contralateral index and thumb fingers are located posterior to the large sulcus, deduced to be the central sulcus. **D** An axial image of functional MRI demonstrates an activated region as hyperintense during hand-grasping, which was therefore surmised to be the hand motor area. The most hyperintense area is a large cortical vein running in the central sulcus. **E** An identical image of **(D)** shows the scalp point over the hand motor area *(arrow)* detected by motor-evoked potentials. **F** Intraoperative cortical recording of somatosensory-evoked potentials following median nerve stimulation. The primary sensory cortical N20 potential is recorded at electrode *4*. There is a phase-reversal between electrodes *3* and *4*, indicating that the central sulcus lies between *3* and *4*. **G** Operative photograph demonstrating the position of the electrodes. *PreCS*, Precentral sulcus; *PreCG*, precentral gyrus; *CS*, central sulcus

even on a standard clinical imager operating at 1.5 T. The rationale for this technique is based on the blood oxygenation level dependent contrast. Recently, the large signal changes observed in fMRI were thought to be caused mainly by inflow effects of the veins. In the present study, the most activated area was a large vein on the sulcus, supporting the current opinion. Although MEP provide a noninvasive method for topographical mapping of the human motor cortex, in our study the entire motor strip, which bends in a complex manner, could not be localized with the mark on the scalp.

We found good agreement between MEG, MRI and MEP as to the gross location of the sensorimotor cortex and its relationship to the lesion. However, there are still some disadvantages of each method in their practical uses. MSI, at present, proves to be the most reliable method for localization of peri-Rolandic lesions.

References

1. Morioka T, Mizushima A, Yamamoto T, Tobimatsu S, Matsumoto S, Hasuo K, Fujii K, Fukui M (1995) Functional mapping of sensorimotor cortex: a combined use of magnetoencephalography, functional MRI, and motor-evoked potentials. Neuroradiology (in press)
2. Morioka T, Yamamoto T, Katsuta T, Fujii K, Fukui M (1994) Presurgical 3-dimensional magnetic source imaging of the somatosensory cortex in a patient with peri-Rolandic lesion. Neurosurgery 34:930–934

Functional MRI of human motor cortex using a conventional MRI system

M. Sasahira [1], M. Niiro [2], A. Haruzono [1], W. Hirakawa [1], T. Asakura [1], T. Fujimoto [2]

[1] Department of Neurosurgery, Faculty of Medicine, Kagoshima University, Kagoshima, Japan
[2] South Japan Health Science Centre, Miyakonojo, Japan

Abstract. Functional MRI of the brain was performed with motor task activation in normal volunteers and a patient with a meningioma using conventional FLASH sequences and a 2.0 T MRI system. A bright signal intensity in the motor cortex was observed in all cases. In the single-slice studies, the right-sided finger task produced an increase of 6.67 ± 4.36% in the signal intensity of the left motor cortex, while the left-sided finger task increased the signal by 6.09 ± 3.34% in the right motor cortex. There were no significant differences between the sides. In the multiple-slice studies, the activated motor cortex was also seen as a bright signal. Preoperative mapping of the meningioma showed that the motor cortex was displaced posteriorly by the tumour. Our clinical study demonstated the possibility of functional MRI with a standard MRI system and conventional FLASH sequences. Useful information can be obtained by preoperative mapping of the motor cortex.

Key words: Functional magnetic resonance imaging – Motor cortex

Functional mapping of the human brain using MRI has developed recently. The basic principle of this method is that deoxyhaemoglobin acts as an endogenous paramagnetic contrast agent. Thus, changes in the concentration of deoxyhaemoglobin lead to alterations in the MR signal on T2*-weighted images [1, 2]. In this study, we evaluated functional MRI of the human bran using a 2.0 T MRI system and conventional FLASH sequences.

Materials and methods

MRI was performed using a 2.0 T superconducting MRI system. Magnetic global shimming of the head was performed, resulting in a magnetic field homogeneity of about 0.1–0.2 ppm. Midsagittal images were obtained (TR/TE = 300/15, 256 × 256 matrix) with a slice thickness of 5 mm. Using the midsagittal image as an anatomic guide, an axial image was obtained through the primary motor cortex using conventional FLASH sequences (TR/TE = 91/60, flip angle = 40°, 128 × 128 matrix, 25 cm field of view, 1 excitation, slice thickness = 5 mm). The total scanning time for each slice was 14 s. For activation studies, single-slice FLASH images were obtained.

Five volunteers and one patient with a meningioma were investigated. The motor task consisted of repetitive finger-to-thumb opposition movements. For single-slice studies, the following sequence of images was obtained: 4 resting images, 4 task images, 12 resting images, 4 task images, 8 resting images. For multi-slice studies, three sets of 4 resting images and 4 task images were obtained. A subtraction image was generated by subtracting the average data obtained during performance of the first task (four images). Changes in signal relative to the pre-stimulation level were also evaluated.

Correspondence to: M. Sasahira, Department of Neurosurgery, Faculty of Medicine, Kagoshima University, 8-35-1, Sakuragaoka, Kagoshima, 890 Japan

Results

Single-slice study

A bright signal intensity was observed in the motor cortex of all subjects. When the subtraction image was superimposed on the proton image, the activated area was almost consistent with the primary motor cortex. The right-sided finger task produced an increase of 1.9–23.5% (6.67 ± 4.36%) in the left motor cortex signal, while the left-sided finger task increased the signal by 1.5–18.2% (6.09 ± 3.34%) in the right motor cortex. There was no significant difference between the two sides.

Multi-slice study

A bright signal intensity was also noted in the motor-cortex. The maximal signal intensity in the activated motor area increased by 11.0% in the left motor cortex and by 8.8% in the right motor cortex. There was no significant difference between the two sides.

Clinical application of functional MRI

In the patient with a convexity meningioma, a multi-slice study was performed. A bright signal intensity area was noted in the parietal cortex just behind the posterior margin of the tumour. The left motor area was compressed posteriorly by this tumour (Fig. 1).

Discussion

The basic principle of functional MRI is that deoxyhaemoglobin acts as an endogenous paramagnetic contrast agent. The change in deoxyhaemoglobin is relatd to the alterations of T2*signal intensity seen with gradient-echo sequences [1, 3].

Functional MRI was initially tried using a high magnetic field (4.0 T) [4] or echo-planar imaging (EPI) [5–7]. Using a high magnetic field strength gives a higher signal-to-noise ratio and better spatial resolution than using a low field strength, while EPI also gives better temporal resolution. However, conventional MR imagers (1.5 or 2.0 T) with conventional gradient echo sequences have been used more recently.

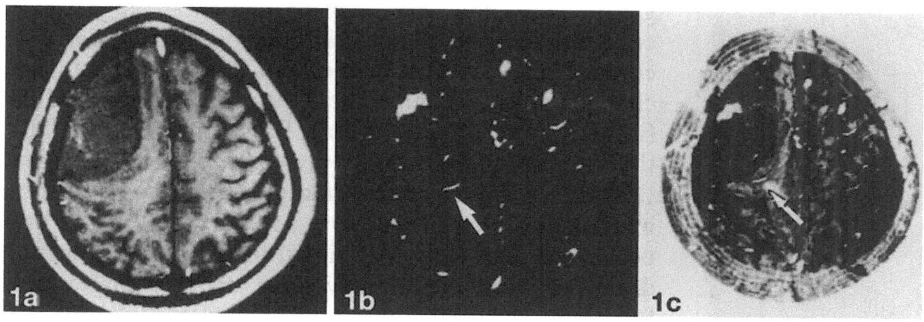

Fig. 1a–c. Clinical application of functional MRI. **a** T1-weighted image of convexity meningioma. **b** Subtraction image. A bright signal is noted in the motor cortex *(arrowhead)*. **c** Subtraction image superimposed on the surface anatomy image. The left motor area was compressed posteriorly by the tumour *(arrowhead)*.

The brightest regions of the brain activity image closely correspond to the areas of the motor cortex that are considered to be involved with finer activity. An approximate 4–21% change in signal intensity was noticed in the published papers. In our study, the activated region was along the sulci of the motor cortex. The right-sided finger task produced an increase of 6.67 ± 4.36% in the left motor cortex, while the left-sided finger task increased the signal by 6.09 ± 3.34% in the right motor cortex. There was no significant difference betwen the two sides.

We tried to use functional MRI for pre-surgical mapping of the motor cortex. In the convexity meningioma, the motor cortex was seen as a bright area osteriorly displaced by the tumour. Jack et al. [8] tested the same trial and demonstrated localized activation of cortical functional mapping by invasive techniques matching the data obtained with functional MRI.

Our results are similar to previously reported data, showing an increased signal intensity of the activated motor area on subtraction images. Functional MRI may also be useful as preoperative mapping of the motor cortex. To obtain high quality images, however, it is necessary to make an effort to improve the signal-to-noise ratio and obtain an statistic distribution image for accurate identification of the activated area.

References

1. Ogawa S, Lee TM, Kay AR et al. (1990) Brain magnetic resonance imaging with contrast dependent on blood oxygenation. Proc Natl Acad Sci USA 87:9868–9872
2. Thulborn KR, Waterton JC, Styles P et al. (1982) Oxygenation dependence of the transverse relaxation time of water protons in whole blood at high field. Biochem Biophys Acta 14:265–270
3. Turner R, LeBihan D, Moonen CT et a. (1991) Echo-planar time course MRI of cat brain oxygenation changes. Magn Reson Med 22:159–166
4. Ogawa S, Tank DW, Menon R et al. (1992) Intrinsic signal changes accompanying sensory stimulation: functional brain mapping with magnetic resonance imaging. Proc Natl Acad Sci USA 89:5951–5955
5. Bandettini PA, Wong EC, Hinks RS et al. (1992) Time course EPI of human brain function during task activation. Magn Reson Med 25:390–397
6. Blamire AM, Ogawa S, Ugurbil K et al. (1992) Dynamic mapping of visual cortex by high-speed magnetic resonance imaging. Proc Natl Acad Sci USA 89:11069–11073
7. Kwong KK, Belliveau JW, Chesler DA et al. (1992) Dynamic magnetic resonance imaging of human brain activity during primary sensory stimulation. Proc Natl Acad Sci USA 89:5675–5679
8. Jack CR Jr, Thompson RM, Butts RK et al. (1993) Sensory motor cortex: correlation of presurgical mapping with functional MR imaging and invasive cortical mapping. Radiology 190:85–92

Inflow effect in functional MRI using gradient-echo at 1.5 T

K. Kikuchi[1], **Y. Ishimaru**[1], **K. Sadamoto**[2], **S. Ohue**[2], **H. Miki**[3], **K. Hamamoto**[3], **E. Yoshitome**[4], **D. Le Bihan**[5]

[1] Department of Radiology, Washokai Sadamoto Hospital, Ehime, Japan
[2] Department of Neurosurgery, Washokai Sadamoto Hospital, Ehime, Japan
[3] Department of Radiology, Ehime University School of Medicine, Ehime, Japan
[4] Yokogawa Medical System, Tokyo, Japan
[5] National Institutes of Health, Bethesda, Maryland, USA

Abstract. On functional MRI (fMRI) the main reason for signal changes is thought to depend on the blood oxygenation level dependent (BOLD) contrast. On fMRI, using the conventional GFE T2* effect, it appears to be mixed with significant blood flow (inflow) signal due to the large flip angle and short TR of the GFE technique. We attempted to discriminate between the susceptibility effects and the inflow effects with presaturation (SAT) methods. A series of 15 sequential images was acquired with a long TE GFE sequence under photic stimulation. We inserted the SAT slab above and below the imaging plane to suppress the unsaturated flowing protons. To alter the inflow effects, we changed the distance between

Correspondence to: K. K. Kuchi, Department of Radiology, Washokai Sadamoto Hospital, 1-3-3 Takahara-cho, Matsuyama-chi, Ehime 790, Japan

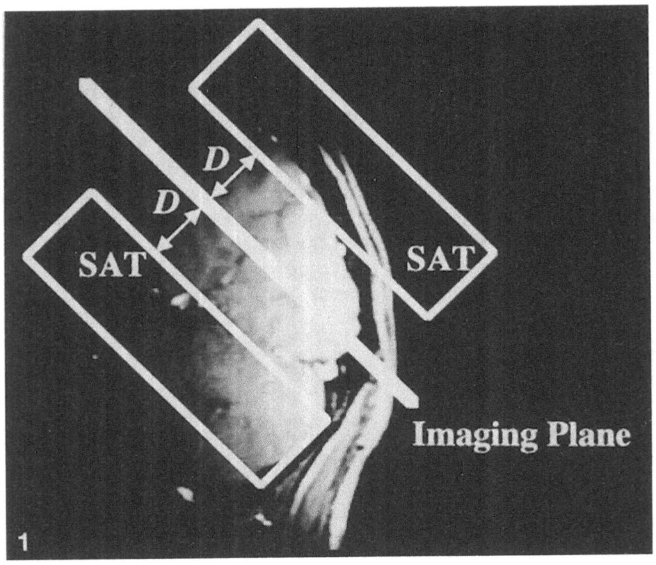

Fig. 1. Image showing orientation of imaging plane and presaturation (SAT) slab

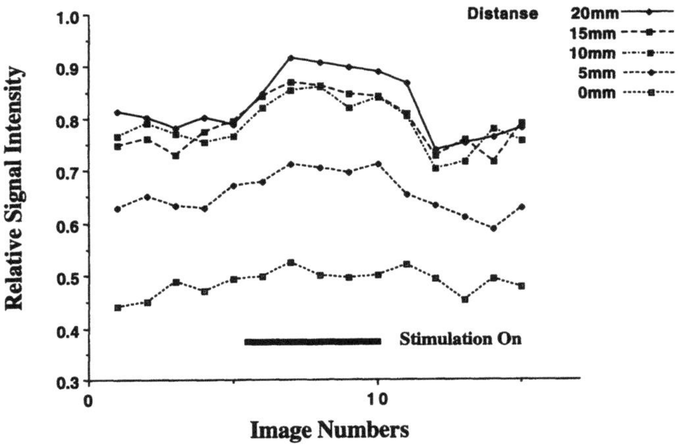

Fig. 2. Time course of relative signal intensity changes in visual cortex with imaging plane and SAT slab separated by distance indicated

the imaging plane and the SAT slab. When the distance was increased, the quantity of signal intensity changes had also increased, and the signal changes were observed even when the imaging plane and the SAT slab were adjacent. Our results show that the signal changes on fMRI with conventional GFE technique are affected by inflow effects and BOLD contrast.

Key words: Functional magnetic resonance imaging – Blood oxygenation level dependent contrast – Inflow effect – Gradient field echo

---

Recently, many studies have been published about functional MRI (fMRI). The main reason for signal changes on fMRI is thought to depend on blood oxygenation level dependent contrast (BOLD) contrast, due to susceptibility difference between deoxyhaemoglobin and oxyhaemoglobin [1]. Other effects have also been suggested to contribute to the signal changes on fMRI. Using the conventional gradient field echo (GFE) T2* effect, signal change appears in part to be due to significant blood flow (inflow) signal due to the large flip angle and short TR of the GFE technique commonly employed for the current fMRI [2, 3]. Inflow effects of large draining veins carrying hyperoxygenated blood from activated regions of brain tissue will affect the MR signal intensity from near the draining veins, which may have no relation to brain function. This could result in misregistration of fMRI; therefore, discriminating between these effects is a substantial problem in fMRI.

In this study, we attempt to discriminate between the susceptibility effects and the inflow effects with presaturation (SAT) methods. We employ the SAT pulse to alter the inflow effects. We hypothesize that the SAT pulse can suppress the MR signal that originates from unsaturated protons flowing into the imaging plane, and when the SAT slab and the imaging plane are adjacent, no unsaturated protons flow into the imaging plane. If the intensity changes are caused by the BOLD contrast, we could observe intensity changes when the imaging plane and SAT slab are adjacent. If the intensity changes are caused by inflow effects, the signal changes are decreased by reducing the distance between the imaging plane and the SAT slab.

Materials and methods

Our studies were carried out on a conventional 1.5 T MR system with a 5 in surface coil. A series of 15 sequential images was acquired with a long TE GFE sequence to obtain T2*-weighted images. Our sequence was the spoiled GRASS (SPGR), TR 93, TE 40 ms, flip angle 25°, slice thickness 5 mm, field of view 25 cm, matrix 128 × 96, band width 7.4 kHz, with flow compensation. After the localized sagittal image, fMRI of the visual cortex was obtained in an oblique image orientation along the calcarine sulcus (Fig. 1). A photic stimulation paradigm (8 Hz flashing light-emitting diode LED) was performed with a goggle. The first 5 images were acquired without LED flashing, the next 5 with flashing, and the last 5 images were again without flashing. We inserted the SAT slab above and below the imaging plane to suppress unsaturated flowing protons. To alter the inflow effects, we changed *D* (the distance between the imaging plane and the SAT slab) from 20 to 0 mm. The SAT slab thickness was 40 mm.

A region of interest (ROI) was placed on the visual cortex to analyse the signal intensity changes. To get rid of a signal intensity reduction originating from the influence of the SAT slab side lobe, we acquired the signal intensity of copper sulphate phantom under the same situation, and calculated the relative signal intensity (RSI): signal intensity of visual cortex divided by phantom signal intensity.

To make a visual estimation, subtraction images were computed from activated images and rest images, and the subtraction images were put on the same location as T1-weighted images.

Results

Figure 2 shows the signal intensity chages of the visual cortex. When *D* was increased, the quantity of signal intensity change also increased. This fact indicated that the signal changes were influenced by the inflow effects. The signal changes were observed, even when the imaging

Table 1. Relative signal intensity changes in visual cortex

Distance between SAT slab and image plane (mm)	Mean relative signal intensity		Signal change (%)
	Stimulation off	Stimulation on	
20	0.797	0.892	11.9
15	0.762	0.848	11.3
10	0.770	0.839	9.0
5	0.643	0.697	8.4
0	0.469	0.505	7.7

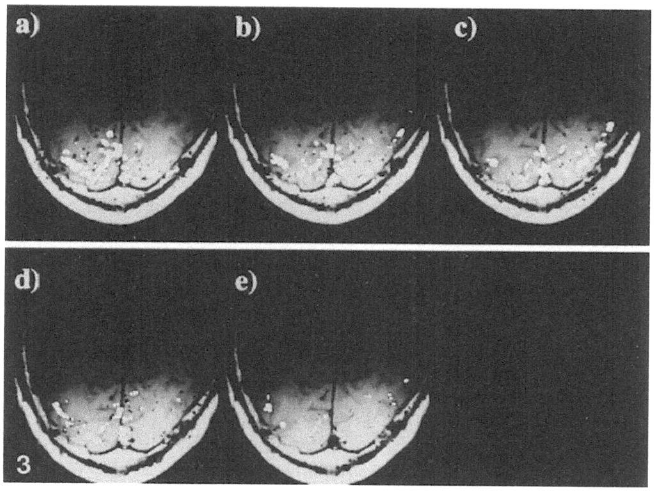

Fig. 3a–e. Superimposition of subtraction images on T1-weighted SE images. The subtraction image is obtained by spoiled GRASS images acquired with the light-emitting diodes off and subtracting the resulting image from corresponding summation of images acquired with the diodes on. The distance between imaging plane and SAT slab was **a** 20, **b** 15, **c** 10, **d** 5, and **e** 0 mm

plane and the SAT slab were adjacent ($D = 0$ mm). This indicated that the signal changes were also influenced by BOLD contrast. The distances between the SAT slab and the imaging plane were 20, 15, 10, 5, and 0 mm; the signal intensity increased by 11.9, 11.3, 9.0, 8.4, 7.7%, respectively (Table 1). On the subtraction image analysis (fig. 3), the area of increased signal intensity was dependent on the quantity of the inflow effects.

Discussion

Our results show that signal changes on fMRI with the conventional GFE technique are affected by the inflow effects and BOLD contrast. We presume that the signal change might be due to the draining veins, so we have to consider misregistration to estimate fMRI. The signal intensity change, demonstrated in the visual cortex, depends on the distance between the imaging plane and the SAT slab. We conclude that the signal changes of fMRI using the conventional GFE technique are caused by both inflow effects and BOLD contrast.

References

1. Ogawa S, Lee TM, Kay AR, Tank DW (1990) Brain magnetic resonance imaging with contrast dependent on blood oxygenation. Proc Nat Acad Sci USA 87:9868–9872
2. Kwong KK, Belliveau JW, Chesler DA, Goldberg IE, Weisskoff RM, Poncelet BP, Kennedy DN, Hoppel BE, Cohen MS, Turner R, Cheng H-M, Brady TJ, Rosen BR (1992) Dynamic magnetic resonance imaging of human brain activity during primary sensory stimulation. Proc Nat Acad Sci USA 89:5675–5679
3. Kim SG, Ashe J, Georgopoulos AP, Merkle H, Ellermann JM, Menon RS, Ogawa S, Ugurbil K (1993) Functional imaging of human motor cortex at high magnetic field. J Neurophysiol 69:297–302

MRI of olfactory structures: normal subjects and patients with olfactory dysfunction

L. M. Levy[1], **A. J. Bartsch**[2], **S. Rajan**,[1], **D. Schellinger**[1], **R. I. Henkin**[2]

[1] Georgetown University Hospital Washington, D.C., USA
[2] The Taste and Smell Clinic, Washington, D.C., USA

Abstract. The visualization of olfactory structures of the human brain during life has been difficult, if not impossible. While visualization of anatomical structures of the visual and auditory systems has been carried out for many years, olfactory structures have not been well defined. With the advent of MRI, it was possible not only to visualize these structures in patients with various disease processes, but also in subjects who did not have expressed abnormalities in olfactory functions. The purpose of this work is to estimate the success of the visualization of olfactory structures in a group of normal subjects and in patients. We also estimated the size of these structures in patients with loss of smell.

Key words: Olfactory bulbs – Olfactory tract – Magnetic resonance imaging

Correspondence to: L. M. Levy

Initial studies using routine radiography and then pneumoencephalography offered a modest attempt to visualize the olfactory structures. CT did not demonstrate these structures well due to the presence of adjacent bone which hampered any systematic approach to study these structures [1]. With the advent of MRI, it was possible not only to visualize these structures in patients with various disease processes, but also in subjects who did not have abnormalities in olfactory functions [2, 3]. It is the purpose of this work to estimate the success of visualization of olfactory structures in a group of normal subjects and in patients. Because it has been commonly accepted that patients with loss of smell have this symptom because of or related to changes in central nervous system (CNS) olfactory structures, we also estimated the size of these structures in patients with loss of smell.

Patients and methods

Patients without smell dysfunction were aged between 4 to 80 years (mean 40 years) and comprised 31 males and 36 females. All patients were studied retrospectively. These patients were referred for examination of the orbits, paranasal sinuses, pituitary, cranial nerves and frontal tumors. Patients with loss or dysfunction of smell included 14 women and 14 men, aged 16–82 years (mean 46 years). Olfactory structures were measured directly from MR images by two of the investigators (R.I.H., A.B.) in a blind manner without any knowledge of the patient's name or status. All measurements were obtained from imagers using a field strength of 1.5 T using coronal T1-weighted studies with section thickness varying from 3 to 6 mm. Routine brain studies were available for each patient and included T1-weighted images with and without gadolinium. Gap size was 0.1 mm for 3- and 4-mm sections, and 0.3 mm for 5- and 6-mm sections.

Results

An evaluation of olfactory structures in coronal sections revealed that olfactory sulci could be identified bilaterally on T1-weighted images in all patients studied. Olfactory bulbs were also identified bilaterally in most patients. Olfactory tracts were less readily identified on thinner sections. We found that while these structures can be seen in a relatively large number of patients, it may be necessary to examine a large number of sections in an appropriate area. For sagittal or coronal sections, the olfactory sulci can be identified in about 75% of patients, bulbs in about 25%, and tracts and transitions in up to 50%.

However, the sulci are observed in only 17% of sections, bulbs in about 5%, and tracts and transitions in 10%. Measurement of olfactory structures on coronal sections indicated no significant difference in size between left and right sides. The olfactory structures tend to be smaller in females than in males. Normal mean bulb length was 7.8 ± 0.5 mm on the left and 8.1 ± 0.2 mm on the right. Our estimates of bulb length are comparable with previously reported measurements, which ranged from 6 to 15 mm [2, 4, 5]. Estimates of bulb width were less variable and also comparable with previous measurements, which ranged from 3 to 7 mm [5]. Estimates of mean olfactory tract width compared well with previous reports of average width of 4.5 mm [5].

Although there was no correlation between olfactory sulcus depth and age, olfactory sulcus width increased with age, consistent with gray matter atrophy. There was also a negative correlation between olfactory bulb width and age, suggesting that as age increased olfactory bulb width decreased, although there was no such trend in the height of the olfactory bulb. A comparison of estimates of olfactory structure size in patients with loss of smell and in control subjects indicated no significant differences in depth or width of bulbs, tracts, or transitions between bulbs and tracts. The mean depth (length) of the olfactory sulci was significantly greater in patients with disturbed olfaction than in controls and the mean width of the right but not the left olfactory sulcus was also greater.

Discussion

These studies indicate that olfactory sulci and bulbs can be seen on MRI in most patients, if appropriate sections are acquired. Olfactory tracts and transitions from bulb to tract are seen less often, in part because of their smaller size. There was a small trend toward a decrease in the width of both left and right olfactory bulbs as age increased, although there was no such trend in their height, correlating with human autopsy studies [6]. The data obtained in patients with loss of smell indicate that they exhibit no consistent differences in size of olfactory structures from controls. Although it is commonly believed that most pathology associated with loss of smell resides in the CNS, olfactory structure size may not be a determining factor in assessing smell loss in patients. While diseases affecting olfactory bulbs or temporal lobes can induce loss of smell, this type of pathology represents only a small fraction of the pathology commonly associated with loss of smell. Most commonly, loss of smell is due to pathology of a biochemical nature which takes place at the olfactory receptor, not in the CNS [7]. The hypothesis of receptor pathology is important in the medical management of these conditions [7]. Thus, a change in focus from an anatomical to a more biochemical one could play an important role in the successful understanding of these disorders and their potential therapy.

References

1. Schellinger D, Henkin RI, Smirniotopoulos JG (1983) CT of the brain in taste and smell dysfunction. AJNR 4:752–754
2. Suzuki M, Takashima T, Kadoya S, Miyayama S, Taira S (1984) MR imaging of olfactory bulbs and tracts. AJNR 10:951–957
3. Klingmueller D, Dewes W, Krahe T, Brecht G, Schweikert HU (1987) Magnetic resonance imaging of the brain in patients with anosmia and hypothalamic hypogonadism (Kallmann's syndrome). J Clin Endocrinol Metab 65:581–584
4. Smail M, Janetta PJ (1981) The cranial nerves: anatomy, pathology, pathophysiology, diagnosis, treatment. Springer, Berlin Heidelberg New York, pp 6–7
5. Lang J (1987) Übergeordnete Systeme. Praktische Anatomie. Springer, Berlin Heidelberg New York, pp 325–326, 447
6. Meurmann OH (1950) Experimental studies of the effect of pathological changes in the nasal mucous membrane on the olfactory bulb. Acta Otolaryngol (Stockh) 38:477–483
7. Henkin RI (1993) Evaluation and treatment of human olfactory dysfunction. In: English G (ed) Otolaryngology. Lippincott, Philadelphia, pp 1–86

Functional MRI of olfaction in normals and patients

L. M. Levy [1], C. S. Lin [2], R. I. Henkin, [2], C. Ariz [1], S. Rajan [1], D. Schellinger [1], D. LeBihan [1]

[1] Georgetown University Hospital Washington, D.C., USA
[2] The Taste and Smell Clinic, Washington, D.C., USA

Abstract. Our purpose was to evaluate the utility of functional MRI (fMRI) in the investigation of olfactory function. fMRI of the brain was performed on 12 healthy subjects and in 5 patients. Coronal sections were selected through the mid- to anterior temporal region of the brain. Significant activation was noted especially in the frontal and temporal lobes. Some of these activated regions corresponded to the orbitofrontal, entorhinal and pyriform cortical areas. Additional regions of activation were also observed in other areas of the frontal and temporal lobes. Imagination of smell produced less activation than active stimulation. Areas of negative activation were also noted in the frontal and temporal lobes. Patients demonstrated either abnormal patterns of activation, or no activation, depending on the nature of their dysfunction. These studies indicate that MRI may be used to demonstrate olfactory cortex activation.

Key words: Functional magnetic resonance imaging – Olfaction

There is presently no method to document objectively whether or not loss of smell is present in patients with olfactory dysfunction. Visualization of olfactory function of the human brain during life has been difficult, if not impossible. Functional visualization of the visual, motor and sensory systems has been recently carried out by MRI, but little has been done on olfactory function [1–4]. Initial nonivasive studies of olfactory structures using CT did not demonstrate these structures well [5]. With the advent of MRI, it was possible not only to visualize the anatomy of these structures in normal subjects and in patients [6, 7], but also possibly to evaluate olfactory function. Because it has been commonly accepted that patients with loss of smell have this symptom related to changes in central nervous system (CNS) olfactory structures, we recently estimated the size of these structures in patients with loss of smell, and found little relationship to the presence of olfactory dysfunction. The purpose of this study was to evaluate the feasibility of using MRI to study olfaction from a functional approach.

Subjects and methods

MRI of the brain was performed on 12 healthy subjects using a 1.5 T imager with a head coil. None of the subjects had clinical evidence of olfactory dysfunction. In addition, 5 patients with hyposmia were also studied. A modified gradient-echo FLASH sequence was used with TE 35 ms, TR 50 ms, flip angle 30°, field of view 325 mm, slice thickness 4 mm, acquisition time per image 5 s. Coronal sections were selected through the mid- to anterior temporal region of the brain. These slices covered the olfactory cortex and olfactory projections: the nucleus accumbens, orbitofrontal cortex and part of the pyriform cortex; and the septal nuclei, amygdaloid complex, pyriform cortex and entorhinal cortex. In some cases, additional views were obtained posteriorly through the hippocampal and posterior entorhinal regions. Olfactory stimulation was performed using an absolute solution of amyl acetate presented 2 cm from the external nares. Two consecutive series of 15 images each (without olfactory stimulation followed by stimulation respectively) were obtained in 3 min. Functional activation images were correlated with high-resolution T1-weighted images for better anatomical localization. Pre- and poststimilation images were compared using Z statistics [8] and analyzing the correlation between stimulus pattern and time course of intensity response. All subjects were examined for age, handedness, and subjective perception of stimulus.

Correspondence to: L. M. Levy

Results

Activation was found to be significant in some regions (Z score greater than 2), and activation ratios were in the range of 2–8%. Significant activation was noted especially at the base of the frontal lobes and in the temporal lobes. Some of these activated regions corresponded to the orbitofrontal, entorhinal and pyriform cortical areas. Additional regions of activation observed in other areas of the frontal and temporal lobes were in the areas of the nucleus accumbens, the septal nuclei, and the amygdaloid complex. Regions of significant activation in the superior portions of the frontal lobes were also noted.

The temporal response to stimulation appeared rapid, occurring within seconds. In addition, stimulation studies repeated immediately after the initial study in 4 subjects showed decreased activation relative to the initial study, suggesting adaption.

The activation showed increased frequency with decreasing Z score values in the 12 healthy subjects: 7 subjects showed activation at Z scores greater than 2.0, 9 at Z scores greater than 1.5, and all 12 at Z scores greater than 1.3. The regions that showed activation included the inferior and lateral frontal regions in 6 cases, the temporal lobes in 8 cases, and the superior frontal regions in 10 cases. There was more activation noted on the left side in the frontal and temporal lobes (all subjects were right-handed). Imagination of smell produced less activation than active stimulation, with differences in the activated sites.

Several regions of decreased signal following stimulation were also observed. These tended to occur in the superior frontal regions, in the midline, at the base of the anterior frontal lobes, and near the medial and superior temporal lobes. Some of these regions were within vessels.

In all the patients with hyposmia, decreased detection of the olfactory stimulus was associated with markedly decreased cerebral activation relative to the normal cases. Both the Z scores and the number of possibly activated regions were significantly decreased.

Discussion

These studies indicate that functional MRI may be used to demonstrate olfactory cortex activation. Significant activation was observed in regions of the frontal and temporal lobes. These correspond to the orbitofrontal, entorhinal and prepyriform cortical areas. Additional regions of activation observed in other areas of the frontal and temporal lobes appear to be in the areas of the nucleus accumbens, the septal nuclei, and the amygdaloid complex, and these results are in agreement with the literature data. Regions of activation in the superior portions of the frontal lobes may also represent cognitive functions associated with olfaction.

Several regions of decreased signal following stimulation were also observed. These may be related to patterns of deactivation within the brain. Regions that were within vessels may refer to blood coming from deactivated regions. In fact, there may be hemodynamic changes that may simulate effects of deactivation, and further research is underway to evaluate those changes further.

Although it is commonly believed that it is in the CNS that most pathology associated with loss of smell resides, smell loss is usually due to pathology of a biochemical nature which takes place at the olfactory receptor, not in the CNS [9, 10]. Assessment of receptor pathology in hyposmia is important in applying therapy, and receptor pathology is amenable to biochemical change after treatment with a broad range of drugs, trace metals and hormones [10]. Thus, a biochemical or functional focus could play an important role in successful understanding of these disorders and their potential therapy.

References

1. Belliveau JW, Kennedy DN, McKinstry RC et al. (1991) Functional mapping of the human visual cortex by magnetic resonance imaging. Science 254:716–719
2. Ogawa S, Menon RS, Tank DW et al. (1993) Functional brain mapping by blood oxygenation level-dependent contrast MRI. Biophys J 64:803–812
3. Turner R, LeBihan D, Moonen CTW, Despres D et al. (1991) Echo planar time course MRI of cat brain oxygenation changes. Magn Reson Med 22:159–166
4. Connelly A, Jackson GD, Frackowiak RSJ et al. (1993) High resolution functional mapping of activated human primary cortex using a clinical MRI system. Radiology 188:125–130
5. Schellinger D, Henkin RI, Smirniotopoulos JG (1983) CT of the brain in taste and smell dysfunction. AJNR 4:752–754
6. Suzuki M, Takashima T, Kadoya S, Miyayama S, Taira S (1989) MR imaging of olfactory bulbs and tracts. AJNR 10:951–957
7. Klingmueller D, Dewes W, Krahe T, Brecht G, Schweikert HU (1987) Magnetic resonance imaging of the brain in patients with anosmia and hypothalamic hypogonadism (Kallmann's syndrome). J Clin Endo Metab 65:581–584
8. LeBihan D, Jezzood P, Turner R, Cuenod C et al. (1993) Analysis of functional MR images with z maps: works in progress. J Magn Reson Imaging 3(P):141
9. Meurmann OH (1950) Experimental studies of the effect of pathological changes in the nasal mucous membrane on the olfactory bulb. Acta Otolaryngol (Stockh) 38:477–483
10. Henkin RI (1993) Evaluation and treatment of human olfactory dysfunction, In: English G (ed) Otolaryngology. Lippincott, Philadelphia, pp 1–86

Functional MRI of memory in transient global amnesia

L. M. Levy, V. N. Starbuck, G. G. Kay, J. Kattah, S. Potolicchio, S. Cohan, C. S. Lin, C. Ariz, D. Schellinger, D. LeBihan

Georgetown University Hospital, Washington, D.C., USA

Abstract. The purpose of this study was to evaluate the feasibility of functional MRI (fMRI) in the investigation of transient global amnesia (TGA). MRI of the brain was performed on normal subjects and a patient with TGA. fMR images were obtained of left temporal and frontal regions of the brain. A 55-year-old woman was studied during a 6-h period of amnesia and again 2 weeks later, when memory had returned to normal. In all cases, memory testing was conducted during fMRI using a version of the Hopkins Verbal Learning Test. During TGA, the patient showed little or no activation during list learning or recognition testing. After her TGA had resolved, she demonstrated normal list learning and recognition. As in the healthy subjects, activation in the temporal region occurred during both list learning and recognition, whereas frontal activation was seen more often during recognition testing.

Key words: Functional magnetic resonance imaging – Memory testing

Correspondence to: L. M. Levy

Recent advances in functional magnetic resonance imaging (fMRI) technology have made it possible to image the brain noninvasively during performance of specific tasks. Using the deoxyhemoglobin contrast method, focal increases in neuronal activity can be detected and localized to specific regions of the brain [1–4]. Although it has been used to study the visual cortex, sensorimotor cortex, language and visual mental imagery in normal subjects, there have been few published studies using fMRI to investigate brain functioning in neurological diseases. In view of the high spatial resolution of MRI, fMRI should be able to provide a detailed views of regions of cortex activated during cognitive tasks.

We used fMRI to study a patient with transient global amnesia (TGA). TGA is characterized by a temporary inability to form new memories, temporary retrograde amnesia, and absence of other neurologic signs [5–7]. The patient was studied during the period of amnesia and 2 weeks after the amnesia had cleared. Auditory verbal memory testing was conducted during fMRI scanning of left temporal and frontal regions. Separate images were obtained during encoding of word list items, and during recognition testing for list items. Free recall and recognition of list items were tested at each session.

Case report

A 55-year-old right-handed woman was admitted via the emergency room for diagnosis and investigation following a period of acute confusion. At the time of the initial test session, she was not oriented to person, place, time or situation. She was not able to provide personal information other than her name and some other vague responses. In spite of this disorientation and confusion, the patient remained calm and fully compliant. The duration of the entire period of TGA was 6 h. The patient returned for follow-up testing 2 weeks later, when she was fully alert, oriented, calm and cooperative. Conventional MRI of the brain on admission and at follow-up were normal.

Materials and methods

MRI of the brain were performed on the patient and on 9 healthy subjects using a 1.5 T imager with a head coil. None of the subjects had clinical evidence of cognitive disfunction. A modified gradient-echo FLASH sequence was used with TE 35, TR 50 ms, flip angle 30°, field of view 325 mm, slice thickness 4 mm, acquisition time per image 5 s. Sagittal images were selected to cover the lateral portion of the frontotemporal region, at 42–49 mm from the midline. In addition, coronal sections, usually three, were selected at the levels of the head of the caudate nucleus, its body and the hippocampus. The functional stimulation pattern involved a 3-min scan of 30 images: 10 at rest, 5 with testing, 5 at rest, 5 with testing, and 5 at rest. Pre- and poststimulation images were compared using Z statistics [8]. The stimulus-pattern versus intensity response was correlated, and the Z scores, activation ratios and activated areas were measured for each activated region. The sites of activation were noted. In addition, activation images were correlated with high-resolution images for better anatomical localization.

All subjects were presented with a modified version of the Hopkins Verbal Learning Test (HVLT) during fMRI sessions. Words from the 12-item word list were continuously read to the subject during the recording periods, allowing the list to be repeated. During the first period (encoding), the subject was asked to listen and try to memorize the word list. During the second period (recognition), the subject was instructed to listen to words from the HVLT recognition list and asked to decide whether each word belonged to the previous (encoding) list. She was not required to make any overt responses during either memory or recognition testing. A different word list from the HVLT was administered at each test session. Following fMRI, free recall and recognition testing were conducted to determine the actual level of performance.

Results

At the initial test session the patient was unable to recall any list items freely. On recognition testing, she correctly identified 8 of the 12 list items and falsely identified 1 nonlist item. Memory testing at the follow-up session revealed a significant degree of recovery: she correctly recalled 8 list items without cueing and identified 11 list items on recognition testing with 3 false-positive identifications. This level of performance reflected a return to normal memory function.

fMRI results from the initial test session during the period of global amnesia showed little or no activation during either list learning or recognition testing. In contrast, fMRI at the 2-week follow-up session revealed several regions of activation, with Z scores ranging from 1.6 to 2.75. Two distinct patterns of activation were observed, as in the normal cases: temporal activation occurred during both list learning and recognition, but frontal activation was seen more prominently during recognition testing.

Discussion

As expected, a significant degree of recovery occurred over the 2 weeks between test sessions. At the initial test session, during the amnesic attack, the patient was unable to learn the word list and generally unable to recognize list items in a recognition format. fMRI at that time showed no activation during the memory test procedure. At the follow-up session, the patient's memory for word-list items had returned to normal. fMRI following recovery of memory functioning demonstrated two clear patterns of activation. During list learning, there was activation localized to the left temporal region. During recognition testing, activation was apparent in the left frontal cortex as well as in the left temporal region. This suggests that encoding and recognition tasks utilize both common and distinct pathways.

This study demonstrates the utility of fMRI as a tool for investigating the neurocognitive manifestations of neurologic conditions such as transient global amnesia. Our results are in agreement with reports that TGA is associated with dysfunction of temporal brain structures, possibly due to changes in perfusion [6, 7]. The present case demonstrates the use of fMRI to track the changes in brain activation associated with recovery of brain function. fMRI also provides a means for better understanding brain-behavior relationships in normal individuals, e.g., the differential activation associated with distinct aspects of memory. Furthermore, this technique can be used to study the changes in brain functioning underlying specific cognitive tasks and neuropsychological tests.

References

1. Belliveau JW, Kennedy DN, McKinstry RC et al. (1991) Functional mapping of the human visual cortex by magnetic resonance imaging. Science 254:716–719

2. Ogawa S, Menon RS, Tank DW et al. (1993) Functional brain mapping by blood oxygenation level-dependent contrast MRI. Biophys J 64:803–812
3. Turner R, LeBihan D, Moonen CTW, Despres D et al. (1991) Echo planar time course MRI of cat brain oxygenation changes. Mag Res Med 22:159–166
4. Connelly A, Jackson GD, Frackowiak RSJ et al. (1993) High resolution functional mapping of activated human primary cortex using a clinical MRI system. Radiology 188:125–130
5. Hodges JR, Warlow CP (1990) Syndromes of transient global amnesia: towards a classification. A study of 153 cases. J Neurol Neurosurg Psychiatry 53:834
6. Matsuda H, Higashi S, Tsuji S, Sumiya H et al. (1993) High resolution Tc-99m HMPAO SPECT in a patient with transient global amnesia. Clin Nucl Med 18:46–49
7. Laloux P, Brichant C, Cauwe F, Decoster P (1992) Tech-99m HMPAO single photon emission computed tomography imaging in transient global amnesia. Arch Neurol 49:543–546
8. LeBihan D, Jezzood P, Turner R, Cuenod C et al. (1993) Analysis of functional MR images with z maps: works in progress. J Magn Reson Imaging 3(P):141

Clinical application of relative quantification in single-Voxel ^{1}H-MRS for brain examination

H. Shimizu[1], K. Sato[1], Y. Ono[1], S. Fujiwara[1], T. Yoshimoto[2], N. Arai[3]

[1] Department of Neurosurgery, Kohnan Hospital, 4-20-1 Nagamachi-minami, Taihaku-ku, Sendai 982, Japan
[2] Department of Neurosurery, Tokohu University, Sendai, Japan
[3] GE Yokogawa Medical Systems, Tokyo, Japan

Abstract. A method of relative quantification using external standards was tested for its usefulness in clinical single-voxel long-TE proton magnetic resonance spectroscopy (MRS). Using *N*-acetyl-L-alanine solution (NALA) as an external standard, the variance of NALA signal intensity over days was 7.4% when different volunteers were placed in the head coil together with the standard. In 12 volunteers' frontal white matter, the calculated normal ranges of *N*-acetyl aspartate (NAA), choline-containing (Cho) and creatine-containing compounds (Cre) to NALA were 3.6 ± 1.0, 2.1 ± 0.8 and 1.5 ± 0.8 (mean $\pm$ 2 SD) respectively. All 14 gliomas showed elevated Cho/NAA ratios, but 7 had normal Cho/NALA ratios. Cho/NALA increased and NAA/NALA decreased with the histological grade, indicating that high-grade gliomas contain more Cho and less NAA. Although changes in T1 and T2 relaxation and water compartments must be taken into account, relative quantification using an external standard is useful in clinical long-TE proton MRS.

Key words: Proton MRS – Brain, relative quantification

The search for a method has been one of the major interests in the field of in vivo magnetic resonance spectroscopy (MRS). Although several recent reports [1–3] deal with methods for absolute quantification in single-voxel proton MRS (^{1}H-MRS) with short TE sequence, long-TE acquisitions are also popular, because of the ease of spectral analysis. ^{1}H-MRS using long TE presents several problems for quantification, such as the heavy influence of T2 relaxation and diffusion changes, and temperature effect. We therefore tested a simple means of relative quantification using an external standard to investigate its clinical usefulness. Since selection and evaluation of an external standard are important in terms of its readiness for clinical use and stability over time, we first performed phantom experiments. The stability and variability of relative quantification within normal individual volunteers were then tested, to estimate the fundamental errors of the method and the normal ranges of each metabolite detectable by proton MRS. The results of clinical application of the method were also presented.

Correspondence to: H. Shimizu

Methods

1.5 T system and a standard headcoil for magnetic resonance (MRI), which produces a homogeneous B1 field [4], were used to perform single-voxel point-resolved spectroscopy (PRESS). The parameters were as follows: spectral width 2500 Hz, 2048 data points, TR 2000 ms, TE 272 ms, and number of averages 128 for external standards and 256 for brain examinations. Volumes of interest (VOI) varied from $13 \times 13 \times 15$ mm to $20 \times 20 \times 20$ mm for both brain and standard measurements. Data processing was performed using software supplied by the manufacturer. Following zero-filling, 2 Hz of exponential filtering, Fourier transformation, manual zero-order phasing and baseline correction. Gaussian fitting was applied to measure areas under four dominant peaks of the spectra, namely N-acetyl aspartate (NAA) at 2.0 ppm, creatine-containing compounds (Cre) at 3.0 ppm, choline-containing compounds (Cho) at 3.2 ppm, and lactate, if any, at 1.3 ppm. The peak area was then divided by the size of the VOI.

Phantom experiments. Lactic acid solution (200 mM) containing 5 mM of $NiCl_2$ and *N*-acetyl-L-alanine solution (200 mM) containing 5 mAM of $NiCl_2$ (NALA) were tested. These concentrations of chemicals were determined through preliminary experiments, so that a sufficient signal-to-noise ratio (SNR > 200:1) and T1 shortening to avoid T1 saturation with current TR were achieved. For a signal intensity of LAC, a double peak was assumed to be a single

Table 1. Summary of gliomas: mean metabolite/standard ratios

	Histological grade			
	I	II	II	IV
Cho/NALA	0.8	2.4	4.6	7.9
Cre/NALA	1.0	1.3	1.5	1.4
NAA/NALA	1.7	2.1	0.9	0.6
Lac/NALA	1.6	1.2	1.8	4.4
Cho/NAA	0.5	1.2	10.0	80.8
Cho/Cre	0.8	2.1	3.4	5.5
Cre/NAA	0.6	0.6	4.3	14.4
Number	1	4	7	2

Cho, choline; NALA, 200 mM *N*-acetyl-L-alanine; NAA, *N*-acetyl aspartate; Lac, lactic acid

peak for curve fitting. For a signal intensity of NALA, a single peak at 1.9 ppm was used. Reproducibility of a single measurement was first tested by performing PRESS five times each on nine LAC or NALA standards. The dependence of the standard position in the headcoil on the stability of the signal was also determined by repeating experiments with the standards around a water bottle phantom placed at different distances from the coil elements. To investigate the possible degradation of LAC and NALA over time, standards were measured repeatedly up to 55 days after preparation. Changes in the peak areas were analysed by taking the ratio to signal intensity of freshly prepared standard at each timepoint.

Experiments in normal volunteers. Normal volunteers were placed in the headcoil with LAC and NALA at the fixed position, which was found to by the above experiment to give the least variation in repeated measurements. The frontal white matter of the volunteer and the standard were measured alternately, to produce several sets of peak ratios of brain metabolite to LAC or NALA standard in 13 normal volunteers. This experiment was repeated every 4 days to confirm the reliability and variation of the method over time.

Clinical application. Fifteen patients with intracranial tumours (15 gliomas and 1 meningioma) were involved in the study, all of whom had given informed consent. The data were analysed by the conventional method (taking ratios of metabolites) and by the present method of relative quantification. The time taken for a study involving three different VOI was about 45 min.

Results

Phantom experiments

The error of measurement was 1.9% (100 × SD/mean) for the LAC and 2.0% for NALA. The best reproducibility was achieved when a standard was placed in such a way as to make an equilateral triangle with neighbouring elements. Repeated measurements of the LAC revealed that the signal decreased linearly with time, by 12% per week. On the other hand, ratios of old NALA/new NALA signals did not show significant increase or decrease over 40 days, with fluctuations of less than 10%. Using NALA as an external standard, the variance of NALA signal intensity over time was 4.4% when a water load standard was placed in the headcoil together with the standard. It increased to 7.4% when different volunteers replace the water standard.

Experiments in normal volunteers

NAA of the brain/LAC or NALA ratios in a single volunteer varied by 2.8–10.4% in a single stage, and the same degree of error was observed for measurements over time. Based on these limitations, normal ranges of NAA, Cho and Cre/std standard ratios could be estimated as 6.4 ± 1.3, 3.6 ± 1.5 and 2.3 ± 1.6 ($n = 9$, mean ± 2 SD, a.u.) respectively, when LAC was used as an external standard. When NALA was used as an external standard, these ranges were 3.6 ± 1.0, 2.1 ± 0.8 and 1.5 ± 0.8 ($n = 12$, mean ± 2 SD), respectively.

Clinical application

All brain tumours showed elevated Cho/NAA ratios, as previously reported. However, 7 out 14 gliomas had a Cho standard (NALA) ratio of no more than the normal range when studied by this method. In these tumours the reduction of the NAA peak was the actual cause of the high Cho/NAA ratio. Table 1 summarises the results of 14 glioma cases in relation to histological grading. Cho standard increased and NAA standard decreased with the histological grade, indicating that high-grade gliomas contain more Cho and less NAA. Lac standard increased abruptly in grade 4 gliomas. The standard ratio did not change significantly with malignancy. When the metabolite ratios were calculated, these changes in individual peaks were not clear.

Discussion

The difference in the stability of signals between the water phantom (4.4%) and the volunteers (7.4%) suggests that changes in the Q-factor of the coil influenced the stability of signal intensity of an external standard by 3%. We considered these variances as a complex of experimental errors attributable to, for example, slight variations in preparation of the standard, slight difference in the shimming, water suppression and data processing (especially baseline correction and line-fitting procedure), and unavoidable limitations of the MR system itself.

As an external standard, NALA seemed to be superior to LAC, since it gave a single peak at 1.9 ppm and the intensity did not change over 40 days.

Our results show that relative quantification in long-TE proton MRS provides more useful data than metabolite ratio analysis only However, since T1 and T2 relaxation and water compartment changes are not corrected in this method, care is needed when pathologic lesions with considerable change in the parameters are studied.

References

1. Ernst T, Kreis R, Ross BD (1993) Absolute quantitation of water and metabolites in the human brain. I. Compartments and water. J Magn Reson 102: 1–8

2. Kreis R, Ernst T, Ross BD (1993) Absolute quantitation of water and metabolites in the human brain. II. Metabolite concentrations. J Magn Reson 102:9–19
3. Kreis R, Ernst T, Ross BD (1993) Development of the human brain: in vivo quantification of metabolites and water content with proton magnetic resonance spectroscopy. Magn Reson Med 30:424–437
4. Hayes CE, Edelstein WA, Schenck JF, Mueller OM, Eash M (1985) An efficient, highly homogeneous radiofrequency coil for whole-body NMR imaging at 1.5 T Magn Reson 63:622–628

Standard terminology for MR image description

G. H. du Boulay [1,2], B. A. Teather [2], D. Teather [2], M. A. Higgott [2], N. P. Jeffery [2]

[1] Institute of Neurology, Queen Square, London, England
[2] Medical Systems Research Unit, De Montfort University, Leicester, England

Abstract. A glossary of descriptive terms for use in structured reporting in magnetic resonance cerebral images is presented. The glossary characterises lesions in terms of lesion types, shape, geometric qualifiers, intensity content, scales of intensity and associated signs. Anatomical definitions, disease terms and user instructions are also provided. Terminology is being utilised to establish statistical databases that may be utilised to identify combinations of image features that assist in differential diagnosis.

Key words: Glossary – Magnetic resonance imaging – Image description language – Structured reporting – Cerebral images

The information in MR images of lesions in the brain is conveyed by shapes, their relationships to one another, their sizes, relative grey levels, anatomical associations and alterations between sequences. Observers try to match what they see with what they remember from previous experience and to interpret it in terms of what they know about neuropathology. In broad terms an experienced neuroradiologist is fairly successful in separating some groups of conditions but has, nevertheless, to accept severe limitations both in his pattern discrimination and in the statistical evaluation of certainty of interpretation. In order to improve the differential diagnostics between a set of similar conditions, a radiologist may laboriously list many detailed characteristics of a substantial group of cases whole final diagnoses have become known. To do this the radiologist must define his descriptive terms and then adhere consistently to them throughout his work. Another radiologist elsewhere, tackling a related question, will rarely be in a position to use the identical terminology because it has not been precisely described in publications and there are no generally accepted rules for lesion description. The result is that the labours of the two are not as mutually supportive as they might be. Common experience and teaching are affected by disagreements about the usage of descriptive terms and unconscious inconsistencies of language.

Correspondence to: G. H. du Boulay

Table 1. Glossary of image description language: further descriptors

Geometric qualifiers
- Margin of whole lesion *Sharp*, or *Graded*
- Area of whole lesion

Intensity content
- Homogeneous or Unstructured heterogeneous

Scales of intensity
- Reference: cerebral or cerebellar white
- Grade: +++, ++, +, iso, –, – –, – – –

Associated or "other" signs include
- Mass effect
- Ventricular dilatation (specify)
- Sulcal compression
- Sulcal widening
- Loss of brain substance

Anatomical locations
- A list too large for this publication, including definitions used or "Lobes"

Disease index
- WHO list

User instructions

Lesion types
- A list which is useful when multiple lesions are present, in order to avoid having to provide detailed descriptions of every one

Correspondences
- This facility keys in the information provided by other sequences about identified parts of lesions.

Methods

Standard terms for image description were incorporated into "BRAINS" [1, 2], a suite of programs for advice in CT diagnosis of cerebral lesions. We have used our experience in CT to define a structured description language for describing both lesions and relevant abnormal signals in MRI. The terminology presented here was developed over a number of years, involving discussions with a range of experienced neuroradiologists [3, 4].

The structured terminology has been incorporated into a prototype image description system. Experience with this computer-based, menu-driven image description system for MRI, supported by comprehensive data capture, has been encouraging. We have evidence from pilot studies of the power of such a system in discriminating between multiple sclerosis and vascular disease [5] and between different stages of HIV encephalitis [6]. The image

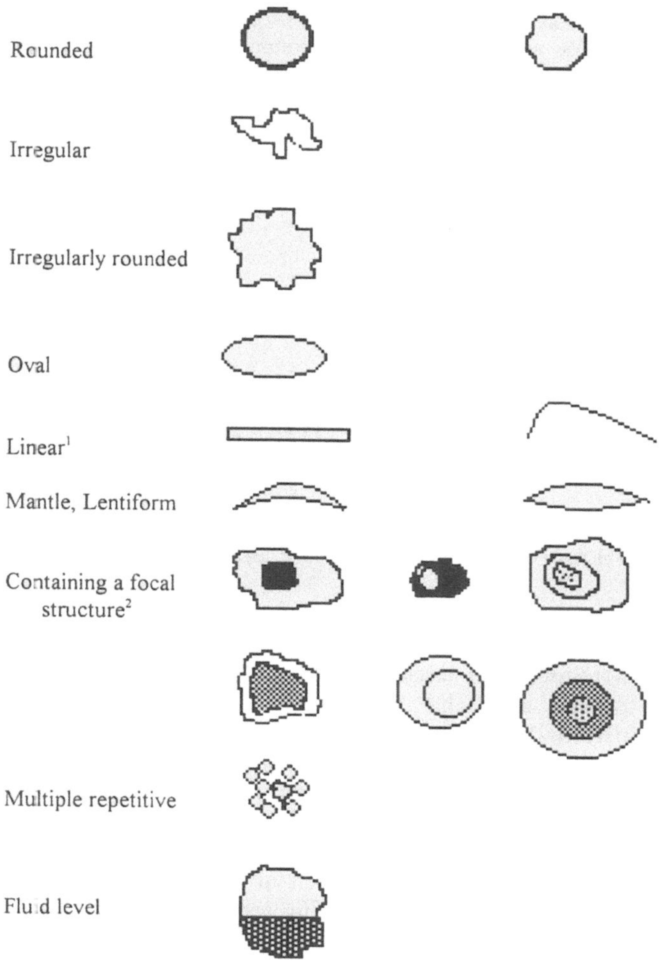

Fig. 1. Glossary of lesion description language – shape.
[1] Linear not more than 4 mm wide and at least 5 times longer than width.
[2] A "focal structure" is an area of the lesion, often, but not always near to its centre, usually well defined around all of its margin, and seeming to represent either the centre of activity of the lesion or the lesion itself as distinct from surrounding oedema. Note that the focal structure can be large and, in some cases, may even represent the majority of the lesion.

description language, although developed over several years, would benefit from further refinement. We wish therefore to expose it to general trial, in particular as a teaching tool, because only in that way could it hope to be made generally acceptable [7, 8].

Results

Most of the descriptive language has been defined in "Help" text for the descriptor system. The short extract from the illustrated glossary shown in Fig. 1, though not quite comprehensive, should convey the way it works. To this list of "SHAPES" must be added a number of other despriptors as listed in Table 1. An example image description is presented in Fig. 2.

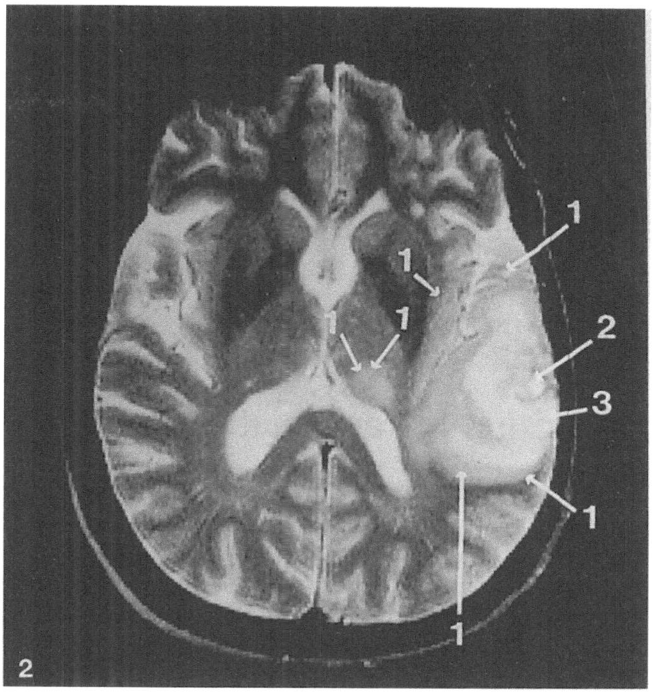

Fig. 2. Example image description.
This lesion (1), in the temporal grey and central and peripheral white matter, also involves the thalamus. It is irregular in outline, and contains a focal structure (2 + 3), which contains a ring structure (3). The centre of the focal structure (2) is unstructured heterogeneous with intensities (compared with cerebral white matter) of – and + and ++ and +++. The ring part of the focal structure has intensities of + and ++ and +++. The remainder of the lesion shows intensities of + and ++. There is mass effect and compression of the cerebral sulci

Discussion

There are many ways of reporting MRI examinations of patients. A full description of the findings is rare because of the time it takes to write and read. Nevertheless the consistent use of such descriptive terms as are thought essential would be useful advance and could be learned early in a neuroradiologist's training.

In a research environment full descriptions come into their own and the statistical analysis of detailed image characteristics, stored by a ready-made (but adaptable) system, has much to offer.

References

1. du Boulay GH, Teather D, Morton BA, Wills KM, Inocent PR, Plummer D (1987) Brains – a computer advisor system to aid in CT scan interpretation and cerebral disease diagnosis. Neuroradiology 29:196–199
2. Teather D, Teather BA, Wills KM, du Boulay GH, Plummer D, Isherwood I, Gholkar A (1988) Evaluation of computer advisor in the interpretation of CT images of the head. Neuroradiology 30:511–517
3. du Boulay GH, Woods AJ, Teather D, Teather BA, Wills KM, Plummer D (1988) Towards an advisor for MRI. Neuroradiology 30:245–251

4. du Boulay GH, Field B, Teather BA, Teather D, Plummer D (1992) The extraction of expert knowledge for MR image acquisition from the published literature. Riv Neuroradiol 5:473–482
5. du Boulay GH, Teather BA, Teather D, Jeffery NP, Higgott MA, Plummer D (1994) Discriminating multiple sclerosis from other diseases of similar presentation – can a formal description approach help? Riv Neuroradiol 7:37–45
6. du Boulay GH, Teather BA, Teather D, Santosh C, Best J (1994) Structured reporting of MRI of the head in HIV. Neuroradiology 37:S 144
7. Jeffery NP, Teather BA, Teather D, Sharples M, du Boulay B, du Boulay GH (1994) Intelligent tutoring for MR image interpretation and the diagnosis of cerebral disease. Neuroradiology 37:S 144
8. Teather D, Teather BA, Sharples M, Jeffery NP, du Boulay B, du Boulay GH (1994) Intelligent tutoring or MR imaging of the head and cerebral disease. Proceedings of the 12th International Congress of the European Federation for Medical Informatics MIE '94, pp 650–653

Algorithm for automatic matching of brain stem atlas to MR images

R. Tadmor[1], **R. Tenny**[1], **M. Furst**[2]

[1] Faculty of Medicine, Tel Aviv University, Tel Aviv 69978, Israel
[2] Department of Electrical Engineering Systems, Faculty of Engineering, Tel Aviv University, Tel Aviv 69978, Israel

Abstract. When lesions are detected on magnetic resonance images (MRI) of the brain stem, it can be difficult to determine exactly which nuclei or fibre tracts are involved. We introduce a user-friendly automatic algorithm that calculates a nonlinear transformation that matches a given anatomical atlas to MR images. A brain stem atlas was constructed from histological serial sections of a human brain stem, in which the auditory nuclei and fibre tracts were traced. The algorithm is based on matching the brain stem outline of MRI sections to the corresponding atlas sections. The estimated transformations are applied to the nuclei and fibre tracts in the atlas and are then superimposed on the MR images. The algorithm was tested on MRI patients with multiple sclerosis (MS) whose ability to judge the laterality of sounds was tested psychoacoustically. Our results indicate that there is a relationship between the type of behavioural abnormality and the location of MS lesions relative to the auditory pathway.

Key words: Magnetic resonance imaging – Brain stem atlas – Auditory pathway – Multiple sclerosis

In magnetic resonance images (MRI) of the human brain obtained with T1- or T2-weighted sequences, the brain stem normally appears as a homogeneous region. However, it is in fact an assemblage of many different fibre tracts and nuclei where each of these carries different information. These nuclei can rarely be differentiated by the naked eye on MRI. Lesions can be visualized when appearing at different signal intensities. In multiple sclerosis (MS), for example, the lesions appear as bright patches on T2-weighted images [1]. Since nuclei and fibre tracts are so close to each other, it is difficult to localize a lesion accurately in the brain stem and its relation to the underlying nuclei.

Correspondence to: M. Furst

Recently, Furst et al. [2] proposed an algorithm for matching MRI sections to a superimposed detailed anatomical atlas that was constructed from a series of histological sections of adult human brain stem. Edges of the brain stem, auditory nuclei, and fibre tracts were manually traced and entered into a computer-aided anatomy system [3]. It was then possible to reconstruct sections in any plane or thickness to correspond to a particular MRI section. Each of the MRI sections was matched to the corresponding section in the atlas. The algorithm required manual registration of the brain stem outline of every MR scan, a time-consuming and inaccurate procedure. In this paper we introduce a user-friendly matching algorithm that requires only minimal interaction by the user.

Materials and methods

For this study 11 MS patients were examined and the brain stem analysed. MRI were obtained on an 1.9 T unit scanner with T2-weighted, spin-echo pulse sequences. Data were collected in 3 planes: axial, coronal and sagittal. Contiguous 5 mm sections were obtained with TR 1500 ms for the sagittal sections and TR 2500 ms for the axial and coronal sections; TE 80 ms was used for all sections. Each of the MRI sections was matched to a corresponding section in the above described atlas while using the matching algorithm.

The algorithm searches for a transformation that can be applied to the anatomical atlas and, as a result, the brain stem outlines of both an MRI section and its corresponding atlas section overlap. Initially, a three-dimensional linear transformation was found from landmarks that were manually indicated, as can be seen on Fig. 1. Three landmarks were denoted in the midsagittal plane (A, B, and C), corresponding to well-defined anatomical structures: the cerebral peduncle, the middle cerebellar peduncle (brachium pontis), and the inferior colliculus. The additional two pairs of landmarks (D, E and F, G), were denoted only for determining the plane of symmetry in both axial and coronal planes. Any coronal or axial section could be used for marking these four landmarks. As a result, two sets of corresponding landmarks were obtained: the first indicated by the user and the second à priori, as marked in the atlas. The two sets were sufficient for calculating a 4×3 matrix that

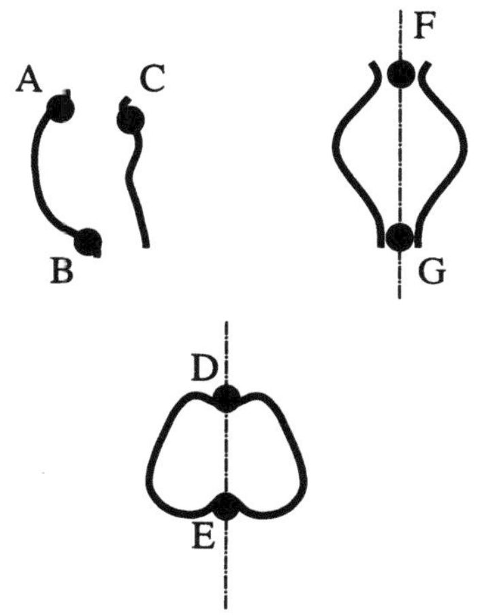

Fig. 1. The seven landmarks indicated on the brain stem in sagittal (*A, B, C*), axial (*D, E*) and coronal (*F, G*) planes

corresponds to a three dimensional linear transformation from the atlas to an individual human brain stem.

Two-dimensional projections of the transformed anatomical atlas were obtained and superimposed on different MR images. For most sections, the linear transformation was not adequate, as the atlas brain stem outlines did not overlap with those on the MR images. It was therefore necessary to search for a transformation that was specific for each section.

For good matching it is essential that both outlines overlap; therefore, a search for a better transformation was based on detecting the brain stem outline on MRI. In some sections, the brain stem outline was very clear, and any edge detection algorithm [4] could be applied to determine the brain stem outline. However, in many sections part of the outline was undetectable because it either merged with other tissues, or partial averaging occurred due to the transition changes in shape.

A special algorithm for delineating the brain stem outline was developed [5], whereby various edges were detected by different threshold techniques. The preferred edge was chosen as the one where the distance to the initial outline was minimal. Comparison between the chosen edge and the initial atlas outline yielded a modified non linear transformation that guaranteed one-to-one mapping for each point in the brain stem, including the outline and inner points [6].

Once the transformation was found, it was applied to the auditory pathway. Figure 2 demonstrates the superimposed auditory pathways (bright dots) on an MRI study in the three different axes.

Results

Figure 2 represents an MR study where MS lesions were detected in all three planes. Some of the lesions overlapped with the auditory pathway, and others did not. As defined in previous studies [1, 3, 7], a lesion is considered to involve the auditory pathway only if it interacts with the same part of the auditory pathway in at least two different perpendicular planes. For the patient whose images are shown in Fig. 2, it was concluded that her MS lesions involved the trapezoid body.

Furst et al. [3] have shown that there is a close correlation between the location of MS lesions relative to the brain stem auditory pathway and the behavioural performances of patients in click lateralization tests. Clicks were introduced to both ears simultaneously, and subjects were asked to indicate where in the head they perceived them: centre, left or right. Different stimuli with interaural time delays (ITD) or level differences (ILD) were presented. Normally, the binaural clicks are perceived everywhere around the head. For small ITD (less than 0.3 ms) and ILD (less than 5 dB) the clicks are perceived to be in the centre. For bigger ITD (between 0.3 ms and 1 ms), or ILD (between 5 and 20 dB), they are lateralized to the right or left.

Of the 11 patients with MS who underwent MRI studies, 5 did not have lesions that involved the brain stem auditory pathways. These patients all performed normally in the lateralization test. Three patients perceived all the binaural clicks from the side only and never in the centre. Those patients had lesions involving the lateral lemniscus. Two patients perceived the binaural clicks with ITD at the centre only. Their performance with clicks with ILD was normal. These patients had lesions involving the trapezoid body.

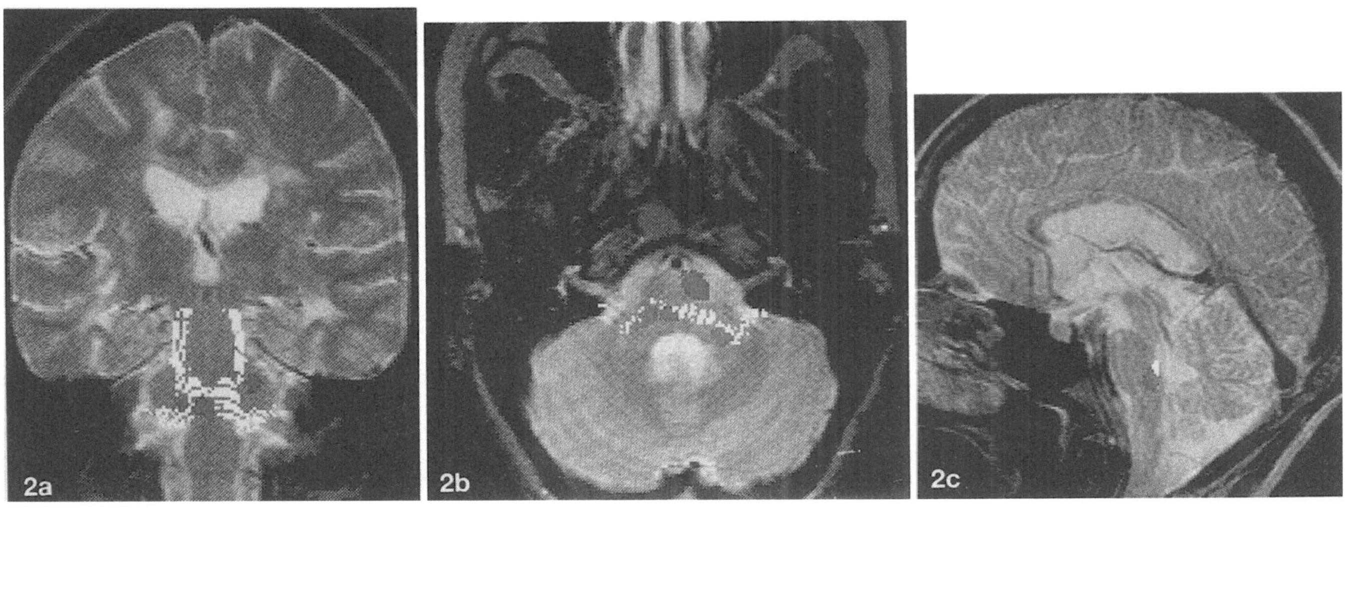

Fig. 2 a–c. Superimposed auditory pathways *(bright dots)* on MRI study with MS lesions *(dark patches)* in the three axes (**a** coronal, **b** axial, **c** sagittal)

References

1. Rumbach L, Armsprach JP, Gounot D, Namer IJ, Chambron J, Warter JM, Collard M (1991) Nuclear magnetic resonance T2 relaxation times in multiple sclerosis. J Neurol Sci 104:176–181
2. Furst M, Levine RA, Korczyn AD, Fullerton BC, Tadmor R, Algom D (1994) Brainstem lesions and click lateralization in patients with multiple sclerosis. Hear Res (in press)
3. Levine RA, Gardner JC, Stufflebeam SM, Fullerton BC, Carisle EW, Furst M, Rosen BR, Kiang NYS (1993) Binaural auditory processing in multiple sclerosis patients. Hear Res 68:59–72
4. Gonzales RC, Woods RE (1992) Digital image processing. Addison-Wesley, Reading, Mass
5. Tenny R (1994) Algorithm for matching brainstem atlas to MR images. M.Sc Thesis, Faculty of Engineering, Tel Aviv University
6. Bookstein F (1978) The measurement of biological shape and shape change (Lecture Notes in Biomathematics). Springer-Verlag, New York
7. Levine RA, Gardner JC, Stufflebeam SM, Fullerton BC, Carisle EW, Furst M, Rosen BR, Kiang NYS (1993) Effects of multiple sclerosis brainstem lesions on sound lateralization and brainstem auditory evoked potentials. Hear Res 68:73–88

MRA

MR Angiography: comparison of time-of-flight, phase-contrast and digital substraction angiography

K. E. W. Eberhardt [1], H. P. Hollenbach [2], U. Böttcher [2], W. J. Huk [1]

[1] Division of Neuroradiology, Department of Neurosurgery, University of Erlangen, Erlangen, Germany
[2] Siemens Medical Engineering Group, Erlangen, Germany

Abstract. We compared two MR angiography (MRA) techniques, time-of-flight (TOF) and phase-contrast (PC), with digital substraction angiography (DSA), in relation to operative findings in 40 patients with cerebrovascular disease. The investigations were performed using a 1.5 T whole-body system. 2D- and 3D-TOF and 2D- and 3D PC sequences were used in sagittal and axial planes. Velocity-encoding of the PC sequence varied between 5 and 100 cm/s, depending on the blood flow velocity. The 3D data-sets were analysed using a maximum intensity projection program. The sensitivity of TOF and PC is comparable with that of DSA in the diagnosis of venous thrombosis. MRA may be superior to DSA in patients with giant aneurysms.

Key words: Magnetic resonance imaging - MR angiography - Time-of-flight - phase contrast - Digital substraction angiography

We compared two MR angiography (MRA) techniques, time-of-flight (TOF) and phase-contrast (PC) angiography, with digital substraction angiography (DSA).

Materials and methods

We compared the diagnostic sensitivity of the two MRA techniques with that of DSA in 40 patients with cerebral vascular disease. Their average age was 53.7 years (17–82 years); there were 22 men and 18 women. The interval between the DSA and MRA ranged from 1 to 12 days (mean 3.6 days). Subsequently 25 patients had surgery and 15, interventional procedures within the next 2–18 days (mean 10.3 days). The investigations were performed using a 1.5 T whole-body system. We compared 2D-(TR/TE/α 22/10/35 ms/ms/deg) and 3D-TOF sequences with a magnetization transfer pre pulse [1, 2] and TONE RF pulse (TR/TE/α 10/11/25 ms/ms/deg) with a 2D-PC sequence (TR/TE/α 76/8-11/15 ms/ms/deg). The flow velocity encoding varied between 5 and 100 cm/s. The measurement time for the 2D-PC sequence was 40 s and that for the 3D-PC, 8 min. The 3D data-sets were analysed using a maximum intensity projection (MIP) program. All patients also underwent DSA examination. The results were compared and evaluated using specific diagnostic criteria and a diagnostic score.

Correspondence to: K. E. W. Eberhardt, Division of Neuroradiology, Department of Neurosurgery, University of Erlangen, Schwabachanlage 6, D-91054 Erlangen, Germany

Table 1

Disease	MRA		DSA
	TOF	PC	
Giant aneurysm	0.25	0.63	0.38
Venous occlusion	0.60	1.00	0.75
AV fistulae	0.50	0.82	0.93
Dissection of carotid artery	1.00	0.75	0.50

Results

PC can be superior to DSA and TOF in diagnosis of giant aneurysms. The diagnostic score (Table 1) of PC (0.63) is higher than that of DSA (0.38) and TOF (0.25). In patients with compression or occlusion of the venous system PC shows revascularisation and collateral circulation better than DSA or TOF (Fig. 1), as reflected in a higher diagnostic score (PC: 1.0; DSA: 0.75; TOF: 0.6). The diagnostic sensitivity to arteriovenous fistule is comparable between DSA and PC (DSA: 0.93; PC: 0.82; TOF: 0.5) (Fig. 2). If the flow velocity does not differ in arteriovenous malformations, DSA is superior to PC (Fig. 3). In dissections of the carotid artery TOF is superior to DSA and PC (TOF: 1.0; PC: 0.75; DSA: 0.5). Only with TOF could pathological details such as the dissection membrane be detected in these patients.

Discussion

MRA can depict flowing spins in two different ways: time-of-flight and phase-contrast. While TOF [2] is based on the inflow of unsaturated spins into the imaging volume, PC relies on flow-induced phase shifts when spins are moving along motion-sensitising gradients. Both techniques have their strengths and weaknesses, and it is important to make proper selections based on their physical properties. Specifically, PC is expected to be more sensitive to slow flow and offers the potential of quantitative flow imaging and direction sensitivity [3]. The PC technique offers very interesting new insights in the diagnosis of vascular lesions [4]. The possibility of flow-velocity and direction-sensitive measurement can make this technique an alternative method for diagnosis of giant aneurysms and arteriovenous fistule. If the neck of giant aneurysms cannot be shown with DSA, PC can help to identify the branches and their relationship to the neck by analysis of the jet effect. In patients with secondary venous occlusion flow-encoded 2D-PC sequen-

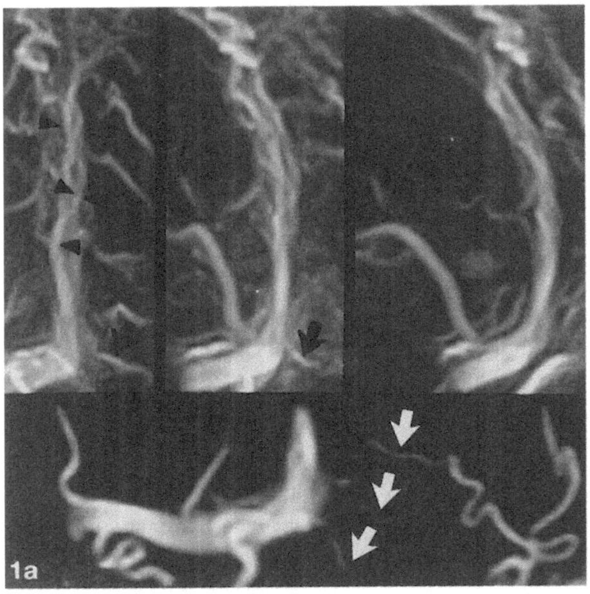
1a

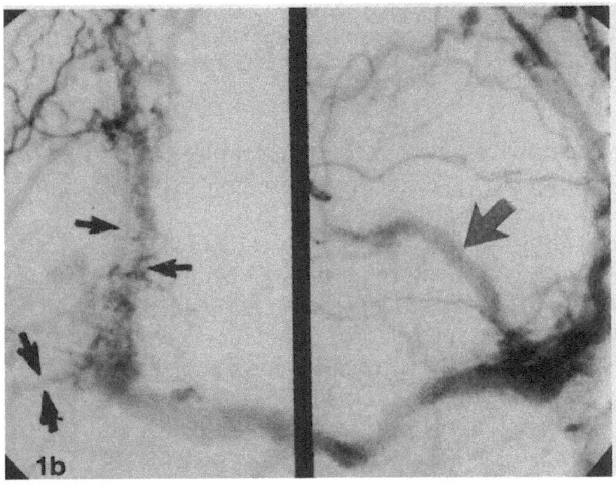
1b

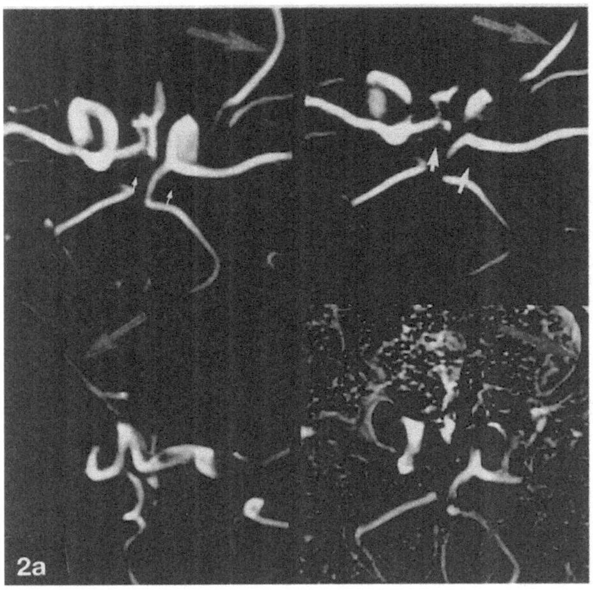
2a

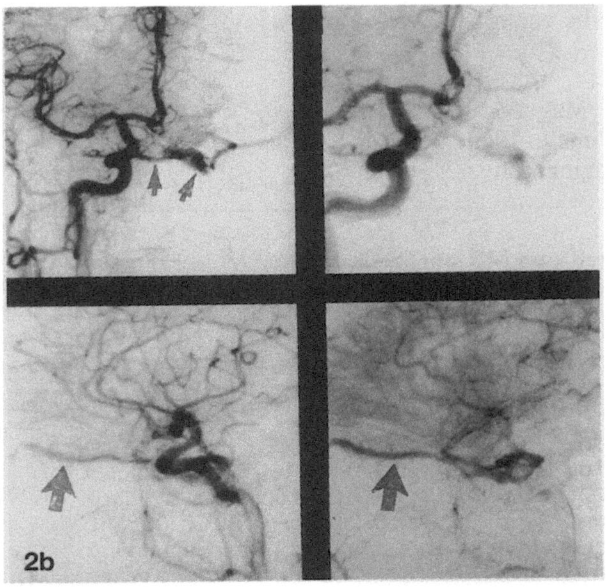
2b

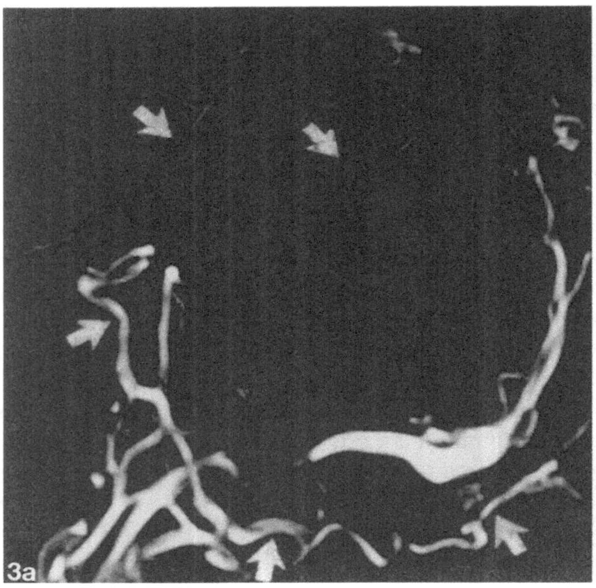
3a

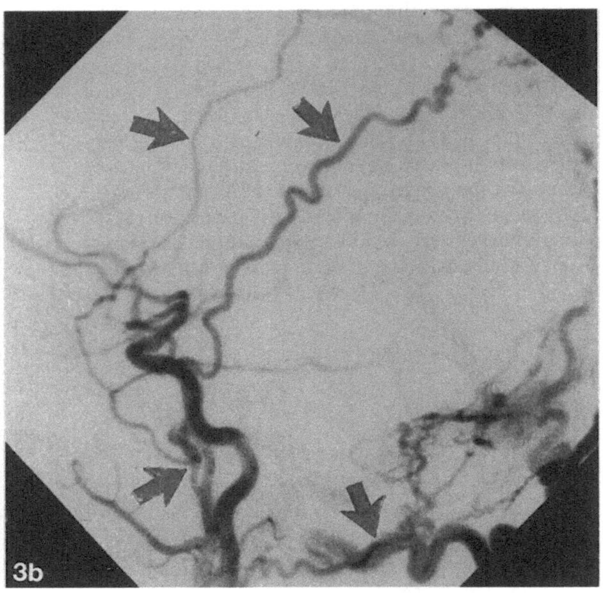
3b

Abb. 1 a, b. Venous occlusion secondary to a dural arteriovenous dural fistula. **a** 2D-PC flow-encoded sequences show revascularisation and collateral circulation of sagittal and transverse sinus *(arrows)* better than **b** DSA

Abb. 2 a, b. Arteriovenous fistula fed by internal and **b** external carotid arteries, draining to contralateral **a** superior orbital vein. Flow velocity-encoded 2D-PC sequences and DSA show the fistule and the dilated vein *arrows*. The vein shows arterial blood flow with an inverted phase signal *(arrowhead)*

Abb. 3 a, b. Dural arteriovenous fistula. **a** 2D-PC flow-encoded sequence and **b** DSA identified the feeding vessels *(arrows)*, the superficial temporal and occipital arteries

ces can show revascularisation and collateral circulation better than any other method. In arteriovenous fistule, small feeding arteries and draining veins can be identified by flow inversion within them using velocity-encoded 2D-PC sequences. TOF [5] can be superior to DSA and PC for vascular lesions with high flow velocities such as arterial dissections, where it can show the dissection membrane directly, due to its high spatial resolution.

References

1. Modic MT, Masaryk TJ, Tkach TA; Ruggieri PM, Dillinger JJ, Ross JS (1993) Three-dimensional time of flight angiography with a specialized gradient head coil. J Magn Reson Imag 3:365–375
2. Edelman RR (1992) Basic principles of magnetic resonance angiography. Cardiovasc Intervent Radiol 15:3–13
3. Edelman RR, Ahn SS, Chien D, Li W, Goldman A, Mantello M, Kramer J, Kleefield J (1992) Improved time of flight MR angiography of the brain. Radiology 184:395–399
4. Smith MA (1990) The measurement and visualization of blood vessel flow. Clin Phys Physiol Meas 11:101–123
5. Turski PA, Grist T (1993) Flow quantification extends MR's neuroapplications. Diagn Imag 15(5):68–77

Flow patterns in the carotid artery bifurcation of patients with cerebrovascular disease on phase-contrast MR angiography

M. Takamura[1], **K. Moritake**[1], **T. Kagawa**[1], **F. Ohta**[1], **H. Kawamitsu**[2]

[1] Department of Neurosurgery, Shimane Medical University, Izumo, Japan
[2] Department of Radiology, Shimane Medical University, Izumo, Japan

Abstract. To measure blood flow patterns in carotid arteries of patients with cerebrovascular diseases and healthy volunteers, we used two-dimensional phase-contrast magnetic resonance angiography (MRA). For 5 healthy volunteers and 11 patients, MRA was performed on the common, internal and external carotid arteries and the vertebral arteries at a level of 20 mm above and 20 mm below the bifurcation of the internal carotid arteries on the axial scans. The flow studies in 38 arteries of healthy volunteers all showed laminar flow, except for one common carotid artery. The flow studies of 8 arteries in patients (except one) showed turbulent flow. Stenosis was detected in all 8 arteries which exhibited conventional cerebral angiography. These results demonstrated usefulness of measuring the flow patterns in the carotid arteries of patients with cerebrovascular disease by phase-contrast MRA.

Key words: MR angiography – Carotid arteries – stenosis

MR angiography (MRA) provides information about the cerebrovascular system without harming the patient [1–3]. It can also measure blood velocity and analyse blood flow patterns if a two-dimensional phase-contrast method is used. Using both a phase-contrast method and a two-dimensional time-of-flight method, we investigated the blood flow patterns in the main cerebral arteries of patients with cerebrovascular disease and of healthy volunteers.

Correspondence to: T. Kagawa, Department of Neurosurgery, Shimane Medical University

Methods

Five normal volunteers (4 men, 1 woman) and 11 patients (6 men, 5 women) were studied. The patients had been diagnosed as having obstructive cerebrovascular disease on the basis of their clinical signs and physical examination. MRA was performed at 1.5 T.

Time-of-flight MRA first was performed. In addition, phase-contrast MRA was performed on the common, internal and external carotid arteries and the vertebral arteries at the level of 20 mm above and 20 mm below the bifurcation of the internal carotid arteries on the axial scans [4, 5]. The middle cerebral arteries were studied in the middle portion of M1 on the sagittal image. The scanning parameters are shown in Table 1.

Phase-contrast MRA offers the ability to scan on speed image rapidly, but can indicate only the magnitude of the velocity, and its vertical, horizontal, anterior and posterior components (Fig. 1). For the study, only the vertical component was investigated. Seventy-five sets of data (which included the velocity and flow patterns) from the 11 patients and 35 sets from the 5 volunteers were examined. The interval between successive R-waves was divided into 16 equal parts by a gated electrocardiogram. The changes in the velocities through one pulsation in all the vessels were examined. At the peak velocity

Table 1. MR angiography parameters

	Time-of flight	Phase-contrast
Flip angle (degrees)	30	30
Repetition time (ms)	33	35
Echo time (ms)	7	9
Velocity encoding (cm/s)		150
Aecqusition matrix		256×128
Pixel size (cm^2)		0.008
Section thickness (mm)		5

Table 2. Comparison of Abnormalities on MRA and conventional angiography

Case	Age (years)	Sex	Stenosis on Conventional angiography	Turbulence on MRA
1	45	F	Rt ICA	Rt ICA
2	63	M	Lt ICA	Lt ICA
3	67	F	Both MCA	Rt MCA
4	45	M	Rt ICA	Both ICA
5	83	M	None	None
6	48	M	None	None
7	55	F	None	None
8	44	F	-	Both ICA
9	36	M	Circle of Willis	Lt ICA
10	57	F	Both ICA	Both ICA
11	68	M	Both ICA	Both ICA

ICA, Internal carotid artery; MCA, middle cerebral artery

observed, the patterns of blood flow were investigated from the centre of the vessels to the sides, as well as anteriorly and posteriorly. However, the blood flow patterns were examined only in the vertical direction for the middle cerebral arteries. For 10 patients, the results were compared with those obtained by cerebral angiography by using the Seldinger method.

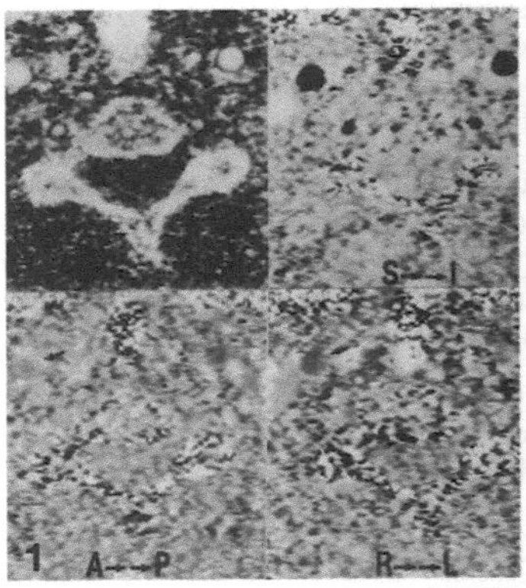

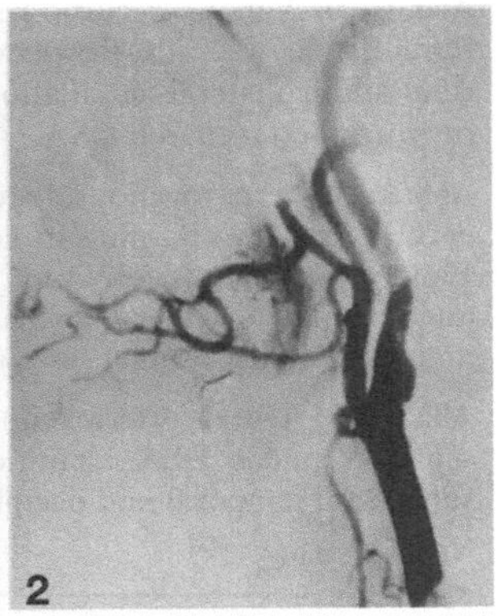

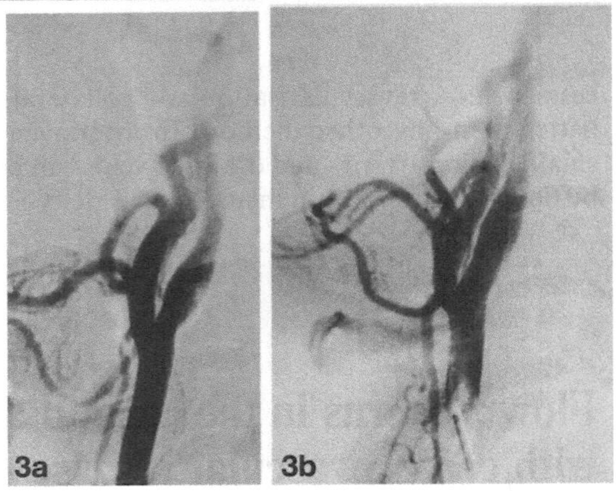

Abb. 1. Phase-contrast MRA: a velocity image can be obtained, in which only velocity is indicated (*A*, anterior; *I*, inferior; *L*, left; *P*, posterior; *R*, right; *S*, superior)

Abb. 2. Conventional angiogram, showing stenosis on the posterior wall at the right internal carotid artery bifurcation

Abb. 3 a, b. Conventional angiogram showing a very mild stenotic plaque on the posterior wall of the **a** right internal carotid artery bifurcation; the left (**b**) is normal

Results

There was no significant difference in the peak velocity for one pulsation between the patients and the normal volunteers.

In 38 of the sections examined (including all except one of the normal volunteers) the velocities exhibited a parabolic distribution, suggesting that there was laminar blood flow in these areas. The results from the 11 patients are shown in Table 2.

In 9 of the 75 vessel sections in the patients, a stenotic change was detected by the Seldinger method. A parabolic pattern by phase-contrast MRA was not detected in eight regions in all patients except for patient, 3 in whom it was not observed in only one region. On the other hand, 2 patients (nos. 4 and 9) demonstrated no stenotic changes by the Seldinger method, nor was there a parabolic pattern by phase-contrast MRA, suggesting the presence of a stenosis. In the other areas, a parabolic pattern was detected. In case 1, a stenotic change with the formation of an ulcer was observed on the posterior wall at the bifurcation of the right internal carotid artery by the Seldinger method and time-of-flight MRA (Fig. 2). The distribution of velocities distal to the stenosis differed from the normal pattern. In case 4, a stenotic change was recognised on the posterior wall of the bifurcation of the right internal carotid artery by the Seldinger method and time-of-flight MRA (Fig. 3). However, there were no abnormal changes in the left internal carotid artery.

The velocity patterns of bilateral carotid arteries differed from the normal pattern.

Discussion

In both cases, the patterns by phase-contrast MRA appeared to be different from a parabolic distribution, suggesting that there is some impediment to blood flow.

It is known that blood flow is in layers in normal vessels [6] and turbulent in stenotic areas [7, 8]. The blood velocity can be determined by the measurement of the phase lag, so one can determine the distribution of velocity in all areas of a vessel.

Phase-contrast MRI could detect an obstruction, which caused a slight morphological change, by detecting alterations in the pattern of velocity distribution. However, these measurements must be performed under suitable conditions to obtain the correct diagnosis.

References

1. Walker MF, Souza SP, Dumoulin CL (1988) Quantitative flow measurement in phase contrast MR angiography. J Comput Assist Tomogr 12:304–314
2. Enzmann DR, Ross MR, Marks MP, Pelc NJ (1994) Blood flow in major cerebral arteries measured by phase-contrast cine MR. AJNR 15:123–129
3. Adler RS, Chenevert TL, Fowlkes JB, Pipe J, Pubin JM (1991) Calculation of pressure gradients from MR velocity data in a laminar flow model. J Comput Assist Tomogr 15:483–488
4. Motomiya M, Karino T (1984) Flow patterns in human carotid artery bifurcation. Stroke 15:50–56
5. Masaryk TJ, Ross JS, Modic MT, Lenz GW, Haacke EM (1988) Carotid bifurcation: MR imaging. Radiology 166:461–466
6. Enzmann DR, Pelc NJ (1991) Normal flow patterns of intracranial and spinal cerebrospinal fluid defined with phase-contrast cine MR imaging. Radiology 178:467–474
7. de Roos A, Reichek N, Axel L, Kressel HY (1989) Cine MR imaging in aortic stenosis. J Comput Assist Tomogr 13:421–425
8. Litt AW, Eidelman EM, Pinto RS, Riles TS, McLachlan SJ, Schwartzenberg ST, Weinreb JC, Kricheff II (1991) Diagnosis of Carotid artery stenosis: comparison of sDFT time-of-flight MR angiography with contrast angiography in 50 patients. AJNR 12:149–154

Measurements of flow velocity of the arteries in head and neck with three-point phase-contrast Magnetic Resonance Angiography

T. Makabe[1], K. Kinoshita[1], T. Itoh[1], S. Asari[1], T. Ohmoto[1], A. Doi[2], E. Yoshitome[3]

[1] Department of Neurological Surgery, Okayama University, Okayama, Japan
[2] Department of Neurosurgery, Okayama Kyokuto Hospital, Okayama, Japan
[3] GE Yokogawa Medical Systems, Tokyo, Japan

Abstract. We compared two- and three-point methods for phase-contrast MR angiography in vitro. The three-point method is an excellent technique by which we can measure the flow velocity of the arteries in the head and neck without careful slice selection.

Phase-contrast MR angiography (MRA) has been shown to be a practical and clinically applicable technique for the imaging of blood flow. We have previously reported about flow velocity and volume in the arteries of the head and neck by means of phase-contrast MRA. This method, however, is somewhat limited in its application to measurement due to the stationary protons. We have now developed a new method by which we can measure the flow velocity of vessels that are thinner than the slice thickness.

This investigation examines flow velocity calibration of three-point phase-contrast MRA with application to flow, both in a flow phantom and in the arteries in the head and neck of volunteers and patients.

Key words: Three-point method – Phase-contrast – Flow velocity – Stationary proton

Correspondence to: T. Makabe, Department of Neurological Surgery Okayama University Medical School. 2-5-1 Shikata-cho, Okayama, 700 Japan.

Materials and methods

Theory

Phase-contrast MRA makes use of the flow-encoding gradient pulses, which impart a velocity-dependent phase shift to the transverse magnetisation of moving spins while leaving stationary spins unaffected. For the purpose of this presentation, we refer to Dumoulin's original theory as the "two-point method".

Images from bipolar flow encoding gradient pulses give vectors Z1 and Z3. These vectors give a phase shift of θ. However, the phase shift of θ is different from the real phase shift of ϕ because it includes the signal of the stationary protons. The three-point method also requires another image, this being given by the null flow encoding gradient. This image gives a vector Z2. When the phase shift θ is not so large, the vector of the signal of the moving protons gives a constant magnitude and the end of the vector lies on a circle whose centre is the vector Z4. So, this three-point method illustrates the real phase shift of θ, generated from only the moving protons (Fig. 1a).

An angiogram is produced by making complex calculations of three successively projected images for which all imaging parameters are identical, except for the magnitude of the flow-encoding gradient (Fig. 1b).

Figure 2a shows the slice selection for the two-point method. The two-point method needs to be selected carefully in case the moving protons overlap with the stationary protons.

Figure 2b shows the slice selection for the three-point method; this method does not required such careful slice selection because the stationary protons are completely suppressed.

Phantom study

Steady-flow studies were performed using a flow phantom that consisted of a vinyl tube. The circulating fluid was physiological saline. We used an agar as the stationary protons (Fig. 3a).

1a

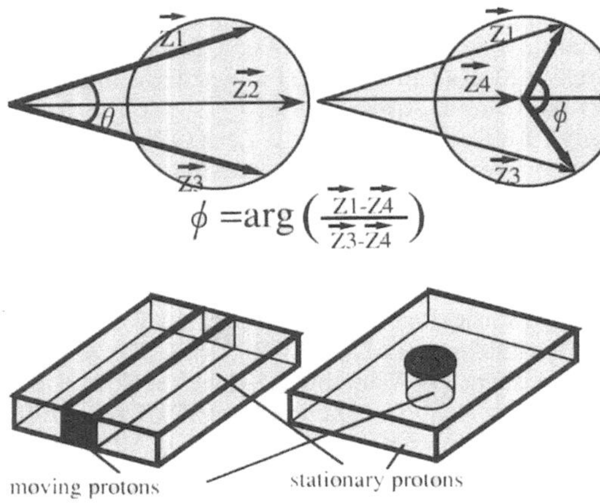

1b

2a

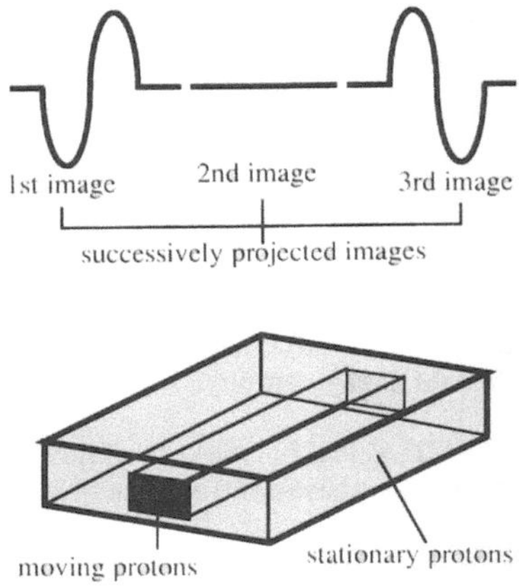

2b

Fig. 1a b. Theory of the three-point method

Fig. 2a, b. Slice selection for the two-point method

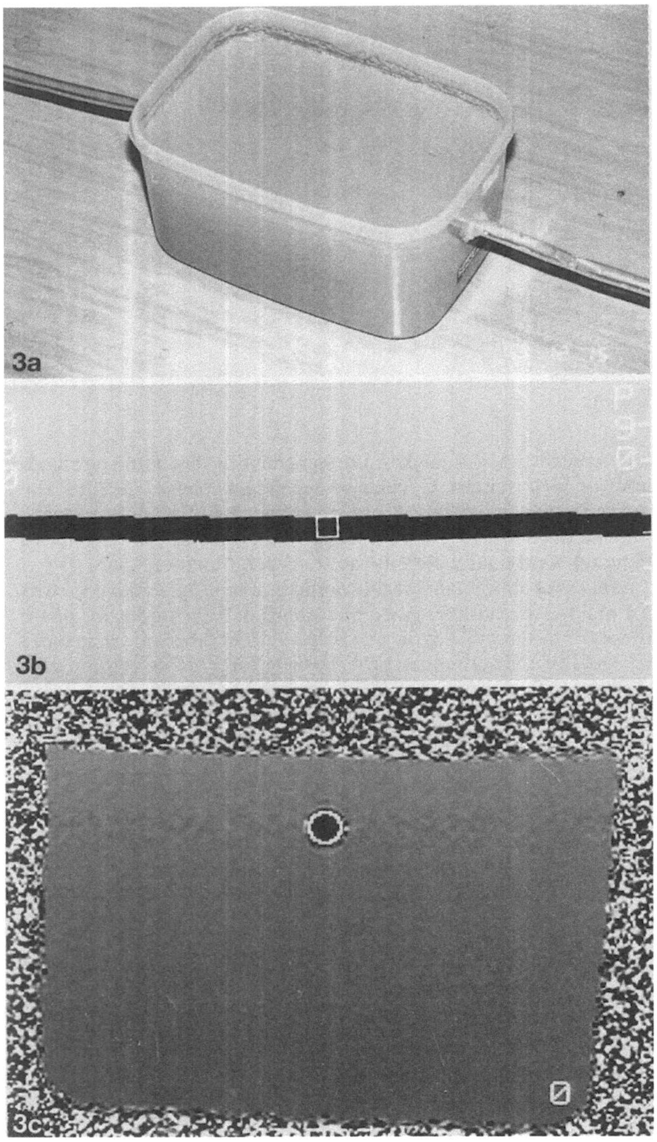

Fig. 3a. Flow phantom. **b** Flow image of the phantom imaged using the three-point method. **c** Flow image using the two-point method

First, the velocity encoding was varied but all other imaging parameters were kept constant. Secondly, the flip angle was varied but all other imaging parameters were kept constant. Thirdly, the flow velocity was varied but all other imaging parameters were kept constant, both with the three-point and the two-point methods.

Results

Figure 3b shows the flow image of the phantom scanned by the three-point method. Figure 3c shows the flow image of the phantom scanned by the two-point method.

Figure 4a shows the relationship between the velocity encoding and the measured flow velocity. The actual mean velocity and the flip angle were fixed and the velocity encoding was varied from image to image. These data show that the velocity encoding needs to be more than twice as great as the mean velocity.

Figure 4b shows the relationship between the velocity encoding and the measured diameter of the vinyl tube. In these conditions, the diameter of the vinyl tube was always less than 9 mm.

Figure 4c shows the relationship between the flip angle and the measured flow velocity. The actual mean velocity and the velocity encoding were fixed, and only the flip angle was varied. When the flip angle was 60°, the measured velocity was closest to the actual mean velocity.

With the flow phantom study, the velocity encoding is required to be more than twice as great as the mean velocity. Also, a position of 60° is suitable for the flip angle for the three-point method.

Two series, comprising six images of the two- and three-point methods of the phantom, were taken in which the flow velocity was varied from image to image but all other imaging parameters were kept constant. The solid line is the "least squares fit" of the data.

The measured flow velocity showed a very good correlation with the actual flow velocity up to 60 cm/s when using both methods, but the three-point method tended to overestimate, while the two-point method tended to underestimate (Fig. 4d).

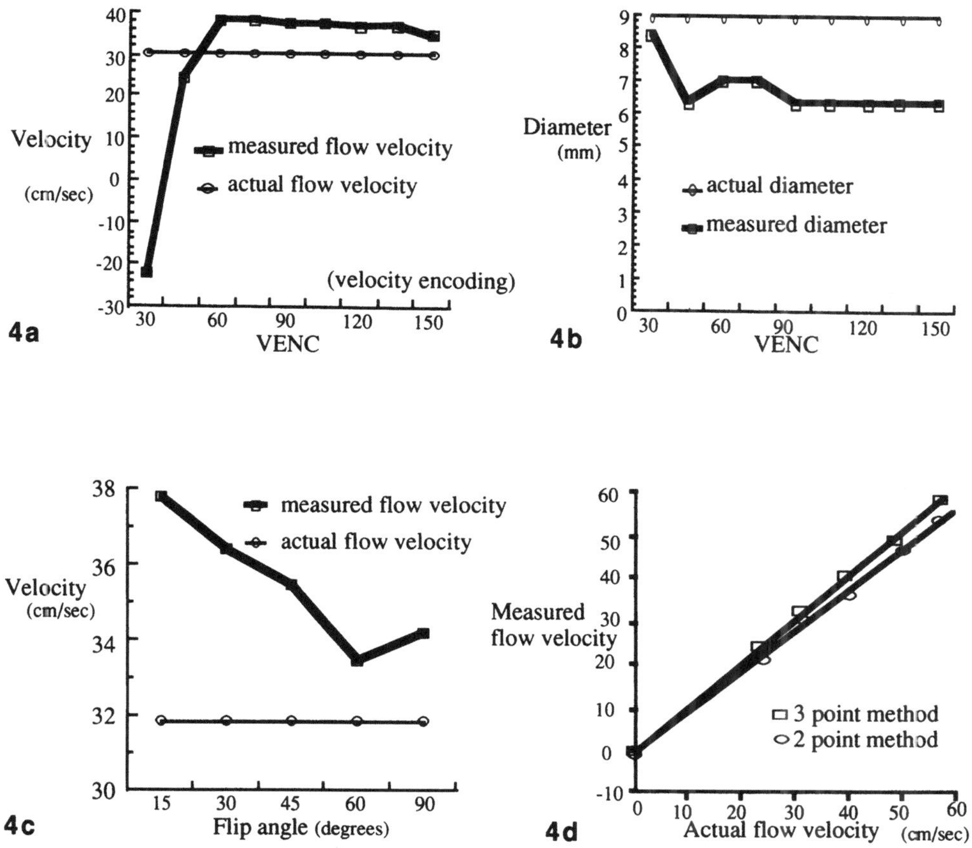

Fig. 4. Relationship between **a** velocity encoding *(VENC)* and measured flow velocity. **b** VENC and measured diameter of the vinyl tube. **c** Flip angle and measured flow velocity. **d** Correlation between measured and actual flow velocity

Discussion

MRA procedures which make use of flow-induced phase shifts have distinct advantages with respect to time-of-flight methods. For example, time-of-flight angiography is not well suited to vessels having slow flow because of the limited life-time of the MR-active bolus. The detectability of slow flow by phase-sensitive techniques, however, is limited only by the strength of flow encoding the magnetic field gradient and the signal-to-noise ratio of the image. In principle, time-of-flight techniques are less sensitive to velocity dispersions within a pixel, but are also less suitable for quantative flow measurements [1–3].

Flow-induced phase shifts occur whenever transverse spin magnetisation moves along a magnetic field gradient. This is because field gradients cause the magnetic field (and hence the resonance frequency) to vary as a function of location. If the gradient is applied for a finite period of time, the temporary change in resonance frequency will result in the accumulation of a phase shift in the transverse magnetisation for both stationary and moving spins. For stationary material this phase shift will be proportional to the position of the spin along the gradient, and can be undone by applying a second gradient pulse having opposite polarity (or the same polarity if used with a refocussing radiofrequency pulse). If the transverse magnetisation moves during the interval between the gradient pulses, however, the phase shift of the first pulse will not be exactly cancelled by the phase shift of the second pulse and the residual phase shift will be proportional to the velocity and higher terms of motion.

This method is limited in the situation of flow measurement because the surrounding stationary protons are incompletely suppressed. (In Fig. 3C, even the area of the air shows some phase shift.)

Using the three-point method, we can measure the flow velocity of even thinner vessels than the slice thickness because the surrounding stationary protons are completely suppressed.

The flow rate measured by the three-point method is somewhat high. The chief source of error is probably signal loss of slow flow near the vessel wall. The three-point method is however more precise than the two-point method.

Acknowledgements. This work was supported in part by GE Yokogawa Medical Systems, Tokyo.

References

1. Cousins JP, Dumoulin CL, Souza SP et al. (1989) A protocol for isolation of carotid and vertebral arteries in MR angiography. AJNR 10:921–922
2. Dumoulin CL (1992) Phase contrast magnetic resonance angiography. Neuroimaging Clin North Am 2:657–676
3. Dumoulin CL, Hart HRJ (1986) Magnetic resonance angiography. Radiology 161:717–720

Cervical MR Angiography using the coronal plane including the origin of the vertebral artery

T. Taoka [1], S. Iwasaki [2], H. Nakagawa [2], A. Fukusumi [2], M. Nakane [2], K. Kichikawa [2], H. Ohishi [3], S. Nakanisi [4], A. Hirai [4]

[1] Department of Radiology, Nara Prefectural Hospital, 1-30-1 Hiramatsu-cho Nara City, Nara 631 Japan
[2] Department of Radiology, Nara Medical University, Nara, Japan
[3] Department of Oncoradiology, Nara Medical University, 834 Shijo-cho Kashihara City, Nara 634, Japan
[4] Hirai Hospital, 70 Ishikawa-cho Kashihara City, Nara 634, Japan

Abstract. Coronal and axial planes in cervical MR angiography (MRA) were compared to determine which plane is more useful in the diagnosis of the vertebral and subclavian arteries. MRA was obtained in 18 patients with symptoms suggestive of arteriosclerosis using a 1.0 T MR unit with a coil designed for cervical MRA. Each artery was classified into categories based on the visualisation of the artery including the branch point of the vertebral artery. The number of cases in which the branch point was visualised was as follows (coronal/axial): right subclavian artery, 18/16; left subclavian artery, 14/16; right vertebral artery, 15/15; left vertebral artery, 12/16. The ability to visualise branch points was a little higher on the axial plane, but the difference was minimal. Considering that coronal MRA can visualise the total length of cervical artery, coronal MRA seems to be better than axial MRA.

Key words: Magnetic resonance angiography – Three-dimensional time-of-flight – Subclavian artery – Vertebral artery

Coronal and axial planes in cervical MR angiography (MRA) were compared to determine which plane is more useful for examination of the vertebral and subclavian arteries especially the origin of the vertebral artery.

Materials and methods

MRA was obtained in 18 patients with symptoms suggestive of arteriosclerosis. A 1.0 T unit with a coil designed for cervical MRA was used [1]. MRA in both planes was acquired by 3D FISP (TR 45 TE 10 FA 15). In coronal plane MRA, field of view (FOV) was 25 cm and slab thickness 64 mm, and in the axial plane, FOV was 20 cm and slab thickness 96 mm. Each artery was classified based on the visualisation of each artery, concentrating upon the origin of the vertebral artery (VA). Group A: The entire length of the arteries was visualised clearly, including the VA origin. Group B: The origin of the VA origin was visualised clearly, but some part of the arteries was not seen clearly. Group C: The origin of the VA origin was not visualised.

Results

The number of cases in which the origin was visualised (group A and B) was (coronal/axial): right subclavian artery, 18/16; left subclavian artery, 14/16; right VA, 15/15; left VA, 12/16 (Figs. 1–3).

For the left subclavian artery and VA, the visualisation of the origin was better with axial plane. For right subclavian arteries, it was better in the coronal plane, and for the right VA, it was equally good in both planes. However, there were minimal differences in visualisation of each artery.

Fig. 1 a b. A 48-year-old man with vertigo. **a** Coronal, **b** Axial MRA. In each plane the whole lengths of both subclavian arteries is visualised, including their origins and so are both vertebral arteries. Each artery on each plane is categorised as group A

Fig. 2 a, b. A 72-year-old man with multiple infarct on MRA. **a** Coronal MRA, **b** axial MRA. On both coronal and axial MRA, the origin of the right subclavian artery is visualised, but the peripheral portion is not (group B). While the whole length of the right vertebral artery, including its branching point, is visualised in the axial plane (group A), the origin is not visualised in the coronal plane *(arrow)* (group C).
The origin of the left subclavian artery is visualised, but the peripheral portion is blurred in both planes (group B). The entire length of the left vertebral artery is clearly visualised icluding its origin on both planes (group A)

Discussion

The origin of the VA is the common site for arteriosclerotic stenosis, and vertebral artery stenosis at this site may be a cause of vertebrobasilar insufficiency [2]. MRA can visualise the origin of the VA without an invasion, and enable an estimation of stenosis [3].

Cervical MRA using the coronal plane has the advantage of visualising the total length of the cervical arteries above the aortic arch. On the other hand, this plane is parallel to the cervical arterial flow and supposed to have a disadvantage from saturation.

On MRA using the axial plane, this plane is perpendicular to the arterial flow and supposed to have better signals from flow. However, it is impossible to describe the total length of the cervical arteries by single scan. So as to acquire an image of the whole length of cervical artery, a multislab is necessary [4].

In this study, visualisation of the branch points was a little higher in the axial plane, but the difference was minimal. It is also important to visualise the whole length of arteries on cervical MRA. Thus the advantages of the coronal plane became greater.

In this study, the advantage of the axial plane on flow direction was not so significant. Considering that coronal MRA can visualise the total length of the cervical artery, coronal MRA seems to be better than axial MRA.

Correspondence to: T. Taoka

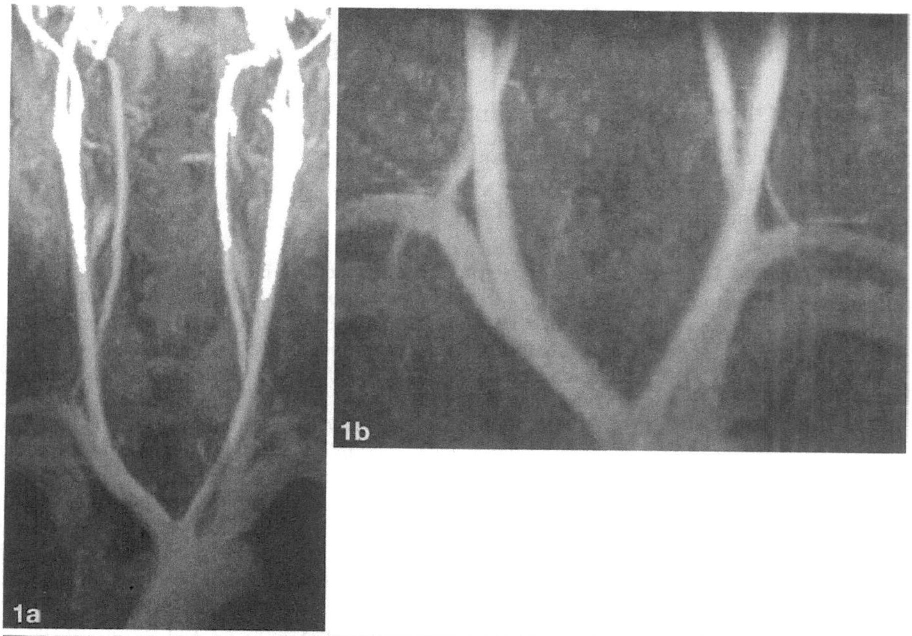

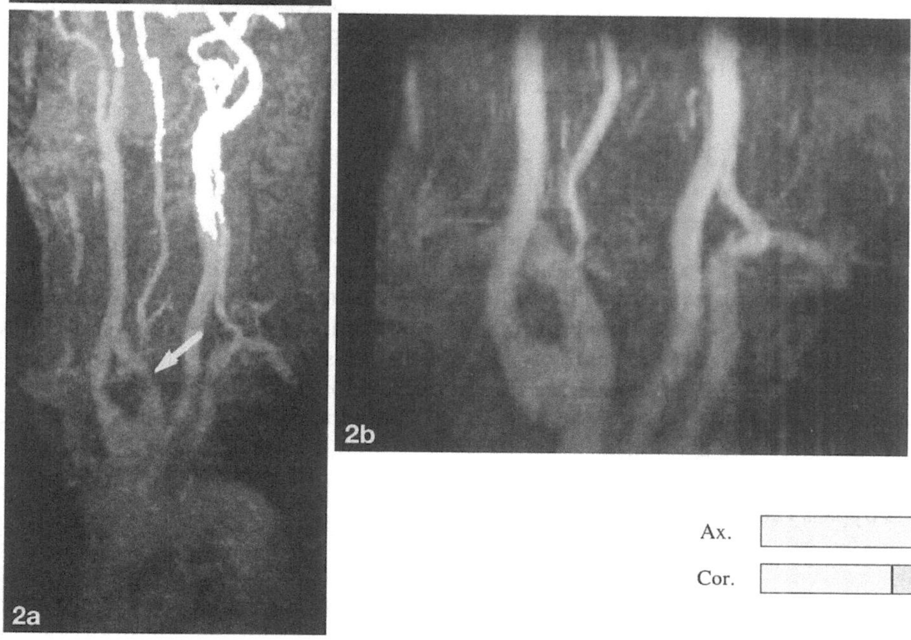

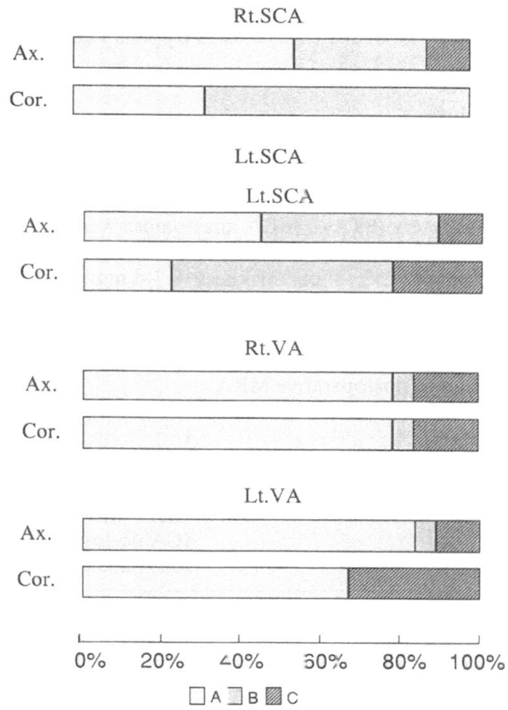

References

1. Anderson CM, Saloner D, Lee RE, Fortner A (1990) Dedicated coil for carotic MR angiography. Radiology 176:868–872
2. Okawar RS, Nibbelink D (1974) Vertebral artery occlusion following hypertension and rotation of the head. Stroke 6:740–742
3. Zawadzki MB, Gillan G (1992) Extracranial carotid magnetic resonance angiography. Cardiovasc Intervent Radiol 15:82–90
4. Furuya Y, Isoda H, Hasegawa S, Takahashi M, Kaneko M, Uemura K (1992) Magnetic resonance angiography of extracranial carotid and vertebral arteries, including their origins. Neuroradiology 35:42–45

Fig. 3. Comparing coronal and axial MRA in visualisation of each artery (*VA*, vertebral artery; *SCA*, subclavian artery)

Correlation between magnetic resonance angiography and cerebral blood flow change in patients who underwent bypass surgery

Y. Kumon [1], **S. Sakaki** [1], **T. Ueda** [1], **K. Kohno** [1], **S. Ohta** [1], **H. Miki** [2], **K. Hamamoto** [2]

[1] Department of Radiology, Ehime University School of Medicine, Ehime 791-02, Japan
[2] Department of Radiology, Ehime University School of Medicine, Ehime, Japan

Abstract. To evaluate bypass function, we examined the relationship between postoperative magnetic resonance angiography (MRA) and postoperative change in cerebral blood flow (CBF) using ^{133}Xe-SPECT in nine patients who underwent bypass surgery. MRA was obtained through the methods of three-dimensional time-of-flight (3D-TOF), and 2D-TOF with selective presaturation and phase contrast. The findings of postoperative MRA were classified into marked, moderate and poor flow groups according to the degree of blood flow supplied via the bypass. Patients in the marked or moderate flow groups exhibited a postoperative improvement in CBF, but those in the poor flow group did not. As postoperative MRA correlated well with postoperative change in CBF in patients who underwent bypass surgery, it was useful for evaluation of bypass function.

Key words: Magnetic resonance angiography – Xenon 133 – Single photon emission computed tomography – Extracranial-intracranial arterial bypass

Magnetic resonance angiography (MRA) is not merely applied to detect stenoses, obstructions and aneurysms in the intracranial arteries [1–3] and to determine whether a bypass graft is patent [1, 4], but also to show information on cerebral blood flow (CBF) as a functional image. We examined the relationship between postoperative MRA and postoperative change in CBF in patients who underwent bypass surgery in order to evaluate bypass function.

Patients and methods

Nine patients [4 internal carotid artery (ICA) occlusion; 4 middle cerebral artery (MCA) occlusion; 1 MCA stenosis] who received superficial temporal artery (STA) – MCA anastomose were examined. Three-dimensional time-of-flight (3D-TOF) MRA (TR 40 ms; TE 4–5 ms; flip angle 25°; slice thickness 0.7–1 mm; matrix 256×256×64 or 256×192×64; NEX 1; slab thickness 0.7–1×64 mm), 2D-TOF MR angiography with selective presaturation (TR 45 ms; TE 8.7 ms; flip angle 60°; slice thickness 1.5 mm; matrix 256×128; NEX 1; slice number 2–128) and phase images from phase-contrast MRA (TR 25–30 ms; flip angle 15–20; slice thickness 1.5 mm; matrix 256×128×64; NEX 1; slab thickness 1.5×32 or 1.5 64 mm; VENC 5–40 cm/s) were obtained with a 1.5 T unit. CBF at rest and under acetazolamide loading were measured quantitatively by ^{133}Xe-SPECT before and after the operation (mean 2.3 months after surgery) with MRA at the same time, and postoperative CBF changes were assessed. The findings of MRA were classified into three groups according to the degree of blood flow supplied from the bypass; the marked flow group, where the M2 and M3 portions of the MCA were supplied from the STA; the moderate flow group, where the M3 portion was supplied and supply to the M2 portion was suspected; and the poor flow group, where only the M3 portion was supplied (Table 1). The relationship between these MRA classifications and CBF change was examined.

Results

Four patients with ICA occlusion and one with MCA occlusion were included in the marked flow group, two patients with MCA occlusion or stenosis in the moderate flow group, and two patients with MCA occlusion in the poor flow group. Patients in the marked (Fig. 1) or moderate flow group exhibited a postoperative improvement in CBF, but those in the poor flow group (Fig. 2) did not.

Discussion

3D-TOF MRA can demonstrate the patency of a bypass by a clear connection of vascular signals between the bypass and the MCA, and by a postoperative increase in the signal intensity of the MCA [1]. However, as it provides only static images, the degree of flow supplied from the bypass to the MCA is difficult to detect. MRA

Table 1. Classification of postoperative MRA

Type	I	II	III
3D-TOF	STA * M3 * M2	STA * M3 * M2	STA * M3
Phase-image selective MRA	STA → M3 → M2	STA → M3 → M2	STA → M3
Lesion	ICA occlusion 4 MCA occlusion 1	MCA occlusion 1 MCA stenosis 1	MCA occlusion 2

Correspondence to: Y. Kumon

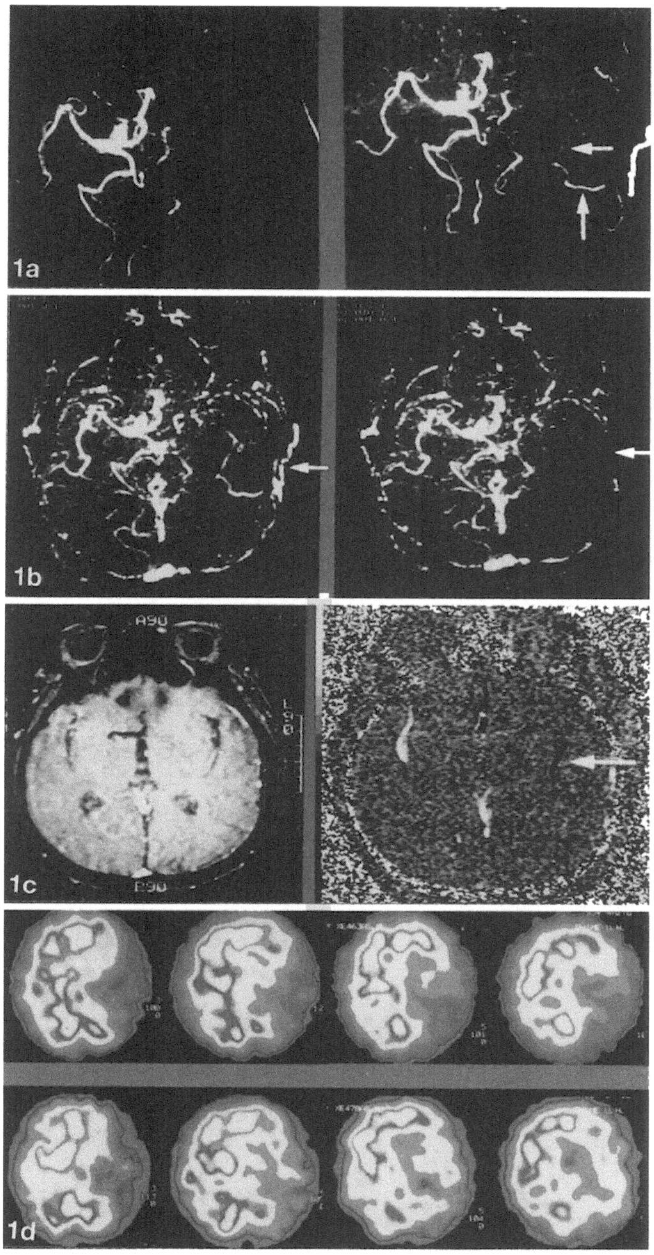

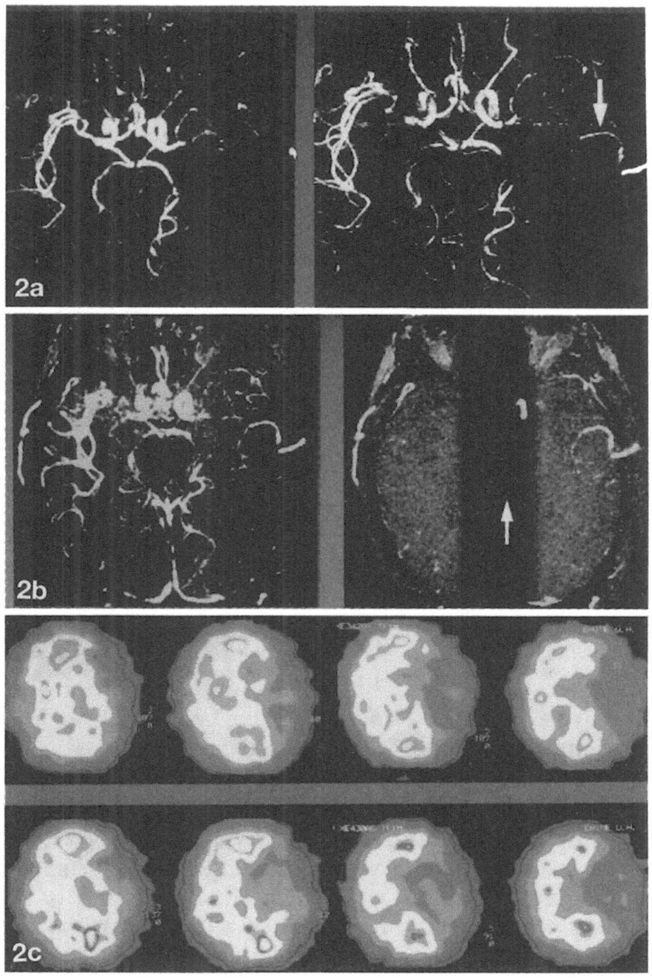

Fig. 1 a d. A patient with occlusion of the left internal carotid artery (ICA) (marked flow group) **a** Preoperative axial 3D-TOF MRA *(left)* shows absence of signal of the left middle cerebral artery (MCA). Postoperative axial 3D-TOF MRA *(right)* demonstrates the patency of left superficial temporal artery (STA)-MCA shunt and appearance of signal of M2 and M3 portions of the left MCA *(arrow)*. **b** Presaturation of left STA *(arrow)* eliminates signal of M2 and M3 portions of the left MCA, indicating that these portions are supplied from the left STA (*left*, before presaturation; *right*, after presaturation). **c** Postoperative axial phase image of phase-contrast MRA demonstrates the retrograde flow of the M2 portion of the left MCA *(arrow)*. **d** Pre- and postoperative ^{133}Xe-SPECT (acetozolamide load) showing the improvement of cerebral blood flow (CBF) in the left frontoparietal region after surgery *(arrow)*

Fig. 2 a–c. A case of occlusion of the left MCA (poor flow group). **a** Preoperative axial 3D-TOF MRA *(left)* shows occlusion of the left MCA and weak signal of the M2 and M3 portions of the left MCA. Postoperative axial 3D-TOF MRA *(right)* demonstrates the patency of the left STA-MCA shunt and an increase in signal of only the M3 portion of the left MCA *(arrow)*. **b** Presaturation of both ICAs and basilar artery *(arrow)* leaves signal of only the M3 portion of the left MCA, indicating that only the M3 portion of the left MCA is supplied from the left STA (*left*, before presaturation; *right*, after presaturation). **c** Pre- and postoperative ^{133}Xe-SPECT (acetozolamide load) showing no improvement of CBF in the left cerebral hemisphere after surgery

with presaturation can show the vascular territory receiving blood from the bypass [2, 4], and phase-contrast MRA can reveal the direction of blood flow [5]. In order to detect the bypass function, we used MRA with a combination of these methods, and classified the patients into three groups according to the degree of blood flow supplied from the bypass. Patients in the marked or moderate flow groups exhibited a postoperative improvement in CBF, but those in the poor flow group did not. Thus, as postoperative MRA correlated well with postoperative changes in CBF in patients who underwent bypass surgery, it was useful to evaluate bypass function.

References

1. Aoki T, Houkin K, Kamiyama H, Iwasaki Y, Abe H, Koiwa M, Kawaguchi S, Kashiwaba T (1993) Diagnosis of intracranial occlusive vascular disease and evaluation of extracranial-intracranial (EC/IC) arterial bypass using three dimensional magnetic resonance angiography (Japanese) No to Shinkei 45:57–62
2. Edelman RR, Mattle HP, O'Reilly GV, Wentz KU, Liu C, Zhao B (1989) Magnetic resonance imaging of flow dynamics in the circle of Willis. Stroke 21:56–65
3. Sevivi RJ, Tsuruda JS, Schmalbrock P (1990) Three-dimensional time-of-flight MR angiography in the evaluation of cerebral aneurysms. J Comput Assist Tomogr 14:874–881
4. Mabuchi S, Nakayama N, Isu T, Harata T, Nanbu T (1994) Evaluation of the patency of an extracranial-intracranial bypass using magnetic resonance angiography with selective presaturation of bypass vessels. Neurol Med Chir (Tokyo) 34:365–370
5. Dumoulin CL, Souza SP, Walker MF, Wagle W (1989) Three-dimensional phase contrast angiography (Japanese). No To Shinkei 45:57–62

Assessment of cerebral blood flow after external-to-internal carotid MR angiography with presaturation

T. Nambu[1], K. Miyasaka[1], Y. Kikuchi[1], T. Isu[2], S. Mabuchi[2]

[1] Department of Radiology, Hokkaido University, N-15 WT Sapporo 060 Japan
[2] Department of Neurosurgery, Kushiro Rosai Hospital, Kushiro, Hokkaido, Japan

Abstract. We studied 27 external-to-internal carotid (EC/IC) bypass tracts in 24 patients using magnetic resonance angiography (MRA). We diagnosed patency of the bypass by comparing MRA with and without selective presaturation on the bypass by comparing MRA with and without selective presaturation on the bypass vessel. Fifteen bypasses in 14 patients were also studied by conventional angiography within a week interval, and patency of the bypass was correctly diagnosed by MRA in all but one case. For further assessment of blood distribution, presaturation on the circle of Willis was set on nine sites in 8 patients, which clarified the anterograde flow distribution. We conclude that MRA using presaturation is a useful, non-invasive assessment of the bypass patency and blood circulation after EC/IC bypass surgery.

Key words: Grafts, patency – Bypass – Magnetic resonance angiography – Presaturation pulse

MR angiography (MRA) has been established as a useful non-invasive method to demonstrate vascular structures. We present our experience in postsurgical assessment of extracranial(EC)-intracranial(IC) bypass surgery using MRA with selective presaturation.

Patients and methods

Twenty-four patients (aged 27–70 years, mean 56) who underwent EC/IC bypass surgery had MRA. Three patients had bilateral bypass surgery. MRA parameters were 3D FISP (TR/TE/excitation = 38/6.8 ms/1, matrix 256 × 192, flip angle 15° FOV 220 mm), using a 1.5 T imager. After a usual MRA examination, an additional scan was performed with a 10-mm-thick presaturation pulse set just on the bypass tract under the scalp. MRA images with presaturation were compared with the images without presaturation. The patency of the bypass was diagnosed when flow signals from middle cerebral artery (MCA) branches disappeared by presaturation (Fig. 1) [1].

Eight patients had another MRA with selective presaturation on the circle of Willis; oblique-sagittal presaturation was set on the upper end of the internal carotid artery (ICA) to cause a loss of anterograde flow signal without spoiling bypass flow signal, or presaturation on the anterior communicating artery (Acom) to confirm the cross-flow from the contralateral ICA.

Table 1. Postsurgical assessment of EC/IC bypass patency using MRA with selective presaturation

Patent bypasses		Obstructed bypasses	
Period of patency	Number	Period of patency	Number
3 weeks	1	<7 days	2
4–6 weeks	5	3–8 weeks	2[a]
3–5 months	3	2 ~ 5 months	1[a]
1–2 years	2	Unknown	5
2–5 years	3		
7–9 years	3		
14 Y	1		

[a] Patients in whom repeated MRA showed the change from "patent" to "obstructed"

Results

Accuracy of MRA diagnosis of graft patency

Fifteen bypass tracts in 14 patients were examined with MRA and conventional angiography within 7 days. Diagnosis of the patency agreed in 14 bypass tracts (10 patent tracts, 4 obstructed tracts). In one case, angiography showed patent but poor flow of the bypass, with a lot of transdural anastomotic vessels through the skull

Correspondence to: T. Nambu

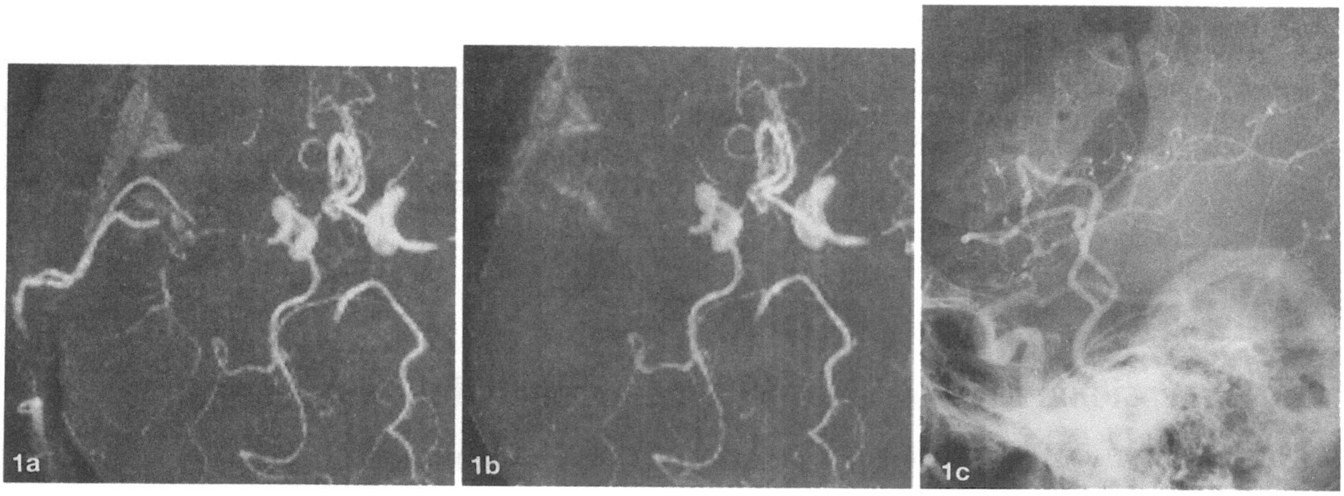

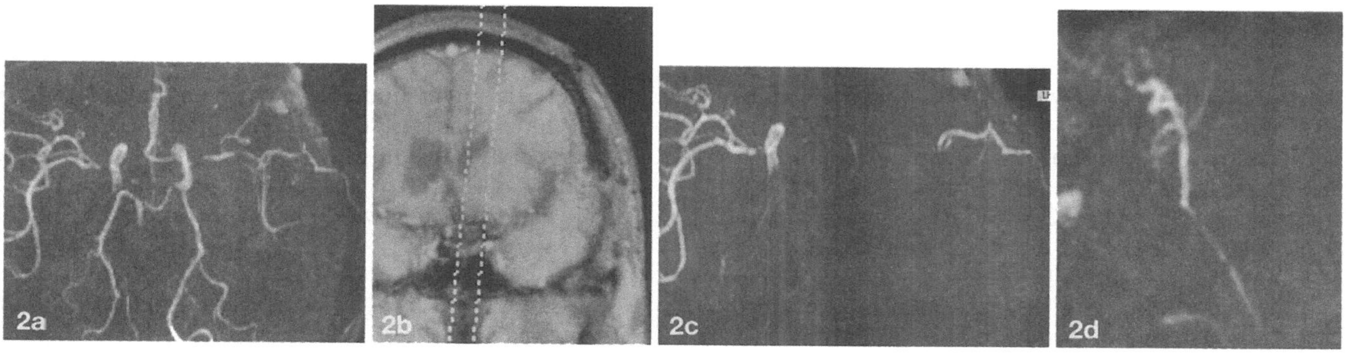

Fig. 1 a–c. A 27-year-old man who had right superficial temporal to middle cerebral artery (STA-MCA) bypass for MCA obstruction due to moyamoya disease. **a** MRA demonstrates obstruction of right MCA. **b** Selective presaturation on bypass vessel demonstrates loss of right MCA signal. **c** Conventional external carotid angiography confirmed patency of bypass

Fig. 2 a–d. A 40-year-old woman who had left STA-MCA bypass for severe MCA stenosis. **a** MRA demonstrates the bypass tract and MCA branches. **b** Method of setting presaturation pulse on distal ICA. **c** MRA with this selective presaturation shows disappearance of anterograde flow, giving a clear, selective image of bypass flow. **d** Selective lateral reconstruction of the left cerebral hemisphere shows clear "bypass image"

base. On MRA, the signal of the MCA branches did not disappear well, so obstruction of the bypass was suspected.

Presaturation on ICA and Acom

In 8 cases, MRA with presaturation pulse on the circle of Willis spoiled anterograde blood flow. In 5 cases with a patent bypass, anterograde flow was proved by stenosed but patent ICA and MCA. In 3 cases with complete ICA obstruction, a presaturation pulse on the Acom proved cross-flow from the contralateral ICA. This technique enabled selective and positive demonstration of collateral flow distribution through the EC/IC bypass (Fig. 2).

Clinical assessment of the patent EC/IC bypass graft

Overall, of 27 bypasses, 9 bypasses were examined with a single MRA study, and 18 bypasses with two or more. In the last examinations, 17 bypasses were found to be patent, while another 10 bypasses were obstructed. Among 10 obstructed cases, 3 bypasses were patent at the initial examination, and follow-up studies diagnosed obstruction between 1 and 2 months, 3 and 5 weeks, and 2 and 5 months respectively (Table 1).

Discussion

EC/IC bypass is a principal treatment of ischaemic cerebral disease, and its postsurgical evaluation is important. Usually MRA can demonstrate collateral tracts through the external cerebral artery [2], but the patency of the anastomosis and bypass flow distribution may occasionally be uncertain. Our MRA method can show collateral circulation by disappearance of flow signal after presaturation on the bypass tract. Presaturation on the ICA or anterior cerebral artery was also helpful in confirming anterograde blood distribution. Disadvantages of this imaging technique include the parietal region not being included in the slab, incomplete demonstration of fine branches and lack of quantitative value. However, in our trial, evaluation of bypass patency was almost accurate in correlation with MRA and conventional angiography, so this MRA method can obviate postsurgical angiography. Selective presaturation on the circle of Willis gives further information about flow direction and distribution [3], and makes it possible to obtain a clear "bypass image".

References

1. Nambu T, Mabuchi S, Itamoto K et al. (1993) Nippon Acta Radiol 53:341–343
2. Kodama T, Ueda T, Suzuki Y et al. (1993) MRA in the evaluation of EC-IC bypass patency. J Comput Assist Tomogr 17:922–926
3. Edelman RR, Mattle HP, O'Reilly GV et al. (1990) Magnetic resonance imaging of flow dynamics in the circle of Willis. Stroke 21:56–65

Two-dimensional time-of-flight MR angiography following surgery

J. Ryterski[1], A. Pytlewski[1], P. Kozłowski[1], R. Poniatowska[1], S. Otto[2], T. Kryst[1]

[1] Department of Neuroradiology, Institute of Psychiatry and Neurology, Warsaw, Poland
[2] Department of Surgery, Medical Academy, Warsaw, Poland

Abstract. Our purpose was to assess the applications of two-dimensional time-of-flight angiography (MRA) after surgical treatment of carotid arteries. Endarterectomy was performed in patients with 50–95% stenosis of internal carotid artery (ICA). Fourteen patients who had been operated upon were examined with 2D TOF sequential angiography using a 0.38 T resistive magnet. Images were reconstructed with the maximum intensity projection method in rotated coronal planes. Additionally, spin-echo MRI of the brain was performed to determine the presence of vascular lesions. In 12 patients who underwent carotid endarterectomy and in 2 patients with vascular grafts, MRA allowed results of the treatment and prognosis to be assessed. In 2 cases, examination showed symptomatic ICA occlusion after endarterectomy. In 3 cases ICA stenosis remained after surgery. In 7 patients normal blood flow was observed. MRA, as a non-invasive diagnostic procedure, is a valuable method to evaluate postsurgical patients because it can depict blood flow in vessels and minimalise health risks for the patient.

Key words: Magnetic resonance angiography – carotid arteries – endarterectomy – vascular graft – magnetic resonance imaging.

In the past 5 years MR angiography (MRA) has become a very reliable method in the evaluation of vascular diseases. Several clinical trials have been published which compare MRA and conventional angiography or non-invasive methods, such as duplex ultrasonography [1–5]. MRA has shown high sensitivity in the detection of lesions in the carotid arteries, but lower specificity in the estimation of vascular lesions, especially in the estimation of the degree of stenosis [6]. Symptomatic patients with $>50\%$ diameter stenosis might undergo endarterectomy [7]. Many studies have concentrated on the evaluation of MRA in the preoperative diagnosis. Our aim was to determine the usefulness of MRA in the postsurgical assessment of carotid arteries, using two-dimensional time-of-flight (2D TOF) MRA.

Correspondence to: J. Ryterski, Department of Neuroradiology, Institute of Psychiatry and Neurology, Al. Sobieskiego 1/9, 02-957 Warsaw, Poland

Patients and methods

MRA was performed in 14 patients (11 males, 3 females; mean age 56 years) who underwent surgical treatment of stenosis of internal carotid artery (ICA). In 12 cases with 50–95% ICA stenosis endarterectomy was performed, and 2 patients had vascular grafts (Fig. 1A). MRA examinations were carried out within 3 months of surgery. MRA was performed with a resistive magnet unit operating at 0.38 T. We used a 2D TOF sequence, with images obtained in the axial plane. The imaging parameters used were as follows: TR 60, TE 12 ms, flip angle 90°, section thickness 1 mm with 0.6 mm overlapping matrix 128 × 256, FOV 20 cm. Approximately 100–150 sections were acquired. Images were reconstructed with maximum intensity projection (MIP) in rotated coronal planes and assessed by two radiologists with experience in both conventional angiography and MRA. To assess the percentage of diameter stenosis criteria employed by The North American Symptomatic Carotid Endarterectomy Trial (NASCET) were used [8]. Stenosis grades were defined as 0–50%, 50–75%, 75–99%, and occlusion. Additionally, spin-echo MRI of the brain was performed using T1-weighted sagittal and coronal images (TR 0.5 s, TE 20 ms) and T2-weighted coronal images (TR 2.0 s, TE 25/80 ms).

Results

Fourteen patients who underwent surgical treatment of carotid arteries were evaluated with MRA. Twenty-eight carotid arteries were studied with MRA. Twelve arteries were normal, 10 had mild stenosis (Fig. 2), 4 had moderate and severe stenoses (Fig. 3), and 2 were occluded (Fig. 3). These results were confirmed by Doppler sonography, except in 2 cases in which significant differences occurred regarding the presence and degree of stenosis. Additional spin-echo MRI of the head disclosed wide ischaemic

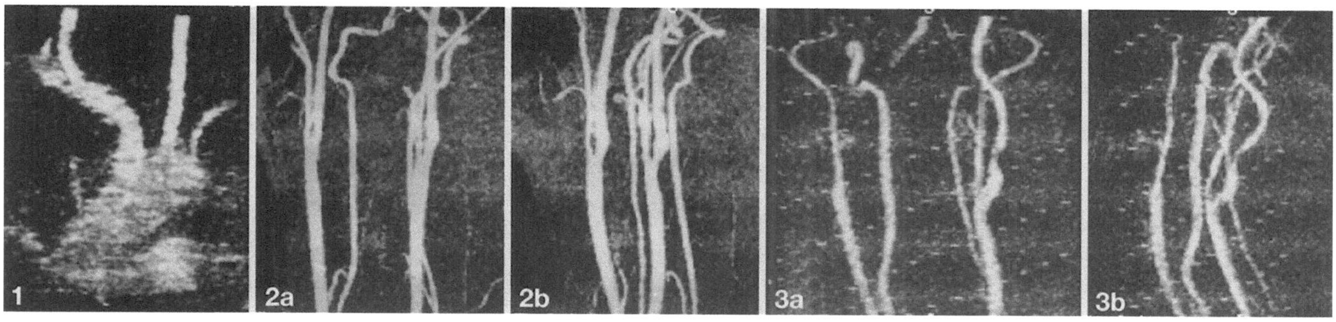

Fig. 1. Artificial, double-coated, veluric vascular graft of the left common carotid artery occlusion of the left vertebral artery

Fig. 2. Mild stenosis of left internal carotid artery (ICA) above bifurcation after endarterectomy. Moderate stenosis of right ICA

Fig. 3. Occlusion of right ICA; moderate stenosis of the left ICA 2 cm above bifurcation

lesions in 3 patients (in parietal and frontal lobes of cerebral hemispheres), diffuse, small and ischaemic lesions in the deep white matter of cerebral hemispheres in 8 cases, and no abnormalities in the brain structures in 3 patients.

Discussion

There is considerable controversy regarding carotid endarterectomy, its benefits and disadvantages, so it is important to minimalise the complications associated with this procedure [7]. Thus, using an accurate non-invasive method of imaging the carotid arteries would be of great benefit to the patient. In centres which are experienced in the technique, Duplex and colour Doppler scanning has achieved a high level of accuracy with sensitivity and specificity varying in various studies from 84% to 93% [3–7]. MRA with additional MRI of the brain offers a more complete evaluation of the carotid and vertebral arteries in conjunction with assessment of brain parenchyma. Technical progress in MRA provides increasing accuracy of this non-invasive method in the evaluation of carotid lesions. With our equipment only 2D TOF sequences could be used for acquisition of MRA, which offers good results at the level of the carotid bifurcation. We consider MRA a valuable non-invasive method to evaluate postsurgical patients, which minimalises health risks for patients.

References

1. Litt AW, Eidelman EM, Pinto RS et al. (1991) Diagnosis of carotid artery stenosis: comparison of 2D time-of-flight MR angiography with contrast angiography in 50 patients. AJR 156:611–616
2. Polak JF, Bajakian RL, OLeary DM, Anderson MR, Donaldson MC, Jolesz FA (1992) Detection of ICA stenosis: comparison of MR angiography, color Doppler sonography and arteriography. Radiology 182:35–40
3. Anderson CM, Saloner D, Lee R, et al (1992) Assessment of carotid artery stenosis by MR angiography: comparison with X-ray angiography and color-coded Doppler ultrasound. AJNR 13:989–1003
4. Polak JF, Kalina P, Donaldson MC, O'Leary DH, Whittemore AD, Mannick JA (1993) Carotid endarterectomy: preoperative evaluation of candidates with combined Doppler sonography and MR angiography. Radiology 186:333–338
5. Mattle HP, Kent KC, Edelman RR, Atkinson DJ, Skillman JJ (1991) Evaluation of the extracranial carotid arteries: correlation of magnetic resonance angiography, duplex ultrasonography and conventional angiography. J Vasc Surg 13:838–845
6. Heiserman JE, Drayer BP, Fram EK, Keller PJ, Bird CR, Hodak JA, Flom RA (1992) Carotid artery stenosis: clinical efficacy of two-dimensional time-of-flight MR angiography. Radiology 182:761–768
7. Anson JA, Heiserman JE, Drayer BP, Spetzler RF (1993) Surgical decisions on the basis of magnetic resonance angiography of the carotid arteries. Neurosurgery 32:335–343
8. Fox J (1993) How to measure carotid stenosis. Radiology 186:316–318

Acetazolamide-enhanced MR angiography of intracranial aneurysms

K. Tsuchiya, Y. Mizutani, T. Seki, J. Hachiya, Y. Furuya

Department of Radiology, Kyorin University School of Medicine, Mitaka, Tokyo, Japan

Abstract. The purpose of our study was to evaluate the enhancing effect of acetazolamide in three-dimensional time-of-flight magnetic resonance angiography (MRA) for the diagnosis of intracranial aneurysms. MRA obtained at 1.5 T before and after acetazolamide administration was compared in a group of five patients without aneurysms and another group of seven patients with seven aneurysms. In each patient, distal arterial branches were more clearly demonstrated on MRA with the administration of acetazolamide than without. Four of the seven aneurysms (mean diameter, 9.0 mm) were better depicted after the acetazolamide infusion. In the remaining three aneurysms (mean diameter, 4.7 mm), no significant change was noted. This method improves the visualisation of distal small arteries and provides better images of relatively large aneurysms.

Key words: Magnetic resonance angiography – Intracranial aneurysm – Acetazolamide – Contrast media

Acetazolamide, a carbonic anhydrase inhibitor, is known to have the effect of increasing regional cerebral blood flow. It has been reported that administration of this agent can lead to improved visualisation of peripheral intracranial arteries and detection of stenosis in the main trunk of major cerebral arteries by three-dimensional (3D) time-of-flight (TOF) magnetic resonance angiography (MRA) [1, 2]. Meanwhile, MRA has been accepted as a useful method for screening intracranial aneurysms [3, 4]. The purpose of this study was to evaluate the enhancing effect of acetazolamide in 3D TOF MRA for the diagnosis of intracranial aneurysms.

Materials and methods

We studied five patients without aneurysms (one male and four females, aged 38–84 years) and another group of seven patients with seven aneurysms diagnosed on conventional cerebral angiography (two males and five females, aged 45–78 years). There were two internal carotid-ophthalmic artery aneurysms, two middle cerebral artery aneurysms, two internal carotid-posterior communicating artery aneurysms and one basilar tip aneurysm. Of these seven aneurysms, one had a previous episode of minor rupture and the remaining six were unruptured. 3D TOF MRA was performed before and 5 min after the intravenous administration of 1 g acetazolamide. MRA was carried out on a 1.5-T unit, using the following parameters: repetition time/echo time 28/4.8 ms, flip angle 25°, field of view 14 cm, slab thickness 60 mm, partitions 64, imaging matrix 256 × 128, number of excitations 2. A direct comparison was made between images before and after the administration of acetazolamide.

Correspondence to: K. Tsuchiya, Department of Radiology, Kyorin University School of Medicine, 6-20-2, Shinkawa, Mitaka, Tokyo, 181, Japan.

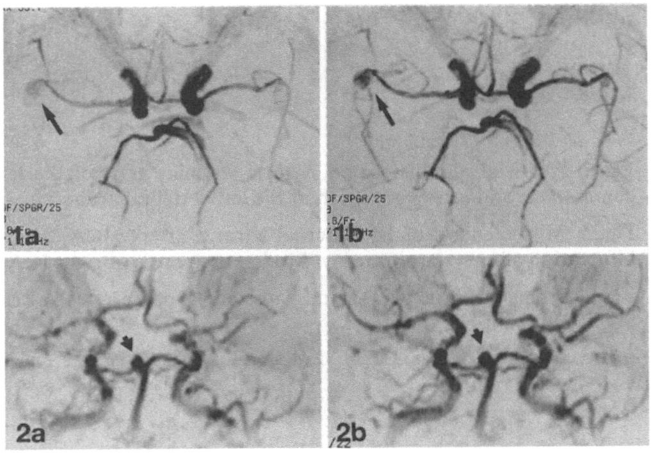

Fig. 1 a, b. Unruptured right middle cerebral artery aneurysm in a 78-year-old woman. 3D time-of-flight MRA before **(a)** and after **(b)** administration of acetazolamide. The aneurysm is more clearly demonstrated after acetazolamide infusion (*arrows*); distal arterial branches are also well demonstrated after acetazolamide infusion

Fig. 2 a, b. 3D time-of-flight MRA before **(a)** and after **(b)** administration of acetazolamide in a 51-year-old woman with an unruptured basilar artery tip aneurysm (*arrows*). No major change in the appearance of the aneurysm is evident after acetazolamide infusion

Results

In all patients of either group, peripheral arterial branches were much more clearly demonstrated on MRA after the administration of acetazolamide. In the group of patients with aneurysms, four of the seven were better demonstrated with an increase in the signal intensity within the dome after infusion of acetazolamide (Fig. 1). The mean diameter of these aneurysms was 9.0 mm. In the remaining three aneurysms, mean diameter 4.7 mm, no significant change in appearance was noted (Fig. 2). Short-term side effects were not recognised after the administration of acetazolamide.

Discussion

Acetazolamide is usually used for the treatment of epilepsy, glaucoma, etc. In nuclear medicine, it is utilised as a test drug for assessing the cerebral vasodilatory capacity of patients with ischaemic cerebrovascular disease in single-photon emission CT. Its effect of increasing regional cerebral blood flow has been shown by clinical studies using Doppler ultrasound [5] and other cerebral blood flow studies [6–8]. Being a carbonic anhydrase inhibitor, this drug raises the level of intracranial carbon dioxide, resulting in an increase of cerebral blood flow. As demonstrated in our patients, the administration of acetazolamide can improve the image quality of MRA [1, 2]. Gadolinium is used for the same purpose. However, it has a drawback in that the dura mater, choroid plexus, venous structures and membranes of the paranasal sinuses are also enhanced.

Results of this study demonstrated that, although not analysed statistically because of our limited series, relatively large aneurysms are well demonstrated after the administration of acetazolamide. We believe that this is attributable to the rise in blood flow within an aneurysm with an increase of the flow in the parent artery. Relatively small aneurysms did not show enhancement with acetazolamide. This is probably because these aneurysms have already presented a high enough signal intensity on MRA before the administration of acetazolamide. As the above-stated haemodynamic effect is suspected, position, size of the neck, and direction of projection of the dome of aneurysms may be factors that influence the enhancing effect of acetazolamide. In this study, we started post-acetazolamide scans 5 min after injection. However, as the effect of acetazolamide reaches its peak about 20 min after injection [5, 6], our starting the post-acetazolamide imaging may have been a little too early.

Most of the aneurysms in this series were unruptured. Acetazolamide is known to increase the regional cerebral blood flow by up to 70–75% [5–7]. The direct haemodynamic effect of acetazolamide on cerebral aneurysms is uncertain. However, we believe that the effect of acetazolamide infusion on patients as a whole is far less than that of conventional angiography. Also, although acetazolamide is a safe agent, it should be kept in mind that some patients complain of dizziness, congestion of the head, light-headedness, and headache [2, 9].

In conclusion, acetazolamide-enhanced 3D TOF MRA provides better images of relatively large aneurysms. We recommend using it when results of conventional MRA are equivocal in the presence of an aneurysm. Additionally, its use is probably of value in follow-up studies of unoperated aneurysms. We do not recommend using this agent in patients with a previous episode of aneurysmal rupture.

References

1. Araki Y, Tanaka H, Ohtani M, Yamamoto H, Yamamoto T, Tsugaguchi I (1992) MR angiography enhanced by sodium acetazolamide (in Japanese). Nippon Act Radiol 52:1605–1607
2. Mandai K, Sueyoshi K, Fukunaga R, Nukada M, Ohtani F, Araki Y, Tsukaguchi I, Abe H (1994) Acetazolamide challenge for three-dimensional time-of-flight MR angiography of the brain. AJNR 15:659–665
3. Sevick RJ, Tsuruda JS, Schmalbrock P (1990) Three-dimensional time-of-flight MR angiography in the evaluation of cerebral aneurysms. J Comput Assist Tomogr 14:874–881
4. Ross JS, Masaryk TJ, Modic MT, Ruggieri PM, Haacke EM, Selman WR (1990) Intracranial aneurysms: evaluation by MR angiography. AJNR 11:449–456
5. Hauge A, Nicolaysen G, Thorensen M (1983) Acute effects of acetazolamide on cerebral blood flow. Acta Physiol Scand 117:233–239
6. Vorstrup S, Henriksen L, Paulson OB (1984) Effect of acetazolamide on cerebral blood flow and cerebral metabolic rate for oxygen. J Clin Invest 74:1634–1639
7. Sullivan HG, Kingsbury TB IV, Morgan ME, Jeffcoat RD, Allison JD, Goode JJ, McDonnell DE (1987) The rCBF response to Diamox in normal subjects and cerebrovascular disease patients. J Neurosurg 67:525–534
8. Rogg J, Rutigliano M, Yonas H, Johnson DW, Pentheny S, Latchaw RE (1989) The acetazolamide challenge: imaging techniques designed to evaluate cerebral blood flow reserve. AJNR 10:803–810
9. Ringelstein EB, Van Eyck S, Mertens I (1992) Evaluation of cerebral vasomotor reactivity by various vasodilating stimuli: comparison of CO_2 to acetazolamide. J Cereb Blood Flow Metab 12:162–168

The usefulness of MR angiography for the long-term follow-up of intracranial arteriovenous malformations

T. Abe [1], Y. Horichi [2], K. Matsumoto [1], H. Ikeda [1], H. Doi [1], T. Iwata [1], T. Hayashi [2]

[1] Department of Neurosurgery, Showa School of Medicine, 5-8 Hatanodai 1, Shinagawa-ku, Tokyo 142, Japan
[2] Department of Neurosurgery, Showa School of Medicine, 5-8 Hatanodai 1, Shigawa-ku, Tokyo 142, Japan

Abstract. We reviewed the MR angiographic studies of 13 patients with intracranial arteriovenous malformations. In those patients treated by transarterial embolisation of the gamma knife, demonstration of the vessels on MR angiography was found to be improved by the use of intravenous gadolinium contrast medium.

Correspondence to: T. Abe

Key words: Magnetic resonance angiography – Brain, arteriovenous malformations – Gadolinium-DTPA

We describe an assessment of the utility of magnetic resonance angiography (MRA) in the follow-up of patients with intracranial arteriovenous malformations (AVMs).

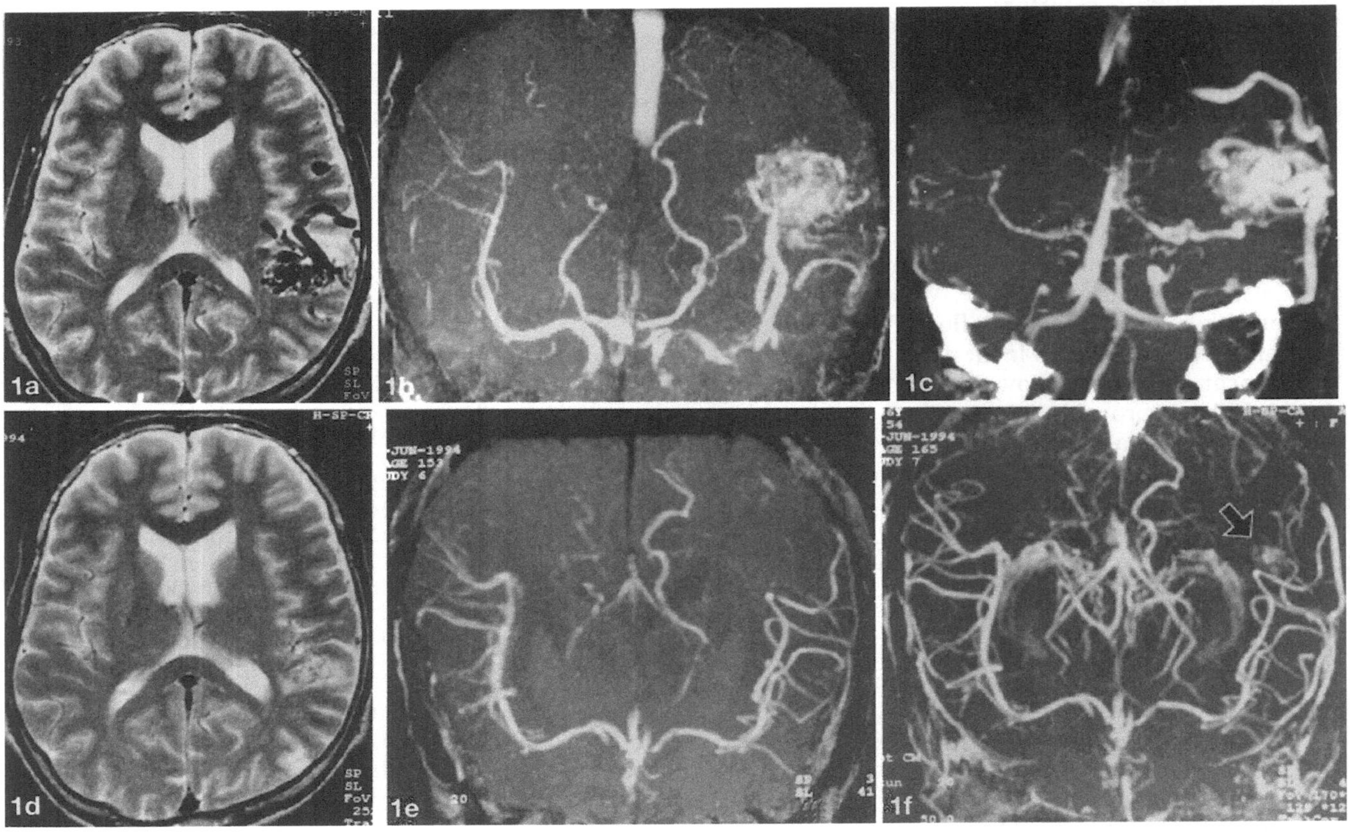

Fig. 1 a–f. Arteriovenous malformation with a nidus approximately 4 cm in diameter in the left temporoparietal region, fed by the middle cerebral artery and draining into the superior sagittal and left transverse sinuses in a 34-year-old man. Before treatment: **a** axial T2-weighted MRI and coronal 3D **(b)** and 2D **(c)** TOF MRA. Thirteen months after combined embolisation and gamma knife treatment the nidus is seen to be smaller on T2-weighted MRI **(d)**, plain **(e)** and contrast-enhanced **(f)** 3D-TOF MRA. The residual nidus *(arrow)* was seen only after administration of Gd-DTPA

Patients and methods

We reviewed the MRA studies of 13 patients (7 men and 5 women, aged 20–50 years, mean 36 years) with AVMs of the brain. MRA was carried out at 1.0 T, using the magnetisation transfer contrast and tilting optimised nonsaturated excitation (TONE) techniques. We used two- and three-dimensional (2D and 3D) time-of-flight (TOF) MRA. Intravenous contrast medium (Gd-DTPA) was used in some cases. Images were generated using maximum-intensity projection processing.

The AVMs had become manifest through intracranial haemorrhage in 5 patients, subarachnoid haemorrhage in 2, epilepsy in 3 and were incidental findings in 3. Two patients had been treated by transarterial embolisation, 2 by the gamma knife, and a further 2 by both methods; 7 patients had not undergone treatment. The duration of follow-up varied from 5 months to 15 years (mean 6 years).

Results

In the untreated patients the 3D-TOF method was excellent for demonstrating small AVMs, while the 2D technique was useful for showing slow flow, as in dilated vessels, and those draining some lesions. In the patients treated by embolisation, the gamma knife or a combination of the two, MRA with Gd-DTPA was found to be most useful for demonstrating the feeding vessels, the nidus, and the peripheral vessels (Fig. 1). In the 5 patients who had a giant nidus to the AVM, visualisation of the vessels was relatively poor.

Discussion

Since MRA is noninvasive and can be performed quickly, it is a useful means of following patients with known intracranial AVMs in the outpatient clinic, but the quality of the results varies from case to case.

Utility of MR angiography in intracranial aneurysms: statistical correlation and surgical benefits of the 3-D time-of-flight method

F. Ikawa[1], T. Uozumi[2], K. Kiya[1], M. Sumida[2], H. Satoh[2]

[1] Department of Neurosurgery, Hiroshima Prefectural Hospital, 1-5-54 Ujinakanda, Minami-ku, Hiroshima, 734, Japan
[2] Department of Neurosurgery, Hiroshima University School of Medicine, Hiroshima, Japan

Abstract. We evaluated the clinical benefit of three-dimensional (3-D) time-of-flight (TOF) MR angiography (MRA) and spoiled GRASS (SPGR) source imaging for intracranial aneurysms. MRA was performed on 40 aneurysms confirmed by cerebral angiography. The findings of MRA and SPGR images were compared with those of conventional angiograms. The size of aneurysms and their necks were statistically compared. The anatomical relationship between aneurysms and parent arteries was evaluated. The size of aneurysms by TOF MRA correlated with conventional angiograms ($r=0.932$). The size of aneurysmal necks by SPGR source imaging ($r=0.956$) correlated better than with TOF MRA ($r=0.844$). In anterior communicating artery aneurysms, the anatomical relationship between the aneurysms and the bilateral A1 and A2 could be clarified by axial images of TOF MRA. In carotid-opthalmic artery aneurysms, SPGR imaging clearly demonstrated the anatomical relationship of the aneurysms with the optic nerve.

Key words: Magnetic resonance imaging – Magnetic resonance angiography – Aneurysm, intracranial

Although magnetic resonance angiography (MRA) has often been used for screening in cerebral aneurysms [1, 2], it has rarely been reported that MRA is used as a source of preoperative information. Anatomical information regarding an aneurysm, including its size, neck size and surgical orientation between the aneurysm and parent arteries, is important in planning a neurosurgical approach.

Materials and methods

A total of 40 aneurysms confirmed by cerebral angiography were imaged by spoiled GRASS (SPGR) imaging and three-dimensional (3-D) time-of-flight (TOF) MRA. There were 13 internal carotid (IC) aneurysms, 10 middle cerebral artery (MCA) aneurysms, 7 anterior communicating artery (A-com) aneurysms, 2 distal anterior cerebral artery (ACA) aneurysms, 4 basilar aneurysms, and 4 vertebral artery (VA) aneurysms, these aneurysms had diameters ranging from 3 to 60 mm. 3-D TOF MRA was performed while the field of view (FOV) was made as small as 11–12 cm to narrow down the interested field. Conventional angiograms, TOF MRA and SPGR images of each aneurysm were compared with one another. The size of the aneurysm, the diameter of its neck, and the anatomical relationship with its parent arteries and nerve were examined and compared on each image. All MR angiograms were independently interpreted by two neurosurgeons in our institute. All MR studies were performed at 1.5 T. The pulse sequence used for the 3-D TOF MRA was a SPGR: TR/TE 35/4.5–4.7; flip angle 20°; thickness 0.7 mm; slab thickness 42 mm (60 sections); FOV 11–12 cm; matrix 256 SSNESSNO× 128; two excitations per phase-encoding step. The imaging time was 9 min 31 s for the 60 sections of TOF MRA. With 3-D TOF sequences, postprocessing maximum intensity projection (MIP) images through the entire imaging volume were automatically generated. This resulted in 19 MIP images perpendicular to the axial imaging plane (projection images) at 10° increments.

Correspondence to: T. Abe

Results

All aneurysms were detected by TOF MRA and SPGR imaging. The size of aneurysms on TOF MRA significantly correlated to those on conventional angiograms. The formula for linear regression was $Y=1.031X\text{-}0.805$ ($r=0.932$, $P=0.0001$). Neck sizes of aneurysms on TOF MRA and SPGR images were compared with those on conventional angiograms. The size of aneurysmal necks on TOF MRA significantly correlated to these on conventional angiograms. The formula for linear regression was $Y=0.648X+0.515$ ($r=0.844$, $P=0.0001$). The size of aneurysmal necks on SPGR imaging sifnificantly correlated to those on conventional angiograms. The formula for linear regression was $Y=0.788X+0.496$ ($r=0.956$, $P=0.0001$). In the source image of SPGR imaging, the necks appeared to be nearly the same size as on conventional angiograms.

There were seven A-com aneurysms. Conventional angiography showed the anatomical relationship with the A1 and A2 segments in all cases when performed in several different directions, but it was difficult to understand the relationship in some cases. Axial TOF MRA alone easily showed the anatomical relationship of aneurysms with bilateral A1 and A2 in four cases. In all cases it was possible to understand which A1 was dominant and the direction of the aneurysms using TOF MRA only. There were three aneurysms located in the IC-ophthalmic artery. In all cases, the anatomical relationship of these aneurysms with the ICA, optic nerve and the ophthalmic artery was readily demonstrated on TOF MRA and SPRG source imaging.

Discussion

MRA can be divided into two types: the phase-contrast (PC) method [3] and the TOF method [4]. In another study [5], we concluded that the TOF method was more useful for demonstrating aneurysms than the PC method, due to its higher spatial resolution and shorter imaging time. Therefore, in this study TOF MRA with a small FOV was used for intracranial aneurysms. Preliminary retrospective studies comparing 3-D TOF MRA with conventional angiograms have yielded promising results [6, 7]. In our study, all aneurysms confirmed by conventional angiography were demonstrated by TOF MRA, i.e. the sensitivity was 100%.

According to our results, as a preoperative examination it is important that the size of an aneurysmal neck be measured with SPGR source imaging. However, the size of aneurysms by TOF MRA and their neck size by SPGR source imaging were useful for operation.

Observation of the aneurysms from the direction of the axial slice provided information not available on conventional angiography. A-com aneurysms have more parent arteries (bilateral A1, A2 and A-com) than aneurysms at other sizes, so to locate these parent arteries by conventional angiography requires a simultaneous evaluation of multiple views. In axial MRA images, however, the relationship between the aneurysms and the parent arteries can be readily observed. In IC aneurysms, TOF MRA was useful when aneurysms compressed the optic nerve or oculomotor nerve, as SPGR source imaging revealed the direction in which nerves were being compressed.

The TOF technique requires only one set of data, thereby avoiding the potential problems induced by eddy currents and patient motion [4, 8]. They require less postprocessing and can be designed to minimize intraboxel phase dispersion [2]. This 3-D TOF technique permits the use of small boxels, motion refocus gradients, and short echo time. All these factors serve to minimize phase dispersion induced by motion and T2* phenomena and thus minimize intravascular signal loss [9]. The major limitations of the 3-D TOF technique include the misrepresentation of high signal stationary tissue (e.g., fatty tissue and methaemoglobin) as flow on the MIP postprocessed image. In this study, we used a small FOV of 11–12 cm and limited the region of interest to the site of the aneurysm such as Willis's ring. We restricted the area of MIP by minimizing the boxel size within the range where the signal to noise ratio was maintained, thus improving the spatial resolution and reducing the FOV.

References

1. Huston J III, Rufenacht DA, Ehman RL, Wiebers DO (1992) Intracranial aneurysms and vascular malformations: comparison of time-of-flight and phase-contrast MR angiography. Radiology 181:721–730
2. Nakagawa T, Hashi K (1994) The incidence and treatment of asymptomatic, unruptured cerebral aneurysms. J Neurosurg 80:217–223
3. Dumoulin CL, Souza SP, Walker MF, Wagle W (1989) Three dimensional phase contrast angiography. Magn Reson Med 9:139–149
4. Pernicone JR, Siebert JE, Potchen EJ, Pera A, Dumoulin CL, Souza SP (1990) Three-dimensional phase contrast MR angiography in the head and neck: preliminary report. AJNR 11:457–465
5. Ikawa F, Sumida M, Uozumi T, Kuwabara S, Kiya K, Arita K, Kurisu K, Satoh H (1994) Comparison of three-dimensional phase-contrast magnetic resonance angiography with three-dimensional time-of-flight magnetic resonance angiography in cerebral aneurysms. Surg Neurol 42:287–292
6. Ross JS, Masaryk TJ, Modic MT, Ruggieri PM, Haacke EM, Selman WR (1990) Intracranial aneurysms: evaluation by MR angiography AJNR 11:449–456
7. Sevick RJ, Tsuruda JS, Schmalbrock P (1990) Three-dimensional time-of-flight MR angiography in the evaluation of cerebral aneurysms. J Comput Assist Tomogr 14:874–881
8. Edelman RR, Wentz KU, Mattle H, Zhao B, Liu C, Kim D, Laub GA (1989) Projection arteriography and venography: initial clinical results with MR. Radiology 172:351–357
9. Schmalbrock P, Yuan C, Chakeres DW, Kohli J, Pelc NJ (1990) Volume MR angiography: methods to achieve very short echo times. Radiology 175:861–865

MR angiography of arteriovenous malformations: usefulness of phase-contrast with different velocity encoding

M. Sumida, T. Uozumi, F. Ikawa, O. Yukawa, K. Migita

Department of Neurosurgery, Hiroshima University of Medicine, 1-2-3 Kasumi, Minami-ku, Hiroshima, 734, Japan

Abstract. To evaluate the usefulness of MR angiography in arteriovenous malformations (AVM) and compare the phase-contrast (PC) with different velocity encoding (VENC) and time-of-flight (TOF) techniques, we prospectively studied 27 patients. In 3, PC was performed before and after embolisation and in 5 before and after radiosurgery. VENC was adjusted to 60 cm/s and 10 or 20 cm/s. PC with VENC 60 cm/s demonstrated main feeders in all cases but could not demonstrate smaller feeders. PC with VENC 10 cm/s demonstrated the nidus, draining veins and varices in all cases. After embolisation and radiosurgery, PC with VENC 10 cm/s clearly demonstrated the reduction or obliteration of the nidus and varix. PC is superior to TOF in demonstrating AVMs and is useful for preoperative diagnosis and follow-up, especially after embolisation and radiosurgery.

Correspondence to: M. Sumida

Key words: Arteriovenous malformation – Magnetic resonance angiography – Phase contrast

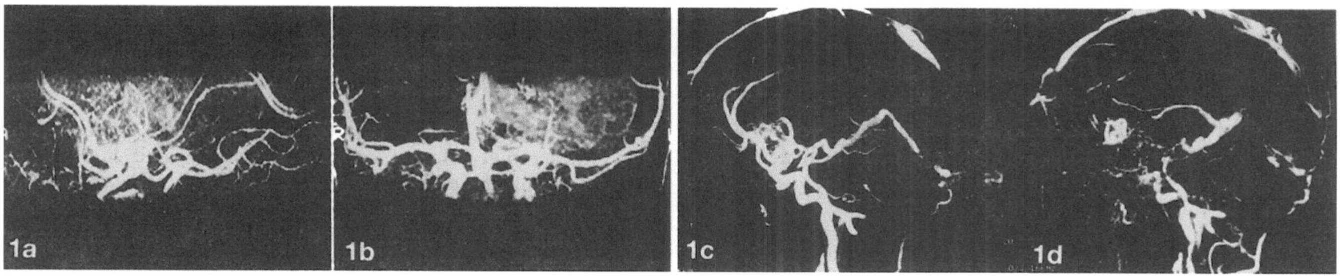

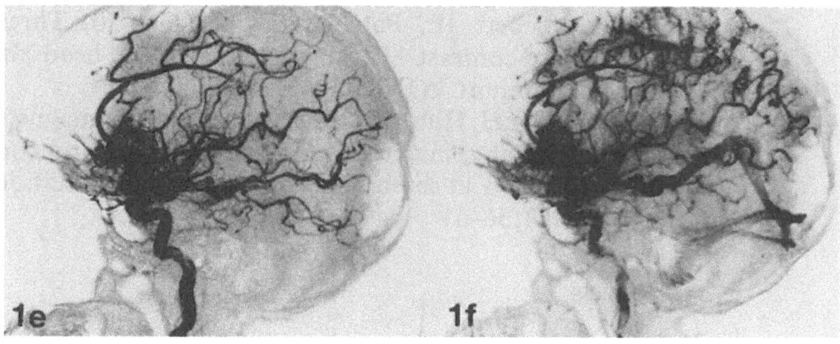

Fig. 1a–f. Arteriovenous malformations (AVMs) in the head of the caudate nucleus with a large haematoma. **a, b** 3D-TOF cannot demonstrate the AVM due to high intensity of the haematoma. **c** 3D-PC with velocity encoding 60 cm/s shows feeders, branches from the anterior communicating artery and part of the nidus. **d** 3D-PC with 20 cm/s shows nidus clearly and drainage to the basal vein of Rosenthal. **e, f** Conventional angiography shows the AVM, as in the 3D-PC images

MR angiography (MRA) techniques are being used more commonly and improving. There are two methods: phase contrast (PC) and time-of-flight (TOF). In general, the 3D-TOF method is more commonly used; however slow flow cannot be detected with this technique. With PC, velocity encoding (VENC) can be changed. We tried to demonstrate arteriovenous malformations (AVMs), including variable flow, with 3D-PC with different VENC and compare them with 3D-TOF.

Patients and materials

We prospectively studied 27 patients before surgery who were diagnosed with AVMs using conventional angiography. In 3 patients, 3D-PC was scanned before and after embolisation and in 5 before and after radiosurgery.

A 1.5 T MR unit was used. All patients were scanned with 3D-PC and 3D-TOF without contrast media. PC was 3D-PC with 2 mm thickness, 256 × 192 or 128 matrix field of view (FOV) 20 cm. VENC was adjusted to 60 cm/s and 10 or 20 cm/s. TOF was 3D-TOF with 0.7 mm thickness and FOV 11 cm. Scan time of both methods was 8–10 min.

Results

3D-PC with VENC 60 cm/s demonstrated main feeders in all cases but could not demonstrate smaller feeders. PC with VENC 10 cm/s demonstrated the nidus, draining veins and varices in all cases. After embolisation and radiosurgery, PC with VENC 10 cm/s clearly demonstrated the reduction or obliteration of the nidus and varices in all cases except one. In this patient, only a small nidus was found during surgery.

3D-TOF demonstrated only main feeders and part of the nidus and did not demonstrate any draining veins in all patients. In 2 patients with haematoma, TOF could not demonstrate any AVM (Fig. 1).

Disussion

MRA generally employs one of two fundamental methods, TOF and PC. PC differs from TOF in a very fundamental way. While TOF relies on flow-related enhancement to identify moving spins [1, 2], the PC technique uses velocity-induced phase shifts to distinguish flowing blood from surrounding tissue [3, 4].

The rapid flow velocity in AVM arterial supply causes wash-in freshly magnetised blood into the imaging volume. This reduces saturation effects and provides an excellent opportunity to visualise the arterial structures. However, the AVM arterial supply frequently becomes geometrically complex with tortuous hypertrophic vessels, producing multiple regions of complex flow with acceleration and turbulence. The limitation of 3D-TOF is its relative inability to visualise the venous drainage of AVMs, due to saturation of the slower flowing venous components. The result may be a loss of signal intensity within these regions of complex flow [5, 6].

PC is superior to TOF in some ways. One of them is the change of VENC as shown in this study. With low-velocity encoding, PC is more sensitive to slow flow and clearly demonstrates veins. Moreover, because the background is well suppressed, PC can demonstrate flow in haematomas, where because of an improved single-to-noise ratio and reduced dispersion, the flow is more clearly shown. However, disadvantages of PC are the longer scan time, lesser spatial resolution, and phase dispersion [7, 8].

Considering these characteristics of PC, AVMs are one of the most appropriate clinical applications of 3D-PC. Repeated MRA examinations are required after embolisation and radiosurgery. MRA is especially useful as it is a noninvasive method. Other lesions which are appropriate to clinical application are venous angioma, carotid cavernous fistula, sinus thrombosis and so on. In comparison with PC, the clinical applications of TOF are aneurysms, and intracranial obstructive lesions such as moyamoya disease. We think it is vital that the characteristics of each MRA method are well understood and used appropriately.

In conclusion, PC is superior to TOF in demonstrating AVMs especially in the nidus and draining veins. PC is useful not only for a preoperative diagnosis but also for follow-up examinations especially after embolisation and radiosurgery.

References

1. Dumoulin CL, Cline HE, Souza SP, et al (1989) Three-dimensional time-of-flight magnetic resonance angiography using spin saturation. Magn Reson Med 11:35–46
2. Wehrli FW, Shirakawa A, Gullberg GT, et al (1986) Time-of-flight MR flow imaging: selective saturation recovery with gradient refocusing. Radiology 160:781–785
3. Dumoulin CL, Hart HR (1986) Magnetic resonance angiography. Radiology 161:717–720
4. Dumoulin CL, Souza SP, Walker MF, et al (1989) Three-dimensional phase contrast angiography. Magn Reson Med 9:139–149
5. Marchal G, Bosnans H, Van Fraeyenhoven L, et al (1990) Intracranial vascular lesions: optimization and clinical evaluation of three-dimensional time-of-flight MR angiography. Radiology 175:443–448
6. Edelman RR, Wentz KU, Mattle HP, et al (1989) Intracerebral arteriovenous malformations: evaluation with selective MR angiography and venography. Radiology 173:831–837
7. Pernicone JR, Siebert JE, Potchen EJ, et al (1990) Three-dimensional phase-contrast MR angiography in the head and neck: preliminary report. AJNR 11:457–466
8. Nussel F, Wegmuller H, Huber P (1991) Comparison of magnetic resonance angiography, magnetic resonance imaging and conventional angiography in cerebral arteriovenous malformation. Neuroradiology 33:56–61

MR angiography in the investigation of venus angiomas

C. C. Lui[1,2], **Y. L. Kuo**[1], **R. J. Lee**[1], **Y. L. Wan**[2], **T. Y. Lee**[1,2]

[1] Department of Diagnostic Radiology, Chang Gung Memorial Hospital, Kaohsiung, Taiwan
[2] Chang Gung Medical College, Kaohsiung, Taiwan

Abstract. We studied eight angiographically proven venous angiomas (malformations) with two-dimensional (2D) time-of-flight (TOF) MR angiography (MRA). In seven cases we could show the caput medusae on unenhanced MRA, but contrast-enhanced MRA gave better vascular detail. Therefore, in uncomplicated or asymptomatic cases, 2D TOF MRA should be the modality of choice when it is considered necessary to image venous angiomas.

Key words: Angioma – Cerebral angiography – Magnetic resonance angiography – Venous malformation

---

Since the advent of MR angiography (MRA), it has been widely used either as a diagnostic or screening test for many cerebrovascular diseases. To date, MRA can show excellent visualization of the dural sinuses, deep and superficial veins [1]. Venous angioma is often diagnosed by the characteristic angiographic features. We attempted to evaluate the role of MRA in the diagnosis of venous angioma.

Materials and methods

We studied eight patients (2 men, and 6 women) with typical conventional angiographic findings of venous angioma (Table 1). All had CT and MRI at 1.5 T before and after intravenous contrast medium. MRA included arteriography [3D time-of-flight (TOF) in 2 cases; 2D TOF in 6] and venography (2D TOF acquired in axial and coronal planes in all cases). Three patients had venography and after intravenous gadolinium contrast enhancement. All were reviewed for the location of the angioma, presence of intramedullary veins, and visualisation of draining veins.

Results

The caput medusae of the angioma could be demonstrated in seven cases on unenhanced MRA (Fig. 1). The draining vein was not well seen in two cases (Fig. 2) due to in-plane flow. Intravenous gadolinium contrast enhancement provided better vascular detail (Fig. 2).

Discussion

The angiographic appearance of venous angiomas is dilated intramedullary veins converging into a large draining vein that reaches the superficial or deep venous system [2]. The venous malformations pass transcerebrally through the white matter. It is believed that the malformation represents an anatomical variant or persistence of the embryological venous drainage of the brain and should therefore be called developmental venous anomalies [3]. It may be associated with other anomaly or vascular malformations (cases 2 and 8) [4]. They may be found in any portion of the brain, but are most common in the frontal lobe and cerebellum [2, 5]. Haemorrhage can occur in venous angioma but is unusual and association with other vascular malformation should be excluded first [4, 6, 7]. However, angiographic study is the gold standard

Correspondence to: C. C. Lui, Department of Diagnostic Radiology, Chang Gung Memorial Hospital, 123 Ta Pei Road, Niao Sung Hsiang, Kaohsiung Country (833), Taiwan

Table 1. Summary of cases

Case	Sex/age (years)	Clinical presentation	Site of Angioma	Other lesions	MRA Technique TR/TE (ms) flip angle°/thickness (cm)	Contrast medium
1	F/16	Seizures	Frontal	–	2D/TOF 45/8.7/60°/1.5	+
2	M/50	Ptosis	Midbrain	Tectal cavernoma	2DTOF 45/8.7/50°/1.5	
3	F/55	Dementia	Cerebellum	–		
4	F/27	Seizures	Cerebellum	–	2DTOF 45/8.7/60°/1.5	
5	F/30	Facial palsy	Cerebellum	Pontine tumour	2DTOF 45/8.7/60°/1.5	
6	F/62	Vertigo	Cerebellum	–	2DTOF 45/8.7/50°/1.5	+
7	F/29	Seizures	Frontotemporal	–	2DTOF 42/8.7/55°/1.5	
8	M/40	Tremor	Temporoparietal	Varix	2DTOF 42/8.7/55°/1.5	+

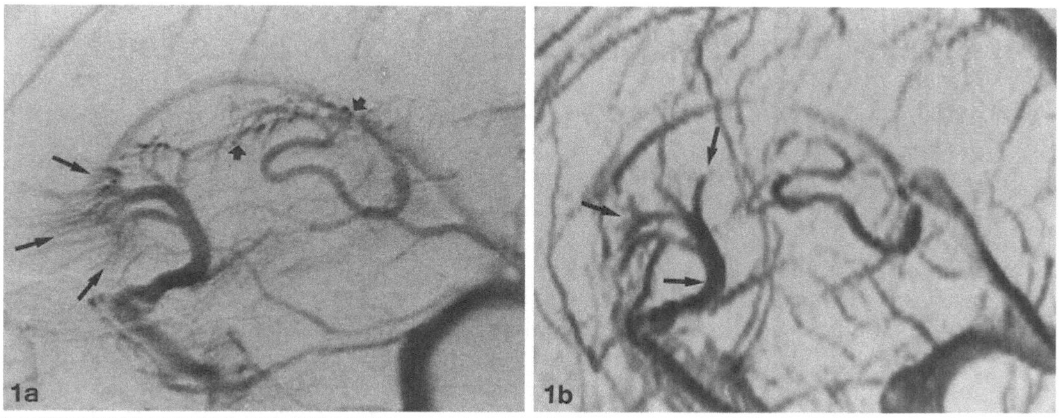

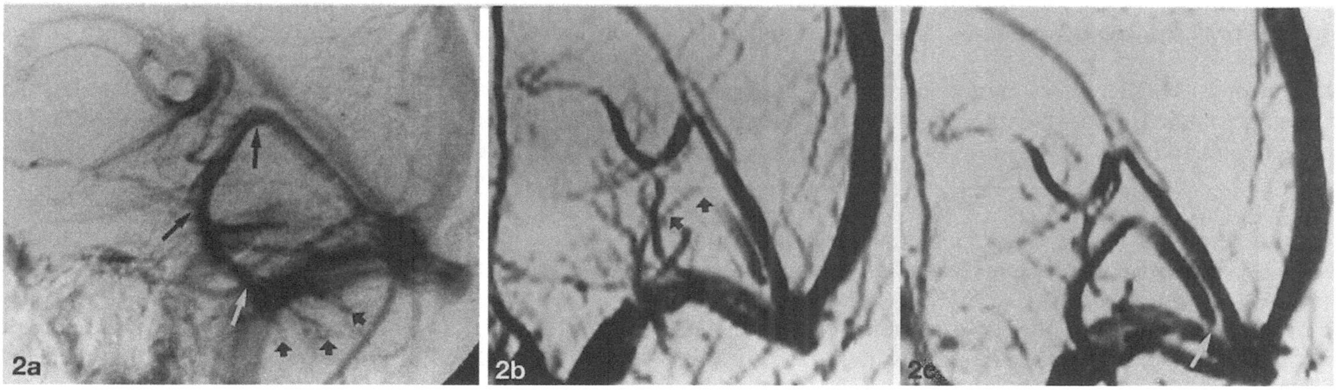

Fig. 1a, b. Case 7, **a** Lateral projection of left carotid angiogram shows two venous angiomas *(arrows)*. **b** MRA shows the caput medusae and the draining vein *(arrows)* of the frontal angioma

Fig. 2a–c. Case 3 **a** Lateral projection of vertebral angiogram shows a venous angioma *(arrows)*. **b** MRA shows part of the draining vein *(arrows)*. **c** After intravenous gadolinium, the angioma and draining vein are more clearly seen, and a focal stenosis just before the dural sinus is shown better than on conventional angiography *(arrow)*

for the diagnosis. It is invasive and surgical intervention is rarely needed for the angioma itself [6, 7]. Because the venous angiomas are low flow and low resistance, these lesions are generally not well demonstrated on 3D TOF MRA [8]. Due to its sensitivity to slow flow, the lesions may be visualized more clearly on 2D TOF MRA, but the in-plane flow can compromise the image quality [1] (Fig. 2b). Intravenous injection of gadolinium can achieve an improvement of vessel detail [9] (Fig. 2).

Since an operation is seldom performed in uncomplicated cases, angiography is the definite diagnosis of venous angioma should one be required. MRA is a good alternative test, and in undertermined cases, intravenous injection of gadolinium is helpful.

References

1. Lindan CE, Wallace RC (1992) Cerebrovascular anatomy on magnetic resonance angiography. Neuroimaging Clin North Am 2:743–752
2. Huang YP, Robbins A, Patel SC (1984) Cerebral venous malformation. In: Kapp JP, Schmidek HH (eds) The cerebral venous system and its disorders. Grune & Stratton, Orlando, pp 373–474
3. Lasjaunias P, Burrows P, Planet C (1986) Developmental venous anomalies (DVA): the so-called venous angioma. Neurosurg Rev 9:233–44

4. Truwit CL (1992) Venous angioma of the brain: history, significance, and imaging findings. AJR 159:1299–1307
5. Uchino A, Imada H, Ohno M (1990) Magnetic resonance imaging of intracranial venous angiomas. Clin Imag 14:309–314
6. Kondziolka D, Dempsey PK, Lunsford DL (1991) The case for conservative management of venous angiomas. Can J Neurol Sci 18:295–299
7. Rigamonti D, Spetzler RF, Medina M, Rigamonti K, Geckle DS, Pappas C (1990) Cerebral venous malformations. J Neurosurg 73:560–564
8. Marchal G, Bosmans H, Van Fraeyenhoven L, Wilms G, Hecke PV, Plets C, Baert AL (1990) Intracranial vascular lesions: optimization and clinical evaluation of three-dimensional time-of-flight MR angiography. Radiology 175:443–448
9. Seiderer M (1994) MR angiography. In: Felix R, Heshiki A, Hosten N, Hricak H (eds) Magnevist monography. Blackwell, Oxford, pp 159–166

Magnetic resonance angiography of developmental venous anomalies (venous angiomas): three-dimensional time-of-flight versus phase contrast

H. Y. Choi[1], **K. M. Shin**[2], **M. H. Kim**[2], **H. C. Park**[2], **H. Y. Kim**[1]

[1] Department of Radiology, College of Medicine, Ewha Womens University, Seoul, Korea
[2] Department of Neurosurgery, College of Medicine, Ewha Womens University, Seoul, Korea

Abstract. We analyse MR angiography (MRA) in eight cases among ten patients demonstrating venous anomaly on MRI. In six of the eight cases contrast-enhanced three-dimensional time of flight (3D TOF) MRA nicely demonstrated both dilated draining and medullary veins. 3D phase-contrast MRA with velocity encoding below 10 cm/s only showed hyperintense dilated draining veins.

Key words: Magnetic resonance imaging – Magnetic resonance angiography – Venous angioma – Developmental venous anomaly

Venous angioma in the brain, a benign developmental anomaly, is very frequently and incidentally discovered on contrast-enhanced CT [1] or MRI studies [2–4]. Our purpose was to find an adequate sequence for magnetic resonance angiography (MRA) and to demonstrate the findings on MRA of venous angiomas. The two major techniques for this purpose are three-dimensional (3D) time-of-flight (TOF) and phase-constrast (PC) MRA.

Patients and methods

We saw ten patients who had a developmental venous anomaly on MRI, examined on a 1.5-T superconducting imager. Eight of these patients underwent MRA with the use of 3D TOF and PC sequences. 3D TOF sequence was used with enhancement in six and without enhancement in five. 3D PC was performed with variable velocity encoding of above 25 cm/s in three and below 10 cm/s in eight patients. For contrast enhancement, gadopentetate dimeglumine was administered at 0.1 mmol/kg. We also used maximum intensity projection and interactive vascular imaging techniques for focussed images.

Correspondence to: H. Y. Choi

Results

The developmental venous anomaly was well demonstrated by MRI images (Fig. 1a) in ten patients. 3D PC images definitely showed dilated draining veins at less than the 10 cm/s velocity encoding in all eight cases (Figs. 1b, 2a). On the other hand, enhanced 3D TOF images showed both dilated draining and medullary veins well in all six patients although the signal intensity of veins was less than that of the arteries (Figs. 1c, 2b). Enhanced 3D TOF MRA correlated nicely with typical conventional angiographic findings (Fig. 1d).

Discussion

Cerebral developmental venous anomalies are encountered as incidental findings in patients with non-specific complaints. Saito and Kobayashi [5] suggested that venous angiomas occur when an accident in embryogenesis results in occlusion or maldevelopment of the normal venous drainage of part of the brain. Lasjaunias et al. [6] have suggested that the name "venous angioma" be changed to "developmental venous anomaly" to reflect this characteristic more precisely.

Previous reports have been explored the efficacy of MRA in depicting intracranial vascular structures. However, to our knowledge, MRA findings of venous angioma have rarely been reported. Truwit [7] briefly described the sequences and Hustone et al. [8] reported one case of MRA finding a venous angioma. Three-dimensional TOF techniques clearly depict high-velocity proximal arteries and the use of gadopentetate dimeglumine has optimized the visualization of venous structures [9]. In contrast, the 3D PC technique permits flexible imaging of fast or slow flow by varying the amount of velocity encoding [8, 9].

In this study, we found that draining veins of developmental venous anomaly were well depicted, low flow-

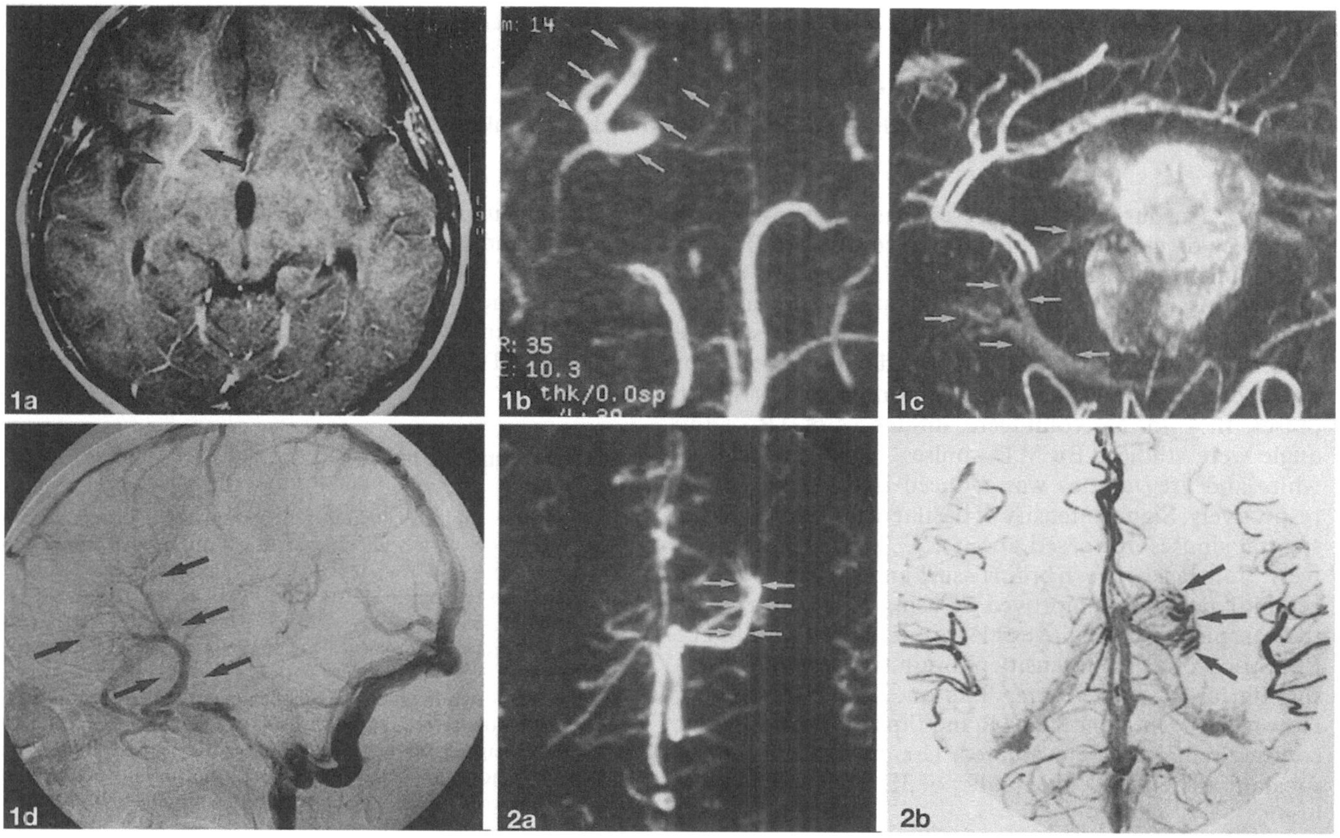

Fig. 1a–d. Twelve-year-old boy with haemorrhagic cavernous malformation. **a** Contrast-enhanced T1-weighted MRI shows enhancing linear draining and medullary veins (*arrows*) near the frontal horn of the right lateral ventricle. **b** Axial PC MRA demonstrates hyperintense draining veins (*arrows*) and appears similar to **a**. **c** Oblique sagittal contrast-enhanced TOF MRA demonstrates "open umbrella configuration" of medullary veins and dilated draining veins (*arrows*) well. Lobulated high-signal "mass" is methaemoglobin in haemorrhagic cavernous malformation. **d** Conventional angiogram, lateral projection, reveals typical radiating collection of medullary veins collecting centrally into large draining veins and terminating in the superficial middle cerebral vein (*arrows*)

Fig. 2a, b. Ten-year-old boy with headache for 4 years. **a** Coronal PC MRA image reveals intense dilated draining vein connecting with fine medullary veins (*arrows*). **b** Contrast-enhanced TOF MRA nicely demonstrates "caput medusae" of medullary veins and draining vein (*arrows*)

encoding velocities of 5–10 cm/s on 3D PC and enhanced 3D TOF can directly depict both the medullary and draining veins because venous structures were of interest. Therefore, if the finding of venous angioma is typical on contrast-enhanced MRI and MRA, further invasive conventional angiographic examination could be avoided.

The most adequate sequences for MRA of venous angiomas were 3D contrast-enhanced TOF for demonstrating both medullary and draining veins and 3D PC with velocity encoding of 10 cm/s for showing hyperintense draining veins.

References

1. Valavanis A, Wellauer J, Yasargil MG (1983) The radiological diagnosis of cerebral venous angioma: cerebral angiography and computed tomography. Neuroradiology 24:193–199
2. Toro VE, Geyer CA, Sherman JL, Parisi JE, Brantley MJ (1988) Cerebral venous angiomas: MR findings. J Comput Assist Tomogr 12:935–940
3. Wilms G, Demaerel P, Marchl G, Baert AL, Plets C (1991) Gadolinium-enhanced MR imaging of cerebral venous angiomas with emphasis on their drainage. J Comput Assist Tomogr 15:199–206
4. Wilms G, Marchal G, Hecke P, Fraeyenhoven L, Decrop E, Baert AL (1990) Cerebral venous angiomas: MR imaging at 1.5 tesla. Neuroradiology 32:31–35
5. Saito Y, Kobayashi N (1981) Cerebral venous angiomas. Clinical evaluation and possible etiology. Radiology 1981; 139:87–94
6. Lasjaunias P, Burrows P, Planet C (1986) Developmental venous anomalies (DVA): the so-called venous angiomas. Neurosurg Rev 9:233–244
7. Truwit CL (1992) Venous angioma of the brain: history, significance, and imaging findings. AJR 159:1299–1307
8. Hustone J III, Rufenacht DA, Ehman RL, Wiebers DO (1991) Intracranial aneurysms and vacular malformations: comparison of time-of-flight and phase-contrast MR angiography. Radiology 181:721–730
9. Chakeres DW, Schmalbrock P, Brogan M, Yuan C, Cohen C (1990) Normal venous anatomy of the brain: demonstration with gadopentetate dimeglumine in enhanced 3D MR angiography. AJNR 11:1107–1118

Intracranial MR angiography: application of magnetisation transfer contrast

T. Kodama, T. Yano, Y. Samejima, K. Watanabe

Department of Radiology, Miyazaki Medical College, 5000 Kihara Kiyotake, Miyazaki, 889-16 Japan

Abstract. The purpose of the present study was to evaluate the effect of magnetisation transfer contrast (MTC) on three-dimensional (3D) time-of-flight (TOF) MR angiography (MRA). All images were acquired with a 1.5-T system using a quadrature head coil. In 23 subjects, single volume 3D TOF MRA was performed with and without MTC preparation pulses using binomial on-resonance pulses. In 4 normal volunteers, influences of TR or flip angle were studied. By MTC pulses, signal intensity of white and grey matter was reduced by 43% and 35%, respectively. Signal intensity of basilar artery and superior sagittal sinuses decreased about 15% and 32%, respectively. Contrast between brain tissues and basilar or middle cerebral artery was improved by using MTC pulses, and the conspicuity of small vessels was improved with MTC. Reduction of signal intensity of brain tissue by MTC was slightly larger with shorter TRs and lower flip angles. However, the influences of TR and flip angles on vascular contrast remain to be evaluated. Use of MTC pulses can substantially enhance the quality of 3D TOF MRA of the brain.

Key words: Magnetic resonance angiography – Magnetisation transfer contrast

Three-dimensional (3D) time-of-flight (TOF) MR angiography (MRA) has proved an effective, noninvasive method for evaluating intracranial blood vessels. When forming projection images of TOF MRA the maximum intensity projection (MIP) algorithm is most often used. In the MIP, the vessel intensity should be about 2 standard deviations above the mean background noise to maintain good vascular contrast the calibre of most vessels is reduced and low-flow details tend to disappear [1]. The purpose of the present study was to study the effect of magnetisation transfer contrast (MTC) on 3D TOF MRA and determine whether MTC could be used to improve the quality of TOF MRA.

Materials and methods

Twenty-three subjects, including 7 normal volunteers, underwent 3D TOF MRA with and without MTC pulses. All images were acquired with a 1.5-T system using a quadrature head coil. The binominal on-resonance pulses were used as MTC pulses with a duration of 1 ms and a |B1| of 21 μT. Magnetisation transfer rates (MTR) of several brain tissues were calculated by: (signal intensity without MTC – signal intensity with MTC/signal intensity without MTC × 100%. Contrasts between brain parenchyma and basilar artery or middle cerebral artery (distal M2 portion) were calculated by: (vessel signal intensity – brain signal intensity/brain signal intensity. In addition, small calibre cerebral arteries were evaluated on MIP images. In 4 normal volunteers, influences of TR or flip angle were evaluated.

Visualisation of the branches of the middle cerebral and posterior cerebral arteries was graded as grade 1: poorly visualised small vessels; grade 2: discontinuous small vessels; grade 3: continuous small vessels; and grade 4: many continuous small vessels.

Results

MTC pulses had greater effect on brain tissues than on blood in basilar arteries (33–43% vs 15%) (Fig. 1) and use of MTC significantly improved the vascular contrast (Fig. 2). The conspicuity of small vessels was improved

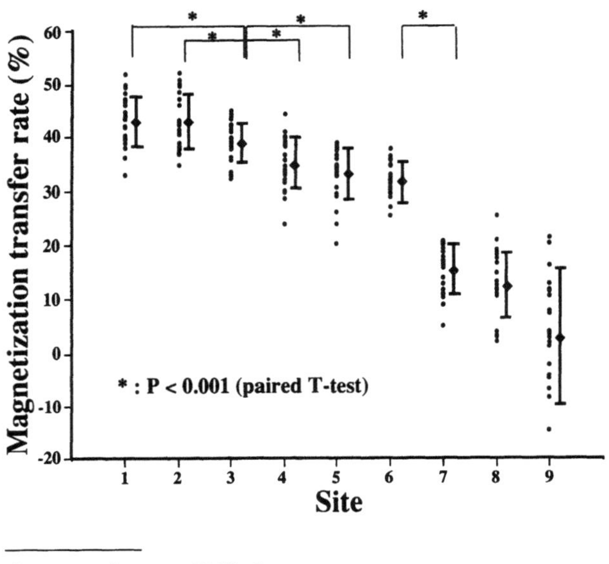

1. Pons 42.7 ± 4.7
2. Corpus callosum 42.7 ± 5.1
3. Thalamus 38.6 ± 3.8
4. Cortex 34.5 ± 4.7
5. Putamen 32.9 ± 4.7
6. SSS 32.0 ± 3.0
7. Basilar a. 15.2 ± 4.5
8. Fat 12.7 ± 6.4
9. CSF 1.8 ± 11.9

(%)

Fig. 1. Magnetisation transfer rate in several tissues (pulse sequence: FE 35/7/20°)

Correspondence to: T. Kodama

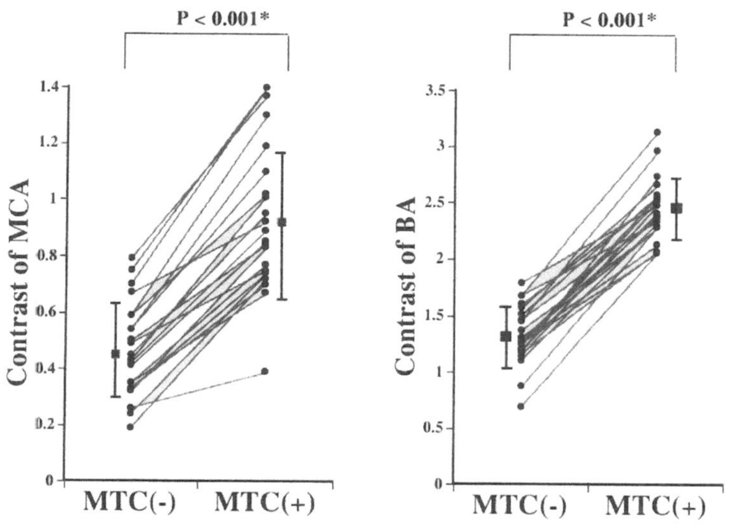

Fig. 2. Contrast between arteries and brain parenchyma (pulse sequence: FE 35/7/20°). Use of magnetisation transfer contrast significantly improved vessel contrast (*$P < 0.001$, paired t-test)

Table 1. Conspicuity of small-calibre cerebral arteries

	with MTC				
	Grade 1	Grade 2	Grade 3	Grade 4	Total
Without MTC					
Grade 1	0	6	2	0	8
Grade 2	0	2	8	4	14
Grade 3	0	0	0	1	1
Grade 4	0	0	0	0	0
Total	0	8	10	5	23 cases

with MTC in 21 of 23 (Table 1). MTR was significantly higher in the white matter (43%) than in the grey matter (33%). MTR of superior sagittal sinuses (32%) was significantly higher than that of basilar arteries. MTR of brain tissues was higher with shorter TR or smaller flip angle, and these phenomena were also observed in vitro studies using cooked egg white. The influences of TRs and flip angles on vacular contrasts in MRA with MTC were similar to those in conventional MRA.

Discussion

Use of MTC significantly improved the contrast between blood vessels and brain parenchyma by suppressing the intensity of the latter [2, 3]. We applied 1-2-1 binomial on-resonance pulses as MTC pulses. The signal intensity of brain parenchyma decreased more than that of blood in vessels and the conspicuity of small vessels was improved with MTC pulses. The signal intensity of arteries is enhanced by the intflow of spins originating outside the quadrature head coil, which is also being used as the radiofrequency transmitter. So the signal intensity of arteries was less suppressed than that of veins. Intensity of fat is reportedly not suppressed by MTC using off-resonance pulses, and hyperintense fat can obscure vascular information [3]. In our study, however, the intensity of fatty tissues decreased about 13% by using MTC pulses probably because binomial pulses were used [4].

References

1. Tsuruda J, et al (1992) Artifacts associated with MR neuroangiography. AJNR 13:1411–1422
2. Edelman RR, et al (1992) Improved time-of-flight MR angiography of the brain with magnetization transfer contrast. Radiology 184:395–399
3. Lin W, et al (1993) Intracranial MR angiography: application of magnetization transfer contrast and fat saturation to short gradient-echo, velocity-compensated sequences. Radiology 186:753–761
4. Yeung HN, et al (1992) Magnetization transfer contrast with periodic pulsed saturation. Radiology 183:209–214

Time-of-flight MR Angiography of the brain: improved vessel visualisation with magnetisation transfer contrast

I. Ikushima, Y. Korogi, Y. Sakamoto, T. Hirai, S. Hamatake, R. Murakami, M. Takahashi

Department of Radiology, Kumamoto University School of Medicine, 1-1-1 Honjo, Kumamoto 860 Japan

Abstract. The signal intensity from brain parenchyma can be suppressed with use of magnetisation transfer contrast (MTC) pulses. The purpose of this study is to evaluate the effects of MTC on vessel visualisation during MR angiography (MRA). The study group consisted of seven healthy volunteers. Three-dimensional time-of-flight MRA was performed with and without MTC. Analysis of vessel-brain signal difference-to-noise ratios (SD/N) was performed. The visualisation of small blood vessels was also estimated. MTC pulses improved the vessel-brain SD/N (mean improvement: 10%) as well as the visualisation of small vessels. This study suggests that MTC has a great value for improving visualisation of small cerebral arteries.

Key words: Time-of-flight magnetic resonance angiography – Magnetisation transfer contrast

Three-dimensional time-of-flight magnetic resonance angiography (3D TOF MRA) is a noninvasive procedure for imaging brain vessels [1, 2]. However, signal intensity of brain tissue interferes with demonstration of small vessels when maximum-intensity projection (MIP) reconstruction is performed. Magnetisation transfer contrast (MTC) is a method for reducing the signal intensity of the brain tissue and to improve the contrast of the small vessels [3, 4]. In this study, we studied the effects of MTC on vessel visualisation in 3D TOF MRA quantitatively and qualitatively.

Material and methods

We investigated seven healthy volunteers (all women) ranging in age from 24 to 29 years. All MRA images were acquired with a 1.5-T superconducting system. The imaging sequence used was 3D-FISP (fast imaging with steady precession) and its parameters included a repetition time of 40 ms, echo time of 7 ms, 20° flip angle, 128 × 256 matrix, 20 cm field of view, and 50 mm excitation volume divided into 64 axial partitions. The MTC pulse used had a duration of 8192 μs, a bandwidth of 250 Hz and a 1.5 kHz off-resonance single radiofrequency pulse. MRA was obtained with and without MTC pulses.

Region of interest analysis was performed for flow signal intensities in the midportion of the M1 segment of the middle cerebral artery and for stationary tissue in the brain tissue posterior to the M1 [5]. Background noise was measured as the standard deviation of the signal intensities in a region of interest positioned outside the brain. Vessel-brain signal difference-to-noise ratios (SD/N) were calculated as (vessel signal intensity – brain signal intensity)/standard deviation of background noise [5].

Correspondence to: I. Ikushima

Table 1. Signal intensity on maximum-intensity projection images

Case	Signal intensity[a]		SD of background[b]	SD/N[c]	SD/N (%)[d]
	Artery	Brain			
1	870/809	354/270	7.0/7.0	74/77	104
2	896/865	360/285	7.0/7.0	77/83	108
3	916/836	357/263	7.0/6.8	80/84	105
4	692/662	336/279	7.5/7.6	48/50	104
5	818/743	350/256	7.0/7.0	67/70	104
6	788/754	366/280	7.2/7.0	59/68	115
7	893/866	372/281	7.2/6.3	72/93	129

[a] Signal intensity without MTC/signal intensity with MTC
[b] Standard deviation of background without MTC/with MTC
[c] Signal difference/noise ratios without MTC/with MTC
[d] Signal difference/noise ratio with MTC)/(signal difference/noise ratios without MTC)%

Table 2. Visualisation scores of small arteries with and without magnetisation transfer contrast (MTC)

Artery	Case 1	2	3	4	5	6	7
Rt. PCoA[b]	x/x[a]	x/x	2/3	x/x	x/x	3/3	2/3
Lt. PCoA	1/3	x/x	2/3	2/2	x/x	3/3	0/2
Rt. P3, P4	0/2	2/2	1/2	1/2	2/3	2/3	2/2
Lt. P3, P4	1/3	2/3	2/3	0/2	1/3	2/3	0/0
Rt. MCA first branch	2/3	3/3	1/3	0/1	1/2	0/1	2/3
Lt. MCA first branch	2/3	2/3	2/3	3/3	3/3	3/3	1/3
Rt. M3, M4	3/2	0/3	1/2	1/3	0/3	0/3	1/2
Lt. M3, M4	1/3	0/3	0/1	2/3	2/3	1/3	0/0
Total scores	10/19	9/17	11/20	9/16	9/17	14/22	8/15

[a] 0, Not seen; 1, vessel just visible; 2, discontinuous; 3, continuous; x, not assessed. Scores without MTC/with MTC are presented
[b] Right, left PCoA, posterior communicating artery; MCA, middle cerebral artery

Visualisation of the small cerebral arteries was also evaluated qualitatively by two radiologists in consensus with a four-point grading system (0: vessel not seen; 1: slightly visible; 2: discontinuous vessel; 3: continuous vessel; x: not assessed).

Results

Quantitative measurements of the signal intensity are summarised in Table 1. In all subjects, the signal intensity of the brain tissue was more suppressed than that of the arteries. The mean SD/N was improved by up to 10% (range: 4–29%) by the addition of the MTC pulse, although it was not statistically significant.

Visualisation of small arteries significantly improved by addition of the MTC pulse, whereas the effects on large

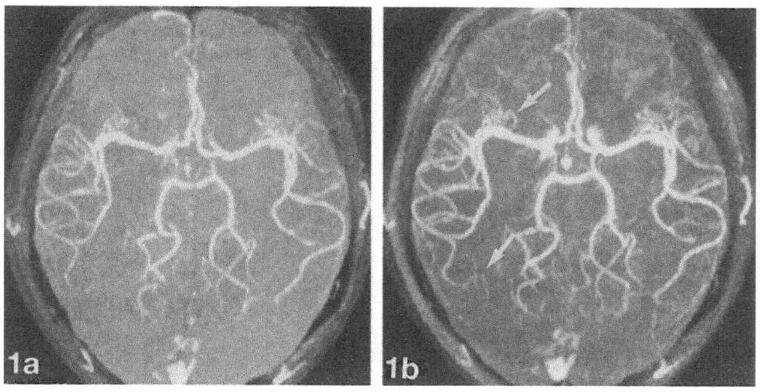

Fig. 1. The 3D TOF MRA axial collapse images of case 5, without (**a**) and with (**b**) magnetisation transfer contrast (MTC) pulse. Visualisation of small peripheral arteries is remarkably improved by addition of MTC (*arrows*)

vessels were minimal (Fig. 1). The mean total grade of vessel conspicuity was 17.9 with MTC and 10.0 without MTC ($P < 0.05$) (Table 2).

Discussion

Conventional 3D TOF MRA has often failed to visualise the slow flow in the small peripheral vessels because the magnetisation of slowly flowing blood becomes saturated. MTC pulse has proved useful in suppressing the signal intensity of background tissues containing a significant amount of bound water, while blood vessels are not suppressed because of a low concentration of bound water. Edelman et al. [5] showed 13% improvement of the vessel-brain SD/N by addition of MTC pulse in one volunteer. Although the MTC pulse they applied had a longer duration than ours, their results were almost consistent with the improvement of the mean vessel-brain SD/N in out study. Since there were significant differences among volunteers, further study with a larger number of cases may be needed. Qualitative evaluation showed marked improvement of small vessel visualisation despite the nonsignificant improvement of the vessel-brain SD/N. Improvement of small-vessel visualisation may depend not only on vessel-brain SD/N, but also on some other factors, such as reductions in motional blurring and spatial averaging [5]. However, it is postulated that slight improvement of the SD/N is enought to achieve better visualisation of small vessels. In conclusion, MTC is of great value in improving visualisation of small cerebral arteries.

References

1. Laub GA, Kaiser WA (1988) MR angiography with gradient motion rephasing. J Comput Assist Tomogr 12:377–382
2. Ruggieri PM, Lsub GA, Masaryk TJ, et al (1989) Intracranial circulation: pulse-sequence considerations in three-dimensional (volume) MR angiography. Radiology 171:785–791
3. Lin W, Tkach JA, Haacke EM, et al (1993) Intracranial MR angiography: application of magnetization transfer contrast and fat saturation to short gradient-echo, velocity-compensated sequences. Radiology 186:753–761
4. Hajnal JV, Baudouin CJ, Oatridge A, et al (1992) Design and implementation of magnetisation transfer pulse sequence for clinical use. J Comput Assist Tomogr 16:7–18
5. Edelman RR, Ahn SS, Chien D, et al (1992) Improved time-of-flight MR angiography of the brain with magnetization transfer contrast. Radiology 184:395–399

Dynamic cerebral gadolinium-enhanced subtraction MR angiography

J. C. Froment[1], P. Douek[2], F. Turjman[1], B. Falise[3], P. Tournut[1]

[1] Hôpital Neurologique et Neurochirurgical P. Wertheimer, Lyon, France
[2] Centre Hospitalier Lyon Sud, Pierre Bénite, Lyon, France
[3] Siemens, Division Médicale, Paris, France

Abstract. Dynamic cerebral GD-enhanced subtraction MR angiography (MRSA) and comparative two-dimensional time-of-flight MRA were performed in 15 patients (17 examinations). MRSA uses a fast Turbo-FLASH sequence (eight consecutive sets), in conjunction with a bolus injection of Gd-DOTA at the end of the second set, and maximum-intensity projection postprocessing of subtracted pre-from-postinjection images. Dural sinuses were well delineated by MRSA. Small arteries were poorly defined. MRSA appeared to be useful for detection of sinus thrombophlebitis, tumoural superior sagittal sinus compression or obstruction, and subtraction of subacute haematoma.

Key words: Magnetic resonance angiography – Contrast media – Gadolinium DOTA – Sinuses, dural

Correspondence to: J. C. Froment, Radiology Department, Hôpital Neurologique et Neurochirurgical P. Wertheimer, BP Lyon Montchat, F-69394 Lyon Cedex, France

The purpose of this study is to evaluate the feasibility of a new cerebral MR angiography technique, which combines fast MRI, gadolinium injection, and subtraction.

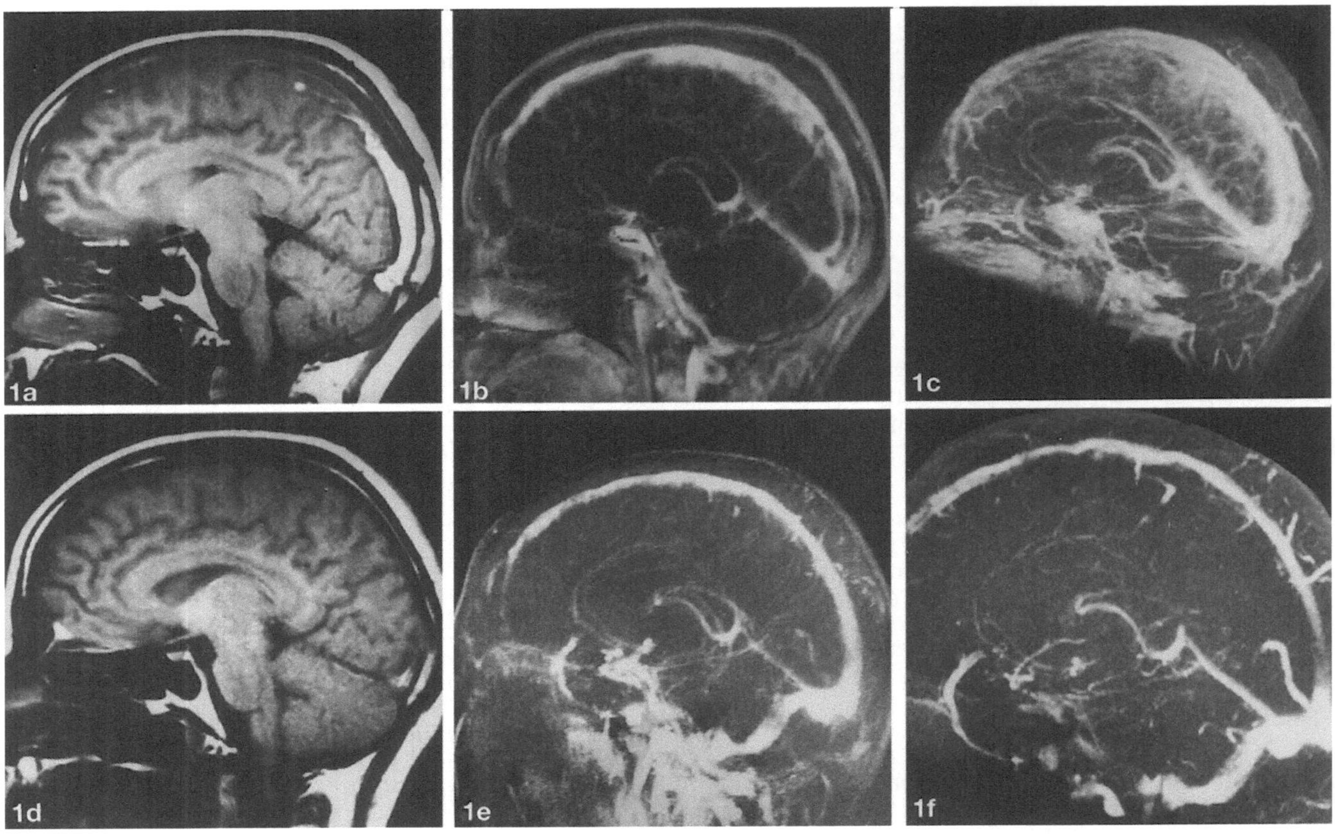

Fig. 1. T1-weighted spin-echo MRI (**a**) shows cerebral thrombophlebitis with hyperintense clot in the superior sagittal sinus in a 23-year-old woman. **b** Gadolinium-enhanced MR subtraction angiography shows low-signal clot within superior sagittal sinus. **c** Time-off-flight MRA poor delineation of the clot. Following treatment, the T1-weighted image (**d**) is normal, and gadolinium-enhanced MR subtraction angiography (**e**) shows normal opacification of the superior sagittal sinus. Time-of-flight MRA (**f**) also shows normal opacification of the sinus; the low signal in its vertical part is an artefact

Materials and methods

Seventeen examinations were performed in 15 patients, 11 females and 4 males, 13–70 years (mean: 43 years), for suspected venous thrombosis (9 cases: 7 negative examinations, 2 patients with venous thrombosis), superior sagittal sinus (SSS) occlusion or compression by tumour (4 cases: 3 negative examinations, 1 patient with SSS compression), or vascular malformation (2 cases: 1 negative examination and 1 patient with an aneurysm of an anterior cerebral artery).

MRI was obtained at 1.5 T. Dynamic contrast-enhanced MR subtraction angiography (MRSA) was performed using a segmented K-space Turbo-FLASH sequence [TR 15.2, TE 5, TI 39 ms, flip angle 40°, 5 slices, thickness 18 mm (for veins) or 6 mm (for arteries), orientation: sagittal > coronal = 20°, field of view 250 mm, matrix size 192×256, 1 acquisition, 8 consecutive sets, acquisition time of one set 20 s]. Two sets of data were acquired without contrast medium; the following sets were collected after an intravenous bolus injection of Gd-DOTA (0.1 mmol/kg, 5 ml/s). On a standard MR console, preinjection stack slices were subtracted from postinjection stack slices. In addition, each preinjection image was subtracted from its corresponding postinjection image; the resulting subtracted images were then postprocessed with a maximum-intensity projection (MIP) algorithm. In each case, comparative contrast-enhanced two-dimensional time-of-flight MRA (TOF MRA) was also performed.

Results

The main cerebral veins and sinuses were well demonstrated by MRSA in all cases, and usually the vertical part of the SSS appeared to be better opacified with MRSA than with TOF MRA. MRSA was superior to conventional TOF MRA in a case of SSS thrombosis (Fig. 1), since the clot was hyperintense and difficult to detect by TOF MRA, but was very clearly defined as a hypointensity within the SSS by MRSA. In a case of parasagittal meningioma, TOF MRA was in favour of a SSS obstruction by the tumour, but MRSA indicated that the SSS was free and only compressed, which was confirmed at surgery.

Arteries were usually poorly defined. A distal aneurysm of the anterior cerebral artery was well shown by MRSA, but the arterial vasculature was better seen with conventional TOF MRA. In case of subacute haematoma, the hyperintense signal of methemoglobin was well subtracted by MRSA, but remained superimposed to the vessels after the MIP postprocessing of TOF MRA; the underlying vessels were better demonstrated by MRSA, while the surrounding ones were better defined with TOF MRA.

Discussion

The principle of the technique is based on the capability of the segmented K-space FLASH sequence to detect the injected contrast medium in the vessels, and on the suppression of the background signal intensity by subtraction.

One disadvantage of MRSA is the need of contrast injection, which ist not mandatory for TOF MRA, but is often used to improve the visualisation of veins. MRSA subtracted images can be obtained only in a selected projection, since to save the time, only a small number of slices are acquired. Small vessels cannot be detected because of the poor spatial resolution, which is the result of fast imaging.

Venous structures were well delineated by MRSA. The vertical part of the SSS is better opacified with MRSA than with TOF MRA, as the sinus is parallel to the MR sections during the TOF MRA acquisition. Intravenous clots are easier to delineate with MRSA since they appear as hypointensities with this technique, but remain hyperintense with TOF MRA. The dynamic information given by MRSA is useful to differentiate tumoural SSS compression from obstruction. Finally, differentiation of vessels from haematoma is easier with MRSA, which erases the hyperintensity of the haematoma by subtracting it, but is limited by the insufficient definition of small vessels; this could be improved by using ultrafast MR machines.

In conclusion, MRSA appears to be a feasible technique. Its main indication could be the opacification of the dural sinuses for the diagnosis of thrombophlebitis or tumoural obstruction. Further evaluation and technical improvements are still required, especially for arterial angiography.

Holograph versus maximum-intensity projection display of neurovascular anatomy and pathology

J. Hunter, C. Ogilvy, R. Schulz, G. Geil, L. Lustrin, A. Wolfe, J. Taveras

Departments of Neuroradiology and Neurosurgery, Massachusetts General Hospital & Voxel, CA 92653, USA

Abstract. We compared the commonly used maximum-intensity projection (MIP) algorithm for extracting information for three-dimensional (3D) rendering with a holographic technique for true 3D volume display. The holographic technique uses all the data generated by magnetic resonance angiography, whereas MIP selects only certain data to create a rendering.

Key words: Holography – Maximum-intensity projection

A hologram, from the Greek meaning "whole message" is a three-dimensional (3D) image formed by the interference of light beams from a coherent light source (laser). The classic way of making a hologram is to split a coherent light beam into two parts, shining the "object beam" on and/or through the object, then recombining the unaltered "reference beam" and the altered "object beam" to create an inteference pattern – the hologram. This interference pattern – recorded on a specially processed high resolution photographic emulsion – is a complex series of light and dark bands which are characteristic for that object. Bright fringes appear where overlapping crests in the light waves reinforce one another, dark fringes when a trough in one cancels a crest in another. When this interference pattern is reilluminated with light of the same wavelength and from the same incident angle, the 3D object is optically reconstructed at its correct location in space, utilizing the intensity and phase information found in the recorded pattern. All of the object points are recreated at their same relative positions so that a volumetric image appears.

Such a hologram cannot be made directly from an MRA data set because there is no "object" for the object beam to shine on. Instead, the data for the first section are laser projected on to a diffuser screen, from where they travel to the photographic emulsion and are holographically recorded as a sectional image seen at the distance of the screen (Fig. 1). The screen then moves back to the interslice distance, the second section is projected, and a hologram of this is recorded superimposed upon the first hologram within the same photographic emulsion. This process is repeated sequentially for every section in the full data set. When viewed, all voxels in all sections are seen at their correct relative positions in three dimensions.

Whilst reconstruction of a hologram normally takes place using a monochromatic laser beam, the novel lightbox technology displayed, enables optical reconstruction of the full aperture hologram to occur using ordinary white light (Fig. 2).

The human visual system uses several depth cues to distinguish the relative positions of objects in a 3D scene. Normally depth cues are additive. These cues are divided into two categories: physical and psychological. Whilst holography can utilize all of the physical and psychological depth cues in its 3D display, 3D renderings of any description rely on the pschological cues alone to trick the

Correspondence to: J. Hunter

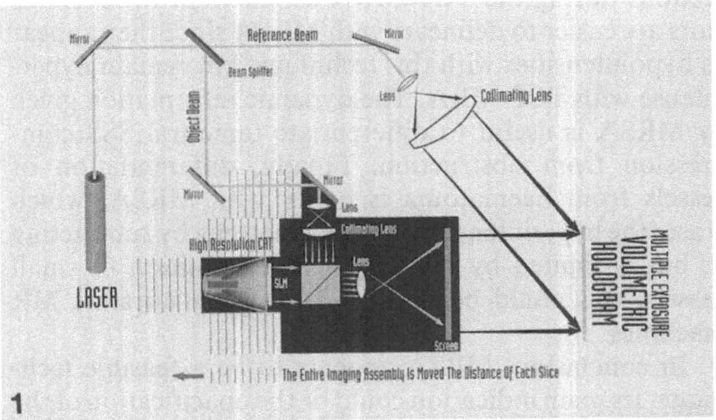

Fig. 1. Diagram of holographic laser camera

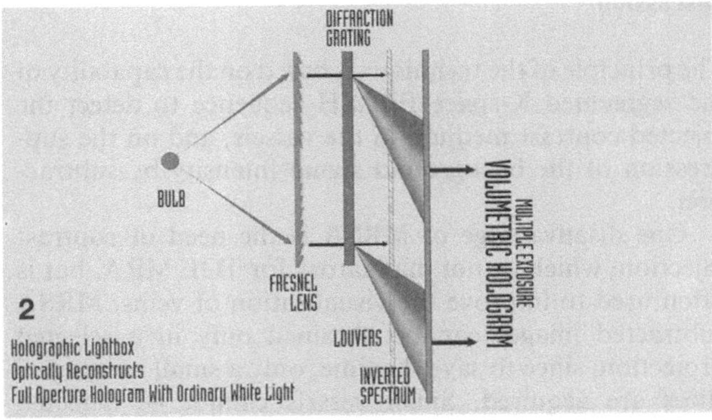

Fig. 2. Diagram of holographic lightbox

mind into thinking that there is true depth to an image which is being displayed on a flat surface.

Maximum-intensity projection (MIP) belongs to the ray-casting class of renderers. Ray-casting techniques work by passing parallel rays from an arbitrarily chosen viewing direction through the full data set. The final intensity value at the viewing plane is calculated according to a set of rules applied to each voxel intersected along the ray. MIP proceeds along the ray and compares values, keeping only the maximum for the final image. MIP is thus comparatively computationally inexpensive and also allows a significant enhancement of the contrast-to-noise ratio (CNR) and to a lesser extent of the signal-to-noise ratio [1].

This enhancement occurs because the MIP algorithm eliminates all but $1/N$th of the full data set, where N is the number of sections of reformations from any one projection. Given a typical 120 slice MRA of the cervical carotids, the MIP algorithm retains less than 1% (1/120) of the acquired data. It selects voxels to retain by assuming that the most diagnostically important will be those which appear brightest from the chosen viewing direction. Different subsets of voxels are selected for different viewing directions [2].

Materials and methods

Holograms were constructed from the raw data sets of MRA performed on 43 individuals with angiographically proven neurovascular pathology. These holograms were then systematically compared with the automatically reconstructed MIPs which consisted of a collapsed MIP in the plane of the data acquisition (usually axial) and a series of "rotated MIPs" (usually lateral) in a plane orthogonal to that of the original data acquisition. All data were acquired using 2D time-of-flight (TOF), 3D phase-contrast (PC) and multiple overlapping thin-slab acquisition (MOTSA) sequences [3]. Comparison was based on the ease of viewing the pathology and of making the diagnosis from the two viewing modes, speed of reading, and attention to the discrimination of small vessels such as the posterior communicating arteries.

Results

Twenty-three aneurysms, 9 atherosclerotic carotid arteries, 1 carotid dissection, 1 case of bilateral carotid pseudoaneurysm, 6 arteriovenous malformations (AVMs), 1 carotid-cavernous fistula, 1 venous sinus thrombosis, 2 cases of middle cerebral artery stenosis and 1 normal angiogram were included in the study. Two patients each had two aneurysms. All patients had conventional angiography.

Greater detail was visible on the holograms of complex vascular malformations, especially in the venous anatomy. The necks and domes of the aneurysms could be more easily and accurately identified by holography when compared with the MIP reconstructions, using angiography as the "gold standard". There were 2 cases in which a posterior communicating artery was visible on the hologram but not seen at all on the MIP images, although reference back to the raw MRA data set confirmed its presence. There was some loss of brightness of small peripheral vessels outside of the region of interest in 2 of the vascular malformations which did not detract from making an accurate diagnosis. Speed of reading a single holographic image was found to be greater than reading a complete set of rotated MIPs, following a short learning curve.

Discussion

Holography produced a faithful representation of the MRA data set without introducing artifacts which might mislead. As anticipated, some small vessels and, interestingly, the venous anatomy of AVMs were more clearly visible on the hologram. In at least one third of the cases where holograms were available preoperatively they gave the neurosurgeon a better understanding of the anatomy of these complex vascular malformations.

There are four possible explanations for the dropout of signal from superficial vessels noted on two of our AVMs, namely windowing; "flat fielding" – in which the brightness of a laser beam is greatest at the center and falls off to the periphery, "chromatic aberration" – where because of imperfections in the optical system there is chromatic breakup of the image at the periphery; and field-of-view

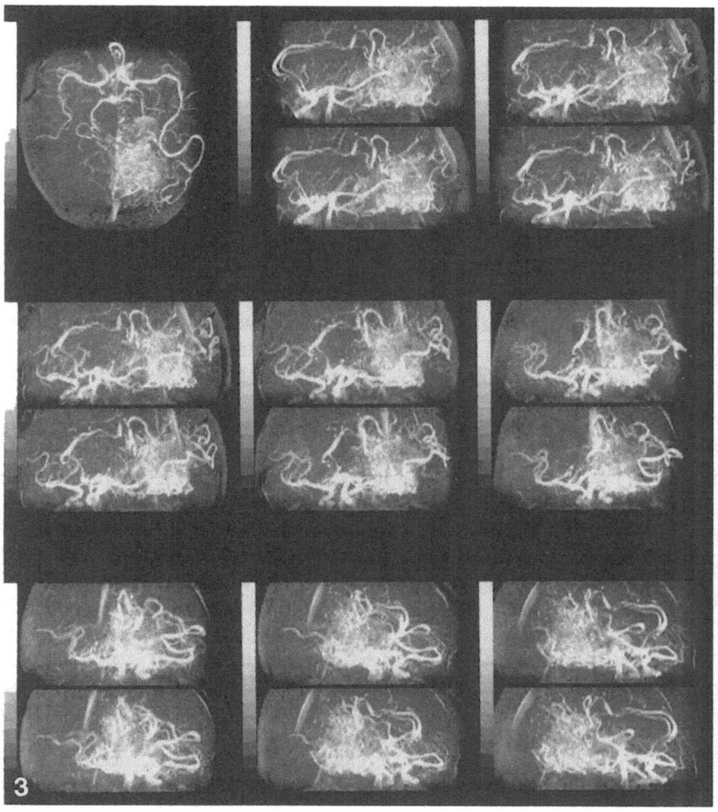

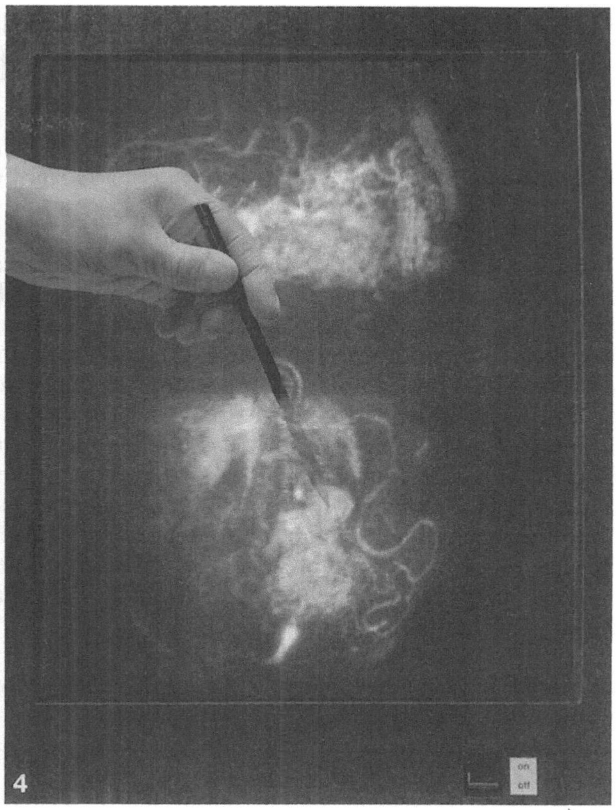

Fig. 3. A 59-year-old man with a diagnosis of arteriovenous malformation (AVM) of the corpus callosum. MRA demonstrated a large left parietal AVM but the collapsed maximum-intensity projection (*top left*) is confusing, as it apparently demonstrates a large left middle cerebral artery branch which turned out to be a branch of the external carotid artery

Fig. 4. The hologram, displayed as a single photograph projected in space, is a composite of left lateral (*top*) and oblique axial (*bottom*) views. The venous pouch is more clearly defined by holography. Holography has been found to be accurate in defining the relationship between feeding arteries, draining veins and the AVM nidus in these complex lesions

considerations restricted by the chosen optics of the system which currently run at a 15 cm deep by 30 cm diameter volume field of view.

It shoud be noted that in the case illustrated, the collapsed MIP was misleading in seemingly superimposing a scalp branch of the external carotid artery onto brain parenchyma as if it were an intrinsic vessel (Figs. 3, 4). The hologram clearly showed there was no connection, and this was confirmed by reference to the individual sections. In fact, difficulty was also encountered in viewing these same vessels on the rotated MIPs, presumably as a result of the ray tracing technique whereby intermediate signal from a vessel will be lost or cancelled out by higher signal along the same ray coming either from superimposed brighter vessels or scalp fat, when performing a 180° lateral rotation.

MIP provides "angiogram-like" images from which lower-intensity features of the vessels may be lost. This leads to an apparent reduction in vessel diameter, an overestimation of blood turbulence or stenosis and a loss of visualization of smaller or slow-flowing vessels. It is, therefore, essential to refer to the raw data set when interpreting MRA. Strategies such as the "restricted MIP", which clips the 3D data set outside of the region of interest before projection in order to minimize background, help to improve the final result.

Holography produces a faithful representation of the MRA whilst offering the benefits of a different viewing perspective, an improvement over the MIP in terms of vessel conspicuity, and better depth discrimination.

The best strategy is to optimize the sequence parameters in order to increase vascular signal and resolution and minimize background noise, as this improves both reconstruction technologies.

References

1. Brown DG, Riederer SJ (1992) Contrast-to-noise ratios in maximum intensity projection images. Magn Reson Med 23:130–137
2. Anderson CM, Saloner D, Tsuruda JS, Shapeero LG, Lee RE (1990) Artifacts in maximum-intensity-projection display of MR angiograms. AJR 154:623–629
3. Blatter DD, Parker DL, Robinson RO (1991) Cerebral MR angiography with multiple overlapping thin slab acquisition, part 1. Quantitative analysis of vessel visibility. Radiology 179:805–810

MR angiography of intracranial tumours using magnetisation transfer contrast and tilted optimised nonsaturating excitation

T. Kadota, H. Nakagawa, C. Kuroda

Departments of Diagnostic Radiology and Neurosurgery, The Centre for Adult Diseases, Osaka, Japan

Abstract. Our findings in 23 patients with intracranial tumours indicate that three-dimensional time-of-flight MR angiography with magnetisation transfer contrast and tilted optimised nonsaturating exertation, with and without Gd-DTPA, can play an important role in providing significant information on the pathological vascular anatomy of brain tumours. 3D MRA obtained noninvasively is valuable for planning clinical treatment and follow-up of the patients with brain tumours, despite a few limitations including the inability to depict small vessels and the restricted region of coverage. With continued technical progress, this might become a valuable alternative to conventional angiography.

Key words: Magnetic resonance angiography – Intracranial tumours – Gadolinium

Preoperative assessment of the pathological vascular anatomy of brain tumours, such as feeding arteries and the relation to the venous system, is indispensable to planning the clinical treatment. High detectability and excellent delineation of the regional extent of brain tumours by spin-echo (SE) (MRI) have been reported. Accepted thought to date, however, is that conventional angiography has provided the most detailed vascular information related to brain tumours.

Recently, significant progress has been made in MR angiography (MRA) techniques that have strongly enhanced the capability of MRA in the noninvasive demonstration of anatomical detail of the vasculature. The quality of MRA considerably improved when a high resolution pulse sequence with magnetisation transfer contrast (MTC) and tilted optimised non-saturating excitation (TONE) became available [1]. Studies of intracranial vascular lesions with use of MRA have been reported [2, 3]. To our knowledge, however, few reports have dealt with its usefulness in brain tumours [4, 5].

The purpose of this study is to present the clinical significance of three-dimensional (3D) time-of-flight (TOF) MRA, acquired both before and after intravenous Gd-DTPA in the study of pathological vasculature for the planning of treatment and follow-up of patients with brain tumours.

Correspondence to: T. Kadota

Patients and methods

We retrospectively studied 29 patients with intracranial tumours (meningioma 13, malignant glioma 5, metastatic brain tumours 11). The patients ranged from 24 to 77 years of age; 13 were men and 16 women.

3D TOF MRA was performed on a 1.5-T imager with a circularly polarised head coil. Data acquisition was performed with the same 3D fast imaging with steady-state precession (FISP) sequence with MTC and TONE, before and after intravenous administration of Gd-DTPA at a dose of 0.1 mmol/kg. Gradient motion refocussing to rephase spins flowing at a constant velocity was applied in the read and section-select directions. A shorter available echo time (TE) of 7.7 ms was used. Other parameter settings for MRA were defined in patients with intracranial lesions other than brain tumours. A short repetition time (TR) of 40 ms and an angle of 20° gave the best contrast between vessels and stationary tissues. MRA acquired in a volume (slab) with a thickness of 56 mm for 64 partitions, along with a matrix size of 512×256 and a field of view of 224 mm, resulting in a small voxel size of $0.43 \times 0.875\ mm^3$. MTC was induced by a Gaussian radiofrequency pulse centered 1.5 kHz off-resonance with a duration of 8 ms and a power of 9.0×10^{-6}T. In order to create TONE effects of reducing the saturation of blood, the flip angle at the middle of the slab had a value of 20°, but increased by a factor of 2 from the entry to the end of the slab of brain tissue.

The images were postprocessed by means of a maximum-intensity projection (MIP) algorithm to create projection views of the intracranial vasculature within the imaging volume.

Results

In all patients with intracranial tumours, multiview TOF MRA acquired before and after intravenous Gd-DTPA made it possible to demonstrate the topographical relationship between the tumours and the surrounding vascular structures, which facilitated treatment.

Meningioma

In 6 of 13 patients with meningiomas, the feeding arteries were recognisable with unenhanced MRA angiograms. The contrast-enhanced MRA was successful in detecting sinus involvement in 5 patients (Table 1).

Malignant gliomas

In all 5 patients with malignant gliomas the feeding arteries were demonstrated by unenhanced MRA. Enhanced contrast MRA showed venous drainage in 4 patients (Table 2). The multiview capabilities of MRA allowed precise definition of these feeding and draining vessels. Displacement of the arteries was shown in all patients. These MRA findings were in good agreement with the surgical findings.

Table 1. MRA findings in patients with meningiomas

Patient	Age (years)/Sex	Tumour site	MRA		
			Feeding artery	Arterial displacement	Dural sinus involvement
1	46/F	Sphenoid ridge	–	+	–
2	57/M	Parasagittal	–	+	–
3	45/F	Cerebral convexity	–	–	–
4	55/F	Parasagittal	MMA, CM	+	Narrowing
5	77/F	Cerebral convexity	MMA	+	–
6	58/M	Fourth ventricle	–	+	–
7	46/M	Cerebellopontine angle	AICA	+	–
8	42/M	Falx cerebri	CM	+	Occlusion
9	67/F	Tentorium	–	+	–
10	66/F	Sphenoid ridge	MMA	+	–
11	52/M	Parasagittal	FP	+	Occlusion
12	51/F	Parasagittal	–	–	Narrowing
13	42/F	Cerebellar convexity	–	+	Narrowing

+, Demonstrated; –, not demonstrated; CM, callosomarginal artery; MMA, middle meningeal artery; AICA, anterior inferior cerebellar artery; FP frontopolar artery

Table 2. MRA findings in patients with malignant gliomas

Patient	Age (years)/Sex	Tumour site	Pathology	MRA		
				Feeding artery	Arterial displacement	Draining vein
1	57/F	Temporal	AA	MCA	+	BV
2	69/M	Occipital	GB	PC	+	–
3	46/F	Frontal	GB	PIFA	+	SC
4	24/M	Cerebellar hemisphere	GB	PICA	+	IH
5	52/F	Temporal-basal ganglia	GB	MCA	+	BV

+, Demonstrated; –, not demonstrated; GB, glioblastoma; AA, anaplastic astrocytoma; MCA, middle cerebral artery; PIFA, posterior internal frontal artery; PICA, posterior inferior cerebellar artery; BV, basal vain; SC, superior cortical vein; IH, inferior hemispheric vein

Metastatic brain tumours

Of 11 patients with metastatic brain tumours, MRA demonstrated feeding arteries in 3 patients and venous drainage in 2.

Discussion

3D TOF MRA has enhanced the capability of MRI to depict the detailed vascular anatomy of the brain. However, there are major shortcomings, including progressive saturation and motion-induced intravoxel dephasing.

Significant attempts were made to overcome these major shortcomings in this study. Relatively thin 3D volumes (slabs) with thickness of 56 mm perpendicular to the direction of the cerebral arteries were primarily used to decrease progressive saturation. A shorter available TE of 7.7 ms was used to decrease the effect of spin dephasing. 3D TOF MRA data in our series are based on a small voxel element of $0.4735 \times 0.875 \times 0.875\ mm^3$. Intravoxel phase dispersion can be minimised through the combination of shorter TEs and the use of a small voxel. MRA before and after intravenous Gd-DTPA, was considered necessary for consistent understanding of the pathological vessels of brain tumours in our study. Rapidly flowing arterial blood is insensitive to progressive saturation on unenhanced MRA and can be shown well. However, the use of Gd-DTPA markedly improves direct visualisation of the venous abnormalities.

Compared with conventional angiography, the major advantage of 3D MRA is its capability to provide multiple views of anatomically detailed vasculature with a single 3D data set. Axial view projections are helpful to detect displacement of deep veins caused by mass effect. Oblique projections are useful in providing information related to sinus involvement by the tumours. Such images are difficult to obtain by conventional angiography, but can be easily obtained by 3D MRA.

One of the major limitations for the full implementation of MRA is the inability to depict small vessels due to poor spatial resolution, which still remains in this improved MRA technique, resulting from spin dephasing caused by marked turbulence of blood flow in small vessels. Another limitation of MRA is that this volume gradient-echo technique covers a limited region of interest for cerebral vascular imaging.

References

1. Edelman RR, Ahn SS, Chien D, et al (1992) Improved time-of-flight MR angiography of the brain with magnetization transfer contrast. Radiology 184:395–399
2. Marchal G, Bosmans H, Van Fraeyenhoven L, et al (1990) Intracranial vascular lesions: optimization and clinical evaluation of three-dimensional time-of-flight MR angiography. Radiology 175:443–448
3. Ross JS, Masaryk TJ, Modic MT, et al (1990) Intracranial aneurysms: evaluation by MR angiography. AJNR 11:449–456
4. Creasy JL, Price RR, Presbrey T, et al (1990) Gadolinium-enhanced MR angiography. Radiology 175:280–283
5. Kadota T, Kuriyama K, Inoue E, et al (1993) MR angiography of meningioma. Magn Reson Imaging 11:473–483

Phase-contrast MR angiography in the diagnosis and follow-up of cerebral sinus and venous thrombosis

E. Keller[1], S. Lessmann[1], J. Gieseke[2], L. Solymosi[1]

[1] Division of Neuroradiology, Department of Radiology, University of Bonn, Bonn, Germany
[2] Philips Medical Systems, Bonn, Germany

Abstract. 3D-phase-contrast MR angiography (PCA) was utilised in 58 patients with suspected cerebral sinus (ST) or venous thrombosis. ST was diagnosed in 16 patients, demonstrating both intraluminal thrombus (on T1-weighted gradient-echo images) and the absence of flow (on phase-subtraction images). In a patient with a thrombosis of the cortical veins only (proven by arterial angiography), asymmetry of the cortical veins was visible, without detection of the thrombus. Of the patients with ST 47% presented with a combination of general symptoms, e.g. headache, and focal neurological signs, e.g. motor and/or sensory deficits, whereas 41% only had one or more general symptoms. A semiquantitative analysis of the demonstration of normal vessels showed that the best results were obtained using a velocity sensitivity of 20 cm/s covering the flow range of both small veins and sinuses. However, assessment of cortical veins and basal sinuses (petrosal and cavernous remains difficult, so that arterial angiography should be used as a supplementary measure in such cases.

Key words: Sinus thrombosis – Cerebral venous thrombosis – Magnetic resonance angiography – Phase-contrast angiography

Early diagnosis or exclusion of sinus (ST) or venous thrombosis is clinically very important in determining the optimal treatment and clinical course of patients. Nowadays, MRI [1, 3] and MR angiography (MRA) [4–6] provide noninvasive alternatives to catheter angiography. Improvements of MRA allow 3D-phase-contrast MRA (PCA) of the entire brain in a tolerable time (12–16 min) and limitations of "inflow techniques" can be overcome. The purpose of this study was to evaluate the optimal PCA parameters, to analyse the image quality, and to compare the results with clinical findings.

Correspondence to: E. Keller

Patients and methods

Eighty MRA examinations were obtained in 58 patients (mean age: 36 years; range: 0–85 years; 18 male, 40 female). After MRI spin-echo T1-weighted sagittal, axial, and T2-weighted axial, 3D-PCA was performed in a coronal view with flied of view 210–230 mm, 110–150 slices, 3/-1.5 mm slice thickness, 205×256 matrix in 12–16 min using a velocity sensitivity (VS) of 30 cm/s (n=28), 10–15 cm/s (n=16) on a 0.5 T (n=68) and 1.5 T (n=12) system. Eleven patients underwent follow-up examinations. The criteria of ST included visualisation of the thrombus in MRA and absence of flow in MRA (Fig. 1). The image quality of normal vessels was analysed semiquantitatively with a four-point rating score comparing three different VS values: 0: not visible; 1: vessel identified but discontinuous, artefacts present; 2: vessel continuous, slight artefact; 3: vessel clearly seen, no artefacts.

Results

The patients with suspected thrombosis presented with eigher general symptoms (GS: headache 50%, papilloedema 28%, changes of consciousness 28%, vomiting 22%) and/or focal neurological signs (FS: motor and/or sensory deficit 45%, dysphasia 16%, seizures 12%). In 16 patients, ST was diagnosed to be located in the lateral sinus (LS) in 53%, the superior sagittal sinus (SSS) in 18%, in SSS + LS in 12% and in SS + LS + straight sinus in 12%. One patient had a thrombosis of the cortical veins only (proven by angiography) with parasagittal oedema MRI and an asymmetry of the bridging veins MRA. The thrombus itself was not visible. In patients with thrombosis, the combination of GS and FS was the most frequent clinical presentation (47%); 24% had one GS, 17% two or more GS and 12% one FS. After heparin treatment, the clinical outcome varied between a complete

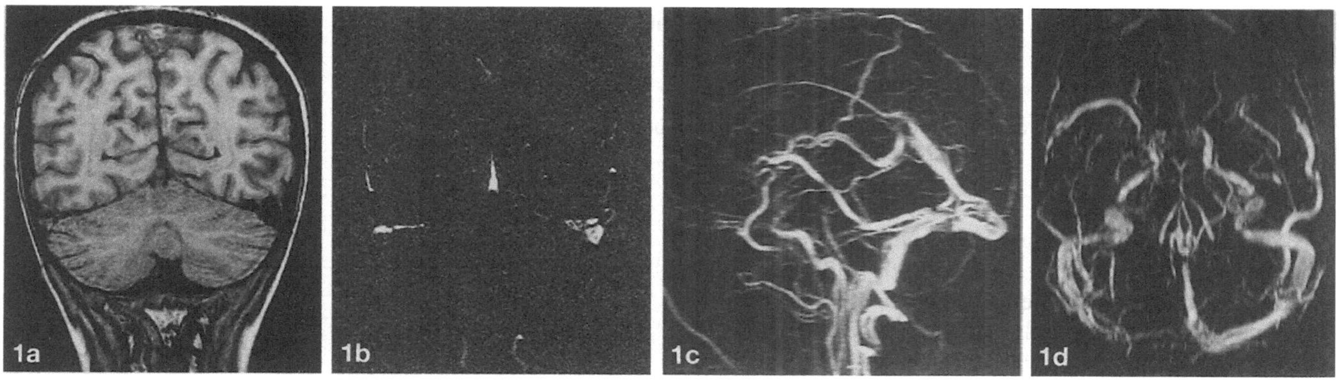

Fig. 1 a–d. 14-year-old patient with acute leukaemia, who developed thrombosis of the superior sagittal (SSS) and right lateral sinus (LS). **a** Iso- to hyperintentense thrombus in the SSS and isointense thrombus in the lower part of the right LS on T1-weighted gradient-echo images. **b** Absence of flow on the corresponding phase-subtraction images. **c** Sagittal maximum-intensity projection (MIP) shows the extent of SSS thrombosis. **d** Axial MIP of the LS demonstrates expansion of thrombus into the right LS

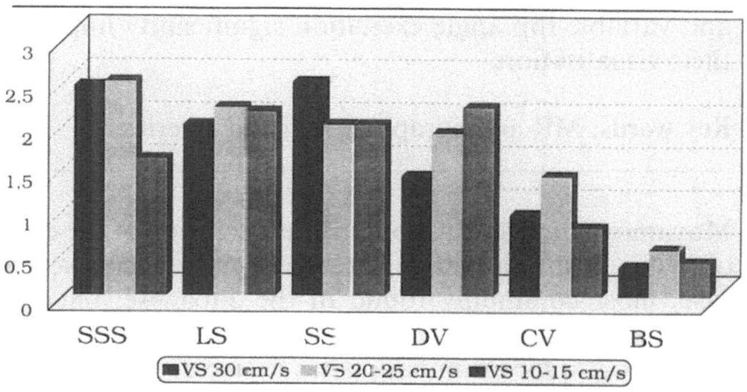

Fig. 2. **a** Depiction of normal vessels **b**Semiquantitative analysis of visibility of veins. *SSS*, superior sagittal sinus; *LS*, lateral sinus; *SS*, straight sinus; *DV*, deep cerebral veins; *CV*, cortical veins; *BS*, basal sinuses (petrosal/cavernous); *VS*, velocity sensitivity

recovery (41%), and minimal (35%) or severe (24%) neurological deficits. No patient died. Eight patients showed haemorrhages and 7 had neurological deficits. The degree of recanalisation was assessed by MRA, detecting a complete ($n = 4$), partial ($n = 4$) or no ($n = 3$) restitution of flow. In 40 patients with normal vessels, the image quality was analysed semiquantitatively. The results are demonstrated in Fig. 2.

Discussion

Initially, patients with cerebral thrombosis often present with unspecific, general symptoms due to the intracerebral hypertension. In the clinical course, additional focal neurological signs may appear and persist. In order to apply optimal anticoagulation therapy, early diagnosis is necessary and MRI/MRA is the noninvasive method of choice for detection of ST and perenchymal lesions. In particular, 3D-PCA provides optimal information about sinus patency and is superior to "inflow techniques". Two image sets (T1-weighted gradient-echo and phase-subtraction images) allow reliable differentiation between thrombosis and flow, and saturation effects cannot occur due to velocity sensitivity in all directions. However, PCA requires an optimal velocity range set by the VS value to prevent aliasing artifacts. In our study, a VS of 20 cm/s was best to cover the flow range of both small veins and sinuses. However, the assessment of cortical veins and basal sinuses (superior inferior petrous and cavernous sinus) remains difficult due to anatomical variations, limitations in spatial resolution and a lack of dynamic information given by angiography. Therefore in such cases arterial angiography should be used as a supplementary method to reach a final diagnosis.

References

1. McMurdy SK, Brant-Zawadzki M, Bradley WG, Chang GY, Berg BO (1986) Dural sinus thrombosis: study using intermediate field strength MR imaging. Radiology 161:83–86
2. Macchi PJ, Grossmann RI, Gomori JM, Goldberg HI, Zimmermann RA, Bilaniuk LT (1986) High field MR imaging of cerebral venous thrombosis. J Comp Assist Tomogr 10:10–15
3. Sze G, Simmons B, Krol G, Walker R, Zimmerman RD, Deck MD (1988) Dural sinus thrombosis: verification with spin echo techniques. AJNR 9:679–686
4. Pernicone JR, Siebert JE, Potchen EJ, Pera A, Dumoulin CL, Souza SP (1990) Three-dimensional phase contrast MR angiography in the head and neck: preliminary report. AJNR 11:457–466
5. Mattle HP, Wentz KU, Edelman RR, Wallner B, et al (1991) Cerebral venography with MR. Radiology 178:453–458
6. Vogl TJ, Bergmann CU, Villringer A, Einhäupl KM, Balzer JO, Steinhoff H, Felix R (1993) Venous MR angiography for the primary diagnosis and follow-up of sinus venous thrombosis. The correlation with the clinical picture and DSA. RöFo 159:78–85

MR angiography of moyamoya disease

A. Mizushima[1], K. Hasuo[1], S. Matsumoto[1], K. Masuda[1], T. Matsushima[2], M. Fukui[2]

[1] Department of Radiology, Kyushu University, 3-1-1 Maidashi, Fukuoka 812, Japan
[2] Department of Neurosurgery, Kyushu University, Fukuoka, Japan

Abstract. MR angiography findings in 33 patients with moyamoya disease were compared with findings of conventional angiography. Steno-occlusive changes tend to be overestimated by three-dimensional time-of-flight (3D-TOF) on lower magnetic field units, but with newer 1.5 T units, 3D-TOF findings compare favourably with angiography. Moyamoya vessels are usually inadequately visualised on 3F-TOF, even at 1.-5 T. Magnitisation transfer and variable flip angle excitation significantly improved their visualisation.

Key words: MR angiography – Carotid arteries

Moyamoya disease, or spontaneous occlusion of the circle of Willis, is an idiopathic cerebrovascular occlusive disease, most commonly found in the Japanese, but also reported in other Asian and Western countries.

Angiographic examination has been essential for diagnosis [1]. The diagnostic criteria consist of bilateral stenoses or occlusion, primarily involving the supraclinoid portions of the internal carotid arteries, extending to the proximal portions of the anterior and middle cerebral arteries and parenchymal, leptomeningeal and transdural collateral formation, most often seen in the basal ganglia, so-called moyamoya vessels (MMV).

The objective of this study was to determine the clinical value of MRA in the diagnosis of moyamoya disease, regarding the two major angiographic criteria and to determine if can be diagnosed without conventional angiography.

Patients and methods

Thirty-three patients (11 males and 22 females, 1–53 years) with angiographically proven moyamoya disease, underwent a total of 83 MRA studies. Most of the patients presented with ischaemic symptoms or seizures, but 2 asymptomatic patients were found in the family study, using MRA.

Three MRI units were used from different manufacturers at different magnetic field strengths (1.5, 1.0, 0.5 T). MRA findings were compared with conventional angiography, performed within 1 month of MRA. Postperative sides of 12 patients were excluded. Several different scanning methods were employed (Table 1). All the patients had 3D-time-of-flight (3D-TOF) MRA without gadolinium. Other scanning methods were used for better visualisation of MMV. These included 2D-TOF, contrast-enhanced 3D-TOF, 3D-TOF with magnetisation transfer and variable flip angle excitation (ramped RF) at 1.5 T, rephase-dephase subtraction at 1.0 T, and 3D phase contrast at 0.5 T. Steno-occlusive changes on both angiography and MRA (3D-TOF) were graded according to the grading of Satoh et al. (Table 2) [2]. MMV in the basal ganglia were also graded in five stages (Table 3).

Correspondence to: A. Mizushima

Table 1. Imaging methods

Field strength (T)	Method	Examinations
1.5	3D-TOF	25
1.5	2D-TOF	11
1.5	3D-TOF with Gd	6
1.5	3D-TOF with MTR	8
1.0	3D-TOF	10
1.0	3D-SUB	10
0.5	3D-TOF	7
0.5	3D-PC	6
	Total	83

TOF, time-of-flight; MTR, magnetisation transfer and ramped radiofrequency; SUB, rephase-dephase subtraction; PC, phase contrast

Table 2. Grading of stenosis or occlusion

1. Slight to moderate stenosis internal carotid artery (ICA), lumen < 10%
2. Severe stenosis of ICA, lumen < 10%
3. Occlusion of anterior (ACA) or middle (MCA) cerebral artery
4. Occlusion of ICA or MCA + ACA with partial preservation of trunk of ACA or MCA
5. Occlusion of ICA or MCA + ACA; no main trunk of ACA or MCA seen

Table 3. Grading of moyamoya vessels (MMV)

Marked	Prominent MMV throughout basal ganglia
Moderate	Intermediate between marked and mild
Mild	MMV clearly visible but limited to a small portion near ICA bifurcation
Minimal	MMV faintly visible near ICA bifurcation
None	MMV not seen

Results

With 3D-TOF MRA, stenosis or occlusion of the internal carotid arteries and/or proximal anterior and middle cerebral arteries were detected on all the 74 sides (Fig. 1). At 0.5 and 1.0 T, most of the stenotic lesions were overestimated with correct estimates being obtained in only about 20%. Using a newer 1.5 T unit, however, the rate of overestimation was reduced to 27% and correct estimates could be made in 67% (Table 4).

Visualisation of MMV by different methods is shown in Table 5. With lower magnetic field units, detection of MMV by 3D-TOF is quite limited. On most sides, MMV are either not detectable or tend to be grossly underestimated when present. In children, well-developed MMV were only partially visualised.

At a higher magnetic field, MMV were fairly constantly visualised by 3D-TOF in most patients, but were often

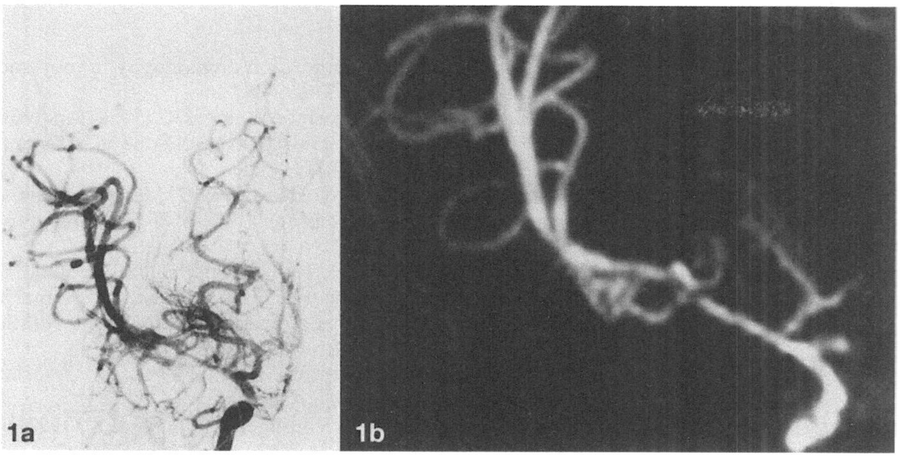

Fig. 1a, b. A 5-year-old boy with moyamoya disease. Moderate stenoses of distal ICA and proximal MCA are seen on both conventional angiography (**a**) and 3D-TOF MRA (**b**)

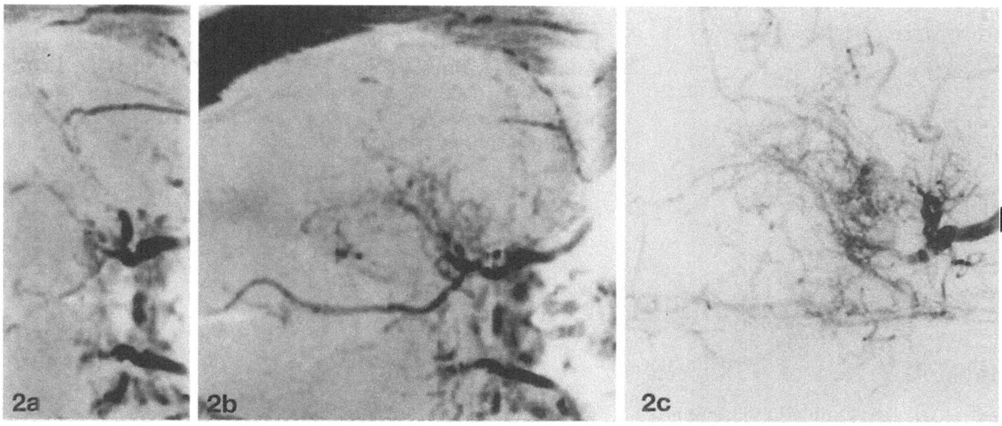

Fig. 2a–c. A 35-year-old woman with previous bypass surgery on the right. Moyamoya vessels on the left are seen only faintly on 3D-TOF (**a**). With magnetisation transfer and ramped RF (**b**), they are much better seen, and correlate well with angiography (**c**)

Table 4. Estimation of stenosis or occlusion by 3D-TOF

Field strength (T)	Sides	Under-estimation (%)	Correct (%)	Over-estimation (%)
1.5	40	2 (5)	27 (68)	11 (27)
1.0	20	0	4 (20)	16 (80)
0.5	14	1 (7)	3 (21)	10 (72)

Table 5. Demonstration of moyamoya vessels

Technique	Sides	Correct (%)	Under-estimation (%)	Not seen (%)
3D-TOF (1.5 T)	40	17 (43)	20 (50)	3 (7)
3D-TOF (1.0 T)	20	1 (5)	14 (70)	5 (25)
3D-TOF (0.5 T)	14	0	9 (65)	5 (35)
3D-TOF (1.5 T) Gd	12	8 (67)	3 (25)	1 (8)
3D-TOF (1.5 T) MTR	10	8 (80)	1 (10)	1 (10)
2D-TOF (1.5 T)	17	14 (82)	3 (18)	0
3D-PC (0.5 T)	12	5 (42)	4 (33)	3 (25)
3D-SUB (1.0 T)	20	8 (40)	12 (60)	0

underestimated. With 3D-phase contrast, and rephase-dephase subtraction methods, visualisation of MMV improved but there were still many cases of non-detection and underestimation.

Intravenous gadolinium can help improve visualisation of MMV, but subcutaneous and intracranial venous signals can degrade the images. A combination of magnetisation transfer and ramped RF can help us to visualise MMV without contrast medium or significant increase in venous signal (Fig. 2).

Discussion

3D-TOF MRA showed steno-occlusive changes on all sides. The degree of stenosis was significantly overestimated in our earlier cases with lower field units. Recent higher magnetic field units with advanced velocity compensation are more accurate with less overestimation of stenosis [3–5], and better correlation with angiography. Even mild stenosis can be accurately demonstrated.

MMV are more difficult to visualise because of their small size and relatively slow flow [3]. They are usually underestimated by 3D-TOF, especially at lower magnetic field strengths. Small vessels that are of high signal intensity on partition images are not infrequently obscured after maximum intensity projection [5].

There are several different techniques to improve visualisation of small and low velocity intracranial arteries [6–8] and we used some of these to demonstrate MMV. 2D-TOF and 3D-rephase-dephase subtraction are more sensitive to low velocity vessels in the basal ganglia, but because of poorer resolution and visualisation of intracranial veins, interpretation of images can be difficult. Moreover, these methods cannot be used to assess steno-occlusive changes. 3D-phase contrast can help visualise. MMVs, if the velocity encoding gradient is properly selected, but MMV that are not very prominent on angiography are often not visualised. Intravenous gadolinium helps visualisation of MMV on 3D-TOF, but increased signals from subcutaneous tissue, and intracranial veins often obscure intracranial pathology. TOF with magnetisation transfer and ramped RF is currently considered to be the best choice. This single scanning method can show both stenosis and MMV. The only drawback of this technique is the prolongation of acquisition time by 40% compared with simple 3D-TOF.

References

1. Takahashi M (1980) Magnification angiography in moyamoya disease. Radiology 136:379–386
2. Satoh S, Shibuya H, Matsushita Y, Suzuki S (1988) Analysis of the angiographic findings in cases of childhood moyamoya disease. Neuroradiology 30:111–119
3. Yamada I, Matsushima Y, Suzukiu S (1992) Moyamoya disease: diagnosis with three-dimensional time-of-flight angiography. Radiology 184:773–778
4. Evans AJ, Richardson DB, Tien R, MacFall JR, Hedlund LW, Heinz ER, Boyko O, Sostman HD (1993) Poststenotic signal loss in MR angiography: effects of echo time, flow compensation, and fractional echo. AJNR 14:721–729
5. Tsuruda J, Saloner D, Norman D (1992) Artifacts associated with MR neuroangiography. AJNR 13:1411–1422
6. Seiderer VM, Bauer WM, Villringer A, Einhaupl K (1990) 3D-MR-Angiographie mit Gd-DTPA. ROFO 152:327–332
7. Edelman RR, Ahn SS, Chien D, Li W, Goldmann A, Mantello M, Kramer J, Kleefield J (1992) Improved time-of-flight MR angiography of the brain with magnetization transfer contrast. Radiology 184:395–399
8. Atkinson D, Brant-Zawadzki M, Gillan G, Purdy D, Laub G (1994) Improved MR angiography: magnetization transfer suppression with variable flip angle excitation and increased resolution. Radiology 190:890–894

MR angiography of cerebral vasospasm in primates

H. Kobayashi[1], T. Tsuji[2], M. Kabuto[1], Y. Handa[1], T. Kubota[1]

[1] Department of Neurosurgery, Fukui Medical School, Fukui, Japan
[2] Department of Neurosurgery, Fukui General Hospital, Fukui, Japan

Abstract. Seven Japanese monkeys were used in this study. Magnetic resonance angiography (MRA), using the time-of-flight (TOF) method, was obtained. After control studies of both MRA and conventional angiography, subarachnoid haemorrhage (SAH) was induced on day 0. Angiography was performed again on day 7 to observe the development of cerebral vasospasm. The reactivity of the vessels to acetazolamide was also observed. Spasm was detected on both MRA and conventional angiography on day 7. MRA after acetazolamide showed dramatic enhanced vasodilatation in both control and spastic arteries on day 7, whereas conventional angiography showed no change.

Key words: Acetazolamide – Cerebral vasospasm – Magnetic resonance angiography – Primate – Subarachnoid haemorrhage

The recently developed magnetic resonance angiography (MRA) provides fine anatomical details of the brain and cerebral vasculature noninvasively [1–3]. The purpose of this study in primates was to observe spastic arteries by MRA and to study the reactivity of the vessel to acetazolamide.

Materials and methods

Seven Japanese monkeys were used in this study. Anaesthesia was induced with ketamine i.m. and maintained by sodium pentobarbital i.p. The animals were intubated, and allowed to breathe spontaneously during conventional angiography and MRA. The animals were then paralysed, and ventilated with a Harvard respirator. Subarachnoid haemorrhage (SAH) was then induced as described elsewhere [4]. Angiography was performed again on day 7 to observe the development of vasospasm. The reactivity of the cerebral vessels to acetazolamide was also observed. MRA was performed on a 1.5 T unit. Three-dimensional time-of-flight (TOF) MRA was obtained with the following sequences: repetition time 53 ms, echo time 6.5 ms, 4 excitations, flip angle 30°, 256 × 192 data matrix, field of view 8 cm, and a single 19.6 mm excitation volume divided into 28 0.7-mm-thick portions. Conventional angiography was also performed both on day 0 before SAH and on day 7. The MRA and conventional angiography were both performed twice a day, immediately before and 10 min after administration of acetazolamide 500 mg i.p.

Correspondence to: H. Kobayashi, Department of Neurosurgery, Fukui Medical School, Matsuoka, Fukui 910-11, Japan

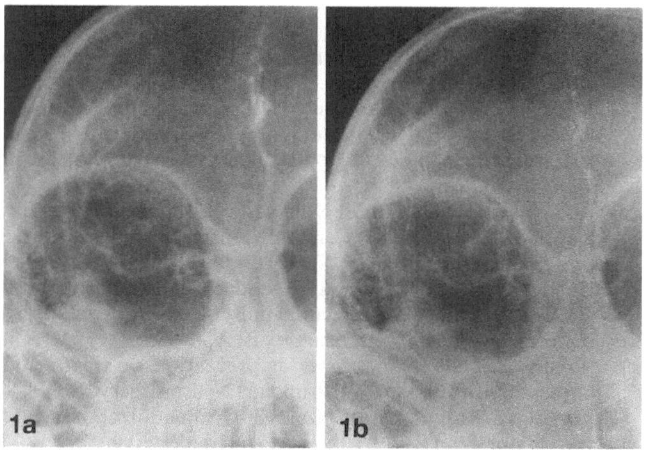

Fig. 1 a, b. Conventional cerebral angiograms (anteroposterior). **a** Baseline injection of right carotid artery. **b** On day 7 after subarachnoid haemorrhage, showing vasospasm

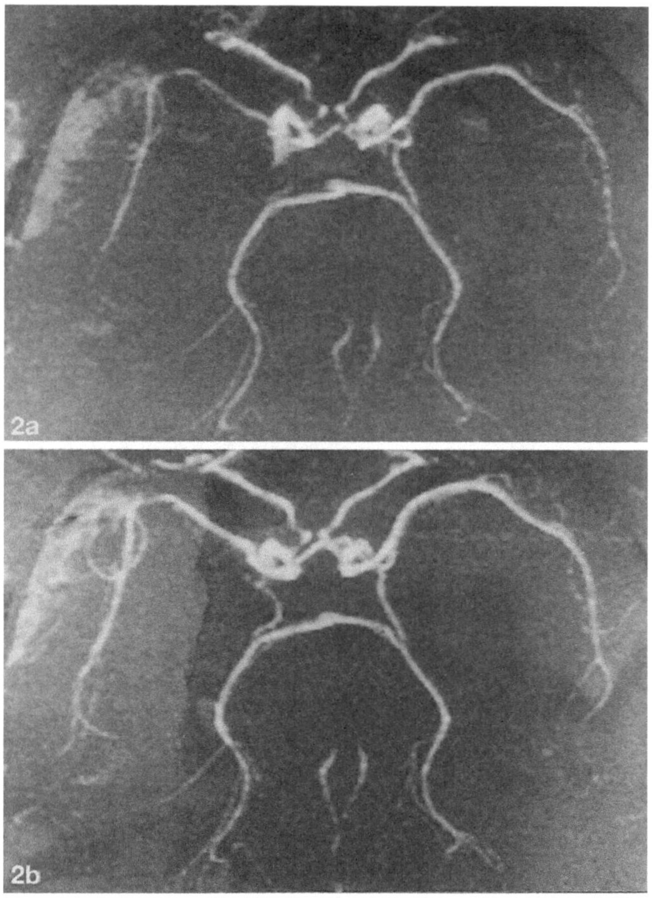

Fig. 2 a, b. Three-dimensional time-of-flight MR angiography on day 7. **a** Before, **b** after acetazolamide administration. The spastic right middle cerebral artery becomes dilated

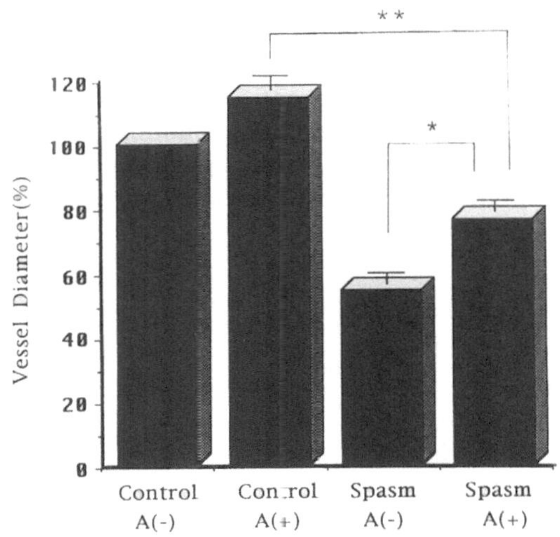

Fig. 3. Diameter of the right middle cerebral artery on MRA. *A(−)* before, *A(+)* after acetazolamide. Significant dilatation of the middle cerebral artery is shown after acetazolamide administration. * $P<0.05$, ** $P<0.01$

Results

There were no significant differences in physiological parameters between day 0 and day 7. The data also showed no significant differences between the results before and after the injection of acetazolamide. All animals had evidence of cerebral vasospasm on both conventional angiography and MRA on day 7, compared with the control angiograms (Figs. 1, 2). the arteries on the clot side were significantly more spastic than those on the other side. The diameter of the right middle cerebral artery (MCA) on TOF MRA decreased to 54% as a result of spasm. Injection of acetazolamide i.p. caused a dramatically enhanced dilatation in both peripheral and proximal spastic arteries. The diameter of the spastic MCA on TOF MRA increased from 54% to 76% after acetazolamide ($P<0.05$) (Fig. 3). Neither control cerebral arteries nor spastic cerebral arteries in the conventional angiograms increased in calibre after i.p. injection of acetazolamide.

Discussion

The pathogenesis of cerebral vasospasm is poorly understood, and it has been hypothesised that several vasoconstrictor substances are putative spasmogens [5–7]. It is generally presumed that ischaemic deficits are caused by reduced blood flow through the narrowed segments of conducting vessels. The diagnostic utility and specificity provided by the use of acetazolamide as a vasodilatatory change were suggested by Vorstrup et al. [8]. Acetazolamide is known to increase cerebral blood flow due to vasodilatation, which occurs through tissue acidosis by inhibition of carbonic anhydrase [8]. The CO_2 reactivity, or acetazolamide effect, occurs primarily in small pial vessels less than 100 μm in diameter. In our study, MRA after acetazolamide showed a dramatically enhanced dilatation of both peripheral and proximal spastic arteries, whereas the conventional angiogram showed no change in the vessel diameters before and after acetazolamide administration. The dramatic apparent dilatation of the spastic artery on MRA after acetazolamide administration was probably secondary to increased signal intensity due to increased blood velocity near the vessel wall.

References

1. Kobayashi H, Hayashi M, Kawano H, Handa Y, Kabuto M, Ishii Y (1989) Magnetic resonance imaging of embolism from intracranial aneurysms. Surg Neurol 32:225–230
2. Lewin JS, Laub G (1991) Intracranial MR angiography: a direct comparison of three time-of-flight techniques. AJNR 12:1133–1139
3. Tsuruda J, Saloner D, Norman D (1992) Artifacts associated with MR neuroangiography. AJNR 13:1411–1422
4. Kobayashi H, Ide H, Aradachi H, Arai Y, Handa Y, Kubota T (1993) Histological studies of intracranial vessels in primates following transluminal angioplasty for vasospasm. J Neurosurg 78:481–486
5. Kobayashi H, Hayashi M, Kobayashi S, Kabuto M, Handa Y, Kawano H, Ide H (1991) Cerebral vasospasm and vasoconstriction caused by endothelin. Neurosurgery 28:673–679
6. Kobayashi H, Ide H, Handa Y, Aradachi H, Arai Y, Kubota T (1992) Effect of leukotriene antagonist on experimental delayed cerebral vasospasm. Neurosurgery 31:550–556
7. Wilkins RH (1987) Attempts at prevention or treatment of intracranial arterial spasm: an update. Neurosurgery 18:808–825
8. Vorstrup S, Brun B, Lassen NA (1986) Evaluation of the cerebral vasodilatory capacity by the acetazolamide test before EC-IC bypass surgery in patients with occlusion of the internal carotid artery. Stroke 17:1291–1298

Detection of delayed cerebral vasospasm by MR angiography

K. Kuwamura[1], M. Saitoh[1], K. Mandai[1], T. Marumoto[1], N. Tamaki[2]

[1] Department of Neurosurgery, Hyogo Prefectural Awaji Hospital, Hyogo, Japan
[2] Department of Neurosurgery, Kobe University, School of Medicine, Kobe, Japan

Abstract. MRA was useful in detecting cerebral vasospasm after subarachnoid haemorrhage. We carried out experiments by performing MRA with a clip placed inside the coil of the imager, and observed neither heat generation nor displacement of the clip.

Key words: Magnetic resonance angiography – Vasospasm – Subarachnoid haemorrhage

In the diagnosis of delayed vasospasm following subarachnoid haemorrhage, conventional angiography is a superb method for delineating morphological changes in blood vessels. However, since angiography is an invasive procedure, single photo emission computed tomography (SPECT) and transcranial Doppler (TCD) are often employed in the assessment of vasospasm. These methods do not provide morphological information directly, and thus the data acquired are unsatisfactory from an anatomical point of view. There have not been many reports concerning the application of magnetic resonance angiographs (MRA) to the diagnosis of cerebral vasospasm. This is presumably due to fears that the strong magnetic field might affect metallic clips or that the metallic clips might generate artefacts. Dujovny et al. [1] reported that the Sugita clip is not affected by a strong magnetic field because it does not contain martensite.

Correspondence to: K. Kuwamura

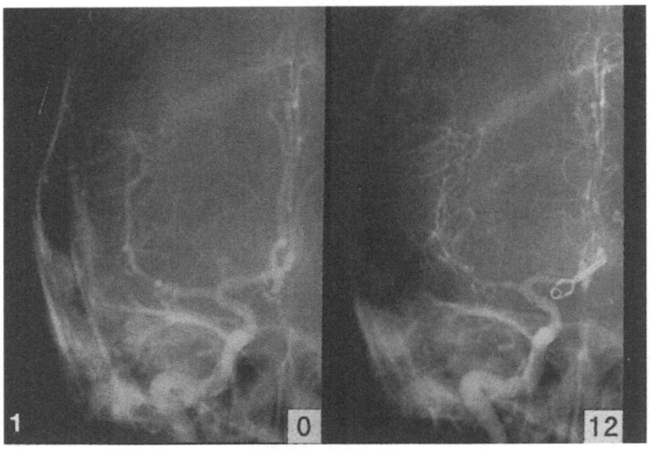

Fig. 1. Case 1. Right carotid angiogram on days 0 and 12. The study shows diffuse vasospasm (compare with day 0)

Methods

We performed a comparative study concerning the relative usefulness of clinical symptoms, cerebral angiography and MRA at 1.5 T in identifying cerebral vasospasm. Most images were obtained using the three-dimensional time-of-flight (3D-TOF) subtraction method. Cerebral angiography (CA) was performed via the femoral artery, before (within 48 h of bleeding) and during (8.9 days on average) the onset of cerebral vasospasm. MRA was performed three times: before, during and after the development of vasospasm. Fourteen of 69 patients with subarachnoid haemorrhage (SAH) underwent both

Table 1. Summary of 14 patients with subarachnoid haemorrhage

Case	Age (years)	Sex	Grade		Site of ruptured AN	Vasospasm		
			H & H	Fisher		Symptomatic	Angiogram	MRA
1	70	F	III	3	Unknown	+	+	+
2	47	M	II	3	Anterior communicating	+	+	+
3	63	F	III	3	Posterior communicating	+	+	+
4	59	F	IV	4	Basilar	+	+	+
5	58	M	III	3	Anterior communicating	+	+	+
6	49	F	II	3	Posterior communicating	+	+	+
7	57	M	IV	3	Internal carotid bifurcation	+	−	−
8	67	F	IV	4	Anterior communicating	+	+	+
9	79	F	III	2	Basilar	−	−	−
10	42	F	III	3	Posterior interior cerebellar	−	−	−
11	50	M	II	2	Middle cerebral	−	+	+
12	44	M	II	3	Anterior communicating	−	−	−
13	72	F	IV	3	Middle cerebral	−	−	−
14	56	F	II	3	Distal anterior cerebral	−	+	+

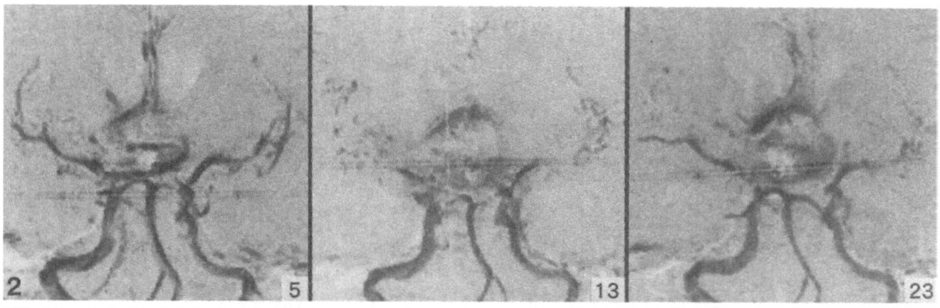

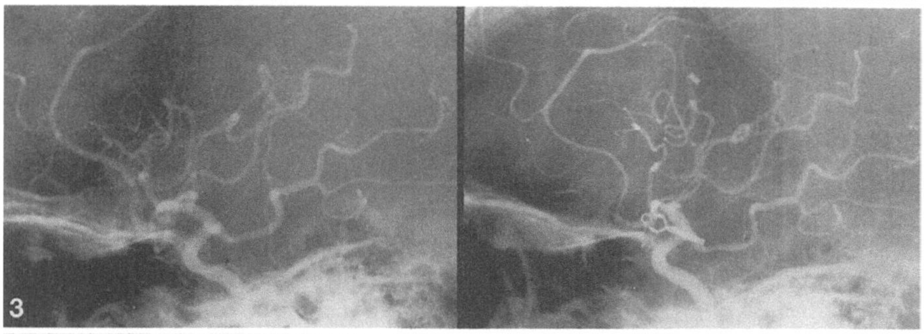

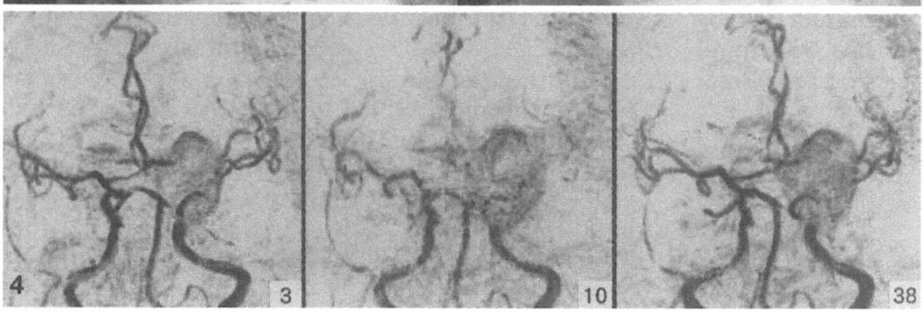

Fig. 2. Case 1. MRA on day 13 shows diffuse spasm in the ACA and MCA territories on both sides

Fig. 3. Case 2. Left carotid angiogram on day 10 shows focal spasm of the A1, A2, M1 and M2 segments comparison with day 0 (*left*)

Fig. 4. Case 2. MRA on day 10 shows spasm of the right A1 and A2 and left A2 and M2 segments. The left A1 and M1 could not be assessed because of artefact caused by an aneurysm clip

CAG and MRA. The findings, with regard to clinical features, CAG and MRA, are listed in Table 1.

Cerebral vasospasm was assessed by comparing cerebral angiograms divided into smaller sections: segments A1 and A2 of the anterior cerebral artery (ACA) and segments M1 and M2 of the middle cerebral artery (MCA) bilaterally. A blood vessel with a diameter of 75% or less than that seen using conventional CAG was judged to have exhibited vasospasm. MRA was also divided into smaller sections for comparison: A1, A2, M1 and M2. On MRA, a blood vessel which was not clearly seen at the time of vasospasm was assumed to exhibit vasospasm. In addition, patients with no evidence of cerebral vasospasm underwent CAG at the presumed time of vasospasm, around day 10. MRA was also performed three times: before, during and after vasospasm.

Results

The compatibilities between the findings of MRA and CAG were 98% in the ACA territory and 91% for the MCA. The territories of 22% of the arteries were not seen on MRA due to artefacts caused by aneurysm clips. However, the total compatibility of MRA and CAG was 94%.

We present two illustrative cases.

Case 1

A 47-year-old man with SAH and an aneurysm on the anterior communicating artery (grade II in the H&H classification and group 3 in the Fisher CT classification). On day 9, the level of consciousness fell to semicomatose. Symptomatic vasospasm was suspected. CAG was performed on day 12, and diffuse vasospasm was seen in the ACA and MCA bilaterally (Fig. 1). MRA (Fig. 2) did not show the A1 and A2 due to artefacts caused by a clip. Inadequate visualisation of A3, M1, M2 and M3 on both sides was confirmed on the examination carried out on day 13. Gradual enhancement of these vessels was observed on day 23.

Case 2

A 49-year-old woman with SAH and a left posterior communicating artery aneurysm (grade II, group 3). Symptomatic vasospasm started from day 5. On day 10, CAG (Fig. 3) showed spasm of the A1, A2, M1 and M2 on the left, and A1 and A2 on the right. Serial MRA (Fig. 4) on days 3, 10 and 38 showed focal spasm of A1 and A2 on the right, and A2 and M2 on the left on day 10.

Discussion

MRA is useful and will become the noninvasive diagnostic tool of choice for detection of vasospasm.

Reference

1. Dujovny M, Kossovsky N (1985) Aneurysm clip motion during magnetic resonance imaging. Neurosurgery 17:543–548

The value of time-of-flight MRA in interventional neuroradiology

A. M. Wang[1], A. N. Shetty[1], F. Y. Tsai[2]

[1] Department of Diagnostic Radiology, William Beaumont Hospital, Royal Oak, 3601 West 13 Mile Road, Royal Oak, MI 48073, USA
[2] Department of Radiology, University of Missouri-Kansas City, School of Medicine, Kansas City, Missouri, USA

Abstract. The clinical value of time-of-flight magnetic resonance was assessed in 16 patients who underwent endovascular treatment for cerebrovascular disease. Because each had a baseline study prior to and a follow-up study after the treatment, the result of the latter could be closely monitored noninvasively. In patients with dural sinus thrombosis, the pretreatment study also provides a guide for planning treatment.

Key words: Cerebrovascular disease – Aneurysm – Arteriovenous fistula – Interventional endovascular treatment – Magnetic resonance angiography

---

Recently, with the improvement of the microcatheter and embolic agents, interventional endovascular embolization procedures for aneurysms and arteriovenous fistulae (AVF) have increased in the past few years [1, 2]. Due to the advancement in neuroimaging techniques, stroke and dural sinus thrombosis can now be reasonably diagnosed early enough to provide an effective interventional thrombolytic treatment [3, 4]. The objectives of this study are: (1) for the embolization technique prior to the treatment to identify the aneurysm and its relationship with the parent vessel, as well as its collateral circulation, and to identify the AVF and its feeding artery and the drainage vein; for thrombolytic treatment to identify the occluded vessels and their relationship to the collateral flow; (2) for the embolization technique after the treatment to determine whether there is residual flow in the parent artery, the aneurysm or AVF, and its collateral circulation; for the thrombolytic technique, to determine the recanalization of the vessels that received thrombolytic treatment. To achieve this goal, a noninvasive alternative is desirable, even though a conventional cerebral angiogram is a gold standard. The preliminary studies indicate the potential utility of time-of-flight (TOF) MR angiography in the untreated [5] and treated aneurysm [6], dural AVF [7] and dural sinus thrombosis [3]. Our initial experience in 16 patients with cerebrovascular disease who underwent interventional endovascular treatment is presented and discussed.

Correspondence to: A. M. Wang

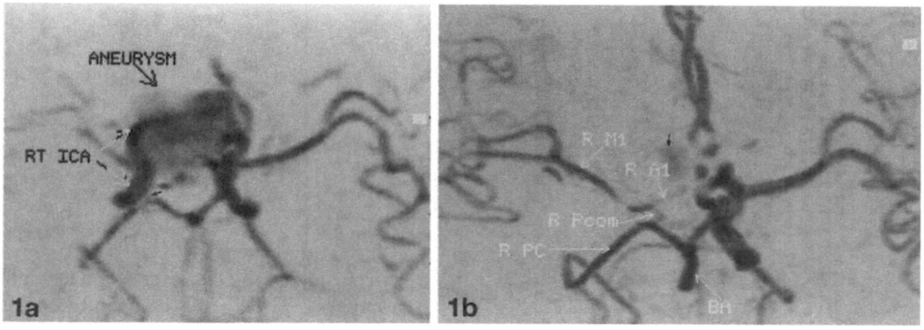

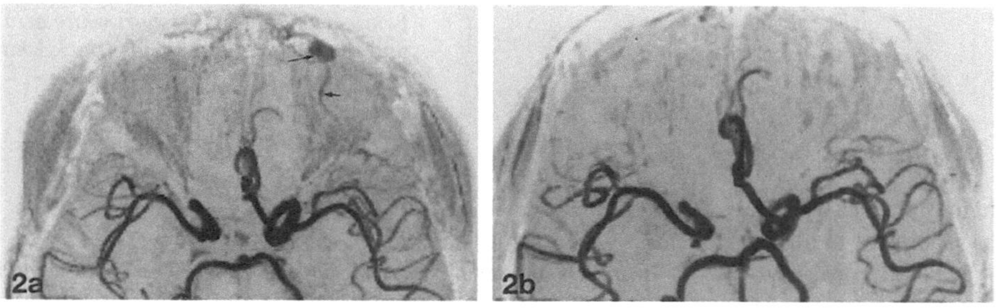

Fig. 1 a, b. A 68-year-old female presented with headache and loss of vision in her left eye. **a** 3D TOF MRA shows a giant aneurysm of the suprachnoid portion of the right internal carotid artery (*RT ICA*). The right posterior communicating artery (*small arrows*) is identified. **b** Three months after balloon occlusion of the aneurysm and the right internal carotid artery, 3D TOF MRA shows occlusion of the aneurysm and the artery with excellent collateral circulation. A small amount of haemorrhage is seen in the aneurysm (*small arrow*). *R*, right; *A1*, anterior; *M1*, middle cerebral artery segments; *Pcom*, posterior communicating artery; *BA*, basilar artery

Fig. 2 a, b. A 38-year-old woman presented with left frontal migraine after a motor vehicle accident. **a** 3D TOF MRA shows an arteriovenous fistula (AVF) between a diploic vein (*arrow*) and the frontal branch of the left superior temporal artery (*short arrow*). **b** One month after endovascular occlusion of the arterial feeder with a platinum coil, 3D TOF MRA shows complete occlusion of the arterial feeder with platinum coil, 3D TOF MRA shows complete occlusion of the AVF. The patient recovered completely, with no more migraine

Patients and methods

Sixteen patients, aged between 4 days and 78 years, were included in this study. Fifteen patients underwent neuroendovascular treatment; one patient was treated at an outside institution. MR studies were performed on a 1.5 T imager. The 3D TOF technique was used for evaluation of cerebral aneurysm or AVF; 2D TOF, along with selective presaturation of arterial flow, was used for evaluation of dural sinus thrombosis. Each patient was studied at least once prior to and once after the treatment.

Results

Giant internal carotid artery aneurysm ($n=3$), carotid cavernous fistula ($n=2$), dural AVF ($n=1$) and dural sinus thrombosis ($n=10$) were found prior to the interventional endovascular treatment. The giant internal carotid artery aneurysms were treated by balloon occlusion of the parent arteries and the aneurysms ($n=3$; one patient was treated at an outside institution). The aneurysms and the parent arteries were occluded with excellent collateral circulation ($n=2$) and demonstrated on 1-month, 3-month, and 6-month follow-up MRI and MRA studies (Fig. 1), and the symptoms were improved. One patient who was treated at an outside institution developed a stroke after the treatment and the follow-up MRI and MRA showed occlusion of the aneurysm and the parent artery as well as ipsilateral middle cerebral artery occlusion and a haemorrhagic infarction. Of two patients with carotid cavernous fistula, one was embolized via the transvenous approach and another patient was embolized via the transarterial approach; both patients' fiustulae were occluded and demonstrated on follow-up MRA and conventional angiographic studies and clinical symptoms were resolved. One patient with traumatic dural AVF was treated by platinum coil embolization through the feeding artery and follow-up MRA showed complete occlusion of the dural AVF (Fig. 2). Ten patients with dural sinus thrombosis were treated with endovascular thrombolytic treatment with urokinase. Follow-up MRA showed complete recanalization ($n=9$) (Fig. 3) and partial recanalization ($n=1$); nine patients recovered completely clinically; one patient did not improve because of a brainstem infarct from the coexisting basilar artery occlusion.

Discussion

Experience in the use of MRA as a diagnostic imaging technique to detect and evaluate cerebral aneurysms, AVF and dural sinus thrombosis has been promising [3, 5, 6]. However, there are not enough data regarding the use of this new diagnostic modality as a noninvasive imaging technique in the evaluation of patients who have under-

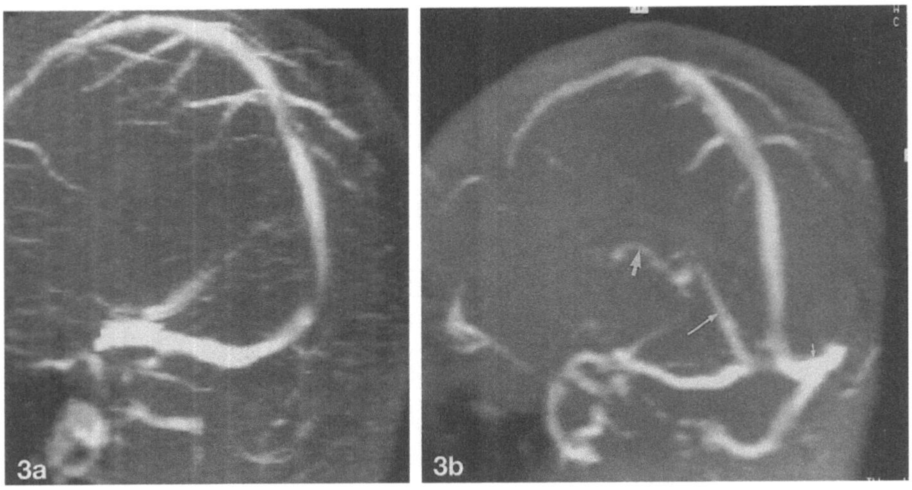

Fig. 3a, b. A 20-year-old woman presenting in coma. **a** 2D TOF MRA shows occlusion of the left lateral and straight sinuses (*LS, SS*) and the deep cerebral veins. **b** 2D TOF MRA 1 week after endovascular thrombosis with urokinase shows recanalization of the SS (*white arrow*), left LS (*short white arrow*) and the deep cerebral veins (*thick white arrow*). The patient recovered completely

gone interventional endovascular treatment. Because the platinum coils and silicon or latex balloon do not produce metallic artifact and the increase of the use of thrombolytic with urokinase, TOF MRA seems to be a very useful noninvasive method for assessing this post-therapy status. The pitfall of using gradient-echo sequences for MRA is the subacute haemorrhage with high signal intensity mimicking patency of the vessel (due to dephasing effect resulting in shortening T1). This can be solved by using a spin-echo pulse sequence in which the hyperintense subacute hemorrhage can be identified or phase-contrast MRA in which only flowing spins in the vessel, resulting in high signal. For monitoring the treatment progress, comparison of the post-treatment TOF MRA with pretreatment TOF MRA is important. In addition, the pretreatment study provides useful information regarding the collateral circulation for embolization and the location of the occluded vessel for thrombolytic treatment.

References

1. Fox AJ, Viñuela F, Pelz DM, et al (1987) Use of detachable balloons for proximal artery occlusion in the treatment of unclippable cerebral aneurysms. J Neurosurg 66:40–46
2. Carasco AE, Aymard A, Gobin P, et al (1993) Selective endovascular treatment of 71 intracranial aneurysms with platinum coils. J Neurosurg 79:3–10
3. Padayachee TS, Bingham JB, Graves MJ, et al (1991) Dural sinus thrombosis: diagnosis and follow-up by magnetic resonance angiography and imaging. Neuroradiology 33:165–167
4. Tsai FY, Higashida RT, Matovich V, Alfieri K (1992) Acute thrombosis of the intracranial dural sinus: direct thrombolytic treatment. AJNR 13:1137–1141
5. Ross J, Masaryk T, Modic M, et al (1990) Intracranial aneurysms: evaluation by MR angiography. AJNR 11:449–456
6. Tsuruda JS, Sevick RJ, Halbach VV (1992) Three dimensional time-of-flight MR angiography in the evaluation of intracranial aneurysms treated by endovascular balloon occlusion. AJNR 13:1129–1136
7. Chen JC, Tsuruda JS, Halbach VV (1992) Suspected dural arteriovenous fistula: results with screening MR angiography in seven patients. Radiology 183:265–281

Low-field 2D-time-of-flight MRA of intracranial and cervical blood vessels as a complementary technique in cerebrovscular ischaemic disease

M. Cellerini, E. Marin, G. Pellicanò, G. Dal Pozzo

Department of Neuroradiology, University of Florence, Florence, Italy

Abstract. We set out to assess the utility of low-field two-dimensional time-of-flight (2D-TOF) MRA of intracranial and cervical blood vessels in patients with conventional MRI findings of cerebrovascular ischaemic disease. We examined 21 patients with stroke syndromes in the acute and subacute phases. Standard MRI cranial examination (spin-echo T1-, spin-density- and T2-weighted images) was followed by a 2D-TOF MRA of intracranial and cervical blood vessels. In 5 patients, a haemodynamic study of the circle of Willis was obtained by means of selective presaturation bands. Cranial MRI showed brain lesions (occlusive infarct, watershed and multifocal leukoencephalopathy). MRA showed findings consistent with steno-occlusion of the internal carotid artery in 14

Correspondence to: M. Cellerini, Sezione Aggregata di Neuroradiologia, Dipartimento di Fisiopatologia Clinica, Università degli Studi di Firenze, Viale Morgagni 85, I-50100 Florence, Italy

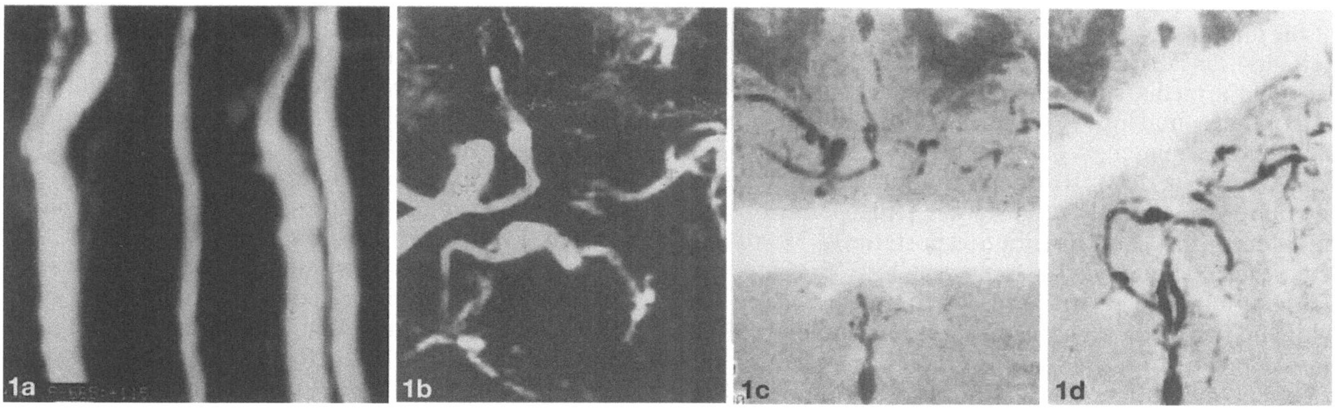

Fig. 1 a–d. Patient with left basal ganglia infarct secondary to internal carotid artery obstruction. 2D-TOF MRA of cervical (**a**) and intracranial (**b**) vessels. Flow signal in left internal carotid artery is interrupted soon after its origin, without distal reconstitution of intravascular signal consistent with obstruction. Axial MRA of circle of Willis with selective presaturation slabs placed on the vertebrobasilar system (**c**) and the right internal carotid system. (**d**) allow demonstration of collateral flow to the compromised territory through the ipsilateral posterior communicating artery

patients, the middle cerebral artery in 4 and the posterior cerebral artery in 1. In 2 patients, MRA was negative. In all but 1 patient, there was a correlation between the side of brain lesions and the side and degree of intravascular signal abnormalities. Selective presaturation of individual vessels of the circle of Willis allowed demonstration of collateral supply to the compromised territory in 3 patients.

Key words: Magnetic resonance imaging – Magnetic resonance angiography – Stroke

Our goal was to assess the role of low-field two-dimensional time-of-flight (2D-TOF) MRA of intracranial and cervical blood vessels in patients with conventional MRI findings consistent with cerebrovascular disease. In particular, we correlated the conspicuity and the distribution of the brain lesions on conventional MRI to the side and degree of the vascular abnormalities shown by MRA.

Patients and methods

The clinical records and imaging studies of 21 patients (12 men, 9 women, mean age 58.8 years) who presented with acute or subacute stroke syndromes were examined retrospectively. Information on the symptoms and their time of onset was obtained from the clinical records. A previous cardiovascular accident was reported in 6 patients. The time between the onset of symptoms nd MRI was less than 48 h in 8 patients (acute phase) and from 3 to 15 days in the remaining patients (subacute phase). All had conventional cranial MRI findings consistent with ischaemic brain lesions (occlusive infarcts, watershed infarcts, multifocal leukoencephalopathy) and underwent MRA of both intracranial and cervical blood vessels.

MRI, and MRA, were performed on a permanent 0.3 T Unit. The standard cranial MRI encompassed spin-echo, sagittal or axial T1-weighted 500/30/2 (repetition time/echo time/excitations) and axial spin-density and T2-weighted (3000–4000/30–110/2) images. On the conventional MRI study, we documented the site, size and characteristics of the cerebrovascular lesions.

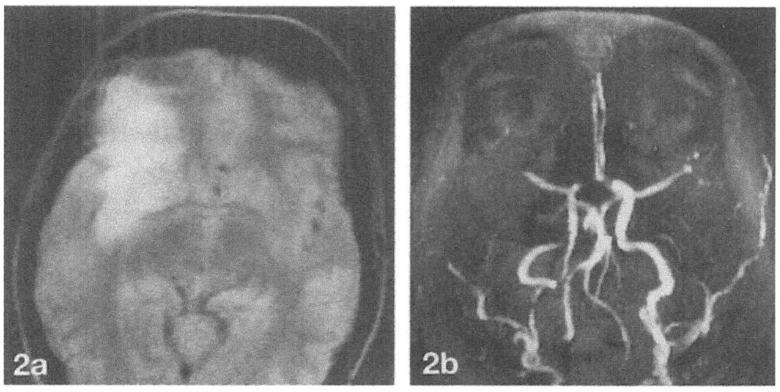

Fig. 2 a, b. Patient with acute occlusive infarct in the territory of the right middle cerebral artery. **a** Large lesion involving cortex and subcortical white matter of the lateral part of the right frontal lobe. **b** 2D-TOF MRA of intracranial vessels. The flow signal in the right middle cerebral artery can be followed only for a short distance. Note absent signal in the distal branches of the right middle cerebral artery in comparison to contralateral vessel

In all patients, MRI was followed by a 2D-TOF MRA of intracranial and cervical blood vessels. The MRA parameters included: 30–60/10/1, 60°–90° flip angle, 256 × 192 matrix, 19–23 cm field of view, 2 mm slice thickness with a 0.5 mm overlap. First moment flow compensation was always employed. The application of presaturation pulses for selective arterial imaging extended the minimum TR to 60 ms. Acquisition time ranged from 8 to 15 min for each MRA. Both axial source and projection (MIP) images were reviewed: the vessels were classified as normal, stenotic or occluded on the basis of the MRA. A focal signal attenuation greater than 50% of the lumen diameter, or a signal void with distal reconstitution of intravascular signal, was considered a stenotic lesion. In the absence of a distal reconstitution of intravascular signal, the lesion was interpreted as an occlusion. The vascular distribution of cerebral lesions as depicted by MRI was compared with MRA.

In 5 patients, presaturation of individual vessels of the circle of Willis was obtained to determine direction of blood flow and the origin of possible collateral circulation to the ischaemic areas.

Results

MRI showed findings consistent with cerebral occlusive infarcts in 16 patients, watershed infarcts in 2 and multifocal leukoencephalopathy in 3. The distribution of occlusive infarcts was as follows: cortico-subcortical areas of the lateral aspect of the frontal and temporal lobes (10 patients), basal ganglia (3 patients), cortico-subcortical areas of the medial surface of the occipital lobe (2 patients) and of the frontal lobe (1 patient). Watershed lesions were in the white matter of parasagittal areas in the border-zones between the anterior and middle cerebral artery distribution anteriorly, and between the posterior and middle cerebral artery distribution posteriorly. Multifocal leukoencephalopathy was unilateral in 2 patients and bilateral in 1 patient with a prevalence of lesions in the white matter of the right hemisphere. On standard MRI, flow in one carotid siphon was not seen in 9 cases.

In patients with occlusive infarcts, MRA showed flow signal consistent with high-grade stenosis and/or obstruction at the origin of the ipsilateral internal carotid artery (9 patients), middle cerebral artery (4) and posterior cerebral artery (1). In 2 patients with infarcts in the territory of the anterior and posterior cerebral arteries respectively, MRA was normal. In patients with watershed infarcts and multifocal leukoencephalopathy, MRA showed abnormalities at the carotid bifurcation consistent with mild to high-grade narrowing. In all cases but one there was a correlation between the side of major brain lesions and the side and degree of abnormalities on MRA.

MRA with presaturation bands for selective arterial imaging allowed demonstration of collateral flow through the circle of Willis in 3 patients with infarcts in the distribution of the middle cerebral artery and ipsilateral internal carotid artery obstruction.

Discussion

MRA is a relatively new, noninvasive vascular imaging technique whose utility for showing carotid bifurcation disease has been demonstrated [1–3]. Furthermore, excellent correlation with conventional angiography has also been demonstrated for the diagnosis of intracranial vascular occlusion [1]. However, these data were obtained on middle to high-field MRI systems. Up to now, limited experience is available on the clinical efficacy of low-field MRA of intracranial and cervical vessels in patients with cerebrovascular disease [4].

Sequential acquisition of 2D data sets with TOF MRA employing first-order flow compensated gradient-echo pulse sequences, thin-slice excitation and presaturation pulses for selective arterial imaging proved adequate for obtaining clinically useful vascular images on a low-field MR systems. However, some pitfalls can occur in the interpretation of MRA. One of the major problems was focal signal loss caused by complex flow phenomena: reduction of the echo delay to the minimum available (10 ms) was unable to eliminate completely phase shift and turbulent dephasing effects that contributed significantly to intravascular signal loss. Furthermore, visualisation of distal branch vessels with low-field MRA is usually poor. This artefact may be overcome by refinement of pulse sequences providing a better signal contrast resolution between flowing and stationary spins.

Although in 9 patients internal carotid artery steno-occlusion could be suspected on standard MRI alone, MRA provided additional information that could not be derived from the standard MR images. In our series, MRA proved to be particularly useful for defining the real extent and degree of steno-occlusive disease; demonstrating patency in dubious or suspected vascular occlusion; and revealing a branch (e.g. middle cerebral artery) rather than a major vessel occlusion (e.g. internal carotid artery) suggested by MRI and vice versa. The high correlation between the distribution of the ischaemic lesions, as depicted by standard MRI, and the vascular abnormalities demonstrated by MRA may be considered a reliable sign that MRA, even at low field strength, can demonstrate the possible cause of the stroke especially in the acute phase. Moreover, in some patients with internal carotid occlusion, MRA was able to define a pattern of collateral flow to the damaged territory. Selective MRA at the level of the circle of Willis, by means of presaturation pulse technique [5], proved to be particularly useful in demonstrating collateral flow through anterior and/or posterior communicating arteries in case of internal carotid occlusion.

References

1. Heiserman JE, Drayer BP, Keller PJ, Fram EK (1992) Intracranial vascular stenosis and occlusion: evaluation with three-dimensional time-of-flight MR angiography. Radiology 185:667–673
2. Masaryk TJ, Modic MT, Ruggieri PM, et al (1989) Three-dimensional (volume) gradient-echo-imaging of the carotid bifurcation: preliminary clinical experience. Radiology 171:801–806
3. Ross JS, Masaryk TJ, Modic MT, Ruggieri PM, Haacke EM, Selman WR (1990) Intracranial aneurysms: evaluation with MR angiography. AJNR 11:449–456
4. Pavone P, Marsili L, Catalano G, et al (1992) Carotid arteries: evaluation with low-field-strength MR angiography. Radiology 184:401–404
5. Edelman RR, Mattle HP, O'Reilly GV, et al (1990) Magnetic resonance imaging of flow dynamics in the circle of Willis. Stroke 21:56–65

Clinical utility of synthesised brain surface imaging: surface anatomy scanning and MR angiography

Y. Ogura[1], K. Katada[2], F. Imai[3], Y. Kato[3], H. Sano[3], T. Kanno[3], M. Nomura[1], G. Takeshita[1], S. Koga[1]

[1] Department of Radiology, School of Medicine, Fujita Health University, Fujita, Japan
[2] School of Health Science, Fujita Health University, Fujita, Japan
[3] Department of Neurosurgery, School of Medicine, Fujita Health University, Fujita, Japan

Abstract. An MRI technique permitting direct, noninvasive display of brain surface structures (surface anatomy scanning, SAS) was developed using T2-weighted images. In this study, synthesised SAS, which combines contrast-enhanced MR angiography and SAS, was used to 50 cases, and the detection rate of lesions and preoperative simulation was evaluated. Synthesised SAS enabled detection of more lesions (94%) than SAS alone (52%). Synthesised SAS has the following advantages: noninvasive visualisation of the brain surface structures (sulci, lesions and veins) and skin markers for surgical planning; practical data acquisition and postprocessing times; preoperative assessment of the suitability for a craniotomy; and minimisation of surgical damage to normal brain tissues and veins.

Key words: Surgical planning - Cerebral cortex - Brain surface mapping - Magnetic resonance angiography

Surface anatomy scanning (SAS) is a noninvasive, practical technique that allows direct display of brain surface structures including sulci, gyri, lesions and major supeficial cerebral veins using MRI. The advantage of SAS is that the brain surface can be imaged in relief using cerebrospinal fluid as a physiological contrast medium [1, 2]. We have developed a synthesised SAS technique that combines SAS and contrast-enhanced MR angiography (MRA), and have applied it to stimulate an operative field.

Methods

The position of the lesion was predicted from data of CT, MRI and angiography, and was marked on the patient's scalp. Scalp markings for craniotomy were also placed by neurosurgical residents and marked by placing water-filled plastic tubes along these markings (Fig. 1).

SAS was obtained using SSFP (steady-state free precession) [3]. The standard imaging parameters were: TR/TE 50/40, flip angle (FA) 60°, 2 excitations. MRA was obtained using two-dimensional time-of-flight (2D-TOF) with injection of Gd-DTPA. The parameters for MRA were TR/TE 100/12, FA 80–120° and 1 excitation. The slabs for SAS and MRA contained 7–14 sequential images with a slice thickness of 5 mm [4]. Total examination time was 7–14 min.

Multistep tilted stereograms of SAS and MRA were reconstructed with maximum intensity projection (MIP), and were overlapped. We evaluated the detectability of the lesions, comparing SAS with synthesised SAS, and the simulation for the surgical design, i.e., the suitability of the skin marker for the operative field on synthesised SAS.

Fifty patients were investigated by synthesised SAS, including 17 with metastatic tumours, 15 with meningiomas and 7 with gliomas. Simulations for operative fields using synthesised SAS with skin markers were performed in 45 cases. The imaging direction was parietal in 28 cases, lateral in 12, and posterior in 10.

Correspondence to: Y. Ogura

Results

In 19 of 50 cases, the lesions were obliterated by large mass effect, with poor visualisation of sulci, and poor discrimination between oedema and tumours. In 5 cases, including a granuloma, an arteriovenous malformation (AVM) and a meningioma, the lesions were not detected with SAS, because the lesion had mildly prolonged T2 (Fig. 1b).

In synthesised SAS, the 19 cases that were not distinguishable from surrounding oedema on SAS were identified, owing to the contrast-enhancement of the lesions. The detectability of lesions using synthesised SAS was 94% (47 of 50 cases), which was superior to that of SAS (52%) (Fig. 1c, d). The 3 cases that could not be detected on synthesised SAS were 2 low-grade astrocytomas and an AVM.

The skin marker positions for operative field were evaluated in 45 cases by synthesised SAS. The locations of the skin markers were adequate in 13 cases (29%), and this was confirmed by operation (Fig. 1e). In 29 of 45 cases (64%), the marker positions were inadequate. All cases were corrected by repeated synthesised SAS. In 3 cases, the positions could not be evaluated, because the lesions had poor enhancement.

Discussion

Since the cerebral cortex has finely mapped functional localisation, the identification of the cortical gyri on radiological images is of great clinical importance. In particular, the motor cortex and central gyrus need to be identified in the operative field to achieve damage to them during operations.

In our previous study, SAS was evaluated for its ability to reveal the relative positions of the gyri, sulci, major superficial cerebral veins and cortical and subcortical lesions [1, 2]. SAS provided limited visualisation of the venous structures and lesions. To overcome the problem with SAS, we have now developed synthesised SAS, using contrast-enhanced MRA and combining it with SAS. On synthesised SAS images, it is possible to display all the brain surface structures including gyri, sulci, skin mark-

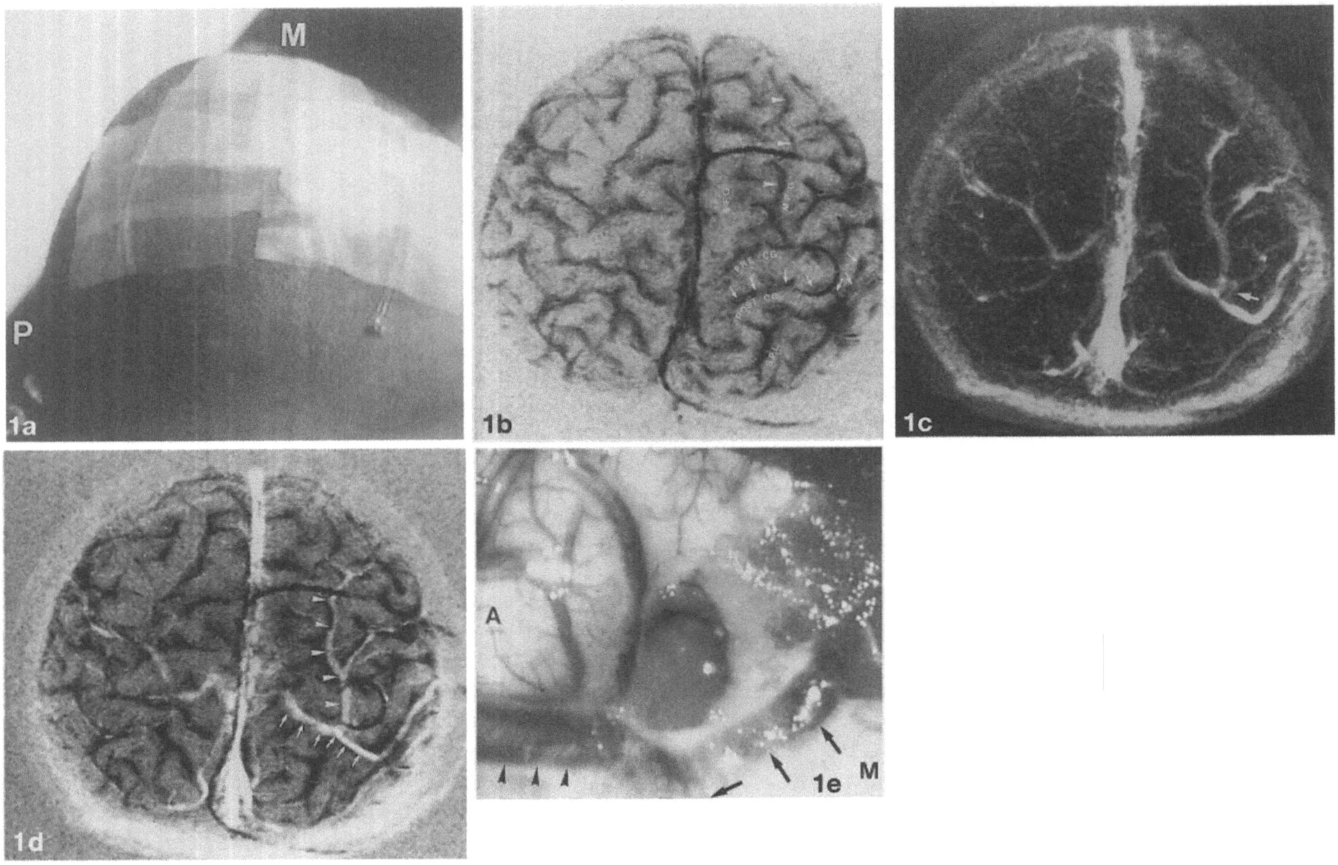

Fig. 1a–e. A 35-year-old man with a granuloma. **a** Skin incision planning: note water-filled plastic tube marker. *M,* medial; *P,* posterior. **b** Surface anatomy scanning (SAS). Important brain surface structures can be observed, including the central sulcus (*arrows*), superior frontal sulcus (*arrowheads*), and skin markings for craniotomy (*square*) and the lesion (*circle*). The latter was not detected because of poor T2 prolongation. *SFG,* superior frontal gyrus; *MFG,* middle frontal gyrus; *PRE CG,* precentral gyrus; *POST CG,* postcentral gyrus; *SPL,* superior parietal lobule. **c** Contrast-enhanced MRA. The enhancing lesion can be detected just under the confluence of superficial veins. **d** Synthesised SAS: surface structures, including sulci, gyri, and veins are displayed on the same images. The lesion lay in the postcentral gyrus. A superficial cerebral vein (*arrows*) was in the postcentral sulcus; another vein (*arrowheads*) in the superior frontal sulcus. **e** Surgical view. The lesion, which could not be identified on the brain surface, was successfully removed through a corticotomy in the postcentral sulcus just behind the confluence of the cortical veins (*arrowheads,* arrows). *A,* anterior; *M,* medial

ings, lesions, and superficial cerebral veins, and to discriminate clearly between subcortical enhanced lesions and surrounding oedema, which had been difficult with SAS alone. In addition, the stereoscopic observation yielded information on the depth of each brain surface structure and allowed precise discrimination of individual brain surface structures. This technique also allows surgeons to check the position for craniotomy before the operation. In addition, because of short scanning time, the position of the skin marker can be corrected by repeated synthesised SAS, if the marker position was inadequate in the previous examination. This helps to minimise the surgical damage due to disorientation in the operative field and the time required for the operation.

Synthesised SAS has the following advantages: noninvasive display of the brain surface structures (sulci, lesions and veins) and skin markers for surgical planning; practical data acquisition and postprocessing times; preoperative evaluation of the suitability for a craniotomy; and minimisation of surgical damage to normal brain tissues and veins.

References

1. Katada K, Takeshita G, Koga S, et al (1987) MR imaging of brain surface structures: surface anatomy scanning (SAS). Radiology [Suppl] 165:303
2. Katada K (1990) MR imaging of brain surface structures: surface anatomy scanning (SAS). Neuroradiology 32:439–448
3. Takane A, Koizumi H (1992) MR imaging of brain surface using steady-state free precession. Magn Reson Med 25:344–348
4. Machida Y, Fujii K, Katada K, et al (1989) Visualisation of brain surface structures with conventional T2-weighted multisection MR images. Radiology [Suppl] 173:355

Vascular

Quantitating blood flow by digital angiography: a gold standard?

G. du Boulay[1], **J. N. H. Brunt**[2], **A. Wallis**[1]

[1] Institute of Neurology, National Hospital, Queen Scare, London WCIN 3DG, England
[2] Clatterbridge Centre for Oncology, Merseyside, England

Abstract. Volume blood flow is measurable from digital data acquired during angiography and can be plotted as it changes throughout a cardiac cycle. The method has now been introduced on a trial basis during some carotid and vertebral studies at the National Hospital, Queen Square. The results, which fall numerically within the range predicted by ^{133}Xe cerebral blood flow methods, reveal patterns consistent with pathological conditions. It is suggested that the method could provide a standard to assist and calibrate ultrasonic flow measurement and magnetic resonance quantitative angiography.

Key words: Digital angiography – Blood flow

Materials and methods

The method has been fully described [1–4]. Calibre of vessels may be measured both by the known magnification factor and densitometrically. Calibre measurements should be corrected by the combined magnification factors previously established for the methods used. A flow curve can then be calculated for the time covered by the captured angiographic series and from this, peak and mean flows for one cardiac cycle are obtainable.

Results

Technical failures, particularly our management of the video recordings, deprived us of usable findings in four cases. The diagnostic categorisation of two patients is doubtful. Two recent cases are not yet fully worked up. The 16 presented in Tables 1 and 2 fall into four main categories. That not all the flow results we wanted were obtainable in every case was sometimes due to the inclusion of too short a length of internal carotid artery in the collimated X-ray window. In others, crossing branches and other sources of noise caused too much uncertainty.

For patients 1 and 5, we have not established the magnification correction factors for calibre. These two results are likely to be slightly understated. Most of the results are consistent with or slightly lower than expectations from ^{133}Xe methods.

Discussion

Normal volumetric cerebral blood flow

133-Xe dilution methods (intra-arterial and inhalation), using biexponential washout curves for fast and slow compartments (mostly grey and mostly white matter) or only recording initial flow, provide measurements biased by the proximity of the detectors to superficial cortical grey matter.

Thus, grey matter flows of 75–113 ml/100 g per min [5] are likely to be accurate, while mean cerebral hemisphere flow of ca. 64 ml/100 g per min is likely to be overestimated.

After correction for both the real proportion of grey and white matter and the distance from the detectors, the true mean hemisphere volumetric blood flow (man, con-

Table 1. Digital quantitative flow measurements in patients

Patient	Clinical signs	Age (years)	Vessel	Mean Calibre (mm)	Flow: ml/min		
					Mean	Peak	Trough
Quasi-normals							
4	Ablated AVM	35	RCC	7.5	119	545	20
			IC	4.8			
7	Proptosis; no intra-cranial pathology		RCC			600–800	35
12	MS; fits; eye pain	47	LCC	7.74	290	600+	
			IC	4.1	184	430	
21	SAH? No pathology	34	LCC	7.7	371	1500	ca.20
			LCC		246	2250	
			IC	4.5	107	400	

AVM, arteriovenous malformation; R, right; CC, common carotid artery; IC, internal carotid artery; MS, multiple sclerosis; L, left; SAH, subarachnoid haemorrhage; V, vertebral artery; ICP, intracranial pressure

Correspondence to: G. du Boulay

Table 2. Digital angiographic flow measurements in patients

Patient	Clinical signs	Age (years)	Vessel	Mean Calibre (mm)	Flow: ml/min Mean	Peak	Trough
Vascular diseases							
1	Cerebral ischaemia; shunted cranio pharyngiom	74	RCC	5 uncorrected	<150	650	
			IC	3	30	70–100	20
3	Carotids occluded?	69	RV	4.7	175	350	0
9	Vertebral stenosis at C6	45	LV	3.2	33	75	20
23	Post-aneurysm clipping	51	LCC	5.8	189	900	0
			IC	5.2			
Arteriovenous malformations							
11	High-flow AVM in thalamus	35	RIC	5.9	404	1300	< 20
14	Largely carotid-supplied, occipital	66	LV	4.4	164	800	< 20
Space-occupying lesions							
2	Sphenoid ridge meningioma	43	RCC	5			0–30
			IC	4.4	95	185	
5	Postoperative cavernoma	22	RCC	6.25 uncorrected	200	750	0
			IC	3.7	100	210	
6	Metastasis raised IC	60	LCC	5.7	250	650	100
10	Cerebral haematoma, obtunded	62	LCC	6.7	118	530	> 20
15	Chordoma	63	RV	4.4	67	170	< 20
22	Probable glioma	37	LCC	7.3	341	1500	ca. 20
			IC	5.9	107	430	0

Table 3. Some ultrasound "flow" measurements from the literature

Ultrasound blood "velocity" and "volumetric flow"

Reference	Method	Site	cm/s	ml/min
[11]	Doppler sonography	IC	Not stated	537
		EC	Not stated	296
		V	Not stated	317
[8]	Doppler sonography	CC	Not stated	444–474
[10]	Transcranial doppler sonography	IC	40[a]	Not stated
Ringelstein (1990)	Transcranial doppler sonography	C1	39	226[b]
		C4	47	355[b]
		C neck	32	378[b]
		V	37	109[b]
[9]	Duplex sonography	MC	102 systolic 50 diastolic	Not stated

[a] Velocities are mean unless otherwise stated
[b] calculated from average calibres
C, IC, EC, CC, carotid, internal, external and common carotid arteries; V, vertebral artery; MC, middle cerebral artery

scious, passive) is likely to lie close to 41 ml/100 g per min [6]. The average adult male and female human brain weight = 1400 g. Therefore, the average total mean brain blood flow (41 × 14) = 574 ml/min. The cross-sectional area of one vertebral artery approximates half of one internal carotid artery. Therefore, expected mean internal carotid artery flow = 191 ml/min (± ca 30%), and expected vertebral artery flow = 96 ml/min (ca 30%).

Ultrasound methods give very different results, as shown in Table 3.[1]

Ultrasound-based volumetric blood flow measurements

Ultrasound-based volumetric blood flow measurements, derived from velocity and calibre measurements, are often unrealistically higher than those attested by 133-Xe and hydrogen-ion electrode studies, and it is recognized [7] that ultrasound "volumetric flow", however clinically useful, is a convention rather than a reading of actuality. Perhaps ultrasound velocity measurements are sometimes biased by the high-speed central arterial stream.

Magnetic resonance angiography

This depends on setting sequence times within an approximately correct range for the velocity of blood within the arteries to be imaged. Ultrasound-derived figures might

[1] Personal calculation, G. du B.

not be the best guide. Good MR angiogram images are, nevertheless, obtained by setting sequences to accommodate velocities for, e.g. the middle cerebral at 50–85 cm/s. If that were really a mean velocity for the whole width of the vessel and the whole cardiac cycle, volumetric flow in the average middle cerebral would be unrealistically high.

An implication of this reasoning is that MR angiography as currently practised may be insensitive to juxtamural and diastolic flow.

Quantitative MR angiography

This may have a role in future, for instance in interventional work. A "gold standard" for calibration of MR measurements is required.

Clinical observations

This pilot study had a rule, notwithstanding the safety of the method, to test only the flow in one neck artery or arterial tree in any patient.

High-flow arteriovenous malformations (AVMs) showed abnormally high mean and peak flows in the neck artery tested, but in them diastolic flow was low.

In patient 3, no patent carotid artery was found. The vertebral artery flow approximated that of one normal carotid.

The lowest vertebral artery flow was in a vessel that exhibited a stenosis at C2 (patient 9).

In patient 2, the sphenoid ridge meningioma was not very vascular and the tumour surrounded the carotid artery. The mean and peak flows were low.

It is noted that high diastolic flows seem to accompany raised intracranial pressure. Indeed, the character of the flow curves may be of considerable interest.

Discussion

This practicable method of obtaining intravascular velocity and volumetric blood flow measurements during angiograms takes 2–4 min for each injected vessel. Currently, analysis of the data takes about 1 h per vessel, but could be greatly accelerated. Software improvements will cut this and improve the quality of information.

It is encouraging to find that the volumetric blood flows measured are in accord with expectations from thoroughly authenticated work using other methods, particularly ^{133}Xe dilution.

The results reflect the clinical conditions of the patients. Ultrasound flow measurement is popular because of its non-invasiveness, but it is not accurate and needs calibration and reassessment.

Our method has many potential uses, not least as a reliable comparison for magnetic resonance blood flow quantitation.

Acknowledgement. We wish to acknowledge with great gratitude the support for this work from John Young's Family Trust.

References

1. Brunt JNH, Boulay GH du, Wallis A, Wicks DAG (1991) Fluid flow measurement in vessels from digital subtraction angiography video recordings. Neuroradiology 33 [Suppl]:456–458
2. Brunt JNH, Hawkes DJ, Seifalian AM, Boulay GH du, Colchester AFC, Wallis A (1992) The measurement of blood flow waveforms X-ray angiography, pts 1,2. Proc Inst Mech Eng 206:73–85; 87–91
3. Colchester ACF, Hawkes DJ, Brunt JNH, Boulay GH du, Wallis A (1986) Pulsatile blood flow measurements with the aid of 3-D reconstruction from dynamic angiographic recordings. In: Bacharach ST (ed) Information processing in medical imaging. Martinus Nijhoff, Dordrecht, pp 247–265
4. Seifalian AM, Hawkes DJ, Colchester AFC, Hobbs KE (1989) A new algorithm for deriving pulsatile blood flow waveforms, tested using simulated dynamic angiographic data. Neuroradiology 31:263–269
5. Wilkinson TMS, Bull JWD, Boulay GH du, Marshall I, Ross J, Russell RW, Symon L (1969) Regional blood flow in the normal cerebral hemisphere. J Neurol Neurosurg Psychiat 32:367–378
6. Munck O, Barenholdt O, Busch (1968) Cerebral blood flow in organic dementia, measured with the xenon-133 desaturation method. Scand J Lab Clin Invest [Suppl] 102
7. Winkler P, Helmke K (1990) Major pitfalls in Doppler investigations with particular reference to the cerebral vascular system. 1. Sources of error, resulting pitfalls and measures to prevent errors. Pediatr Radiol 20:219
8. Matsumoto M, Sekimoto H, Griya Y, Matsumoto M, Tsuchia H, Takasaki M, Takizawa S (1992) Simultaneous cardio-cerebral ultrasonic measurement technique for assessing the interrelationship between cardiac and cerebral circulations in elderly subjects: a preliminary study. Ultrasound Med Biol 18:45–49
9. Schweizer J, Oehmichen F (1992) Erfahrungen bei der Anwendung der farbkodierten intrakraniellen Duplexsonographie. VASA 21:299–302
10. Sorteberg W, Langmoen TA, Lindgaard K-F, Nornes H (1990) Side-to-side differences and day-to-day variations of transcranial Doppler parameters in normal subjects. J Ultrasound Med 9:403–409
11. Yoshimura S, Furuhata H, Suzuki N, et al (1982) Non-invasive and quantitative measurement of volume flow-rate in internal and external carotid and vertebral arteries by ultrasound. J Jpn Coll Angiol 22:191–198

Reperfusion effects on the capillary network: an experimental study

W. Reith[1], M. Forsting[1], L. Klimaschewski[2], S. Heiland[1], J. Weber[1], A. Thron[3], K. Sartor[1]

[1] Departments of Neuroradiology, University of Heidelberg, Heidelberg, Germany
[2] Department of Anatomy, University of Heidelberg, Heidelberg, Germany
[3] Department of Neuroradiology, Rheinisch-Westfälische Technische Hochschule, Aachen, Germany

Abstract. Reperfusion during the early stage of cerebral ischaemia reduces infarct size and would be an ideal treatment for this disease. However, experimental studies on ischaemia of the brain have revealed that a transient of the cerebral circulation is followed by an impaired recirculation. The aim of our study was to correlate microangiography with histological and ultrastructural findings in transient forcal cerebral ischaemia. In 32 male Wistar rats, transient focal cerebral ischaemia was induced by endovascular occlusion of the middle cerebral artery (MCA). Twelve animals underwent perfusion fixation for light and electron microscopy while 20 rats were prepared for microangiography. Microangiograms obtained after 2 h of MCA occlusion, and then 2 or 22 h of reperfusion showed a reduction in the number of capillaries. On light and electron microscopy the endothelial cells appeared markedly swollen, resulting in narrowing of the lumina of the capillaries. In this model of transient ischaemia, reperfusion was only partial and a combination of tissue oedema and endothelial swelling caused blockage of the capillaries. Influenced and worsened by other factors, this might be one of the main problems with thrombolytic therapy.

Key words: Focal ischaemia – Reperfusion – No-reflow phenomenon – Microangiography – Thrombolysis

Reperfusion during the early stage of cerebral ischaemia reduces infarct size [1, 2] and would be an ideal treatment for this disease. Thrombolytic therapy with tissue plasminogen activator leading to recirculation in the territory of the initially occluded vessel has been proven effective in acute myocardial infarction, and thus hopes for salvaging ischaemic brain tissue in the same way have arisen [3, 4]. Clinical pilot studies in acute cerebral ischaemia underline the concept that recanalization is positively correlated with better clinical outcome [5]. Experimental studies have shown that reperfusion can salvage ischaemic tissue [6]. Controversies concern the influence of leucocytes responsible for the postischaemic hypoperfusion [3]. The aim of our study was to correlate microangiographic findings with histological and ultrastructural findings after transient focal cerebral ischaemia.

Correspondence to: W. Reith, Department of Neuroradiology, Kopfklinikum, University of Heidelberg Medical School, Im Neuenheimer Feld 400, D-69120 Heidelberg, Germany

Supported in part by the Deutsche Forschungsgemeinschaft (Ku 294/18-1), Germany

Materials and methods

Focal ischaemia was induced using the suture occlusion model [1]. Reperfusion was achieved by withdrawing the suture after 2 h. Twelve animals underwent perfusion fixation for light and electron microscopy after 2 h of middle cerebral artery (MCA) occlusion, and then 2 or 22 h of reperfusion; 20 were prepared for microangiography at the same time points. Rats were randomly assigned to one of these groups.

For microangiography the rats were transcardially perfused with a mixture of 20% barium sulphate and gelatin; microangiograms were assessed both macroscopically and microscopically. The perfusion-fixed rat brains were investigated by light and electron microscopy. Small tissue blocks were taken from corresponding areas of the frontoparietal cortex and the lateral segment of caudoputamen on both the abnormal and normal side of the brain. Semi-thin (1 μm) and ultra-thin (90 nm) sections were cut with an ultramicrotome and stained with Richardson's solution for light microscopy, and with uranyl acetate in maleate buffer as well as lead citrate for electron microscopy.

Results

In control animals with permanent MCA occlusion, microangiograms were devoid of vessels in the ischaemic area. After 2 h of MCA occlusion and then 2 or 22 h of reperfusion, a rarefaction in capillary density was seen in the nonischaemic, normal perfused hemisphere (Fig. 1). By light microscopy, typical necrotic changes were observed in infarcted areas including shrunken, triangular shaped neurons with intensely stained nuclei as well as swollen and hyperchromatic glial nuclei. Vacuolar degeneration occurred throughout the neuropil. The arterioles and capillaries showed distinct changes in all three groups. The most obvious finding was a marked reduction in the number of intact capillaries in the ischaemic regions (Fig. 2). This was due to a collapse of the vessels, not to any kind of thrombotic occlusion; only very rarely were leukocytes detected in small blood vessels. On the ultrastructural level, endothelial denudation from the basement membrane, signs of endothelial damage with swollen cytoplasm and condensed nuclear chromatin, and smooth muscle cell fragmentation of irregularly shaped arterioles were observed frequently (Fig. 3). Similar endothelial changes as in the arterioles could be found in most collapsed capillaries. In correspondence with microangiographic observations, pial arteries descending into the cortex showed a wide lumen in the upper cortical layer but a narrowed lumen in deeper layers. No morphological changes were noted in the nonischaemic hemisphere.

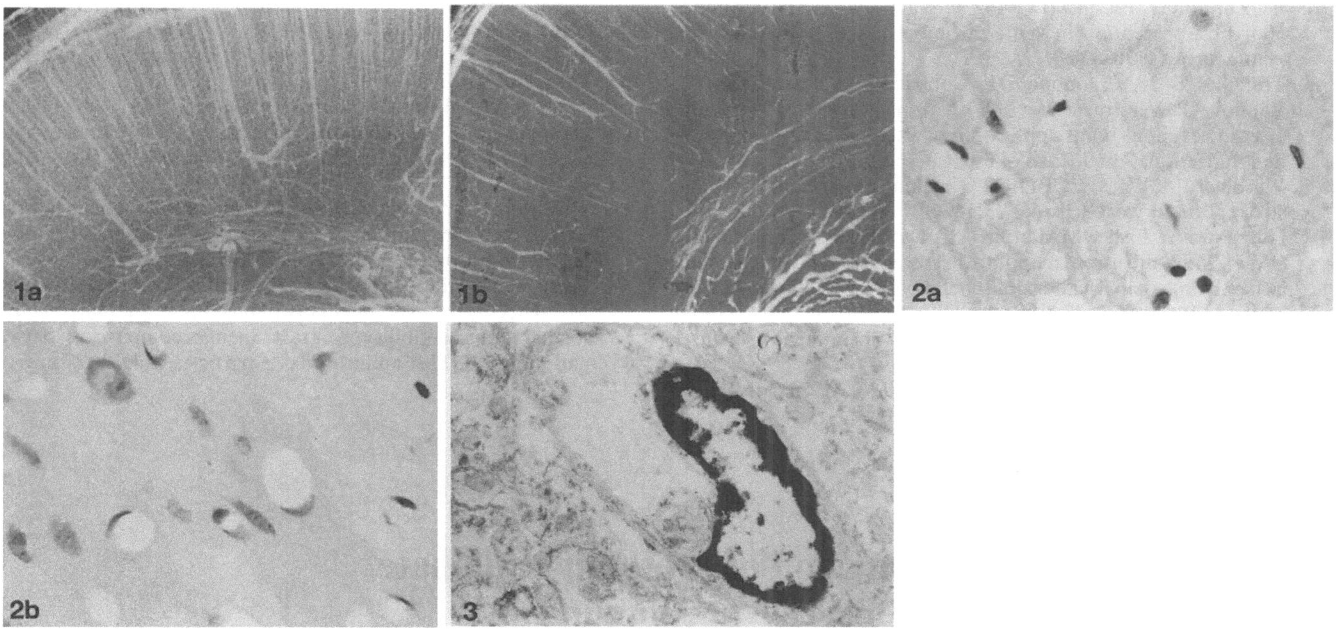

Fig. 1. The frontoparietal cortex of the nonischaemic hemisphere revealed excellent filling fo the arteries, arterioles and the capillaries (**a**) whereas the ischaemic hemisphere showed rarefication of the capillary density in the middle cerebral artery territory with patchy nonfilling (**b**)

Fig. 2. Light microscopic examination showed typical necrotic changes in infarcted areas (**a**) including shrunken, triangular shaped neurons with intensely stained nuclei and swollen, hyperchromatic glial nuclei. Vacuolar degeneration occurred throughout the neuropil. The most obvious finding was a marked reduction of intact capillaries in the ischaemic regions in comparison to the nonischaemic hemisphere (**b**)

Fig. 3. Electron micrograph of a small artery in a rat subjected to 2 h of reperfusion after 2 h of occlusion. Endothelial denudation from the basement membrane, signs of endothelial damage (swollen cytoplasm, condensed nuclear chromatin) and smooth muscle cell fragmentation of irregularly shaped arterioles were frequently observed

Discussion

After recirculation following 2 h of occlusion we observed in microangiograms a rarefaction in capillary density and a marked reduction of infarct capillaries in the ischaemic regions due to a collapse of capillaries. Experimental studies on ischaemia of the brain have revealed that a transient arrest of the cerebral circulation is followed by an impaired recirculation. Ames et al. [7] called this observation "no-reflow phenomenon". The nature of the perfusion defects following focal cerebral ischaemia and reperfusion remains largely undefined. Several explanations exist including endothelial swelling, endothelial luminal membrane tags, perivascular oedema [8–10]. Nishigaya et al. [11], using the same rat stroke model, found that recirculation following ischaemia worsened arterial changes and increased brain oedema; they considered the small arteries in ischaemic lesions to be the major sites from which oedema fluid exuded during recirculation.

Our findings support the hypothesis of the no-reflow phenomenon as a cause of microvascular damage after reperfusion due to a combination of endothelial swelling and perivascular oedema. Knowing the pathophysiology after restortion of blood flow is important for the developmental of novel therapeutic strategies for acute ischaemic stroke. The key findings of our work was that reperfusion occurred only in part and that a combination of tissue oedema and endothelial swelling caused blockage of the smaller capillaries, while the larger arterioles appeared more resistant. We believe the phenomenon of rarefaction of the capillaries to be a mechanical problem, which is caused by the early cytotoxic oedema. Influenced and worsened by other factors, this might be one of the main problems with thrombolytic therapy. Thrombolysis often succeeds in reopening large arteries, but (consistently) fails to reopen the microvasculature. Since plasma reaches the capillaries [12] even if they are blocked by red and white blood cells and cell fragments, a solution of this problem seemed to be to combine thrombolysis with the use of cytoprotective agents, such as calcium channel blockers and radical scavengers. Without therapeutic intervention the rarefaction of capillaries seemed to be irreversible, since no morphological changes were observed after 2 and 22 h of reperfusion, respectively.

References

1. Minematsu K, Fisher M (1992) MK-801 reduces extensive infarction after suture middle cerebral artery occlusion in rats. Neurology
2. Kaplan B, Brint S, Tanabe J, Jacewicz M, Wang XJ, Pulsinelli W (1991) Temporal thresholds for neocortical infarction in rats subjected to reversible focal ischemia. Stroke 22:1032–1039

3. del Zoppo GJ, Pessin MD, Mori E, Hacke W (1991) Thromboebolytic intervention in acute thrombotic and embolic stroke. Semineurol 11:368–384
4. Tranches B Jr, Chamone DF, Cobbaert C, Werf F van de, Vanhove P, Verstraete M (1991) Coronary recanalization rate after intravenous bolus application of alteplase in acute myocardial infarction. Am J Cardiol 68:161–165
5. Wardlaw JM, Warlow CP (1992) Thrombolysis in acute ischemic stroke: does it work? Stroke 23:1826–1839
6. Hasegawa Y, Fisher M, Latour LL, Dardzinski BJ, Sotak CH (1994) MRI diffusion mapping of reversible and irreversible ischemic injury in focal brain ischemia. Neurology (in press)
7. Ames A, Wright RL, Kowada M, Thurston JM, Majno G (1968) Cerebral ischemia. II. The no-reflow phenomenon. Am J Neuropathol 52:437–453
8. Harrison MJG, Sedal L, Arnold J, Russel R (1975) No-reflow phenomenon in the cerebral circulation of the gerbil. J Neurol Neurosurg Psychatry 38:1190–1193
9. Leaf A (1973) Cell swelling: a factor in ischemic tissue injury. Circulation 48:455–458
10. Dietrich WD, Bush R, Yoshida S, Ginsberg MD (1987) Histopathological and hemodynamic consequences of complete versus incomplete ischemia in the rat. J Cereb Blood Flow Metab 7:300–308
11. Nishigaya K, Yoshida Y, Sasuga M, Nukui H, Ooneda G (1991) Effect of recirculation on exacerbation of ischemic vascular lesions in rat brain. Stroke 22:635–642
12. Reith W, Forsting M, Vogler H, Heiland S, Sartor K (1994) Early MR detection of experimentally induced cerebral ischemia using magnetic susceptibility contrast agents: comparison between gadolinium-DTPA and iron oxide particles. AJNR (in press)

Selective intra-arterial infusion of protamine sulphate for transient blood-brain barrier opening in rats

M. Tsuura, T. Terada, K. Nakai, T. Itakura, N.Komai

Department of Neurological Surgery, Wakayama Medical College, bancho-27 Wakayama city, Wakayama, Japan, 640

Abstract. To determine the appropriate dose of protamine sulphate (PS) for blood-brain barrier (BBB) opening and its effect, commercially available 1% PS solution was administered into the internal carotid artery of the rats. The degree of BBB disruption was evaluated as a blue stain in the brain following intravenous injection of 2% Evans's blue solution. Three rats were observed for 1 week after 1 ml of PS infusion to examine neurological signs. The following results were obtained: at least 1.0 ml of PS was necessary for BBB opening in this rat model; 1.0 ml of PS opened the BBB transiently for approximately 60 min and no BBB changes were detected 90 min after PS injection; PS-infused rats did not show any neurological deficits. Intra-arterially infused 1.0 ml PS opened the BBB for approximately 60 min. Superselective intra-arterial infusion of PS may provide a useful method for delivering the chemical agent into the brain.

Key words: Blood-brain barrier – Intra-arterial infusion – Protamine sulphate

Protamine sulphate (PS) has been known to change negative charges of the luminal surface of the endothelium and vascular permeability. To determine the appropriate dose and the effect of PS for blood-brain barrier (BBB) opening, commercially available PS solution was administered into the internal carotid artery (ICA) of rats, and the degree of BBB opening was evaluated.

Correspondence to: M. Tsuura

Materials and methods

Operative procedures

Male Sprague-Dawley rats weighing 250–400 g were anaesthetized with intraperitoneal pentobarbital. A PE-25 tube was inserted into the femoral vein for application of Evans blue (EB) solution. The right external and internal carotid arteries were exposed through a midline neck incision. After a microcatheter was inserted from the external carotid artery to the internal carotid artery for PS injection, the commercially available 1% PS solution was infused through the catheter for 1 min. After a varied time delay, 2 ml/kg of 2% (EB), which binds to serum albumin in vivo, was administered intravenously to evaluate the degree of the BB opening. The rats were sacrified 30 min after EB administration, and the blue stain in the brain was classified into two groups: no BBB opening (–) (no blue stain detected), and BBB opening (blue stain detected in the right middle cerebral artery territory).

Dose of PS for BBB opening

Three different doses of PS solutions (0.35, 0.5 and 1.0 ml) were administered into the ICA of the rats ($n = 5$ in each dose). Thirty minutes after PS infusion, 2% EB (2 ml/kg) was injected through the femoral vein. Sixty minutes following the EB injection, the rats were sacrified and the blue stain in the brain was evaluated. In three rats, 1.0 ml of 0.9% saline was administered instead of PS as a control study, and the BBB opening was evaluated as well.

Period of BBB opening after PS infusion

After the 1.0 ml of PS had been infused, 2% EB was injected, with a varied time delay: immediately after ($n = 3$), 30 min after PS ($n = 4$), 60 min after ($n = 4$), and 90 min after PS infusion ($n = 5$). The rats were sacrified 60 min after EB administration, and the colour of the brain was classified into two groups: BBB opening and no BBB opening.

Changes in neurological signs

In three rats, 1.0 ml of PS solution was infused into the internal carotid artery. Then the catheter was removed and the insertion point of the external carotid artery was ligated. The rats were awakened and kept for 1 week. 1 week after the operation, neurological signs (paresis and activity) were evaluated.

Results

Dose of PS for BBB opening

All the rats in which 0.25 ml or 0.5 ml of PS was infused failed to induce BBB opening in this model. Only 1.0 ml of PS infusion resulted in BBB opening, which was detected as a blue-stained area in the right middle cerebral artery territory. According to these results, at least 1.0 ml of PS solution was necessary for BBB opening in this model, when this commercially available PS solution was used. A saline infusion as a control study did not induce any BBB disruption.

Period of BBB opening after PS infusion

The reversibility of BBB opening caused by 1.0 ml of PS solution was evaluated in this rat model. Both immediately and 30 min after the PS solution was infused, all the rats had blue stain in the right middle cerebral artery territory. When EB solution was administered 60 min after the PS infusion, three out of four rats showed BBB disruption and blue stain was not detected in one of the four rats. However, when EB solution was administered 90 min after PS infusion, no blue stain was detected in any of the five rats. According to these results, 1.0 ml of PS solution probably opened the BBB transiently for approximately 60 min.

Changes in neurological signs after transient BBB opening

All of the three rats that survived for 1 week showed no motor paresis. Although the activity of the rats decreased for 1 or 2 days after the PS infusion, the activity recovered 1 week after the operation.

Discussion

Protamine sulphate (PS) is a polycation and has been known to change negative charges on the endothelial surface and vascular permeability in the various organs [1, 2].

In our results, at least 1.0 ml of PS solution was required to disrupt the local BBB in the rat brain. The effect was transient and continued for approximately 60 min. Accordingly, the appropriate dose of the PS solution can be used to open the local BBB in this model. However, there seem to be some problems in using PS solution to disrupt the BBB, especially in humans. For instance, this dose of PS solution for BBB opening in rats is a considerably large dose per body weight. Maybe a higher concentration of the PS solution is more practical, but highly concentrated solution seems to induce brain oedema in animal experiments and may cause endothelial damage resulting in vascular occlusion [3–5]. Since the PS solution we used did not cause neurological signs 1 week later and induced BBB opening for only a short time, the dose seems to be safe for use, though detailed histological and electrophysiological examinations will be necessary in the future. In addition, if superselective intra-arterial infusions are applied, it will be less dangerous, because the PS solution disrupts only local BBB in the brain and may be smaller in volume.

Apart from BBB disruption due to intra-arterial infusion, many other methods for delivering the chemical agents into the local area of the brain have been developed. Sterotactic injection of the chemical agents, or implantation of the micropellet containing the chemical agents, is one of these methods that may be widely used. However, as the sterotactic approach requires surgical procedures and destroys a part of the brain tissue, superselective intra-arterial delivery of the chemical agent to the local brain tissue may be less invasive and more useful.

References

1. Strausbaugh LJ (1987) Intracarotid infusions of protamine sulfate disrupt the blood-brain barrier of rabbits. Brain Res 409:221–226
2. Vehaskari VM, Chang CT, Stevens JK, Robson AM (1984) The effects of polycations on vascular permeability in the rats. J Clin Invest 73:1053–1061
3. Hardebo JE, Kahrstrom J (1985) Endothelial negative surface charge areas and blood-brain barrier function. Acta Physiol Scand 125:495–499
4. Nagy Z, Peters H, Huttner I (1983) Charge-related alternations of the cerebral endothelium. Lab Invest 49:662–671
5. Westergren I, Johansson BB (1991) Dixyradine, a phenothiazine derivative, can prevent brain oedema induced by intracarotid injection of protamine sulfate. Acta Neurochir (Wien) 113:171–175

Multiplanar MRI of cerebral infarcts along the distribution of the basal perforating arteries

S. Takahashi[1], K. Ishii[1], K. Matsumoto[1], S. Higano[1], N. Kurihara[1], H. Fukasawa[2], K. Sakamoto

[1] Department of Radiology, Tohoku University School of Medicine, Sendai, Japan
[2] Division of Pathology, Research Institute of Brain and Blood Vessels, Akita, Japan

Abstract. Multiplanar magnetic resonance (MR) images of 77 discrete infarcts in the basal grey matter region from 71 patients were reviewed for their distribution and extent, in correlation with the distribution of perforating arteries on cadaver microangiograms. On MRI, the distribution and extent of lesions in the supply area of individual groups of arteries, as determined on axial images, conformed well to the distribution of each group of arteries. This would be expected from the relevant findings on coronal and sagittal microangiograms. Multiplanar MRI enabled precise evaluation of involved vascular territories of cerebral infarcts in the basal grey matter region.

Key words: Magnetic resonance imaging – Basal perforating arteries – Infarction

The basal grey matter is supplied by different groups of perforators (Fig. 1) [1, 2]. This study illustrates multiplanar MRI of infarcts in those regions and correlates their appearances with cerebral angiographic findings of the same patients, where available. We also correlate the extent and location of infarctions on multiplanar MRI with the anatomical distributions of perforating arteries seen on microangiograms of unrelated cadavers.

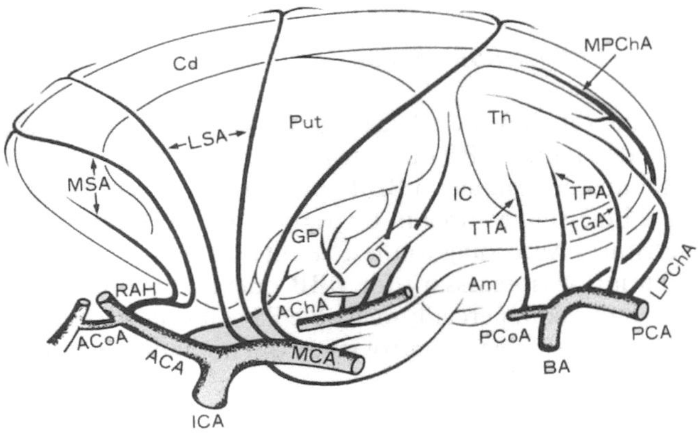

Fig. 1. Diagram of the basal perforating arteries (adapted from [1]). *ACA*, anterior cerebral artery; *AChA*, anterior choroidal artery; *ACoA*, anterior communicating artery; *Am*, amygdala; *BA*, basilar artery; *Cd*, caudate nucleus; *GP*, globus pallidus; *IC*, internal capsule; *ICA*, internal carotid artery; *LPChA*, lateral posterior choroidal artery; *LSA*, lateral striate arteries from middle cerebral artery; *MCA*, middle cerebral artery; *MPChA*, medial posterior choroidal artery; *MSA*, medial striate arteries; *OT*, optic tract; *PCoA*, posterior communicating artery; *PCA*, posterior cerebral artery; *Put*, putamen; *RAH*, recurrent artery of Heubner; *TGA*, thalamogeniculate arteries; *Th*, thalamus; *TPA*, thalamoperforate arteries; *TTA*, thalamotuberal arteries

Materials and methods

Seventy-one patients with 77 discrete infracts in the basal grey matter who had had at least two-plane MRI of the brain were selected. Axial images were obtained in all and were used to determine the precise locations of individual infarcts. MRI was obtained with 1.5 T and 0.5 T MR units.

We assessed the precise location and extent of each infarct, as depicted on coronal and sagittal MRI, to find out whether or not

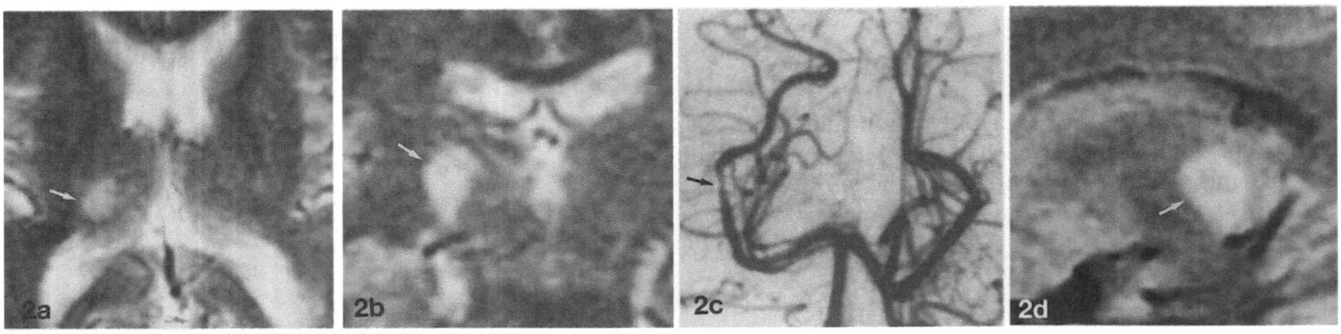

Fig. 2a–d. MRI of a patient with Déjérine-Roussy syndrome, demonstrating an infarct in the region of the right TGA. Axial (**a**) and coronal (**b**) T2-weighted and sagittal proton-density-weighted (**c**) images reveal an infarct in the posterolateral portion of the right thalamus (*arrow*). **d** Vertebral angiogram shows stenosis of the ambient segment of the posterior cerebral artery (*arrow*), from which the TGA originates

Correspondence to: S. Takahashi, Department of Radiology, Tohoku University School of Medicine, 1-1 Seiryomachi, Aoba-ku, Sendai 980, Japan

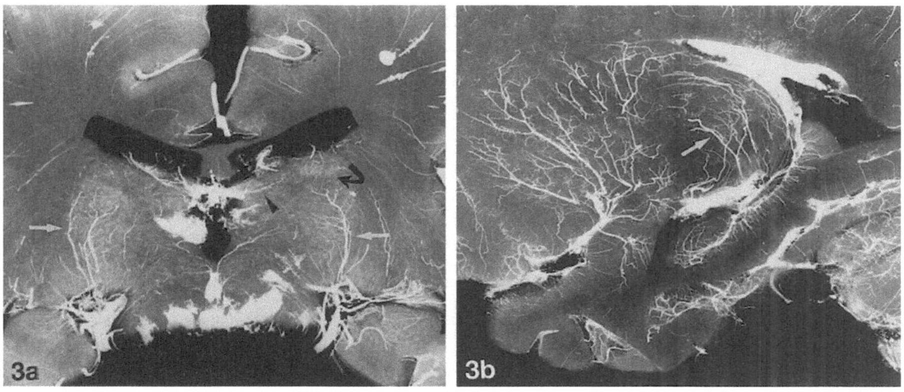

Fig. 3a, b. Microangiograms showing the TGA and choroidal arteries (reprinted from [3]. **a** Coronal microangiogram through the ambient segment of the posterior cerebral artery shows the TGA (*arrows*), entering the brain between medial and lateral geniculate bodies to give a large capillary blush in lateral thalamus. Medial and lateral narrow blushes are caused by the MPChS (*double arrowheads*) and the LPChA *curved arrows,* respectively. **b** Sagittal microangiogram shows the TGA (*arrows*) supplying the lateral thalamus

these findings corresponded to the distribution of the vessels in the coronal and sagittal planes, as determined from multiplanar microangiograms of unrelated cadavers [2, 3]. In addition, the extent of the infarct on the MRI was correlated with the findings on cerebral angiograms obtained in 46 patients.

Results

There were discrepancies in 28 infarcts. The regions of the medial and lateral striate arteries, the anterior choroidal artery, the thalamotuberal, thalamoperforate and thalamogeniculate arteries, the medial and the lateral posterior choroidal arteries were affected in 9, 21, 8, 6, 14, 13, 2 and 4 patients, respectively. The precise location and extent of individual infarcts, seen on coronal and sagittal MRI, conformed well to the distribution of each group of arteries, as determined from coronal and sagittal microangiograms (Figs. 2, 3). From cerebral angiograms obtained from 46 patients with 52 infarcted lesions, angiographic findings were judged to be consistent with the extent of 24 infarcts visualized on MRI.

Discussion

In conclusion, there may be a reciprocal relationship between the sizes of areas supplied by various groups of arteries, depending on the degree of development of individual groups of arteries. However, a general knowledge of the relationship between vessels and deep structures of the brain, as seen on axial, coronal, and sagittal sections, will be helpful in interpreting MRI findings and will aid in conducting a detailed neurological examination in a patient with an infarct in the deep grey matter of the cerebrum. We also believe that this knowledge would aid in the interpretation of cases with intracerebral haemorrhage, arteriovenous malformation, moyamoya disease, and tumours of the basal grey matter of the cerebrum.

References

1. Aitken HF (1928) Diagram of the arterial circulation of the basal ganglia. N Engl J Med 199:1084
2. Takahashi S, Goto G, Fukasawa H, Kawata Y, Uemura K, Suzuki K (1985) Computed tomography of cerebral infarction along the distribution of the basal perforating arteries. 1. Striate arterial group. Radiology 155:107–118
3. Takahashi S, Goto G, Fukasawa H, Kawata Y, Uemura K, Yaguchi K (1985) Computed tomography of cerebral infarction along the distribution of the basal perforating arteries. Thalamic arterial group. Radiology 155:119–130

Gadolinium-DTPA-enhanced MRI in transient cerebral ischaemia: experimental study

S. Nagahiro[1], Y. Ushio[1], M. Sumi[2], M. Takahashi[2]

[1] Department of Neurosurgery, Kumamoto University Medical School, Kumamoto, Japan
[2] Department of Radiology, Kumamoto University Medical School, Kumamoto, Japan

Abstract. The influence of transient ischaemia on cerebrovascular permeability was studied sequentially in rats by magnetic resonance imaging with contrast enhancement using gadolinium-DTPA. Unilateral intraluminal occlusion of the internal carotid and middle cerebral arteries, lasting from 5 min to 5 h, was performed. Parenchymal enhancement of the striatum and the cerebral cortex on the ischaemic side, due to disruption of the blood-brain barrier, was seen in rats subjected to 1–5 h of ischaemia; it was detected earlier in rats subjected to longer periods of ischaemia. Enhancement of the lateral ventricle due to disruption of the blood-cerebrospinal fluid barrier at the choroid plexus and enhancement of the ipsilateral anterior cerebral artery appeared transiently in the early reperfusion stage (6 h and 1 day) in rats subjected to 15 min–5 h of ischaemia.

Key words: Blood-brain barrier – Blood-cerebrospinal fluid barrier – Cerebral ischaemia – Magnetic resonance imaging – Contrast enhancement

The changes in gadolinium-DTPA (Gd-DTPA) enhancement on magnetic resonance imaging (MRI) following transient cerebral ischaemia have not been adequately determined, because clinical studies have included patients with various diseases (thrombosis and embolism), varying degrees of permanent and transient ischaemia, and different time courses of ischaemia. Therefore, we studied a rat model of transient focal ischaemia, using MRI with Gd-DTPA.

Materials and methods

Male Wistar rats weighing 240–270 g were used. We employed the reversible focal ischaemia model of Koizumi et al. [1] and Longa et al. [2]. Unilateral internal carotid and middle cerebral arteries were transiently occluded by inserting a nylon thread into the carotid artery and removing it after intervals ranging from 5 min to 5 h. Contrast-enhanced MRI using a 7.05 T system was performed 6 h, 1 day and 7 days after occlusion. T1-weighted images were obtained, with a 1.2-mm slice thickness at the strial level before and after the administration of Gd-DTPA (0.2 mmol/kg) via the tail vein. At the end of the experiment, the brains were subjected to histological examination.

Correspondence to: S. Nagahiro, 1-1-1 Honjo, Kumamoto 860, Japan

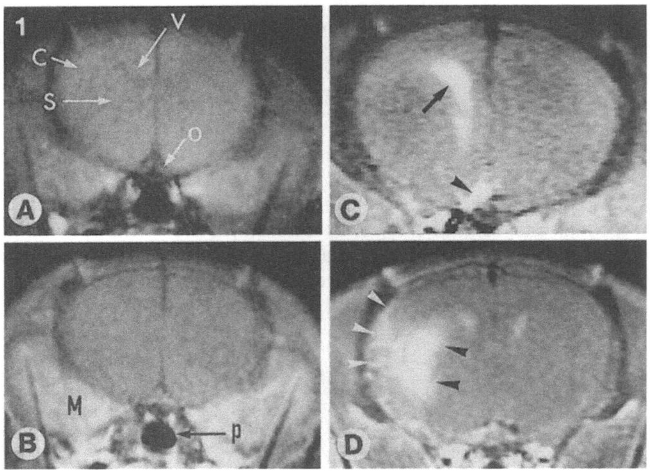

Fig. 1 A–D. T1-weighted coronal images at the level of the striatum before (**A**) and after (**B–D**) intravenous Gd-DTPA. **A** Control rat. *C*, cerebral cortex; *S*, striatum; *V*, lateral ventricle; *O*, optic nerve. **B** Same rat. Intracranial structures do not enhance, but extracranial soft tissues do show enhancement. *M*, Muscle; *P*, pharynx. **C** Image obtained 6 h after ischaemia in a rat subjected to 1 h of ischaemia. The lateral ventricle (*arrow*) and interior frontal region along the anterior cerebral artery (*arrowhead*) enhance on the affected side. **D** Image obtained on day 7 in rat subjected to 3 h of ischaemia, showing parenchymal enhancement in the lateral striatum (*black arrowheads*) and cerebral cortex of the middle cerebral artery territory (*white arrowheads*)

Results

Three patterns of enhancement were observed on the ischaemic side: (1) parenchymal enhancement in the lateral striatum and cortex, (2) enhancement of the lateral ventricle and surrounding areas (venticular enhancement), and (3) enhancement of the frontal base corresponding to the anterior cerebral artery (vascular enhancement) (Fig. 1).

Parenchymal enhancement was seen in the 1- to 5-h ischaemia groups; it was detected earlier in the animals subjected to longer periods of ischaemia (Table 1). Histologically, the urea of parenchymal enhancement showed ischaemic changes, including tissue necrosis and ischaemic neuronal damage accompanied by gliosis, indicative of BBB disruption following ischaemia. In this model, the threshold ischaemic time that did not produce significant BBB disruption on MRI was 30 min.

Ventricular enhancement was seen in the early reperfusion stage in rats subjected to 15 min–5 h of ischaemia (Table 1). Gd-^{14}C-DTPA autoradiograms in rats subjected to 1 h of ischaemia demonstrated accumulation of the

Table 1. Time-course of parenchymal, ventricular, and vascular contrast enhancement on T1-weighted images following transient focal ischaemia

Duration of ischaemia (cases)	Parenchymal enhancement			Ventricular enhancement			Vascular enhancement		
	6 h	Day 1	Day 7	6 h	Day 1	Day 7	6 h	Day 1	Day 7
5 min (5)	0[a]	0	0	0	0	0	0	0	0
15 min (6)	0	0	0	3	0	0	2	0	0
30 min (6)	0	0	0	5	0	0	5	5	0
1 h (6)	0	1	5	6	4	0	5	4	0
2 h (5)	0	5	5	4	3	0	4	5	0
3 h (5)	1	5	5	2	3	0	4	5	0
5 h (4)	4	4	4	2	1	0	4	3	4

[a] Columns show the number of animals with contrast enhancement

tracer in the choroid plexus, the walls of the lateral ventricle, and the surrounding brain tissue on the ischaemic side. This appeared to be due to increased permeability of the blood-cerebrospinal fluid barrier, rather than BBB disruption.

Ventricular enhancement was also seen in the early reperfusion stage (Table 1). Enhancement of the ipsilateral anterior cerebral artery may have been due to intimal injury caused by insertion of the nylon thread.

Discussion

Study of Gd-DTPA-enhanced MRI in a rat model of experimental cerebral ischaemia was useful for the sequential, non-invasive evaluation of the regional dynamic changes in cerebrovascular permeability following ischaemia.

References

1. Koizumi J, Yoshida Y, Nakazawa T, Ooneda G (1986) Experimental studies of ischaemic brain oedema. Jpn J Stroke 8:1–7
2. Longa EZ, Weinstein PR, Carlson S, Cummins R (1989) Reversible middle cerebral artery occlusion without craniectomy in rats. Stroke 20:84–91

Studies of the effect of persistent plasma flow in focal cerebral ischaemia, using different MRI contrast media*

W. Reith[1], S. Heiland[1], M. Forsting[1], H. Vogler[2], K. Sartor[1]

[1] Department of Neuroradiology, University of Heidelberg Medical School, Kopfklinikum, Im Neuenheimer Feld 400, D-69120 Heidelberg, Germany
[2] Department of Contrast Media Research, Schering AG, D-1000 Berlin, Germany

Abstract. Fast magnetic resonance imaging (MRI) techniques, with a bolus application of contrast media, allow us to visualize cerebral perfusion. When using these techniques, normal perfusion is characterized as a sharp signal drop following bolus application of the contrast medium, related to the susceptibility effect. Theoretically, no signal drop should be observed in ischaemic brain regions. However, most published data on dynamic MRI in cerebral ischaemia do show a signal reduction even in ischaemic brain tissue. We wanted to investigate whether this signal reduction was related to the molecular weight of the contrast medium. Using an endovascular occlusion model, focal cerebral ischaemia was induced in ten Wistar rats. As contrast media we used gadolinium-DTPA (Gd-DTPA) and macromolecular superparamegnetic iron particles (SPIO). No signal reduction occurred in the ischaemic hemisphere when using iron oxide particles, but a significant signal reduction of 12% with a significantly delayed mean transit time occurred when using Gd-DTPA. Our observation of partial, delayed signal reduction when using Gd-DTPA might be explained by persistent capillary plasma flow. A second reason might be that small Gd-DTPA molecules are able to pass the capillaries, whereas the macromolecular SPIO particles, like red blood cells, are unable to do so. It remains to be

* Supported in part by the Deutsche Forschungsgemeinschaft (Ku 294/18-1), Germany

Correspondence to: W. Reith

determined for how long after vessel occlusion this kind of residual flow persists and whether it can be used for therapeutic interventions.

Key words: Perfusion imaging - Contrast media - Cerebral ischaemia

Fast susceptibility-weighted magnetic resonance imaging (MRI) techniques, following a bolus administration of paramagnetic or superparamagnetic contrast media, allow us to monitor cerebral perfusion [1]. When using these techniques, normal perfusion is characterized as a sharp signal drop following bolus application of the contrast medium related to the susceptibility effect. Theoretically, no signal drop should be observed in ischaemic brain tissue [2]. We wanted to investigate whether this signal reduction depends on the molecular weight (MW) of the contrast medium.

Materials and methods

Using an endovascular model, focal cerebral ischaemia was induced in ten male Wistar rats. For occlusion of the middle cerebral artery (MCA), the common cerebral artery (CCA) and the external artery (ECA) were exposed through a midline neck incision. The distal CCA and the ECA were first ligated with a 4-0 suture, and a 4-0 monofilament nylon suture (length 40 mm), whose tip had been rounded by heating, was then inserted through an arteriectomy of the common carotid artery (CCA). The suture was gently advanced into the ICA to a point approximately 17 mm distal to the carotid bifurcation. Mild resistance to this advancement indicated that the suture had entered the anterior cerebral artery (ACA), thus occluding the origins of the MCA and the posterior communicating artery. Within 60 min of MCA occlusion, all animals were examined on a 2.0 T experimental MR unit. The contrast-enhanced perfusion MRI studies were performed using a T2-weighted FLASH sequence (TR 25, TE 21 ms, flip angle 20°, acquisition matrix 128 × 256, field of view 10 cm × 10 cm, slice thickness 3 mm, Δt 1.6 s). We used a coronal slice through the optic chiasm. Administration of the contrast medium was begun after the third image. As contrast agents we used gadolinium-DTPA (Gd-DTPA), with a molecular weight of 590 d, and macromolecular superparamagnetic iron oxide particles (SPIO), with a molecular weight of 300000 D. After an IV bolus injection of Gd-DTPA (0.3 mmol/kg), 20 images were acquired within 32 s. This protocol was repeated 5 min later to study the effects of SPIO (0.03 mmol/kg). The signal intensity was quantified by placing regions of interest (ROI) in identical areas of the ischaemic and non-ischaemic hemispheres. This way, the relative concentration of the contrast agent in the brain

$$C_s(t) = -\ln(S(t)/S_0).$$

was calculated, where S_0 is the mean signal intensity in the ROI measured before bolus application. This conversion allowed us to calculate the parameters rrCBV (relative regional cerebral blood volume) and MTT (mean transit time), defined as

$$\text{rrCBV} = \int C_s(t)\,dt$$

and

$$\text{MTT*} = \frac{\int t \cdot C_s(t)\,dt}{\int C_s(t)\,dt}.$$

and calculated by numerical integration. The upper integration limit was set to 16 s after bolus injection to eliminate the effects of the second pass of the bolus, which was observed more than 17 s after bolus injection. Immediately after the MRI examination, the animals were prepared for microangiography. All rats were transcardially perfused with a mixture of 20% barium sulphate and gelatine 8:2 (10). After dehydration and embedding in paraffin, microangiograms were made of each tissue block. Microangiograms were analyzed both macroscopically and microscopically to correlate the areas of perfusion deficits on MRI with the state of the vascular network.

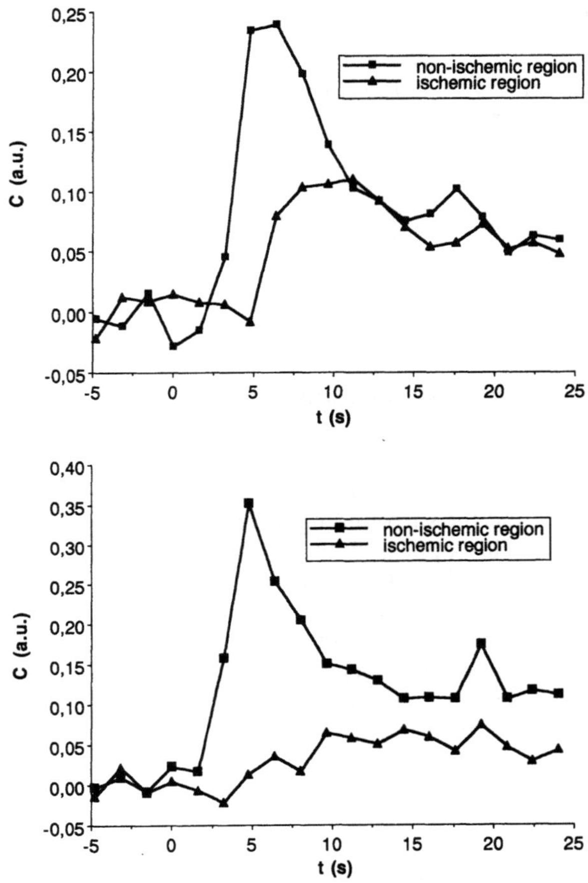

Fig. 1. Time density curves of the non-ischaemic hemisphere showed a first signal drop (MTT) 5.88 s (gadopentetate dimeglumine) (*top*) and 5.36 s (iron oxide) (*bottom*) after contrast medium injection. Using superparamagnetic iron particles, there is almost no signal decrease in the ischaemic area, whereas there is a reduced and delayed (but significant) signal decrease in the same ischaemic area when using paramagnetic Gd-DTPA

Results

All MRI examinations were performed 45–60 min after vessel occlusion. As expected, the initial, conventional T2-weighted spin-echo images were normal in all animals; specifically, we did not observe any early signs of cerebral ischaemia. In the non-ischaemic hemisphere, the time-signal intensity curves (Fig. 1) showed a mean transit time of 5.8 s in Gd-DTPA and 5.4 s in SPIO, and a signal reduction of 21% (Gd-DTPA) and 30% (SOIO). No signal reduction occurred in the ischaemic hemisphere when using SPIO, but a significant signal reduction of 12% with a significantly delayed MTT (7 s) occurred when using Gd-DTPA. The relative decrease in the rrCBV in the ischaemic region was 47% (Gd-DTPA) and 100% (SPIO).

Discussion

We demonstrated that both magnetic-susceptibility contrast media, the intravascular superparamagnetic iron particles and the lanthanide chelate gadopentetate dimeglumine, provide a sensitive imaging method for the early differentiation of ischaemic from normally perfused brain tissue. The dosages of both contrast media used in this study are the same for humans (gadopentetate dimeglumine) and are considered to be safe (iron oxide particles). Our observations of partial, delayed signal reduction when using Gd-DTPA might be explained by persistent capillary plasma flow. A second reason might be that the small Gd-DTPA molecules are able to pass the capillaries, whereas the macromolecular SPIO, like red blood cells, are unable to pass. It remains to be determined how long after vessel occlusion this kind of plasma flow persists and whether it can be used for therapeutic interventions.

References

1. Villringer A, Rosen BR, Belliveau JW, et al (1988) Dynamic imaging with lanthanide chelates in normal rat brain: contrast due to magnetic susceptibility effects. Magn Reson Med 6:164–174
2. Runge VM, Kirsch JE, Wells JW, Woolfolk CE (1993) Assessment of cerebral perfusion by first-pass, dynamic, contrast-enhanced, steady-stae free-precission MR imaging: an animal study. AJR 160:593–600

Studies of cerebral perfusion by dynamic, contrast-enhanced, T2*-weighted MRI in patients with acute cerebral infarcts

S. Ohue[1], K. Kusunoki[1], H. Ichikawa[1], H. Watanabe[1], M. Saito[1], K. Sadamoto[1], K. Kikuchi[2], Y. Ishimaru[2], Y. Kumon[3], S. Sakaki[3]

[1] Department of Neurosurgery, Washokai Sadamoto Hospital, 1-3-3 Takewara, Matsuyama, Ehime, 790 Japan
[2] Department of Radiology, Washokai Sadamoto Hospital, 1-3-3 Takewara, Matsuyama, Ehime, 790 Japan
[3] Department of Neurosurgery, Ehime University School of Medicine, Ehime, Japan

Abstract. Dynamic, contrast-enhanced, T2*-weighted magnetic resonance imaging (MRI) was used to assess cerebral perfusion in 5 normal volunteers and 13 patients with acute cerebral infarcts. A dynamic study was performed, using a spoiled GRASS pulse sequence and a long echo time with 1.5T MR system. After four images were obtained, a bolus of 0.1 mmol/kg of gadolinum DTPA (Gd-DTPA) was administrated intravenously. In normal subjects, symmetrical sequential patterns that showed loss of signal intensity were observed after intravenous injection of Gd-DTPA. In 5 out of 13 patients with infarcts, perfusion defects were clearly demonstrated as areas without signal loss. In 5 patients, there was less magnitude of the peak reduction in signal intensity. In 4 patients, the time to peak of signal reduction was delayed. Only 3 patients had normal dynamic curves. The dynamic study using T2-weighted imaging was useful for assessing cerebral perfusion in patients with acute cerebral infarcts.

Key words: Magnetic resonance imaging – Perfusion – Gadolinium – Cerebral infarcts

When a compact bolus of paramagnetic contrast (e.g. gadolinium chelates) is administered intravenously, it produces local magnetic field inhomogeneity. This susceptibility effect can be recognized as a transient signal intensity loss on T2*-weighted images (T2*-WI). Recently, dynamic, contrast-enhanced, T2*-weighted imaging has been used to study cerebral haemodynamics [1–4]. We applied this method to cerebral pathology in normal volunteers and to patients with acute cerebral infarcts.

Correspondence to: S. Ohue

Materials and methods

We examined 3 healthy subjects and 13 patients with acute cerebral infarcts within 24 h of the onset of cerebral ischaemia. None of the subjects showed any areas of abnormal signal intensity on spin-echo (SE) images. Magnetic resonance imaging (MRI) was performed using a conventional 1.5 T MR system with a spoiled GRASS (SPGR) sequence and a long echo time. A series of T2-WIs were recorded before, during, and after a bolus injection of 0.1 mmol/kg gadolinium-DTPA (Gd-DTPA). The imaging parameters were as follows: TR 61, TE 30 ms, flip angle 10 or 20°, 0.75 or 1 excitations, slice thickness 10 mm field of view 24 cm. The dynamic study was analysed by two methods: subtraction image, calculated with the SPGR images before and after the injection, and time intensity curve, obtained from a region-of-interest (ROI) measurement.

Results

In normal volunteers (Fig. 1), signal intensity was symmetrically reduced after Gd-DTPA administration. The time to peak reduction in signal intensity was around 20 s

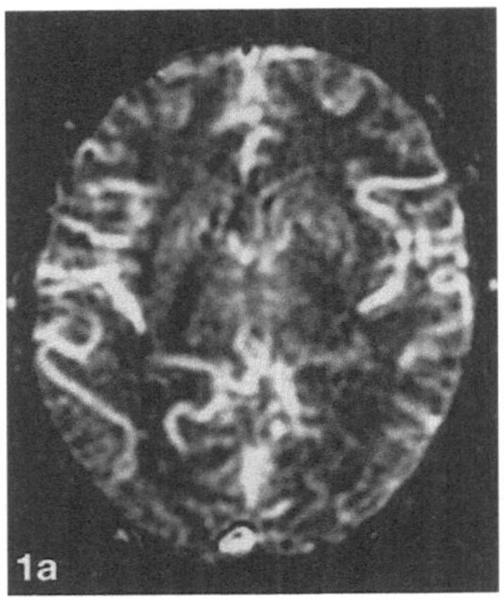

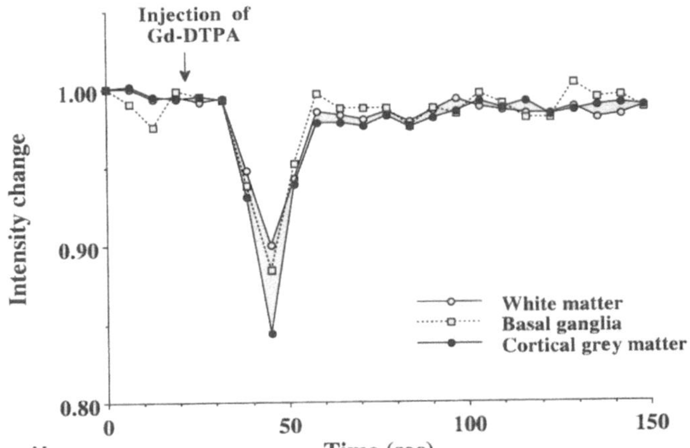

1b

Fig. 1a, b. Dynamic T2*-weighted images of a healthy subject. **a** Subtraction image calculated with the images before Gd-DTPA injection and at a peak of Gd-DTPA-induced signal reduction. **b** Mean time intensity curves from the regions of interest (ROI) in the cortical grey matter, white matter and basal ganglia

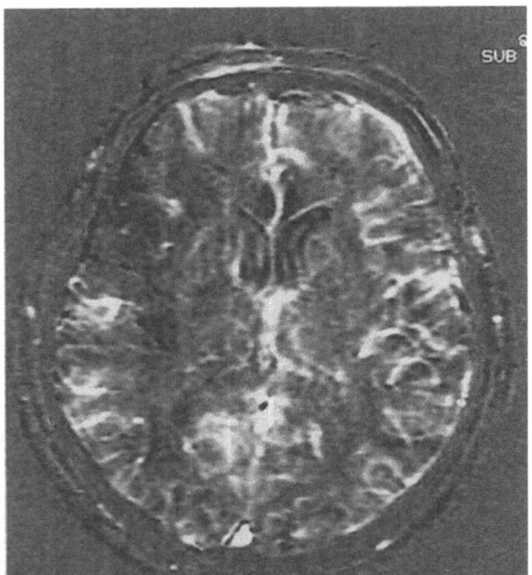

Fig. 2. Dynamic MRI in case 1 with occlusion of the M2 segment of the right middle cerebral artery; subtraction image calculated with the images before Gd-DTPA injection and 20 s after injection

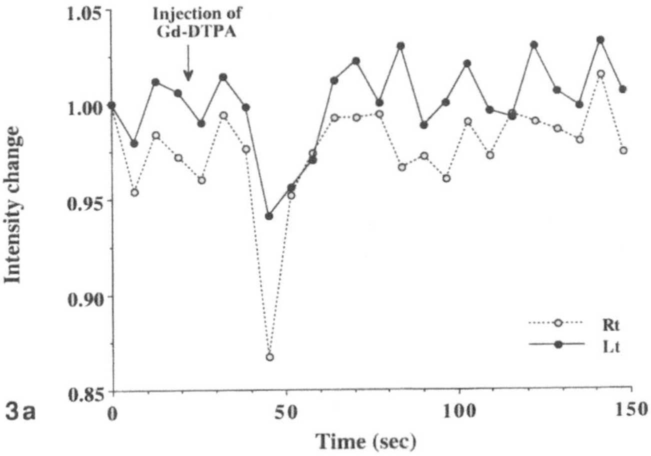

3a

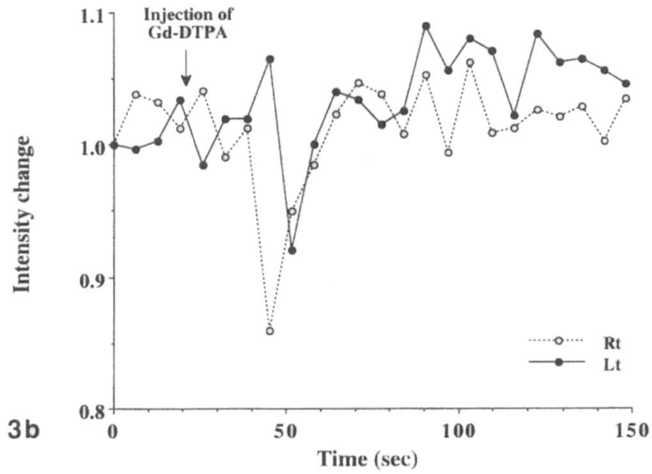

3b

Fig. 3a, b. Dynamic MRI in case 12 with stenosis of the M1 segment of the left middle cerebral artery. Time intensity curves from ROI in the basal ganglia (**a**) and frontal lobe (**b**)

after the injection. The mean peak value was -16% in the cortical grey matter, -10% in the white matter and -12% in the basal ganglia.

The results in patients with infarcts are summarized in Table 1. In 5 of 13 patients, the lesions of perfusion defects were clearly demonstrated as areas without signal loss on the subtraction images (Fig. 2). A mild decrease in signal attenuation was observed in 5 patients, and a delay in the time to peak of signal reduction in 4 patients (Fig. 3). Only 4 patients showed normal dynamic curves.

Discussion

Dynamic, contrast-enhanced, T2*-weighted MR imaging has been reported to be useful in the study of patients with subacute and chronic infarcts [1–4], intracerebral haematoma [1], and brain tumour [1, 4]. In patients with subacute and chronic ischaemia, the area of infarction was shown to be more apparent and extensive on the dynamic images than on SE images [2]. Moseley et al. [5] demonstrated perfusion deficits on dynamic T2*-WI within

Table 1. Results in 13 patients with acute infarcts

Case	Age (years) sex	Stroke type	Angiography	Time from onset (h)	Defect on subtraction image	Attenuation of peak value	Delay of time to peak
1	65/M	Minor	M2 occlusion	2	+	Severe	+
2	69/F	Minor		3	–	mild	–
3	62/F	Major	M1 occlusion	4	+	Severe	+
4	54/M	TIA	IC stenosis	6	–	Mild	–
5	68/M	TIA		6	–	None	–
6	56/F	RIND		8	–	None	–
7	63/M	RIND	IC occlusion	11	–	Mild	–
8	66/F	Minor	M1 stenosis	11	+	Severe	–
9	62/M	Major	IC occlusion	12	+	Severe	+
10	67/M	RIND		15	–	Mild	–
11	66/M	RIND	IC occlusion	17	–	None	–
12	72/F	TIA	M1 stenosis	23	–	Mild	+
13	40/M	Minor		24	+	Severe	–

TIA, Transient ischaemic attack; RIND, reversible ischaemic neurological defect; M1, M2, segments of middle cerebral artery; IC, internal carotid artery

minutes of experimental occlusion of the middle cerebral artery in cats, even when no abnormality was evident on SE images. Therefore, we applied dynamic MRI to the change of cerebral perfusion in patients with acute infarcts who had no abnormal intensity areas on SE images. In 10 out of 13 patients, evidence of ischaemic lesions was clearly demonstrated on dynamic, T2*-weighted MRI; perfusion defects were seen, mild decrease in signal attenuation in 5 and delay in the time to peak reduction, in 4 patients. Only 3 patients had normal dynamic curves. Dynamic, T2*-weighted MRI was thus useful for studying cerebral perfusion in patients with acute cerebral infarcts. This technique provided the possibility of early therapeutic intervention, such as thrombolytic therapy, in patients with acute stroke.

References

1. Edelman RR, Mattle HP, Atkinson DJ, Hill T, Finn JP, Mayman C, Ronthal M, Hoogewoud HM, Kleefield J (1990) Cerebral flood flow: assessment with dynamic contrast-enhancement T2*-weighted MR imaging at 1.5T. Radiology 176:211–220
2. Warach S, Li W, Ronthal M, Edelman RR (1992) Acute cerebral ischemia: evaluation with dynamic contrast-enhanced MR imaging and MR angiography. Radiology 182:41–47
3. Tzika AA, Massoth RJ, Ball WS, Majumdar S, Dunn RS, Kirks DR (1993) Cerebral perfusion in children: detection with dynamic contrast enhanced T2*-weighted images. Radiology 187:449–458
4. Guckel F, Brix G, Rempp K, Deimling M, Rother J, Georgi M (1994) Assessment of cerebral blood volume with dynamic susceptibility contrast enhanced gradient-echo imaging. J Comput Assist Tomogr 18:344–351
5. Moseley ME, Kucharczyk J, Mintorovithch J (1990) Diffusion-weighted imaging of acute stroke: correlation with T2-weighted and magnetic susceptibility-enhanced MR imaging in cats. AJNR 11:423–429

Does circulation from the unaffected carotid artery in children with unilateral moyamoya disease prevent progression of the basal network?

L. Borota, R. Bajic, S. Domonji, B. Prstojevic, P. Petrovic

Department of Neuroradiology, Institute of Neurosurgery, University Clinical Centre, Belgrade, Serbia, Yugoslavia

Abstract. Our aim was to clarify some factors influencing the occurrence and development of the basal network in children with unilateral moyamoya disease. We studied eight children with unilateral stenosis or occlusion of the carotid artery and/or its branches. All patients were studied angiographically by the standard Seldinger technique, and divided into two groups according to the findings: the first group included patients without a basal network, whereas the second one included patients with a basal network. We concluded that if the process leading to stenosis or occlusion is not constantly progressive, and if perfusion from the unaffected internal carotid artery is effective, basal moyamoya network will not develop, and that slow development of the basal network in children with unilateral moyamoya disease may be the result of the

Correspondence to: L. Borota

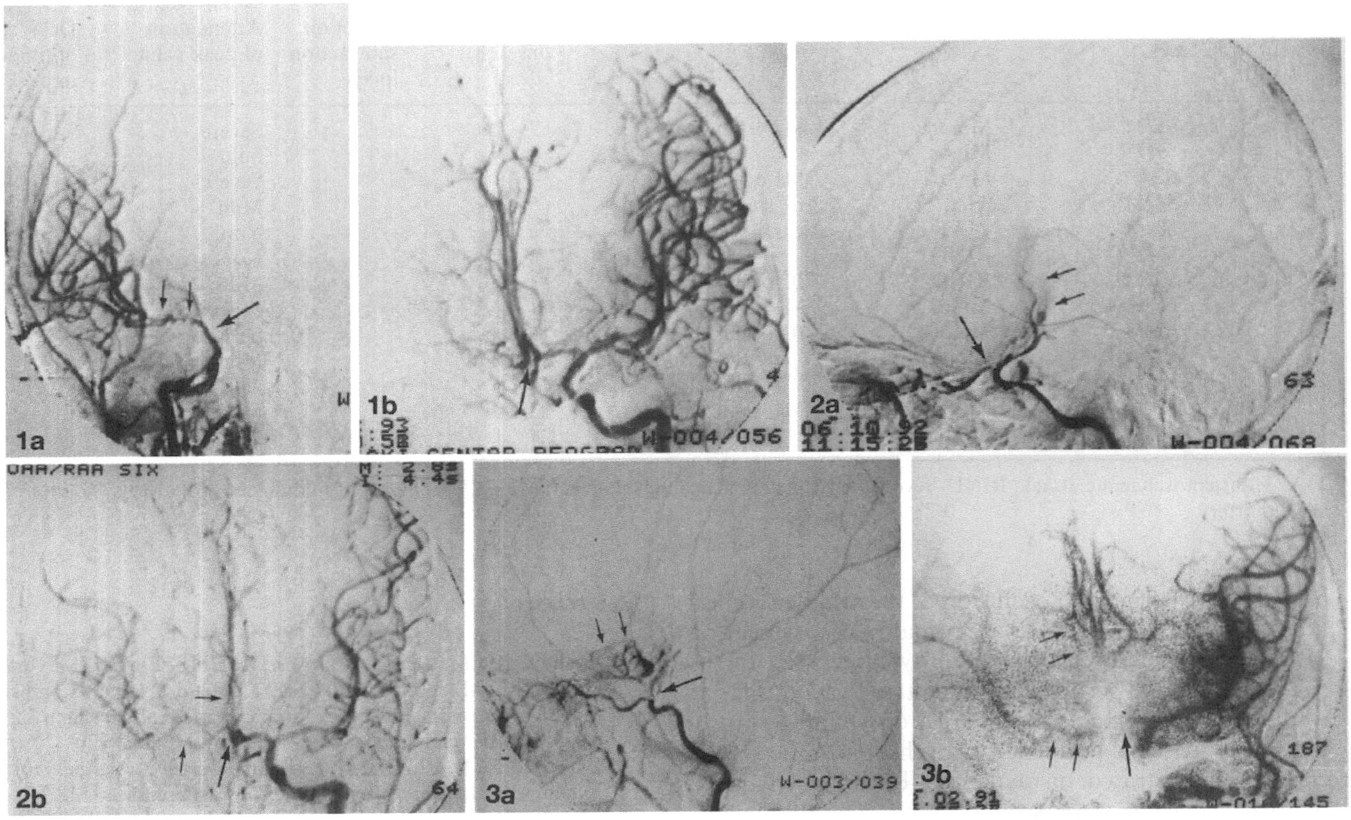

Fig. 1a, b. Case 1. **a** Stenosis of the termination of the right ICA (*arrow*) and stenosis of right middle cerebral artery (*small arrows*). **b** Collateral flow via anterior communicating artery (*arrow*)

Fig. 2a, b. Case 7. **a** Subocclusion of the right ICA above the origin of ophthalmic artery (*arrow*) and thalamic moyamoya network (*double arrows*). **b** Collateral flow via the anterior communicating artery (*arrow*) and the narrowed lumen of the right middle and anterior cerebral arteries (*small arrows*)

Fig. 3a, b. Case 8. **a** Occlusion of the right ICA above the origin of the opthalmic artery (*arrow*) and ethmoidal moyamoya network (*double arrows*). **b** Collateral flow via the anterior communicating artery (*arrow*) and the narrowed lumen of the right middle and anterior cerebral arteries (*small arrows*)

protective effect of perfusion via the anterior communicating artery from the unaffected internal carotid artery.

Key words: Collateral circulation – Moyamoya disease

Parenchymal anastomoses connect the lenticulostriate, thalamoperforating, thalamogeniculate and choroidal arteries enabling a collateral pathway in cases of progressive reduction of the lumen of the anterior cerebral arteries, and play a special role in patients with moyamoya disease [1]. Our aim was to clarify some factors influencing the occurrence and development of the basal network in children with unilateral moyamoya disease.

Patients and methods

We studied eight patients admitted to hospital because of symptoms dominated mainly by hemiparesis of different degrees (Table 1). Unilateral stenosis or occlusion of the internal carotid artery (ICA) or its branches was diagnosed in all patients. All were examined by transfemoral injection of both carotid arteries and the vertebrobasilar system. The external and internal carotid arteries were catheterised selectively in some patients.

Patients were divided in two groups: those without and those with a basal moyamoya network.

Results

In the first group stenoses or occlusions of the ICA and(or its main branches were seen (Figs. 1, 2). The angiographic findings are summarised in Table 2.

In one patient of the second group, the right ICA was almost occluded, whereas in the other it was obliterated just above the origin of the ophthalmic artery. These patients showed development of thalamostriate or ethmoidal moyamoya vascular networks (stage II), narrowed anterior and middle cerebral arteries (stage III), and marked collateral blood flow from the opposite ICA (Fig. 3).

Discussion

According to the classification of Hilal [2], occlusions of the blood vessels at the base of the brain may be divided into two groups: occlusions with or without a dense

Table 1. Clinical data

Patient	Sex	Age (years)	Clinical picture
1st group			
1	F	11	Headache, hemiparesis, motor aphasia
2	M	7	Headache, hemiparesis, motor aphasia
3	M	16	Headache, hemiparesis
4	F	8	Headache, hemiparesis
5	F	4	Hemiparesis
6	M	16	Hemiparesis, motor aphasia
2nd group			
7	M	4	Headache, hemiparesis
8	F	13	Headache, hemiparesis

Table 2. Main angiographic findings

Patient	Stenosis			Occlusion			Cross-filling
	ICA	ACA	MCA	ICA	ACA	MCA	
1st group							
1	+		+		A1		to ACA
2	+	+	+				to ACA
3	+				A1		to ACA
4	+	A1	M1				to ACA, MCA
5	+						to ACA, MCA
6				+			to ACA,MCA
Total	5	2	3	1	2		
2nd group							
7	+						to ACA, MCA
8				+			to ACA, MCA
Total	1			1			

ACA, MCA, anterior and middle cerebral arteries; ICA, internal carotid artery

vascular moyamoya network. In the group without a vascular network, the supraclinoid segment of the internal carotid artery is occluded or stenosed to a variable degree, while the proximal part of the artery is somewhat reduced in diameter to adapt to a decreased flow. The middle cerebral artery is nearly always affected. The anterior cerebral artery may be spared, or its involvement limited to a few millimeters from its origin. If communicating arteries are not involved, cross-filling from the unaffected arteries is present [2]. The appearances of the ICA and its main branches in the first four patients of the first group almost completely correspond to those mentioned above.

According published data, the follow-up of patients with such changes in the ICA and its branches usually shows recanalisation of the occluded vessels, although in some cases worsening of the angiographic picture is noted [2–4].

In patient 5, the ICA was stenosed along its length up to the origin of the ophthalmic artery. This picture is seen in congenital hypoplasia of the ICA with preserved intracranial circulation [2].

Complete occlusion of the ICA at the siphon, seen in the last patient of the first group, may be caused by dissection, arteritis or embolism as previously published [5, 6].

According to the data cited above, pathological processes which cause changes in the ICA and its branches, seen in patients of our first group, are mainly reversible or stationary with preserved collateral circulation through the communicating arteries of the circle of Willis. On the other hand, the pathological process, not yet fully understood, which causes changes to the "carotid fork" in patients with a basal moyamoya network, is permanently progressive and unstoppable [7–9]. On the basis of data from the literature mentioned above, and our own results, we conclude that if the process leading to stenosis or occlusion is not constantly progressive, and if perfusion from the unaffected ICA is effective, a basal moyamoya network will not develop.

In the classical, bilateral form of moyamoya disease, a pathological process permanently progresses, causing a simultaneous stenosis of the supraclinoid segment of both ICAs. As the blood flow decreases, the lumen of the anterior and middle cerebral arteries begins to reduce from the 3rd stage, according to the classification of Suzuki. In the 5th stage of the disease these arteries do not fill [7, 8]. A basal moyamoya network appears as a result of a slow occlusive process affecting the circle of Willis, particularly the supraclinoid segment of the ICA [2, 10, 11]. In the 1st stage of the disease, a basal moyamoya network is not present. In the 2nd stage a moyamoya network appears as a "puff of smoke" above the sella turciea. The 3rd stage is characterised by an enormously developed moyamoya network. From the 4th stage, a basal network begins to disappear [7, 8]. In the patients of the second group, the lumen of the anterior and middle cerebral arteries corresponds to the 3rd stage, whereas the shape of the basal network corresponds to the 2nd stage of the disease.

Some results indicate that the perfusion of the affected hemisphere of the brain in children with unilateral moyamoya disease is significantly better than that in children with bilateral moyamoya [12]. It is obvious that better perfusion of the affected hemisphre is a consequence of the preserved colateral blood flow from the unaffected ICA. Since the lumen of the main cerebral arteries reflects the degree of stenosis, whereas the basal network reflects the degree of perfusion in the 2nd and 3rd stage of moyamoya disease, we have come to another conclusion: the slow development of the basal network in children with unilateral moyamoya disease may be the result of the protective effect of perfusion via the anterior communicating artery from the unaffected ICA.

References

1. Djang W, Gray L, Drayer B (1992) Ultracranial occlusive vascular disease. In: Taveras J, Ferruci J (eds) Radiology – diagnosis, imaging, intervention, vol 3. Lippincott, Philadelphia, pp 1–23
2. Hilal SK (1974) Arterial occlusive disease in infants and children. In: Newton TH, Potts DG (eds) Radiology of the skull and brain – angiography. St. Louis, pp 2286–2310
3. Gold AP, Carter S (1976) Acute hemiplegia of infancy and childhood. Pediatr Clin North Am 23:413–433

4. Livet MO, Raybaud CA, Pinsard N (1980) Aspects diagnostique des occlusions artérielles cérébrales de l'enfant. Ann Pédiatr 27:277–285
5. Harwood Nash DC, McDonald P, Argent W (1971) Cerebral arterial disease in children. An angiographic study of 40 cases. Am J Roentgenol 111:672–686
6. Raybaud CA, Livet MO, Jiddane M, Pinsard N (1985) Radiology of ischaemic stroke in children. Neuroradiology 27:567–579
7. Suzuki J, Kodama N (1971) Cerebrovascular "moyamoya" disease. Angiology 22:223–236
8. Suzuki J, Takaku A (1969) Cerebrovascular "moyamoya" disease. Arch Neurol 20:288–299
9. Picard L, Levesque M, Crouzet G (1974) The "moyamoya" syndrome. J Neuroradiol 1:47–133
10. Kono S, Oka K, Sueshi K (1990) Histopathologic and morphometric studies of leptomeningeal vessels in moyamoya disease. Stroke 21:1044–1050
11. Drayer BP, Djang WT (1992) Physiological considerations in extra- and intracranial vascular disease. In: Taveras JM, Ferrucci JT (eds) Radiology – diagnosis, imaging, intervention, vol 3. Lippincott Philadelphia, pp 1–10
12. Kuwabara Y, Ichiou Y, Otsuka M, et al (1990) Cerebral hemodynamic change in the child and the adult with moyamoya disease. Stroke 21:272–277

Anomalous origin of the parieto-occipital artery, associated with moyamoya disease: case report

A. Uchino[1], Y. Aiko[2], K. Yamabe[2], H. Aibe[1], C. Kuromatsu[2], M. Tanaka[1]

[1] Department of Radiology, Kyushu Kosei-Nenkin Hospital, Kitakyushu, Japan
[2] Department of Neurosurgery, Kyushu Kosei-Nenkin Hospital, Kitakyushu, Japan

Abstract. We report an anomalous origin of the parieto-occipital artery, associated with moyamoya disease. The left anterior choroidal artery was markedly hyperplastic and supplied the parieto-occipital branches of the left posterior cerebral artery.

Key words: Anterior choroidal artery – Posterior cerebral artery – Parieto-occipital artery – Moyamoya disease

Moyamoya disease is relatively frequently associated with cerebral aneurysms [1]. It is also infrequently found in conjunction with cerebral arterial anomalies, such as cerebral arteriovenous malformations (AVMs) [2–4] and persistent trigeminal arteries [5–7].

Takahashi et al. [8] observed hyperplastic anomalies of the left anterior choroidal artery (AChA) in 2.3% of their subjects, and only 2 out of 25 hyperplastic AChA supplied the parieto-occipital branches of the posterior cerebral artery (PCA). To our knowledge, there has been no report of moyamoya disease being associated with this type of hyperplastic AChA.

Case report

A 13-year-old boy experienced transient paresis of both arms, which occasionally occurred while he was singing. Clinically, he was suspected of having moymoya disease; therefore, magnetic resonance MRI with MR angiography (MRA) was performed. MRA showed the typical appearance of moyamoya disease (Fig. 1). Selective cerebral angiography was performed prior to surgery, and the presence of moyamoya disease was confirmed. A left internal carotid arteriography demonstrated a markedly hyperplastic AChA, which supplied not only the choroidal branches, but the parieto-occipital branches of the left PCA. The posterior communicating artery (PCoA) was hypoplastic; it supplied only the perforating branches (Fig. 2). A left vertebral arteriography revealed normal blood supplies consisting of temporal branches of the left PCA (Fig. 3). The anomalously originating parieto-occipital branches and the normally supplied temporal branches anastomosed at their ambient segments.

Correspondence to: A. Uchino, Department of Radiology, Sga Medical School, 5-1-1 Nabeshima, Saga 849, Japan

Discussion

Moyamoya disease is an intracranial arterial occlusive disease of unknown etiology, and it is most prevalent in Japan [9]. Since there is a relatively high familial incidence (7%), important hereditary components have been suggested in the pathogenesis of this disease [10]. Moyamoya disease has reportedly been associated with cerebral arterial diseases, such as aneurysms [1]. AVMs [2–4], and persistent trigeminal arteries [5–7]. Kato et al. [11] reported a case of moyamoya disease where the right occipital artery arose from the right internal carotid artery (ICA). Ueda et al. [12] reported a case of anomalous origin of the anterior cerebral artery, associated with moyamoya disease. Except for cerebral aneurysms, these cerebral arterial abnormalities are considered congenital in origin. It is well known that hyperplastic AChAs may supply temporo-occipital lobes [13]. However, as in our patient, a hyperplastic AChA that supplies the parieto-occipital lobes is rare (018%) [8]. There are two reports of cases whose AChA originated from the ICA proximal to the PCoA [14, 15]. We initially misdiagnosed our patient, in that he was thought to have had an anomalous arrangement of the origins of his AChA and PCoA. However, we noted that the patient had a rare type of hyperplastic AChA with a hypoplastic PCoA. The association of moyamoya disease with this type of hyperplastic AChA is considered incidental.

According to Suzuki and Takako's classification [9], our patient had stage-3 moyamoya disease. In stage 4, the

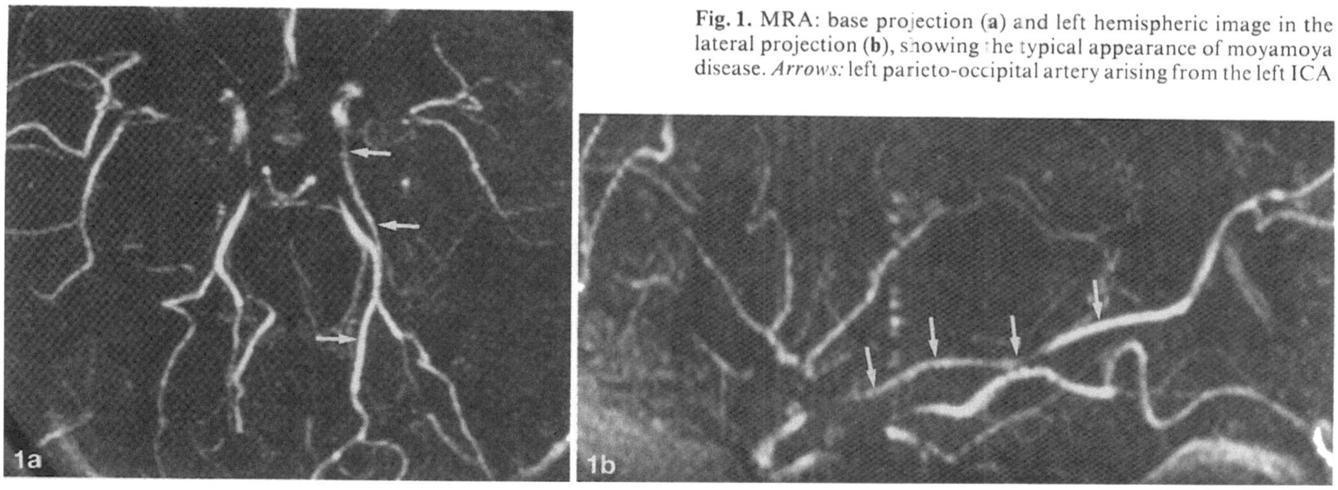

Fig. 1. MRA: base projection (**a**) and left hemispheric image in the lateral projection (**b**), showing the typical appearance of moyamoya disease. *Arrows:* left parieto-occipital artery arising from the left ICA

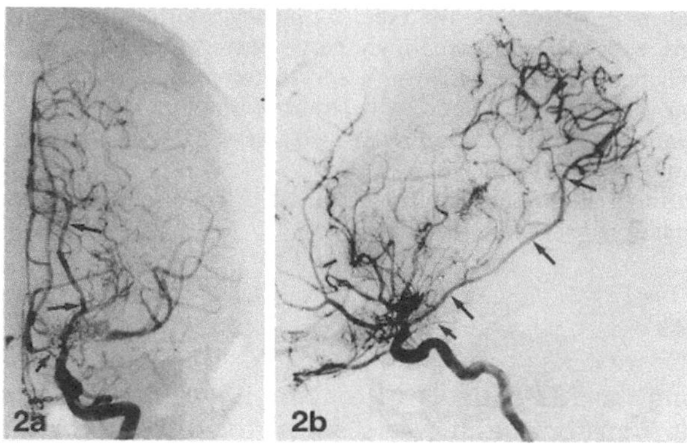

Fig. 2. Anteroposterior (**a**) and lateral (**b**) projections of left internal carotid angiogram: stage 3 moyamoya disease is confirmed. *Long arrows:* left parieto-occipital artery supplied by the markedly hyperplastic AChA. *Short arrows:* hypoplastic left PCoA

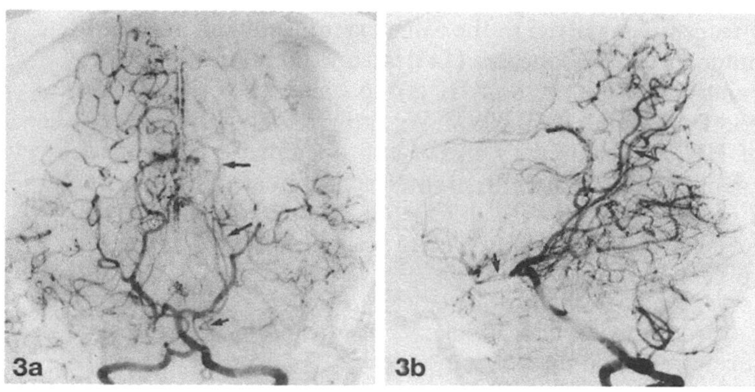

Fig. 3. Townes (**a**) and lateral (**b**) projections of left vetrebral angiogram. The left parieto-occipital artery is faintly opacified (*long arrows*), indicative of an anastomosis with the temporal branch of the left PCA. *Short arrows:* left PCoA

occlusion of the ICA extends to the origin of the PCoA. Therefore, in our patient the hyperplastic AChA may have been involved relatively early, causing ischaemic strokes in his left parieto-occipital lobe.

References

1. Kodama N, Suzuki J (1978) Moyamoya disease associated with aneurysm. J Neurosurg 48:565–569
2. Kayama T, Suzuki S, Sakurai Y, Nagayama T, Ogawa A, Yoshimoto T (1986) A case of moyamoya disease accompanied by an arteriovenous malformation. Neurosurgery 18:465–468
3. Lichtor T, Mullan S (1987) Arteriovenous malformation in moyamoya syndrome: report of three cases. J Neurosurg 67:603–608
4. Okada T, Kida Y, Kinomoto T, Sakurai T, Kobayashi T (1990) Arteriovenous malformation associated with moyamoya disease: case report. Neurol Med Chir (Tokyo) 30:945–948
5. Kwak R, Kadoya S (1983) Moyamoya disease associated with persistent primitive trigeminal artery: report of two cases. J Neurosurg 59:166–171
6. Tan E-C, Takagi T, Nagai H (1991) Intracranial carotid artery occlusion with telangiectasia (moyamoya disease) associated with persistent primitive trigeminal artery: case report. Neurol Med Chir (Tokyo) 31:800–803
7. Chen S-T, Liu Y-H (1993) Moyamoya disease associated with bilateral persistent primitive trigeminal arteries: report of a case. J Formosan Med Assoc 92:385–387
8. Takahashi S, Suga T, Kawata Y, Sakamoto K (1990) Anterior choroidal artery: angiographic analysis of variations and anomalies. AJNR 11:719–729
9. Suzuki J, Takaku A (1969) Cerebrovascular "moyamoya" disease: disease showing abnormal, net-like vessels in base of brain. Arch Neurol 20:288–299
10. Kitahara T, Ariga N, Yamaura A, Makino H, Maki Y (1979) Familial occurrence of moyamoya disease: report of three Japanese families. J Neurol Neurosurg Psychiatry 42:208–214
11. Kato Y, Kurokawa T, Hasuo K, Matsushima T (1985) Moyamoya disease with a developmental anomaly of the mesenchyme. Eur J Pediatr 144:93-95
12. Ueda T, Kikuchi H, Karasawa J, Nagata I, Naruo Y, Hashimoto K (1986) Anomalous origin of anterior cerebral artery associated with occlusive cerebrovascular disease. Neurol Med Chir (Tokyo) 26:409–413 (Jpn)
13. Takahashi M, Arii H, Tamakawa Y (1980) Anomalous arterial supply of temporal and occipital lobes by anterior choroidal artery: angiographic study. AJNR 1:537–540
14. Hara N, Koike T, Akiyama K, Toyama M (1989) Anomalous origin of anterior choroidal artery. Neuroradiology 31:88
15. Moyer DJ, Flamm ES (1992) Anomalous arrangement of the origins of the anterior choroidal and posterior communicating arteries: case report. J Neurosurg 76:1017–1018

Haemorrhagic transformation of acute cerebral ischaemia on CT

S. Bastianello, D. Toni, M. L. Sacchetti, M. Fiorelli, M. Rasura, C. Argentino, L. M. Fantozzi, C. Fieschi, L. Bozzao

Department of Neuroradiology, University of Rome "La Sapienza", Viale dell'Università 30, I-00185 Rome, Italy

Abstract. In a continuous series of 132 patients with ischaemic stroke studied in the acute phase, we assessed the occurrence and CT appearances of haemorrhagic transformation (HI) related to clinical outcome. Fifty-seven patients (43%) developed HI (only 3 had parenchymal haemorrhage). On the first CT, early signs of an ischaemic lesion were more frequent in HI (93%) than in non-HI (20%) ($P<0.0001$). Patients with early CT low-density showed a worse outcome in 74% of cases (17 dead and 33 poor outcome) compared with patients with a negative CT scan on admission, of whom 59% had a good outcome ($P<0.0002$). Clinical outcome in the HI patients group was impaired to the same extent, showing a worse outcome in 78% of cases (14 dead and 30 poor outcome) compared with the non-HI group of which 57% had a good outcome ($P<0.0002$). We showed a high frequency of HI in patients with stroke and documented that the haemorrhagic transformation of ischaemic stroke did not directly influence the clinical outcome, while early CT ischaemic signs may be the main predictors of both HI and clinical outcome.

Key words: Cerebral ischaemia – Haemorrhagic transformation – Computed tomography

While the radiological features and incidence of haemorrhagic infarction (HI) are reported in several studies, the clinical consequences of haemorrhagic transformation of an ischaemic stroke are not well established [1, 2]. Although it occurs in 40–70% of cases of an embolic stroke [3, 4], HI has been considered a sign of potential neurological disaster and has prompted a reluctance to use anticoagulants or thrombolytic agents in the acute phase [5–8]. In a continuous series of patients with a first-ever ischaemic hemispheric stroke, admitted to hospital within 5 h of the event and not given thrombolytic agents, we aimed to determine: the incidence of HI; the pathophysiological mechanisms of HI; the early clinical and laboratory predictors of HI; and any possible relationship between HI and the clinical outcome.

Patients and methods

We studied 132 patients with acute ischaemic stroke (mean age 66.4 years). All underwent CT within 5 h of the onset of symptoms; CT was repeated at 5–7 days and at 1 month in surviving patients. Autopsies were taken into consideration in patients who died.

Early CT findings were as follows: normal CT; slight lowdensity [9, 10] (SL); dense middle cerebral artery [11, 12].

CT examinations at 5–7 days and/or autopsy data (in 7 cases), allowed us to determine the type, frequency and location of HI. Lesions with clear areas of highdensity were considered as HI, whether petechial, spotty (Fig. 1), and scattered (Fig. 2) or parenchymal (Fig. 3) with blood collections within an area of low attenuation [13, 14]. At this time we also assessed the site and size of brain parenchymal damage.

During a 30-day follow-up we evaluated the case fatality ratio and functional status of survivors.

Results

Among the 132 patients with acute ischaemia, haemorrhagic transformation was seen on the 1-week CT and autopsy examinations in 57 (43%) of cases. HI was

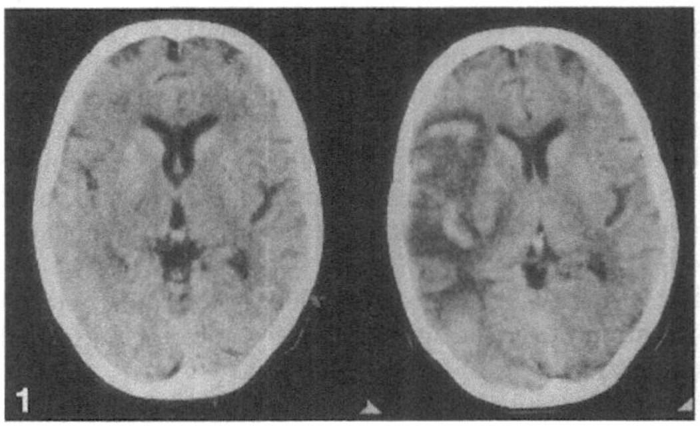

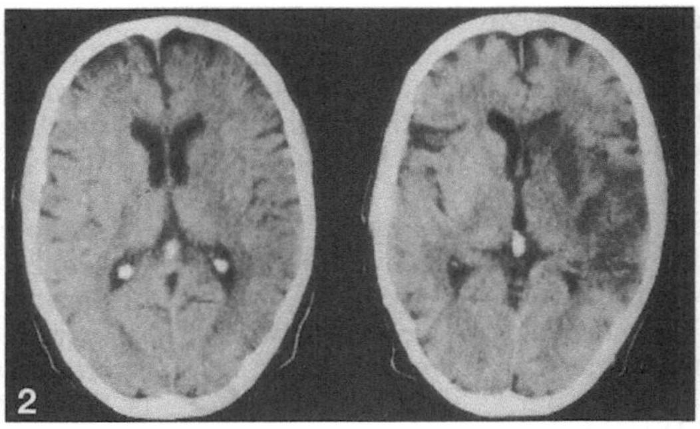

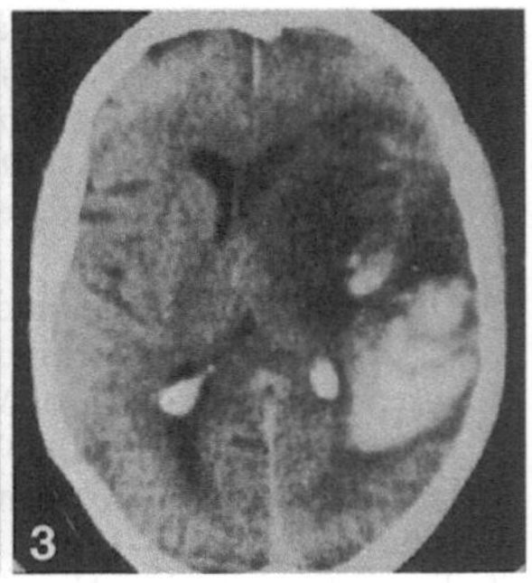

Fig. 1. First (*left*) and 5-day (*right*) CT documenting a spotty haemorrhagic infarct. Spotty dense areas are well seen within the ischaemic temporal lobe (*right*); early CT signs of ischaemic infarction were present previously (*left*)

Fig. 2. First (*left*) and 7-day control (*right*) CT. Petechial haemorrhagic transformation, consisting of small, punctate dense areas within the ischaemic lesion, is present on the second study. Deep and superficial early CT signs were present in the acute phase

Fig. 3. A large, confluent, dense blood clot within the infarct, with ventricular shift and sulcal effacement is shown on CT 2 days after the onset of symptoms; slight deep and superficial lowdensity was evident at the same level on CT in the acute phase (not shown)

Correspondence to: S. Bastianello

Table 1. Early CT findings (within 5 h)

	Haemorrhagic infarction (57)	Nonhaemorrhagic infarction (75)
Early lowdensity	53 (93%)	15 (20%)
Dense middle cerebral artery	28 (49%)	7 (9%)

$P<0.0001$

Table 2. Outcome in patients with and without haemorrhagic transformation a 1 week CT or autopsy

	Haemorrhagic infarction (57)	Nonhaemorrhagic infarction (75)
Dead	14 (25%)	8 (11%)
Poor outcome	30 (53%)	24 (32%)
Good outcome	13 (22%)	43 (57%)

$P<0.0002$

pethechial in all but 3 patients in whom a parenchymal haemorrhage was observed. Of the 75 non-HI cases, 10 had a negative 1-week CT.

Early CT findings of ischaemic damage were seen in 68 of 132 cases (52%) and in 53 of 57 patients with HI (93%). A dense middle cerebral artery was observed in 28 of 57 of the HI group (49%), and in 7 of 75 of the non-HI patients (9%) ($P<0.0001$) (Table 1).

Of the patients with HI, 14 (25%) died, 30 (53%) had a poor outcome and only 13 (22%) had a good outcome; of the non-HI patients 8 (11%) died, 24 (32%) had a poor outcome and 43 (57%) a good outcome ($P<0.0002$) (Table 2).

Clinical outcome in patients with low density on the early CT was also impaired; 17 (25%) died, 33 (49%) had a poor outcome and 18 (26%) a good outcome; among the patients with a normal CT on admission 5 (8%) died, 21 (33%) had a poor outcome and 38 (59%) a good outcome ($P<0.0002$).

Discussion

Reported rates of HI vary from 54% to 78% in autopsy [3, 15] and 39–50% in CT studies [4, 14]. Using CT, we found HI in 57 of 132 (43%) consecutive acute ischaemic stroke patients who were not treated with thrombolytic agents; this was about the same rate as we reported previously in a small series [14].

Haemorrhagic transformation of a bland infarct results form an ischaemic insult of sufficient degree to damage the endothelial vascular wall and restoration of blood flow into the injured vascular territory. Reperfusion of an ichaemic brain area can occur from 3–4 days to 2 weeks from the stroke [16], through reopening of major vessels which were formerly occluded [11, 12, 14] or by development of collateral blood supply via leptomeningeal anastomoses [17, 18].

The value of early CT signs as regards the clinical course is widely discussed [14, 19]. In the 57 patients who subsequently developed HI, early low density on CT was present in 93%, strongly predicting haemorrhagic transformation of the ischaemic stroke.

The worst clinical outcome seems not to be related to haemorrhagic transformation but to early CT low density, as in previous studies [14, 17, 19], confirming that HI is rather common in thrombo-embolic ischaemic stroke.

In 3 patients we observed parenchymal HI, simulating a parenchymal haematoma, with rapid worsening of clinical status, and in 2 cases death occurred. It remains unsettled whether these parenchymal haemorrhages represent a severe form of bleeding from late reperfusion, or rupture of one or more injured capillaries, but certainly they do not represent the common form of haemorrhagic transformation of ischaemic stroke.

References

1. Ott BR, Zamani A, Kleefield J, Funkenstein HH (1986) The clinical spectrum of hemorrhagic infarction. Stroke 17:630–637
2. Fisher M, Zito JL, Siva A, DeGirolami U (1984) Hemorrhagic infarction: a clinical and CT study. Stroke 15:192
3. Jorgensen L, Torvik A (1969) Ischemic cerebrovascular disease in an autopsy series, part II. J Neurol Sci 9:285–320
4. Yamaguchi T, Minematsu K, Choki J, Sawada T, Ikeda M (1984) Clinical and neuroradiological analysis of thrombotic and embolic cerebral infarction. Jpn Circ J 48:50–58
5. Pessin MS, Estol CJ, Lafranchise EF, Caplan LR (1991) Safety of anticoagulation in hemorrhagic infarction. Stroke 41:346
6. Pessin MS, Del Zoppo GJ, Estol CJ (1990) Thrombolytic agents in the treatment of stroke. Clin Neuropharmacol 13:271–289
7. The rT PA/Acute Study Group (1991) An open safety/efficacy trial of rT PA in acute thrombolytic stroke: final report. Stroke 22:153
8. Von Kummer R, Forsting M, Sartor K, Hacke W (1991) Intravenous plasminogen activator in acute stroke. In: Hacke W, Del Zoppo GJ, Hirschberg M (eds) Thrombolytic therapy in acute ischemic stroke. Springer New York Berlin Heidelberg, pp 161–167
9. Tomura N, Uemura K, Inugami A, Fujita H, Higano S, Shishido F (1988) Early CT finding in cerebral infarction. Radiology 168:463–467
10. Bozzao L, Bastianello S, Fantozzi LM, Angeloni U, Argentino C, Fieschi C (1989) Correlation of angiographic and sequential CT findings in patients with evolving cerebral infarction. AJNR 10:1215–1222
11. Tomsick TA, Brott TG, Chambers AA, et al (1990) Hyperdense middle cerebral artery sign on CT: efficacy in detecting middle cerebral artery thrombosis. AJNR 11:473–477
12. Bastianello S, Pierallini A, Colonnese C, et al (1991) Hyperdense middle cerebral artery CT sign. Comparison with angiography in the acute phase of ischaemic supratentorial infarction. Neuroradiology 33:207–211
13. Yamaguchi T, Hayakawa T, Kikuchi H, Abe T (1991) Thrombolytic therapy in embolic and thrombotic cerebral infarction: a cooperative study. In: Hacke W, Del Zoppo GJ, Hirschberg M (eds) Thrombolytic therapy in acute ischemic stroke. Springer New York Berlin Heidelberg, pp 168–174
14. Bozzao L, Angeloni U, Bastianello S, Fantozzi LM, Pierallini A, Fieschi C (1991) Early angiographic and CT findings in patients with hemorrhagic infarction in the distribution of the middle cerebral artery. AJNR 12:1115–1121
15. Adams RD, Van der Eecken HM (1953) Vascular disease of the brain. Annu Rev Med 14:213–252

16. Hart RG, for Cerebral Embolism Study Group (1986) Timing of hemorrhagic transformation of cardioembolic stroke. In: Stober T, Schimrigk K, Ganten D, Sherman DG (eds) Central nervous system control of the heart. Nijhoff, Boston, pp 229–232
17. Bozzao L, Fantozzi LM, Bastianello S, Bozzao A, Fieschi C (1989) Early collateral blood supply and late parenchymal brain damage in patients with middle cerebral artery occlusion. Stroke 6:735–740
18. Van der Eecken HM, Adams RD (1953) The anatomy and functional significance of the meningeal arterial anastomoses of the human brain. J Neuropathol Exp Neurol 12:132–157
19. Horowitz SH, Zito JL, Donnarumma R, Patel M, Alvir J (1991) Computed tomographic – angiographic findings within the first five hours of cerebral infarction. Stroke 22:1245–1253

Spontaneous intracerebral haematomas: value of dynamic CT in predicting aetiology

N. Khandelwal[1], E. Chandra[1], S. N. Mathuriya[2], R. K. Vasishta[3], V. K. Kak[2], S. Suri[1]

[1] Department of Radiodiagnosis, Postgraduate Institute of Medical Education and Research, Chandigarh-160012, India
[2] Department of Neurosurgery, Postgraduate Institute of Medical Education and Research, Chandigarh-160012, India
[3] Department of Pathology, Postgraduate Institute of Medical Education and Research, Chandigarh 160012, India

Abstract. Thirty patients with spontaneous intracerebral haematoma (ICH) were studied by dynamic computed tomography (CT) and cerebral angiography. The prospective predictive value of dynamic CT in demonstrating the underlying aetiology in ICH was evaluated. Dynamic CT correctly predicted 90% of aneurysms, 100% of arteriovenous malformations and 100% of normal studies, as compared to angiography. It can obviate angiography in patients where dynamic CT does not show any vascular abnormality.

Key words: Dynamic computed tomography – Angiography – Lobar haematoma – Spontaneous haematoma

Spontaneous intracerebral haematoma (ICH) refers to all varieties of bleeding in the cerebral parenchyma in which trauma or other exogenous factors do not play an essential part [1]. It constitutes a major neurosurgical problem, and its incidence varies from 10 to 32% of all cerebrovascular strokes [2]. The various aetiological factors include arterial hypertension, aneurysm, angioma, neoplasm, coagulopathy, collagen vascular disease, cortical vein and/or dural sinus thrombosis [3]. Cerebral angiography was the main investigation used to diagnose these conditions prior to the advent of computed tomography (CT) [4]. The indications for cerebral angiography in spontaneous ICH are less clear as compared with subarachnoid haemorrhage (SAH), as the majority are caused by systemic diseases and managed conservatively [5]. There are scant reports dealing with the diagnosis of underlying aetiology in spontaneous ICH [5, 6]. The aim of this prospective study was to utilize the potential of dynamic CT in predicting the underlying aetiology in spontaenous ICH, excluding hypertensive bleeding, and to define a clear indication for angiography in this clinical setting.

Correspondence to: N. Khandelwal

Table 1. Site of haematomas

Site	Patients
Supratentorial	
Temporal	7
Parietal	8
Frontal	5
Frontoparietal	1
Temporoparietal	3
Occipital	1
Basal ganglia (including thalamus)	3
External capsule	1
Infratentorial	
Cerebellum	1
Total	30

Materials and methods

Thirty patients (19 males and 11 females) ranging age from 14 to 62 years and admitted with spontaneous ICH between 1990 and 1994, were studied prospectively. All hypertensive patients with haemorrhage in the thalamus, putamen, internal capsule and cerebellum were excluded from this study. CT was carried out to confirm the diagnosis of ICH, and its location, size and associated SAH and intraventricular heamorrhage IVH were recorded. A dynamic CT was carried out, covering the circle of Willis and the region of haematoma, followed by conventional CT of the head. Cerebral angiography was carried out in all patients except one, and the findings were correlated with those of the dynamic CT. A surgical procedure was performed in 23 patients, and a histopathological examination was carried out in 15 of these.

Results

Twenty-nine patients had supratentorial haematomas ranging from 2 to 8 cm in diameter. Only one patient had an infratentorial haematoma, measuring 4.1 cm in diameter. The location of the haematomas is shown in Table 1. The dynamic CT, angiographic, surgical and histopatho-

Table 2. Dynamic CT, cerebral angiography, surgical and histopathological findings

	Dynamic CT	Angiography[a]	Surgery	Histopathology
Aneurysm	9	10	8	0
Arteriovenous malformation	10	9	8	8
Others	0	0	1 (tumour)	1 (tumour)
Normal	11	10[a]	6	6

[a] Angiography was not performed in one patient

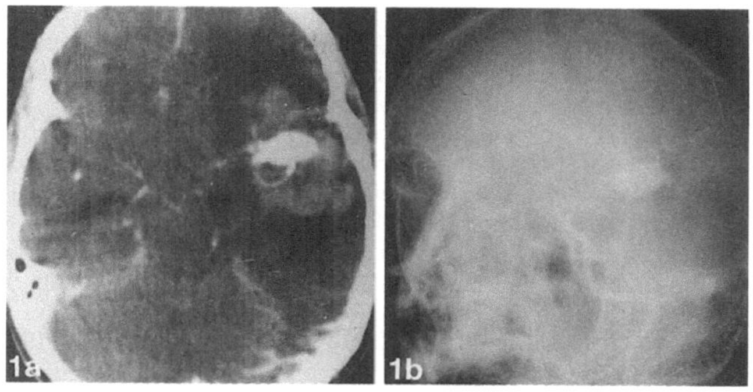

Fig. 1. a Contrast-enhanced CT showing an aneurysm inside the intracerebral haematoma. **b** Angiography confirms an aneurysm

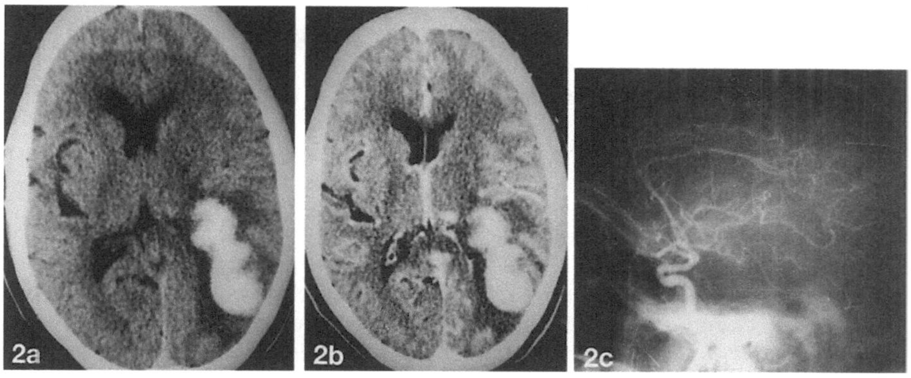

Fig. 2. a CT showing lobar haematoma. **b** Dynamic CT shows not vascular abnormality. **c** Cerebral angiogram (lateral view) showing normal vascular pattern

logical findings are shown in Table 2. Of the ten aneurysms demonstrated on cerebral angiography, dynamic CT demonstrated all but one, which was 4 mm in diameter (Fig. 1). Eight of these aneurysms were clipped surgically. One patient had a mycotic aneurysm and was treated conservatively. The other patient died of a rebleed prior to surgery. All the nine arteriovenous malformations (AVMs) were demonstrated on dynamic CT. In one patient, a diagnosis of AVM was made on dynamic CT, but angiography was normal. Surgical excision of the lesion proved it to be a glioma. Cerebral angiograms in 11 patients, where dynamic CT did not reveal any vascular abnormality, were normal (Fig. 2). Angiography was not carried out in one patient, and surgical evacuation of the ICH was performed on the basis of dynamic CT findings. A histopathological examination in six of these patients did not reveal any abnormal findings.

Discussion

Hypertension is the most common aetiological factor for spontaneous ICH, accounting for 50% of all strokes [5]. There are specific sites for bleeding to occur in hypertensive patients, viz. putamen, thalamus, internal capsule and cerebellum. Lobar haematomas may be seen in a minority of these patients.

Several publications describe the predictiveness of aneurysms, based on the location of SAH with or without associated ICH by CT [6–10]. However, only a few reports are available predicting the underlying pathology in spontaneous ICH [5, 6].

In the present study, dynamic CT prospectively predicted 90% of aneurysms, 100% of AVMs and 100% of normal studies, when compared to cerebral angiography. In one patient, cerebral angiography demonstrated a 4-mm anterior communicating artery aneurysm, which was missed on dynamic CT. Dynamic CT misinterpreted a case of glioma as an AVM. Dynamic CT correctly predicted all the AVMs, including the flow-related and intranidal aneurysms.

Seven patients were hyperintensive at the time of presentation with lobar haematomas. Two patients had saccular aneurysms, two had AVMs, and two had normal angiography. None of the patients with a negative dynamic CT had any angiographic abnormality. The present study demonstrates a higher diagnostic yield of angiography in hypertensive patients who had haemorrhages outside the basal ganglia as also reported in a previous study [11].

References

1. Russell DS (1954) The pathology of spontaneous intracerebral haemorrhage. Proc R Soc Med 47:689–704
2. Ojeman RG, Heros RC (1983) Spontaneous brain hemorrhage. Stroke 14:468–475
3. Weisberg LA (1986) Thalamic hemorrhage. Clinical CT correlations. Neurology 36:1382–1386

4. Picard L, Roland J, Lepoire J, Montant J, et al (1980) The role of angiography in the neuroradiological diagnosis of intracerebral hematomas. In: Pia HW, Langmaid C, Herski J (eds) Advances in diagnosis and therapy. Springer, Stuttgart, pp 171–176
5. Laissy JP, Normand G, Monroc M, Duchateau C, Alibert F, Thiebot J (1991) Spontaneous intracerebral hematomas from vascular causes. Predictive value of CT compared with angiography. Neuroradiology 33:291–295
6. Hayward RD, O'Reilly GVA (1976) Intracerebral haemorrhage. Accuracy of computerized axial scanning in predicting the underlying pathology. Lancet I:1–4
7. Scotti G, Ethier R, Melançon D, Terbrugge K, Tchang S (1977) Computed tomography in evaluation of intracranial aneurysms and subarachnoid hemorrhage. Radiology 123:85–90
8. Van Gijn J, Van Dongen KJ (1982) The time course of aneurysmal hemorrhage on CT. Neuroradiology 3:153–156
9. Ghoshhajra K, Scotti, Marasco J, Baghai-Naiini P (1979) CT detection of intracranial aneurysms in subarachnoid hemorrhage. AJR 132:613–616
10. Liliequist B, Lindqvist M, Valdimarsson E (1977) Computed tomography and subarachnoid hemorrhage. Neuroradiology 14:21–26
11. Gilbert JT, Jose B, Harold PA, Wendy RKS (1987) The predictive value of arteriography in nontraumatic intracerebral hemorrhage. Stroke 17:881–883

Parenchymal manifestations of acute cerebrovenous occlusion

F. Y. Tsai, A. M. Wang, V. B. Matovich, M. Lavin, B. Berberian, W. Yuh

UMKC-Trumsa Medical Center, 2301 Holmes St. Kansas City, MO 64108, USA

Abstract. We report our experience with 29 patients with acute dural sinus and/or deep venous thrombosis, correlating their clinical presentation to their radiologic findings, and using dural sinus pressure to gauge severity and staging.

Key words: Dural sinus thrombosis – Venous infarction – Urokinase – Cerebral edema – Thrombolysis

Materials and methods

This report concerns 29 patients referred from January 1989 to May 1993. Intradural sinus pressure was measured before, during and after thrombolysis. All patients had cerebral angiography and/or venography to confirm the diagnosis. Dural sinus venography was performed via the percutaneous transfemoral vein approach, using a 5F angiographic catheter as a guide. A no. 18 Tracker catheter (preferably with multiple side-holes) was then advanced into the dural sinus, coaxially, through the 5F guiding catheter. We prefer to perform transverse sinus venography from the contralateral transverse sinus across the torcular herophili. This technique is easier than the retrograde approach through the ipsilateral sinus and allows us to measure intrasinus pressure.

Results

Patients fell into one of five stages of increasing severity, based on cross-sectional imaging findings. Stage I patients had no evidence of brain swelling or cerebral edema (6 patients). Stage II patients had only brain swelling without focal edema (5 patients), while stage III patients did have focal edema (7 patients). Stage IV patients had evidence of paranchymal hemorrhage (5 patients) and stage V patients had massive edema and hemorrhage (6 patients).

Correspondence to: F. Y. Tsai

Discussion

CT and MR findings in cerebrovenous and dural sinus thrombosis have been reported previously; however, the reports were primarily focused upon chronic or subacute cases [1–3]. Venous occlusive disease may be confused with arterial infarcts or hemorrhage, delaying the appropriate treatment and having potentially fatal consequences [4–11]. We have found more brain parenchymal changes from acute dural sinus thrombosis than previously described [12–15]. We divide the stages of acute venous occlusion into five. These stages directly correlate with the dural sinus pressure, which we measured when dural sinus venography was performed. Intradural sinus pressure will rise after occlusion of the dural sinus distally [14, 15]. The early stages of acute thrombosis may not exhibit any brain parenchymal changes. CT or MRI without intravenous contrast medium may not show any abnormality in stage I, or only slight hyperdensity or increased intensity (Fig. 1); MR venography may be more sensitive to occlusion. The elevated pressure will induce venous congestion as venous drainage is restricted. The extracellular water content increases and leads to brain swelling and cerebral edema [14, 15]. Stage II patients did manifest brain swelling. We measured dural sinus pressure in two patients in stage II, as 20 mm Hg and 28 mm Hg (normal is less than 10 mm). These patients did have obliteration of cerebral sulci and the sylvian fissure. This picture may be confused with acute middle cerebral artery occlusion. The presence of the abnormalities described above for stage 1 will aid differentiation. At this stage, even though MRI or CT does show some brain swelling, clinical signs and symptoms are often more striking. Our stage II patients were very drowsy or obtunded.

In stage III, the thrombosis leads to more apparent parenchymal changes and cerebral edema (Fig. 2). At this stage, all our patients were comatose. The pressure within the dural sinuses also increased significantly, to 33–

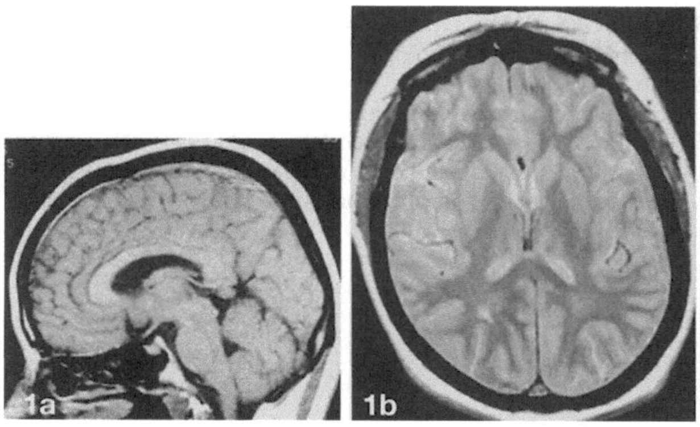

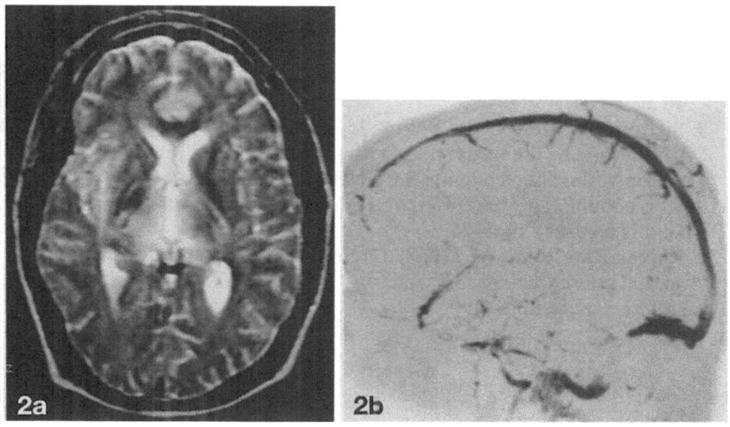

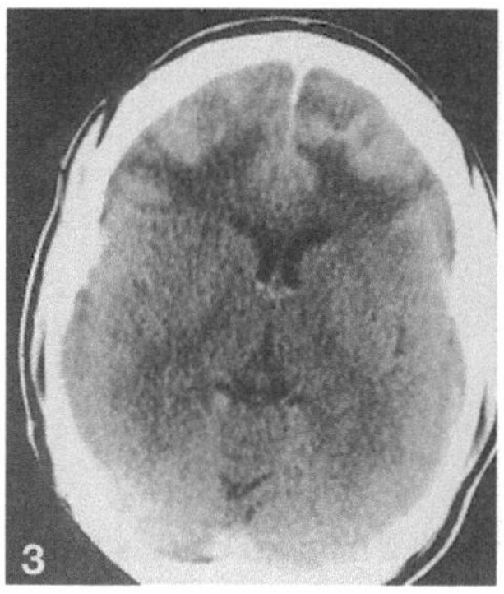

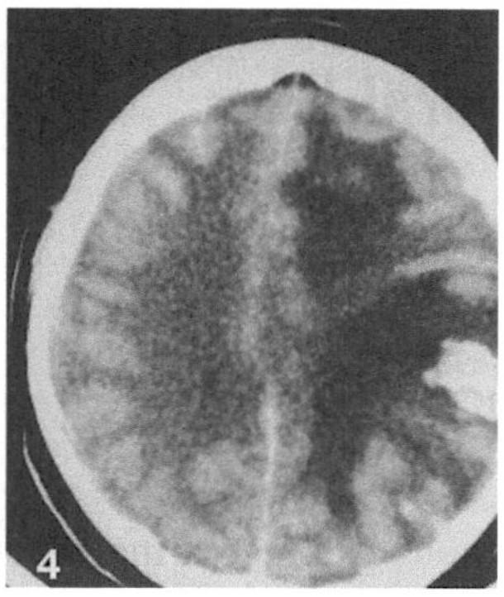

Fig. 1 a, b. Stage I. **a** Sagittal T_1-weighted MRI shows increased intensity in the sagittal sinus from the thrombus. **b** Proton density MRI shows no parenchymal abnormality, but isointensity in the sagittal sinus

Fig. 2 a, b. Stage III. **a** T_2weighted MRI shows extensive edema in the thalamus, with increased intensity secondary to deep vein and dural sinus thrombosis. **b** 2-D time-of-flight MR venography shows occlusion of the deep veins and straight sinus and thrombosis of the sagittal sinus above the torcula

Fig. 3. Stage IV. Contrast-enhanced CT showed a filling defect in the front of the sagittal sinus, due to thrombosis. Extensive edema is seen in the frontal lobes with early cortical hemorrhage

Fig. 4. Stage V. CT shows extensive edema and hematoma in the left paretal lobe

42 mmHg. Up to this stage, however, the blood-brain barrier is intact. The increased extracellular water is probably interstitial rather than vasogenic or cytotoxic. In stage IV, patients had cerebral edema and small hemorrhages, with pressures of 48–51 mmHg. The examples clearly demonstrate that the progression of parenchymal change is directly related to the intradural sinus pressure. If the dural sinus pressure gets high enough, the capillary intraluminal pressure will exceed the integrity of the capillary wall, resulting in hemorrhage. The final stage of venous or dural sinus occlusive disease is massive edema and/or hematoma. This stage is invevitably fatal. Patients with massive cerebral edema and hemorrhage had arteriography only (their high pressures were inferred from the imaging appearance). The increments of dural sinus pressure appear to increase about 10 mm Hg in each stage.

The progression of change in brain parenchyma has an essentially linear relationship to the dural sinus pressure. The other factor that may influence this progression is the duration of the obstruction. The severity of the injury associated with increasing pressure is different in acute versus chronic elevation [15]. The pressure may be very high in chronic obstruction compared to that seen in outpatients with acute thrombosis. The clinical presentation may also be influenced by this factor. The slow onset of symptoms in these patients correlated with less parenchymal change. The stages of cerebral venous occlusive disease have prognostic implications. Stages I–III are not associated with cell death, so the parenchymal changes can be entirely reversed, although this result may require timely intervention. Stage IV disease, however, is associated with true infarction and a small hemorrhage may occur (Fig. 3). Improvement is possible with appropriate therapy, however, some changes may be irreversible. Venous pressures high enough to reach stage V result in generalized disruption of the blood-brain barrier and inadequate cellular perfusion. Stage V means significant, irreversible infarction (Fig. 4) and is inevitably fatal. We believe that acute dural sinus and deep venous thrombosis may lead to various stages of venous occlusive disease, with the degree of severity depending on the degree of venous congestion, as measured by dural sinus pressure.

References

1. Virapongse C, Cazenave C, Quisling R, Sarwar M, Hunter S (1987) The empty delta sign: frequency and significance in 76 cases of dural sinus thrombosis. Radiology 162:779–785
2. Theron A, Wessel K, Linden D, Schroth G, Dichgans J (1986) Superior sagittal sinus thrombosis: neuroradiological evaluation and clinical findings. J Neurol 233:283–288
3. Tsuruda JS, Shimakawa A, Pelc NJ, Saloner D (1991) Dural sinus occlusion: evaluation with phase-sensitive gradient-echo MR imaging. AJNR 12:481–488
4. Vogl TJ, Bergman C, Villringer A, Einhaupl K, Lissner J, Felix R (1994) Dural sinus thrombosis: value of venous MR angiography for diagnosis and follow-up. AJR 162:1191–1198
5. Bousser MG, Chiras J, Bories J, Castaigne P (1985) Cerebral venous thrombosis: a review of 38 cases. Stroke 16:199–213
6. Angelov A (1989) Intracranial venous thrombosis in relation to pregnancy and delivery. Pathol Res Pract 185:843–847

7. Gettelfinger DM, Kokmen E (1977) Superior sagittal sinus thrombosis. Arch Neurol 34:2–6
8. Estanol B, Rodriguez A, Conte G, Aleman JM, Loyo M, Pizzuto J (1979) Intracranial venous thrombosis in young women. Stroke 10:680–684
9. Sindou M, Mercier P, Bokor J, Brunon J (1980) Bilateral thrombosis of the transverse sinuses: microsurgical revascularization with venous bypass. Surg Neurol 13:215–220
10. Krayenbuhl HA (1967) Cerebral venous and sinus thrombosis. Clin Neurosurg 14:1–24
11. Kalbag RM, Woolf AL (1967) Cerebral venous thrombosis: with special reference to primary asceptic thrombosis. Oxford University Press, London, pp 237–250
12. Tsai FY, Higashida RT, Matovich VB, Alfieri KM (1992) Acute thrombosis of the intracranial dural sinus: direct thrombolytic treatment. AJNR 13:1137–1141
13. Sandhu AS, Johns D, Albertyn LE (1991) Deep cerebral vein thrombosis. Neuroradiology 33 [Suppl]:241–243
14. Yuh WTC, Simonson TM, Wang AM, et al (1994) Venous sinus occlusive disease: MR findings. AJNR 15:309–316
15. Tsai FY, Wang AM, Matovich VB, et al (1994) MR staging of acute dural sinus thrombosis: correlation with venous pressure measurements and implication for treatment and prognosis. AJNR (in press)

Arteriovenous malformations of the temporal lobe: clinical and angiographic characteristics

F. Turjman[1], T. F. Massoud[2], G. Duckwiler[2], J. Sayre[2], G. Guglielmi, F. Viñuela[2]

[1] Department of Radiology, Hôpital Neurologique, 59 Boulevard Pinel, F-69003 Lyon, France
[2] UCLA Medical Center Endovascular Therapy, Los Angeles, California, USA

Abstract. Arteriovenous malformations (AVMs) located in the temporal lobe appear with clinical and angioarchitectural characteristics that are different from those in other lobar locations. The purpose of this work was to determine these characteristics. Between 1987 and 1990, 27 patients with pure temporal AVMs were referred to our institution for endovascular therapy. The clinical presentation – hemorrhage, epilepsy or other, including progressive neurological deficit and headache – and the following angioarchitectural parameters: characteristics of the venous drainage, type of nidus and presence of aneurysms, were studied. These characteristics were evaluated on selective and superselective angiograms. A clinical presentation of epilepsy was found to correlate with a temporal location of the AVM ($P=0.05$). Three angioarchitectural characteristics were found with a higher rate in the temporal location than in other lobar locations: presence of fistula 52% vs 44%, presence of venous stenosis 66% vs 58%, and presence of varix 66% vs 58%. The presence of fistula was the only statistically significant parameter. These characteristics have potential therapeutic implications for endovascular therapy.

Key words: Arteriovenous malformation – Endovascular therapy – Angioarchitecture – Location

Cerebral arteriovenous malformations (AVMs) frequently involve the temporal lobe. In this series of 100 patients with AVM, 27 had purely temporal AVMs. We noted that the angioarchitecture of temporal AVMs seemed to differ from that of AVMs at other cerebral locations. Willinsky et al. [1] have reported a "kinking" of temporal AVM venous drainage at the tentorium. The goal of this work is to study various parameters of the angioarchitecture of temporal AVMs and compared them with those at other locations, in order to verify this hypothesis.

Correspondence to: F. Turjman

Materials and methods

Twenty-seven patients with pure temporal AVMs were referred to our institution between 1987 and 1990 for endovascular embolisation. We reviewed the clinical details and cerebral angiograms of these patients retrospectively. Patients ranged in age from 8 to 82 years. There were 55 male and 45 female patients. Clinical presentation was one of epilepsy (47% of patients), hemorrhage (40%), or other (13%), including headaches and progressive neurological deficits.

In all patients, superselective angiograms were obtained in orthogonal planes following catherisation of various pedicles of the malformation. The following vascular characteristics were evaluated on these angiograms: type of nidus, characteristics of venous drainage, and presence of aneurysms.

The type of nidus was determined as plexiform (presence of a network of dilated abnormal vessels between feeding arteries and draining veins), purely fistulous (direct communication between feeding artery and draining vein), and mixed [2, 3]. Five parameters of venous drainage were considered: deep or superficial, number of draining veins, number of large draining veins, presence of varix or varices, presence of venous stenosis. A varix was defined as a markedly ectatic vein [4] and venous stenosis [5] as a reduction of 50% or more of the vein diameter. A Chi-square test was performed to identify which characteristics were correlated with a temporal location of the AVM. The level of significance was $P=0.05$.

Results

A statistically significant correlation was found between temporal location of the AVM and a clinical presentation of epilepsy ($P=0.05$). A higher rate of the three following

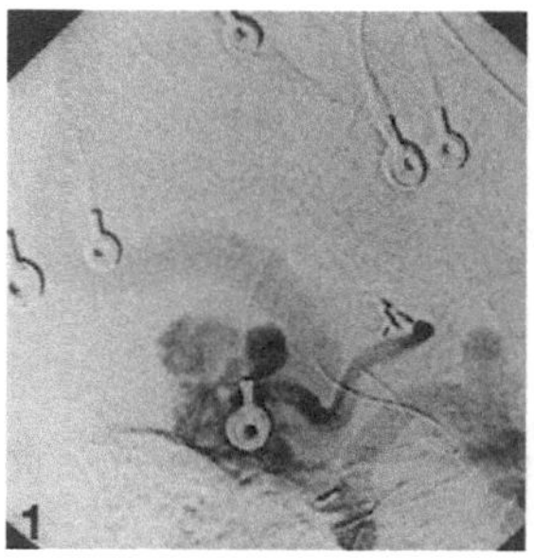

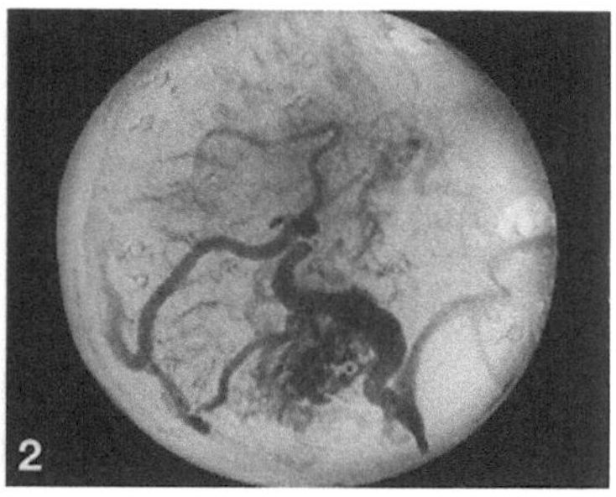

Fig. 1. Right temporal arteriovenous malformation: superselective angiogram after microcatherization of a temporal posterior artery shows a direct fistula within the nidus

Fig. 2. Right lateral angiogram, venous phas of right temporal AVM: impairment of the venous drainage with varix and venous stenosis is demonstrated

angiographic characteristics was demonstrated for temporal AVM than for AVM at other lobar locations: presence of fistula inside the AVM nidus (52% vs 44%), presence of venous stenosis in the venous drainage (66% vs 58%) and presence of varix (66% vs 58%). Amongst these three angio-architectural characteristics the presence of fistula was the only statistically significant parameter ($P=0.04$)

Discussion

Epilepsy is usually the second most common clinical presentation of AVMS, the most common being hemorrhage [6–8]. Our data indicate a correlation between epilepsy and a temporal location of an AVM – findings also obtained by Yeh et al. [9].

We were able to demonstrate a high rate (52%) of intranidal fistulae. These fistulae are more frequent in temporal locations than in any other lobar locations. The presence of direct arteriovenous communication without an intervening arterial network (fistula) may be suspected on a conventional angiogram when there is a combination of asymmetrical enlargement of an arterial feeder with a large varix. They are usually present within a nidus. Viñuela et al. [3] have emphasized the important potential therapeutic implications of this finding. Sudden occlusion of one or more of these fistulae may produce sudden hemodynamic changes in the surrounding AVM, which can lead to postembolization hemorrhage of the AVM. The possibility of hemorrhage can be reduced by staging the embolization.

Difficulties in temporal AVM surgery have been emphasised by several groups. They usually identify two groups in this particular location, medial and external temporal AVM. The external temporal AVMs are usually easier to remove surgically.

Heros [10] reported three malformations in obscure locations on the medial aspect of the temporal lobe involving the choroidal fissure and lying adjacent to the basal ganglion and internal capsule; he specifically noted the difficulties in exposing these lesions during surgery. Drake [11] reported six medial temporal lobe AVMs and their surgical management. Stein [12] described surgical techniques for AVMs located on the medial aspect of the hemisphere. Amongst them, three were located in the amygdaloid nucleus and uncus, and four in the parahippocampal fusiform gyrus region.

Conclusion

The study of the angioarchitecture of temporal AVMs using superselective angiography demonstrated a significantly higher rate of fistulae than in other locations. The presence of these direct AV communications in association with nidus is important for the endovascular therapist. The therapeutic occlusion of fistulae using the usual mixture may lead to inadvertent occlusion of the venous side, carrying a risk of post-embolization bleeding. We believe that these fistulae must be demonstrated with special attention during superselective angiography in temporal AVMs. When they are present, the time allowed for polymerization of the embolization mixture must be adapted.

References

1. Willinsky R, Lasjaunias P, Terbrugge K, Pruvost P (1988) Brain arteriovenous malformations: analysis of the angioarchitecture in relationship to hemorrhage (based on 152 patients explored and/or treated at the hospital Bicêtre between 1981 and 1986). J Neuroradiol 15:225–237
2. Lasjaunias P, Manelfe C, Chui M (1986) Angiographic architecture of intracranial AVMs and fistulas: pretherapeutic aspects. Neurosurg Rev 9:253–263
3. Viñuela F (1986) Identification of an arteriovenous fistula in arteriovenous malformations (abstract). AJNR 7:553
4. Viñuela F, Drake CG, Fox AJ, Pelz DM (1987) Giant intracranial varices secondary to high-flow arteriovenous fistulae. J Neurosurg 66:198–203
5. Viñuela F, Nombela F, Roach MR et al (1985) Stenotic and occlusive disease of the venous drainage system of deep brain AVM's. J Neurosurg 63:180–184
6. Brown RB Jr, Wiebers DO, Forbes GS (1990) Unruptured intracranial aneurysms and arteriovenous malformations: frequency of intracranial hemorrhage and relationship of lesions. J Neurosurg 73:859–863
7. Crawford PM, West CW, Chadwick DW, Shaw MDM (1986) Arteriovenous malformations of the brain: natural history in unoperated patients. J Neurol Neurosurg Psychiatry 49:1–10
8. Stein BM (1984) Arteriovenous malformations of the medial cerebral hemisphere and the limbic system. J Neurosurg 60:23–31
9. Yeh HS, Kashiwagi S, Tew JM Jr, Berger TS (1990) Surgical management of epilepsy associated with cerebral arteriovenous malformations. J Neurosurg 72:216–223
10. Heros RC (1982) Arteriovenous malformations of the medial temporal lobe. Surgical approach and neuroradiological characterization. J Neurosurg 56:44–52
11. Drake CG (1979) Cerebral arteriovenous malformations: considerations for and experience with surgical treatment in 166 cases. Clin Neurosurg 26:145–208

Venous restrictive disease in cerebral arteriovenous malformations

S. C. Patel[1,2], T. Burke[1], V. Chundi[1], W. Sanders[1], J. Landi[1], B. Mehta[1], G. Malik[2]

[1] Section of Neuroradiology, Henry Ford Hospital, 2799 W. Grand Blvd., Detroit, MI 48202, USA
[2] Department of Neurosurgery, Henry Ford Hospital, 2799 W. Grand Blvd., Detroit, MI 48292, USA

Abstract. In a review of 151 patients with cerebral anterovenous malformations we found venous stenosis or occlusion in 69 cases (46%); involving the deep or superficial systems with approximately equal frequency. Although patients with uniquely deep venous drainage tended to have bled, there was no clear evidence that venous restrictive changes promoted hemorrhage.

Key words: Cerebral, arteriovenous malformations – Venous occlusion – Venous stenosis – Hemorrhage

The morbidity and mortality of brain arteriovenous malformations (AVM) are often related to the occurrence of hemorrhage. Many morphological factors are implicated in increased incidence of hemorrhage in patients with AVM. These include large size of the nidus, deep location of the AVM, central venous drainage, intranidal aneurysm, venous stenosis, and occlusion, and presence of a single draining vein only for AVM [1–3]. It is presumed that most of the hemorrhages in AVM occur as a result of the rupture of the AMV nidus near the venous end [2]. For this reason, the venous system of the AVM is being increasingly scrutinized for morphological changes. Due to increased intraluminal pressure transmitted through the arteriovenous shunt of the AVM nidus, the draining veins undergo morphological changes that result in tortuosity, elongation, and irregularity of the venous walls, probably resulting from the endothelial damage. The increased incidence of stenosis and occlusion of the draining veins in AVM is probably the result of a combination of these morphologic changes. It has been postulated that venous restriction might alter the natural history of AVM, possibly increasing the risk of intracranial hemorrhage [4–6]. Recently, the increased incidence of morbidity and mortality following endovascular therapy and/or surgical excision of AVMs has been found in patients with venous restrictive disease in AVM [5]. To evaluate the incidence of stenotic and occlusive process involving the venous system in arteriovenous malformations, we are reporting our experience with 151 patients.

Materials and methods

Retrospective reviews of the cerebral angiograms of 230 patients were carried out. Seventy-nine patients were excluded because of incomplete angiography on medical records and 151 patients with AVMs were reviewed. All patients had magnification cerebral angiography; the medical records were checked for documentation of hemorrhage on presentation in each case. The following lesion characteristics were evaluated by angiography: location, type (pial or mixed pial-dural), volume of the nidus (AP diameter × height on the lateral projection × transverse diameter on frontal projection), arterial aneurysm (berry or flow-related), flow dynamics (slow or fast), pattern of venous drainage (superficial, deep or combined superficial and deep), number of draining veins (single or multiple), and venous abnormality, such as stenosis, occlusion, venous aneurysm or venous wall irregularity.

Correspondence to: S. C. Patel

Results

Of the 151 patients, 78 patients were male and 73 patients were female: the age was 11–74 years. One hundred and twenty-eight patients (85%) had pial arteriovenous malformation, while 23 (15%) had mixed pial-dural arteriovenous malformation. Seventy patients presented with intracranial hemorrhage, while 42 patients had history of headache or AVMs that were discovered incidentally. Thirty-two patients had seizure disorder. Six patients presented with subarachnoid hemorrhage as the result of a congenital berry aneurysm rupture documented at surgery. Venous stenosis and occlusion were seen in 69 of the 151 patients (46%). Venous stenosis-occlusion was present in 42% (29 of 69 patients) and involved the deep venous system. Venous stenosis-occlusion involving the superficial venous system was seen in 40 of the 69 patients (58%). Venous aneurysms were seen in 39 patients, while venous wall irregularity was seen in only 31 patients. Hemorrhage was seen in 70 patients in the entire group of 151 patients. In the venous stenosis-occlusion group, hemorrhage was only seen in 33 patients, while the incidence of hemorrhage in the nonstenotic group was only 41% (37 of 90 patients). There was no statistically significant difference in the incidence of hemorrhage between the venous stenosis-occlusion group and nonstenotic group.

The pattern of venous drainage of the arteriovenous malformation, venous drainage associated with stenosis and its relation with hemorrhage was also evaluated. Twenty-five percent (39 of 151 patients) had deep venous drainage of arteriovenous malformation. In this group, 67% (26 of 39 patients) showed evidence of hemorrhage. Forty-eight percent of the total sample (72 of 151 patients) showed superficial venous drainage. Of these patients, 38% (28 of 72 patients) showed evidence of hemorrhage. Twenty-six percent (40 of 151 patients) had combined (both superficial and deep) venous drainage. Of the patients in this group, 38% (16 of 39 patients) showed evidence of hemorrhage. Chi-square analysis revealed that here is an statistically significant correlation between deep venous drainage and hemorrhage; patients with deep venous drainage thus appeared to be at a greater risk of hemorrhage than those with combined venous drainage or superficial venous drainage ($P<0.01$).

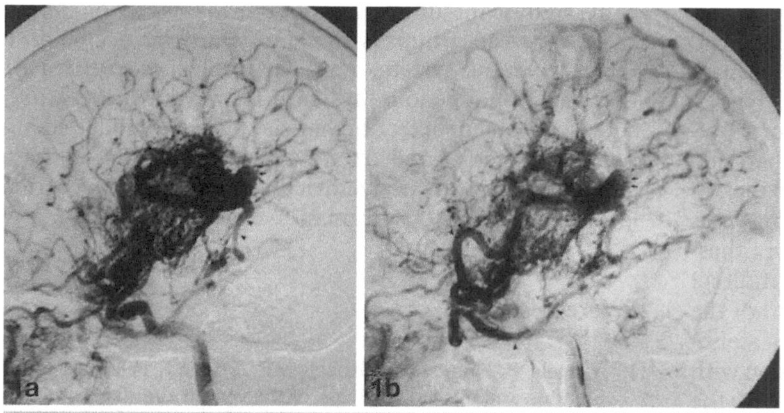

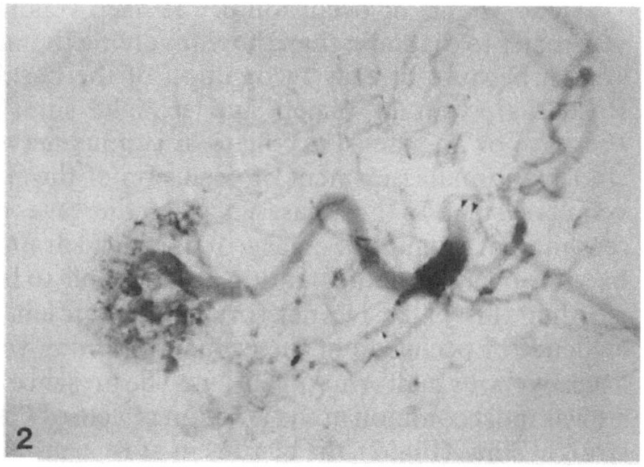

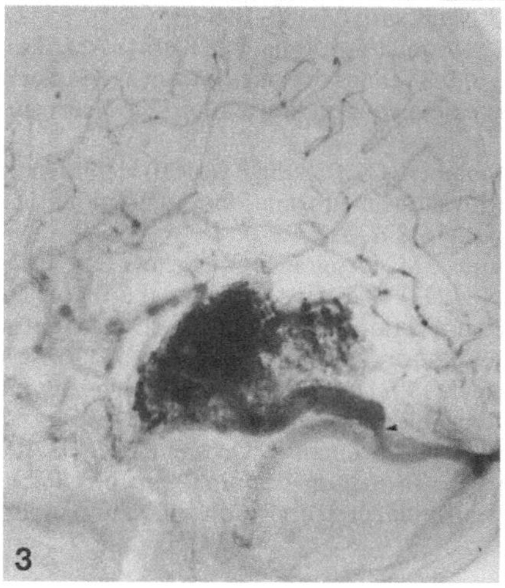

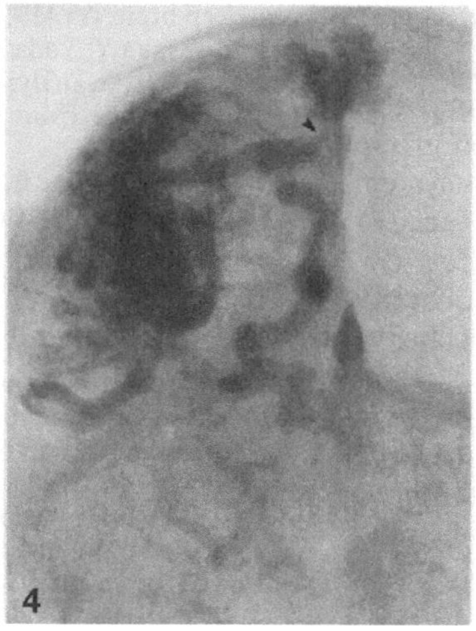

Fig. 1a, b. Internal carotid angiogram showing large thalamic and basal ganglion AVM. There is complete occlusion of the vein of Galen *(small arrows)* with retrograde opacification of the basal vein of Rosenthal and extensive collateral venous channels *(arrowheads)*.

Fig. 2. Carotid angiogram of basal ganglion AVM. There is high-grade stenosis of the junction of the vein of Galen and straight sinus *(large arrowheads)*. Extensive venous collaterals *(small arrows)* and retrograde opacification of the basal veins of Rosenthal *(small arrowheads)*

Fig. 3. Carotid angiogram showing a moderate size temporal lobe AVM and high-grade stenosis *(arrowheads)* of the large draining vein at its junction with the transverse sinus

Fig. 4. Carotic angiogram showing parietal AVM with high-grade stenosis *(arrowhead)* of the draining vein at its junction with the superior sagittal sinus

Those patients with deep venous drainage and superficial venous drainage were compared for venous stenosis and their relationship to hemorrhage. Fifty-five percent (16 of 29 patients) with stenosis of the deep venous drainage showed evidence of hemorrhage whereas 43% (17 of 40 patients) with stenosis of superficial venous drainage showed evidence of hemorrhage. Approximately 41% (37 of 90 patients) presented with hemorrhage without stenosis which was statistically insignificant. The location of AVM was also correlated with incidence of hemorrhage in relationship of venous stenosis to hemorrhage. Sixty-nine percent of the total sample (44 of 151 patients) had lobar arteriovenous malformation. Forty-two percent of these patients (44 of 104 patients) showed evidence of hemorrhage at presentation. Forty-seven percent of these patients with hemorrhage (49 of 104 patients) demonstrated evidence of venous stenosis, and 45% (42) of these showed evidence of hemorrhage. Seventeen percent of the patients (26 of 151 patients) presented with deep-seated AVMs (basal ganglia, thalamus, intraventricular and/or periventricular). Of this group, 69% (28 of 26 patients) presented with hemorrhage. Sixty-two percent of patients with deep-seated AVMs (16 of 26 patients) also demonstrated evidence of venous stenosis. Fifty-six percent of the patients (9 of 16 patients) with similar venous stenosis demonstrated hemorrhage. Eleven percent of the total group (16 of 151 patients) demonstrated infratentorial arteriovenous malformation. Of this group, 44% (7 of 16 patients) presented with hemorrhage. Twenty-five percent (4 of 16 patients) showed evidence of venous stenosis, 50% (2 of 4 patients) of those patients with venous stenosis of an infratentorial AVM demonstrated evidence of hemorrhage at presentation.

Discussion

The incidence of venous restrictive disease in our series is quite high, approaching 46%. The incidence of stenotic lesions was higher (58%) in the superficial system than in the deep venous system (42%).

Stenosis and/or occlusion of the deep venous system was easier to diagnose than those involving the superficial system because of easy recognition of the basal vein of Rosenthal, vein of Galen and straight sinus (Fig. 1). Presence of an extensive collateral venous network precludes optimal assessment of occlusion of the superficial venous system. In those cases in which there was extensive recruitment of multiple enlarged superficial draining veins by arteriovenous malformation, it is possible to hypothesize that this extensive network may represent indirect evidence of occlusion of the primary draining vein of the arteriovenous malformation nidus. The presence of stenosis was most common at the junction of vein of Galen with straight sinus (Fig. 2), the basal vein of Rosenthal with the vein of Galen and the superficial cortical vein with the dural venous sinuses, such as the transverse sinus and the superior sagittal sinus (Figs. 3, 4). The elaborate network of venous collaterals in the stenotic and occlusion group involving both the deep and the superficial venous system indicate a gradually evolving process. Surgical and/or endovascular intervention might abruptly alter flow dynamics, which may be the cause of increased morbidity and mortality due to a phenomenon known as occlusive hyperemia, as suggested in recent reports [4, 5].

A review of the statistics on the incidence of hemorrhage revealed no statistically significant differences between the stenotic and/or occlusion group and the nonstenotic occlusion group. In fact, the incidence of hemorrhage was slightly higher in the nonstenotic occlusion group. The Chi-square analysis failed to show any statistically significant differences in the incidence of hemorrhage between groups with stenotic and/or occlusion of the deep venous system, the superficial venous system and the combined venous system. However, there was a significant incidence of higher risk of hemorrhage identified in the deep-seated arteriovenous malformation (basal ganglia, thalamus, periventricular and/or intraventricular) with deep venous drainage.

References

1. Viñuela F, Nombela L, Roach MR, Fox AJ, Pelz DM (1985) Stenotic and occlusive disease of the venous drainage system of deep brain AVM's. J Neurosurg 63:180–184
2. Miyasaka Y, Yada K, Ohwada T, Kitahara T, Kurata A, Irikura K (1992) An analysis of the venous drainage system as a factor in hemorrhage from arteriovenous malformations. J Neurosurg 76:239–243
3. Marks MP, Lane B, Steinberg GK, Chang PJ (1990) Hemorrhage in intracerebral arteriovenous malformations: angiographic determinants. Radiology 176:807–813
4. Al-Rodhan NRF, Sundt TM, Piepgras DG, Nichols DA, Rufenacht D, Stevens LN (1993) Occlusive hyperemia: a theory for the hemodynamic complications following resection of intracerebral arteriovenous malformations. J Neurosurg 78:167–175
5. Wilson CB, Hieshima G (1993) Occlusive hyperemia: a new was to think about an old problem. J Neurosurg 78:165–166
7. Young WL, Kader A, Pile-Spellman J, Ornstein E, Stein BM (1994) Arteriovenous malformation draining vein physiology and determinants of transnidal pressure gradients. Neurosurgery 35:389–396

Arteriovenous malformations of the brain: risk of first bleeding, rebleeding and related risk factors in 168 untreated patients

S. Perini [1], G. Talamini [2], A. Pasqualin [3], M. G. Pecoraro [1], R. Da Pian [3], A. Benati [1]

[1] Department of Neuroradiology, City Hospital, Verona, Italy
[2] Department of Biostatistics and Epidemiology, Medical Clinics Institute, University of Verona, Italy
[3] Department of Neurosurgery, City Hospital, Verona, Italy

Abstract. A long-term follow-up study of 168 patients with untreated arteriovenous malformations (AVMs) who were admitted to the neurosurgical departments of Verona and Padua was conducted to evaluate the risk of bleeding and rebleeding of the cerebral AVMs. Two different prospective (historical) trials were performed in two groups of patients. The risk of first bleeding was evaluated in a first group of 71 patients who had never bled before: mean bleeding risk was 2.8% per year. The risk of rebleeding was evaluated in a second group of 107 patients who had had one previous haemorrhage: the risk of bleeding was 3.5% per year. In 41 patients who had survived a second haemorrhage, a 7.7% mean risk of a third haemorrhage was observed. The risk of death was 1.3%, 1.6% and 3%, respectively, in the three groups.

Key words: Arteriovenous malformations – Intracranial haemorrhage – Risk of haemorrhage – Natural history – Risk of bleeding

Correspondence to: S. Perini, Servizio di Neuroradiologia, Ospedale Maggiore, Piazale Stefani 1, I-37126, Verona, Italy

The aim of the present study was to evaluate the risk of bleeding and rebleeding in patients with untreated arteriovenous malformations (AVMs), to identify anatomical and clinical parameters affecting the severity of bleeding, and to compare our results with recent data in the literature [1–4].

Materials and methods

A group of 168 untreated patients admitted to the Neurosurgical Departments of Verona and Padua from 1952 to 1993 with the diagnosis of cerebral AVM was selected and analysed in a long-term follow-up study. In all cases, diagnosis was obtained by angiography and (in more recent ones) by CT and MRI. Patients had been diagnosed as untreatable or had refused surgical or neuroradiological treatment. Follow-up evaluation was achieved during a median period of 15 years (range 1–40) and was continued until surgery, embolization or death.

Our group comprised 96 males (57%) and 72 females (43%); mean age at diagnosis was 31.69 years (min 2, max 69). The early symptoms were a haemorrhage in 58% of cases and seizures in 38%; headache or other symptoms were present in 4% of cases. The sites of the lesions were as follows: frontal 10 (6%); rolandic 31 (18.4%); posterior parietal 14 (8.5%); occipital 11 (6.5%); temporal 27 (16%); posterior limbic 11 (6.5%); callosal-cyngular 21 (12.5%); insular 5 (3%); basal ganglia 25 (15%); cerebellar 10 (6%); brainstem 1 (0.6%); other 2 (1%).

The size of the AVM was evaluated on the angiogram on the basis of its volume. The group of 168 patients was subdivided into four volume subgroups: (a) small AVMs < 10 ml: 64 (38%); (b) medium AVMs, 11–20 ml: 34 (20.5%); (c) large AVMs, 21–50 ml: 49 (29%); (d) giant AVMs, > 50 ml: 21 (12.5%).

The risk of haemorrhage was evaluated in our population (168 patients) following two different prospective (historical) trials, one to evaluate the risk of first bleeding and the other to assess that of rebleeding. The follow-up period started at angiography, which was performed in every patient for the diagnosis of cerebral AVM (and complemented in more recent cases with CT and MRI); in all cases the end-point was haemorrhage. The mortality rate and death risk were also evaluated in both trials.

The risk of bleeding (first haemorrhage) was evaluated in a group of 71 patients (group 1) diagnosed before any haemorrhage and observed from angiography to the first bleeding during a median follow-up periof of 8.5 years (range 1–29).

The risk of rebleeding was established in a group of 107 patients (group 2), including the patients diagnosed by angiography at first haemorrhage (97 cases) and those out of the first group who survived the first haemorrhage (10 cases). The patients were observed to evaluate the risk of a second haemorrhage during a median follow-up period of 15 years (range 2–40). We considered as rebleeding any haemorrhage occurring at least 6 months after the first. The risk of third bleeding was evaluated in a subgroup of 41 patients out of the group of 52 patients who survived a second haemorrhage; the remaining 11 patients were lost to follow-up for surgery and/or embolisation, and 1 died during the follow-up for causes unrelated to AVM. The risk of third bleeding was evaluated during a median follow-up period of 10.8 years (range 1–32).

Age, sex, clinical symptoms at onset, AVM volume and site, feeding arteries, concomitant aneurysms and drainage veins were evaluated as possible risk factors and related to the bleeding and rebleeding rates. Venous drainage was classified as superficial or deep, and its extent classified into 4 grades: (1) single non-ectatic vein; (2) single ectatic vein with or without other non-ectatic veins; (3) multiple ectatic veins with or without huge venous dilatation; (4) extensive hemispheric drainage.

Statistical analysis was performed according to Kaplan and Meier survical curves and the Cox model for study of the Odds ratio. Our study is not free of selection bias or from censored data related to "drop-out", death from unknown causes or successive therapy in subjects previously untreated.

Results

In group 1 (71 patients) haemorrhage occurred in 17 of 71 cases (24%); 50% of patients bled during a 17.6-year period, with a mean bleeding risk of 2.8% per year (Fig. 1); death was observed in 5 of 71 cases (7%) and was related in all cases to first haemorrhage; 19% of patients died during a 16-year period, with a mean mortality risk of 1.2% per year (Fig. 4).

In group 2 (107 patients), a second haemorrhage occurred in 61 of 107 cases (57%); 10% of patients rebled during the first year; 5% during the second year; 50% during a 14-year period, which means an approximate mean rebleeding risk of 3.5% per year (Fig. 2). In this group, 9 of 107 patients (8.5%) died because of the second haemorrhage and 28 of 107 (26%) died during the follow-up period of causes related to the AVM; 50% of these patients died during a 28.8-year period, with a mean mortality risk of approximately 1.6% per year (Fig. 4). In the subgroup of 41 patients available for evaluation of the risk of third haemorrhage, a third bleeding was observed in 32 of 41 cases (78%); 22.5% bled during the first 2 years; 50% of patients had a third haemorrhage during a 6.5-year period with an approximate mean rebleeding risk of 7.7% per year (Fig. 3). Death due to third bleeding occurred in 14 of 41 (35%), and 18 of 41 patients (44%) died during the follow-up period of causes related to AVM; 50% of patients died after a 16.7 year period with a mean mortality risk for third bleeding of 3% per year (Fig. 4).

Overall censored data related to drop-out were as follows: drop-out, 8; death from unknown causes, 14; subsequent therapy in previously untreated patients, 39.

In the analysis of risk factors, the variables considered (age, sex, symptoms at onset, location of the AVM, type and number of arterial feeders, concomitant aneurysms, deep or superficial draining veins) did not significantly influence bleeding or rebleeding rates. The analysis of relative risk by Cox model gave an statistical trend for the variable "AVM volume > 20 ml" as a risk factor for a first haemorrhage ($P < 0.056$), and for the variable "extensive venous drainage" as a risk factor for a second haemorrhage ($P < 0.043$). Subsequent analysis with survival curves did not confirm these trends.

Discussion

On the basis of our results, the mean risk of a first bleeding from a brain AVM is 2.8% and the rebleeding risk, 3.5% per year (10% during the 1st year and 5% during the 2nd year after rebleeding). In our study the mean risk of first bleeding is basically the same as that reported by Graf (2%–3% per year), Crawford (risk of SAH 2% per year) and Brown (2.2% per year). A moderate increase in risk was observed during the 1st and 2nd year afer a haemorrhage (10% and 5%) compared with Graf's results (6% in the 1st year and then 2% per year). Moreover, our rates are lower than those reported by Ondra (bleeding and rebleeding risk of 4% per year). The average risk of a third bleeding in our series is 7.7% per year (13% in the 1st year after rebleeding). This underlines an important increase in the risk of haemorrhage compared with the other two groups of patients. Although a selection bias undoubtedly exists for this group of patients, who had not undergone any treatment and whose clinical condition was severe, we believe that the risk of a third haemorrhage is considerably

1
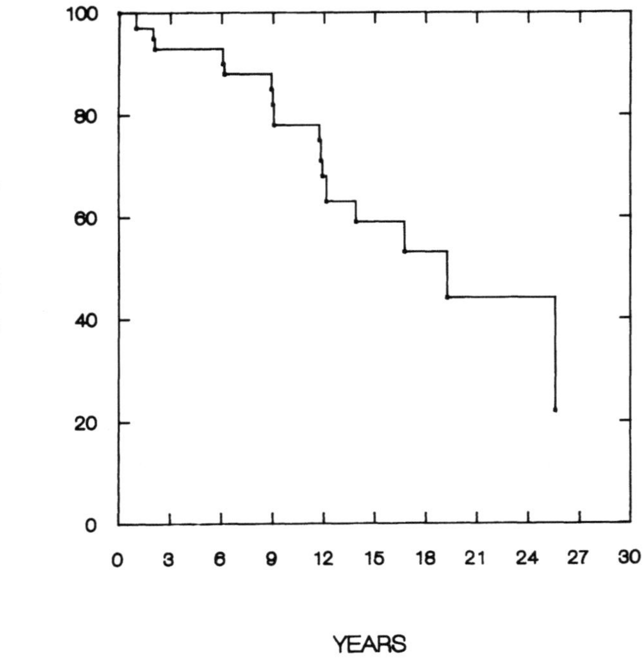

2
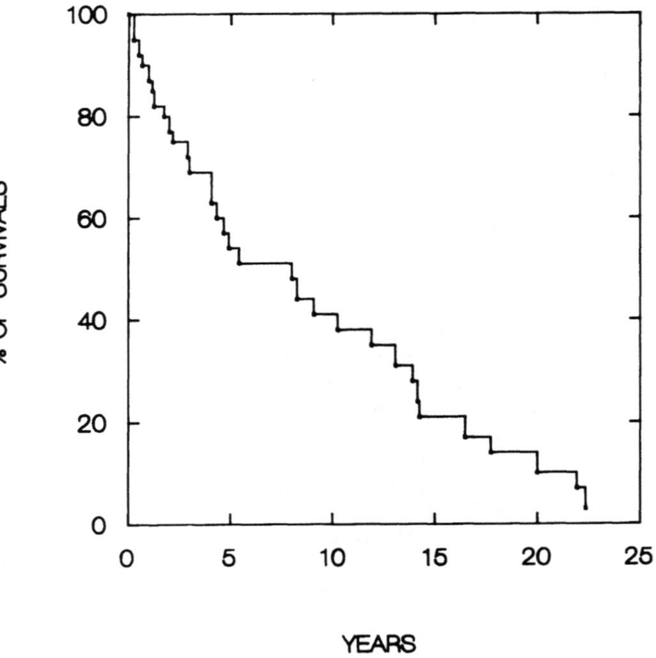

3
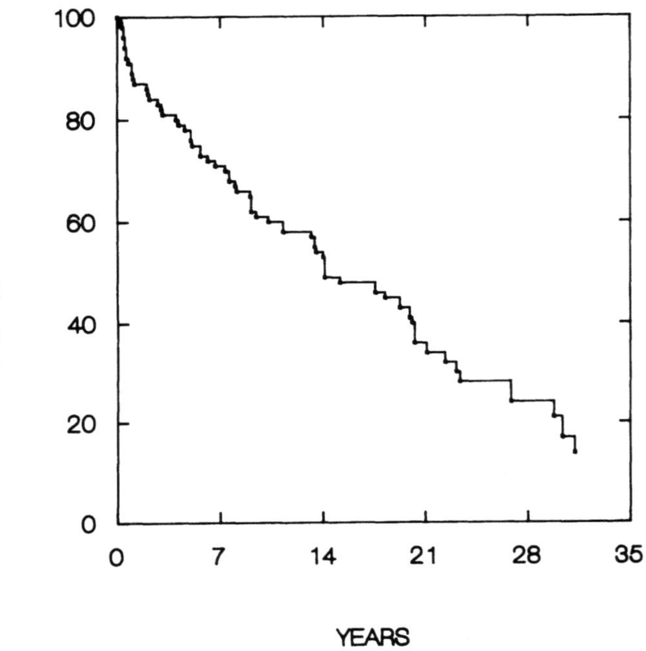

4
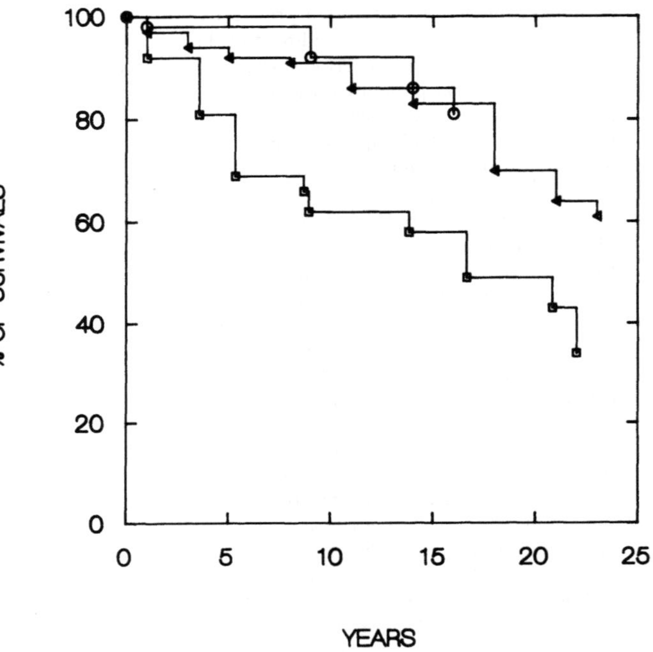

Fig. 1. Risk of first bleeding. The slope shows a basically straight trend; 50% of patients had a bleeding in 17.6 years

Fig. 2. Risk of second bleeding. The survival curve shows a basically straight trend with the exception of a steeper initial slope corresponding to a higher rate of rebleeding in the 1st year

Fig. 3. Risk of third bleeding. The survival curve has two slopes: the first is steeper because of a very high bleeding rate during a 6.5 year period (50% of patients bled); the slope then becomes more gradual

Fig. 4. Risk of death. The mortality risk does not differ significantly between the first and second groups (*circles* and *triangles*), while a considerable increase in risk is evident in the third *(squares)*

higher than previously thought (only Crawford reports a 58% risk of a further haemorrhage within 15 years in a group of patients who had previously experienced more than one haemorrhage).

The risk of death for groups 1, 2 and 3 in the present study was 1.2%, 1.6% and 3%, respectively (Ondra: 1%). The increased risk of bleeding in the second group in comparison with the first (3.5% vs. 2.8%), does not imply a similar increase in mortality risk. In fact, we observed a remarkable increase in the risk of death (3%) in our third group, confirming the severity of recurrent haemorrhage in the prognosis of brain AVMs. Our results are based on a small number of patients (41). Definitive conclusions on this point will be subject to the evaluation of a larger group of patients for risk of a third haemorrhage.

Acknowledgements. We are grateful to Professor S. Mingrino, Head of the Neurosurgical Department of the University of Padua for allowing us access to his archives.

References

1. Graf CJ, Perret GE, Torner JC (1983) Bleeding from cerebral arteriovenous malformations as a part of their natural history. J Neurosurg 58:331–337
2. Crawford PM, West CR, Chadwick DW, Shaw MDM (1986) Arteriovenous malformations of the brain: natural history in unoperated patients. J Neurol Neurosurg Psychiatry 49:1–10
3. Brown RD Jr, Wiebers DO, Forbes G, O'Fallon WM, Piepgras DG, Marsh R, Maciunas RJ (1988) The natural history of unruptured intracranial arteriovenous malformations. J Neurosurg 68:352–357
4. Ondra SL, Troupp H, George ED, Schwab K (1990) The natural history of symptomatic arteriovenous malformations of the brain: a 24 year follow-up assessment. J Neurosurg 73:387–391

Effect of presence and removal of angiomas on regional cerebral blood flow, as assessed by stable xenon CT

D. Van Roost[1], J. Schramm[1], L. Solymosi[2]

[1] Neurochirurgische Universitätsklinik Bonn, Germany
[2] Neuroradiologie, Radiologische Universitätsklinik, Bonn, Germany

Abstract. In 19 patients with a cerebral arteriovenous malformation (AVM), the regional cerebral blood flow (rCBF) was assessed by means of xenon-enhanced CT (Xe/CT) before and after resection of the AVM. Each assessment comprised an acetazolamide challenge in order to check the cerebrovascular reserve capacity. Scanning through the AVM was purposely avoided, but a single brain slice at the level of the basal ganglia was examined. Five regions of interest (ROIs) in grey matter of the AVM-bearing hemisphere were compared with the corresponding contralateral regions. Interhemispherical differences exceeding 20% of the contralateral value, in either the positive or the negative direction, were considered as significant. AVM-related (AVM-R) and AVM-non-related (AVM-NR) ROIs were looked at separately. Before surgery, very different rCBF patterns were found, including a normal rCBF as well as a reduced or an increased rCBF, in AVM-R, or AVM-NR, or both. After AVM removal, an rCBF increase in AVM-R is relatively rare, whereas an rCBF decrease is a relatively frequent event. A fall in rCBF to a level of impaired reserve capacity correlates with the occurrence of a postoperative neurological deficit.

Key words: Arteriovenous malformation – Cerebral blood flow – Computed tomography – Xenon Surgery

An AVM can lead to changes in the rCBF, the most likely of which are expected to be steal phenomena and a hypoperfusion [1], while luxury perfusion is also a theoretical possibility. The vascular territory that shares its supply with the AVM should be the most susceptible to such changes. Reverse changes of the rCBF after surgical or endovascular treatment of an AVM are equally well imaginable. In 19 patients, we studied the rCBF and its postulated changes before and after angioma excision.

Correspondence to: D. Van Roost, Neurochirurgische Universitätsklinik, Sigmund-Freud-Strasse 25, D-53127 Bonn, Germany

Patients and methods

Nineteen patients with a mean age of 38 (range 17–66 years) were examined. They presented mainly with seizures or with an intracerebral haemorrhage and harboured AVMs at different locations and varying in size and in configuration of their arterial feeders and venous drainage. According to the grading scale of Spetzler and Martin [2], which reflects the risk at surgery, 6 AVMs each corresponded to grade 1 and 2 respectively, 5 AVMs corresponded to grade 3 and 1 AVM to grade 4. For the assessment of rCBF, we used the method of stable-xenon CT (Xe/CT), consisting of an Anzai-Sogyo closed inhalation system and a Siemens Somatom DRH computer tomograph The specific parameters were a xenon concentration of 28% vol and a combined wash-in/wash-out measurement of 4 min each. Each XE/CT study comprised measurement at rest and again after Diamox (acetazolamide) challenge. The latter causes powerful cerebral vasodilatation and enables the cerebrovascular reserve capacity to be checked [3].

Because the recording of more than one brain slice per study was problematic from a technical point of view with our equipment, we purposely did not choose the single studied slice through the AVM nidus, but through morphologically unaffected brain. Indeed, even if the methodological problem of ROIs that only encompass blood vessel lumina is disregarded, we were not interested in the perfusion of the angiomatous vessel lumina but rather in the perfusion of the brain tissue at distance from the AVM. We were especially interested in the brain that is supplied by the same large vessels as the AVM, whether by transient or by parallel arteries. Therefore, we preferentially selected the single measurable brain slice at the basal ganglia level, where the image discloses all supratentorial vascular territories at a glance. Five ROI in grey matter of the AVM-bearing hemisphere were compared with the corresponding contralateral regions; these were the thalamus, the head of the caudate nucleus, and the territories of the anterior, middle and posterior cerebral arteries. In most cases, the study was performed shortly before surgery (9–10 days) and repeated 1–4 weeks after surgery. Xe/CT studies provided absolute rCBF values expressed in ml/100 g brain tissue per min. The interpretation of the figures was not always simple, however.

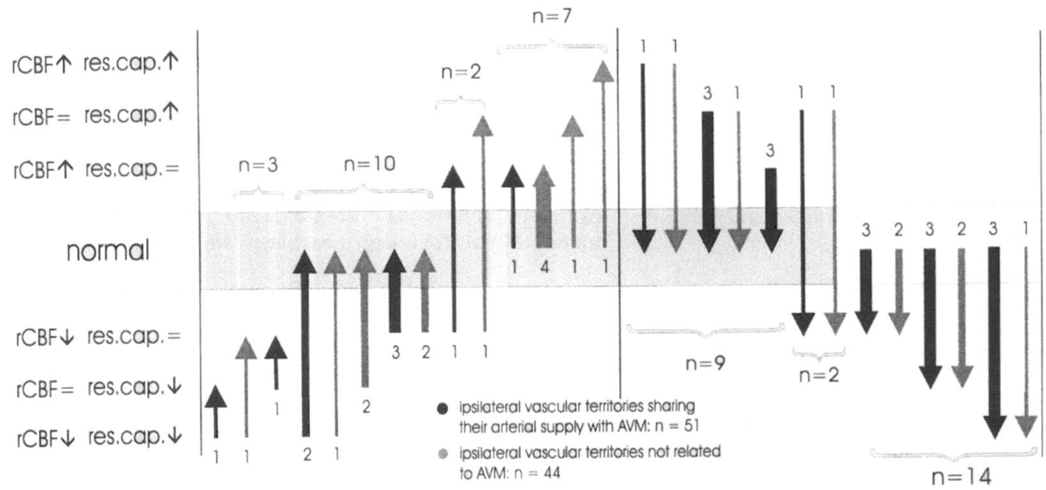

Fig. 1. Changes of rCBF and reserve capacity in surgically treated AVM patients, pre- and postoperatively (tail and head of *arrows*, respectively). The *arrows* thus represent the different types of change that occurred, the *figures* and the *thickness* of the *arrows* indicating the number of ROIs in which they were observed. The total number of ROIs studied in 95, divided into 51 AVM-related and 44 AVM-non-related ROIs. The *arrows* represent only those ROIs in which the rCBF was not normal, either pre- or postoperatively. Res. cap, Reserve capacity

From studies in normal volunteers, we learned that there was a definite decline in cerebral blood flow with age, although with broad normal ranges, and there was quite some variation in cerebral blood flow over time. For this reason, we did not compare the absolute rCBF figures, but concentrated on comparison of interhemispherical differences exceeding 20% in either direction. We believe that only clear-cut asymmetries between the hemispheres within one study can be considered as indicative for pathology.

Results

Figure 1 summarises the results. Out of a total of 95 ROIs, only those with pre- or postoperative rCBF aberrations were displayed. ROIs that share their supply with the AVM (AVM-R, $n=51$) and those that do not (AVM-NR, $n=45$) were considered separately. Each arrow represents a number (1–4) of ROIs: the initial (preoperative) rCBF and the final (postoperative) rCBF. Preoperative hypoperfusion was found in 15 of the 95 ROIs, 8 of which were in AVM-R and 7 in AVM-NR. Impaired reserve capacity occurred in 4 AVM-R and in 4 AVM-NRs. Postoperatively, the rCBF recovered and reached normal values in 5 AVM-R and 5 AVM-NR. In 1 AVM-R and 1 AVM-NR preoperative hypoperfusion gave way to postoperative hyperperfusion. Preoperative hyperperfusion was found in 11 of the 95 ROIs, 8 of which were in AVM-R and 3 in AVM-NR. Postoperatively, the rCBF decreased to normal values in 7 AVM-R and in only 2 AVM-NR. The rCBF changed from better to worse than normal in 1 AVM-R and 1 AVM-NR. In 14 ROIs, 9 of which were in AVM-R and 5 in AVM-NR, the rCBF dropped from normal to lowered values. In particular, a postoperative rCBF at a level of impaired reserve capacity was found to correlate with the occurrence of a new neurological deficit. In two cases, such a hypoperfusion was due to postoperative vasospasms, as proven by Doppler sonography. In these two cases, the showed, irrespective of its preoperative level, rCBF a downward change in all 5 ipsilateral ROIs. In non-vasospastic cases, a hypoperfusion with impaired reserve capacity was confined to AVM-R.

Xe/CT discloses very different patterns of rCBF in AVM patients before surgery, including a normal rCBF as well as a reduced or an increased rCBF, in AVM-R or AVM-NR ROIs, or in both. A postoperative rCBF increase in an AVM-R ROI ($n=9/51$, 18%) was less frequent than in an AVM-NR ROI ($n=13/44$, 30%), whereas conversely, a decrease of rCBF was more frequent in an AVM-R ROI ($n=17/51$, 33%) than in an AVM-NR ROI ($n=8/44$, 18%). A postoperative drop of rCBF to a level of impaired reserve capacity correlated with the occurrence of a new neurological deficit. This was observed in 6 of 51 AVM-R ROIs (12%) and, in association with vasospasm only, for 3 of 44 AVM-NR ROIs (7%).

References

1. Okabe T, Meyer JS, Okayasu H, Harper R, Rose J, Grossman RG, Centeno R, Tachibana H, Lee YY (1983) Xenon-enhanced CT CBF measurements in cerebral AVMs before and after excision. J Neurosurg 59:21–31
2. Spetzler RF, Martin NA (1986) A proposed grading system for arteriovenous malformations. J Neurosurg 65:476–483
3. Tarr RW, Johnson DW, Rutigliano M, Hecht ST, Pentheny S, Jungreis CA, Horton JA, Yonas H (1990) Use of acetazolamide-challenge xenon CT in the assessment of cerebral blood flow dynamics in patients with arteriovenous malformations. AJNR 11:441–448

Haemodynamics of cerebral arteriovenous malformations investigated by dynamic CT

M. Takeshita [1], M. Izawa [1], T. Ishii [1], H. Onda [1], M. Kagawa [1], K. Takakura [1], M. Toyoda [2], N. Kobayashi [2]

[1] Department of Neurosurgery, Neurological Institute, Tokyo Women's Medical College, Kawada-cho 8-1, Shinjuku-ku Tokyo 162, Japan
[2] Department of Neuroradiology, Tokyo Women's Medical College, Tokyo, Japan

Abstract. The nidal haemodynamics of cerebral arteriovenous malformations (AVMs) are unclear. We studied them by dynamic CT. Using dynamic CT and gamma-variate curve fitting, appearance times (AT), mean transit times (MTT; first moment transit times) and peak times (PT) were determined for the nidus of an AVM in 33 patients, including 14 patients with haemorrhagic and 19 with epileptic episodes. The nidus of patients with haemorrhagic episodes demonstrated statistically delayed PT ($P<0.01$) and MTT ($P<0.02$) compared with those of patients with epileptic episode. There was, however, no statistical difference between the AT of the nidus in both groups. These results suggest that partial intravascular thrombosis caused by haemorrhage may lead to prolonged MTT and PT.

Key words: Cerebral arteriovenous malformation – Dynamic computer tomography – Haemodynamics

Recent advances in CT have made it possible to study local haemodynamics by estimating the flow of contrast medium through brain tissue with rapid-sequence scanning immediately after the administration of a bolus of contrast material. The present study investigates the usefulness of dynamic CT in studying the nidal haemodynamics of arteriovenous malformations (AVMs) determining flow parameters. We also study the relationships between nidal size, flow parameters and symptoms.

Materials and methods

A total of 33 patients (22 men and 11 women, aged 32.4 ± 14.4 years) with AVMs were studied with dynamic CT. All were in the chronic phase (more than 2 months after the onset of symptoms). The first scan of the dynamic study was started simultaneously with the start of the intravenous injection of 50 ml iodinated contrast medium by autoinjector at the rate of 8 ml/s through the antecubital vein. The study was performed at one level, with a 5 mm section thickness, through the centre of the lesion, as determined by a prior static CT examination. The dynamic scanning time was 2 s, with a 2 s interscan delay, and a total of 16 scans (in all, 31 segmental scans) were performed for each patient. The region of interest was outlined so as to enclose the nidus of the AVM. To prepare the functional image (Fig. 1), mean transit time (MTT) peak time (PT) were obtained from a gamma-variated curve by the method of Thompson et al. [1] (Fig. 2). The patients were divided into groups with haemorrhagic or epileptic episodes to examine the relation between these flow parameters of the nidus, the size of the AVM and symptoms and signs.

Correspondence to: M. Takeshita

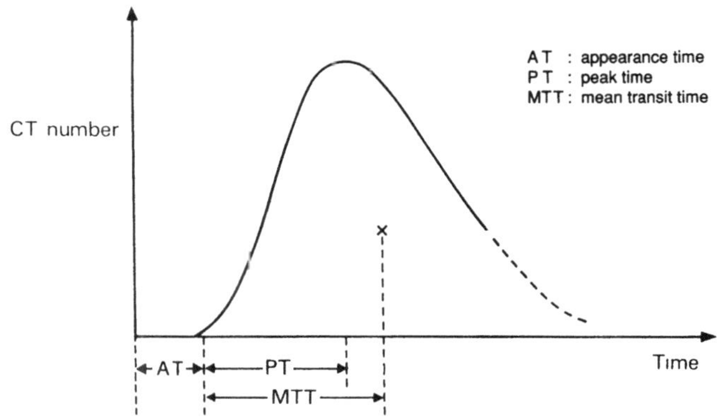

Fig. 1. Gamma-variate fitted time-concentration curve and parameters. AT (appearance time), time from the start of injection to that of curve appearance; *PT* (peak time), time from curve appearance to that of peak appearance; *MTT* (mean transit time), centre of gravity of the shape of the gamma-variate function curve

Results

There were 14 patients in the haemorrhagic episode group and 19 in the epileptic episode group. There was no statistical difference between the nidal maximum diameter between these groups. The nidal MTT and PT of patients with haemorrhagic episodes were 8.91 ± 2.58 and 7.76 ± 2.35 s, and those of patients with epileptic episodes 7.53 ± 2.59 and 6.55 ± 1.83 s. The nidus of patients with haemorrhagic episodes demonstrated statistically delayed PT ($P<0.01$) and MTT ($P<0.01$) and MTT ($P<0.02$) compared with those of patients with epileptic episodes (Fig. 3). The nidal appearance time (AT) in patients with haemorrhagic episodes was 6.50 ± 3.05, that of patients with epileptic episodes 5.94 ± 2.39 s. There was, however, no statistical difference between the AT of the nidus in the two groups.

Discussion

The nidal haemodynamics of AVMs remain controversial despite various methods and many new techniques. Although recent studies of AVMs have focussed attention on the venous drainage [2] and its importance in the pathophysiology of haemorrhage, factors contributing to intracerebral haemorrhage include deep venous drainage pathways having frequent occlusion or stenosis [3], and turbulent venous flow [4] which leads to enhanced platelet and aggregation and thrombosis [5]. There was no statistical difference between the nida maximum diameter

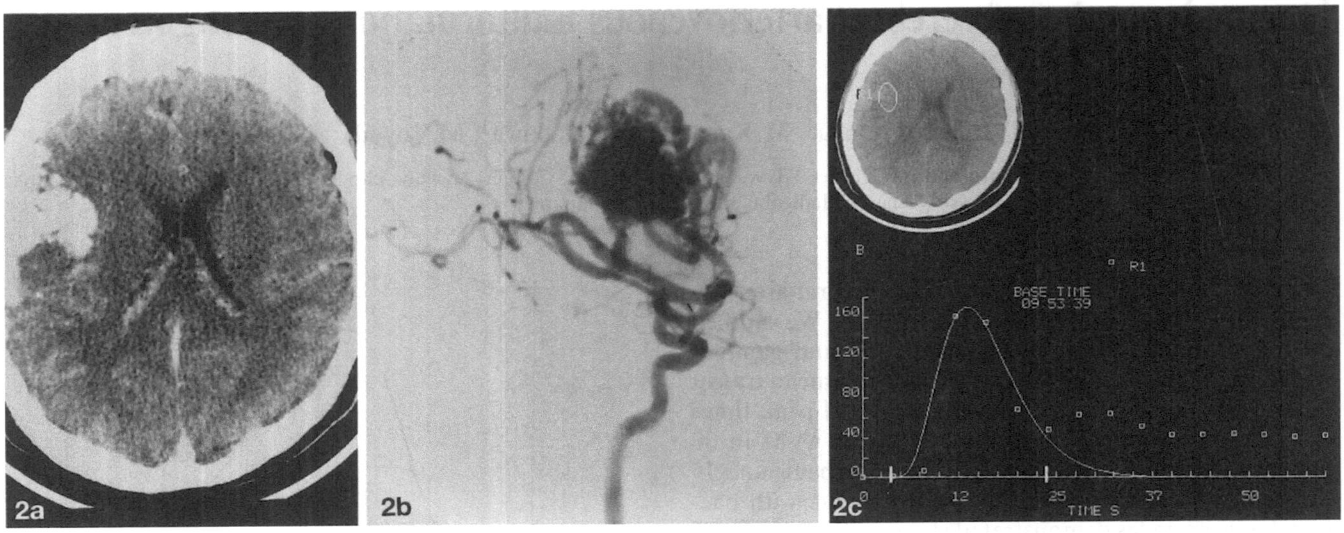

Fig. 2a–c. A 34-year-old man with a left AVM who had an epileptic episode. **a** Contrast-enhanced CT demonstrating anoval high density in the left frontal area. **b** Lateral projection left internal carotid angiogram showing left middle cerebral artery supply to the AVM. **c** Gamma-variate fitted time-concentration curve in a region of interest over the nidus

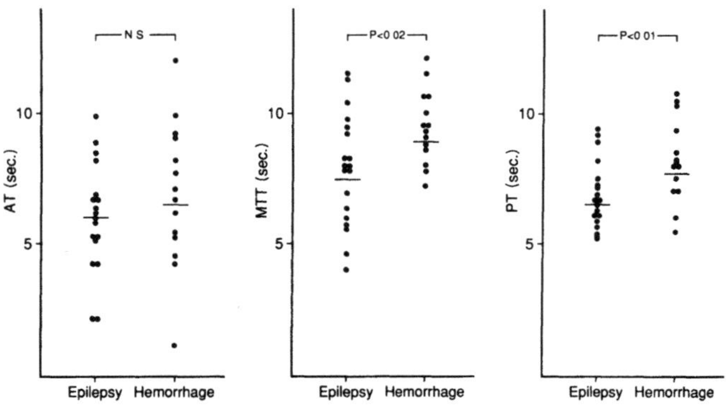

Fig. 3. Comparison of AT, MTT and PT in patients with epilepsy and haemorrhage

in our two groups. In this study using dynamic CT, the nidus of patients with haemorrhagic episodes demonstrated statistically delayed PT and MTT compared with that of patients with epileptic episodes. There was, however, no statistical difference between AT of the nidus in the two groups. These results suggest that partial intravascular thrombosis caused by haemorrhage may lead to prolonged MTT and PT.

References

1. Thompson HK, Starmer CF, Whalen RE et al. (1964) Indicator transit time considered as a gamma variate. Circ Res 14:502–515
2. Miyasaka Y, Yada K, OhwadaT et al. (1992) An analysis of the venous drainage system as a factor in haemorrhage from arteriovenous malformations. J Neurosurg 76:239–243
3. Viñuela F, Nombela L, Roach MR et al. (1985) Stenotic and occlusive disease of the venous drainage system of deep brain AVMs. J Neurosurg 63:180–184
4. Nornes H, Grip A, Wikeby P (1979) Intraoperative evaluation of cerebral hemodynamics using directional Doppler technique. I. Arteriovenous malformation. J Neurosurg 50:145–151
5. Sutherland GR,King MR, Drake CG, et al. (1988) Platelet aggregation within cerebral arteriovenous malformations. J Neurosurg 68:198–204

Cerebral haemodynamics and metabolism in patients with dural arteriovenous fistulae: positron emission tomography

T. Iwama, N. Hashimoto, S. Yoshimura, Y. Takagi, K. Kazekawa, K. Sampei, S. Nishi, Y. Goto, T. Tsukahara

[1] Department of Neurosurgery, National Cardiovascular Centre, 5-7-1 Fujishirodai, Suita, Osaka 565, Japan

Abstract. Cerebral haemodynamics and metabolism were studied in seven patients with dural arteriovenous fistulae (DAVF) using positron emission tomography (DAVF) (PET). Cerebral haemodynamics were impaired in five patients with extensive fistulae. In two severe cases, reduction of cerebral blood flow (rCBF), oxygen metabolism ($rCMRO_2$) and elevation of cerebral blood (rCBV) volume were significant. On angiograms, patients with significant elevation of rCBV showed sinus occlusion (4/5 cases). Patients with significant reduction of rCBF showed retrograde flow into cortical veins and delayed cerebral circulation time (2/2 cases). Radical resection or transvenous embolisation of the involved sinus was performed in three haemodynamically impaired cases. Postoperative PET showed improvements of rCBV and rCBF in all the cases, which also improved clinically. Our results indicate the efficacy of radical treatment of this disease, not only from the clinical but also from haemodynamic and metabolic points of view.

Key words: Dural arteriovenous fistula – positron emission tomography – Cerebral circulation, treatment

Although dural arteriovenous fistula (DAVF) is a relatively uncommon lesion, reports of this disease have increased with the progress of neuroradiological technology [1–5]. Although the symptoms of DAVF are well known, aetiology and pathophysiology of this disease are still uncertain. Sinus occlusion is often demonstrated on angiograms and impairment of venous return is pointed out [1, 3–5]. Impairment of cerebral circulation caused by disturbed venous return is thought to be the key to the pathophysiology of this disease, but cerebral haemodynamics have not been fully evaluated in patients with DAVF [3]. In the present study, we investigated the haemodynamics and oxygen metabolism in seven patients with DAVF using positron emission tomography (PET) to elucidate the correlations among clinical symptoms, angiographic findings and haemodynamic/metabolic data. In five patients who were treated by intravascular and/or direct surgery, the efficacy of the treatments was evaluated from the point of cerebral haemodynamics and metabolism.

Materials and methods

Table 1 shows a summary of clinical and angiographic findings in seven patients with DAVF who were examined by PET. The affected sinus was the transverse/sigmoid sinus (TSS) in four, the superior sagittal sinus (SSS) and TSS in two and the marginal sinus in one patient. Each of the two patients with a DAVF at the SSS and TS had status epilepticus and dementia. Of the other five patients, four presented progressive tinnitus and one dizziness. Five patients (cases 1-5) underwent intravascular and/or direct surgery. Postoperative (PET) was performed at 1-3 months after treatment.

With PET regional cerebral blood flow (rCBF), regional cerebral blood volume (rCBV), regional cerebral metabolic rate of oxygen ($rCMRO_2$) and regional oxygen extraction fraction (rOEF) were measured by the ^{15}O-labelled gas inhalation steady-state method.

Results

Significant reduction of rCBF, $rCMRO_2$ and elevation of rCBV were seen in the two patients with DAVF at the SSS and TSS (cases 1 and 2). In these two patients, angiography demonstrated sinus occlusion and delayed cerebral circulation time. Elevation of rCBV with mild reduction of rCBF was observed in another three patients with DAVF at the TSS. Of these three patients, one patient

Table 1. Clinical and angiographic summary of seven patients with dural arteriovenous fistula (DAVF)

Case	Age (years) sex	Symptoms	Site of fistula	Sinus occlusion	Retrograde flow via cortical vein	Delayed cerebral circulation
1	55/M	Status epilepticus	TSS, SSS	Yes	Yes	Yes
2	64/M	Dementia	SSS, TSS	Yes	Yes	Yes
3	70/F	Tinnitus	TSS	Yes	Yes	No
4	56/M	Tinnitus	TSS	Yes	No	No
5	70/M	Dizziness	TSS	No	No	No
6	56/M	Tinnitus	Marginal sinus	No	No	No
7	61/F	Tinnitus	TSS	No	Yes	No

SSS, Superior sagittal sinus; TSS, transverse sinus

Correspondence to: T. Iwama

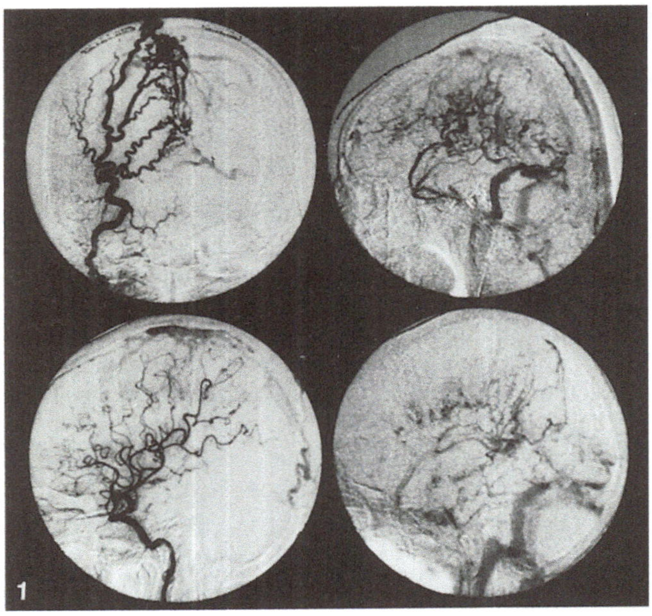

Fig. 1. Case 2. *Top:* Anteroposterior projection of left occipital artery injection *(left)*, demonstrating a dural arteriovenous fistula at the superior sagittal sinus (SSS), which drains in a retrograde fashion via cortical veins *(right)*, lateral projection. *Bottom:* Lateral projection of left internal carotid injection, arterial *(left)*, *venous (right)*, phases, showing delayed circulation and absence of venous return via the SSS

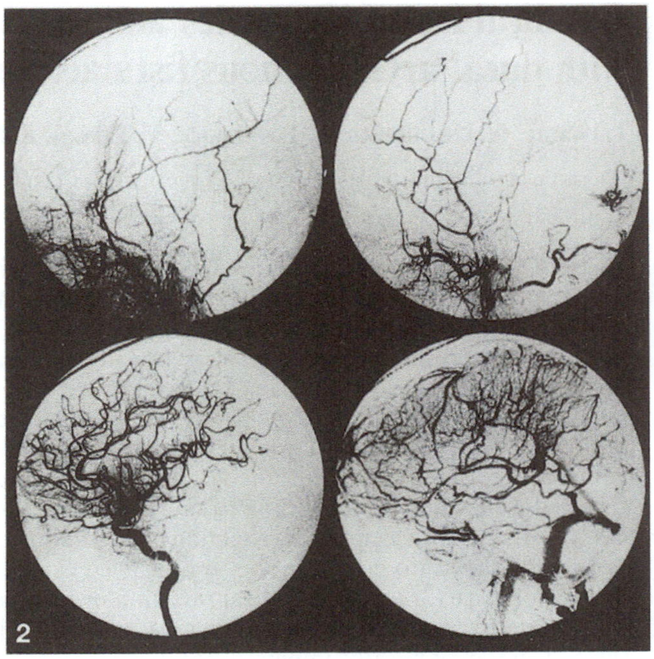

Fig. 2. Case 2 (following treatment). *Top:* Lateral projections of right *(left)* and left *(right)* external carotid angiograms show disappearance of fistula on the SSS. A small shunt remains at the left transverse sinus. *Bottom:* Lateral views of left internal carotid angiogram demonstrate improvement of cerebral circulation. Cortical veins are opacified well, indicating improvement of venous return

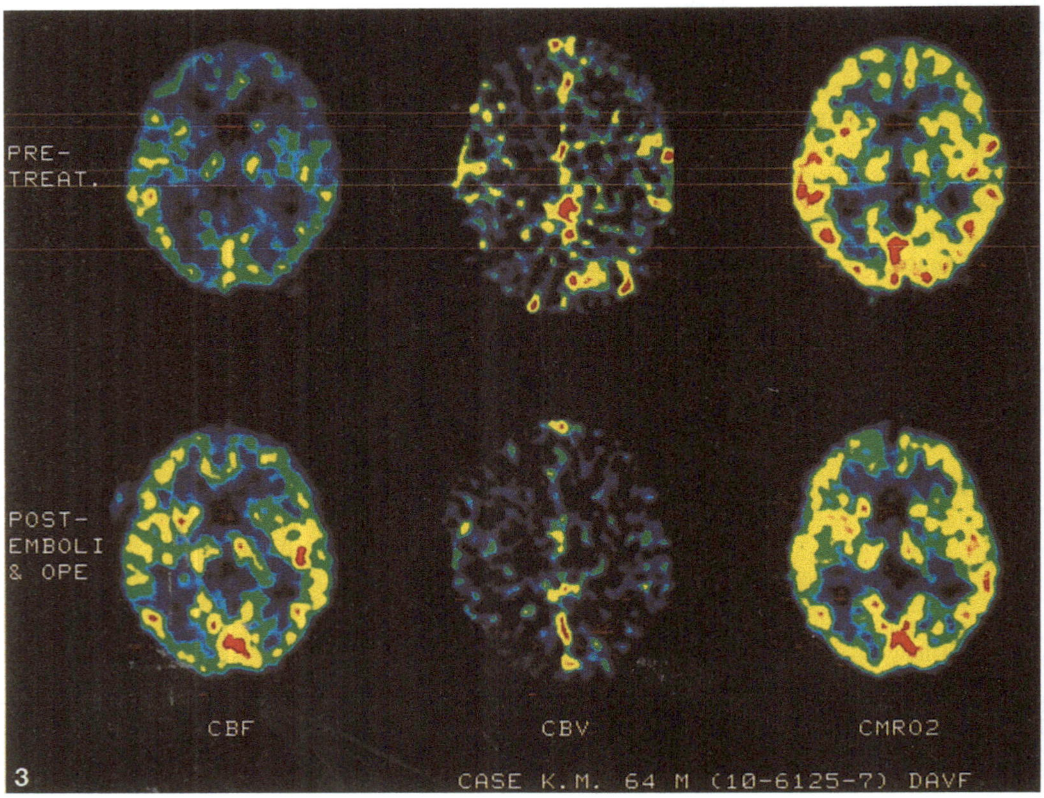

Fig. 3. Case 2. *Top:* PET indicates diffuse reduction in rCBF and elevation of rCBV. *Bottom:* Increase in rCBF and decrease in rCBV are confirmed after treatment. Regional CMRO2 was improved postoperatively in the basal ganglia, although unchanged on this slice

Table 2. Haemodynamic and metabolic data in seven patients with DAVF

Case	rCBF	rCBV	RCMRO$_2$	rOEF
1	24.6	8.3	1.21	0.55
2	24.1	6.0	2.84	0.58
3	42.1	5.4	2.63	0.38
4	31.4	5.8	2.76	0.44
5	28.9	5.4	2.37	0.49
6	30.5	4.5	3.11	0.56
7	49.2	4.6	3.39	0.43

showed sinus occlusion and retrograde flow via cortical veins, and one showed sinus occlusion; the third showed no abnormality and venous return. In the other two patients, no abnormalities were demonstrated in the haemodynamic/metabolic values (Table 2).

In two patients (cases 2 and 4) who underwent surgical resection of the affected sinus improvements of rCBV and rCBF were confirmed postoperatively. In the patient with DAVF at the SSS and TSS who was manifested as dementia (case 2), rCMRO$_2$ was increased and dementia was fully improved after surgery (Figs. 1-3). In the patient with DAVF at the SSS and TSS who presented with status epilepticus (case 1), reduction of rCBV and increase of CMRO$_2$ were achieved and convulsion was controllable after transvenous embolisation of the affected sinus. In the other two patients who underwent transarterial embolisation of the feeding arteries, although clinical symptoms disappeared, haemodynamic abnormalities were unchanged after the treatments.

Discussion

A study of cerebral haemodynamics and metabolism is considered important for understanding pathophysiology and selecting therapeutic modalities in patients with DAVF [3]. In our series of seven patients, clinical symptoms and angiographic findings were correlates well with grades of impairment of cerebral hamodynamics and metabolism. Namely, in cases with global cerebral dysfunction and delayed cerebral circulation, significant reduction of rCBF and rCMRO$_2$ as well as elevation of rCBV were confirmed by PET. In contrast, cases in which cerebral circulation was not delayed showed only elevation of rCBV and with mild reduction of rCBF, even if venous return was partially disturbed by sinus occlusion. From the point of views of cerebral haemodynamics and metabolism, radical treatment, i.e. surgical resection [2, 3] or transvenous embolisation [4] of the affected sinus, is recommended to improve cerebral haemodynamics and symptoms in a case with severe impairment of venous return. Haemodynamics data, especially rCBF and rCBV, are useful indicators not only for understanding the pathophysiology but also for elucidating the efficacy of treatment in patients with DAVF.

References

1. Houser OW, Beker HL Jr, Rhoton AL Jr, Okazaki H (1972) Intracranial dural arteriovenous malformations. Radiology 105:55-64
2. Sundt TM Jr, Piepgras DG (1983) The surgical approach to arteriovenous malformations of the lateral and sigmoid sinuses. J Neurosurg 59:32-39
3. Kawaguchi T, Fujita S, Yamada H, Nishida Y, Mori E (1988) Hemodynamics before and after the total removal of a dural arteriovenous malformation of the posterior fossa. Surg Neurol 30:457-461
4. Halbach VV, Higashida RT, Hieshima GB, Mehringer CM, Hardin CW (1989) Transvenous embolization of dural fistulas involving the transverse and sigmoid tissue. AJNR 10:385-392
5. Lalwani AK, Dowd CF, Halbach VV (1993) Grading venous restrictive disease in patients with dural arteriovenous fistulas of the transverse/sigmoid sinus. J Neurosurg 79:11-15

Sex and age of patients with multiple aneurysms of cerebral blood vessels

R. Bajic, L. Borota, S. Domonji, B. Prstojevic, S. Milosevic, V. Vuckovic

Department of Neuroradiology, Institute of Neurosurgery, University Clinical Centre, Belgrade, Serbia Yugoslavia

Abstract. The aim of this study was to determine the sex and age distributions of patients with multiple aneurysms, to obtain new data which might be useful in investigating the aetiology of multiple aneurysms. The study included 72 patients in whom multiple intracranial aneurysms were revealed angiographically by standard Seldinger's method and digital subtraction angiography. The patients were divided into three groups according to the number of aneurysms. The first group included 39 women (average age 45.9 ± 11.8 years) and 14 men (average age 44.4 ± 9.7 years). The second group comprised 8 women (average age 39.6 ± 3.7 years) and 5 men (average age 49.4 ± 7.2 years) and the third 4 women (average age 47.5 ± 10.3 years) and 2 men (average age 40.5 ± 2.7 years). The female-to-male ratio did not significantly differ among the groups. There was no significant difference between the average ages of men and women in the first and third groups. In the second group, however, the women were significantly younger than the men ($P < 0.02$).

Correspondence to: L. Borota

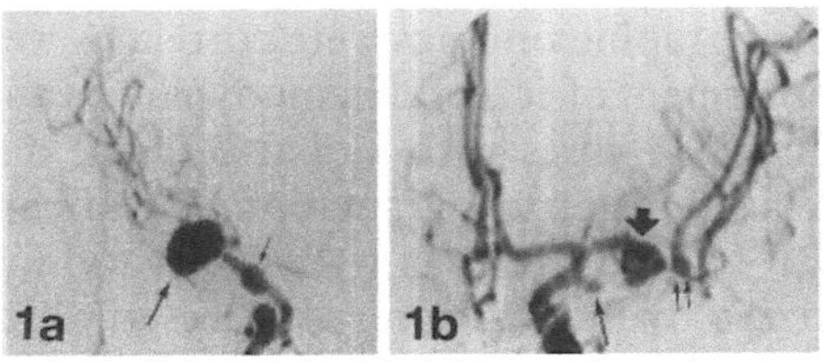

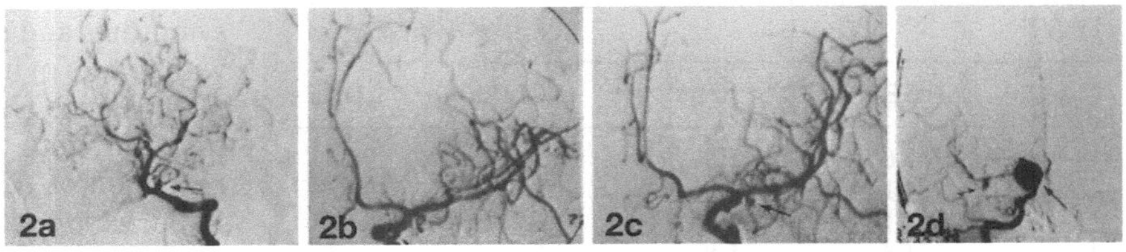

Fig. 1. Aneurysms on **a** eight internal carotid *(small arrow)* and middle cerebral *(arrow)* arteries and **b** left internal carotid *(small arrow)* and proximal *(arrow)* and more distal *(double arrow)* middle cerebral arteries in one man

Fig. 2. Aneurysms on **a** left posterior inferior cerebella, **b** internal carotid, **c** middle cerebral and **d** right internal carotid *(large arrow)* and middle cerebral *(small arrow)* arteries in one woman

The observation that women with three aneurysms are significantly younger than similarly afflicted men, calls for investigation of sex and age factors.

Key words: Intracranial multiple aneurysm – Sex – Age – Aneurysm, aetiology

Multiple intracranial aneurysms are of special interest to both neuroradiologists and neurosurgeons, because of the many difficulties in diagnosis and therapeutic treatment. Moreover, the prognosis of patients with multiple aneurysms is much worse than that of patients with a solitary aneurysm. Multiple aneurysms are relatively common, with a frequency of about 19% of all diagnosed aneurysms [1].

The aetiology of aneurysms, both solitary and multiple, is not yet fully understood. Since age and sex are often cited as possible aetiological or risk factors in the development of intracranial aneurysms [2], we analysed sex and age distribution in our patients in the hope of obtaining new data that might be useful for investigating the aetiology of multiple aneurysms.

Patients and methods

We included 72 patients in our study. All were admitted to hospital because of the clinical picture of a ruptured intracranial aneurysm. Presence of blood in the subarachnoid space was revealed by either lumbar puncture or CT. In all patients, four-vessel study was performed by the standard Seldinger's procedure of a transfemoral approach to the branches of the aortic arch.

All patients were divided into three groups according to the number of aneurysms: the first group comprised patients with two aneurysms; the second of patients with three aneurysms, and the third of patients with four or more. Statistical differences in age were determined by Student's *T*-test.

Results

The first group included 39 women (average age 45.9 ± 11.8 years and 14 men (average age 44.4 ± 9.7 years). The second group consisted of 8 women (average age 39.6 ± 3.7 years) and 5 men (average age 49.4 ± 7.2 years) and the third comprised 4 women (average age 47.5 ± 10.3 years) and 2 men (average age ± SD 2.7 years).

The most interesting results were angiograms of one man and one woman with as many as five aneurysms located predominantly on the internal carotid artery and its branches (Fig. 1, 2).

Analysis of the age distribution demonstrated that there was no statistical difference in the female-to-male ratio among the groups; nor did male patients and female patients in different groups differ in their mean ages. In addition, there was no statistical difference between the average age of men and women in the first and third groups. Surprisingly, in the second group, the women were significantly younger than the men ($P < 0.002$). All female patients in this group were premenopausal.

Discussion

The majority of saccular aneurysms appear between the ages of 40 to 60 years. It is generally accepted that aneurysms affect women more frequently than men, with a female-to-male ratio of 3:2. Before the age of 40, aneurysms are a predominantly male disease, whereas after 40, the majority of patients are women [1–4]. It is obvious from these data that age and sex play a considerable part in the pathogenesis of intracranial aneurysms.

There are many results indicating that degenerative processes following ageing are important in the development of intracranial aneurysms. For example, a vessel proximal to an aneurysm often contains atheromatous plaque [1, 5, 6]. Furthermore, long-lasting high pressure and haemodynamic stress at the level of the arterial fork may contribute to the development of aneurysm [6]. Animal models, based on the induction of high arterial pressure in cynomolgus monkeys, clearly show that permanent high pressure may cause a cerebral blood vessel aneurysm [7, 8]. It is logical that an aneurysm is more likely to appear if long-lasting high arterial pressure is combined with pre-existing congenital defects on the blood vessel wall [1]. However, some workers point out that maldevelopmental errors have not been scientifically demonstrated in patients with aneurysms. Of course, patients with connective tissue disorders are predisposed to the development of aneurysms [6].

Analyses of clinical features showed that there were many differences between male and female patients with aneurysms of cerebral blood vessels. Both single and multiple aneurysms appear more frequently in female patients [3, 4, 10]. Some results indicate that location of intracranial aneurysms differs between men and women.

Recurrent bleeding is more common in women, as is the occurrence of spasm and consecutive cerebral infarcts in female patients [3, 9]. Nevertheless, female patients have some advantages. In our second group of patients, women were significantly younger than men and, according to the data published so far, their prognosis is better [11].

In spite of the obvious relationship between sex and the appearance of intracranial aneurysms, we did not find a satisfactory explanation for this phenomenon in the available literature.

After we had analysed our results, it was thought that hormonal activity might be of special importance for the development of intracranial aneurysms in women. Women in the second group are significantly younger than men in the same group, their mean age being the lowest of all the groups and they all are premenopausal. Moreover, in all the groups, the number of women was much larger than the number of men. These results indicate that in the age/sex combination, age is a dominating aetiological factor in male patients, whereas sex is a dominating aetiological factor in female patients.

Since we have only one statistically significant result, we suggest that it would be necessary to confirm our results by a study based on a larger group of patients with special attention to female patients with hormonal disorders. Also, it may be useful to design an experimental model that will disclose hormonal influences on the development of aneurysms of the cerebral blood vessels.

References

1. Viñuela F, Fox AJ (1992) intracranial arterial aneurysm. In: Taveras JM, Ferrucci JT (eds) Radiology - diagnosis - imaging - intervention, vol 3. Lippincott, Philadelphia, pp 9–17
2. Ostergaard JR (1989) Risk factors in intracranial saccular aneurysms. Aspects on the formation and rupture of aneurysms, and development of cerebral vasospasm. Acta Neurol Scand 80:81–98
3. Locksley HB (1966) Report on the Cooperative Study of intracranial Aneurysms and Subarachnoidal Hemorrhage, section 5, part I: Natural history of subarachnoid hemorrhage, intracranial aneurysms and arteriovenous malformations. J Neurosurg 25:219–231
4. Wilson FM, Jaspan T, Holland IM (1989) Multiple cerebral aneurysms - a reappraisal. Neuroradiology 31:232–236
5. Stehbens WE (1975) Ultrastructure of aneurysms. Arch Neurol 32:798–806
6. Stehbens WE (1990) Pathology and pathogenesis of intracranial berry aneurysms. Neurol Res 12:29–34
7. Kim C, Kikuchi H, Hashimoto N, Hazama F, Kataoka H (1989) Establishment of the experimental conditions for inducing saccular cerebra aneurysms in primates with special reference to hypertension. Acta Neurochir (Wien) 96:132–136
8. Kim C, Kukuchi H, Hashimoto N, Hazama F (1989) Histopathological study of induced cerebral aneurysms in primates. Surg Neurol 32:45–50
9. George B, Zerah M, Mourier KL, Gelbert F, Reizine D (1989) Ruptured intracranial aneurysms. The influence of sex and fibromuscular dysplasia upon prognosis. Acta Neurochir (Wien) 97:26–30
10. Cheng PT, Chang CN (1991) Aneurysmal subarachnoid hemorrhage. Report of 219 cases in Chang Gung Memorial Hospital. Chang-Keng-I-Hsueh 14:149–155
11. Matsuda M, Shiino A, Handa J (1990) Sequential changes of cerebral blood flow after aneurysmal subarachnoid haemorrhage. Acta Neurochir (Wien) 105:98–106

A case of de novo aneurysm rupture

H. Ikeda[1], T. Abe[1], T. Kawamata[1], S. Asamoto[1], T. Fujimoto[2], T. Iwata[1], Y. Fukushima[2], K. Matsumoto[1]

[1] Department of Neurosurgery, Showa University School of Medicine, Tokyo, Japan 142 1-5-8 Hatanodai Shinaga
[2] Department of Neurosurgery, Showa University Fujigaoka Hospital, Tujigaoka, Kanagawa

Abstract. We report a case of ruptured aneurysm arising de novo from a previously angiographically normal vessel.

Key words: Aneurysm - intracranial

De novo aneurysms are those which are demonstrated to arise from a previously normal vessel. We report a case in which an aneurysm of this type gave rise to subarachnoid haemorrhage (SAH).

Correspondence to: H. Ikeda

Case report

A 49-year-old right-handed woman who suffered (SAH) was admitted to hospital. She was not hypertensive, despite smoking and had a history of SAH 10 years previously. At that time, she had a sudden onset of severe headache. CT revealed SAH, and four-vessel cerebral angiography confirmed a single aneurysm at the anterior communicating artery (Fig. 1) On the third day after her ictus, the aneurysm was clipped. She fully recovered and was discharged in June 1983.

The patient remained well until August 1993, when she collapsed after the sudden onset of a severe headache. She was transferred to our hospital with a Glasgow Coma Scale score of 14 and no hemiparesis. CT revealed SAH and four-vessel cerebral angiography showed an aneurysm at the origin of the posterior communicating artery (Fig. 2). The aneurysm was clipped and she was discharged.

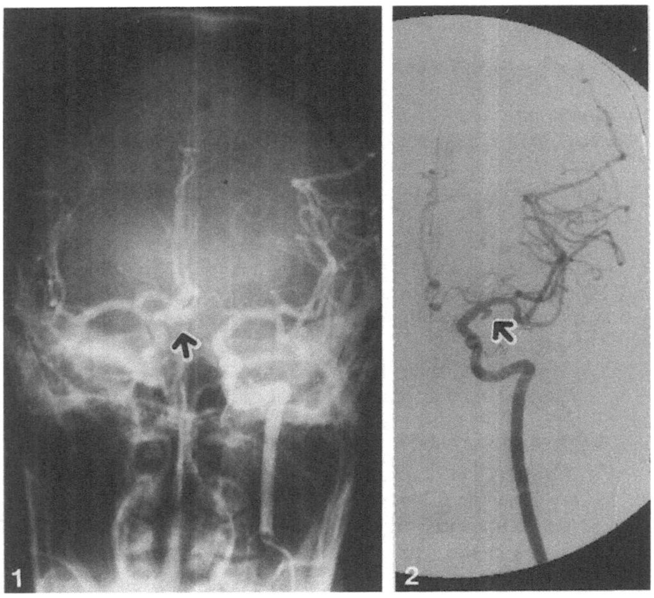

Fig. 1. April 1983: left internal carotid angiogram reveals an aneurysm *(arrow)* on the anterior communicating artery and no other aneurysm

Fig. 2. August 1993: angiography reveals a new aneurysm at the origin of the posterior communicating artery *(arrow)*

Discussion

This case demonstrates the development and rupture of a de novo aneurysm over a 10-year period in a normotensive woman. Rupture of a de novo aneurysm is rare [1–5]. Rinne and Hernesniemi [4] recently reported the rate of de novo aneurysm formation to be 1.1% [4]. The mean interval to the diagnosis of a de novo aneurysm was 11.4 years (range 2–34 years) in the previous literature [4], which is consistent with our case.

References

1. Koeleveld RF, Heilman CB, Klucznik RP, Shucart WA (1991) De novo development of an aneurysm: case report. Neurosurgery 29:756–759
2. Miller CA, Hill SA, Hunt WE (1985) De novo aneurysm. A clinical review. Surg Neurol 24:173–180
3. Misra BK, Whittle IR, Steers AJW, Sellar RJ (1988) De novo saccular aneurysms. Neurosurgery 23:10–15
4. Rinne JK, Hernesniemi JA (1993) De novo aneurysms: special multiple intracranial aneurysms. Neurosurgery 33:981–985
5. Sasaki T, Tominaga M, Miyamoto K, Tsunoda S, Hiasa Y (1993) Clinical studies of the de novo aneurysms. Neurosurgery 32:512–517

Large intracranial aneurysm studied by three-dimensional MRI

N. Kurihara [1], S. Takahashi [1], S. Higano [1], K. Matsumoto [2], K. Sakamoto [1]

[1] Department of Radiology, Tohoku University School of Medicine, Seiryo-machi, Aoba-ku, Sendai, 985 Japan
[2] Department of Radiology, Miyagi Cancer Center, Miyagi, Japan

Abstract. We tried to study large intracranial aneurysms by contrast-enhanced three-dimensional (3D) MRI. Contrast-enhanced, axial (or coronal), 3D-FLASH images were obtained followed by 2D partitions and other perpendicular images reformatted in 11 patients. 3D-MRI showed the aneurysm, adjacent vessels and surrounding neural structures simultaneously, and delineated the exact relationship between them. It also demonstrated the exact size and shape of the aneurysm and the intra-aneurysmal constitution (both the thrombosed portion and patent lumen). Except in a precavernous/cavernous internal carotid aneurysm, we could identify the aneurysm neck well by observation from three different directions. After embolisation, signal intensities of the aneurysm and its parent artery decreased.

Key words: Aneurysm intracranial – Three-dimensional MRI

Correspondence to: N. Kurihara

Magnetic resonance imaging (MRI) has played an important role in diagnosing intracranial aneurysms, principally via routine spin-echo (SE) imaging and MR angiography (MRA) [1, 2]. However, SE images may not delineate the aneurysm neck because of poor spatial resolution. MRA cannot always demonstrate large aneurysms clearly because intra-aneurysmal turbulence and slow flow decrease their signal. Given these clinical limitations of SE images and MRA, we attempted to obtain three dimensional (3D)-MR images to evaluate large intracranial aneurysms.

Patients and methods

Eleven patients (9 women and 2 men) were examined. They had relatively large intracranial aneurysms, the diameter of which ranged from 13 to 53 mm (mean 29 mm). The aneurysm involved the precavernous/cavernous internal carotid artery in 6 patients, the supraclinoid ICA in 1, the M1 portion of the middle cerebral artery (MCA) in 1, the basilar artery tip in 2, and the ambient segment of the posterior cerebral artery (PCA) in 1.

3D-MRI was performed on a 1.5 T system using FLASH with the following parameters; TR/TE 40/6 ms, flip angle 35°, field of view

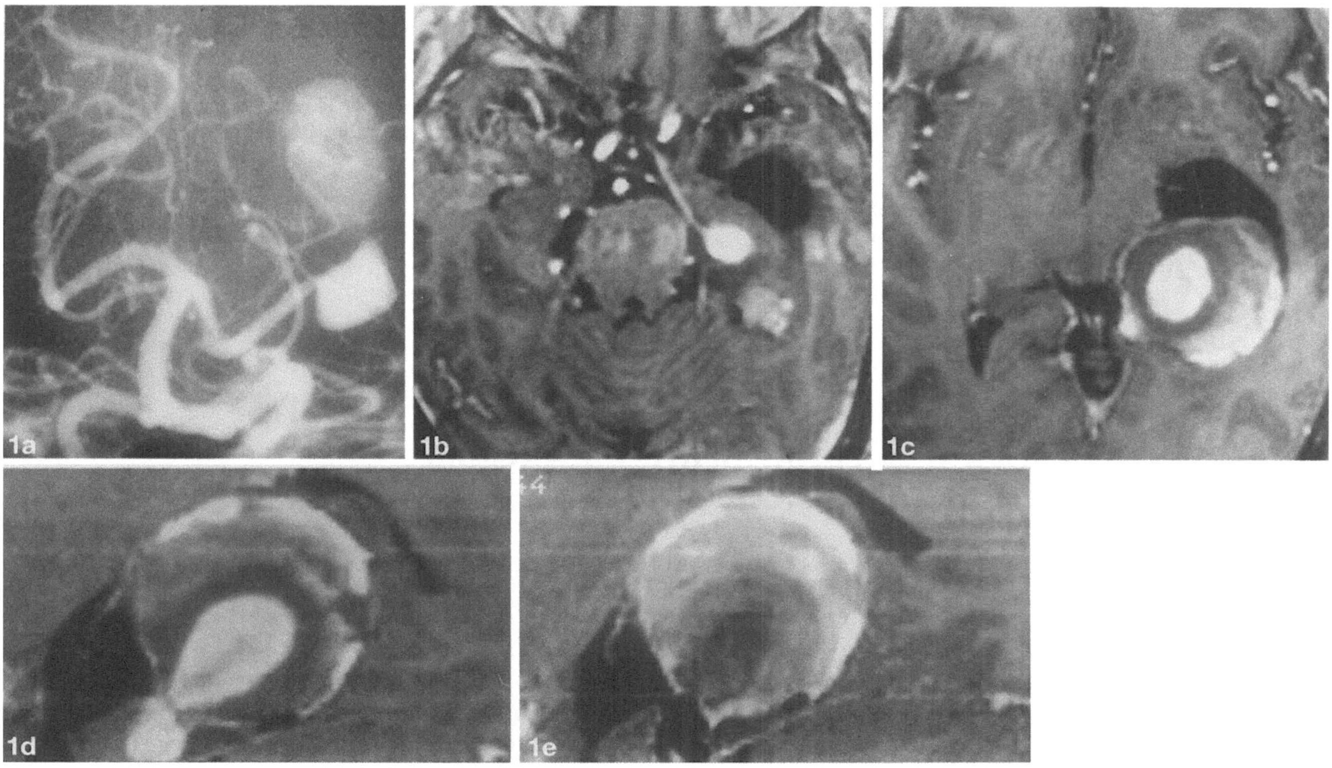

Fig. 1a–c. A left posterior cerebral artery (PCA) aneurysm in a 60-year-old woman. **a** Left vertebral angiogram shows the aneurysm with a large daughter lesion arising from the ambient segment of the PCA. **b** 3D partition axial image clearly reveals the neck of the aneurysm in the left ambient cistern. **c** Image slightly above **b**. Daughter lesion accompanies the lamellar thrombosed portion surrounding the patent lumen. This lesion traps and widens the temporal horn of the left lateral ventricle. **d** Sagittal reformat shows the overall shape. Intraluminal low-intensity band is probably caused by turbulence. **e** Sagittal reformat after embolisation demonstrates the disappearance of luminal enhancement, suggesting thrombosis

24 cm, slab thickness, 64 mm, 64 partitions, slice thickness 1 mm, matrix 256×256 and 1 excitation. Gd-DTPA 0.1 mmol/kg was administered intravenously for clear delineation of vessels. Initially the 3D imaging data were acquired in the axial (9 patients) and coronal (2 patients) planes followed by 2D partitions of 1 mm thickness. Then we obtained other perpendicular images (coronal/sagittal or axial/sagittal) with a multiplanar reconstruction method (slice thickness 1 mm or 1.9 mm). We observed the original 2D partitions and reformatted images carefully. Four patients after embolisation and 1 after surgery were examined in the same way.

Results

3D-MRI showed the aneurysm, adjacent vessels and surrounding neural structures simultaneously and delineated the exact relationship between them (Fig. 1).

3D-MRI demonstrated both the thrombosed portion and the patent lumen. The latter was recognised as an enhanced region, but conventional angiography showed only the patent lumen.

We could identify the aneurysmal neck as a transitional enhanced portion between the patent lumen of the aneurysm and its parent artery in 7 cases by 3D-MRI (precavernous/cavernous ICA 2/6, others 5/5).

After embolisation, signal intensities of the aneurysm and its parent artery became lower than those of pre-embolisation. However, in 1 case, no signal difference was noted.

Discussion

The advantage of 3D-MRI is to demonstrate the detailed relationship between the aneurysm and surrounding neural structures as well as the mass effect caused by it. It could also discern the exact size and shape of the aneurysm and the intra-aneurysmal constitution. This information is potentially of great use to the neurosurgeon in pre-operative planning.

We could identify the aneurysm neck in 7 cases by 3D-MRI. This rate of identification was equal to that of conventional angiography. However, observation from three different directions gave us more reliable information regarding the neck and its relation to surrounding arteries. The four aneurysms whose neck could not be identified were all in the cavernous ICA. The possible reasons for poor delineation of the neck include enhancement of the cavernous sinus; homogenously high-intensity aneurysms; broad necks.

MRA has been recently used for examining patients after embolisation therapy [3]. 3D-MRI also seems to be useful as a noninvasive method for assessing the aneurysm after embolisation, which demonstrates a decrease in signal intensity in the aneurysm and parent artery. However, we must be careful, because subacute thrombosis may reveal no signal change.

References

1. Olsen WL, Brant-Zawadzki M, Hodes J, Norman D, Newton TH (1987) Giant intracranial aneurysms: MR imaging. Radiology 163:431–435
2. Sevick RJ, Tsuruda JS, Schmalbrock P (1990) Three-dimensional time-of-flight angiography in the evaluation of cerebral aneurysms. J Comput Assist Tomogr 14:874–881
3. Turuda JS, Sevick RJ, Halbach VV (1992) Three-dimensional time-of-flight angiography in the evaluation of intracranial aneurysms treated by endovascular balloon occlusion. AJNR 13:1129–1136

Aneurysm associated with caroticocavernous fistula

A. P. Karapurkar[1], **R. Ramakantan**[1]

[1] Departments of Neurosurgery and Radiology, Seth G. S. Medical College and K. E. M. Hospital, Bombay, India

Abstract. Of the 52 patients with caroticocavernous fistulae (CCF) seen in our department, 11 had an associated aneurysm of the internal carotid artery (ICA). Of these, 3 followed trauma, the other 8 were spontaneous in origin. One patient has an aneurysm on the trigeminal artery. Unless a balloon can be placed in the aneurysm, the ICA must be occluded to prevent rupture or rapid enlargement of the aneurysm after the CCF has been treated.

Key words: Corticocavernous fistula – Aneurysm – Trauma

We noted an unusually high incidence of aneurysm [1–4] in patients with caroticocavernous fistulae (CCF). We therefore decided to review our case material to determine the frequency and significance of this association.

Materials and methods

Of the patients with CCF seen in our department, 11 had an additional aneurysm on the cavernous or supracavernous internal carotid artery (ICA). The CCF and aneurysm followed trauma in 3 and and were spontaneous in 8. All the spontaneous CCF were found in females, their ages ranging from 12 to 45 years, average 28 years. Of the 3 CCF which followed trauma, 1 was separate from the fistula, on the supraophthalmic portion of the ICA. Two were on the cavernous segment. Of the spontaneous aneurysms, 3 followed possible cavernous sinus thrombosis. The other causes were berry aneurysm in 2 and atherosclerosis in 3. One patient had a persistent trigeminal artery aneurysm, seen only after the CCF was treated. The post-traumatic supraclinoid aneurysm was also overlooked on the pre-embolisation angiogram.

Results

In 2 patients a balloon could be placed in the aneurysm. This included the patient with the trigeminal artery aneurysm. In 6 patients the ICA was occluded after treating the fistula. In 3 patients no treatment was offered. One of these died soon after the angiogram. In the other the CCF regressed spontaneously and the aneurysm was asymptomatic. She is being followed up carefully.

Discussion

In all patients with CCF, diagnostic workup should include complete angiography with cross-compression to evaluate the circle of Willis. In patients having a CCF with an associated aneurysm, it may be necessary to occlude the ICA unless a balloon can be placed in the aneurysm.

References

1. Alpers BJ, Schlezinger NS (1951) Bilateral internal carotid aneurysms involving cavernous sinus. Arch Ophthalmol 46:403–407
2. Enomoto T, Sato A (1977) Carotid-cavernous sinus fistula caused by rupture of a primitive trigeminal artery aneurysm. J Neurosurg 46:373–376
3. Picard L, Renard M et al. (1970) Aspects radioanatomiques des ruptures de la carotide intracranienne. J Radiol 51:217–222
4. Rougeire J, Guilmet D (1973) Carotid aneurysm. Neurochirurgie 19:649–654

Correspondence to: A. P. Karapurkar

Enhancement of intracranial arterial walls

S. Aoki [1], I. Shirouzu [1], Y. Sasaki [1], T. Okubo [1], N. Hayashi [1], T. Machida [1], E. Hoshi [2], K. Suzuki [2], N. Funada [3], T. Araki [1], Y. Sasaki [1]

[1] Department of Radiology, Faculty of Medicine, University of Tokyo, 7-3-1 Hongo, Bunkyo-ku, Tokyo 113, Japan
[2] Department of Radiology, Tokyo Metropolitan Komagome Hospital, Tokyo, Japan
[3] Department of Pathology, Tokyo Metropolitan Komagome Hospital, Tokyo, Japan

Abstract. We studied intracranial arterial wall enhancement in relation to atherosclerosis. The intracranial vertebral arteries of 30 patients and the carotid arteries of 62 patients were studied using spin-echo MRI with contrast medium and presaturation. We graded arterial wall enhancement as follows: 1, no significant enhancement; 2, faint or thin enhancement; 3, definite and thick enhancement.

Enhancement of both arteries correlated with age ($P<0.05$). Arterial wall enhancement is related to ageing and probably due to neovascularity of atherosclerotic plaques. It should be considered separately from dissection, luminal enhancement, and other flow-related enhancement. In addition, it may open a new window through which to assess intracranial atherosclerosis and other vascular diseases.

Key words: Magnetic resonance imaging – Cerebral blood vessels – Atherosclerosis – Contrast enhancement – Arteries

In some elderly patients we found intracranial arterial wall enhancement on MRI using relatively high resolution. Intracranial arteries usually lack vasa vasorum, but vasa vasorum develop with atherosclerosis [1, 2]. We postulate that arterial wall enhancement on MRI may be related to atherosclerosis and the development of vasa varorum.

Materials and methods

We studied the vertebral arteries (VA) of patients (aged 21–93 years) and the carotid arteries (ICA) of 62 patients (aged 20–88 years), using relatively high resolution MRI spin-echo (600/15, field of view 15 cm, slice thickness 3 mm, matrix 256 × 192, with spatial presaturation (5 cm-thick pulses on both cranial and caudal portions of the scan field) and i.v. Gd-DTPA (0.1 mmol/kg). We staged wall thickness and enhancement of the intracranial arteries as follows (Fig. 1): 1, no significant enhancement of the arterial wall; 2, faint enhancement might be seen, but with a broken ring; 3, definite thick, circumferential enhancement of the arterial wall. The correlation between the results of this staging and patient age was calculated using Spearman's rank correlation (r_s). We also performed a histological study of the intracranial vertebral arteries at autopsy. EVG and factor-VIII-related antigen staining were carried out in 5 patients, who were not studied by MRI.

Results

Figures 2 and 3 show wall enhancement according to age. Age and staging correlate well (VA: $r_s=0.365$, $P=0.047<0.05$, ICA: $r_s=0.638$, $P=0.00<0.05$). Among patients over the age of 60, 11 of 22 (50%) VA and 10 of 25 (40%) ICA showed stage 3 enhancement.

Histological examination revealed a small number of fine capillaries at the surface of the adventitia of the vertebral artery in 2 patients without significant atherosclerosis. In 2 patients with moderate atherosclerosis, neovascularity in the form of small capillaries was observed in the media and intima as well as the adventitia.

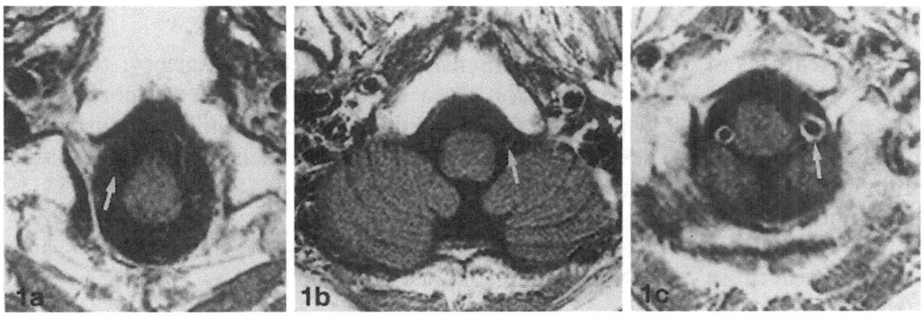

Fig. 1. **a** Stage 1 appearance of vertebral artery in a 20-year-old man. The wall of the vertebral artery shows no evidence of enhancement or thickening. The site of the vertebral artery *(arrow)* can be recognized with difficulty as an area of flow void within the low signal of the cerebrospinal fluid **b** Stage 2 appearance of vertebral artery in a 60-year-old man. The wall of the vertebral artery shows thin, faint, focal enhancement *(arrow)*. **c** Stage 3 appearance of vertebral artery in a 73-year-old woman with multiple infarcts. The wall of the vertebral artery shows thick, intense, circumferential enhancement *(arrow)*

Correspondence to: S. Aoki

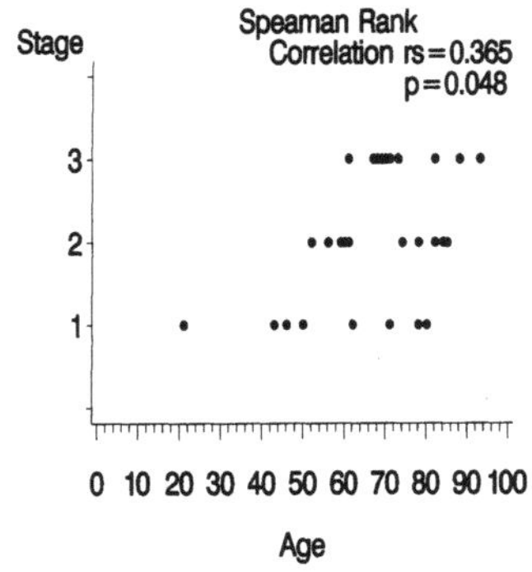

Fig. 2. Enhancement of the vertebral artery wall according to age

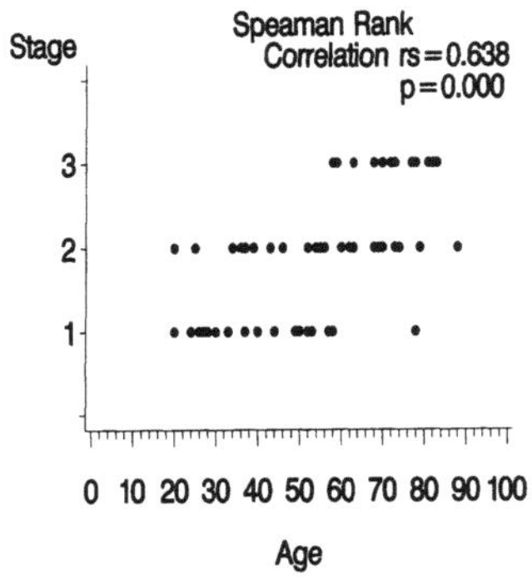

Fig. 3. Enhancement of the carotid artery wall according to age

Discussion

Although enhancement of the arterial wall is a common finding in elderly patients (50% in vertebral, 40% in carotid arteries of those over 60 years of age in our series), no report has referred to enhancement of the intracranial arterial wall. This is probably due to the fact that the laminar flow and other flow-related enhancement and artefacts obscure wall enhancement with routine MRI pulse sequences.

Intravascular enhancement of the cerebral artery due to slow flow has been emphasized in acute cerebral infarction [3, 4]. This "intravascular enhancement" and our "wall enhancement" are two different phenomena that reflect different pathophysiological backgrounds and should be considered separately, although complete differentiation in actual images might be difficult.

Direct visualization of atheromatous plaques of the intracranial artery may open a new window on cerebrovascular diseases. Angiography shows only the lumen of vessels, and there has been no diagnostic method by which to evaluate the intracranial arterial wall. High-resolution, inflow-saturated MRI may play a role in intracranial large vessels by providing information on atherosclerosic changes.

References

1. Liszczak T, Black P, Versos V, Zervas N (1984) The microcirculation of cerebral arteries: a morphologic and morphometric examination of the major canine cerebral arteries. Am J Anat 170:223–232
2. Clower B, Sullivan D, Smith R (1984) Intracranial vessels lack vasa vasorum. J Neurosurg 61:44–48
3. Sato A, Takahashi S, Soma Y et al. (1991) Cerebral infarction: early detection by means of contrast-enhanced cerebral arteries at MR imaging. Radiology 178:433–439
4. Lazar E, Russell E, Cohen B et al. (1992) Contrast-enhanced MR of cerebral arteritis: intravascular enhancement related to flow stasis within areas of focal ectasia. AJNR 13:271–276

MRI of vertebrobasilar disecting aneurysms: diagnostic value and pitfalls of spin-echo sequences

K. Matsumura, M. Matsuda, J. Handa

[1] Department of Neurosurgery, Shiga University of Medical Science, Seta-tsakinowa-cho, Ohtsu, F520-21, Japan, Ohtsu, Japan

Abstract. Magnetic resonance imaging (MRI) features of 12 cases with vertebrobasilar dissecting aneurysms (VBDA) were compared with those of 80 cases with non-dissecting aneurysms (NDA). Seven patients with VBDA showed an eccentrically narrowed true lumen adjacent to the semilunar clot in the false lumen. Such findings were also found in patients with thrombosed NDA. However, the segment of the mural haematoma was longer in those with VBDA. An intimal flap was detected in only 3 cases of VBDA. Two patients with VBDA showed only iso- or high signal intensity of the vertebral artery; therefore, differentiation from obstruction of the vertebral artery was difficult. Flow-dependent spatial misregistration, seen adjacent to the normal vessels, sometimes mimics intramural haematoma.

Key words: Dissecting aneurysm – Vertebrobasilar system – Magnetic resonance imaging

Correspondence to: K. Matsumura

Although the diagnosis of intracranial dissecting aneurysm relies mostly on cerebral angiography, recent reports

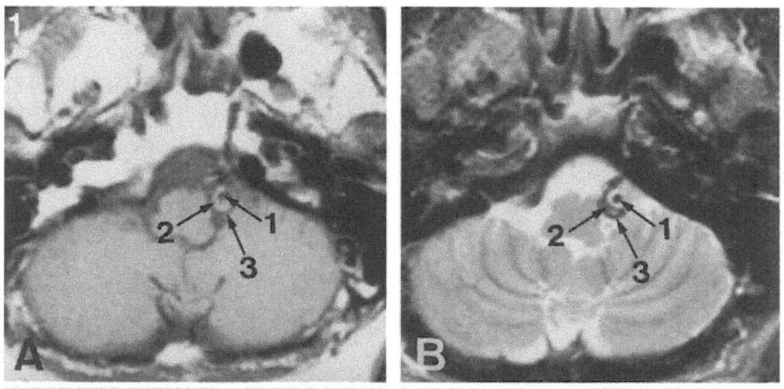

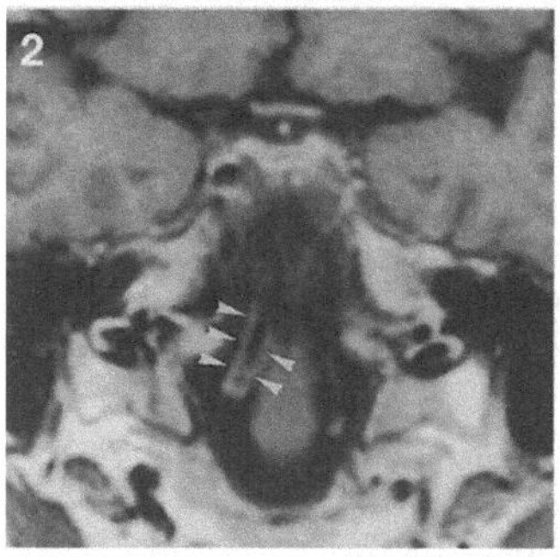

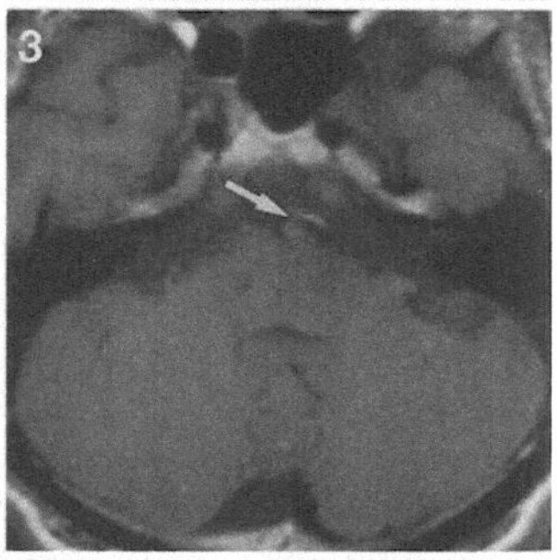

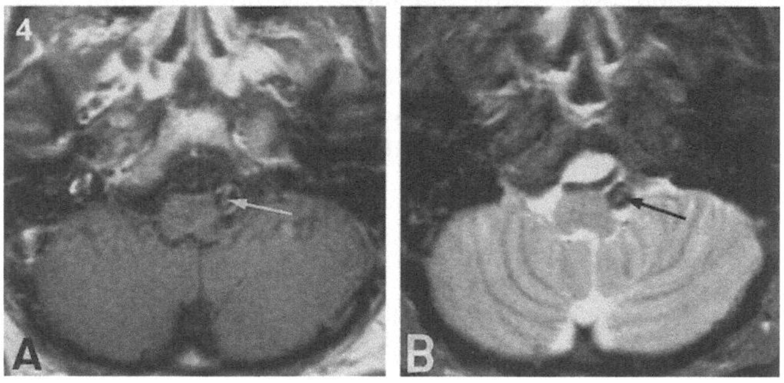

Fig. 1 A, B. Dissecting aneurysm of the left vertebral artery. T1 **(A)** and T2 weighted **(B)** axial images show eccentric signal void indicating true lumen *(1)* and semilunar haematoma consists of haemosiderin deposits showing low signal intensity with both pulse sequences *(3)*

Fig. 2. Dissecting aneurysm of the right vertebral artery. Long segment of true lumen is enclosed by thrombosed false lumen *(arrowheads)* on coronal T1-weighted image with contrast enhancement

Fig. 3. Flow-dependent misregistered signal *(arrow)* is seen adjacent to the normal vertebral artery

Fig. 4 A, B. Dissecting aneurysm of the left vertebral artery. Linear structure in the arterial lumen corresponding to an intimal flap *(arrow)* is shown on T1 **(A)** and T2-weighted **(B)** images

have proved the usefulness of magnetic resonance imaging (MRI) for demonstration of such lesions [1–4]. We studied the MRI features of intracranial vertebrobasilar dissecting aneurysms (VBDA), and compared them with those of non-dissecting aneurysms (NDA).

Patients and methods

Twelve cases of VBDA and 80 of NDA were studied. In all patients the diagnosis was confirmed by cerebral angiography. The MRI studies were performed at 1.5 T. Pulse sequences consisted of T1-weighted images, 500–600/20–30/1–2 (TR/TE/ excitations) and dual-echo proton-density and T2-weighted images, 1800–2700/30–110/1–2. Sections 5 mm thick were obtained in axial, coronal or sagittal planes.

Results

In patients with VBDA, cerebral angiography showed a double lumen in 5, a string sign in 8 and retention of contrast medium in the venous phase in 6.

On MRI, 7 patients with VBDA showed an eccentrically narrowed signal void adjacent to the semilunar haematoma in the false lumen (Figs. 1, 2, 3). These findings were also found in partially thrombosed NDA. In some cases, flow-dependent spatial misregistration was seen as a bright line adjacent to the normal vessels (Fig. 3). This flow artefact was sometimes difficult to distinguish from the intramural clot. Three patients with VBDA showed a linear or curvilinear structure in the arterial lumen corresponding to an intimal flap (Fig. 4). Flow-related enhancement indicating slow blood flow in the false lumen was seen in 3 cases of VBDA. Two patients with VBDA demonstrated only iso- or high signal intensity in the vertebral artery, findings similar to those of arterial occlusion.

Discussion

In this study, the most common MRI feature of VBDA was the eccentrically narrowed true lumen adjacent to the semilunar haematoma in the false lumen. Such findings were also found in patients with partially thrombosed NDA. However, the mural haematoma of VBDA was prone to have a longer segment with band-like shapes along the arterial lumen [3].

The intimal flap separating the arterial lumen and flow related enhancement in the false lumen are thought to be the most reliable signs for the diagnosis of DA [1–3]. However, only a few cases demonstrated these findings in this study. The limited spatial resolution of MRI may fail to delineate such tiny lesions.

It should be taken into consideration that flow-dependent spatial misregistration sometimes showed features similar to the VBDA [5]. Knowledge of this artefact is important to avoid misinterpretation of normal vessels as VBDA.

In conclusion, although MRI on spin echo sequences provides useful information for diagnosis of DA, the findings are not necessarily specific. Differentiation of DA from thrombosed NDA, arterial occlusion or flow artefact of normal vessels is sometimes difficult. Careful interpretation of both MRI and cerebral angiograms is necessary for an accurate diagnosis of VBDA.

References

1. Iwama T, Andoh T, Sakai N, Iwata T, Hirata T, Yamada H (1990) Dissecting and fusiform aneurysms of vertebro-basilar systems. MR imaging. Neuroradiology 32:272–279

2. Kitanaka C, Tanaka J, Kuwahara M, Teraoka A (1994) Magnetic resonance imaging study of intracranial vertebrobasilar artery dissections. Stroke 25:571–575
3. Mizutani T, Aruga T (1992) "Dolichoectatic" intracranial vertebrobasilar dissecting aneurysm. Neurosurgery 31:765–773
4. Quint D, Spickler EM (1990) Magnetic resonance demonstration of vertebral artery dissection. Report of two cases. J Neurosurg 72:964–967
5. Larson TC III, Kelly WM, Ehman RL, Wehrli FW (1990) Spatial misregistration of vascular flow during MR imaging of the CNS: cause and clinical significance. AJNR 11:1041–1084

MRI of vertebral artery dissection: the value of standard spin-echo imaging

V. Kähärä, A. Lamminen, O. Salonen

[1] Department of Radiology, Helsinki University Hospital, Haartmaninkatu 4, 00260 Helsinki, Finland

Abstract. We describe a case in which vertebral artery dissection responsible for a Wallenberg's syndrome was clearly identified on spin-echo MRI.

Key words: Arteries, vertebral, dissection, magnetic resonance, infarction

Reliable angiographic findings (double lumen or intimal flap) in vertebral artery dissection have been confirmed on MRI in only a few cases [1–3]. MRI can reveal an intramural haematoma directly as a semilunar area of high signal causing narrowing of the residual eccentric signal void of the lumen [4, 5].

In arterial dissection, blood penetrates the layers of the arterial wall; the injured intima predisposes to the development of thrombosis and embolisation. Dissection of the carotid arteries is three times as common as that of the vertebral arteries. The incidence of dissection is proportionally higher in young patients suffering from brain infarction.

Angiographic studies show arterial stenosis or occlusion; an intimal flap or double lumen may be seen and a pseudoaneurysm may develop. The most frequent level of vertebral artery dissection is the C1–2 level. Intracranially, bleeding from the dissection may lead to subarachnoid haemorrhage. Vertebralartery dissection has been proved to be the most frequent cause of Wallenberg's syndrome [6].

Case report

A 47-year-old previously healthy man experienced a sudden onset of headache on the right. Clinically, a classical Wallenberg's syndrome was seen: right Horner's syndrome, multiple cranial nerve palsies, limb ataxia on the right and paraesthesiae of the contralateral limbs. MRI at 1.0 T showed a subintimal crescent of increased signal in the wall of the right vertebral artery (Fig. 1) on all spin-echo pulse sequences, adjacent to a narrow area of flow void, indicating the remaining arterial lumen. The sagittal plane was most demonstrative (Fig. 2); the findings were diagnostic of dissection. In the lower brain stem, on the right, high signal was seen on T2-weighted images (Fig. 3), indicating a localised infarct.

Conventional angiography verified a concentric stenosis of the right vertebral artery at the level of the foramen magnum (Fig. 4); the left vertebral artery and carotid arteries were normal.

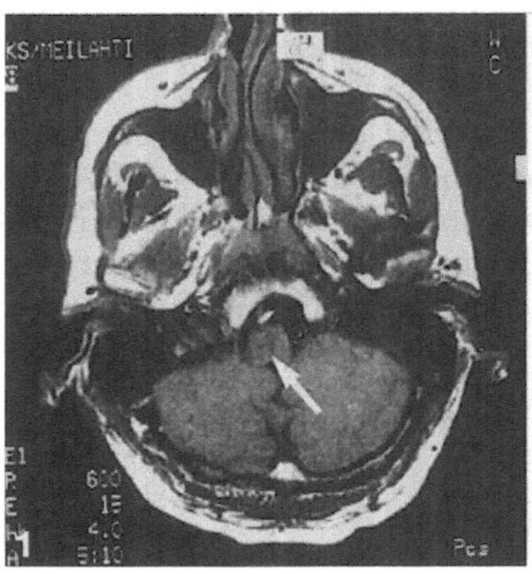

Fig. 1. Haematoma causing narrowing of the residual signal void representing the arterial lumen

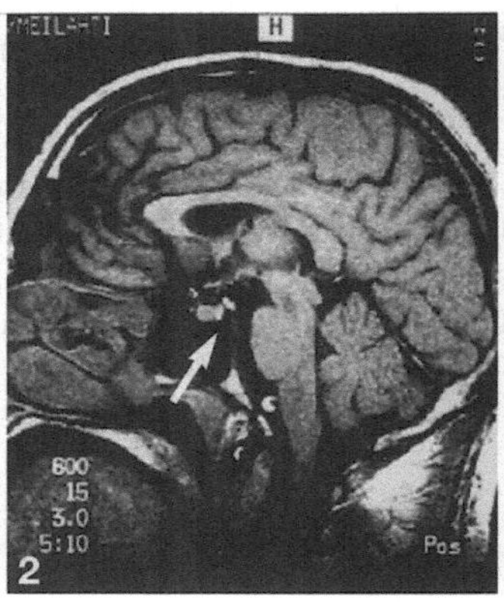

Fig. 2. The haematoma is seen as a subintimal crescent of increased signal in the wallof the right vertebral artery

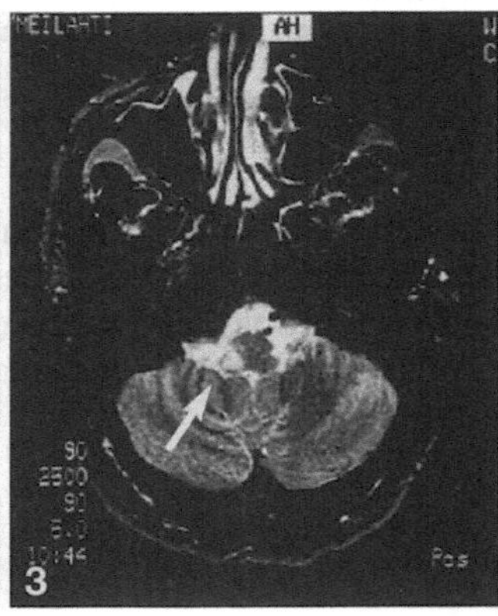

Fig. 3. In the lower brain stem, on the right, a high signal zone on a T2-weighted image indicates a localised infarct

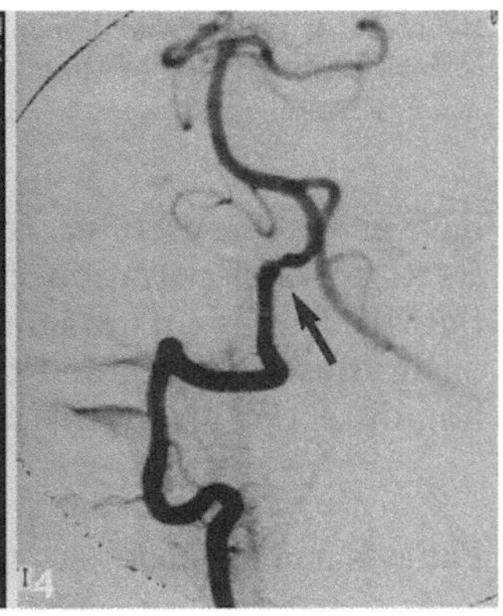

Fig. 4. Angiography verified a concentric stenosis of the right vertebral artery

Correspondence to: V. Kähärä

Discussion

Standard spin-echo sequences are a valuable non-invasive method for the diagnosis and localisation of vertebral artery dissection.

References

1. Yamaura A, Watanabe Y, Saeki N (1990) Dissecting aneurysms of the intracranial vertebral artery. J Neurosurg 72:183–188
2. Kunze ST, Schiefer W (1971) Angiographic demonstration of a dissecting aneurysm of the middle cerebral artery. Neuroradiology 2:201–206
3. Yonas H, Agamanolis D, Takaoka Y, White RJ (1977) Dissecting intracranial aneurysms. Surg Neurol 8:407–415
4. Quint DJ, Spickler EM (1990) Magnetic resonance demonstration of vertebral artery dissection: report of two cases. J Neurosurg 72:964–967
5. Gelbert F, Assouline E, Hodes JE et al. (1991) MRI in spontaneous dissection of vertebral and carotid arteries: 15 cases studies at 0.5 tesla Neuroradiology 33:111–113
6. Hosoya T, Watanabe N, Yamaguchi H, Kubota H, Onodera Y (1994) Intracranial vertebral artery dissection in Wallenberg syndrome. AJNR 15:1161-1165

Absence of the internal carotid artery: report of three cases

N. Hatsuda[1], **Y. Miyamoto**[1], **S. Nakasu**[1], **T. Okada**[2], **M. Kidooka**[2], **J. Handa**[1]

[1] Department of Neurosurgery, Shiga University of Medical Science, Seta Otsu, F520-21 Japan
[2] Division of Neurosurgery, Dai-ni Okamoto Hospital, 54-14 Ishizuka, Shinmei, Uji-shi F611 Japan

Abstract. Three cases of absence of the internal carotid artery are reported, one of bilateral and two of unilateral absence. Angiography demonstrated total non-filling of the internal carotid artery, and no bony carotid canal was disclosed on skull base CT, which proved very useful in the diagnosis of absence of the internal carotid artery. It is difficult, however, to differentiate agenesis from aplasia by solely radiological findings.

Key words: Internal carotid artery – absence, agenesis – Congenital anomaly

Congenital absence of the internal carotid artery (ICA) is rare, and bilateral absence much rarer. We report three cases of this anomaly, one case with bilateral and two with unilateral absence.

Case reports

Case 1

A 40-year-old man came to our outpatient clinic complaining of sudden onset of headaches. CT showed a mass in the pontine cistern, which enhanced with i.v. contrast medium. On angiography, both ICAs and carotid canals were absent. Angiography revealed bilateral absence of the ICA, and the middle cerebral and anterior cerebral arteries were supplied from the vertebral arteries via the posterior communicating arteries (Fig. 1). Basilar ectasia was present. Skull base CT and MRI showed a lack of bony carotid canals (Fig. 2A).

Case 2

A 52-year-old woman suffered a subarachnoid haemorrhage. Lumbar puncture revealed xanthochromic cerebrospinal fluid. The source of subarachnoid haemorrhage was not confirmed. Absence

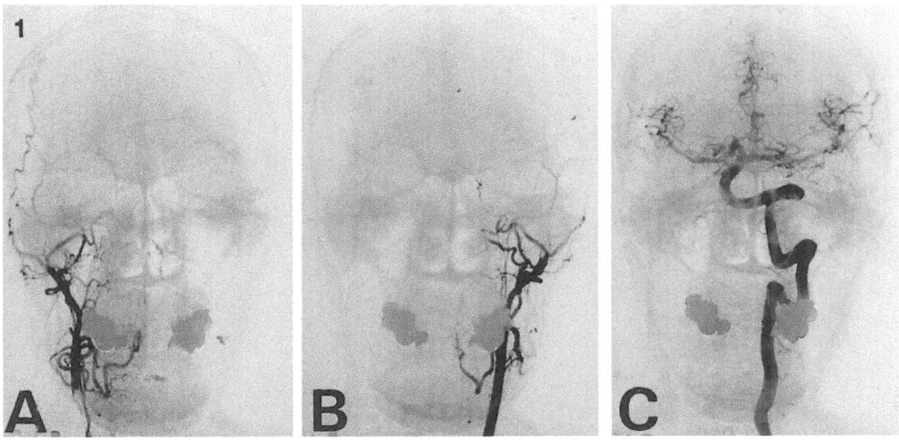

Fig. 1A–C. Case 1. Bilateral common carotid angiography demonstrating no filling of internal carotid arteries. Left vertebral artery injection filled both middle and anterior cerebral arteries via the posterior communicating arteries. **A** right **B** left common carotid **C** artery injections

Correspondence to: N. Hatsuda

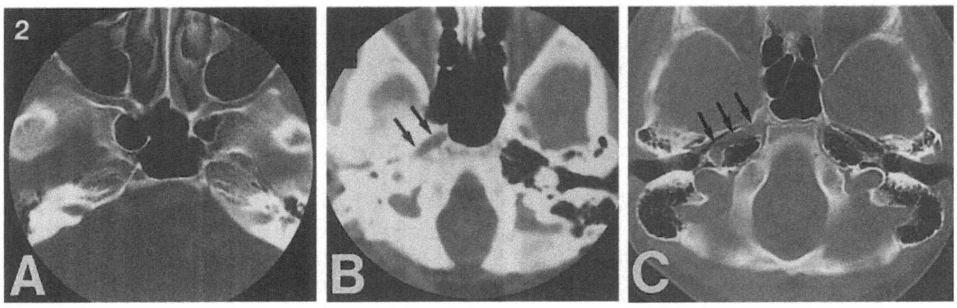

Fig. 2A–C. Skull base CT showing absence of the bony carotid canal. **A** Bilateral absence (case 1). **B, C** right bony carotid canal is visible *(arrows)*, but not the left. **B** Case 2 **C** Case 3

of the left ICA and the ipsilateral bony carotid canal was recognised radiologically (Fig. 2B). After conservative therapy, she was discharged.

Case 3

An 11-year-old boy was admitted for his generalised seizures. He had had headache and occasional vomiting for 5 years. Neurological examination was normal, but slow waves were detected in both fronto-temporal areas on the EEG. Radiological studies disclosed absence of the left ICA and the ipsilateral bony carotid canal (Fig. 2C), and a medium-sized retrocerebellar arachnoid cyst.

Discussion

Since the first report by Tode, more than 90 cases of absence of the ICA have been reported in the literature. Unilateral absence was reported in 73 cases (absence of the right ICA in 25 cases, absence of the left ICA in 47, and the side not stated in 1), and bilateral absence in 21 cases [1].

It is thought that absence of the ICA is caused by a congenital developmental anomaly of the pharyngeal arteries during the 4–12 mm embryonal stage.

The term "absence" includes both aplasia and agenesis. Agenesis of the ICA means a total lack of the ICA, and if a vestige or a portion of the ICA remains, it is termed "aplasia" [2]. However, it is occasionally difficult to differentiate agenesis and aplasia radiologically. Angiography and skull base CT demonstrate absence of the ICA, but they do not necessarily definitely exclude the presence of a vestige or a part of the ICA.

Absence of the internal carotid artery is often associated with other vascular anomalies. Cerebral aneurysm has been found in 33% of patients with unilateral absence of the ICA, and in 23% of cases of bilateral absence [3]. The haemodynamics would be different in unilateral and bilateral absence of the ICA. In bilateral absence, each cerebral hemisphere is supplied almost equally via each posterior communicating artery, but in unilateral absence, the involved cerebral hemisphere is supplied via the ipsilateral posterior communicating artery and via the anterior communicating artery. Bilateral absence of the ICA is often associated with an ectatic basilar artery.

References

1. Cali RL, Berg R, Rama K (1993) Bilateral internal carotid artery agenesis: a case study and review of the literature. Surgery 113:227–233
2. Lie TA (1968) Congenital anomalies of the carotid arteries. An angiographic study and a review of the literature. Excerpta Medica, Amsterdam, pp 35–51
3. Sunami N, Kunisio S, Yamamoto Y, Suga M, Asari S (1986) Bilateral agenesis of the internal carotid arteries. Neurol Surg (Tokyo) 14:809–814

Neoplasms

Magnetisation transfer contrast using fast spin-echo: application to tissue characterisation of intracranial tumours

M. Sasaki[1], **Y. Tamakawa**[1], **S. Ehara**[1], **A. Ogawa**[2]

[1] Centre for Radiological Sciences, Iwate Medical University, Uchimaru 19-1, Morioka 020, Japan
[2] Department of Neurosurgery, Iwate Medical University, Uchimaru 19-1, Morioka 020, Japan

Abstract. The magnetisation transfer (MT) effect on intracranial tumours on multislice fast spin-echo (FSE) images was studied for possible tissue characterisation. On multislice FSE images, attenuation of the signal intensity of tumour tissue and of normal brain tissue attributable to MT effect was compared. The rate of MT effect (MTR) was obtained by subtracting the signal intensity on multislice FSE images from single-slice images. The MTR of brain tumours was lower than that of normal brain tissue. In particular, high-grade gliomas and meningiomas had a relatively high MTR, while cavernous haemangioma and neurinomas had a relatively low MTR. An estimation of MT effect was easily accomplished by obtaining multislice and single-slice FSE images, and this may help differentiate brain tumours.

Key words: Magnetisation transfer contrast – Fast spin-echo – Brain neoplasm – Magnetic resonance imaging

Because multislice fast spin-echo (FSE) has a magnetisation transfer (MT) effect [1–4], we can easily evaluate the MT effects of brain tumours simply by adding single-slice FSE images. To investigate the possibility of tissue characterisation of intracranial tumours, we obtained their MT rate (MTR) using multislice and single-slice FSE images.

Materials and methods

We examined 18 patients with intracranial tumours (21–78 years old, 7 men and 11 women) using a 1.5-T superconductive MR unit. The types of tumours were glioma (4 cases), metastases (3), cavernous haemangioma (1), meningioma (6), neuroma (6), and pituitary adenoma (1).

The pulse sequence was FSE 3000/17, 102/1 TR/effective TE/excitation). Echo-train length was 16 and echo-spacing was 17 ms. Slice thickness was 5 mm with 2.5 mm interslice gaps. The frequency offset between neighbouring slices was 977 Hz. Acquisition time was 1 min. After nine multislice images including the tumour, a single section was obtained at the centre of the previous scan. Transmit and receive gains were fixed. The MTR was calculated from the signal intensity of the tumours on the two types of proton-density-weighted images.

Results

The MTR of tumour tissues were lower than those of normal grey and white matter (Table 1). Among intra-axial tumours, the MTR of high-grade gliomas was relatively higher than that of low-grade gliomas. The MTR of cavernous haemangioma was very low compared with those of other tumours. Metastatic brain tumours showed various MTRs.

Among extra-axial tumours, the MTR of meningiomas (Fig. 1) was lower than that of neurinomas (Fig. 2), although there was some overlap in the MTR.

Table 1. Magnetisation transfer rate of intracranial tumours

Tumour	Magnetisation transfer rate (MR)[a]	
	Cases	Mean ± S.D.
Glioma Low-grade	2	0.21 ± 0.05
High-grade	2	0.32 ± 0.03
Metastasis	3	0.31 ± 0.04
Cavernous haemangioma	1	0.08
Meningioma	6	0.29 ± 0.02
Neuroma	3	0.21 ± 0.04
Pituitary adenoma	1	0.23
White matter	18	0.39 ± 0.01
Grey matter	18	0.33 ± 0.03

[a] MR = (MS − MM)/Ms, where Ms is signal intensity on single slice images and MM signal intensity on multi-slice images

Discussion

The mechanism of MT effect on multislice FSE images is different from that on conventional MT-added images. On multislice FSE images, radiofrequency (RF) pulses of other slices play a part in the off-resonance presaturation RF with different offset frequency. Therefore, the MT effect on multislice FSE images depends on echo-train length (ETL) and number of slices [1, 2, 4]. Factors influencing the offset frequency, such as the interslice gap, can also alter MT effects [1, 2, 4]. In this study, we used the largest ETL and the maximum number of slices on multislice FSE images to enhance the MT effect. It made signal attenuation of white matter as high as 39% compared with single-slice FSE images. However, interslice gaps should remain relatively large (50%) to avoid direct saturation effect of neighbouring slices [2].

Proton-density-weighted images are known to be useful in evaluating MT effect, because it is related to longitudinal magnetisation. FSE images using early-echo as effective TE have strong artefacts related to point spread function, such as blur and pseudo-edge enhancement, especially when large ETL or large echo-spacing is used [1]. To avoid such artefacts, we used two contrast

Correspondence to: M. Sasaki

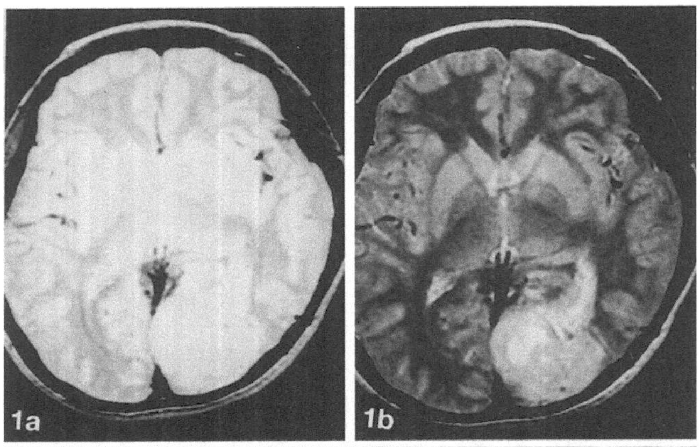

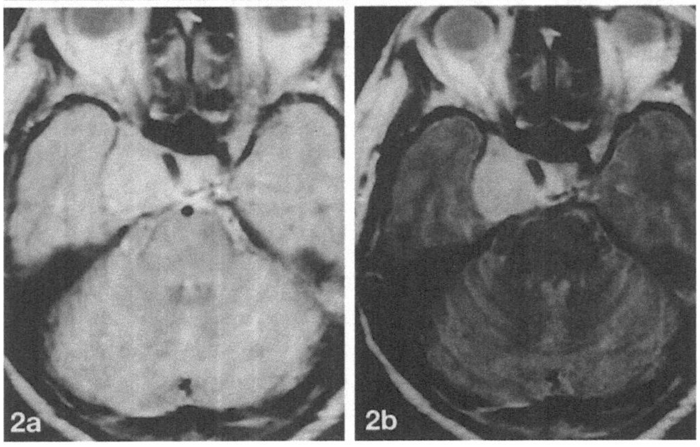

Fig. 1. **a** Single-slice and **b** multislice proton-density-weighted images of a 21-year-old woman with a menigioma. Window width and level are fixed in both images. On the multislice image, signal attenuation of the tumour, as well as of normal brain tissue, is evident. MT rate of the tumour: 0.27

Fig. 2. **a** Single-slice and **b** multislice proton-density-weighted images of a 62-year-old woman with a parasellar neuroma. Signal attenuation of the tumour is less evident on the multislice image **(b)** than on the single-slice image **(a)**. MT rate of the tumour: 0.16

FSE, in which echo trains are split in two, to make two kinds of images [5]. Using this method, we can successfully obtain proton-density-weighted images with a strong MT effect and with less artefacts.

Recently, conventional MT images have been applied for tissue characterisation of the tumour tissue [5]. It has been reported that high-grade gliomas and meningiomas have strong MT effects, and that the MT effects of the tumour tissue reflect the amount of nuclear material in the tumour cells, and the content of collagen. The results of this study correspond to those of the previous study, so the MT effect of the tumour tissue on FSE may be determined by the same factors as on conventional MT sequences, in the same fashion.

MT rate measurement using FSE is a simple and time-saving technique, and it may play some role in the differential diagnosis of intracranial tumours.

References

1. Listerud J, Einstein S, OutwaterE, Kressel HY (1992) First principles of fast spin-echo. Magn Reson Quarterly 8:199–244
2. Constable RT, Anderson AW, Zhong J, Gore JC (1992) Factors influencing contrast in fast spin-echo MR imaging. Magn Reson Imaging 10:497–511
3. Melki PS, Mulkern RV (1992) Magnetization transfer effects in multislice RARE sequences. Magn Reson Med 24, 189–195
4. Sasaki M, Sone M, Ehara S, Tamakawa Y, Ogawa A (1994) Magnetization transfer contrast effect on multislice fast spin-echo (in Japanese). Japn J Magn Reson Med 14:125–131
5. Lundbom N (1992) Determination of magnetization transfer contrast in tissue: an MR imaging study of brain tumors. AJR 159:1279–1285

Contrast manipulation of human brain tumours by magnetisation transfer and paramagnetic contrast medium

C. C. Chen[1], **J. W. Chai**[1], **W. C. Shen**[1], **J. H. Chen**[1], **C. M. Chiang**[1], **S. K. Lee**[1], **H. N. Yeung**[2]

[1] Department of Radiology, Taichung Veterans General Hospital, Taichung, Taiwan
[2] Institute of Biomedical Sciences, Academia Sinica, Taipei, Taiwan

Abstract. We studied 20 patients with intracranial tumours (meningioma, astrocytoma, pituitary adenoma and adenocarcinoma metastasis with MTC (magnetisation transfer contrast) using binomial-pulse saturation at 1.0 T before and after intravascular Gd-DTPA. Our goal was to evaluate the use of MTC (alone and combination with Gd-DTPA) as a potential means of enhancing lesion contrasts in brain tumours. Our preliminary results, based on the image intensity attenuation measured quantitatively, indicate that MTC with (and without) Gd-DTPA cannot be used to differentiate tumour type. However, perifocal oedema in intra-parenchymal tumours is generally found to have a smaller intensity attenuation ratio than that in extra-parenchymal tumours. This observation, if verified

Correspondence to: C. C. Chen, Department of Radiology, Taichung Veterans General Hospital, 169, Sec. 3 Chung-Kung Rd. Taichung, Taiwan

by further study or other means, may be used for better delineation of the fringe area of the tumour than is possible with conventional MRI techniques.

Key words: Magnetic resonance imaging – Magnetisation transfer contrast – Brain, neoplasm

Magnetisation transfer contrast (MTC) (1) is a technique that attracted a lot of interest when it was first discovered owing to its potential clinical impact on the diagnosis of a variety of diseases. Recently, this intrigue seems to have waned considerably (with the notable exception of workers at extremely low fields [2]), on account of the general sentiments, expressed by many who had conducted clinical trials, that MTC fails to reveal any diagnostic information that has not already been found on conventional T1 and/or T2-weighted MRI (with, and sometimes without, the contrast medium Gd-DTPA). In our view, MTC is a complex phenomenon; therefore, before the detailed mechanism of how it works is understood and sufficient evidence documenting its clinical efficacy is accumulated, neither the initial high expectations nor the premature disillusionment are really justified. In this study, we would like to contribute our own experience with MTC for the study of various forms of brain tumours at 1.0 T (and without) the intravascular agent Gd-DTPA.

Methods and materials

Experiments in MTCA require selective presaturation of the immobile components in tissues. There are, in general, two methods of presaturation: continuous off-resonance radiofrequency (RF) irradiation (1) and binomial pulse train (3, 4). For mid- to high-field clinical MRI systems, it is impractical to apply RF power for long periods, which precludes continuous RF irradiation as a viable alternative, leaving binomial pulses as the method of choice for the present study. The main advantage of binomial pulses is the ease of implementation. The major drawback is that its attenuation of signal intensity is often contaminated by T2 decay during the RF-on period. In this study, the presaturation consists of a train of biphasic pulses with a width of 2 ms (4 ms total) followed by a delay of 13 ms. The field amplitude of the presaturation RF pulse was 6.9 mT, while the number of the binomial composites varied from 8 to 12 in the train. After the pre-saturation pulse train, a standard spin-echo sequence was used to image a transaxial or coronal section of the subject's brain. The image acquisition parameters were: slice thickness, 5 mm; FOV 21 cm; data matrix size, 256 × 128 (with half-Fourier in phase-encoding); TE, 30 ms; TR, 2 S; and accumulation, 2. The scan time for each data point was 4 min.

Results

The patient sample number in this study is 20. They can be categorised into four tumour groups, namely, meningioma, astrocytoma, pituitary adenoma, and metastatic adenocarcinoma. The breakdown of patients into the tumour types, and the overall statistical results are summarised in Table 1, which, it must be noted, gives only an overall picture in the form of easily understandable statistics, at the risk of oversimplification. There are many nuances and variations (caused by biological variability and/or other factors) that would require much more space to be clarified.

Table 1. Average image intensity ratio: with/without saturation, after 12 binomial pulses

Tumour	Cases	Before Gd-DTPA		After Gd-DTPA	
		mean	+ S.D.	mean	+ S.D.
Astrocytoma	9	48%	+ 10%	53%	+ 8%
Meningioma	4	39%	+ 3%	47%	+ 8%
Metastatic adenocarcinoma	4	53%	± 10%	57%	± 7%
Pituitary adenoma	3	46%	+ 13%	46%	+ 12%

Discussion

We can summarize our major results in terms of providing answers to our questions:

1. Do MTC images alone contribute results that are clinically unique? In other words, without Gd-DTPA, does MTC offer any additional diagnostic information to conventional T1- or T2-weighted images? Three experienced and impartial radiologists compared the films of MTC images with conventional MRI and found the answer to this question, in most cases, to be yes.
2. More importantly, can MTC, either by itself or in combination with Gd-DTPA, be used to differentiate tumour types based on the image intensity attenuation measured quantitatively? Based on the results shown in Table 1, with the possible exception of meningiomas (in which case, the sample size is too small to make the result statistically significant), the answer is negative.
3. Is MTC capable of differentiating tumours from perifocal oedema? While the answer to this question, based on our results thus far, is inconclusive (owing mainly to lack of good controls rather than technical drawbacks of the method itself), the image intensity attenuation ratio measured in intra-parenchymal tumours is much lower than that measured in extra-parenchymal tumours. This observation may serve as a possible demarcation of the region, normally characterised by conventional MRI as perifocal oedema, of the fringe area of a tumour cell of astrocytoma and/or metastasizing adenocarcinoma or demyelination. This interesting observation can be explained by the fact that freely mobile oedema protons tend to be structurally and dynamically different from their counterparts in the more restricted tumour cell membranes. We feel that this is the most promising area MTC can contribute to. More work needs to be done before this issue can be resolved conclusively.
4. Finally, can the application of a T1 contrast agent in conjunction with MTC add any valuable clues to the diagnosis? In principle, the application of Gd-DTPA will cause T1 shortening in tumours that are highly perfused, and as a result, one expects a significant decrease of the post-contrast MTC effect. Table 1, however, shows this

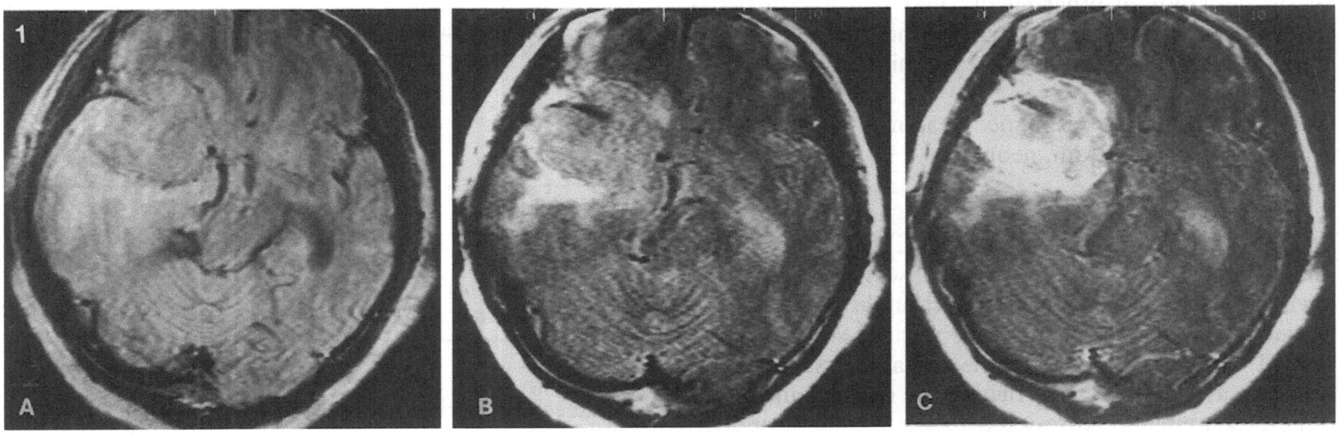

Fig. 1. A–C. MTC of patient with meningioma. Unenhanced images **A** without and **B** with MT and **C** contrast-enhanced image with MT. In **B**, both normal brain tissue and tumour show signal intensity loss; but when MTC is combined with Gd-DTPA (**C**) the contrast between normal brain and tumour is further enhanced by the usual signal loss in the normal brain, while the corresponding attenuation in the tumour is lessened because of the T1 shortening of free water protons by the paramagnetic agent

effect only unequivocally in meningioma (Fig. 1). In all three other cases, its effect is either borderline or absent (as in pituitary adenoma).

References

1. Wolff SD, Balaban RS (1992) Magnetization transfer contrast (MTC) and tissue water proton relaxation in vivo. Magn Reson Med 10:135–144
2. Lundbom N (1992) Determination of magnetization transfer contrast in tissue: an MR imaging study of brain tumours. AJR 159:1279–1285
3. Yeung HN, Aisen AM (!992) Magnetization transfer contrast with periodic pulsed saturation. Radiology 183:209–214

Differential diagnosis of intracranial tumours using in vitro magnetic resonance spectroscopy

Y. Kinoshita[1], **A. Yokota**[1], **Y. Koga**[2]

[1] Department of Neurosurgery, University of Occupational and Environmental Health, 1-1 Iseigaoka Yahatanishi-ku, Kitakyushu, Japan
[2] Chemistry, University of Occupational and Environmental Health, 1-1 Iseigaoka Yahatanishi-ku, Kitakyushu, Japan

Abstract. The diagnostic utility of magnetic resonance spectroscopy (MRS) in intracranial tumours was investigated using in vitro high-resolution spectra. We examined 59 surgically excised samples of brain tumours and 4 non-neoplastic lobectomised brains. Glioblastoma can be distinguished from metastatic brain tumour by the total creatine and glycine peak, medulloblastoma from ependymoma by the taurine peak and neurinoma from meningioma by the inositol peak on ^{1}H-MRS. The phosphomonoester peak may be useful in distinguishing pituitary adenoma, malignant lymphoma and meduloblastoma from other tumours by ^{31}P-MRS. MRS may provide additional information when the differential diagnosis of tumours by MRI is difficult.

Key words: Magnetic resonance spectroscopy – Glycine – Inositol – Phosphorylethnolamine

Correspondence to: Y. Kinoshita

Magnetic resonance imaging (MRI is useful for the anatomical localisation of intracranial tumours. However, its diagnostic specificity for tumours is poor. In vivo magnetic resonance spectroscopy (MRS) is expected to aid in the diagnosis by characterising brain tumours. The aim of this study was to determine the characteristic in vitro MR spectra of various brain tumour extracts and to provide a better interpretation of the spectra obtained in vivo MRS.

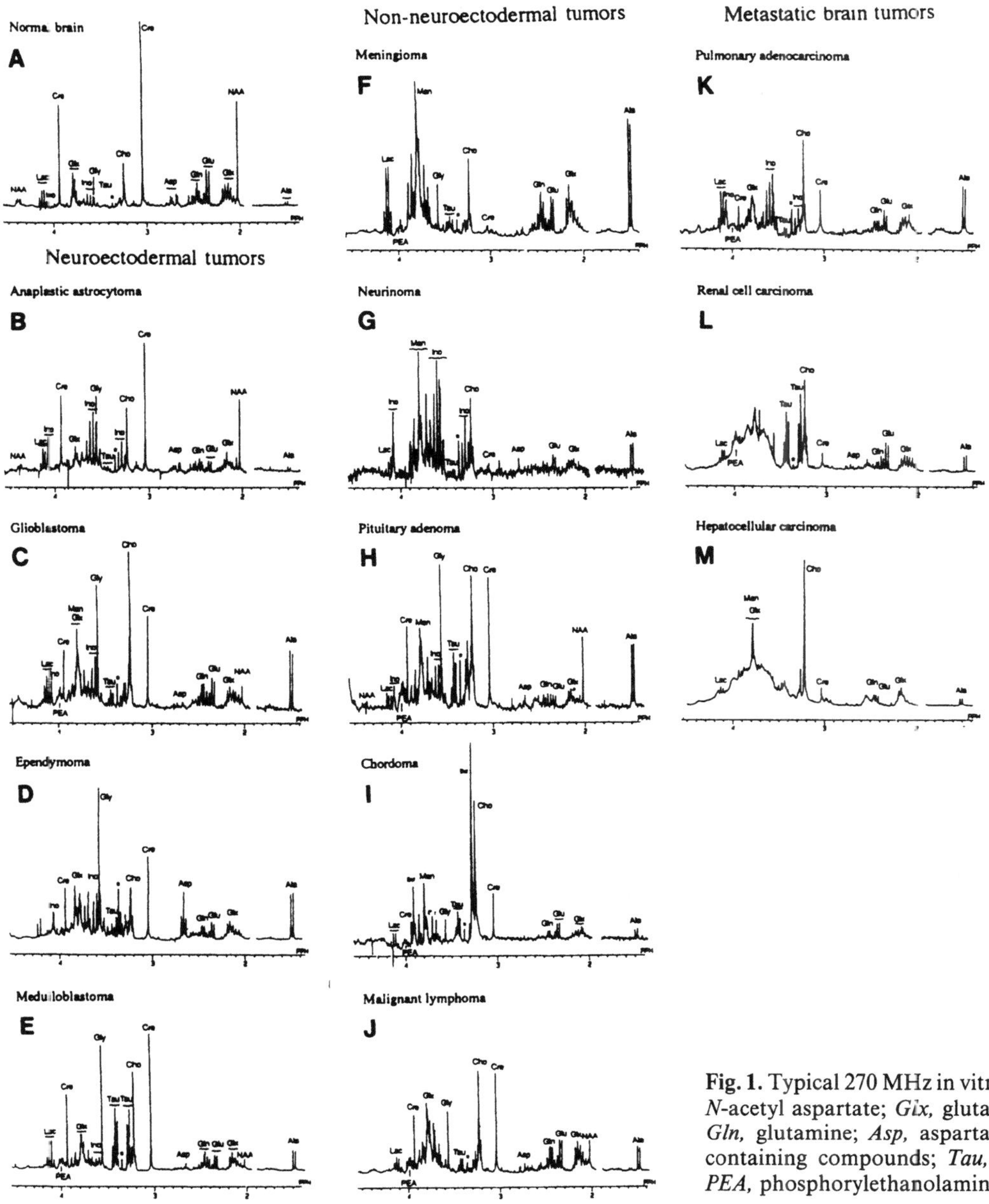

Fig. 1. Typical 270 MHz in vitro ^{1}H-MR spectra. *Ala,* alanine; NAA, *N*-acetyl aspartate; *Glx,* glutamate and glutamine; *Glu,* glutamate; *Gln,* glutamine; *Asp,* aspartate; *Cre* total creatine; *Cho,* choline-containing compounds; *Tau,* taurine; *Gly,* glycine; *Ino,* inositol; *PEA,* phosphorylethanolamine; *Bet,* betaine; *Man,* mannitol

Materials and methods

We examined 59 samples of intracranial tumours and 4 normal brains (Tab. 1). All specimens were removed at surgery, frozen immediately in liquid nitrogen, and stored at −80°C. Perchloric acid extracts were prepared and neutralised. ^{1}H-MR spectra of the extracts were obtained with a 270 MHz (6.3 Tesla) nuclear MR spectrometer [1–3]. Phosphorylethanlamine (PEA) was also analysed using an automated high-speed amino acid analyser [4].

Results

The spectrum of each extract contained signals from a wide range of metabolites, and each of the various intracranial brain tumours showed a different spectrum (Tab. 1, Fig. 1). *N*-Acetylaspartate (NAA) was unequivocally demonstrated in normal tissues. NAA is present in the millimolar range in nervous tissue, but in contrast, is very low in non-nervous tissue. The NAA peak was hardly detected in extramedullary tumours. The clinical significance of total creatine (Cre) on ^{1}H-MR spectra is unknown, but Cre was preserved in high amounts in relatively neuroectodermal tumours and low in non-neuroectodermal tumours. Cre may be related to the origin of brain tumours. Glycine was increased in neuroectodermal tumours. We reported a prominent peak of glycine in astrocytic tumours [2]. This peak at 3.56 ppm might be useful for the differential diagnosis of glial tumours from other brain tumours (Fig. 2). Choline-containing compounds were especially prominent in metastatic hepatocellular carcinoma. Taurine was increased in medulloblastoma, which suggests that medulloblastoma may be distinguished from ependymoma by this peak. Alanine was increased in glioblastoma, meningioma and pituitary adenoma. Inositol was increased in brain tumours, especially in neurinoma. The reason for

Table 1. Metabolite concentrations (μmol/100 g wet weight; mean ± SEM) in normal cerebral cortex and in intracranial tumours

Pathology/Number	N-acetyl-aspartate	Total Creatine	Choline containing compounds	Glycine	Taurine	Alanine	Inositol	Phosphoryl-ethanol-amine
Cerebral cortex 4	555.6 ± 32.9	1076.3 ± 102.7	64.3 ± 10.1	82.2 ± 19.7	153.2 ± 29.1	91.9 ± 18.9	174.3 ± 17.0	115.6 ± 12.3
Neuroectodermal tumours								
Astrocytoma 6	180.8 ± 27.7	780.9 ± 84.1	68.6 ± 6.5	91.3 ± 15.5	169.0 ± 16.7	101.0 ± 20.3	364.7 ± 94.2	116.7 ± 7.3
Anapl. astrocytoma 4	110.2 ± 43.4	564.8 ± 89.0	132.6 ± 7.9	269.5 ± 76.1	227.7 ± 47.7	52.4 ± 17.9	479.6 ± 97.6	226.0 ± 34.4
Glioblastoma 12	40.6 ± 10.9	365.9 ± 40.7	119.2 ± 29.8	501.7 ± 43.9	214.9 ± 42.0	325.8 ± 31.1	333.9 ± 72.5	215.2 ± 34.3
Ependymoma 1	ND	445.8	88.4	677.9	304.8	324.2	502.8	95.8
Medulloblastoma 1	40.3	888.4	205.8	913.5	1930.0	225.2	184.8	498.6
Non-neuroectodermal tumours								
Meningioma 13	ND	145.9 ± 23.2	81.3 ± 11.1	160.3 ± 21.1	358.6 ± 106.8	310.4 ± 42.2	184.7 ± 39.3	177.7 ± 22.1
Neuroma 6	ND	72.9 ± 15.2	124.5 ± 23.7	75.0 ± 6.9	215.6 ± 28.4	156.0 ± 28.4	873.1 ± 142.5	191.9 ± 23.7
Craniopharyngioma 3	ND	86.2 ± 14.5	15.7 ± 9.1	85.6 ± 23.6	128.0 ± 31.0	138.3 ± 32.1	104.6 ± 66.3	77.4 ± 18.4
Chordoma 4	ND	151.6 ± 63.5	110.2 ± 41.6	166.3 ± 44.3	315.6 ± 115.0	131.2 ± 34.5	267.0 ± 141.4	231.2 ± 75.6
Malig. lymphoma 2	51.2 ± 5.7	160.8 ± 37.0	74.3 ± 0.4	197.6 ± 13.3	201.1 ± 11.7	117.1 ± 2.7	160.9 ± 76.2	434.8 ± 18.5
Pituitary adenoma 2	147.9 ± 147.9	311.6 ± 176.6	132.6 ± 18.8	245.1 ± 245.1	853.6 ± 64.9	272.3 ± 80.3	327.6 ± 56.7	465.5 ± 122.9
Metastatic tumours								
Pulmonary adenocarcinoma 3	ND	102.7 ± 12.0	101.4 ± 18.1	136.6 ± 13.6	236.6 ± 26.7	140.7 ± 30.8	337.5 ± 40.1	208.0 ± 18.5
Renal cell carcinoma 1	ND	72.8	72.8	93.7	786.2	103.2	NQ	288.7
Hepatocellular carcinoma 1	ND	212.8	572.2	166.8	117.7	142.7	NQ	226.3

ND not detected, *NQ* not quantifiable

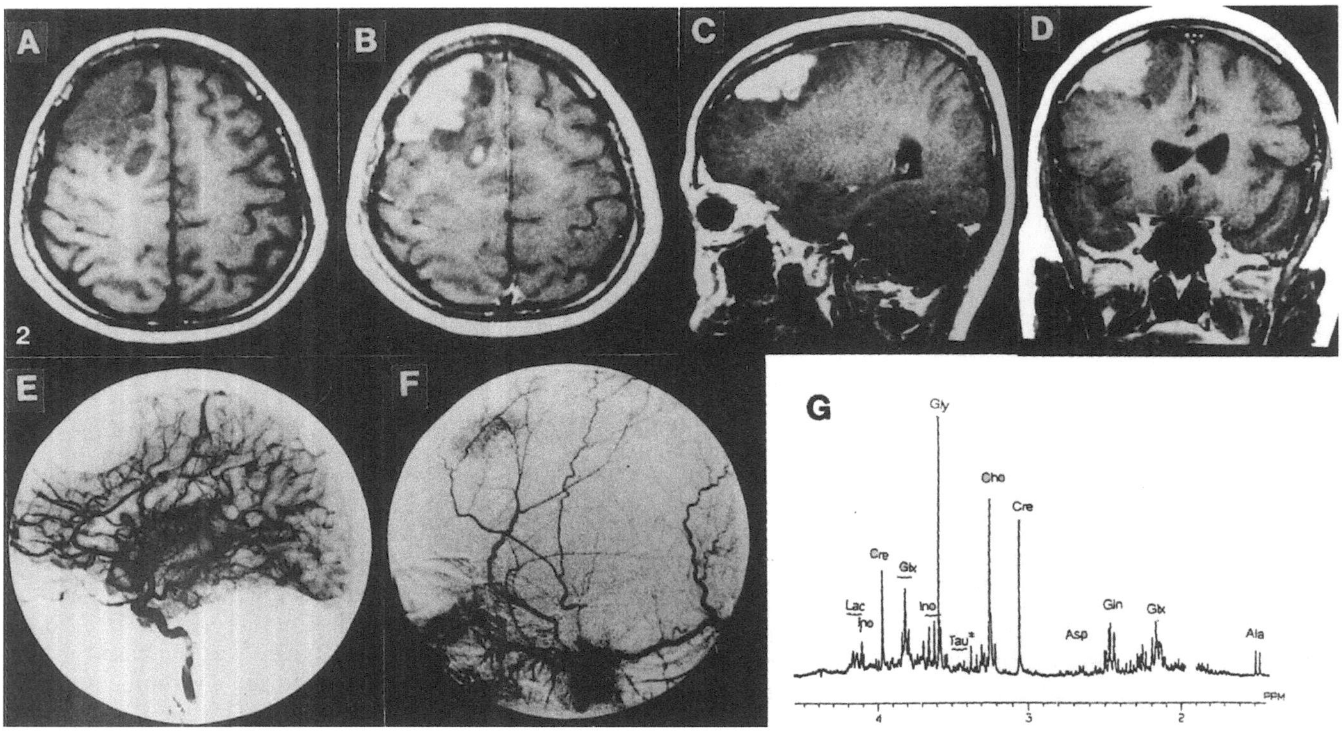

Fig. 2A–G. Axial T1 **(A)**, and contrast-enhanced **(B–D)** MRI right internal **(E)** and external **(F)** angiograms showed an extra-axial tumour, probably a meningioma. In vitro high-resolution ^{1}H-MRS of the surgical specimen **(G)** demonstrated some characteristics of glioma. Pathological examination showed anaplastic astrocytoma. Abbreviations as in Fig. 1

the high inositol content in neurinoma is unknown, but the prominent peak of inositol on MR spectra should be useful for the differential diagnosis of neurinoma from meningioma. PEA content was particularly high in pituitary adenoma, malignant lymphoma and medulloblastoma. PEA is the major constituent of the phosphomonoester (PME) peak of ^{31}P-MR spectrum of the brain [5]; the

PME peak therefore may be useful in distinguishing pituitary adenoma, malignant lymphoma and medulloblastoma from other tumours in ^{31}P.MRS [4].

Discussion

MRS may provide additional information when the differential diagnosis of tumours by MRI is difficult.

References

1. Petroff OAC, Ogino T, Alger JR (1988) High-resolution proton magnetic resonance spectroscopy of rabbit brain: regional metabolite levels and postmortem changes. J Neurochem 51:163–171
2. Kinoshita Y, Kajiwara H, Yokota A, Koga Y (1992) Protonmagnetic resonance spectroscopy of astrocytic tumors: an in vitro study. Neurol Chir (Tokyo) 33:350–359
3. Kinoshita Y, Kajiwara H, Yokota A, Koga Y (in press) Proton magnetic resonance spectroscopy of brain tumors: an in vitro study. Neurosurgery
4. Kinoshita Y, Yokota A, Koga Y (in press) Phosphorylethanolamine content in human brain tumors. Neurol Med Chir
5. Gyulai L, Bolinger L, Leigh JS, Barlow C, Chance B (1984) Phosphorylethanolamine – the major constituent of the phosphomonoester peak observed by ^{31}P-NMR on developing dog brain. FEBS Lett 178:137–142

^{31}P chemical shift imaging of intracranial tumours

M. Sasahira[1], K. Uchimura[1], K. Terada[1], N. Moriya[1], M. Niiro[1], A. Haruzono[1], W. Hirakawa[1], T. Asakura[1], T. Fujimoto[2]

[1] Department of Neurosurgery, Faculty of Medicine, Kagoshima University
[2] South Japan Health Science Centre, Miyakonojou, Japan

Abstract. Chemical shift imaging is useful to obtain spectra of multiple contiguous voxels simultaneously and to demonstrate detailed mapping of metabolites. ^{31}P magnetic resonance (MR) spectra of intracranial tumours are different from those of normal brain tissue. Low concentrations of total ^{31}P, phosphocreatine (PCr) and phosphodiesters (PDE) were observed. Glioblastoma and malignant lymphoma showed a high concentration of phosphomonoester (PME). Glioblastoma, metastatic tumour, malignant lymphoma, epidermoid and chondrosarcoma showed a high concentration of inorganic phosphorus (Pi). Metabolite images demonstrated the extension of the abnormal intensity area, which was correlated with the extension of the tumour. Calculated images (Pi/PCr, PME/PDE) were also useful for demonstrating tumour extension. A transient increase in Pi and acidic pH were noted after treatment.

Key words: ^{31}P chemical shift imaging – Phosphorus metabolism – Intracellular pH – Therapeutic monitor – Brain tumour

^{31}P magnetic resonance spectroscopy (MRS) provides information on phosphorus metabolism in vivo noninvasively, which can be related to tissue energetics, phospholipid metabolism and intracellular pH [1]. The technique used here, three-dimensional chemical shift imaging (3D-CSI), differs from the single-voxel method in that spectra are obtained from multiple contiguous voxels simultaneously [2]. We tried to study tumour metabolism and response to therapy using 3D-CSI.

Correspondence to: M. Sasahira

Materials and methods

3D-CSI was performed on 31 patients with intracranial tumours (5 astrocytomas, 9 glioblastomas, and 1 ependymoma, 3 metastatic tumours, 1 malignant lymphoma, 9 meningiomas, 2 epidermoids, 1 chondrosarcoma). All studies were performed on a clinical 2.0 T MR system. Data acquisition of 3D-CSI was as follows: TR 2 s, matrix 8 × 8, 12 excitations, voxel size 3.1 × 3.1 × 4 cm [2]. The spectra and intracellular pH of the tumours were compared with those of contralateral normal brain tissue. The pH was derived from the chemical shift of inorganic phosphate (δPi) with reference to phosphocreatine (PCr = 0 ppm) and obtained with the use of the formula $pH = 6.77 + \log [(\delta Pi - 3.29)/(5.68 - \delta Pi)]$. The spectral changes after chemo- and radiotherapy were also evaluated.

Results

The ^{31}P spectra of brain tumours were significantly different from those of normal brain tissue. Low concentrations of total ^{31}P, phosphocreatine (PCr) and phosphodiester (PDE) were observed. Glioblastoma and malignant lymphoma showed high concentrations of phosphomonoester (PME). Glioblastomas, metastatic tumours, malignant lymphoma, epidermoids and chondrosarcoma showed high concentrations of Pi. Metabolite images demonstrated the extension of the abnormal inten-

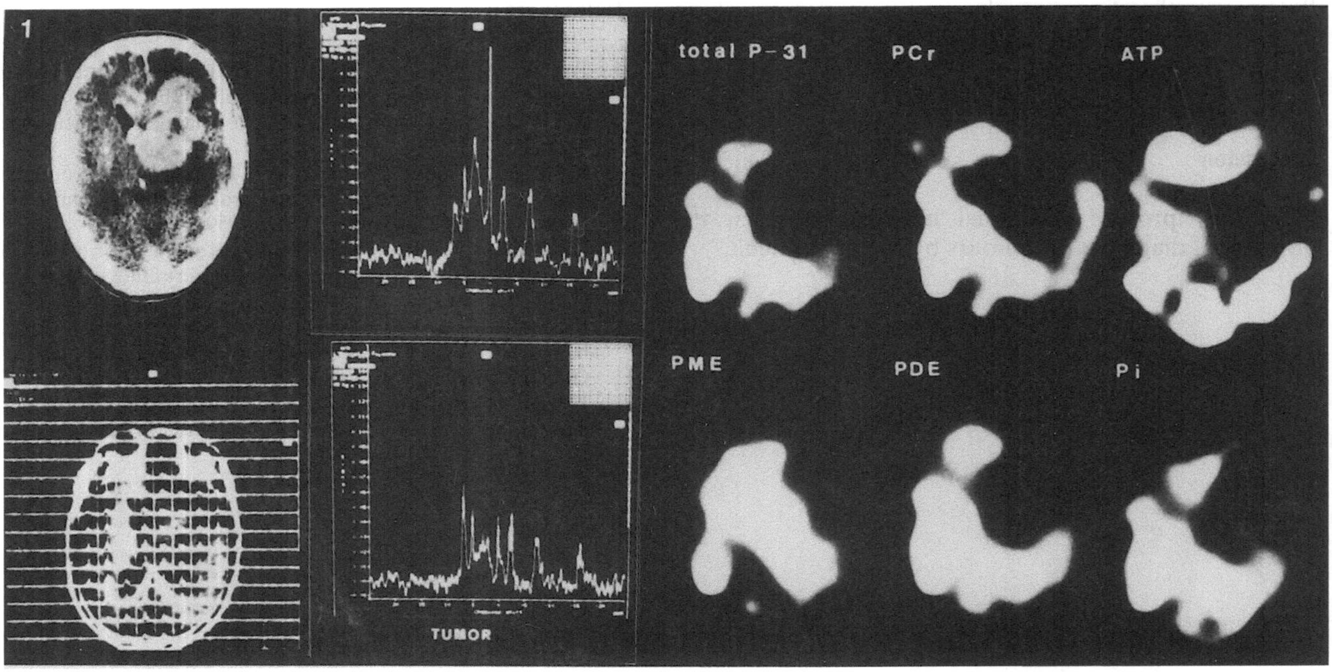

Fig. 1. Glioblastoma in right frontothalamic region, extending to left frontal lobe. Tumour ^{31}P spectrum showed low concentrations of PCr, PDE, and ATP, and high concentrations of Pi and PME. Tumour was seen as a low signal intensity area in the total ^{31}P, PCr, ATP, and Pi and PDE images. PME and Pi images showed high intensity within the tumour. The area of low signal intensity in the PCr image is consistent with the area of tumour and perifocal oedema

sity area, which correlated well with the extension of the tumour (Fig. 1). The tumour pH was more alkaline than that of normal brain tissue. Spectral changes after chemo- and radiotherapy were also detected. Total ^{31}P decreased after treatment. A transient increase of Pi was noted after an intra-arterial injection of ACNU. The tumour pH reverted to normal after treatment.

Discussion

^{31}P MRS provides useful information on brain energy metabolism [1]. CSI techniques provide spectra of multiple contiguous voxels simultaneously and demonstrate the detailed mapping of metabolites [2]. Since 1988, we have been clinically applying ^{31}P CSI to neurosurgical diseases [3–9].

^{31}P MR spectra of brain tumours are significantly different from those of normal brain tumours. Low concentrations of total ^{31}P, PCr and PDE were observed. Glioblastoma and malignant lymphoma showed high concentrations of PME. Glioblastoma, metastatic tumours, malignant lymphoma, epidermoid and chondrosarcoma showed high concentrations of Pi. These findings suggest an anaerobic metabolism and an increase in membrane repair and/or synthesis, associated with the increased growth rate of tumour cells [10]. Metabolite images demonstrated the extension of the abnormal intensity area, which correlated well with the extension of the tumours. Calculated images (Pi/PCr, PME/PDE) are also useful for demonstrating tumour extension. The ^{31}P spectra obtained after therapy showed various changes. Malignant lymphoma showed a dramatic change i.e. a normal pattern of ^{31}P spectra. The decrease in total ^{31}P after treatment may reflect the decreased activity of tumour cells. The acidic pH shift may be associated with overproduction of lactate as a result of tumour necrosis. A transient increase in Pi after an intra-arterial injection of ACNU reflects the necrosis of tumour cells.

In conclusion, ^{31}P CSI yielded metabolic information on brain tumours and was a useful clinical tool for monitoring brain tumour therapy.

References

1. Bottomley PA (1989) Human in vivo NMR spectroscopy in diagnostic medicine: clinical tool or research probe? Radiology 170:1–15
2. Fujimoto T, Tsuji T, Nakano T et al. (1994) Study of normal brain using phosphorus-31 chemical shift imaging. Jpn J Magn Reson 14:1–10
3. Asakura T, Sasahira M, Uchimura K et al. (!991) Clinical evaluation of the cerebral energy metabolism with ^{31}P chemical shift imaging. Prog CT 13:509–520
4. Niiro M, Asakura T, Nakamura K et al. (1990) ^{31}P chemical shift imaging of epileptic brains. Prog CT 12:493–503
5. Sasahira M, Uchimura K, Okada A et al. (1990) ^{31}P spectroscopic imaging of brain tumors. Prog CT 12:59–66
6. Sasahira M, Uchimura K, Yatsushiro K et al. (1990) Early detection of cerebral infarction by ^{31}P spectroscopic imaging. Neuroradiology 32:43–46

7. Sasahira M, Uchimura K, Asakura T et al. (1991) ^{31}P chemical shift imaging of hypertensive intracerebral hematoma. Neuroradiology 33 [Suppl]:358–359
8. Sasahira M, Asakura T, Uchimura K et al. (1992) ^{31}P chemical shift imaging of brain tumors and cerebrovascular disease. Prog CT 14:517–531
9. Uchimura K (1990) A clinical study on the energy metabolism and intracellular pH in human brain with cerebral infarction – detection by ^{31}P-chemical shift imaging and ^{31}P-magnetic resonance spectroscopy. Med J Kagoshima Univ 42:223–244
10. Asakura T, Sasahira M, Uchimura K et al. (1994) ^{31}P magnetic resonance spectroscopy and ^{31}P chemical shift imaging of human brain tumors. Med J Kagoshima Univ 46:29–39

Noninvasive characterisation of intracranial tumours by in vivo proton magnetic resonance spectroscopy

M. Harada[1], M. Tanouchi[1], H. Nishitani[1], H. Miyoshi[2], K. Bandou[3], S. Kannuki[3]

[1] Department of Radiology, School of Medicine, University of Tokushima, 3-18-15, Kuramoto-cho, Tokushima, 770 Japan
[2] Department of Radiological Technology, School of Medical Science, University of Tokushima, 3-18-15 Kuramoto-cho, Tokushima, 770 Japan
[3] Department of Neurosurgery, School of Medicine, University of Tokushima, 3-18-15 Kuramoto-cho Tokushima, 770 Japan

Abstract. We studied the possibility of tissue characterisation of intracranial tumours by localised proton magnetic resonance spectroscopy (^{1}H-MRS). Twenty-six newly diagnosed tumours were examined by in vivo ^{1}H-MRS. The *N*-acetyl aspartate/choline (NAA/Cho ratio of grade 2 astrocytomas was relatively higher than that of those of grade 4. The choline/creatine (Cho/Cr) ratio of meningiomas was considerably higher than that of gliomas of all grades. We found only 2 cases of ependymoma, and the Cho/Cr ratio in both was lower than that in other gliomas. We considered that ^{1}H-MRS can be used to differentiate grade 2 from grade 4 in most cases of astrocytoma by the NAA/Cho ratio, though a few cases will overlap. Meningioma can easily be separated from glioma, and the results of our study suggest that ependymoma has a characteristic pattern.

Key words: Proton magnetic resonance spectroscopy – Brain tumour – Meningioma – Ependymoma

Proton magnetic resonance spectroscopy (^{1}H-MRS) can show biochemical changes in tissue noninvasively and much has been published concerning the utility of this method. We have already reported that ^{1}H-MRS of brain abscesses differs appreciably from that of glioblastoma and that this method is useful in revealing the biochemical status of tissue [1]. We conducted ^{1}H-MRS on patients with primary intracranial tumours and studied the possibility of tissue characterisation of these tumours by ^{1}H-MRS.

Correspondence to: M. Harada

Methods

The 26 patients in this study all underwent tumour resection. A pathological diagnosis was obtained in all patients. 15 of the tumours were astrocytomas, including 6 grade 2, 1 grade 3 and 9 grade 4 (glioblastomas); 4 were diagnosed as meningioma; other tumours were oligodendroglioma (2 cases), ependymoma (2), craniopharymgioma (1) and a brain abscess (1).

Proton MRI and MRS were carried out at 1.5 Tesla with a head coil using the PRESS sequence. The measurement condition was as follows: TR 1500, TE 270 ms, CHESS pulse for water suppression, volume of interest (VOI) 15.6 ml, sum of free induction decays 200. Spectral processing included zero-filling and phase-correction without smoothing function. The VOI was placed on the centre or the contrtast-enhancing area of the tumour.

Signal intensity ratios were used for a quantified comparison as below: NAA/Cho ratio = intensity of NAA(*N*-acetyl aspartate)/intensity of choline (Cho) NAA/Cr ratio = intensity of NAA/intensity of creatine and phosphocreatine (Cr) Cho/Cr ratio = intensity of choline/intensity of creatine and phosphocreatine.

Lactate was not estimated because its tensity was highly variable depending on the measurement area and it was sometimes difficult to distinguish from the signal of lipid.

Results

Figure 1 shows the NAA/Cho ratio in the cases of glioma. The ratio of grade 2 tumours was higher than that of the other grades. The ratio of grade 4 tumours was variable and those of 2 cases were at the same level as those of grade 2. However, in the other 7 cases of grade 4 the ratio was lower than that of grade 2, and a statistically significant difference ($P < 0.01$) was found between them. Oligodendroglioma and grade 3 gliomas had almost the same value.

Figure 2 shows the NAA/Cr ratio in the cases of glioma; the dispersion of the NAA/Cr ratio of grade 4 was a little wider than that of the NAA/Cho ratio, but the same tendency was found as described above for the NAA/Cho ratio.

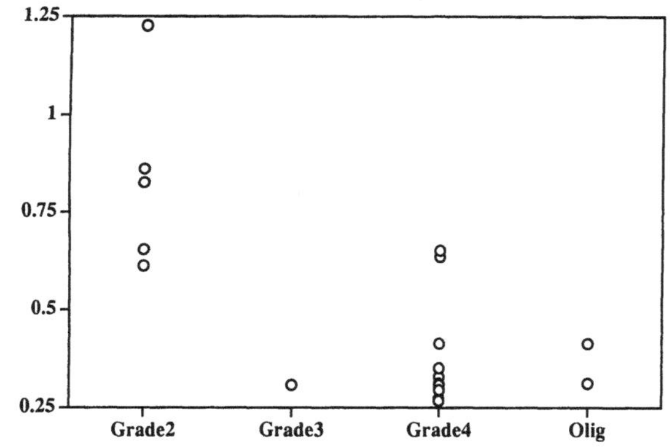

1

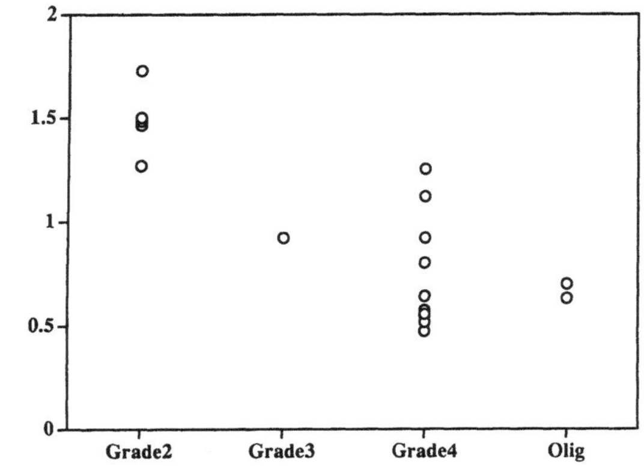

2

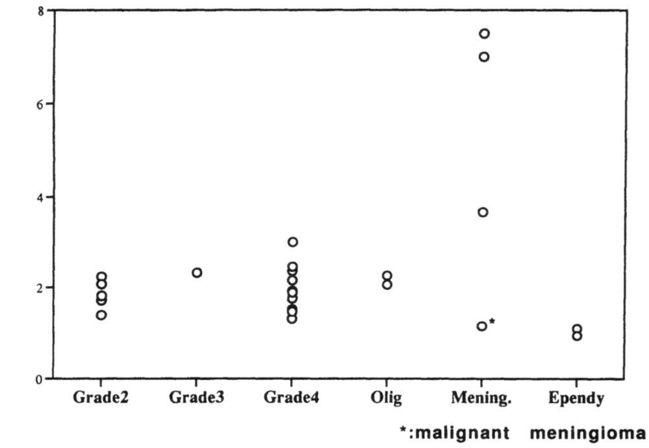

3

Fig. 1. NAA/Cho ratio of gliomas. *Grades 2, 3, 4,* astrocytomas; *Olig,* oligodendroglioma

Fig. 2. NAA/Cr ratio of gliomas. Grades as in Fig. 1

Fig. 3. Cho/Cr ratio of all intracranial tumours in this study. *Mening,* meningioma; *Ependy,* ependymoma

In most cases of meningioma, the intensity of NAA was very low or not recognised. The Cho/Cr ratio was used for the comparison of all groups of brain tumours (Fig. 3). This ratio in meningiomas was remarkably higher than that in the other groups of tumours except for 1 case, which was diagnosed as malignant meningioma and exhibited diffuse invasion of the cerebral parenchyma. In all grades of astrocytoma and oligodendroglioma; we found no differences in the Cho/Cr ratio. Although there were only 2 cases of ependymoma, their Cho/Cr ratio was lower than that of the other groups of glioma.

Discussion

Gill et al. [2] conducted in vitro proton MR spectroscopic studies of intracranial tumours and reported that the NAA/Cr ratio differed significantly in all grades from its value in normal white matter and the Cho/Cr ratio differed significantly in grade 4 tumours from its value in the other grades [2]. They also conducted an in vivo MRS study of a small number of cases and reported that the spectra in vivo were consistent with the in vitro results from the same patients. However, their measurement was conducted with a large volume (64 ml) and the sequence was a little different from ours. We found that the only difference in astrocytoma was in the NAA/Cho ratio between grade 2 and grade 4. The level of Cho/Cr ratio was also mostly the same in all grades of astrocytoma and oligodendroglioma. These results suggest that a decrease in NAA would be dominant in grade 4 and changes of choline would be not so large. Though these results are a little different from those of Gill et al., [2] heterogenity in the tumour and contamination from normal or oedematous parenchyma could not be assessed in either their study or ours. Tumour heterogeneity and contamination from surrounding parenchyma makes spectral interpretation difficult and obscure. However, both studies suggest that low-grade astrocytoma has different biochemical characteristics from high-grade astrocytoma. Furthermore, we also suggested that typical meningioma showed a characteristic ^{1}H-MRS pattern if there was no contamination from other tissues. Our 2 cases of meningioma had the lowest Cho/Cr ratio of all the tumours, and its ratio may be useful for the diagnosis of ependymoma. However, a large number of studies should be conducted to determine its diagnostic usefulness.

References

1. Harada M, Tanouchi M, Miyoshi H, Nishitani H, Kannuki S (1995) Brain abscess observed by localized proton magnetic resonance spectroscopy. Magn Reson Imaging (in press)
2. Gill SS, Thomas DGT, Bruggen NV, Gadian DG, Peden CJ, Bell JD, Cox IJ, Menon DK, Iles RA, Bryant DJ, Coutts GA (1990) Proton MR spectroscopy of intracranial tumours: In vivo and In vitro studies. J Comput Assist Tomogr 14:497–504

MRI contrast enhancement in glioblastomas: its pathological significance

A. Bozzao[1], M. Gallucci[1], G. Calvisi[2], T. Ventura[2], R. J. Galzio[3], A. Ricci[3], B. Orlandi[1], A. Costanzi[1]

[1] Department of Radiology, University of L'Aquila, I-67100 L'Aquila, Italy
[2] Department of Pathology, ULSS L'Aquila, I-67100 L'Aquila, Italy
[3] Department of Neurosurgery, Teramo Hospital, Teramo, Italy

Abstract. Gd-DTPA enhancement was found to correlate with hypercellular, hypervascular areas in 12 glioblastomas, when in vivo and post surgical MRI and pathological examinations were performed. True cysts may demonstrate contrast enhancement on MRI; this was evident in cases in which newly formed vessels were shown inside or near the cyst. Necrotic areas and cystic necrosis did not show any contrast enhancement on MRI.

Key words: Brain neoplasm – Histopathological correlations – Magnetic resonance imaging

The diagnostic accuracy of MRI in imaging brain neoplasms goes far beyond the possibility of confirming the presence of tumours. High sensitivity and specificity are improved by intra venous injections of contrast medium. Paramagnetic contrast media accumulate in the most vascularised neoplastic areas, depending on the alteration of the blood-brain barrier (BBB). However, at least to our knowledge, a comparison between the sites of enhancement and histopathology has never been performed. The aim of our study was to obtain a direct evaluation of the sites of enhancement in nine glioblastomas, by comparing MR examinations of contrast-enhanced specimens with histopathology.

Patients and methods

Twenty-one patients harbouring brain neoplasms were enrolled in the study. They all showed MRI findings suggesting the diagnosis of high-grade tumours. Each patient was submitted to an enhanced MRI within 1 week before surgery. During the surgical procedure a standard dose (0.1 mmol/kg) was injected intravenously 15 min before ligation of the vessels supplying the tumour. The specimens

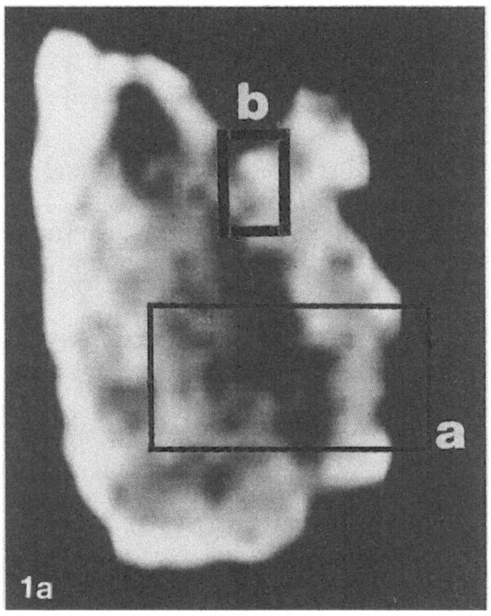

Fig. 1a. MRI of the surgical specimen. In area *a*, a low-signal area is observed between two zones of high signals; **b** histology of the same region shows colliquative necrosis, corresponding to the low-signal area, surrounded by areas with high neoplastic cellularity which gave high signal on MRI. Area *b* gives low signal, with high signal at its margins, as in *a*; histology **c** shows haemorrhagic necrosis *(arrows)* attributable to the MRI high signal, surrounding a larger necrotic area giving low signal on MRI

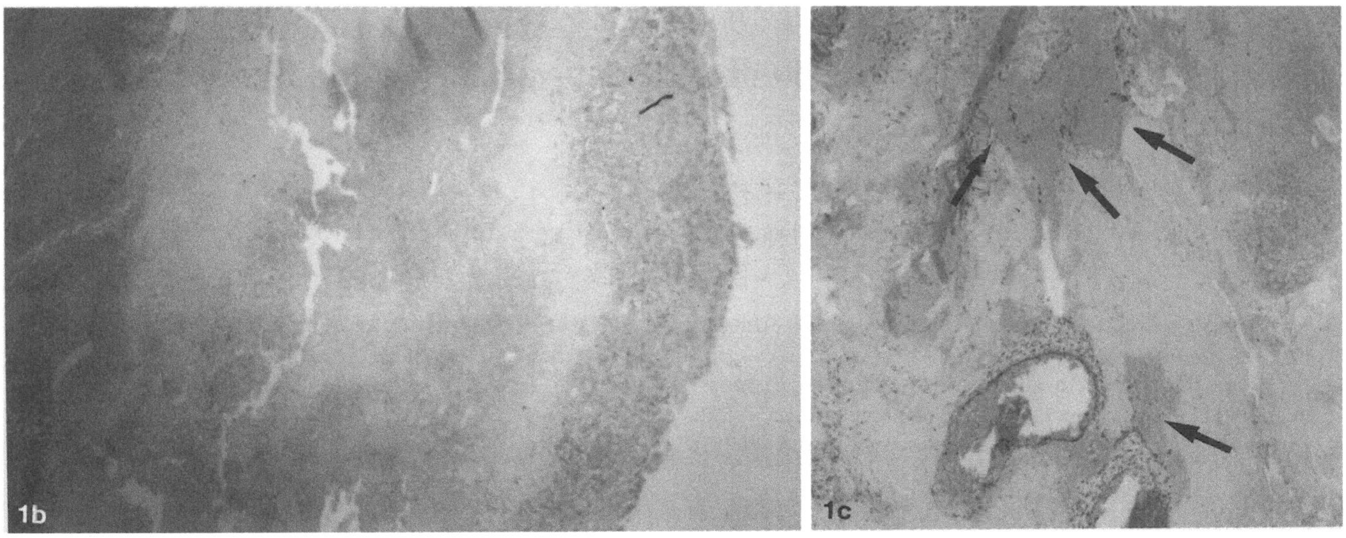

Correspondence to: A. Bozzao

were imaged by MRI within 4 h of surgical removal, then fixed and microscopically evaluated. In 7 cases the poor quality of the material did not allow a pathological study, and in 5 the histological diagnosis was something other than glioblastoma (3 grade-astocytomas and 2 metastases). Nine glioblastomas were finally assessed.

Results

In all specimens these areas of high signal intensity, in the in vivo and post surgical MRI, corresponded to zones of highly anaplastic tumour cells (Fig. 1). Tight vascularisation was also observed, showing the features of high-grade tumour vessels. Alterations were observed both at the endothelial level and in the glial cells surrounding the vessels, which appeared highly anaplastic. Two sharply circumscribed high signal areas corresponded, in the histological specimens, neoplastic cysts, with diameters raging from 6 mm to 2 cm. These cysts showed clear-cut margins and a fibrinoid content. Within the cysts, blood vessels were observed. Those areas in which plain in vivo MRI showed a hyperintense signal on short TR/TE images corresponded to zones of haemorrhagic necroses (Fig. 1). Haemorrhagic degeneration was also found at the edges of the specimens close to the site of the surgical cut. In those areas in which postsurgical MRI did not show enhancement, mostly low-grade or normal glial cells were found on pathological evaluation. These areas were indistinguishable on MRI from those of non-haemorrhagic necroses, which demonstrated the same signal intensity.

Discussion

Contrast enhancement inside specific areas of a brain neoplasm is due to two factors, which are not necessarily related to the tumour malignancy: the integrity of the BBB and interstitial space [1–5]. Our study emphasizes the concept, well known from other studies, performed in animals, that the enhancement inside a brain neoplasm is related to the grade of cellular anaplasia and to the presence of newly formed blood vessels. Neoplastic cysts may also show enhancement. This was observed in two cases in which pathological evaluation demonstrated the presence of vessels close to or inside the cyst. Diffusion may also be the cause of Gd-DTPA accumulation inside the cyst. No enhancement was observed in those areas corresponding to necrotic tissue. This finding is extremely relevant if we consider that the grading of a brain neoplasm is mostly dependent on the presence of necroses. Also relevant is the observation concerning the lack of utility of contrast-enhanced MRI in the correct identification of the tumour margins. Neoplastic cells have been clearly identified far distant from the enhanced areas albeit, in most cases, with a low grade of anaplasia.

References

1. Pollay M, Roberts PA (1980) BBB: a definition of normal and altered function. Neurosurgery 6:575–585
2. Stewart PA, Hayakawa K, Farral CL et al. (1987) Quantitative study of micro vessels ultra structure in human peritumoral brain tissue. Evidence for BBB defect. J Neurosurg 67:697–705
3. Long DM (1970) Capillary ultra structure and the BBB in human malignant brain tumors. J Neurosurg 32:127–144
4. Schmiedl UP, Kenney J, Maravilla KR (1992) Kinetics of pathologic BBB permeability in an astrocytic glioma using contrast-enhanced MR. AJNR 13:5–14
5. Yamada K, Ushio Y, Hayakawa T et al. (1982) Quantitative autoradiographic measurements of BBB permeability in the rat glioma model. J Neurosurg 57:394–398

The effect of time delay on the enhancement pattern of malignant intracranial neoplasms

G. Krol, W. Mason, R. DeLaPaz, B. O'Malley

[1] Department of Radiology and Neurology, Memorial Sloan-Kettering Cancer Center, New York, NY 10021, USA

Abstract. We compared routine spin-echo MR images obtained 15 and 30 min after intravenous contrast medium in 85 patients with suspected intracranial tumors. The delayed images showed more extensive enhancement in the majority of cases. However, no additional lesions were shown.

Key words: Magnetic resonance imaging – Contrast enhancement – Neoplasm

Magnetic resonance imaging (MRI) is the primary modality used for the assessment of improvement or progression of intracranial disease. This is particularly true in patients with brain neoplasms who are undergoing preoperative assesment of the extent of disease or periodic MRI studies following surgery, radiation treatment of chemo-

Correspondence to: G. Krol

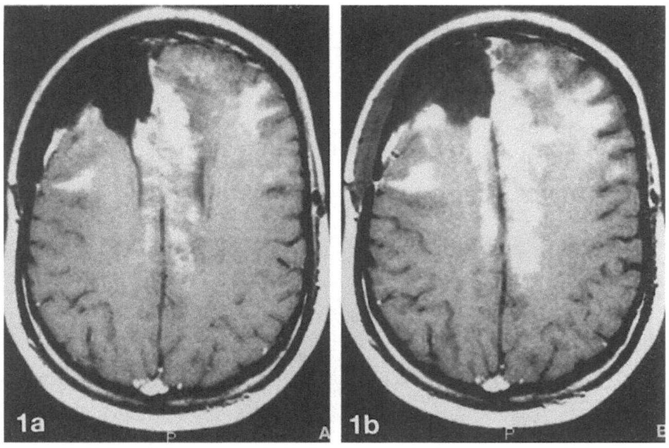

Fig. 1. A patient with diffuse enhancing mass in the left frontoparietal region as a result of recurrent glioblastoma. **(A)** Although the extent of the enhancing component could not be measured, the area of enhancement appears to be significantly larger on the delayed study **(B)**

therapy. The key elements of imaging, the extent and intensity of contrast enhancement, appear to be dose-, technique- and time-dependent. The aim of this investigation was to assess the value of delayed imaging in patients with known or suspected intracranial neoplasms.

Materials and methods

We performed 95 MRI examinations on 85 patients with proven or suspected primary or secondary malignant brain neoplasms. Contrast-enhanced sequences included immediate and delayed spin-echo T1-weighted acquisitions in the axial plane 15–30 min apart. Both series were then photographed in the same format and magnification. MRI studies showing abnormal enhancement consistent with malignant processes were assessed for extent of disease by side-by-side comparison by three neuroradiologists. One investigator (WM), blinded to the type of the study, performed surface area measurements of the enhancing component on all images that showed the lesion. One to four representative corresponding sections through the lesion equator were chosen for comparison. The difference in surface area was expressed as a percentage of the lower value. The thickness of the peripheral enhancement in ring lesions was measured directly. Unmeasurable lesions (because of marked irregularity of enhancement) were compared by side-by-side viewing only.

Results

Twenty-four patients had normal studies and four had brain tumours which were nonenhancing by both immediate and delayed techniques. Two patients, subsequently diagnosed as having meningiomas, were excluded from the study. Of 65 studies in 58 patients with abnormal parenchymal enhancement, the delayed technique was judged (by viewing) to reveal more extensive involvement in 37 (57%) (Fig. 1). The discrepancy in favour of delayed imaging was still larger with the use of surface area measurements n 48 of 57 measurable lesions – 84%. In 29 ring-enhancing or ring component-containing lesions, the peripheral enhancement of the wall was thicker in 21 (72%) and an increase of central intensity was noted in 15 (52%). The delayed technique did not demonstrate any pathology in patients with normal routine MRI or reveal any additional parenchymal lesions in patients with single to multiple metastases. No additional information was provided by delayed imaging in 4 patients with nonenhancing tumors.

Discussion

The intensity of contrast enhancement of parenchymal lesions of the brain, which occur at the sites of a damaged blood brain barrier, is (among other factors) time-dependent. Early experimental studies predicted the useful imaging time after an intravenous dose to be within 60 min after injection. A quantitative correlation of tissue intensity of various intracranial lesions plotted against time revealed that the maximum intensity was achieved when scanning was delayed to at least 8.5 min after the injection. The present investigation confirms that, indeed, in a clinical setting a more complete enhancement of neoplastic tissue is observed when scanning is delayed. This phenomenon appears to be quite prominent in enhancing primary tumours of irregular configuration, which demonstrate the most significant increase in size of the enhancement on a delayed study. Ring lesions commonly demonstrate increased central intensity and thickening of the peripheral ring. Therefore, standardization of technique across the imaging surveilance period is an important factor to avoid a possible erroneus assessment of extent or intensity of enhancement. It is unlikely that this technique will demonstrate any additional lesions in patients with single or multiple metastases, or reveal any enhancement in nonenhancing tumours, compared to a standard technique.

Cystic glioma with spontaneous rupture

A. Uchino[1], K. Yamabe[2], Y. Aiko[2], H. Aibe[1], C. Kuromatsu[2], M. Tanaka[1]

[1] Department of Radiology, Kyushu Kosei-Nenkin Hospital, Kitakyushu, Japan
[2] Department of Neurosurgery, Kuyushu Kosei-Nenkin Hospital, Kitakyushu, Japan

Abstract. We report an unusual cystic anaplastic astrocytoma that ruptured spontaneously. There is no other report of such a ruptured glioma. However, we believe that cystic gliomas have a greater tendency to rupture than previously believed.

Key words: Cystic brain tumour - Spontaneous rupture - Glioma - Computed tomography - Magnetic resonance imaging

The tumours of the glioma group occur more frequently than any other primary intra-axial brain tumour. However, to our knowledge, there are no reports of a ruptured cystic glioma in the literature. All the ruptured intracranial tumours previously reported have been extra-axial tumours, including dermoids [1–3], an epidermoid [4], teratomas [5, 6], and a craniopharyngioma [7].

Case report

A 46-year-old man complained of headaches of gradually progressive intensity. CT without contrast medium, obtained at another hospital, showed a large low density mass in the right temporal lobe (Fig. 1a, b). On emergency admission to our hospital, the patient also complained of dysarthria and left homonymous hemianopia.

However, these symptoms and signs and his persistent headaches resolved spontaneously without treatment. Three days later, MR imaging with contrast medium revealed a ring-like enhanced cystic mass indicative of a cystic glioma. There was no evidence of intratumour haemorrhage. The posteromedial portion of the cyst wall was very thin. The size of this mass decreased slightly during a 3-day period (Fig. 2). Follow-up CT with contrast medium 6 days later, demonstrated that the cystic mass had collapsed (Fig. 3a, b). The anterolateral portion of the cyst wall was irregularly enhanced, with a so-called garland-shaped appearance suggestive of a malignant glioma. However, the posteromedial portion of the cyst wall was not enhanced.

Surgery was performed using a right frontotemporal free bone-flap craniotomy. The mass contained a slightly yellowish water-soluble fluid. The posteromedial part of the cyst wall was very thin, and a minute perforation was discovered at the cyst wall. Cerebrospinal fluid (CSF) was exuding into the cystic mass from the choroidal fissure via the minute perforation. The mass was subtotally removed, and histopathological examination revealed it to be an anaplastic astrocytoma. The patient was referred for radiotherapy.

Discussion

Extra-axial brain tumours are usually surrounded by CSF. Therefore, a cystic mass with a thin wall may rupture when pressure within the cyst increases. However, a cystic

Correspondence to: A. Uchino, Department of Radiology, Saga Medical School, 5-1-1 Nabeshima, Saga 849, Japan

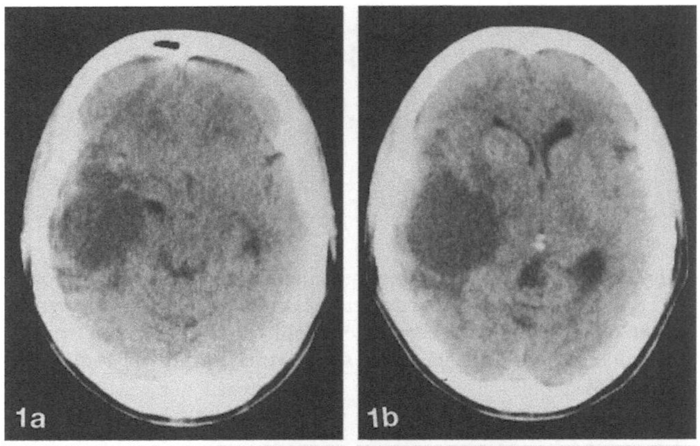

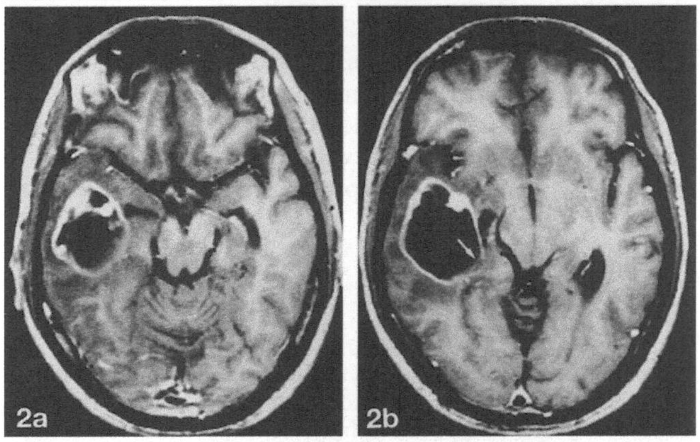

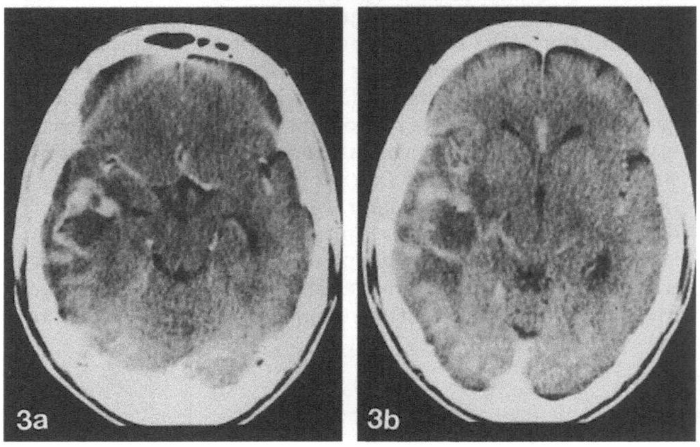

Fig. 1. Axial CT reveals a large low density mass in the right temporal lobe. There is a prominent mass effect, resulting in a midline shift

Fig. 2. Contrast enhanced T1-weighted MRI 3 days later than Fig. 1 shows a ring-enhancing cystic mass indicative of a cystic glioma. The posteromedial portion of the cyst wall (*arrow*) is very thin. The size of the mass has decreased slightly

Fig. 3. Contrast-enhanced CT obtained 9 day after Fig. 1 demonstrate that the size of the mass has decreased

glioma is an intra-axial brain tumour, which is surrounded by the brain parenchyma, or at least by the pia mater. Therefore, a cystic glioma cannot be expected to rupture easily. In the patient reported here, the posteromedial part of the cyst wall was very thin and was located at the surface of the choroidal fissure. As surgically confirmed, a minute perforation developed, presumably due to increased pressure in the cyst. In the event of intratumour heamorrhage, pressure in the cystic tumour simultaneously increases. It is well known that gliomas bleed relatively frequently [8]. In our patient, however, there was no evidence of intratumour haemorrhage.

Patients with a ruptured dermoid usually experience headache and transient ischaemic attacks [2]. Since the content of a dermoid consists of fatty fluid, chemical meningitis frequently develops after its rupture. Using CT or MRI, a ruptured dermoid can be diagnosed easily on demonstrating fat globules throughout the ventricular system and subarachnoid spaces [1–3].

Cystic gliomas contain water-soluble fluid. Thus, when a cystic glioma ruptures, the mass effect of the cystic lesion is decreased, as in our patient, resulting in the spontaneous resolution of clinical symptoms without the development of chemical meningitis. Neither abnormal density nor abnormal intensity is observed in the CSF on CT or MRI. Therefore, the evidence of rupture of cystic gliomas may be obscured and overlooked. We believe that cystic gliomas have a greater tendency to rupture than was previously believed. Subarachnoid dissemination of tumour cells may develop after the spontaneous rupture of a high-grade cystic glioma. Therefore, we should be alert to the size of a cystic tumour during serial CT or MRI.

References

1. Smith AS, Benson JE, Blaser SI, Mizushima A, Tarr RW, Bellon EM (1991) Diagnosis of ruptured intracranial dermoid cyst: value of MR over CT. AJNR 12:175–180
2. Wilms G, Casselman J, Demaerel P, Plets C, Haene ID, Baert AL (1991) CT and MRI of ruptured intracranial dermoids. Neuroradiology 33:149–151
3. Ohkubo T, Sasaki Y, Aoki S, Machida T, Kokubo T (1991) MRI of spontaneously ruptured dermoids in the middle cranial fossa. Neuroradiology 33 [Suppl]:311–312
4. Laster DW, Moody DM, Ball MR (1977) Epidermoid tumors with intraventricular and subarachnoid fat: report of two cases. AJR 128:504–507
5. Ghoshhajra K, Baghai-Naiini P, Hahn HS, Pena CE, Hayat S (1979) Spontaneous rupture of a pineal teratoma. Neuroradiology 17:215–217
6. Kadota Y, Ito M, Wachi A, Sato K (1993) MRI detection of ruptured malignant teratoma in the third ventricle. Neuroradilogy 35:254–255
7. Tokiwa K, Nakayama K, Miyasaka Y, Matsumori K, Beppu T, Asao T (1984) Cystic craniopharyngioma with spontaneous shrinkage of the cyst. Neurol Med Chir (Tokyo) 24:954–957
8. Kondziolka D, Bernstein M, Resch L, Tator CH, Fleming JFR, Vanderlinden RG, Schutz H (1987) Significance of hemorrhage into brain tumours: clinicopathologica study. J Neurosurg 67:852–857

CT and MRI of multicentric oligoastrocytoma

K. Watanabe[1], K. Mineura[1], M. Kowada[1], T. Goto[2], K. Watanabe[2]

[1] Neurosurgical Service, Akita University Hospital, Akita 010, Japan
[2] Southern Thoku Research Institute for Neuroscience, Kooriyama, Fukushima 963, Japan

Abstract. We report a rare biofrontal multicentric oligoastrocytoma shown by CT and MRI in a 37-year-old man hospitalised for generalised convulsions.

Key words: Glioma, multicentric-oligoastrocytoma – Computed tomography – magnetic resonce imaging

Multicentric gliomas are relatively uncommon and usually found histologically to be glioblastomas or anaplastic astrocytomas [1]. We report a rare bifrontral multicentric oliogoastrocytoma.

Correspondence to: K. Watanabe, Akita University Hospital

Case report

A 37-year-old man was admitted with generalised convulsions. On admission, neurologica examination showed no abnormalities.

CT revealed three separate low-density lesions with calcification (Fig. 1). One was in the right frontal lobe and the remaining two lesions in the anterior and lateral parts of the left frontal lobe. The right-sided lesion enhanced to some extent with i.v. contrast medium. These three lesions had low signal intensity on T1-weighted MRI and high signal intensity on T2-weighted images (Fig. 2) These lesions were shown to be separate on axial and coronal images (Fig. 3). A carotid angiogram showed a tumour stain in the right frontal lobe through the early and late phases. The patient underwent subtotal excision of the right frontal tumour and an exploratory biopsy of one left frontal tumour. The left frontal tumour was found to be an oligoastrocytoma, composed of cells with characteristic perinuclear halos and astocytes with less pleomorphism. The histological features of the right frontal tumour were similar, except for a higher frequency of astrocytes (Fig. 4). Following radiotherapy (whole brain 30 Gy, tumour 20 Gy), the patient was discharged without any significant neurological deficit. He is alive, without tumours recurrence, 35 months after surgery.

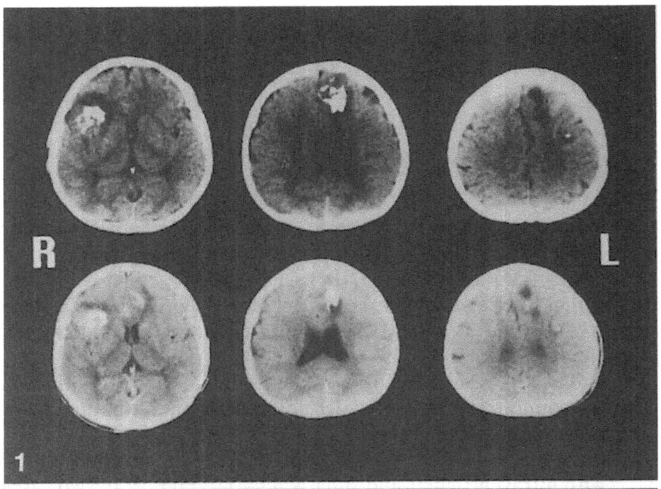

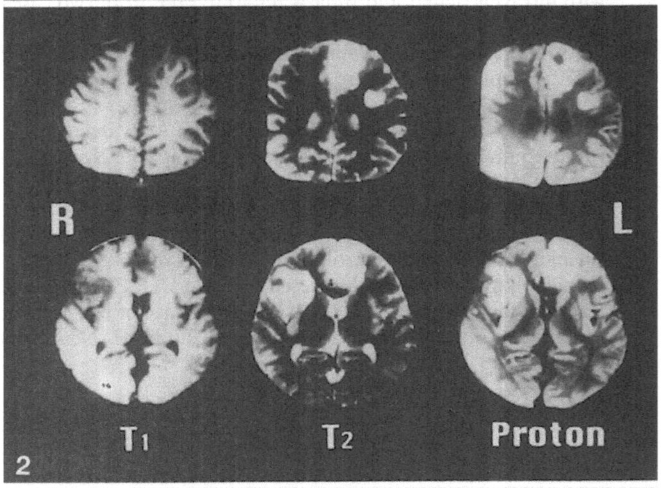

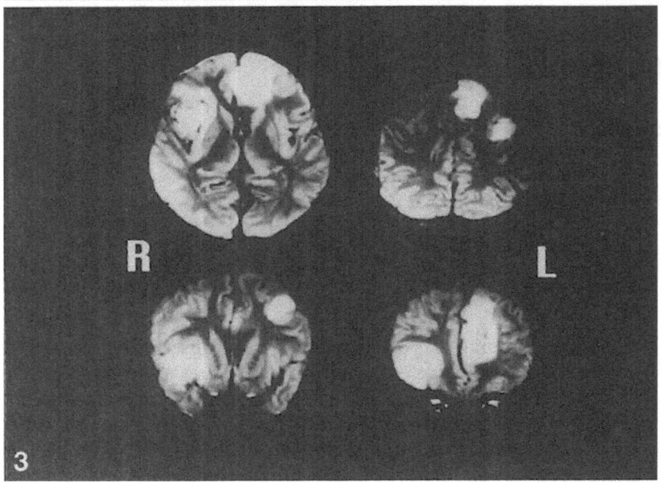

Fig. 1. CT before (*top*) and after (*bottom*) i.v. contrast medium showing three separate low-density lesions with calcification. The right-sided lesion enhanced to some extent

Fig. 2. T1-weighted MRI showing three low signal intensity areas and T2-weighted images showing them to give high signal

Fig. 3. *Top*, axial; *bottom*, coronal; T2-weighted MRI demonstrating three distinctly separate lesions

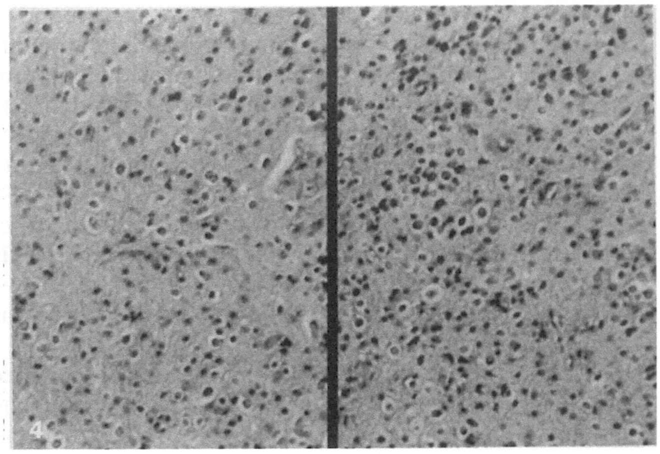

Fig. 4a, b. Surgical specimens. **a** Left frontal tumour, showing cells with characteristic perinuclear halos and astrocytes with less pleomorphism. **b** Right frontal tumour, showing similar findings but with more astrocytes. H & E × 200

Discussion

Russell and Rubinstein [2] suggested the following classification for multiple gliomas: spread via commissural or other pathways; spread via cerebrospinal fluid channels; local metastasis; and multicentic glioma. Multicentric glioma needs extensive, detailed histological examination. In the present case, no continuity between the lesions was detected by neuroradiological imaging, although the lesions have a similar histological pattern. Neither symptoms of meningeal dissemination nor local recurrence have been noted during a relatively long follow-up time of 35 months. The present case was therefore categorised as multicentric glioma.

Multicentric glioma comprises approximately 2.5% of all gliomas [2] and usually has similar histology, which mostly includes glioblastoma or anaplastic astrocytoma [3, 4]. Benign gliomas such as oligodendroglioma or oligoastrocytoma are very rare. Lorentzen [5] and Ogasawara et al. [6] reported multicentric oligodendroglioma respectively, and four cases had different histologies including oligodendroglioma and glioblastoma [3, 7–9]. With regard to oligoastrocytoma, only one case of different histology including oligoastrocytoma and microcystic astrocytoma was reported by Solomon et al. [1]. Our case is a very rare case of multicentric oligoastrocytoma.

References

1. Solomon A, Perret GE, McCormick WF (1969) Multicentric gliomas of the cerebral and cerebellar hemispheres. J Neurosurg 31:87–93
2. Russell DS, Rubinstein LJ (1959) Pathology of tumours of the nervous system. Arnold, London, pp 152–153
3. Batsdorf U, Malamud N (1963) The problem of multicentric gliomas. J Neurosurg 20:122–136
4. Courville CB (1936) Multiple primary tumors of the brain: review of the literature and report of twenty-one cases. Am J Cancer 26:703–731

5. Lorentzen KA (1950) Histological report on a case of ologodendroglioma malignum in the cerebral hemisphere with metastatic extension to the cerebellum. Acta Psychiatr Neurol Scand 25:241–250
6. Ogasawara H, Kiya K, Uozumi T, Sugiyama K, Kawamoto K, Ohta M (1990) Multiple oligodendroglioma. Neurol Med Chir (Tokyo) 30:127–131
7. Nonaka N, Kuratsu J, Miura G, Matsukado Y (1983) Multicentric gliomas, Neurol Chir (Tokyo) 23:751–754
8. Züloch KJ (1941) Das Oligodendrogliom. Z Neurol Psychiatr 172:407–482
9. Köhlmeier W (1943) Über multizentrisch entstandene Oligodendrogliome. Z Neurol Psychiatrie 175:385–402

Effects of intracarotid recombinant human tumour necrosis factor-α on kinetics of glucose metabolism in malignant gliomas

T. Sasajima[1], K. Mineura[1], H. Shioya[1], J. Sasaki[1], M. Kowada[1], N. Tomura[2], J. Hatazawa[3], T. Ogawa[3], K. Uemura[3]

[1] Neurological Service, Akita University Hospital, Akita, Japan
[2] Department of Radiology, Akita University Hospital, Akita, Japan
[3] Department of Radiology and Nuclear Medicine, Akita Research Institute for Brain and Blood Vessels, Akita 010, Japan

Abstract. Two cases of malignant gliomas were studied with positron emission tomography (PET) following three courses of intracarotid recombinant human tumour necrosis factor-α (TNF). In an untreated case, PET revealed two lesions characterised by glucose hypermetabolism and high perfusion. In the frontal hypermetabolic lesion, the metabolic rate of glucose (kinetic CMRGI), influx (k_1), phosphorylation (k_3) and circulation were depressed after the first injection and increased beyond the pretreatment level after the third treatment. In contrast, k_1 and k_3 decreased in the temporal lesion, so that the kinetic CMRGI remained unchanged during the follow-up period. In the second patient, who had received radiochemotherapy 3 months before, the kinetic CMRGI, rate constants and circulation of the tumour were lower than those for the contralateral cortex. No appreciable changes

Table 1. Quantitative measurement of kinetic CMRGI, rate constants and circulation following intracarotid TNF in case 1

	Kinetic CMRGI (mg/100 ml per min)			k_1 (/min)			k_2 (/min)			k_3 (/min)			CBF (ml/100 ml per min)			CBV (ml/100 ml)		
	F	T	N	F	T	N	F	T	N	F	T	N	F	T	N	F	T	N
Before	5.8	7.0	6.8	0.060	0.066	0.069	0.050	0.070	0.095	0.042	0.059	0.081	49.5	43.6	41.7	5.6	6.1	3.1
After																		
1st treatment	2.7	6.7	7.0	0.051	0.072	0.062	0.066	0.056	0.073	0.022	0.046	0.086	42.9	44.0	42.5	3.1	5.6	3.4
3rd treatment	6.4	6.6	6.5	0.076	0.077	0.065	0.144	0.098	0.096	0.083	0.056	0.073	96.4	44.9	39.0	5.7	5.5	3.3

FT; Frontal and temporal hypermetabolic lesions; N, normal cortex

Table 2. Quantitative measurement of kinetic CMRGI, rate constants and circulation following intracarotid TNF in case 2

	kinetic CMRGI (mg/100 ml per min)		k_1 (/min)		k_2 (/min)		k_3 (min)		CBF (ml/100 ml per min)		CBV (ml/100 ml	
	Tumour	Normal	Tumour	Normal	Tumour	Normal	Tumour	Normal	Tumour	Normal	Tumour	Normal
Before	2.8	5.0	0.055	0.065	0.090	0.084	0.033	0.063	23.2	34.8	2.1	2.6
After												
1st treatment	2.9	4.3	0.057	0.066	0.112	0.107	0.035	0.048	25.8	38.1	2.5	2.8
3rd treatment	2.6	4.4	0.054	0.060	0.098	0.094	0.036	0.066	19.9	34.1	1.7	2.7

Normal, Normal cortex

Correspondence to: J. Hatazawa

were noted in any value of the tumour after the therapy. The clinical application of intracarotid TNF combined with other therapy, based on an understanding of glucose metabolism and circulation, will enhance therapeutic effectiveness.

Key words: Malignant glioma - Recombinant human tumour necrosis factor-α - Positron emission tomography - Glucose metabolism - Rate constants

Intracarotid recombinant human tumour necrosis factor-α (TNF) has been applied to the treatment of recurrent and progressive malignant gliomas [1]. TNF is a cytokine showing a variety of biological activities, such as cytotoxic effects and damage to tumour vessels. We have studied the effects of intracarotid TNF on the kinetic cerebral metabolic rate of glucose (CMRGI) and rate constants, as well as circulation, using positron emission tomography (PET) in two patients with malignant gliomas.

Materials and methods

A 48-year-old man presented with mild left hemiparesis; gadolinium-enhancing lesions were seen in the right frontal and temporal regions on MRI. The patient underwent an exploratory biopsy 6 weeks before intracarotid TNF. Specimens were histologically diagnosed as malignant astrocytoma. The second patient was a 61-year-old woman, who was diagnosed with a malignant glioma based on neurological and neuroradiological findings. The patients had received intra-arterial ACNU and focal radiation of 60 Gy 3 months before intracarotid TNF. MRI showed an enhancing lesion in the right temporal lobe. These patients received an intracarotid injection of a 3×10^4 U/M^2 dose of TNF 3 times over a 2-week period.

PET studies were performed the day before, and 24 h after the first injection, and 2 weeks after the third injection. Regional cerebral blood flow (CBF) and blood volume (CBV) were measured using $H_2{}^{15}O$ and $C^{15}O$ tracers. The rate constants of tracer transport from blood to brain (k_1), reverse transport from brain to blood (k_2) and phosphorylation (k_3) were estimated by a non-linear fitting analysis using dynamic scanning after an intravenous injection of ^{18}F-fluorodeoxyglucose (FDG). The kinetic CMRGI was calculated by Phelp's equation with the rate constants and a lumped constant of 0.52. The rate constants and kinetic CMRGI images were calculated using the real-time weighted integration method. Details of the procedure have been published previously [2].

Results

Changes in the kinetic CMRGI, rate constants and circulation are summarised in Tables 1 and 2. In the first case, PET revealed 2 lesions demonstrating glucose hypermetabolism and high perfusion. In the frontal hypermetabolic lesion, kinetic CMRGI, k_1, k_3 and circulation were

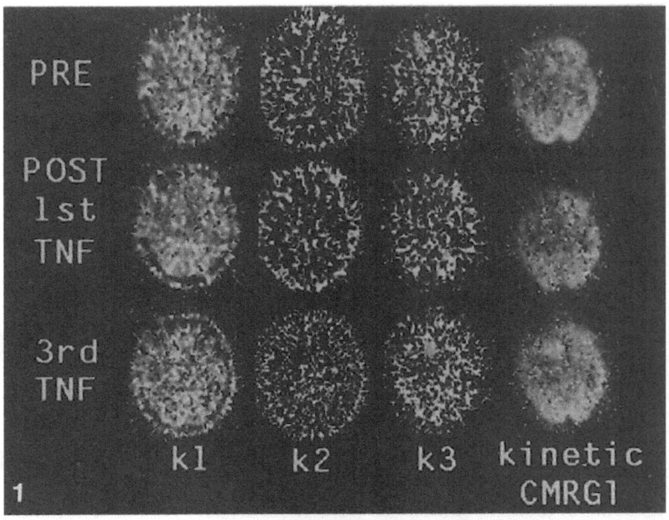

Fig. 1. Case 1. PET 13 mm below intercommisural line. Hypermetabolic lesion in right frontal lobe *(top row)*. Kinetic CMRGI, influx (k_1) and phosphorylation (k_3) fell after first injection *(middle row)* and rose beyond the pretreatment level after the third treatment *(bottom row)*

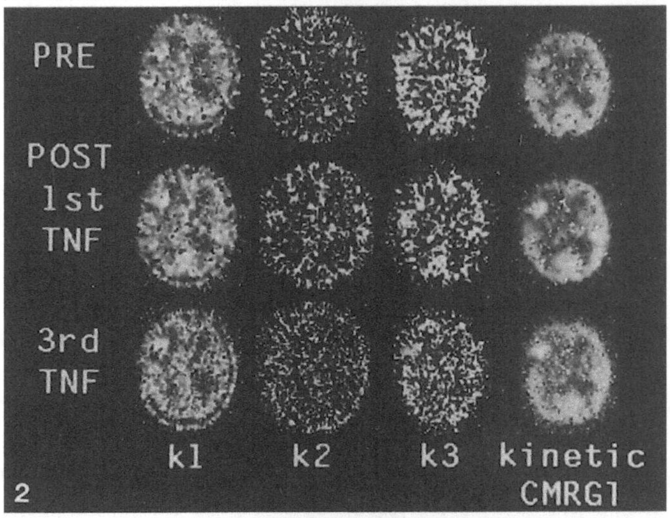

Fig. 2. Case 1. PET images 13 mm above the intercommisural line. The hypermetabolic temporal lesion had high influx (k_1) and phosphorylation (k_3) *(top row)*. Kinetic CMRGI remained unchanged, whereas increase influx and decreased phosphorylation were observed after treatment

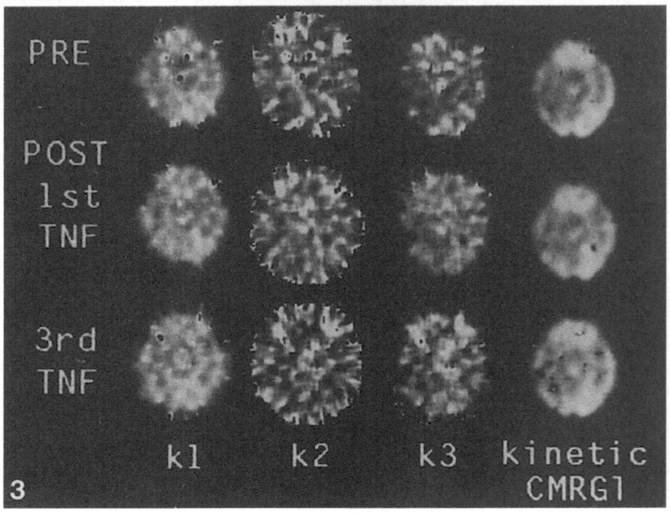

Fig. 3. Case 2. PET showed low glucose metabolism associated with low influx (k_1) and phosphorylation (k_3) in the temporal lesion before treatment top row. Neither tumour nor normal cortex demonstrated obvious changes after treatment

depressed after the first injection, and subsequently increased beyond the pretreatment level after the third treatment (Fig. 1). In contrast, k_1 increased and k_3 decreased in the temporal lesion, so that kinetic CMRGl remained unchanged during the follow-up period (Fig. 2). No appreciable changes were noted in the normal cortex. In the second case, kinetic CMRGI, the rate constants and circulation of the tumour were lower than those for the contralateral cortex. Neither the tumour nor normal cortex demonstrated obvious changes in either value before or after the therapy (Fig. 3). Du ring the 4 months since the therapy, these patients have been free of symptoms without evidence of tumour regrowth on MRI.

Discussion

We used dynamic FDG-PET and analysed glucose phosphorylation and transport. In the first case, k_3 decreased in the frontal and temporal hypermetabolic lesions after the first injection. The reduction in k_3 reflected a primary effect of TNF on the phosphorylation of the tumour. The increase in k_1, however, led to no apparent change of kinetic CMRGI in the temporal lesion. Two weeks after the third treatment, both k_3 and the kinetic CMRGI were higher than pretreatment level in the frontal lesion. This augmentation may indicate tumour progression; patients with increased glucose metabolism after chemotherapy exhibited rapid tumour growth [3]. In our study k_1 changed variedly in relation to circulation in the frontal and temporal lesions. Some authors have reported a heterogeneous response of circulation in experimental tumours. Preferential reduction of circulation is present in the central part of murine tumours [4]. TNF impairs peripheral tumour circulation prior to global reduction in rodent tumours [5]. Detailed analysis of phosphorylation and transport provides additional information regarding glucose metabolism.

In the second case, the glucose metabolism and circulation remained at a low level during the follow-up period. Previous radiochemotherapy may reduce tumour glucose metabolism and circulation. The therapeutic effects of radiochemotherapy on tumour metabolism and circulation have been reported [3, 6]. The low glucose metabolism and phosphorylation in the tumour predicted an inactive behaviour of the tumour. Clinical application of intracarotid TNF combined with other treatment based on an understanding of glucose metabolism and circulation will enhance therapeutic effectiveness in patients with gliomas.

References

1. Yoshida J, Wakabayashi T, Mizuno M, Sugita K, Yoshida T, Hori S, Mori T, Sato T, Karashima A, Kurisu K, Kiya K, Uozumi T (1992) Clinical effect of intra-arterial tumor necrosis factor-α for malignant glioma. J Neurosurg 77:78–83
2. Iida H, Bloomfield PM, Miura S, Kanno I, Murakami M, Uemura K, Amano M, Tanaka K, Hirose Y, Yamamoto S (in press) Effect of real-time weighted integration system for rapid calculation of functional images in clinical positron emission tomography. IEEE Trans Med Imaging
3. Langen KJ, Roosen N, Kuwert T, Herzog H, Kiwit JCW, Kops ER, Muzik O, Bock WJ, Feinendegen LE (1989) Early effects of intra-arterial chemotherapy in patients with brain tumours studied with PET: Preliminary results. Nucl Med Commun 10:779–790
4. Van de Wiel PA, Bouma GJ, Van der Pijl A, Weitenberg ES, Lam AW, Bloksma N (1990) Effect of tumour necrosis factor and lipid A on functional and structural vascular volume in solid murine tumours. Br J Cancer 62:718–723
5. Kluge M, Elger B, Engel T, Schaefer C, Seega J, Vaupel P (1992) Acute effects of tumor necrosis factor α or lymphotoxin on global blood flow, laser Doppler flux, and bioenergetic status of subcutaneous rodent tumors. Cancer Res 52:2167–2173
6. Mineura K, Yasuda T, Kowada M, Ogawa T, Shishido F, Uemura K (1987) Positron emission tomographic evaluation of radiochemotherapeutic effect on regional cerebral hemocirculation and metabolism in patients with gliomas. J Neurooncol 5:277–285

Positron emission tomography in the differential diagnosis of neurosarcoidosis and cerebral gliomas

K. Mineura [1], T. Sasajima [1], M. Kowada [1], T. Ogawa [3], J. Hatazawa [3], K. Uemura [3]

[1] Neurosurgical Service, Akita University Hospital, Akita, Japan
[2] Department of Radiology, Akita University Hospital, Akita, Japan
[3] Department of Radiology and Nuclear Medicine, Akita Research Institute for Brain and Blood Vessels Akita 010, Japan

Abstract. We describe a case of neurosarcoidosis, with positron emission tomography (PET) findings. Regional cerebral circulation and oxygen metabolism increased in a frontal sarcoid lesion showing as a contrast-enhancing high-density area on CT. Glucose metabolism also increased in the lesion. This increased metabolism is a useful landmark in the differential diagnosis of neurosarcoidosis and cerebral gliomas.

Key words: Positron emission tomography – Neurosarcoidosis – Oxygen metabolism – Glucose metabolism – ^{18}F-Fluorodeoxyglucose

Correspondence to: T. Ogawa

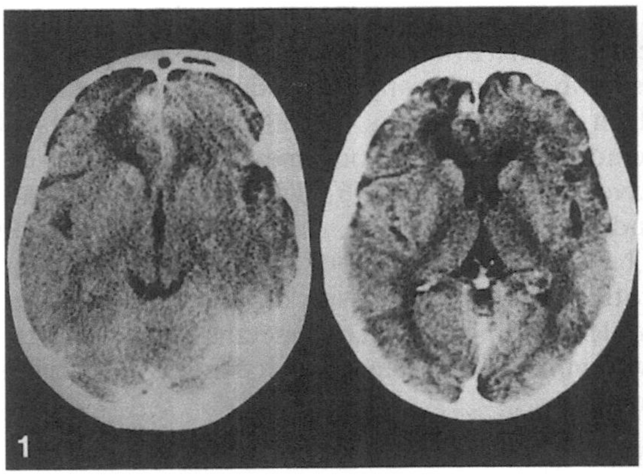

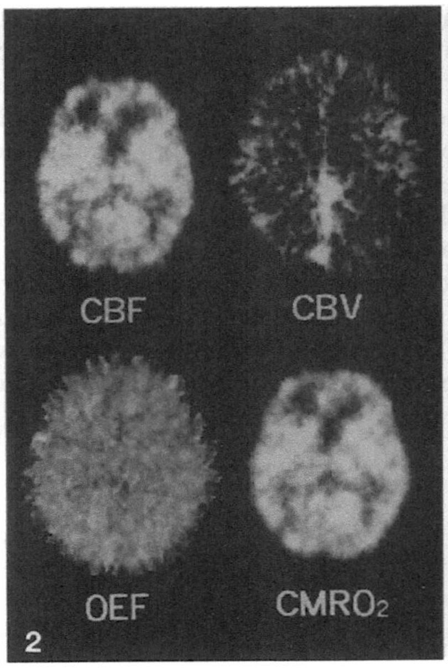

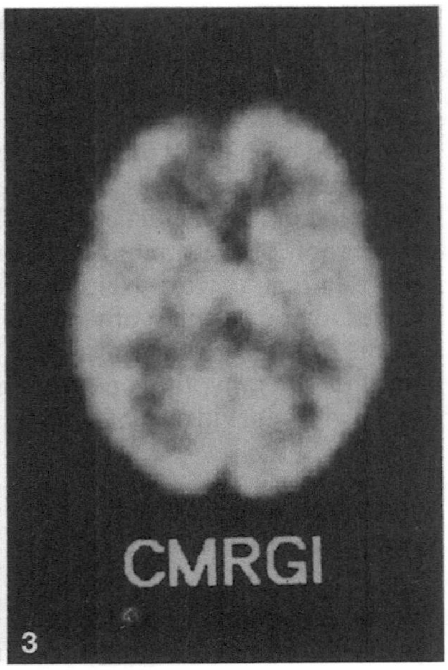

Fig. 1. Contrast-enhanced CT **a** before and **b** after treatment showed an enhancing mass adjacent to the falx, with a surrounding low density area. The mass decreased slightly in size after steroid treatment

Fig. 2. All parameters except for rOEF were reduced in the right frontal enhancing lesion. rOEF was comparable to that of the grey matter. *CBF,* cerebral blood flow; *CBV,* blood volume; *OEF,* oxygen extraction fraction; *CMRO₂,* metabolic rate of oxygen

Fig. 3. PET using ^{18}F-fluorodeoxyglucose showed high uptake in the frontal lesion. *CMRG1,* metabolic rate of glucose

Neurological involvement occurs in 5% of patients with sarcoidosis [1]. Isolated cases of central nervous system (CNS) sarcoidosis without systemic disease have been reported [2, 3]. Neurological manifestations vary widely and relate to the sites of involvement such as cranial nerves, basal meninges, and hypothalamic-pituitary axes, or cerebral parenchyma. CT findings depend on the types of CNS involvement and can be single intracranial mass lesions, multiple enhancing lesions, hydrocephalus and extra-axial mass lesions [4, 5]. These findings mimic those of brain tumours. MRI has a higher sensitivity to anatomical abnormalities of neurosarcoidosis than CT [6, 7]. These interventions, however, often make it difficult to differentiate neurosarcoidosis from other CNS disease. Little is known about the blood flow and metabolism of neurosarcoidosis. We present blood flow and metabolism studies using positron emission tomography (PET) in a patient with neurosarcoidosis.

Case report

A 49-year old man had been treated medically for pulmonary sarcoidosis and undergone iridectomy for resultant glaucoma due to chorioretinitis. He developed generalised convulsions and was admitted for further medical examination.

CT showed a contrast-enhancing mass with a surrounding low density area, adjacent to the falx in the right frontal region (Fig. 1). PET was performed using $C^{15}O_2$, $C^{15}O$, $^{15}O_2$ to measure the regional cerebral blood flow (rCBF), blood volume (rCBV), oxygen extraction fraction (rOEF), and metabolic rate of oxygen ($rCMRO_2$). Circulatory and metabolic parameters such as rCBF, RCBV, $rCMRO_2$ increased in the contrast-enhancing lesion, while these parameters were reduced in the surrounding low density area. The rOEF remained unchanged as normal grey and white matter, indicating a matched increase or reduction of blood flow and oxygen metabolism (Fig. 2).

Biopsy specimens provided a diagnosis of sarcoid granuloma. CT performed months after the initiation of steroid treatment (prednisolone, 30 mg/day) showed a shrinkage of an enhancing mass and surrounding low density area (Fig. 1, right). At that time, PET was performed using ^{18}F-fluorodeoxyglucose as well as $C^{15}O_2$, $C^{15}O$, $^{15}O_2$. The rCBF, rCBV, $RCMRO_2$, and rCMRG1 remained as high as the grey matter, although those slightly decreased due to the effects of surgery or steroid treatment. The metabolic rate of glucose (rCMRG1) in the medial frontal sarcoid lesion also increased to a similar level in the grey matter, whereas the surrrounding and anterior frontal areas showed a depression of FDG uptake, probably owing to oedema or as the effect of surgery (Fig. 3). Such increase in rCBF, rCBV, $rCMRO_2$, and rCMRG1 seem to be pathognomic in the haemocirculation and metabolism of neurosarcoidosis.

The convulsions were well controlled by anticonvulsants and steroids. The dose of steroids was decreased in stages and stopped 6 months after the initiation of steroid treatment. Clinical remission has continued for about 10 years since the PET study. Changes in circulatory and metabolic parameters may imply benefit from steroid therapy in the present case.

Discussion

The preoperative and accurate diagnosis of neurosarcoidosis may be difficult even with modern imaging techniques. We have addressed this issue using PET. In the present case, sarcoidosis primarily affected the frontal meninges, where miliary nodules were formed. The nodules comprised noncaseating sarcoid granulomas. The inflammatory process was granulomatous or lymphoplasmocytic. The granulomatous process can spread into the surrounding brain tissue. The pathologic condition may be similar to a chronic inflammation.

PET showed high rCBF and $rCMRO_2$ in the contrast-enhancing lesion, whereas these parameters were depressed in the surrounding lesion, suggesting oedematous change. The rOEF in the contrast-enhancing lesion remained equal to that in the contralateral grey matter. rCMRG1 also showed a high value even after steroid treatment. PET has been clinically applied to the diagnosis of cerebral gliomas. The rOEF and $rCMRO_2$ are consistently low in cerebral gliomas, whereas rCMRG1 relates to the degree of malignancy [8]. Therefore, the present results indicate that such increases in rCBF, rCBV, $rCMRO_2$, and rCMRG1 seem to be pathognomic in the haemocirculation and metabolism of neurosarcoidosis, a chronic inflammatory disease, and different from those in tumour tissue. Functional PET may supplement anatomic imaging in the diagnosis of neurosarcoidosis.

References

1. Scott TF (1993) Neurosarcoidosis: progress and clinical aspects. Neurology 43:8–12
2. Cahill DW, Salcman M (1981) Neurosarcoidosis: a review of the rarer manifestations. Surg Neurol 15:204–211
3. Cariski AT (1981) Isolated CNS sarcoidosis. JAMA 245:62–63
4. Brooks BS, Gammal TE, Hungerford GD, Acker J, Trevor RP, Russel W (1982) Radiologic evaluation of neurosarcodosis: role of computed tomography. AJNR 3:513–521
5. Ketonen L, Oksanen V, Kuuliala I, Somer H (1986) Hypodense white matter lesions in computed tomography of neurosarcoidosis. J Comput Assist Tomogr 10:181–183
6. Miller DH, Kendall BE, Barter S et al. (1988) Magnetic resonance imaging in central nervous system sarcoidosis. Neurology 38:378–383
7. Sheraman JL, Stern BJ (1990) Sarcoidosis of the CNS: comparison of unenhanced and enhanced MR images. AJR 155:1293–1301
8. Mineura K, Yasuda T, Kowada M, Shishido F, Ogawa T, Uemura K (1986) Positron emission tomographic evaluation of histological malignancy in gliomas using oxygen-15 and fluorine-18-fluorodeoxyglucose. Neurol Res 8:164–168

Cerebral oligodendroglioma: MRI versus histopathological grading

C. G. Choi [1], K. H. Chang [1], M. H. Han [1], J. G. Chi [2], M. C. Han [1]

[1] Department of Radiology, Seoul National Universtiy Hospital, 28 Yongon-Dong, Chongno-Gu, Seoul 110-744, Korea
[2] Department of Pathology, Seoul National University Hospital, 28 Yongon-Dong, Chongno-Gu, Seoul 110-744, Korea

Abstract. We analysed 46 MRI and 37 CT studies in 46 patients with cerebral oligodendrogliomas, to correlate MRI features with histological grading of the tumours. The tumours were pathologically graded as low (16) or intermediate (12), or anaplastic (18) oligodendroglioma. Each MRI criterion, including tumour size, presence or absence of calcification, cyst formation, haemorrhage, oedema, and contrast enhancement, was analysed with respect to the histological grading of the tumours. Among the various imaging features, peritumoral oedema and contrast enhancement were significantly more common in patients with anaplastic tumours than in patients with low-grade tumours. It is concluded that the presence of both peritumoral oedema and contrast enhancement is highly suggestive of anaplastic oligodendroglioma.

Key words: Brain neoplasm – Oligodendroglioma – Magnetic resonance imaging

MRI studies of oligodendrogliomas are rare [1, 2]. There is controversy about the significance of tumour enhancement on CT or MRI in predicting anaplastic tumours [1, 3]. It is not certain whether MRI can predict histological grading of oligodendrogliomas or not. It this study, we have evaluated cerebral oligodendrogliomas with MRI in 46 patients and assessed the correlation between MRI features and histological grading of the tumour.

Correspondence to: Choong Gon Choi, at the present address: Department of Diagnostic Radiology, Asan Medical Center, 388-1, Poongnab-dong Songpa-Gu, Seoul, Korea 138-040

Materials and methods

Forty-six patients with cerebral oligodendroglioma were included in this study, aged between 18 and 64 years (mean 41 years). Standard MRI was obtained as follows: proton-density and T2-weighted spin-echo images in the axial plane and T1-weighted images in the sagittal plane. Contrast-enhanced coronal or sagittal t1-weighted images were obtained in all patients. CT were obtained in 37 patients prior to MRI. All images were reviewed by two observers (C.G.C., K.H.C.) together, without knowledge of the histological grading. The MRI studies were reviewed with special attention to tumour size (small or large with the criteria of 5 cm diameter), the presence or absence of tumour enhancement, peritumoral oedema, calcification, cyst formation and intratumor haemorrhage. Histological specimens of all cases were reviewed by a neuropathologist (J.G.C.) and graded as low (16) or intermediate (12) grade or anaplastic (18) oligodendroglioma with the criteria of cellularity, endothelial proliferation, necrosis, mitosis and pleomorphism [4]. The score test for trends was used in the statistical analysis of the data.

Results

We summarise MRI findings in each subgroup of histological grading and statistical data in Table 1. Peritumoral oedema was only observed in the anaplastic group (6/18,

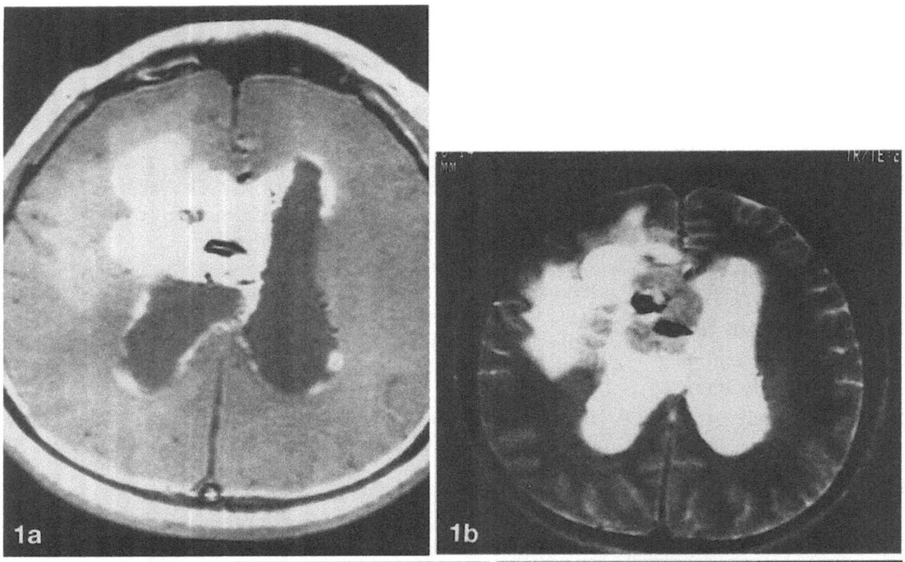

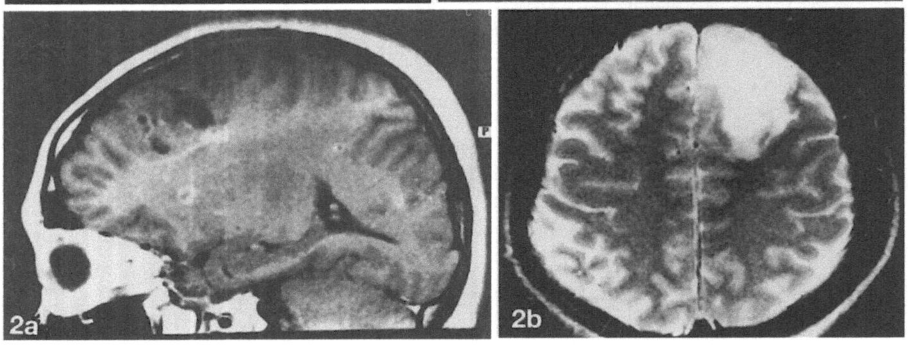

Fig. 1 a, b. Anaplastic oligodendroglioma with both peritumoral oedema and contrast enhancement. **a** Contrast-enhanced T1-weighted axial MRI shows a solid enhancing mass in deep right frontal area. Tumour invasion into the lateral ventricle and CSF seeding are seen. **b** T2-weighted image shows definite high-signal oedema surrounding the mass. Calcification within the mass is seen as low signal

Fig. 2 a, b. Low-grade oligodendroglioma without contrast enhancement or peritumoral oedema. **a** Contrast-enhanced T1-weighted sagittal MRI reveals no definite enhancement of the tumour in the superficial portion of the left frontal lobe. **b** The tumour shows high signal on a T2-weighted axial image but no peritumoural oedema

Table 1. MRI findings and histopathological grading

Histological MRI findings	Low n-= 16 (%)	Intermediate $n = 12$ (%)	Anaplastic $n = 18$ (%)	P-value
Oedema	0/16 (0)	1/12 (8)	6/18 (33)	0.007
Cyst	7/16 (44)	6/12 (50)	11/18 (64)	0.315
Haemorrhage	0/16 (0)	1/12 (8)	1/18 (6)	0.447
Tumour > 5 cm	7/16 (44)	9/12 (75)	13/18 (72)	0.095
Calcification on CT	3/11 (27)	5/8 (62)	6/18 (33)	0.892
Contrast enhancement	0/14 (0)	4/10 (40)	16/17 (94)	0.001

33%) and in one case of an intermediate-grade tumour with intratumoral haemorrhage. Contrast enhancement was seen in 94% (16/17) of the anaplastic group and in 40% (4/10) of the intermediate group, but was not seen in the low-grade group (0/14). The six anaplastic tumours with peritumoral oedema showed contrast enhancement. Among the various imaging features, peritumoral oedema and contrast enhancement were significantly more common in patients with anaplastic tumours (Fig. 1) than in patients with lower grade tumours (Fig. 2). There was significant correlation between these MR findings (peritumoral oedema, contrast enhancement) and pathological grading. However, other criteria such as tumour size, calcification, cyst formation, and haemorrhage, proved not to correlate significantly with pathological grading.

Discussion

Similar to the results of CT studies [1, 3], there was a strong trend for high-grade tumours to enhance on MRI. In the present study, prominent peritumoral oedema as another criterion suggestive of anaplastic tumour is a difference from the results of CT studies [1, 3]. This difference is thought to be caused by the different threshold for the presence of peritumoral oedema. It is not possible to discriminate peritumoral oedema from tumour infiltration itself on either CT or MRI, especially in tumours with poorly defined margins. However, finger-like projections of hyperintensity along white matter tracts on T2-weighted images represent vasogenic oedema. Our results suggest that the presence of either prominent peritumoral oedema or tumour enhancement is favourable for anaplastic tumours or intermediate-grade tumours (Table 1). The presence of both peritumoral oedema and tumour enhancement is likely to be predictive of anaplastic tumours. Both peritumoral vasogenic oedema and enhancement of a tumour are related to the disruption of the blood-brain barrier of capillaries within the tumour [5, 6]. MRI can demonstrate the possible anaplastic portion of the tumour that is appropriate for biopsy procedure and lead to a correct histological diagnosis and grading. The enhancing portion of the tumour should be included in the histological specimens of suspected oligodendrogliomas. We believe that the presence of both peritumoral oedema and contrast enhancement of tumours on MRI is highly suggestive of anaplastic tumours.

References

1. Lee YY, Tassel PV (1989) Intracranial oligodendrogliomas: imaging findings in 35 untreated cases. AJR 152:361–369
2. Tice B, Barnes PD, Goumnerova L, Scott RM, Tarbell NJ (1993) Pediatric and adolescent oligodendrogliomas. AJNR 14:1293–1300
3. Vonofakos D, Marcu H, Hacker H (1979) Oligodendrogliomas. CT patterns with emphasis on features indicating malignancy. J Comput Assist Tomogr 3:783–788
4. Smith MT, Ludwig CL, Godfrey AD, Armbrustmacher VW (1983) Grading of oligodendrogliomas. Cancer 52:2107–2114
5. Sage MR (1982) Blood-brain barrier: phenomenon of increasing importance to the imaging clinician. AJR 138:887–898
6. Long DM (1970) Capillary ultrastructure and the blood-brain barrier in human malignant brain tumors. J Neurosurg 32:127–144

Imaging features and pathological correlations of intracranial oligodendroglioma

X. B. Xie[1], K. H. Fang[1], S. T. Zhong[2]

[1] Department of Radiology, Sun-Yat-sen University of Medical Sciences, Guangzhou, People's Republic of China, 510080
[2] Department of Pathology, Sun-Yat-set University of Medical Sciences, Guangzhou, People's Republic of China, 510080

Abstract. We compared and analysed the CT findings of 75 pathologically proven oligodendrogliomas with those of 81 pathologically proven astrocytomas. The results suggest that there is a close correlation between CT findings and pathological findings and that CT can allow prediction of the diagnosis of oligodendroglioma in most cases, owing to some features that are different from those of astrocytomas, especially calcification. MRI is better for defining tumour extent but not for making a specific diagnosis.

Key words: Oligodendroglioma - X-ray comuted tomography - Pathology

Oligodendroglioma is a less common glioma than astrocytoma [1]. The aims of this study were: to assess to what extent CT can facilitate differentiation of oligodendroglioma from astrocytoma preoperatively; to discuss the pathological basis of CT features of oligodendroglioma on light and electron microscopy; and to assess the role of MRI in diagnosing oligodendroglioma.

Methods and materials

Seventy-five pathologically proven cases of oligodendroglioma were reviewed. Of these, 68 cases involved the cerebral hemisphere, 3 the lateral ventricle and 4 the cerebellum. All patients underwent CT, 10 also MRI. The CT findings were compared with those of 68 pathologically proven cases of astrocytoma. CT-pathological correlations in types of cerebral tumour (grades I, II) were closely studied by light microscopy in 12 cases and by electron microscopy in 5.

Correspondence to: X. B. Xie

Results

In these two types of cerebral glioma, CT findings were as follows:

1. An isodense or slightly dense mass was seen in 60.3% (41/68) of oligodendrogliomas and 29.4% (20/68) of astrocytomas ($P < 0.01$).
2. Little or no oedema was present in 76.4% (52/68) of oligodendrogliomas and 48.6% (33/68) of astrocytomas ($P < 0.01$).
3. Tumour calcification was noted in 77.9% (53/68) of oligodendroglioma and 16.2% (8/68) of astrocytomas ($P < 0.01$). Calcification was seen as a stripe and/or clump in 72.1% (49/68) of oligocendrogliomas and only 5.8% (4/68) of astrocytomas.
4. Little or no contrast enhancement was detected in 79.4% (54/68) of oligodendrogliomas and 35.5% (24/68) of astrocytomas ($P < 0.01$).
5. Peripheral white matter involvement with skull erosion was observed in 14.7% (10/68) of oligodendrogliomas and in no case of astrocytoma ($P < 0.01$).
6. Cystic change was present in 30.9% (21/68) of oligodendrogliomas and 45.6% (31/68) of astrocytomas ($P > 0.05$).

However, comparison of 4 cerebellar oligodendrogliomas and 10 astrocytomas revealed no significant differences between the tumours on CT except that the former were more commonly isodense (2/4) and the latter more often of low density (7/10). In our comparison of 3 lateral ventricular oligodendrogliomas and 3 astrocytomas there were again no significant differences on CT findings except that the former included one markedly calcified tumour and one of the latter had only minimal calcification.

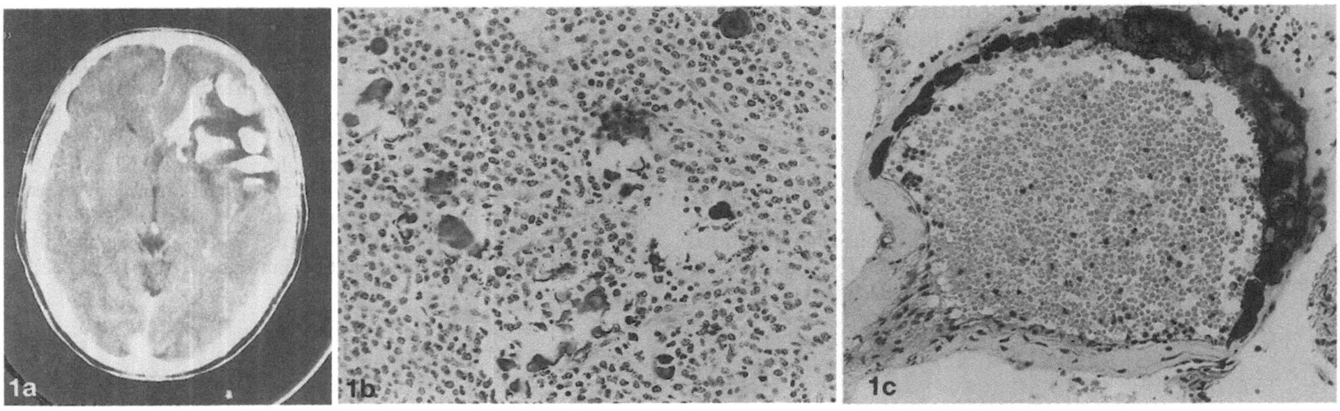

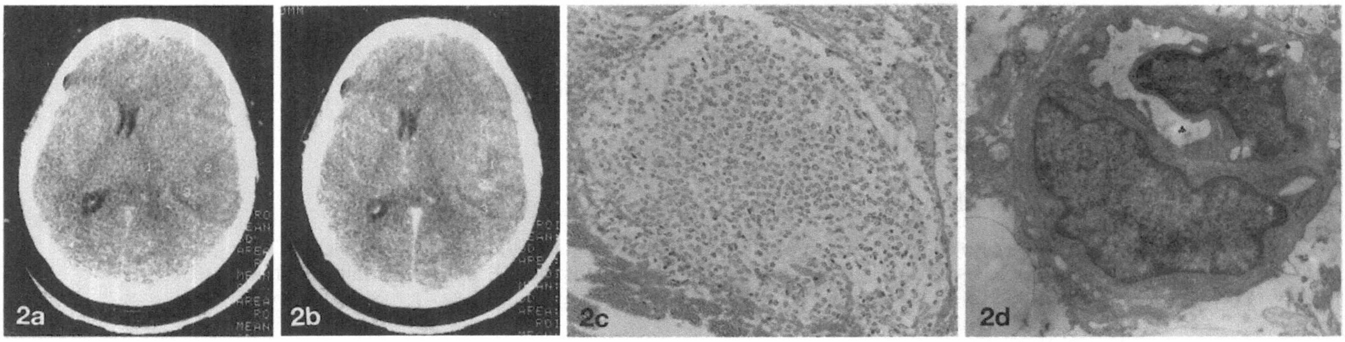

Fig. 1 a–c. Oligodendroglioma of left frontal lobe. **a** CT shows stripes and clumps of calcification in a low-density mass. **b, c** Light microscopy– **b** numerous calcific bodies; (HE, 5 × 10) **c** calcification of a blood vessel wall (HE, 5 × 10)

Fig. 2 a–d. Oligodendroglioma of left temporal lobe. **a** CT shows an isodense mass with minimal oedema. **b** There is only faint contrast enhancement. **c** Light microscopy (HE 5 × 10) shows rich tumour cells and sparse interstitial tissues. **d** Electron microscopy shows close interendotheliocytic linkages and intact basilemma, with only minimal defect at the glial membrane

Table 1. Results of blinded review of tumours

Diagnosis	Radiologist A			Radiologist B		
	Correct	Incorrect	%	Correct	Incorrect	%
Oligodendroglioma	24	4	85-7	24	4	85.7
Astrocytoma	24	4	85.7	21	7	75.0
Total	48	8	85.7	45	11	80.3

Light microscopy showed hypercellularity in 10 of 12 oligodendrogliomas and in 3 of 12 astrocytomas. Correspondingly, 8 of the 12 oligodendrogliomas were isodense or slightly dense, while only 2 of 12 astrocytomas showed this characteristic on unenhanced CT. Hypovascularity was seen in 9 of 12 oligodendrogliomas and 4 of 12 astrocytomas, corresponding to the observation that little or no contrast enhancement was seen in 11 of 12 oligodendrogliomas and in only 6 of 12 astrocytomas. We found that 71.7% (38/53) of the calcific deposits in 53 cases of oligodendroglioma occurred along the blood vessel walls and their surrounding tissues, especially those cases in which the calcium appeared as stripes on CT (Fig. 1).

Electron microscopy showed that endotheliocytes and interendotheliocytic linkages were normal in 4 of 5 oligodendrogliomas, whereas they were swollen and loose in 4 of 5 astrocytomas, corresponding to the observation that little or no contrast enhancement was seen in 4 of 5 oligodendrogliomas in only 1 of 5 astrocytomas (Fig. 2).

The first-choice diagnosis of oligodendroglioma was recorded at the time of initial CT in 45.3% (34/75). Using the method of blinded review, CT studies of 28 cases of oligodendroglioma and 28 of astrocytoma were interpreted by one senior neuroradiologist (A) and one junior neuroradiologist (B) independently, using the data analysed above. The results are summarised in Table 1.

In the 10 cases of oligodendroglioma examined by MRI, T1-weighted images showed low signal intensity in 4 cases and mixed signal in 6; T2-weighting showed higher signal intensity in all cases. In comparison with CT, 6 cases showed relatively clearer tumour margin than on CT, especially the 2 with Gd-DTPA enhancement. But in 2 cases no calcification was seen, despite positive CT findings, and 2 cases had no bone erosion which was visible on CT.

Discussion

Oligodendroglioma is often confused with the more common astrocytoma or even another tumour preoperatively [2, 3]. A correct diagnosis was made on the basis of the original CT reports in only 45.3% of the 75 patients in our series. The accuracy of CT in predicting a diagnosis of oligodendroglioma is not satisfactory, as has been noted previously [4].

Although our CT studies show that there are many similarities in the CT findings in cases of oligodendroglioma and of astrocytoma, they also show that there are many relative dissimilarities and that a combination of these may be characteristic of oligodendroglioma. Using these criteria, the accurate diagnosis rate in a blinded reading test was 85.7% and 80.3% for senior and junior neuroradiologists respectively. We therefore believe that it is possible to make the correct diagnosis in most cases of oligodendroglioma using the combination of these CT features, except for tumours of the lateral ventricles or cerebellum [5, 6].

Our studies also show that there is a close correlation between CT features and pathological findings in oligodendroglioma. The isodensity or slightly high density of this tumour on CT is concordant with the hypercellularity seen pathologically in the same cases. The scant contrast enhancement is concordant with the hypovascularity on light microscopy and normal capillary endotheliocytes and interendotheliocytic joins on electronic microscopy in the same cases. The characteristic calcification of this tumour on CT is also concordant with pathological findings. We found that calcification often occurred in the blood vessel walls and their surrounding tissues. We believe that this pattern of calcification on histopathology may be the cause of characteristic "stripes" of calcification on CT.

As regards MRI, we suggest that it is better than CT for defining tumour extent but not for making a specific diagnosis for oligodendroglioma.

References

1. Lee RR et al. (1989) Intracranial oligodendrogliomas: imaging finding in 35 untreated cases. AJR 152:301
2. Kazner E et al. (1982) Computed tomography in intracranial tumors: differential diagnosis and clinical aspects. Springer, Berlin Heidelberg New York
3. Chin HW et al. (1980) Oligodendrogliomas: a clinical study of cerebral oligodendrogliomas. Cancer 45:1458
4. Burger PC et al. (1987) Clinicopathologic correlations in the oligodendroglioma. Cancer 59:1345
5. Holladay FP et al. (1980) Cerebellar oligodendroglioma in child. Neurosurgery 6:552
6. Dolinskas CA et al. (1987) CT characteristics of intraventricular oligodendroglioma. AJNR 8:1077

Three unusual locations of subependymoma, with emphasis on MRI

C. Hoeffe [1], M. Boukobza [1], M. Polivka [2], J. P. Guichard [1], F. Laffite [1], D. Reizine [2], J. J. Merland [1]

[1] Department of Neuroradiology and Therapeutic Angiography, Hôpital Lariboisière, 10 rue Ambroise Paré, F-75010 Paris, France
[2] Department of Pathology, Hôpital Lariboisière, 10 rue Ambroise Paré, F-75010 Paris, France

Abstract. Spinal cord subependymomas (SE), either intramedullary (IM) or extramedullary (EM) are rare, as are multiple SE. We describe one case of each of these unusual presentations diagnosed mainly with MRI. On MRI, the masses were well demarcated, heterogeneous or homogenous, isointense or giving low signal relative to normal white matter on T1-weighted images and high signal on T2-weighted images. These masses demonstrated either no enhancement or pronounced heterogeneous enhancement. Gross total removal was performed in two cases. The IM SE recurred 7 years after surgery.

Key words: Subependymoma – Magnetic resonance imaging – Gadolinium – Spinal cord

Most subependymomas (SE) involved the cerebral ventricles (particularly the lateral ventricles). We describe unusual presentations of SE, histologically proven and explored by MRI and Gd-DTPA enhanced MRI. MRI examinations were reviewed and correlated with operative and pathological findings.

Correspondence to: M. Boukobza

Case Reports

Case 1: A 27-year-old man was admitted because of the acute onset of torticollis and paresis of the left arm. Cerebral angiogram showed the lesion to be avascular. MRI performed on a 0.5 T unit revealed an enlarged cord from the level of C4-C5 to the level of medulla oblongata, with a solid portion and what appeared as superior and inferior cystic portions. The surgeon thought that a complete removal had been achieved. Seven years later, a paresis of the patient's left arm progressively occurred, and MRI showed an enlargement of the medulla extending from the level of the medulla oblongata to the level of C6. Enhanced images demonstrated no enhancement of the lesion (Fig. 1).

Case 2: A 66-year-old man presented with neck pain, vertigo and unstable gait. MRI performed on a 1.5 T unit showed a mass arising from the level of C1, posterior to the medulla, extending cranially, uplifting and displacing to the left cerebellar peduncles and hemispheres. Post Gd-DTPA enhanced images showed irregular enhancement with a reticulated appearance. The tumour was heterogeneous with central non-enhancing foci probably representing cystic changes or necrosis (Fig. 2). Cerebral angiogram showed no abnormal blush but revealed a displacement to the inside of the PICA, suggesting an extramedullary tumour. During intervention, an extramedullary mass was found and easily dissected from the surrounding tissue. No recurrence was observed on MRI 3 years later.

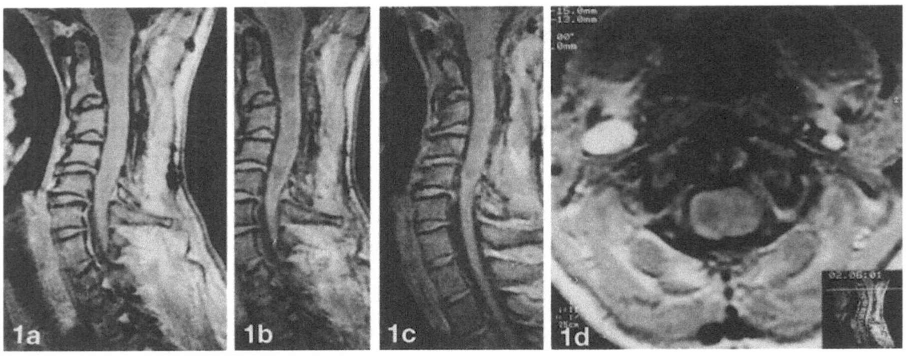

Fig. 1 a–d. Intramedullary subependymoma (SE). **a** Sagittal T1-weighted image (1986) shows an enlargement from the level of the medulla oblongata to C4, with ill-defined areas of low signal. **b–d** Recurrence (1993). Sagittal image shows enlargement of the medulla, extending from the medulla oblongata to C6. **c** There is no abnormal contrast enhancement **d** Axial T1-weighted image shows intramedullary low signal mass relative to normal cord, which does not enhance with contrast medium

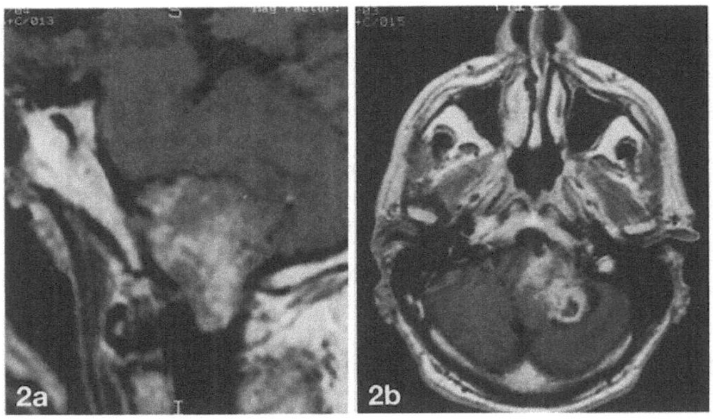

Fig. 2 a, b. Contrast-enhanced sagittal T1-weighted images in **a** sagittal and **b** axial planes demonstrate a mass with irregular enhancement, with a reticulated appearance. This contrast enhancement clearly demarcates neoplasm from surrounding tissues and helps to distinguish this extramedullary lesion from the neuraxis

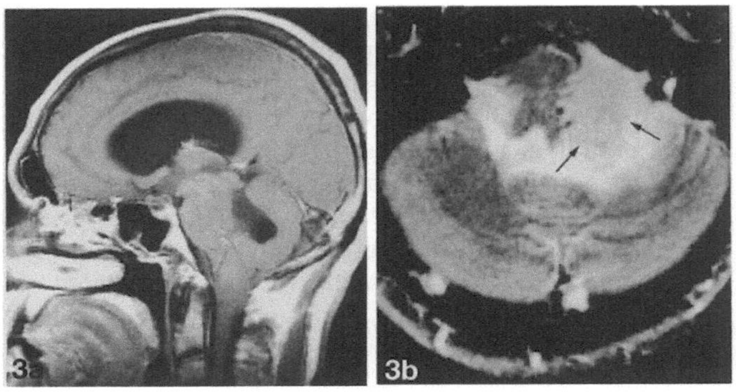

Fig. 3 a, b. Multiple SEs. **a** Contrast-enhanced sagittal image shows a small nonenhancing homogeneous mass arising from the floor of the fourth ventricle. **b** Axial T2-weighted image demonstrates one of the two other tumours: poorly defined, rather homogeneous, giving high signal (but lower than CSF), and surrounded by mild oedema

Case 3: A 53-year-old patient was admitted with recent progressive gait disturbance. MRI examination revealed a small non-enhancing mass arising from the floor of the fourth ventricle and two other lesions, isointense to white matter on T1-weighted images and hyperintense on T2-weighted images, simulating oedema, and non-enhanced on postcontrast images. One of these lesions extended from the level of C1 cranially to the cerebellopontine angle and then through the enlarged foramen of Luschka, and the other was located in the right cerebellopontine angle cistern, invaginating through the foramen of Luschka (Fig. 3). At surgery, these masses were found and another one located on the membrana tectoria, which had been missed on MRI. The spinal cord mass was extramedullary and difficult to dissect from the surrounding structures.

Discussion

The benign nature of this tumour is well known, although we do not know whether spinal cord SE is as benign as intracranial SE [1, 2]. Considering the small number of reported cases, no recurrence has been observed. In our series, it is noteworthy that a recurrence was seen 7 years after apparent total removal. Seven cases of IM SE imaged with MRI have been reported. Four of the reports mentioned MRI without further details [2–5], and only two gave a precise analysis [1, 6]. Two cases of EM spinal SE have been reported to date [7, 8], and Chason [9] reported multiple SE. Our cases of totally subarachnoid extramedullary lesions, hardly separated from (case 2) or with dense adherence to the medulla (case 3), support the heterotopic cell origin theory already described [8]. In most cases, the multiplanar imaging capability of MRI was valuable in assessing the location and the extension of these tumours. In only one case was a small lesion on the membrana tectoria missed. The signal of these lesions was predominantly iso- or hypointense to normal white matter on T1-weighted images and hyperintense on T2-weighted images, and heterogeneous in half the cases. These findings are commonly encountered throughout the literature, except for two reports mentioning an unexplained high signal of the lesion on T1- weighted images [9, 10]. Signal heterogeneity had various aetiologies, verified on histology, such as necrosis, vessels, cysts; in one case the cystic appearance observed at MRI corresponded to areas of the lesion that were well detached from the parenchyma. Margins were well defined in one case, ill defined in one and moderately well defined in one. The question of the appearance of SE after administration of IV Gd-DTPA remains undecided throughout the literature. Among the four spinal SE studied after administration of Gd-DTPA, half showed mild enhancement or none at all and half demonstrated marked enhancement. Considering our three cases, only one demonstrated a marked enhancement, with a reticulated appearance. The lesions in the two other cases did not enhance.

Although there are few data on spinal SE, they seem to exhibit the same features as their intracranial counterparts: when confronted with a nonenhancing or minimally enhancing lesion one must consider the diagnosis of SE. MRI is particularly helpful in evaluation of the location, extent, size and relationships of these unusual forms of SE.

References

1. Pagni C, Canavero S, Giordana MT, Arnetoli (1992) Spinal intramedullary subependymomas: case report and review of the literature. Neurosurgery 30:115–117
2. Vaquero J, Martínez R, Vegazo I, Ponton P (1989) Subependymoma of the cervical spinal cord. Neurosurgery 24:625–627
3. Guha A, Resh L, Tator CH (1989) Subependymoma of the thoracolumbar cord. Case report. J Neurosurg 71:781–787
4. Salvati M, Raco A, Artico M, Artizzu S, Ciapetta P (1992) Subependymoma of the spinal cord. Case report and review of the literature. Neurosurg Rev 15:65–69
5. Lee KS, Angelo JN, McWorther JM, Davis CH Jr (1987) Symptomatic subependymoma of the cervical cord. Report of two cases. J Neurosurg 67 128–131
6. Nakasu S, Nakasu Y, Saito A, Handa J (1992) Intramedullary subependymoma with neurofibromatosis. Report of two cases. Neurol Med Chir 32:275–280
7. Boykin FC, Cowen D, Iannucci CAT, Wolf A (1954) Subependymal glomerate astrocytomas. J Neuropathol Exp Neurol 13:30–49
8. Matsumura A, Hori A, Spoerri O (1988) Spinal subependymoma presenting as an extramedullary tumor. Case report. Neurosurgery 23:115–117
9. Chason JL (1956) Subependymal mixed gliomas. J Neuropathol Exp Neurol 15:461–470
10. Roeder MB, Jinkins JR, Bazan C (1994) Subependymoma of filum terminale: MR appearance. Case report. J Comput Assist Tomogr 18:129–130

Imaging in gangliogliomas: a review of 8 cases

B. M. Berberian, F. Y. Tsai, A. E. Segal, C. Chen, A. M. Wang

Radiology, UMKC, Human Medical Center, 230/Holmes, Kansas City MO 64108, USA

Abstract. With MRI, ganglioglioma may be confused with other intracranial tumors, or not identified. The purpose of this paper is to describe the imaging patterns found in eight cases of biopsy proven ganglioglioma and to help resolve confusion about the diagnosis.

Key words: Ganglioglioma – Brain tumors – Grey matter tumor

Ganglioglioma is a rare primary central nervous system (CNS) lesion, with a reported incidence of between 0.4% and 7.6% of all primary brain neoplasms. The tumor is slow-growing, usually benign and composed of both neuronal and glial elements, with the glial components rarely demonstrating neoplastic proliferation. Ganglioglioma occurs most frequently in children and young adults in the temporal lobe; however, no part of the CNS is exempt. The tumor is treated surgically and carries a relatively good prognosis, with postoperative survival as long as 20 years in some cases; accurate diagnosis is thus essential [1, 2].

Materials and methods

Our eight patients are shown in Table 1. All patients presented with new-onset seizure disorder. All lesions involved grey matter. Four lesions were in the temporal lobe (Fig. 1), two in the parietal lobe, one in the frontal lobe (Fig. 2), and one was multicentric, involving the temporal lobe, right parahippocampal gyrus and hypothalamus, with midline extension into the third ventricle (Fig. 3). The lesions showed contrast enhancement in all eight patients, cystic components in six, definite calcification in three, and equivocal calcification in one.

Table 1. Summary of patients with ganglioglioma

Age (years)	Sex	Site of tumor
5	F	Left temporal lobe; hypothalamus; right parahippocampal gyrus
5	F	Right medial temporal lobe
11	M	Left parietal lobe
11	F	Right temporal lobe
16	F	Right posterior temporal lobe
17	F	Left posterior parietal lobe
32	F	Left temporal lobe
37	F	Left frontal lobe

Discussion

Since gangliogliomas are cortical tumors, small tumors may show only minimally increased attenuation on noncontrast-enhanced CT, and appear as CSF density on T2-weighted MRI. These tumors could be missed if MRI is performed without contrast. Tampieri et al. [3] reported that MRI failed to show the tumor in 2 of their 19 cases and we speculate that this may have arisen because studies were performed without contrast medium. Similarly, Altman [4] demonstrated two cass with hyperdensity on unenhanced CT, and no appreciable contrast enhance-

Correspondence to: F. Y. Tsai

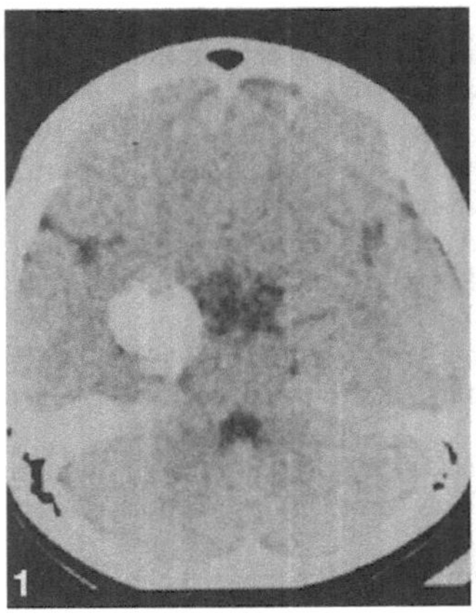

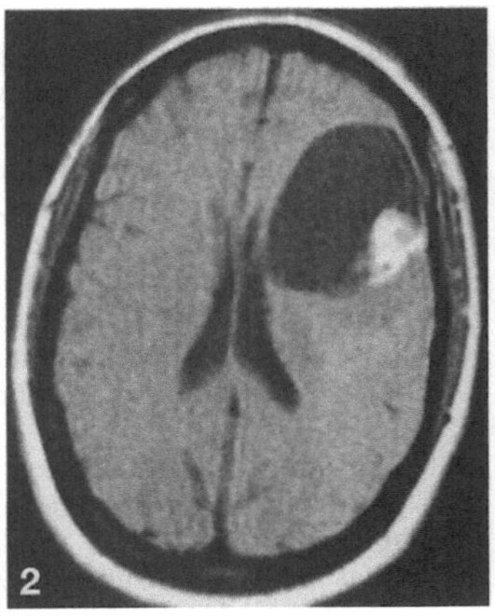

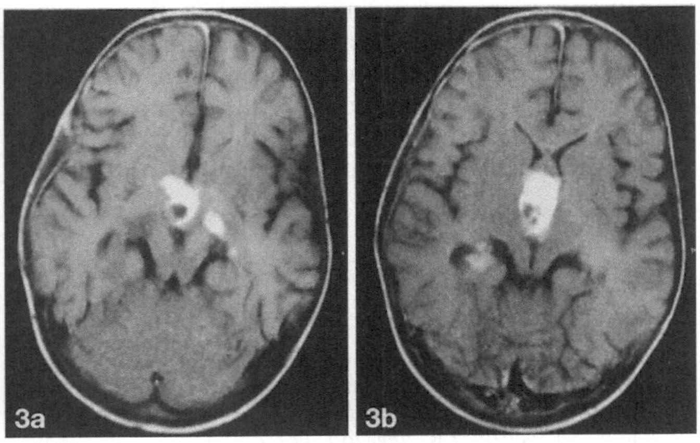

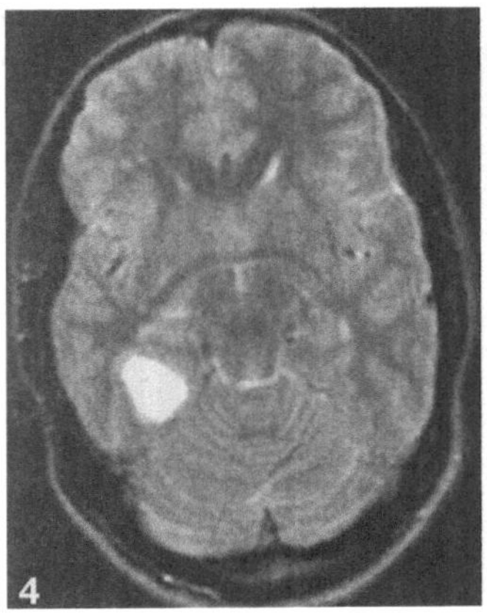

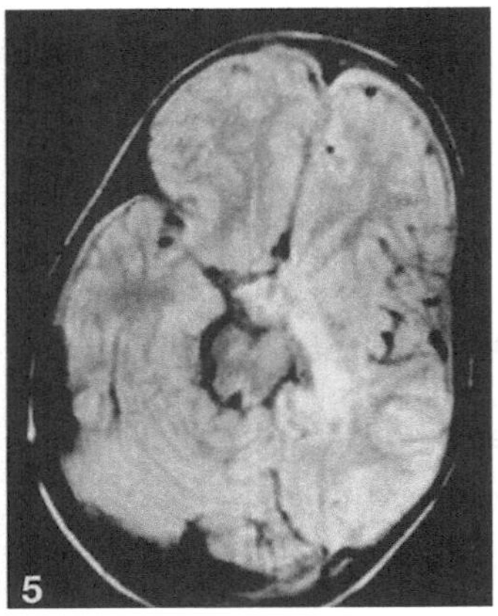

Fig. 1. An 11-year-old girl. CT shows a densely calcified mass in the medial right temporal lobe, without associated edema

Fig. 2. A 37-year-old woman. Contrast-enhanced axial T1-weighted image shows a left frontal cystic mass with an enhancing nodule in the cortical grey matter peripherally, minimal compression on the left lateral ventricle, and effacement sulci

Fig. 3a, b. A 5-year-old girl. Contrast-enhanced T1-weighted images show **a** partially cystic enhancing midline hypothalamic mass, a second enhancing mass in the left medial temporal lobe, without edema, and **b** an enhancing tumor nodule in the right parahippocampal gyrus grey matter with distortion of the ambient cistern and trigone

Fig. 4. A 16-year-old boy. T2-weighted image shows a mass in the right posterior temporal lobe, with mild adjacent cortical distortion

Fig. 5. Same patient as Fig. 3. Proton density image shows a left medial temporal lobe mass with adjacent cortical distortion and effacement of the left suprasellar cistern. Cortical distortion may be the only finding with small grey matter lesions

ment and an area of relatively short T2 relaxation in the left frontal lobe on MRI. Had these lesions been smaller, and had MRI been performed without contrast medium, these tumors could have been overlooked. Cortical grey matter distortion in the absence of an enhancing nodule may be the only clue to the presence of a small tumor (Figs. 4, 5).

Tien et al. [5] reported a case of ganglioglioma with leptomeningeal and subarachnoid spread, a feature that could be confused with metastatic disease. Van Tassel et al. [6] claim that multicentric glioma may mimic metastatic disease on CT, and describe criteria for differentiation including large, solidly enhancing lesions without central necrosis and lesions deep in the hemisphere. Similarly, in our case of multicentric tumor, an enhancing cortical grey matter nodule away from a corticomedullary junction may be a clue to the correct diagnosis.

The patient's age can be a potential source of confusion in the diagnosis of ganglioglioma. The series reported by Castillo et al. [2] included patients in their sixth, seventh and eighth decades. Only postoperatively were these patients correctly diagnosed as having gangliogliomas. A large cystic ganglioglioma with an enhancing nodule could be confused with other intracranial neoplasms, especially in the posterior fossa and temporal lobe. The other types of gliomas tend to have enhancement in white matter, rather than grey matter as in ganglioglioma. A contrast-enhancing cortical grey matter nodule is a hallmark of ganglioglioma.

References

1. Russell DS, Rubenstein LJ (1959) Pathology of tumors of the nervous system, 5th edn. Williams and Wilkins, Baltimore, pp 260–269
2. Castillo M, Davis PC, Takei Y, Hoffman JC Jr (1990) Intracranial ganglioglioma: MR, CT and clinical findings in 18 patients. AJR 154:607–612
3. Tampieri D, Moundjian R, Melauson D, Ethier R (1991) Intracerebral gangliogliomas in patients with partial complex seizures: CT and MR imaging findings. AJNR 12:749–755
4. Altman NR (1988) MR and CT characteristics of ganglioglioma: a rare case of epilepsy in children. AJNR 9:917–921
5. Tien RD, Tuori SL, Pulkingham N, Burger PC (1992) Gangliogliomas with leptomeningeal and subarachnoid spread: results of CT, MR and PET imaging. AJR 159:391–393
6. Van Tassel P, Lee YY, Bruner JM (1988) Synchronous and metachronous malignant gliomas: CT findings. AJNR 9:725–732

Imaging of malignant rhabdoid tumor of brain

M. Hardjasudarma[1], M. Fowler[1], B. Willis[2], W. Stewart[1], J. Lecky[1], R. McClellan[1], H. Hollenberg[1]

[1] Department of Radiology, Louisiana State University Medical Center, Shreveport, La., USA
[2] Department of Pathology, Louisiana State University Medical Center, Shreveport, La., USA
[3] Department of Surgery (Neurosurgery), Louisiana State University Medical Center, Shreveport, La., USA

Abstract. Malignant rhabdoid tumor is a very uncommon, highly malignant neoplasm that primarily affects infants and children. Its most common site of origin is the kidney. Primary origin in the brain, as in this case report of a 4-year-old girl, is rare. The imaging characteristics on CT and MRI are those of a large, malignant mass, with hemorrhage, cystic or necrotic areas, irregular enhancement, and surrounding edema. This child's tumor was highly vascular, and massive hemorrhage complicated the surgery. There may thus be a place for preoperative embolization. The tumor has a tendency for relapse at the primary site and rapidly progressive leptomeningeal metastases.

Key words: Rhabdoid tumor, malignant – Brain – Magnetic resonance imaging

Malignant rhabdoid tumor is one of the least common and most deadly neoplasms of early life. Most originate in the kidney, but extrarenal locations are known. This is a case of primary cerebral involvement.

Case report

A 4-year-old girl presented with progressive right upper extremity monoparesis, and a right central seventh nerve palsy of recent onset. CT and MRI (Fig. 1) showed a large, enhancing left cerebral hemispheric mass containing areas of hemorrhage and necrosis. Angiography demonstrated a highly vascular tumor, primarily supplied by posterior branches of the middle cerebral artery. At surgery a large brain tumor was removed. The procedure was complicated by massive hemorrhage. Gross pathology: small cystic areas and occasional punctate hemorrhages. Histology: Areas of high and sparse cellularity. Large areas of necrosis, some of which contained loose fibrous tissue. The tumor cells varied from polygonal to spindle shaped to stellate, and tended to form whorls of interlacing bundles in the more spindled areas. The nuclei were generally rounded or oval with prominent nucleoli. Some of the more polygonal cells contained discrete globular masses adjacent to the filaments. Immunoperoxidase stains directed against neuron-

Fig. 1. **a** before, **b** after contrast medium T1-weighted (500/20 images; **c** T2-weighted (3500/90) image. There is a very large mass involving the left temporal and frontal lobes, basal ganglia and thalamus. It contains a small hematoma (**a**; *arrow*) and necrotic centers. The tumor is mostly iso-hypointense on T1-weighting and iso-hyperintense to grey matter on T2-weighting. Marked, irregular enhancement is shown

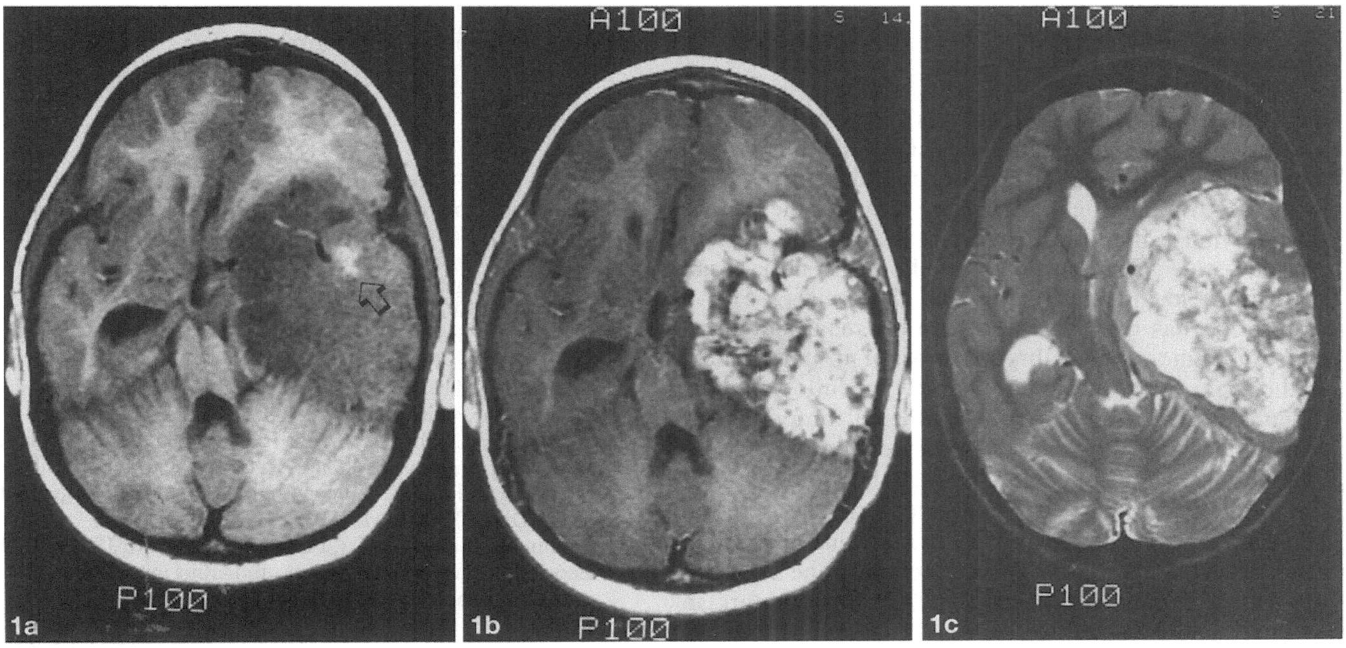

Correspondence to: M. Hardjasudarma, Department of Radiology, Louisiana State University Medical Center – Shreveport, Shreveport, LA 71130-3932, USA

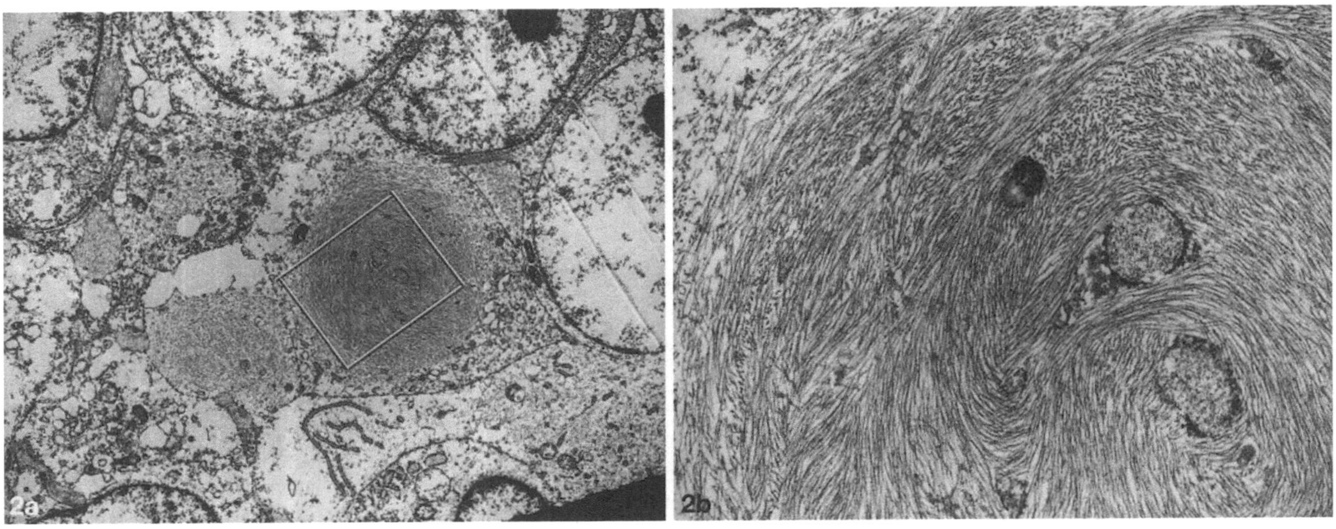

Fig. 2a, b. Electron micrographs of tumor cells revealing the characteristic whorls of microfilaments adjacent to the nuclei. (Original magnification: **a** 3,000×; **b** 20,000×. **b** Magnification of the area enclosed by the *rectangle in* **a**)

specific enolase, S-100, vimentin and keratin were positive. Antibodies against desmin, synaptophysin and glial fibrillary acidic protein failed to stain. Electron microscopy: In addition to the above, the globular masses seen by light microscopy were composed of microfilaments that frequently trapped a few cytoplasmic organelles. Frequent bundles of microfilaments were also seen in other portions of the cytoplasm (Fig. 2). Postoperatively, the patient made a good recovery and was referred to a pediatric oncology hospital. Abdominal and renal ultrasound were normal, without evidence of any masses. Preradiation chemotherapy was instituted. However, tumor recurrence in the chiasmatic cistern was found 3 months postoperatively.

Discussion

This tumor primarily affects infants and young children, and has a male preponderance. It is highly malignant, with a mortality rate > 80% [1]. It most commonly arises in the kidney. Extrarenal sites of origin are rare, and include the liver, thymus, chest wall, paravertebral region, uterus, prostate, the soft tissues of the shoulder, neck, arm, perineum and inguinal region, and the brain [2–5]. An association has been observed between renal malignant rhabdoid tumors, and embryonal types of primary tumors in the central nervous system, namely medulloblastoma, pineoblastoma, primitive neuroepithelial tumor, malignant subependymal giant cell astrocytoma and medulloepithelioma [4, 6]. Congenital primary rhabdoid tumor of the brain, with massive replacement of the cerebral hemispheres by tumor and hydrocephalus, has been reported [7]. Although originally thought to be a variant of Wilm's tumor, the description of these tumors in extrarenal sites has led to debates concerning the cell of origin. Velasco et al. [7], who reported a tumor that stained positively against vimentin, concluded that they might arise from arachnoidal cells. Biggs et al. [8] described a similar tumor that stained positively against both vimentin and cytokeratin and concluded that the tumor was showing early epithelial differentiation [8]. Ota et al. [9] concluded that the cell of origin might be neuroblastic. It seems likely that this tumor arises from primitive pluripotential cells, possibly of neural crest or ectomesenchymal origin. Imaging findings of malignant rhabdoid tumors of the brain have been described as large malignant mass(es), with significant edema and mass effect, areas of hemorrhage and cysts or necrosis, and strong but non-uniform enhancement [2, 3]. These nonspecific findings also apply in our case. Interestingly, to date, all unifocal cerebral cases have affected the left hemisphere [2]. Rapid deterioration is the norm, with relapse at the primary site and development of rapidly progressive leptomeningeal metastases [2]. Angiographically, the tumors are very vascular. In selected instances, presurgical embolization of the main arterial feeders may decrese intraoperative hemorrhage.

References

1. Weeks DA, Beckwith JB, Mierau GW, Luckey DW (1989) Rhabdoid tumor of kidney. Am J Surg Pathol 13:439–458
2. Hanna SL, Langston JW, Parham DM, Douglass EC (1993) Primary malignant rhabdoid tumor of the brain: clinical, imaging, and pathologic findings. AJNR 14:107–115
3. Ho PSP, Lee WH, Chen CY, Chou TY, Wang YC, Sun MJ, Liou WY (1990) Primary malignant rhabdoid tumor of the brain: CT characteristics. J Comput Assist Tomogr 14:461–463
4. Jakate SM, Marsden HB, Ingram L (1988) Primariy rhabdoid tumor of the brain. Virchows Arch [A] 412:393–397
5. Sotelo-Avila C, Gonzalez-Crussi F, deMello D, Vogler C, Gooch WM, Gale G, Pena R (1986) Renal and extrarenal rhabdoid tumors in children: a clinicopathological study of 14 patients. Semin Diagn Pathol 3:151–163
6. Bonnin JM, Rubinstein LJ, Palmer NF, Beckwith JB (1984) The association of embryonal tumors originating in the kidney and in the brain. Cancer 564:2137–2146
7. Velasco ME, Brown JA, Kini J, Ruppert ES (1993) Primary congenital rhabdoid tumor of the brain with neoplastic hydranencephaly. Child's Nerv Sys 9:185–190
8. Biggs PJ, Garen PD, Powers JM, Garvin AJ (1987) Malignant rhabdoid tumor of the central nervous system. Hum Pathol 18:332–337

Pathological study of dural enhancement (flare sign) on MRI of meningiomas

H. Nakau[1], T. Miyazawa[1], K. Tsuchiya[3], K. Shima[1], T. Shirotani[1], H. Chigasaki[1], S. Tamai[2]

[1] Department of Neurosurgery, National Defense Medical College, Saitama, Japan
[2] Department of Laboratory Medicine, National Defense Medical College, Saitama, Japan
[3] Department of Radiology, Kyorin University School of Medicine, Tokyo, Japan

Abstract. The purpose of this study was to clarify the pathological features and clinical significance of the dural enhancement (flare sign) on contrast-enhanced T1-weighted MRI. Tumour cell nests were observed on pathological examination in the dura mater in three of nine cases whose preoperative MRI showed the flare sign. Since we cannot exclude the possibility that tumour cell nests exhibiting this sign were present in the dura mater, our findings suggest that the dura mater surrounding meningiomas should be resected as widely as possible.

Key words: Flare sign – Meningioma – Magnetic resonance imaging – Meningeal sign – Dural tail sign

---

In 1989, Wilms et al. [1] first described meningeal enhancement surrounding meningiomas on T1-weighted MRI obtained with gadolinium (Gd)-DTPA enhancement.

This finding has been called the "dural tail sign" [2], "meningeal sign" [3] and "flare sign" [4]. In order to clarify the clinical significance of and the pathological features associated with this sign, we analysed the pathological findings in nine cases of meningioma showing this sign on preoperative MRI.

Material and Methods

Between 1987 and 1993, 56 patients with meningiomas underwent surgical resection in our institute. Twenty-seven (61%) of 44 cases examined preoperatively with contrast-enhanced MRI exhibited the flare sign. The enhancing dura mater surrounding the tumour was resected in 9 of 44 cases. No patient had previously undergone intracranial surgery. We used 1.5T units for these studies.

We diagnosed flare sign on MRI using the criteria given by Aoki et al. [4]: firstly, linear enhancement presence was along the dura mater from the tumour margin; secondly, enhancement was greater than that on the contralateral side or in distant regions in the midline; thirdly, findings were noted in two different planes; and finally, findings were noticed by three independent observers. The flare sign was diagnosed when all of these criteria were met.

Results

Table 1 summarises the nine cases examined. Connective tissue proliferation in the dura mater was found on pathological examination in each case. Vascular proliferation was observed in only three cases. Tumour invasion of the dura mater was found in four cases. Tumour cell nests were observed 4.5 mm from the edge of the tumour in case 9. In one of the nine cases, a cluster of meningothelial cells was observed. In only two cases were both vascular proliferation and tumour invasion found in the same specimen. Figure 1 shows a representative case.

Discussion

Several studies have previously been made of the histopathological findings associated with the flare sign. The most common interpretation of this sign is that it represents connective tissue proliferation of the dura mater with vascular proliferation [1, 4, 5]. Although we also found connective tissue proliferation in each case we examined, hypervascularity was confirmed in only three of our nine cases. Alternatively, other researchers have suggested that

Table 1. Clinical and pathological findings in nine patients

Case	Age (years)	Sex	Site	Histological type	Connective tissue proliferation	Vascular proliferation	Tumour invasion	Cell clusters
1	73	F	Falx	Transitional	++	–	–	–
2	55	F	Convexity	Transitional	++	–	–	–
3	62	M	Tentorial	Transitional	++	–	–	–
4	69	M	Convexity	Meningotheliomatous	++	–	–	–
5	72	M	Convexity	Fibroblastic	++	+	–	+
6	46	F	Sphenoid Ridge	Meningotheliomatous	++	+	+	–
7	48	M	Convexity	Transitional	++	+	+	–
8	51	F	Falx	Transitional	++	–	+	–
9	84	F	Convexity	Meningotheliomatous	++	–	+	–

Correspondence to: H. Nakau, Department of Neurosurgery, ISDF Central Hospital, 1-2-24 Ikejiri, Setagaya-ku, Tokyo T154, Japan

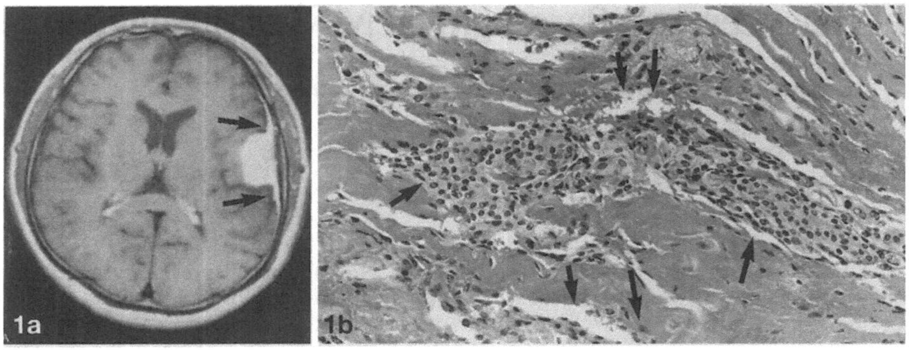

Fig. 1 a, b. Case 7. A 48-year-old man with a 3-month history of headache. **a** T1-weighted MR image after Gd-DTPA administration demonstrates a convexity meningioma with the flare sign (*arrows*). The tumour was a transitional-type meningioma. **b** Both marked invasion of tumour (*arrows*) and vascular proliferation (*arrow heads*) were observed in the marginal dura mater. Haematoxylin and eosin stain

extension of extravascular space, due to increased vascular permeability of dural vessels, might be responsible for this sign [6]. Another possible mechanism, adherence of neoplastic fibrous sheets to the inner surface of the dura mater has been reported by other authors [1, 5, 7]. Some authors believe that the flare sign is due to abnormally thickened arachnoid tissue [5].

The most important aspect of the flare sign from the neurosurgical standpoint is whether tumour cell nests are present in the marginal dura when the flare sign is present. In a review of the literature, we found that a few authors have reported the absence of tumour cells in dura mater that exhibited contrast enhancement [4, 6]. However, most researchers have reported the presence of neoplastic tissue displaying enhancement in marginal dura mater [1, 2, 5]. Since we cannot exclude the possibility that tumour cell nests exhibiting the flare sign were present in the dura mater, our findings suggest that the dura mater surrounding meningioma should be resected as widely as possible.

References

1. Wilms G, Lammens M, Marchal G, Calenbergh FV, Plets C, Fraeyenhoven LV, Baert AL (1989) Thickening of dura surrounding meningiomas. J Comput Assist Tomogr 13:763–768
2. Goldsher D, Litt AW, Pinto RS, Bannon KR, Kricheff II (1990) Dural "tail" associated with meningiomas on Gd-DTPA-enhanced MR images. Radiology 176:447–450
3. Schorner W, Schubeus P, Henkes H, Lanksch W, Felix R (1990) "Meningeal sign": a characteristic finding of meningiomas on contrast-enhanced MR images. Neuroradiology 32:90–93
4. Aoki S, Sasaki Y, Machida T, Tanioka H (1990) Contrast-enhanced MR images in patients with meningioma. AJNR 11:935–938
5. Larson JJ, Tew JM, Wiot JG, Courten-Myers GM (1992) Association of meningioma with dural "tails"; surgical significance. Acta Neurochir (Wien) 114:59–63
6. Sekiya T, Manabe H, Iwabuchi T, Narita T (1992) The dura mater adjacent to the attachment of meningiomas; its enhanced MR imaging and histological findings (in Japanese). Neurol Surg 20:1063–1068
7. Brovich B, Doron D (1986) Recurrence of intracranial meningiomas: the roll played by regional multicentricity. Neurosurgery 64:58–63

MRI of hemorrhagic meningiomas

C. S. Zee, M. Tan, P. M. Colletti, W. D. Boswell

University of Southern California School of Medicine, Department of Radiology, LAC + USC Imaging Science Center, 1744 Zonal Avenue, Los Angeles, CA 90033, USA

Abstract. MRI is an excellent imaging modality for showing hemorrhagic meningiomas. Our high incidence of hemorrhage associated with meningioma (3.7%) is probably secondary to the greater sensitivity of MRI imaging in detection of hemorrhage. Malignant, angioblastic, and fibroblastic meningiomas have a greater "relative bleeding tendency" than other histological types.

Key words: Meningioma – Hemorrhage

Correspondence to: C. S. Zee

Spontaneous hemorrhage occurs in approximately 5% of cases of intracranial gliomas [1] and 15% of intracranial metastatic neoplasms [2]. By contrast, hemorrhage into meningiomas is relatively rare. Oldberg's series of 832 gliomas contained 31 (3.7%) with hemorrhage [3], whereas in Cushing and Eisenhardt's series no meningiomas exhibited hemorrhage [4]. Zimmermann and Bilaniuk [5] found only 8 cases of neoplasm in 107 autopsy studies for intracranial hemorrhage and none were meningiomas.

We found 65 cases of hemorrhage associated with intracranial meningioma in the literature [6–9]. The tumors may present with subarachnoid, intracerebral or

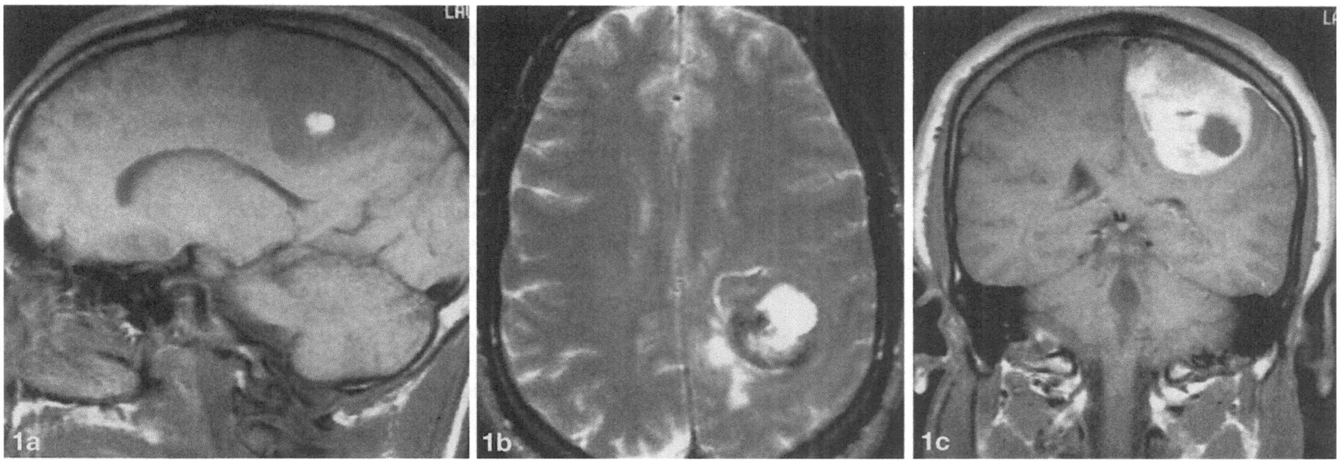

Fig. 1a–c. Convexity meningioma. **a** Sagittal T1-weighted image shows a low signal intensity mass with broad-bases attachment to the calvarium. A focal area of high signal within the mass is consistent with subacute hemorrhage. **b** Axial T2-weighted image shows a cystic mass. The fluid within the cyst is of high signal intensity. The solid component is of low signal intensity, as is the area of hemorrhage. **c** Coronal T1-weighted contrast-enhanced image shows an enhancing mass with a dural tail and a cyst within it

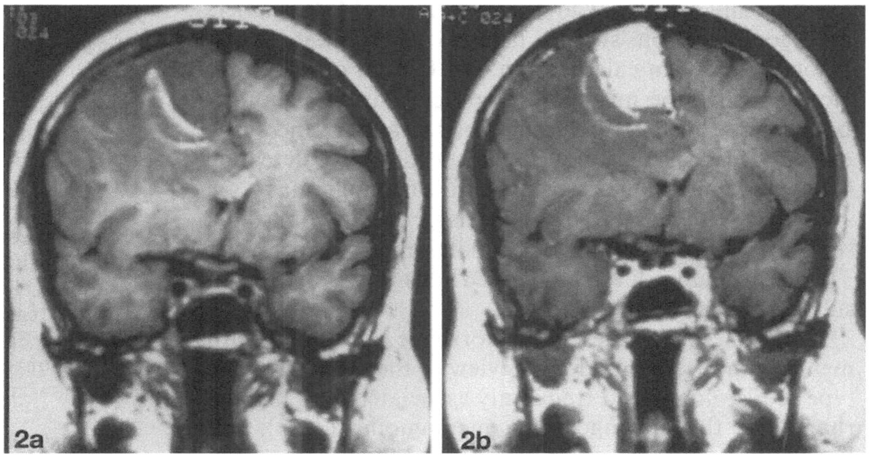

Fig. 2a, b. Parasagittal meningioma. **a** Coronal T1-weighted image shows a low signal intensity mass in the parasagittal region with adjacent high signal intensity, consistent with hemorrhage on the surface of the tumor and subarachnoid hemorrhage. **b** Contrast-enhanced image shows an enhancing mass with broad-based attachment to the calvarium and falx

intratumoral hemorrhage. We present 5 cases of hemorrhagic meningiomas demonstrated on MRI and proven at surgery.

Materials and methods

A total of 133 patients with intracranial meningiomas were examined and 5 hemorrhagic meningiomas were found. The clinical history, MRI findings, and histological features of these 5 meningiomas were reviewed in detail.

Results

A review of the literature revelaed a total of 65 cases of hemorrhagic meningiomas in addition to the 5 cases in our series. The histopathological findings of these 70 cases are as listed in Table 1. The histopathology of our 5 cases was meningothelial (2), angioblastic (2) and malignant (1) meningiomas. According to the review of literature, the most common histological types of meningiomas with hemorrhage were meningothelial and angioblastic types.

Table 1. Histological types of 70 hemorrhagic meningiomas

Meningothelial	25
Unspecified	13
Angioblastic	11
Fibroblastic	10
Malignant	5
Transitional	4
Psammomatous	1
Mixed	1

Discussion

Intracranial hemorrhage in association with meningiomas is infrequent. A total of 13 cases of hemorrhagic meningioma was reported in 1976 [7]. With the advent of CT, more cases of hemorrhagic meningioma were reported [6, 8, 9]. Russell and associates [8], reported 6 cases of meningioma associated with microscopic intratumoral hemorrhage in a series of 131 cases, but only in 3 was the hemorrhage significant enough to cause discernible CT changes. Acute

Table 2. Relative bleeding tendency of different types of meningioma

Histology	Proportion bleeding	Proportions of types of meningioma [10]	Relative bleeding tendency
Malignant	5 (7%)	14 (1%)	7
Angioblastic	11 (16%)	97 (8%)	2
Fibroblastic	10 (14%)	82 (7%)	2
Meningothelial	25 (36%)	749 (63%)	0.57
Transitional	4 (6%)	255 (21%)	0.29
Other and Unspecified	15 (21%)	-	-
Total	70	1197	

hemorrhage exhibits as areas of high density on CT and can be easily detected. Careful assessment of CT numbers and configuration should help to differentiate acute hemorrhage from calcification. On CT, an old isodense clot can easily be mistaken for other sources of nonenhancing low density, such as necrosis, scarring, and cystic changes. For this reason, CT is not sensitive for detecting subacute hemorrhage associated with meningiomas.

With MRI we found 5 hemorrhagic meningiomas in a series of 133 cases, a higher proportion than previously. This is probably due to increased sensitivity of MRI to subacute hemorrhage.

Only 65 other cases of hemorrhage associated with meningioma were found in a review of the literature. The type of histology most frequently associated with hemorrhage was the meningothelial meningioma (36%), followed by angioblastic (16%), fibroblastic (14%), and malignant (7%) types. By relating data from the series of hemorrhagic meningiomas to data obtained from a large series of meningiomas with reported incidence of histopathological types, it is possible to calculate an approximate "relative bleeding tendency" for a given histopathological type of tumor [6]. Angioblastic meningiomas represented 8% of the 1197 surgically verified meningiomas reported by Jellinger and Slowik [10]. However, 16% of the meningiomas associated with hemorrhage reported in the present study were angioblastic. This gives angioblastic meningioma a relative bleeding tendency of 2.0. Using the same method of calculation the relative bleeding tendency for transitional meningioma is 0.29, for meningothelial 0.57, for fibroblastic 2, and for malignant 7 (Table 2).

The exact mechanisms causing meningiomas to bleed are not completely understood. Several hypotheses include endothelial proliferation with obliteration of the vessels and distal necrosis [11], distortion and distension of the blood vessel caused by tumor growth [12], foci of abnormal vessels with the tumor [13], or direct vascular invasion by the meningioma.

Although hemorrhage associated with meningioma is rare, one should keep in mind the possibility of a meningioma in the differential diagnosis of a hemorrhagic lesion. Accurate diagnosis of the hemorrhagic meningioma can facilitate proper surgical treatment.

Acknowledgement. The authors wish to thank Kelly Stewart for transcribing the manuscript.

References

1. Leeds NE, Elkin CM, Zimmerman RD (1984) Gliomas of the brain. Semin Roentgenol 19–27
2. Manclybur TI (1977) Intracranial caused by metastatic tumors. Neurology 27:650
3. Oldberg E (1933) Hemorrhage into gliomas: a review of 832 consecutive verified cases of glioma. Arch Neurol Psychiatry 30:1061–1073
4. Cushing H, Eisenhardt L (1983) Meningiomas - their classification, regional behavior, life history and surgical end results. Thomas, Springfield, p 785
5. Zimmerman RA, Bilaniuk LT (1980) Computed tomography of acute intratumoral hemorrhage. Radiology 135:355
6. Helle TL, Conley FK (1980) Haemorrhage associated with meningioma: a case report and review of the literature. J Neurol Neurosurg Psychiatry 43:725–729
7. Modesti LM, Binet EF, Collins G (1976) Meningiomas causing spontaneous intracranial hematomas. J Neurosurg 45:437–440
8. Russell EJ, George AE, Kricheff II, Budzilovich G (1980) Atypical computed tomographic features of intracranial meningioma. Radiology 135:673–682
9. Martínez-Lage JF, Poza M, Martínez M, et al (1991) Meningiomas with hemorrhagic onset. Acta Neurochir 110:129–132
10. Jellinger K, Slowik F (1975) Histological subtypes and prognostic problems in meningiomas. J Neurol 208:279–298
11. Globus JH, Sapirstein M (1942) Massive hemorrhage into brain tumor. JAMA 120:348–352
12. Zülch KJ (1968) Neuropathology of intracranial hemorrhage. Prog Brain Res 30:151–165
13. Gruszkiewicz J, Doron Y, Gellei B, Peyer E (1961) Massive intracerebral bleeding due to supratentorial meningioma. Neurochirurgia (Stuttg) 12:107–111

Tumour aggressiveness determined by kinetic analysis of glucose metabolism in meningiomas

H. Shioya[1], K. Mineura[1], T. Sasajima[1], M. Kowada[1], H. Iida[2], T. Ogawa[2], J. Hatazawa[2], K. Uemura[2]

[1] Neurosurgical Service, Akita University Hospital, Akita, Japan
[2] Department of Radiology and Nuclear Medicine, Research Institute for Brain and Blood Vessels, Akita, Japan

Abstract. We measured kinetic rate constants and kinetic glucose metabolic rate (kinetic-rCMRGI) using dynamic positron emission tomography, as well as autoradiographic rCMRGI (arg-rCMRGI), in seven patients with meningiomas. The kinetic rate constants were analysed according to the three-compartment model of ^{18}F-fluorodeoxyglucose. Tumour k_1 and k_2 values markedly increased in all examined cases, which suggested high permeability of the blood-tumour barrier. Six patients showed tumour k_3 values lower than those of the contralateral grey matter, whereas one patient showed a higher value. The latter patient suffered from tumour recurrence a relatively short time after surgical resection. Discrepancy between kinetic- and arg-rCMRGI was noted in some patients, probably because of high k_1 and k_2 values. Kinetic analysis of the rate constants is useful for elucidating the detailed metabolic process of glucose.

Key words: Meningioma – Positron emission tomography – ^{18}F-fluorodeoxyglucose

Intracranial meningiomas are usually considered as benign tumours and are curable with surgical removal. However, aggressive behavior or tumour recurrence occasionally occurs. The glucose metabolic rate (rCMRGI) of intracranial meningiomas is correlated with tumour recurrence and tumour growth [1]. Most previous studies concerning glucose metabolism [1-3] have used the specified rate constants of normal brain tissue in order to calculate autoradiographic rCMRGI (arg-rCMRGI). In the present study, we measure kinetic rate constants and kinetic-rCMRGI using dynamic positron emission tomography (PET), as well as arg-rCMRGI, in patients with meningiomas.

Table 1. Clinical features

Case	Age (years)	Sex	Tumour location	Histology
1	44	F	Planum sphenoidale	Meningothelial
2	47	F	Left frontal	Meningothelial
3[a]	50	F	Left sphenoid ridge	Meningothelial
4	50	F	Right sphenoid ridge	Angiomatous
5	57	F	Left parietal	Meningothelial
6	60	M	Left falx	Angiomatous
7	67	F	Right falx	Fibrous

[a] Recurrent tumour

Materials and methods

Seven patients with meningiomas, one male and six females aged from 44 to 67 years with a mean age of 54 years, were studied prior to surgical intervention (Table 1). Histological diagnosis was as follows: four cases of meningothelial type, two cases of angiomatous type and one fibrous type. One meningioma was a recurrence.

PET was performed with the Headtome III or IV. The rate constants of tracer transport from blood to brain (k_1), reverse transport from brain to blood (k_2), and phosphorylation (k_3) were analysed according to the three-compartment model of ^{18}F-fluorodeoxyglucose (FDG) (Fig. 1) [4]. Kinetic-rCMRGI was measured using the rate constants obtained from dynamic analysis developed by Sasaki et al. [5], and arg-rCMRGI was calculated using the rate constants of normal brain tissue determined by Phelps et al. [6]. For the quantitative analysis, regions of interest (ROI) on PET images were delineated on the tumour and the contralateral grey matter. The ROI were 64–100 pixels (256–400 mm^2) in size.

Results

The quantitative data of kinetic analysis are summarised in Table 2, and representative cases are shown in Figs. 2–4. Tumour k_1 and k_2 values markedly increased in all

Table 2. Kinetic rate constants and glucose metabolic rates (mean ± SD)

Region of interest	k_1 (min^{-1})	k_2 (min^{-1})	k_3 (min^{-1})	Kinetic rCMRGI (mg/100 ml/min)	Autoradiographic rCMRGI (mg/100 ml/min)
Tumour	0.098 ± 0.041*	0.214 ± 0.079*	0.036 ± 0.014	3.52 ± 1.03	4.20 ± 0.84
Grey matter	0.052 ± 0.015*	0.114 ± 0.009*	0.046 ± 0.014	3.96 ± 0.82	4.77 ± 0.99

* Significantly different from the values of the contralateral grey matter at (P=0.01, (Student's t-test)

Correspondence to: H. Shioya, Neurosurgical Service, Akita University Hospital, 1-1-1 Hondo, Akita-shi, 010 Japan

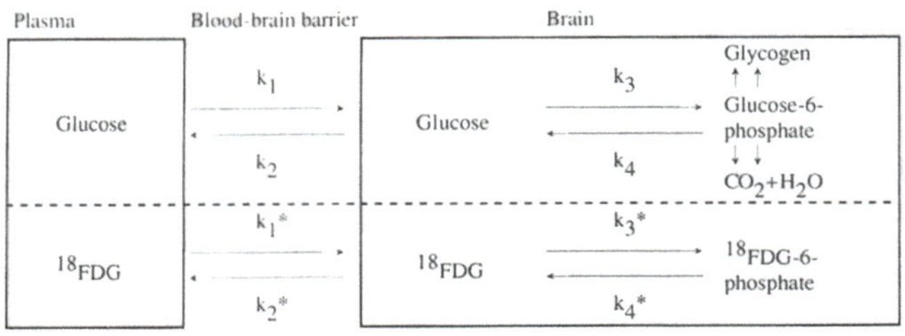

Fig. 1. Three-compartment model developed by Sokoloff et al. [4]

examined cases, which suggested high permeability due to lack of blood-brain barrier. Statistically significant differences were found in these values (k_1, k_2) between the tumour and the contralateral grey matter ($P<0.01$ by Student's t-test). Tumour k_3 values were lower than those of the contralateral grey matter in all cases but one. The remaining one patient, showing an increased tumour k_3 (0.054 min^{-1}), suffered from tumour recurrence within 1 year of extensive resection (Simpson's grade IV) (Fig. 3). Thus, increased k_3 indicated high activity of proliferation. Although kinetic- and arg-rCMRGI were matched in most patients, discrepancy between kinetic- and arg-rCMRGI was noted in some patients (Fig. 4) who showed high k_1 and k_2 values.

Discussion

Glucose is a principal source of energy in the metabolism of brain tissue. rCMRGI of intracranial meningiomas is related to tumour proliferation [1]. In addition, the accumulation of FDG is correlated with proportion of the cells in S + G2M phases of the cell cycle [7]. Enhanced glucose metabolism measured by FDG uptake therefore implicates proliferating activity of tumours. rCMRGI was, however, calculated using the rate constants of normal brain tissue [1–3].

We measured kinetic rate constants and kinetic-rCMRGI using dynamic PET in seven patients with meningiomas. The high k_1 value indicated an increased blood flow due to neovascularisation in the tumour tissue. Such characteristic circulation corresponds to angiographic and pathological findings of hypervascularity in meningiomas. One tumour with a high value of k_3 rapidly after surgical resection, whereas the other tumours, with low values, showed no tumour regrowth. Tumour k_3, an indicator of hexokinase activity, reflected activity of proliferation.

The rate constants may be variable and dependent on pathological characteristic of tumours, i.e. hypervascular

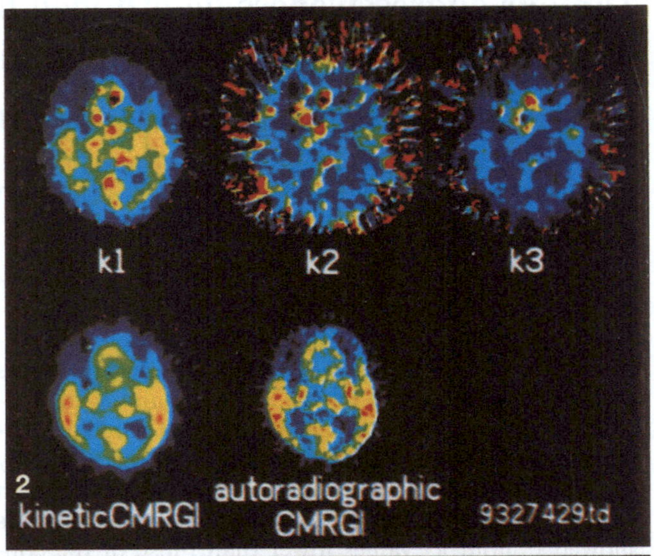

Fig. 2. Case 1. Planum sphenoidale meningioma in a 44-year-old woman. Tumour k_1 and k_2 were higher than in the contralateral grey matter, whereas k_3 and kinetic-rCMRGI were lower

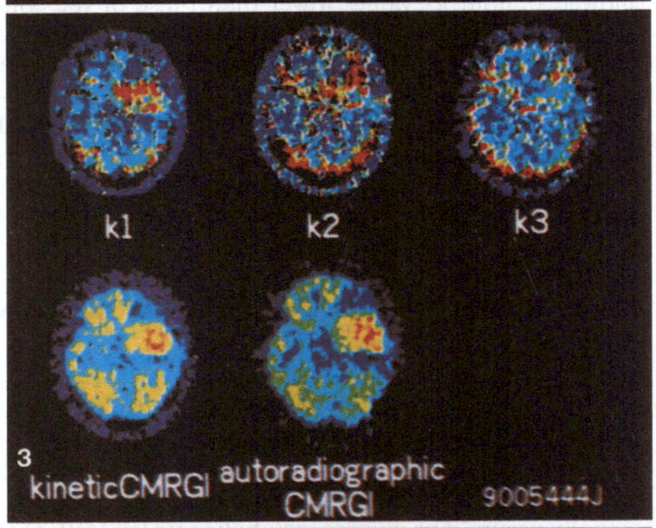

Fig. 3. Case 3. Left sphenoid ridge meningioma in a 50-year-old woman. Although tumour k_1 and k_2 were increased, k_3 and kinetic-rCMRGI were similar to those of the contralateral grey matter

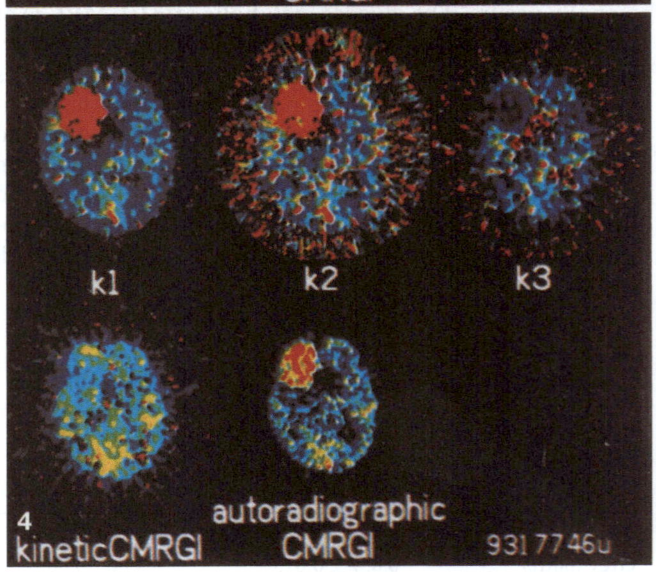

Fig. 4. Case 4. Right sphenoid ridge meningioma in a 50-year-old woman. Discrepancy between kinetic- and arg-rCMRGI was noted; k_3 and kinetic-rCMRGI were lower than those of the contralateral grey matter

tumour tissue such as meningiomas. Further studies on kinetic analysis will provide additional information on glucose metabolism in meningiomas.

References

1. DiChiro G, Hatazawa J, Katz DA, Rizzoli HV, De Michele DJ (1987) Glucose utilization by intracranial meningiomas as an index of tumor aggressivity and probability of recurrence: a PET study. Radiology 164:521–526
2. DiChiro G, DeLaPaz RL, Brooks RA, Sokoloff L, Kornblith PL, Smith BH, Patronas NJ, Kufta CV, Kessler RM, Johnston GS, Manning RG, Wolf AP (1982) Glucose utilization of cerebral gliomas measured by ^{18}F-fluorodeoxyglucose and positron emission tomography. Neurology 32:1323–1329
3. Kuwabara Y, Ichiya Y, Otsuka M, Miyake Y, Gunasekera R, Hasuo K, Masuda K, Takeshita I, Fukui H (1988) High [^{18}F] FDG uptake in primary cerebral lymphoma: a PET study. J Comput Assist Tomogr 12:47–48
4. Sokoloff L, Reivich M, Kennedy C, des Rosiers MH, Pettignew KD, Sakurada O, Shinohara M (1977) The [^{14}C] deoxyglucose method for the measurement of local cerebral glucose utilization. J Neurochem 28:897–916
5. Sasaki H, Kanno I, Murakami M, Shishido F, Uemura K (1986) Tomographic mapping of kinetic rate constants in the fluorodeoxyglucose model using dynamic positron emission tomography. J Cereb Blood Flow Metab 6:447–454
6. Phelps ME, Huang SC, Hoffman EJ, Selin C, Sokoloff L, Kuhl DE (1979) Tomographic measurement of local cerebral glucose metabolic rate in humans with (F-18) 2-fluoro-2-deoxy-D-glucose: validation of method. Ann Neurol 6:371–388
7. Minn H, Joesuu H, Ahonen A, Klemi P (1988) Fluorodeoxyglucose imaging: a method to assess the proliferative activity of human cancer in vivo. Cancer 61:1776–1781

Usefulness and limitations of 3D-CT angiography for operation of meningiomas

T. Miyazawa[1], K. Tsuchiya[2], T. Kaji[3], S. Ishihara[1], H. Nawashiro[1], H. Takiguchi[1], A. Shimizu[1], K. Shima[1], H. Chigasaki[1]

[1] Department of Neurosurgery, National Defense Medical College, Tokorozawa, Saitama, Japan
[2] Department of Radiology, National Defense Medical College, Tokorozawa, Saitama, Japan
[3] Department of Radiology, Kyorin University, Mitaka, Tokyo, Japan

Abstract. The usefulness of contrast-enhanced three-dimensional angiograms of meningiomas for neurosurgical investigation was determined in eight patients. Imaging was performed with helical scanning. Contrast medium was injected intravenously with a power injector before and after initiation of scanning. Although 3D-CT was undoubtedly useful in grasping the three-dimensional anatomical relationship between the tumour and major blood vessels preoperatively, it was difficult to use the findings obtained with 3D-CT to predict the degree of adhesion between major blood vessels and the tumour.

Key words: Three-dimensional computed tomography – Meningioma – Neurosurgery – Adhesion

Contrast-enhanced three-dimensional computed tomography (3D-CT) has been reported to be useful for the demonstration of cerebral aneurysms, meningiomas and other intracranial lesions [1–3]. However, few studies have considered the usefulness of 3D-CT for neurosurgical investigation of cases of meningioma. In the present study, we attempted to determine the usefulness and limitations of 3D-CT angiography and practical operative studies.

Correspondence to: T. Miyazawa, Department of Neurosurgery, National Defense Medical College, Namiki 3-2, Tokorozawa-shi, Saitama-ken, 359 Japan

Materials and methods

Eight patients in whom meningiomas were located in close proximity to the major cerebral blood vessels forming the circle of Willis were studied to determine the usefulness of contrast-enhanced 3D-CT for neurosurgical investigation.

Section thickness was 2 mm at intervals of 1 mm. Helical scanning was performed (1 s per scan; 140 kV, 100 mA or 120 kV, 150 mA). The speed of the movement of the table was 2 mm/s, and scanning time was 30 s. Consequently, the scanned area extended 6 cm along the patient's long axis. Scanning began 25 s after injection and continued for about 1 min. We injected non-ionic contrast medium intravenously at 2 ml/s for 25 s before the start of scanning. Three-dimensional reconstruction was performed using a surface rendering method with a lower threshold of 55 Hounsfield units.

The surgeon's impression of the degree of adhesion between the major blood vessels and tumour was recorded after operation.

A representative case

A 66-year-old woman was admitted with diploia and impairment of visual acuity. Truncal ataxia and nystagmus were observed. T1-weighted MRI performed after Gd-DTPA administration demonstrated left tentorial meningioma. On T2-weighted MRI, the internal carotid, middle cerebral and basilar arteries were found to be compressed and stretched due to mass effect of the tumour (Fig. 1a). An anteroposterior vertebral angiogram also showed displacement of the posterior cerebral and basilar arteries due to mass effect of the tumour (Fig. 1b). Although MRI was helpful in visualising the relationship between blood vessels and tumour, the three-dimensional relationships between these structures were difficult to

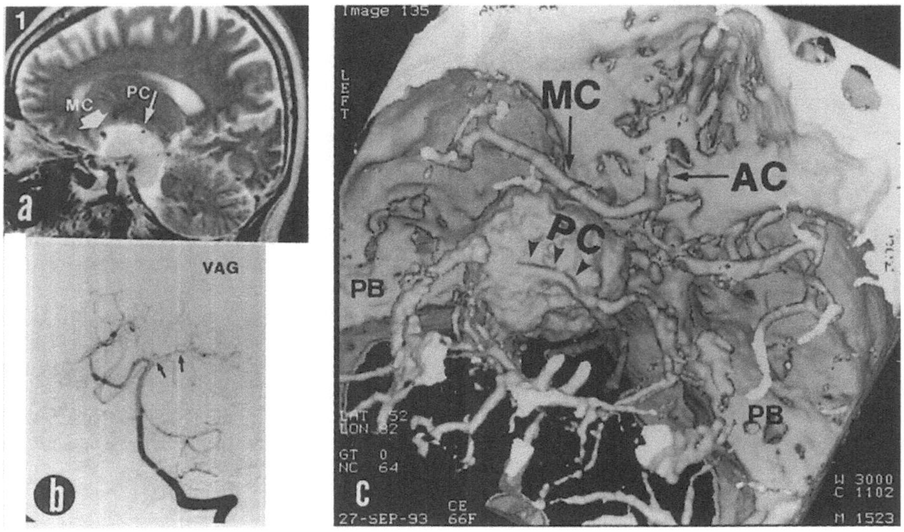

Fig. 1. a T2-weighted image demonstrates enhancement of major blood vessels by a tentorial meningioma. **b** Anteroposterior projection of vertebral angiogram. The posterior cerebral artery *(arrows)* was compressed and stretched by the tumour. **c** 3D-CT. The posterior cerebral artery appears encased or even infiltrated by tumour. *AC* Anterior cerebral artery; *MC* middle cerebral artery; *PC* posterior cerebral artery; *PB* petrous bone

determine. On the other hand, the posterior cerebral artery appeared to be engulfed by the tumour on 3D-CT, but the middle cerebral artery did not (Fig. 1c). During operation, the posterior cerebral artery was dissected away from the tumour with some difficulty but without any injury. By the end of surgery, all major blood vessels were free of tumour.

Discussion

Tsuchiya et al. [2] summarised the advantages and disadvantages of 3D-CT as follows: (1) 3D-CT permits clear visualisation of the anatomical relationship between the tumour and bony structures; (2) it is useful for grasping the three-dimensional relationship between tumour and adjacent major arteries forming the circle of Willis, but does not permit visualisation of perforating arteries: (3) it depicts abnormal venous structures on the surface of tumour; (4) enhancement of the main venous system and choroid plexus sometimes hamper diagnosis with 3D-CT.

Thus, 3D-CT is very useful for discerning the three-dimensional anatomical relationship between tumour and major blood vessels preoperatively; as stated by Tsuchiya and Makita [3]. In our study, the degree of adhesion between tumour and major blood vessels could not be predicted in all eight cases. We must recall that the findings of contrast-enhanced 3D-CT are influenced by the procedure used, the CT density (Hounsfield unit) and the schedule of administration of contrast material. For prediction of surgical difficulties using 3D-CT, higher resolution than that currently available will be required.

References

1. Aoki S, et al. (1992) Cerebral aneurysms: detection and delineation using 3D-CT angiography. AJNR 13:1115–1120
2. Tsuchiya K, Yoshida H, Makita K (1992) Three-dimensional CT angiography of cerebral aneurysms. Jpn J Clin Radiol 37:1617–1620
3. Tsuchiya K, Makita K (1994) Contrast-enhanced three-dimensional computed tomography of meningiomas. Progr Comput Imag 16:27–30

Needle displacement during stereotactic biopsy of a meningioma: a case report

S. Bastianello, A. Paolillo, A. Santoro, P. Ciappetta, R. Delfini, L. M. Fantozzi, P. Baroni, G. P. Cantore, L. Bozzao

Division of Neuroradiology, Department of Neurosciences, University of Rome "La Sapienza", Viale dell'Università 30, I-00185 Rome, Italy

Abstract. Histological diagnosis of brain tumours based on neuroradiological imaging is not always easy. A biopsy procedure may be necessary in selected cases to achieve a correct diagnosis and to apply an adequate therapy. We observed a young man with a rounded mass located in the right temporal lobe. Diagnosis was not possible by CT, MRI and angiography. We therefore decided to perform a brain biopsy using a sterotactic procedure. Histological examination of the fresh biopsy cylinder yielded a diagnosis of papilloma of the choroidal plexus. CT performed after the sterotactic procedure showed the biopsy track outside the tumour, not reaching the target but ending medial to the lateral ventricle, thus documenting procedure failure. This could have been due to displacement of the needle, possibly by a solid mass, during the stereotactic procedure. A new target was calculated and the biopsy repeated. The histological diagnosis was meningioma. The patient was submitted to open brain surgery and a solid meningioma was revealed.

Key words: Stereotactic brain biopsy, failure

Histological diagnosis of brain tumours based on neuroradiological imaging, is not always easy. A biopsy procedure may be necessary in selected cases to achieve a correct diagnosis and to institute appropriate therapy [1]. Stereotactic brain biopsy has become a well-established method for diagnosing brain tumour, complications occur in a very limited proportion of cases and usually comprise bleeding, oedema and focal seizure. The rate of operative mortality is low, ranging from 0.2 to 0.1% [1-4].

Brain biopsy will become a common diagnostic procedure in qualified centres; the occurrence of procedure failure should be kept in mind. We report a worrying case of brain meningioma.

Case report

A 33-year-old man, complaining of headaches and nausea presented after an isolated episode of partial complex seizure. Neurological examination showed a mild right hemiparesis and blurred optic disc.

CT and MRI, performed before and after contrast medium injection, revealed a rounded mass located in the right temporal lobe with sulcal effacement and ventricular shift; markedly heterogeneous contrast enhancement was present. Angiography documented pathological vascularisation inside the mass.

Correspondence to: S. Bastianello

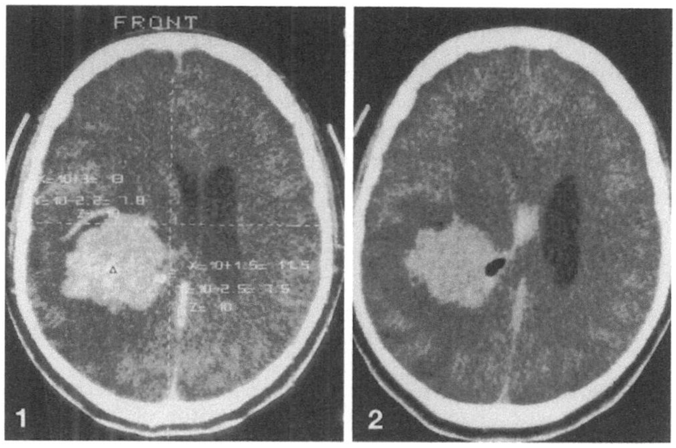

Fig. 1. CT before biopsy procedure showing a rounded mass in the right temporal lobe; the co-ordinates of the target (*arrow*) are indicated

Fig. 2. CT after stereotactic biopsy showed the needle track outside the tumour, not reaching the target but ending medial to the lateral ventricle, where a little gas was evident, documenting procedure failure. A small intraventricular blood collection was also present

Definite diagnosis was not possible by CT, MRI and angiography, and we decided to perform a brain biopsy using a stereotactic procedure.

The Leksell stereotactic system was used and the x, y, and z coordinates were calculated (Fig. 1) [5].

Histological examination of the fresh biopsy cylinder yielded a diagnosis of papilloma of the choroidal plexus. CT performed after the stereotactic procedure showed the biopsy track outside the tumour, not reaching the target but ending medial to the lateral ventricle documenting procedure failure (Fig. 2). This could have been due to this displacement of the needle during stereotactic procedure, possibly by a solid mass. The target was calculated anew and the biopsy repeated. The histological diagnosis was meningioma. The patient was submitted to open brain surgery and a solid meningioma was revealed.

Discussion

Stereotactic biopsy has been described as a diagnostic procedure necessary for anyone dealing with neurooncology [2, 6], though its role is still debated, especially in relationship to the direct surgical approach and concerning the possibility of diagnostic error [6, 7].

When intracranial tumours, whether benign or malignant, are treated, it is generally accepted that, where possible, a histological diagnosis should be established [8, 9]. Moreover, as in other fields of diagnostic pathology, histological examination is of genuine utility in the classification and grading of brain tumours [8].

Based on our experience, we consider sterotactic biopsy a highly accurate and resolutive diagnostic technique.

Although cerebral stereotactic biopsy represents a useful diagnostic procedure, we have to consider some limits.

Concerning neoplastic cerebral mass lesions, the well-known morphological heterogeneity, in particular of gliomas, means that there is a real possibility of making an inaccurate diagnosis from small tissue specimens obtained with sterotactic biopsy; this represents the real limit of this procedure [2, 8, 10, 11]. Moreover, technical mistakes in calculating the coordinates and in reaching the target may occur.

In our case, the blunt point of the needle generally used during brain biopsy was diverted by the solid lesion.

References

1. Voges J, Schroder R, Treuer H, et al (1993) CT-guided and computer-assisted stereotactic biopsy. Acta Neurochir (Wien) 125:142–149
2. Feiden W, Steude U, Bise K, Gundish O (1991) Accuracy of stereotactic brain tumor biopsy: comparison of the histologic findings in biopsy cylinders and resected tumor tissue. Neurosurg Rev 14:51–56
3. Apuzzo LJM, Chandrasoma PT, Cohen D, et al (1987) Computed imaging stereotaxy: experience and perspective related to 500 procedures applied to brain masses. Neurosurgery 20:930–937
4. Chandrasoma PT, Smith MM, Apuzzo MLJ (1989) Stereotactic biopsy in the diagnosis of brain masses: comparison of results of biopsy and resected surgical specimens. Neurosurgery 24:160–165
5. Lunsford LD, Leksell D (1988) The Leksell system. In: Lunsford LD (ed) Modern stereotactic neurosurgery. Nijhoff, Dordrecht
6. Burger PC, Vogel FS (1982) Surgical pathology of the nervous system and its coverings, 2nd edn. Wiley, New York
7. Scerrati M, Rossi GF (1984) The reliability of stereotactic biopsy. Acta Neurochir (Wien) [Suppl] 33:201–205
8. Gullotta F (1981) Morphological and biological basis for the classification of brain tumors. With a comment on the WHO-Classification 1979. In: Krayenbuhl H (ed) Advances and technical standards in neurosurgery, Vol 8. Springer, Vienna New York
9. Kleihues P, Volk B, Anagnostopoulos J, Kiessling M (1984) Morphologic evaluation of stereotactic brain tumor biopsies. Acta Neurochir (Wien) [Suppl] 33:171–184
10. Colombo F, Casentini L, Zanusso M, Danirli D, Benedetti A (1988) Validity of stereotactic biopsy as a diagnostic tool. Acta Neurochir (Wien) [Suppl] 42:152–156
11. Edner G (1981) Stereotactic biopsy of intracranial space occupying lesions. Acta Neurochir (Wien) 57:213–234

MRI of primary central nervous system lymphoma

B. C. Chu, Y. Kikuchi, K. Miyasaka

Department of Radiology, Hokkaido University School of Medicine, K-15 N-7, Kita-ku, Sapporo, Japan

Abstract. Six patients (four women, two men, aged 41–65 years) with histologically proven primary central nervous system lymphoma (PCNSL) underwent 1.5-T MRI examination. T1-weighted, T2-weighted and gadolinium-DTPA-enhanced images were obtained. All patients had follow-up studies. PCNSL may show a spreading pattern and cerebrospinal fluid dissemination in addition to the already known features.

Key words: Lymphoma, central nervous system – Magnetic resonance imaging

Primary central nervous system lymphoma (PCNSL) is rare, but increasing in frequency, not only in immunarompromised patients. MRI appears useful for both diagnosis and follow-up. We present a review of the MRI findings.

Materials and methods

Six patients with histologically proven PCNSL underwent MRI: four were women and two men, aged 41–65 years. All had non-Hodgkin's lymphoma of diffuse large-cell type according to the working formulation. No evidence of AIDS was found in any of the patients. Two patients had undergone stereotactic biopsy or partial craniectomy at the time of the MRI study. Gadolinium-DTPA was employed to increase contrast. Cerebrospinal fluid (CSF) was obtained by lumbar puncture in one patient to analyse the cytology. All patients had follow-up studies so that the spreading pattern could be delineated.

MRI was performed with a 1.5-T magnet. Spin-echo pulse sequences were used in all patients. Axial T1-weighted images were obtained with 500–740/15 (TR/TE). Proton density and T2-weighted images were obtained with 2400–3300/90 and 2400–3100/15-28 separately. Supplementary sagittal view were used for midline lesions.

The location, number and contour of the lesions were noted. The signal intensity of each lesion was described as high, low or isointense relative to grey matter. Oedema and mass effect were graded as mild, moderate or marked. The internal texture of each lesion was characterised as homogenous or heterogeneous after intravenous gadolinium-DTPA.

Results

The clinical and MRI features are summarised in Table 1. On initial examination, total of 15 lesions were noted in the six patients. Two had only one lesion, one had two, one three and two four. Twelve lesions had slightly low to iso-intensities on T1-weighted images and high intensities on T2-weighted images. The other 3 lesions had high signal

Correspondence to: B. C. Chu

Table 1. Clinical and MRI features

Case	Age (years)	Sex	Presenting symptoms follow-up period	Lesions		Signal characteristics		Contrast enhance-ment	Oedema	Mass effect
				Num-ber	Location	T1-weighted	T2-weighted			
1	52	F	Headache	2	Caudate nucleus/frontal	H/H	H + L/H	E/E	Moderate	No
			3 months	2	Caudate nucleus/frontal	H/H	L/SH	E/E	No	No
2	62	F	Dementia	3	Frontal/genu corpus callosum/basal ganglia	H/H SH	H + L/I/H	E/E/E	Marked/no/mild	Mild/no/no
			3 months	3	Frontal/genu corpus callosum/basal ganglia	L/L/I	H/L/SH	E/E/E	Moderate/no/mild	No
3	65	F	Headache	4	Bilateral, temporal/frontal/wall lateral ventricle	L, I/L/I	H, I/H/I	E, E/E/E	No	No
4	46	M	Facial nerve palsy	1	Parasellar	I	SH	E	No	No
			4 months	5	Parasellar/Septum pellucidum/lateral ventricle/fourth ventricle/medulla oblongata			E		
			9 months	1	Spinal cord at C2–4	I	H	E	Moderate	Mild
5	41	M	Coma	4	Bilateral parietal and frontal	L	H	E	Mild	No
6	44	F	Vertigo	1	Cerebellar hemisphere, middle peduncle	I	H	E	Mild	No
			3 months	3	Both cerebellar hemispheres, basal ganglia	I	H	E	Mild	No

H, High; L, low; I, isointense; SH, slightly high; H + L, high and low; E, homogeneous enhancement; HE, heterogeneous enhancement; RE, ring enhancement

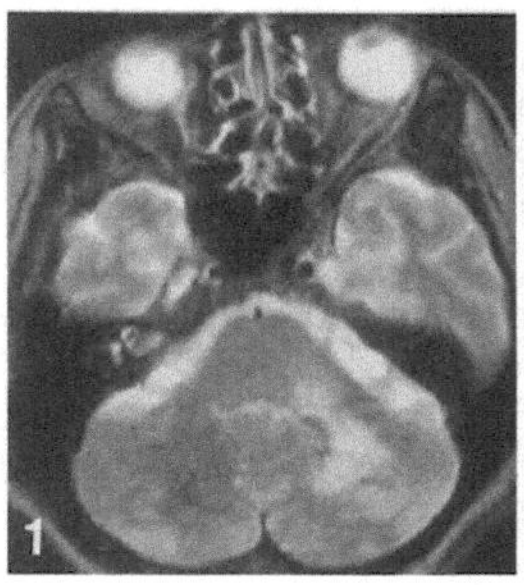

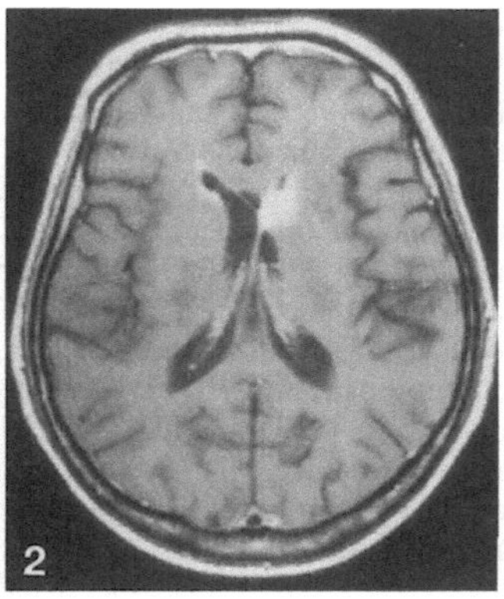

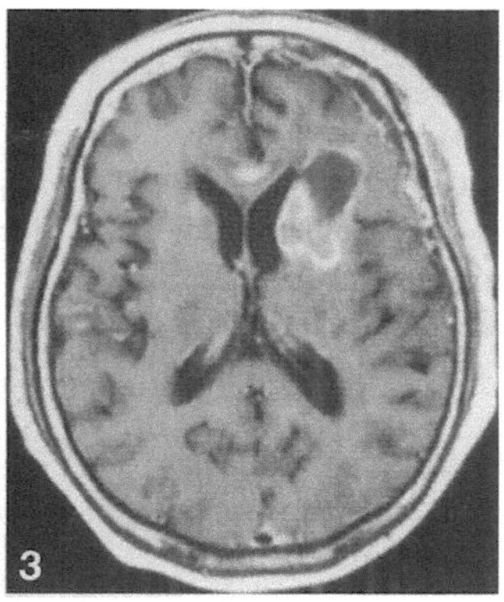

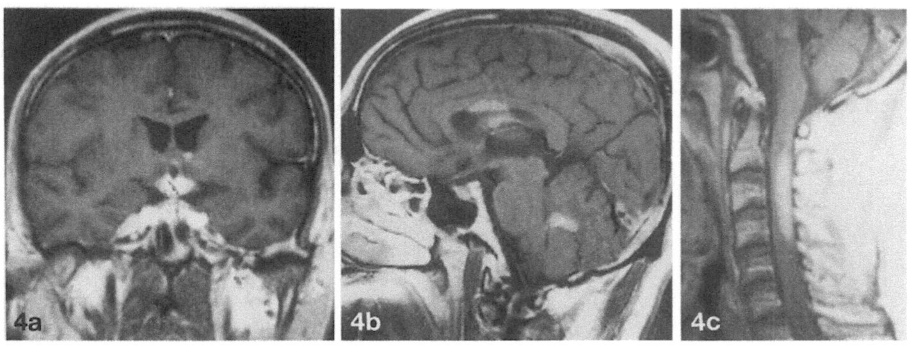

Fig. 1. T2-weighted image: High-signal lesion in the cerebellar hemisphere and middle cerebellar peduncle in a 44-year-old woman

Fig. 2. A 52-year-old woman with lesions in the left caudate nucleus and on the wall of the right frontal horn. Both lesions are hyperintense on this T1-weighted image, after biopsy

Fig. 3. A 72-year-old woman with lesions in the genu of the corpus callosum, right basal ganglia and left frontal lobe. Thelesion on the left enhanced heterogeneously. The loco-signal portion is associated with partial craniectomy

Fig. 4. a Homogeneously enhancing lesions were found in the parasellar region study in a 45-year-old man. **b** Homogeneously enhancing lesions in the third and fourth ventricle were seen 4 months later. **c** A further enhancing lesion developed posteriorly in the spinal cord at C2–4 level 9 months after the initial study

intensities on both T1- and T2-weighted images. Fourteen lesions showed homogeneous enhancement after gadolinium-DTPA injection. Four patients had mild to marked oedema. Two had mild mass effect. One patient had a lesion in the left cerebellar hemisphere and the left middle cerebellar peduncle (Fig. 1). One patient had one lesion in the left caudate nucleus and another abutting the wall of the right frontal horn (Fig. 2). One patient had one lesion in the genu of the corpus callosum in addition to two lesions in the basal ganglia and frontal lobe (Fig. 3). These two lesions gave high signal intensities on T1- and T2-weighted images.

On follow-up studies, two patients developed new lesions. One had developed four lesions in the septum pellucidum, lateral ventricle, fourth ventricle and medulla oblongata (Fig. 4) 4 months after an initial lesion was detected in the parasellar region. Nine months later, MRI of the cervical spine revealed a homogeneously enhancing lesion in the posterior portion of the spinal cord at C2–4, interpreted as dissemination.

Discussion

PCNSL is a rare disorder compromising less than 2% of brain tumours, but an increase in its incidence has been reported in recent years, particularly among immunocompromised patients such as allograft recipients and AIDS patients [1, 2]. MRI may provide detailed delineation of the number and extent of PCNSL in both the brain and the spinal cord [3–5].

The lesions of PCNSL are found to be slightly hypointense on T1-weighted images and slightly hyperintense on proton density and T2-weighted images, relative to grey matter. The observed mild T2 prolongation is probably related to dense cell packing within these tumours, leaving little interstitial space for accumulation of water. Nevertheless, two lesions in our series had high signal intensities on T1- and T2-weighted images, possibly due to haemorrhage resulting from stereotactic biopsy or partial craniectomy.

In general, the lesions of PCNSL induce mild to moderate oedema and mass effect. Typical lesions were sharply demarcated round, oval or very occasionally grey-like masses surrounded by a small rim of oedema. Peritumoural oedema with PCNSL is less than that seen with comparably sized metastatic carcinomas or malignant gliomas [6]. We found disproportionate mass effect on the adjacent structures. This is believed to be a typical feature of PCNSL [6] and may be helpful in differentiating PCNSL from metastatic lesions.

Contrast-enhancement is associated with a focal disturbance of the blood-brain barrier caused by perivascular extension. According to the classical concept, PCNSL originates in the periadventitial cells of the leptomeningeal vessels, invading the adjacent cerebral tissue at a later stage, extending into the perivascular space of the perforating vessels, and finally involving even deep hemispheric structures [7]. The enhancement is generally homogeneous. However, heterogeneous enhancement is also described [3]. Ring enhancement is often associated with AIDS, in particular when the patient has toxoplasmosis [7]. One patient in our series was noted to have ring enhancement, caused in this case by radiation necrosis.

Dissemination through the CSF can be seen in tumours such as medulloblastoma, ependyblastoma, glioblastoma and germinoma. Although the CNS has neither lymphatic circulation nor endogeneous accumulations of lymphoid tissue, intracranial lymphoma may indeed disseminate to the spinal cord, probably because of the leptomeningeal involvement. The latter results in a multifocal pattern that can involve both the brain and the spinal cord. This pattern of involvement most often occurs in secondary or recurrent PCNSL, but is unusual as the initial manifestation of PCNSL. Since lymphomas often spread aggressively within the CNS, but rarely extend outside, the occurrence of these tumours as primary tumours in such an organ system raises the question of the source of these neoplasms.

References

1. O'Neill BP (1989) Primary central nervous system lymphoma. Mayo Clin Proc 64:1005–1020
2. Miyasaka K, Kato C (1991) Central nervous system malignant lymphoma (in Japanese). Imaging Diagn 11:886–895
3. Hochberg FH, Miller DC (1988) Primary central nervous system lymphoma. J Neurosurg 68:835–853
4. Lyons MK, O'Neill BP, Marsh WR, Kurtin PJ (1992) Primary spinal epidural non-Hodgkin's lymphoma: report of eight patients and review of the literature. Neurosurgery 30:675–679
5. Greco A, Jelliffe AM, Maher EJ, Leung AWL (1988) MR imaging of lymphomas: impact on therapy. J Comput Assist Tomogr 12:785–791
6. Schwaighofer BW, Hesselink JR, Press GA, Wolf RL, Healy ME, Berthoty DP (1989) Primary intracranial CNS lymphoma: MR manifestations. AJNR 10:725–729
7. Jiddane M, Nicoli F, Diaz P, Bergvall U, Vincentelli F, Hassoun J, Salamon G (1986) Intracranial malignant lymphoma: report of 30 cases and review of the literature. J Neurosurg 65:592–599

Hepatoma metastatic to the head and brain

M. S. Chou[1], M. B. Lin[1], M. L. Wang[1], G. C. Liu[1], T. C. Tsai[1], J. F. Tsai[2]

[1] Department of Radiology, Kaohsiung Medical College, 100 Shih-Chuan 1st Road, Kaohsiung, Taiwan
[2] Department of Internal Medicine, Kaohsiung Medical College, 100 Shih-Chuan 1st Road, Kaohsiung, Taiwan

Abstract. The imaging features in 12 adult patients with histologically documented hepatocellular carcinoma (HCC) and head and brain metastasis are presented. Usually, the metastatic lesions showed as an isodense tumour mass on CT and high density following i.v. contrast. There were 6 patients (50%) with evidence of tumour haemorrhage. HCC should be considered in the differential diagnosis of metastatic lesions of the head and brain, particularly when evidence of haemorrhage appears in the image study.

Key words: Hepatocellular carcinoma – Metastasis – Brain

Hepatocellular carcinoma (HCC) is one of the most common cancers around the world [1–3]. The major risk factors include male sex, advancing age, cirrhosis and chronic hepatitis B and C virus infection [1–3]. Differences are seen in HCC incidence worldwide, due to aetiological factors prevalent in various regions. In Taiwan, the annual incidence of HCC was 18.6/100000 in 1988 [4]. HCC comprised 21.8% of an autopsy series of 570 malignant tumours in Taiwan [5]. Although up to 50–78% of HCC have extrahepatic metastases, HCC metastasis of the brain and head is rare [6–8]. This report presents 12 cases of HCC with head and brain metastasis, with special reference to the neuroradiological features.

Materials and methods

We retrospectively reviewed 12 cases of HCC with brain or head metastases in 10 men and 2 women aged 35–61 years (median 47 years). The time from diagnosis of HCC to metastasis ranged from 3 to 30 months (median 15 months) in 10 patients. Two patients were verified as having metastatic HCC after operation of the head or brain. The diagnosis of HCC was pathologically confirmed. CT, with and without intravenous contrast medium was performed in all patients, MRI at 0.5 T in one patient. Two patients had cerebral angiography.

Results

There were three types of involvement, according to the compartment of the head: seven patients had cerebral hemisphere lesions in the territory of the cortical arteries, three had calvarial involvement and two had paranasal sinus involvement. Almost all the lesions showed up on imaging as highly enhancing soft tissue masses except those with haematoma. The metastatic lesions usually showed up as an isodense tumour mass on CT, with high density following contrast medium. Hypervascular tumour masses were seen in the two patients who underwent angiography. Six patients (50%) had imaging evidence of haemorrhage, five on CT and one on MRI.

Correspondence to: M. S. Chou

Discussion

In this study, the most common metastatic lesions were those involving haematogenous spread to the brain parenchyma, usually affecting the area of the hemisphere over the territory of a cortical artery. CT scan usually reveals an isodense tumour mass with moderate or high-degree peripheral oedema and the contrast-enhanced scan reveals high density as in other metastases (Fig. 1). Evidence of haemorrhage was noted in four of these seven patients, most of whom presented with a stroke-like syndrome (Fig. 2). Tumours which have a high propensity to develop haemorrhage are metastatic choriocarcinoma, melanoma, bronchogenic carcinoma, and renal cell carcinoma [9]. For a metastatic HCC to present with haemorrhagic stroke is rare, and no more than five such cases have been reported in the literature [6, 7]. Though the exact mechanism of haemorrhage is not clear, there are several factors which may contribute to the high incidence [10–12]. As a primary tumour, metastatic HCC is hypervascular with many fistulous vessels within the mass. As shown in one of our cases (Fig. 2), haemorrhage may also occur at the margin of tumour where aggressive invasion occurs, with necrosis developing thereafter. Systemic hypocoagulopathic state may be another contributing factor.

Calvarium metastasis, is usually considered to arise from haematogeneous spread via the venous route to the diploic vein. In a survey of 19 cases of HCC with central nervous system metastasis, there were four cases with calvarium involvement [13], usually presenting as an extradural mass, sometimes penetrating through the dura mater. Our three patients with calvarial involvement included one (Fig. 3) with a multiple epidural mass that was confirmed to be a metastasis of HCC after operation.

In patients with paranasal sinus, skull base or orbital involvement, the favoured metastatic route is haematogenous spread via the paravertebral venous plexus. The literature reviewed showed only three patients with HCC metastasis to a paranasal sinus [8, 14]. In our series, two patients displayed involvement of maxillary sinus, ethmoid sinus, orbit, and infratemporal fossa. Further extension of the mass to sphenoid sinus and anterior cranial fossa was noted in one of the two cases (Fig. 4) who was confirmed to have metastatic HCC only after operation. Both patients had once suffered from intractable nasal bleeding. Angiography revealed hypervascular tumour stains in both patients. Evidence of methaemoglobulin spots was noted on T1-weighted images in the patient who underwent MRI.

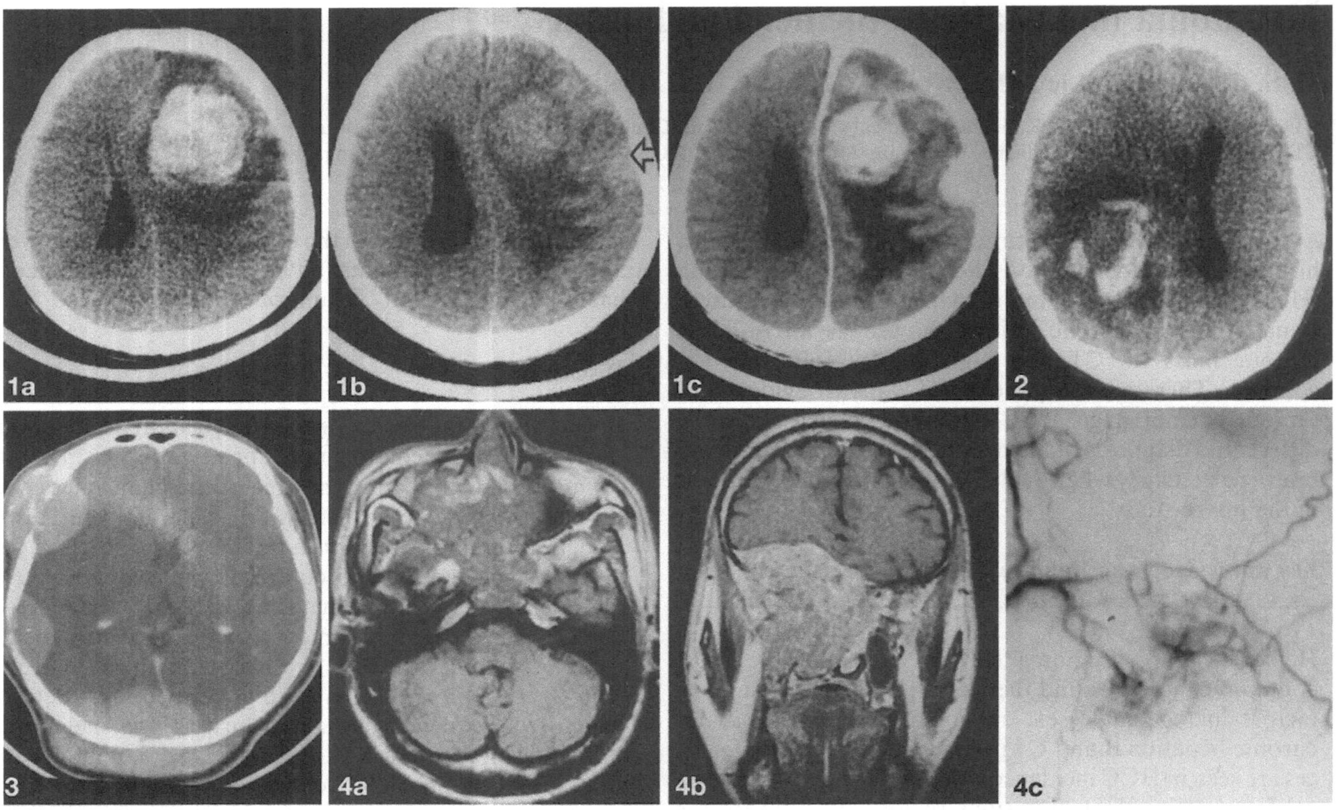

Fig. 1 a–c. A 57-year-old man presented with a stroke during a course of therapy for primary hepatoma. **a** CT shows haematoma in the left frontal lobe. **b** Nine months after operation, CT shows an isodense tumour in the left frontal lobe. Oedema is not present around a smaller mass (*arrow*), which suggests seeding of tumour cells in the CSF. **c** Contrast-enhanced image shows high density

Fig. 2. A 43-year-old woman diagnosed as having hepatoma for 4 months, presented with acute onset of right hemiparesis. CT reveals haemorrhage at the margin of an isodense mass, suggesting aggressive invasion

Fig. 3. A 56-year-old man had bulging of the scalp over occipital region for 9 months. Then 3 months later another two masses in the right frontotemporal region were noted. These proved to be metastatic HCC. A bone-window image shows destruction of the calvarium and epidural tumour

Fig. 4 a–c. A 38-year-old man suffered numbness and swelling of the right upper face for 3 months. MRI revealed a huge mass involving the maxillary, ethmoid and sphenoid sinuses and anterior cranial fossa. **a** Axial T1-weighted image shows scattered high signal, suggesting subacute haematoma. **b** Contrast-enhanced coronal image shows a high-intensity mass. **c** Angiogram reveals multifocal tumour stain

Although the radiological appearance of head and brain metastases of HCC is non-specific, they should be included in the list of differential diagnoses, particularly when there is evidence of haemorrhage from the mass.

References

1. Dibiscegli AM, Rustgi VK, Hoofnagle JH, et al (1988) Hepatocellular carcinoma. Ann Intern Med 108:390–399
2. Tsai JF, Chang WY, Jeng JE, et al (1994) Hepatitis B and C virus infection as risk factors for liver cirrhosis and cirrhotic hepatocellular carcinoma. Liver 14:98–102
3. Tsai JF, Jeng JE, Ho MS, et al (1994) Hepatitis B and C virus infection as risk factors for hepatocellular carcinoma in Chinese: a case-control study. Int J Cancer 56:619–621
4. Department of Health, ROC (1991) Health statistics: vital statistics of the Republic of China. Department of Health, Taipei, p 33
5. Lai YH, Lin WSJ (1976) A pathological study of primary carcinoma of the liver. Thesis for Masters degree, Institute of Pathology, School of Medicine, National Taiwan University
6. Okuda K (1976) Clinical aspect of hepatocellular carcinoma – analysis of 134 cases. In: Okuda K, Peter RL (eds) Hepatocellular carcinoma. Wiley, New York, pp 428–430
7. Ilde DC, Sherlock P, Winawer SJ, Fortner JG (1974) Clinical manifestations of hepatoma – a review of 6 years at a cancer hospital. Am J Med 56:83–91
8. Chang YC, Chen RC (1979) Craniospinal and cerebral metastasis of primary hepatomas: a report of 7 cases. J Formosan Med Assoc 78:594–604
9. Mandybur TL (1977) Intracranial hemorrhage caused by metastatic tumor. Neurology 27:650–655
10. Todo T, Noguchi M, Manaka S (1988) Metastatic hepatoma presenting as intracranial hemorrhage. No To Shinkei 40:919–924
11. Lee JP, Lee ST (1988) Hepatocellular carcinoma presenting as intracranial metastasis. Surg Neurol 30:316–320
12. Henson RA, Ulrich H (1982) Cancer and the nervous system. Blackwell, Oxford, pp 452–454
13. Friedman HD (1991) Hepatocellular carcinoma with central nervous system metastasis: a case report and literature review. Med Pediatr Oncol 19:139–144
14. Waxman JS, Seife B, Waxman M (1985) Hepatocellular carcinoma presenting as sphenoid sinus metastasis. Mount Sinai J Med 52:221–224

Advantages of surgical resection of brain metastasis from lung cancer

Y. Matsushita, H. Katoh, K. Shima, H. Chigasaki

Department of Neurosurgery, National Defense Medical College, Namiki 3-2, Tokorozawa, Saitama, 359 Japan

Abstract. The advantage of surgical resection of metastatic brain tumours is controversial. We reviewed the survival time of 28 patients with brain metastasis from lung cancer. In the patients who underwent surgical resection of metastatic brain tumours, the survival time of the 15 patients with radiation was significantly longer than that of the 10 other patients. Also, the survival time of the 10 patients who underwent surgical resection in the original site of lung cancer was significantly longer than that of the other 15 patients. Survival time was longer in the patients who underwent both surgical resections of metastatic brain tumour and postoperative radiotherapy and in those who underwent surgical resection of both metastatic brain tumour and the primary lung cancer. We emphasise the advantage of surgical resection of both metastatic brain tumour and primary lung cancer and postoperative radiotherapy in the treatment of brain metastasis from lung cancer.

Key words: Metastatic brain tumour – Lung cancer – Postoperative radiotherapy

The advantage of surgical resection of metastatic brain tumours is controversial. In recent years, MRI has been a useful tool for detecting the presence of small metastasis. We reviewed the survival time of patients with metastatic brain tumours from lung cancer which were diagnosed by MRI from 1985 to 1992.

Patients and methods

The patients were 25 men and 3 women with ages ranging from 23 to 78 years. The metastatic brain tumours were confirmed by MRI in all patients. We found one lesion in 10 patients, two lesions in 8 patients and three or more lesions in 10 patients. Twenty-five patients underwent surgical resection of the metastatic tumours (SR+). We performed total resection of metastatic brain tumours in 16 patients and subtotal resection in 9 patients. Fifteen patients were treated with postoperative radiotherapy and 8 with postoperative chemotherapy. The other 3 patients were not treated with surgical resection of the metastatic brain tumours (SR-), but 2 of them were treated with both radiotherapy and chemotherapy. The original lung cancer was resected in 10 patients: 9 from the SR+ group and 1 from the SR- group (Table 1). We confirmed the survival time of patients by telephone research.

Results

In the SR+ group, the survival time of the patients with radiation (8.7 ± 6.3 months) was significantly longer than that of the other patients (3.5 ± 3.2 months; $P < 0.05$) (Fig. 1). Also, the survival time of the 10 patients who underwent surgical resection of the primary lung cancer (10.1 ± 6.8 months) was significantly longer than that of the other 15 patients (4.3 ± 3.7 months; $P < 0.05$) (Fig. 2).

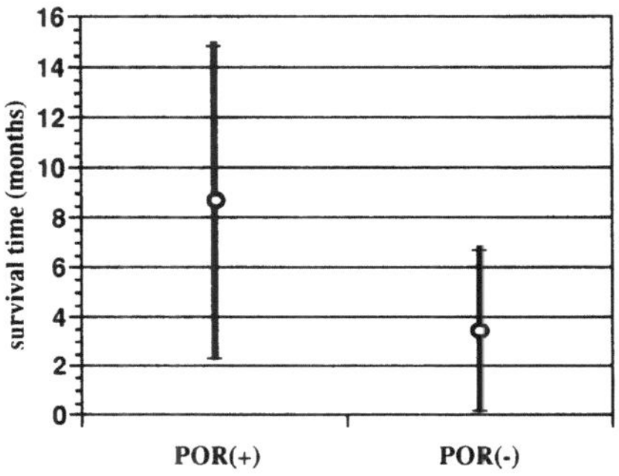

Fig. 1. Relationship between postoperative radiation therapy and survival time. In patients treated by surgical resection, survival time was significantly longer in those who had postoperative radiation ($P < 0.05$). POR(+), Radiotherapy; POR(−), no radiotherapy

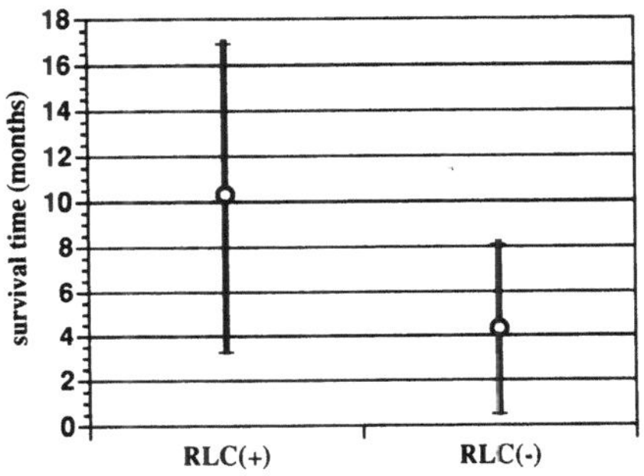

Fig. 2. Relationship between surgical resection of lung cancer and survival time. In patients treated by surgical resection of metastatic brain tumour, survival time of patients who underwent surgical resection of the primary lung cancer was significantly longer ($P < 0.05$). RLC(+), Resection of lung cancer; RLC(−), no resection

Discussion

MRI is more sensitive than CT in the detection of metastatic brain tumours. Previously, patients found to have solitary metastatic brain tumour on CT underwent surgical resection, but since 1984 we have used as indication for operation the detection of metastatic brain tumours by MRI. In this review, we found two or more metastatic brain tumours and resected as many tumours as possible. In the SR+ group, the survival time of patients with radiation was significantly longer than that of the other patients, and the survival time of the 10 patients who underwent surgical resection of the primary lung cancer was significantly longer than that of the other 15 patients

Correspondence to: Y. Matsushita

Table 1. Summary of 28 patients with metastases from lung cancer

Case	Sex	Age (years)	Number of tumours	Resection	Surgery to primary tumour	Radiation	Chemo-therapy	Survival time (months)	Pathology
1	Male	57	1	Total	+	+	–	9	Adeno carcinoma
2	Male	58	1	Subtotal	+	+	–	4	Large cell
3	Female	50	2	Total	+	+	+	15	Adeno carcinoma
4	Male	60	2	Subtotal	+	+	–	4	Adeno carcinoma
5	Male	49	2	Total	+	+	–	11	Adeno carcinoma
6	Female	23	1	Total	+	–	–	10	Adeno carcinoma
7	Male	78	1	Total	+	–	–	1	Squamous
8	Male	43	1	Total	+	+	–	16	Squamous
9	Male	51	2	Subtotal	+	+	–	7	Large cell
10	Male	76	1	Total	+	+	–	24	Squamous
11	Male	56	2	Total	–	+	+	3	Squamous
12	Male	63	3	Subtotal	–	+	+	1	ND
13	Male	70	3	Subtotal	–	–	+	7	Small cell
14	Male	49	4	Subtotal	–	+	+	2	Adeno carcinoma
15	Female	55	2	None	–	+	+	13	Small cell
16	Male	63	2	None	–	+	+	8	Small cell
17	Male	64	3	Total	–	–	–	2	ND
18	Male	57	3	Subtotal	–	+	–	3	Adeno carcinoma
19	Male	47	3	Subtotal	–	–	+	5	Adeno carcinoma
20	Male	67	1	None	–	–	–	2	Adeno carcinoma
21	Male	66	3	Total	–	–	–	6	Squamous
22	Male	69	1	Subtotal	–	+	–	2	Squamous
23	Male	65	3	Total	–	+	+	12	Small cell
24	Male	74	4	Total	–	+	+	12	Small cell
25	Male	62	1	Total	–	–	–	1	Small cell
26	Male	79	2	Total	–	–	–	1	Squamous
27	Male	35	1	Total	–	–	–	1	ND
28	Male	61	3	Total	–	+	–	7	ND

in the SR+ group. In "the generation of MRI", we consider the best therapy for metastatic brain tumours from lung cancer to be surgical resection, including both the lung cancer and as many metastatic brain tumours as possible, and postoperative radiation even if two or more lesions are detected by MRI.

Preoperative localization of intracranial tumors using a co-ordinate grid

G. Krol, J. Galicich, R. DeLaPaz, B. O'Malley

Memorial Sloan-Kettering Cancer Center, 1275 York Avenue, New York, NY 10021, USA

Abstract. Preoperative localization of intracranial tumors using a grid technique is a quick, efficient and cost-effective method facilitating intraoperative identification of tumors and planning of craniotomy.

Key words: Magnetic resonance imaging – Localization

Identification of parenchymal brain tumor during surgery may be difficult, particularly if the lesion is small or does not extend to the cortical surface. The intraoperative approach can be facilitated considerably by preoperative MRI localization. The procedure is performed using a co-ordinate grid which allows estimation of the target approach to the central aspect of the lesion as well as the outline of its periphery in reference to the cranial vault. Although more sophisticated methods of tumor demonstration and localization are presently available, a grid technique offers simple and relatively accurate preoperative assessment of tumor location and planning of the extent of the craniotomy incision.

Material and methods

Preoperative localization was carried out in 53 patients with primary (20) and secondary (33) brain tumors. Forty-four patients had single

Correspondence to: G. Krol

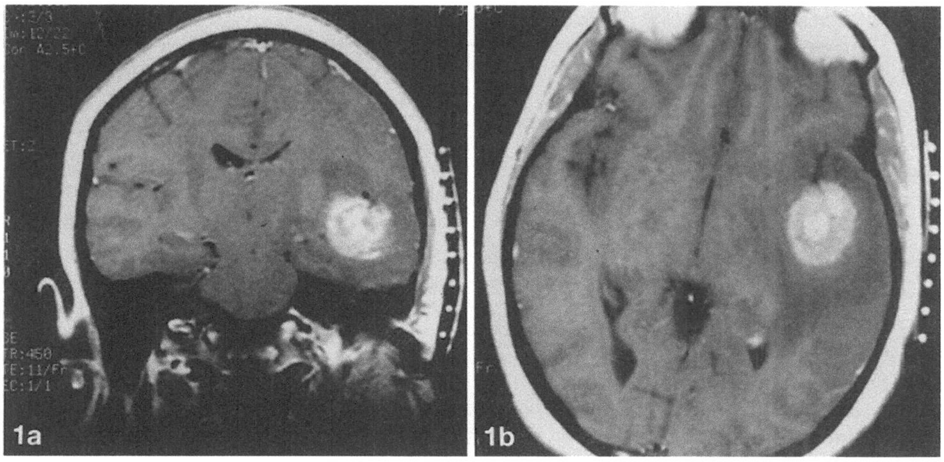

Fig. 1a, b. Left hemispheric lesion. The entry point corresponds to segments 4 (coronal view, **a**) and 4 × 5 (axial view, **b**)

lesions. Of the 9 patients with multiple lesions, 5 had two and four had three metastases. In 51 patients, localization of a single lesion was performed. In 10 of these cases, three-dimensional reconstruction of MRI data was performed. Double localization (using two separate grids simultaneously for two lesions) was done in 2 patients. The size of the lesions (longest diameter) varied from 1 cm to over 9 cm, with the greatest number (17) measuring between 2 and 3 cm.

In preparation for localization, T1- and T2-weighted images are performed and a rough estimate of the location of the lesion is made. An appropriate area of the skull is shaved and the grid placed over the general area of the tumor in such a way that the elements of the grid are parallel to the intended axis of the image plane. The grid is then securely taped to the head and contrast-enhanced images are obtained in three planes. Subsequently, two images in different planes, depicting the lesion in such a way that it is possible to draw a perpendicular line from the centre of the lesion to the inner table, are selected. The intersection of the two appropriate elements of the grid is then marked on the patient's scalp (Fig. 1).

Discussion

The method of grid localization allows for geometric projection of the centre and/or periphery of the parenchymal lesions on the cranial vault. This is beneficial in 2 ways: the shortest approach to the lesion can be chosen (central target), and the extent of craniotomy incision can be planned (peripheral outline). Precise estimation of the location of the intracranial process with reference to the grid and precise marking of the scalp are particularly important with lesions of subcentimetre size which do not involve the cortical surface. There is rather a wide spread of the size of the lesions for which localization is requested. This can be explained by the fact that, although the lesion may be quite extensive, an initial neurosurgical approach may need to be targeted to a particular part of the lesion (such as a cystic component or the part which extends closest to the surface).

The success of the procedure depends upon good patient cooperation and careful observance of the technique. It is important that the grid elements are placed firmly along the skin surface of the scalp and there is no motion of the grid between imaging and skin marking. Intraoperative localization should also assume an approach along the line extending from the centre of the lesion and perpendicular to the inner table of the craniotomy flap. It is important to discuss the surgical approach with the neurosurgeon prior to localization.

3D images are helpful in depicting relationship of the tumor to the grid and localized entry point. It is possible to identify important cortical surface elements along the intended approach route on a good-quality reconstruction.

Ultrasound-guided biopsy in the diagnosis of cerebral lesions: indications and limits

P. Lunardi, M. Acqui, F. Puzzilli, M. Neroni, A. Fortuna

Department of Neurological Sciences, Chair of Neurosurgery, 2nd Rome University, "La Sapienza", Rome, Italy

Abstract. On the basis of our experience, we briefly report the limits and indications for ultrasound-guided biopsy in the diagnosis of supratentorial cerebral lesions. We used Berger's apparatus in 68 cases. Mortality was nil and morbidity minimal. In some cases where a cyst was associated with the tumour, drainage of the liquid component through the biopsy needle produced relief of the neurological symptoms. Histological diagnosis was achievable in more than 90% of the cases; only two cases required another, CT-guided biopsy. The average time

Correspondence to: L. Pierpaolo, Neurochirurgia, Viale dell'Università 30a, I-00185 Rome, Italy

employed was 56 min, much shorter than the time necessary for performing CT-guided biopsy. Therefore, ultrasound-guided biopsy seems to be the method of choice for the diagnosis of supratentorial brain lesions. The limits of this procedure are a lesion size of less than 15 mm and a critical localisation requiring extreme topographic accuracy.

Key words: Brain tumours – Biopsy – Ultrasound

Before the advent of CT a number of techniques for identifying and removing a biopsy target had been described in the neurosurgical literature, on the basis of angiographic, pneumoencephalographic and radioisotopie images of the lesion. The introduction of CT revolutionised this procedure and CT-guided stereotactic biopsy, though complex and slow to perform, became the method of choice for the histological diagnosis of supposedly malignant intracranial lesions for which major surgery bore high risks of mortality or morbidity.

More recently, the development of ultrasonographic "B mode real-time" techniques has provided another, simpler method of visualising endocranial lesions and thereby identifying a possible biopsy target: ultrasound-guided biopsy. The diagnostic accuracy and speed of performance of this procedure in cerebral lesions has undergone further improvements; a reduction in the bulk of the ultrasound transducer and the possibility of calculating needle depth and angulation with absolute precision.

This technical progress has principally been due to the work of Berger [1] and Tsutsumi et al. [2] who devised surgical sets for ultrasound-guided biopsy, consecutive in the former and simultaneous in the latter. Nevertheless, not all of the difficulties that may be encountered in this type of biopsy have been resolved, particularly when the lesion is very small or situated in structures that demand millimetric "spatial discrimination".

As these aspects are still controversial, we decided to review our case-series of intracranial lesions diagnosed by ultrasound-guided biopsy in an attempt to evaluate the indications and limits of this method.

Materials and methods

During the last 4 years we performed 68 biopsies employing the ultrasound-guided technique (Table 1), in 41 males and 27 females ranging in age from 14 to 72 years (average 45.6). In 42 cases the lesion affected the left hemisphere, in 17 the right hemisphere and in 9 it was in the midline. The site was subcortical in 44 cases, deep (basal nuclei) in 14 and the corpus callosum in 10.

With reference to CT or MRI, a burr hole 22 mm in diameter was made via a small skin incision under local anaesthesia (general anaesthesia was only used in one mentally-disturbed 14-year-old boy). The set for ultrasound-guided biopsy described by Berger was mounted and the lesion visualised by transdural ultrasonography. The equipment used was a B-mode real-time scanner with rotating 5 MHz transducer, 1 cm in diameter.

A biopsy target was identified on the lesion, calculating the depth and best angle for introduction of the needle. A small dural incision was then made and, once the leptomeninx had been coagulated, a Sedan biopsy needle inserted: this is a blunt needle at the tip of which there is a lateral slit. The trocar also has a lateral slit at its tip, and by inserting the needle with the two slits aligned, the brain tissue can be aspired via the slit in the hollow end of the trocar. This is then rotated so that the fragment of tissue is cut off by a guillotine-like movement and can be extracted once the trocar has been removed.

Once 5 or 6 biopsy samples had been taken at different depths, an ultrasound scan was repeated to exclude surgical complications. Finally, the dural incision was covered with Surgical and the soft tissues sutured. On average, this surgical procedure lasted 56 min.

Table 1. Clinical data

Sex	male	41
	female	27
Age (years)		14–72
Site of lesion	left cerebral hemisphere	42
	right cerebral hemisphere	17
	midline	9
Position	subcortical	44
	basal nuclei	14
	corpus callosum	10

Table 2. Histological diagnoses obtained

Malignant glioma	42
Low-grade glioma	8
Metastasis	11
Lymphoma	3
Abscess	3
Encephalitis	1

Results

Operative mortality was nil and histological diagnosis was possible in 66 cases (97%). In 2 cases the biopsy sample contained normal brain tissue and the procedure was therefore repeated using a CT-guided technique. In 6 cases there was a cyst associated with the tumour and during the ultrasound-guided procedure the cyst was also drained and there was a clear improvement in the patients' clinical conditions. Lastly, 2 patients' condition worsened due to increased perilesional oedema in one and to subcortical haemorrhage in the other: both resolved with appropriate medical treatment.

Table 2 shows the histological diagnoses. In 3 cases (2 of lymphoma and 1 of encephalitis) the patient was HIV-positive.

Discussion

While intraoperative visualisation of cerebral lesions by ultrasonography became common in the early 1980s, the development of the "B-mode real-time" technique [3–6] has enabled its application to biopsy procedures.

In addition to correct visualisation of the lesion, another fundamental requirement of the biopsy procedure is to automatically maintain the needle at the optimal angle [7]. While this has always been easy to achieve using the apparatus for CT-guided biopsy, for the ultrasound technique it has been necessary to create smaller transducers and particular surgical sets that allow them to be fixed to the skull in order to maintain optimal angulation of the needle.

Our use of Berger's set gave very good results due to its simple application and use. It allows a so-called "consecutive" biopsy; firstly the transducer is applied to visualise the lesion; then it is removed and the biopsy needle mounted on the basis of the coordinates established by the transducer. The advantage of this method is that only one burr hole is necessary. The drawback is the lack of real-time monitoring of the needle penetrating the lesion, however, this limitation is overcome by the possibility, once the target has been visualised, of perfect needle positioning [8].

Despite these technical advances, ultrasound-guided biopsy still presents some limitations. One of these is the reduced spatial resolution of ultrasonography in comparison to other imaging methods (CT, MRI). In fact, both lateral and depth resolution are influenced not only by parameters such as the shape and size of the transducer and pulse length, but also by the frequency used [7]: the greater the frequency used, the better the lateral resolution but the poorer the depth resolution. Therefore, because it requires a compromise between lateral and depth resolution, optimal spatial resolution is not possible using a single wavelength [9]. Moreover, hyperechoic perilesional oedema often makes it difficult to identify the borders of the lesion [9, 10].

In cases where a marked angulation of the needle is indispensible, there may be "shadow" artefacts caused by the bony edges of the burr hole. In very deep-seated lesions, it may also be difficult to calculate the exact size of the lesion, and if the lesion does not fall within the area of the acoustic lens, the resulting images may be larger than the actual lesion.

Another cause of magnified images in deep-seated lesions, may be the fact that the distance between the ultrasound beam emitted and the reflected echo increases as the distance covered by the beam itself increases. Artefacts may also be caused by phenomena of diffraction or repetition that give origin to "phantom" images or "specular" images without an anatomical basis. Such artefacts preclude a millimetric distinction of the biopsy target making ultrasound-guided biopsy difficult to perform for small lesions or for lesions situated in highly functional areas [9, 11, 12].

In our series, one anatomical limitation in the use of ultrasound-guided biopsy involved the difficulties in mounting Berger's set and orientng the transducer in the posterior cranial fossa. The presence of the occipital musles and orientation of the occipital squama make it difficult to perform these manoeuvres under local anaesthesia. However, despite these limitations, ultrasound-guided biopsy doubtless has some advantages [1, 9, 11–13]. Above all it is reliable; for supratentorial lesions larger than 1.5 cm diameter, ultrasound visualisation is sufficient for correct needle positioning and histological diagnosis is possible in almost all cases.

It is simple and quick to perform: in our series it took, on average, 56 min as opposed to 256 min for CT-guided biopsy [12]. It is also a low-cost method because, unlike CT-guided biopsy, no extra equipment or staff are required to exclude any surgical complications other than those used for the identification and localisation of the target. In our experience, these features (simple performance and no other structures apart from the operating theatre involved) were particularly important when biopsy was performed for lesions secondary to HIV infection, as it reduced the risk of transmitting the disease to a minimum.

It is likely that further technical advances in the shape and size of the transducers and surgical sets and a careful choice of the frequencies used, will broaden the indications for this procedure: while in the past the number of CT-guided biopsies performed in our division was equivalent to the number of ultrasound-guided ones, their proportion is currently 1 to 6.

References

1. Berger MS (1986) Ultrasound-guided stereotaxic biopsy using, new apparatus. J Neurosurg 65:550–554
2. Tsutsumi Y, Andoh Y, Sakaguchi J (1989) A new ultrasound-guided brain biopsy technique through a burr hole. Technical note. Acta Neurochir (Wien) 96:72–75
3. Chandler WF, Knake JE, McGillicuddy JE, Lillihei KO, Silver RM (1982) Intraoperative use of real-time ultrasonography in neurosurgery. J Neurosurg 57:157–163
4. Dohrmann GJ, Rubin JM (1981) Use of ultrasound in neurosurgical operations: a preliminary report. Surg Neurol 16:362–366
5. Gooding GAW, Boggan JE, Bank WO, Beglin B, Edwards MSB (1980) Sonography of the adult brain through surgical defect. AJNR 2:449–452
6. Marshall LF, Jennet B, Langfit TW (1974) Needle biopsy for the diagnosis of malignant glioma. JAMA 228:1417–1418
7. Van Velthoven V, Auer LM (1990) Practical application of intraoperative ultrasound imaging. Acta Neurochir (Wien) 105:5–13
8. Roux FX, Constants JP, Ciolaca C, Meder JF, Sermet A (1986) Ultrasonographie en temps réel. Neurochirurgie 32:553–558
9. Auer LM, Van Velthoven V (1990) Intraoperative ultrasound imaging in neurosurgery. Springer, Berlin Heidelberg New York
10. Shetter AG, Beryuccini TV, Pittman HW (1977) Closed needle biopsy in the diagnosis of intracranial mass lesions. Surg Neurol 8:341–345
11. Lunardi P, Acqui M, Maleci A, Di Lorenzo N, Fortuna A (1992) Ultrasound-guided brain biopsy: a personal experience with emphasis on its indications. Surg Neurol 39:148–151
12. Di Lorenzo N, Esposito V, Lunardi P, Delfini R, Fortuna A, Cantore F (1991) A comparison of computerized tomography-guided stereotactic and ultrasound-guided techniques for brain biopsy. J Neurosurg 75:763–765
13. Sommer FG, Filly RA, Minton MJ (1979) Acoustic shadowing due to refractive and reflective effects. AJR 132:973–977

Complications of radiotherapy for brain tumours: MRI detection of haemorrhagic lesions

M. Suzuki[1], T. Takashima[1], M. Kadoya[1], F. Ueda[1], H. Nishijima[1], K. Ikeda[2], T. Yamashima[2], J. Yamashita[2]

[1] Department of Radiology, Kanazawa University School of Medicine, 13-1 Takaramachi, Kanazawa, 920 Japan
[2] Department of Neurosurgery, Kanazawa University School of Medicine, 13-1 Takaramachi, Kanazawa, 920 Japan

Abstract. On follow-up MRI of patients undergoing postoperative brain radiotherapy, markedly hyperintense and/or hypointense lesions were observed on T2-weighted images which were hypointense or hyperintense on T1-weighted images. They were compatible with subacute on chronic haemorrhage and were probably radiation-induced. Special attention should be paid to the presence of these lesions.

Key words: Brain, radiation injury – Haemorrhage – Magnetic resonance imaging

Cerebral radiation injury has been classified into three groups: acute, early delayed and late [1, 2]. Radiation necrosis is the most common clinically recognised form of focal radiation injury. Woo et al. [3] reported focal haemorrhagic injury after irradiation. They found abnormal teleangiectatic vessels at the periphery of the haematoma. Valk and Dillon [1] observed five cases of radiation-induced focal haemorrhage on MRI. We have seen three patients with focal haemorrhagic lesions after irradiation for brain tumours. In this report, we describe the MRI findings of haemorrhagic lesions that are probably radiation induced.

Materials and methods

Three patients, boys aged 12, 13 and 15 years, had undergone postoperative radiotherapy following excision of medulloblastoma or ependymoma 7, 7, and 5 years previously, respectively. Three to thirteen studies were performed in each patient for evaluation. Axial T1- and T2-weighted images were selected in each study. Signal abnormalities were assessed in each case.

Results

A total of nine lesions were observed on the MRI studies. Seven lesions were hypointense on T1-weighted images and markedly hypointense on T2-weighted images (Fig. 1), while two lesions were markedly hyperintense on both T1-weighted images and T2-weighted images with markedly hypointense rim on T2-weighted images (Fig. 2). All lesions were compatible with subacute to chronic haemorrhage. Five lesions were not seen on the initial postoperative MRI study but appeared on the following study. All were in the radiation field selected 5–7 years previously. Radiation dose was 39–52.2 Gy. In one patient with subacute haemorrhage, an operation was performed. Haematoma with anomalous vessels was pathologically confirmed (Fig. 2).

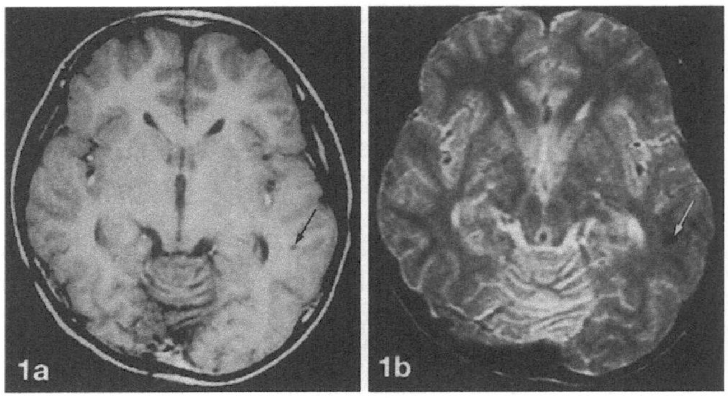

Fig. 1 a, b. Axial T1- and T2-weighted images 5 years after operation. A small low-signal area is seen in the posterior temporal lobe (*arrow*) in **a** which gives markedly low signal in **b** (*arrow*)

Discussion

Cerebral radiation injury has been classified into acute, early delayed and late groups [1]. Late injury occurs a few months to 10 years or more after radiation therapy. Woo et al. [3] reported a patient with apoplectic intracerebral haemorrhage from delayed cerebral necrosis. Autopsy revealed numerous dialted thin-walled vascular channels arranged in a telangiectatic pattern at the periphery of the haematoma, in association with typical features of late radiation necrosis. Valk and Dillon [1] reported five cases of radiation-associated focal haemorrhage on MRI. The patients had been treated with conventional doses of radiation. MRI showed subacute to chronic haemorrhagic changes.

In our cases radiation dose was 39–52.2 Gy, equal to conventional dose. All lesions occurred within the irradiated volume of brain. They were subacute to chronic haemorrhagic lesions, as were those in Valk and Dillon's cases. These lesions showed MRI findings similar to those in cryptic vascular malformations. However, five lesions were not seen on the initial MRI study but appeared on the following study. These lesions were probably radiation induced. With or without symptoms, radiation-induced focal haemorrhagic lesions appeared in follow-up MRI of patients undergoing postoperative brain raadiotherapy. Special attention should be paid to the possible presence of these lesions.

Correspondence to: M. Suzuki

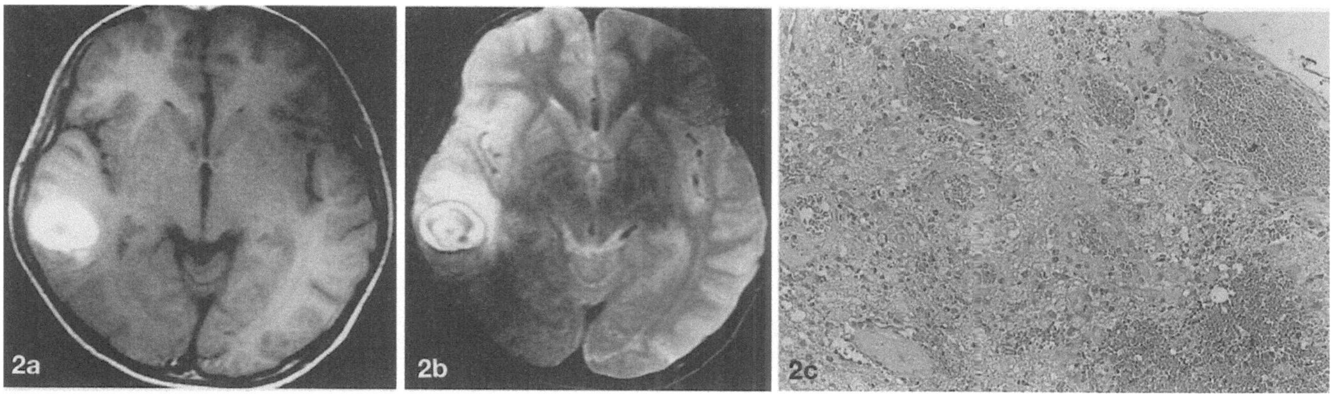

Fig. 2a–c. Axial T1- and T2-weighted images 7 years after operation. A lesion in the right temporal lobe and is compatible with a subacute haematoma. Histopathological specimen (haematoxylin and eosin): multiple dilated, anomalous vessels are seen at the periphery of the haematoma

References

1. Valk PE, Dillon WP (1991) Radiation injury of the brain. AJNR 12:45–62
2. Kramer S, Lee KF (1974) Complications of radiation therapy: the central nervous system. Semin Roentgenol 9:75–83
3. Woo E, Chan YF, Lam K, et al (1987) Apoplectic intracerebral hemorrhage: unusual complication of cerebral radiation necrosis. Pathology 19:95–98

Degenerative diseases

Radiological detection of proven Alzheimer's disease during life using CT evidence of minimum medial temporal lobe thickness

A. J. Molyneux[1], K. A. Jobst[2], N. J. Hindley[2], A. D. Smith[3]

[1] Department of Neuroradiology, Radcliffe Infirmary Trust, Oxford, England
[2] Oxford Project to Investigate Memory and Ageing (OPTIMA), Radcliffe Infirmary Trust, Oxford, England
[3] University Department of Pharmacology, University of Oxford, England

Abstract. The diagnosis of Alzheimer's disease (AD) cannot be made definitively in life. The only reliable diagnosis is by neuropathological examination of the brain. We have followed a series of 200 patients with clinical evidence of dementia using serial temporal lobe-oriented; 58 of these patients have now died, and neuropathological examination of the brain has been performed on all except 2. An age-matched control group of 75 subjects without clinical evidence of dementia was also examined in the same way. Temporal lobe-oriented 2 mm sections were obtained and the minimum thickness of the medial temporal lobe (MTMTL) structures measured. AD was histopathologically confirmed in 44 patients. In this group the mean MTMTL was 7.0 mm (SD 2.1 mm, mean age 78 years). In the control group without dementia the MTMTL was 13.6 mm (SD 2.3 mm, mean age 79 years). When the MTMTL is plotted as multiples of the median for age, its measurement from temporal lobe-oriented CT becomes a reliable predictor of AD, with a detection rate of 92% and a false-positive rate of 5%. There were 20 patients with proven AD and 47 controls who had undergone two or more studies. The rate of reduction in the MTMTL (1.89 mm/year, SD 1.72 mm) was significantly greater than in the control group (0.21 mm/year, SD .75). The measurement of the MTMTL is, with practice, straightforward. The rate at which the MTMTL declines may be important in prognosis and therapy.

Key words: Senile dementia of Alzheimer type – Alzheimer's disease – Computed tomography – Dementia – Histopathology

The definitive diagnosis of Alzheimer's disease (AD) on clinical grounds is not possible. Numerous brain-imaging modalities have been used in attempts to improve diagnostic accuracy. However, the need for histopathological verification has meant that few series have been able to correlate clinical assessments, imaging findings and necropsy data. The pathological changes in AD are most pronounced in the medial temporal lobe structures and include high densities of plaques and tangles, and neuronal loss giving rise to marked temporal lobe shrinkage [1]. Conventional CT performed either parallel to, or at positive angle to the orbito-meatal line, does not provide optimum imaging of the temporal lobe structures, particularly the medial temporal lobe. The medial temporal structures can be well demonstrated by tilting the gantry down the long axis of the temporal lobe. This has been shown in a number of studies [2]. Volumetric studies using MRI have also revealed medial temporal lobe atrophy in patients with senile dementia of Alzheimer type (SDAT) [3]. However, all these studies are based on the clinical diagnosis of SDAT and therefore cannot predict an accurate incidence of atrophy in AD, since between 12% and 35% of these clinical diagnoses may be incorrect in patients with dementia [4].

Patients and methods

The Oxford Project to Investigate Memory and Ageing (OPTIMA) is a prospective, longitudinal study of patients with dementia or memory impairment, together with age-matched controls without evidence of cognitive deficit [5]. All subjects are studied in detail and followed at annual intervals until death [6]. This has resulted in the largest prospective study to date of serially imaged subjects with proven AD. Investigations include CT scanning with both axial and temporal lobe-oriented views, the latter using 2 mm contiguous slices at an angle 20° caudad to the orbitomeatal line, representing a line drawn between the top of the mastoids and the top of the hard palate on the lateral topogram, as previously described [5]. A topogram with the correct gantry angle is demonstrated in Fig. 1, and appearances in a non-demented control aged 66 years and with no histological evidence of central nervous system (CNS) disease are shown in Fig. 2. The equivalent view in a case of AD is demonstrated in Fig. 3.

Scans are examined for evidence of cortical atrophy, whether generalised or focal, and other significant pathology. Numerous anatomical measurements are made from the scans. The MTMTL was found to be the most sensitive correlate of subsequently proven AD. The measurements are made at the level of the brain stem, midway through the medial temporal lobe, from the hard copy image using the linear scale on the scan and callipers. If the patient is straight in the scanner the same slice on both sides is measured; however, in some patients, where there is asymmetry of the head in the gantry, different slices are measured on the left and right to obtain equivalent sections. The MTMTL itself represents the distance between the medial aspect of the temporal horn of the lateral ventricle and the cerebrospinal fluid (CSF) within the cistern at the level of the brain stem, as previously described [5]. Partial volume effects may need to be taken into account but are minimised by using 1.5- or 2-mm-thick contifuous sections. The procedure is conducted by two observers blind to the patient's identity. Interobserver reliability was high [5]. The neuropathological diagnosis of AD is made according to strict Khachaturian criteria.

Results

The mean MTMTL, expressed as the multiple of the median (MoM) for age in controls, for the 75 controls, 44 patients with AD and 10 other patients with dementia is

Correspondence to: A. D. Smith, Department of Pharmacology, University of Oxford, Oxford OX2 6HE, England

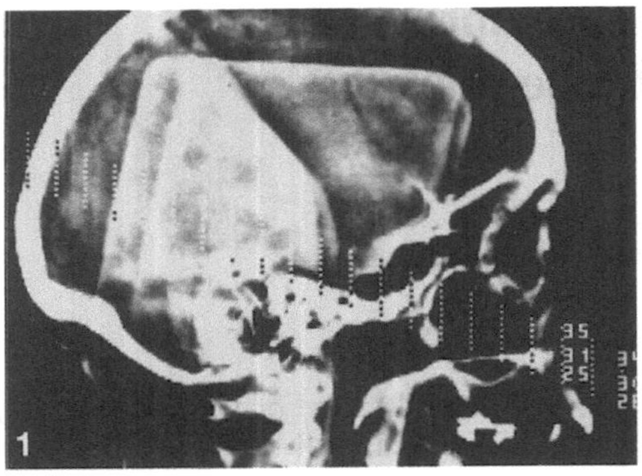

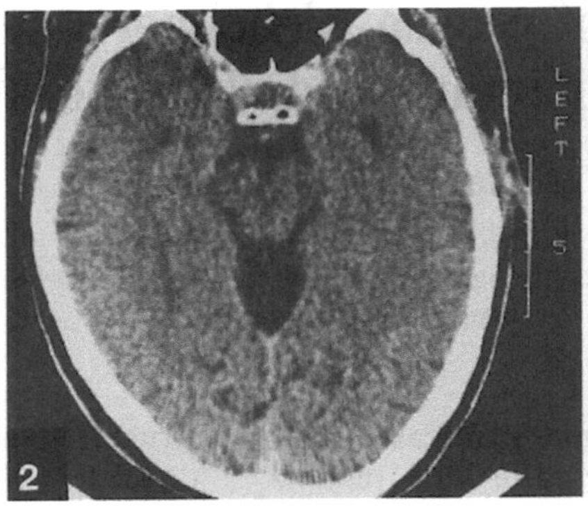

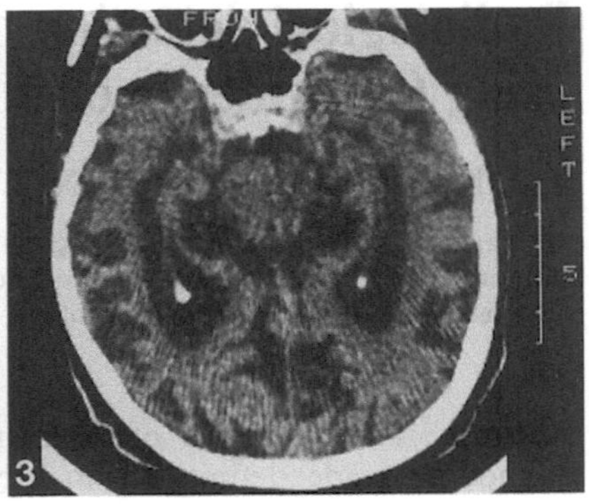

Fig. 1. Lateral "topogram" showing temporal lobe orientation

Fig. 2. Temporal lobe-oriented CT in a control aged 66 with no brain pathology at necropsy

Fig. 3. Temporal lobe-oriented CT in a 66-year-old patient with necropsy-confirmed AD

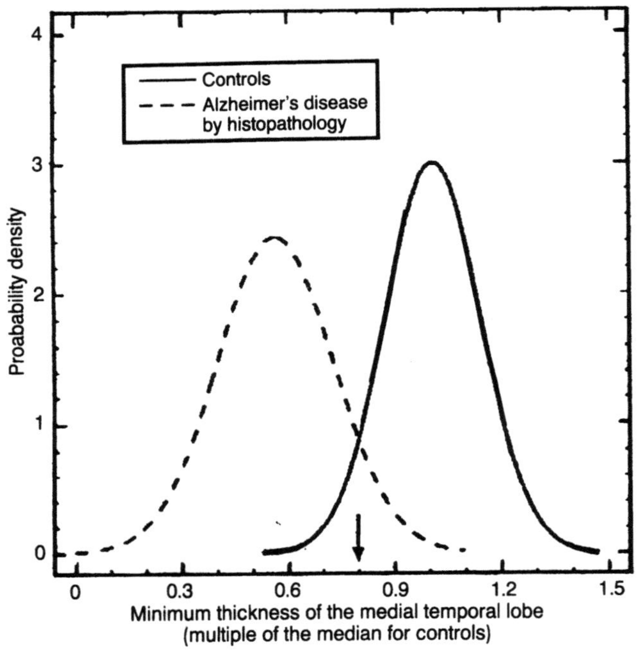

Fig. 4. Calculated Gaussian distributions for minimum thickness of medial temporal lobe in multiples of the median for controls (MoM). *Arrow,* cut-off value (<0.79 MoM), which should yield an expected false-positive rate of 5% and detection rate of AD of 92%

Table 1. Minimum thickness of medial temporal lobe (MTMTL) measured from CT scans in patients with Alzheimer's disease (AD), other dementias, and controls

Group[a]	No.	Mean (SD) MMSE score	Minimum thickness of medial temporal lobe, as mean (SD) MoM
AD (cases)	44	9.3	0.56 (0.16)*
Controls (no dementia)	75	28 (2)	1.0 (0.13)
Other dementias	10	14 (5)	0.85 (0.24)**

MoM, multiple of mean; MMSE, Mini mental state exam
* $P<0.001$ for difference from controls (t-test; distributions are gaussian; cf. Table 2)
** $P<0.002$ for difference from AD, but *not* from controls ($P>0.06$, Mann Whitney)
[a] All 54 patients with dementia and 2 controls have come to necroscopy. Other dementias = multi-infarct (2). Creutzfeldt-Jakob disease, progressive supranuclear palsy, Parkinson's disease, normal pressure hydrocephalus, glioma, hypoperfusion/post-ischaemic damage to hippocampi, no detectable CNS lesions

given in Table 1. The mean MTMTL in patients with AD was 7.0 mm (SD 2.1; range 2–11 mm; mean age 78 years), whilst for the 75 controls it was 13.6 mm (SD 2.3 mm; range 10–19 mm; mean age 70 years). Normal distribution curves plotting MTMTL as MoM for cases of AD and controls clearly differentiate the two groups (Fig. 4). This shows that a cut-off of 0.79 MoM would yield a false-positive rate of 5% for a detection rate of 92% for AD [5]. In the 20 AD patients who had two or more annual CT studies in life the change in the MTMTL differed markedly from that in the 47 comparable controls: 15.1% per year (95% CI 10.0–20.2%) for confirmed AD, as against 1.5% (95% CI 0.2–2.8) for controls (Table 2) [7].

Table 2. Rate of atrophy of medial temporal lobes

	Age at first CT (years)	CAMCOG score at CT	Annual rate of decline in CAMCOG (points per year)	Minimum thickness of medial temporal lobe at first scan (mm)	Annual rate of atrophy of medial temporal lobe (mm)
Controls (47)	68.4 (65.4, 71.4)	97.0 (95.5, 98.5)	-0.7 (1.5, -1.1)	14.6 (14.1, 15.2)	0.21 (0.02, 0.39)
Dementia of Alzheimer type (61)	73.1 (71.1, 75.2)	54.9 (51.9, 61.8)	12.9 (10.2, 15.6)*	10.1 (9.4, 10.9)*	1.55 (1.24, 1.86)[a]
Confirmed Alzheimer's disease (20)	76.2 (72.9, 79.4)	44.8 (30.8, 58.4)*	18.8 (9.7, 26.1)	9.4 (8.1, 10.8)*	1.89 (1.25, 2.54)[a]

Mean (95% CI). * Significantly different from controls ($P<0.0001$, U-test)

Discussion

Whilst the use of CT alone is not diagnostic of AD, these data from our cohort indicate that the MTMTL is a better predictor of AD than is reported for the routine application of clinical criteria alone [4, 5]. There is debate as to whether AD is an inevitable consequence of ageing or represents a true disease process. Our evidence of a dramatic difference in the rates of atrophy between cases of AD and controls supports the latter view, which is endorsed by recent neuroanatomical work [8]. For there to be any progress in understanding and modifying the course of the condition, accurate identification of patients is essential. The advent of a relatively simple and accurate noninvasive test with a high sensitivity and specificity has been of substantial vàlue in the clinical management of our patients. Pasquier et al. have recently confirmed its reproducibility in the clinical setting [9]. Similar results have been achieved with MRI [3]. However, this modality can be difficult to use in patients with dementia because of their restlessness. Furthermore, MRI is more expensive and less available world-wide than CT. We believe this technique could be easily adopted for the examination and better diagnosis of this group of patients.

Acknowledgements. We would like to thank participants in the study, their families, and referring physicians. We are particularly grateful to Elizabeth King and the research nurses for their expert management of the patients, to Drs. Margaret Esiri, James Morris, Catherine Joachim and Brendan McDonald for pathological diagnoses and to Drs. James Byrne, Philip Anslow and the Neuroradilogy staff for their support. This research is supported by a grant from Bristol-Myers Squibb. Fig. 4 and Table 1 are reproduced with perimission of the Lancet, Ltd (from [5]); as is Table 2 [7].

References

1. Braak H, Braak E (1991) Neuropathological staging of Alzheimer-related changes. Acta Neuropathol 82:239–259
2. George AE, Leon MJ de, Stylopoulos LA, et al (1990) CT diagnostic features of Alzheimer's disease: importance of the choroidal/hippocampal fissure complex. AJNR 11:101–107
3. Jack CR, Petersen RC, Obrien PC, et al (1990) MR-based hippocampal volumetry in the diagnosis of Alzheimer's disease. Neurology 42:183–188
4. Kukull WA, Larson EB, Reifler BV, et al (1990) The validity of 3 clinical diagnostic criteria for Alzheimer's disease. Neurology 40:1364–1369
5. Jobst KA, Smith AD, Szatmari M, et al (1992) Detection in life of confirmed Alzheimer's disease using a simple measurement of medial temporal lobe atrophy by computed tomography. Lancet 340:1189–1193
6. King EM, Smith A, Jobst KA (1992) Autopsy: consent, completion and communication in Alzheimer's disease research. Age Ageing 22:209–214
7. Jobst KA, Smith AD, Szatmari M, et al (1994) Rapidly progressing atrophy of medial temporal lobe in Alzheimer's disease. Lancet 343:829–830
8. West M, Coleman PD, Flood DG, Troncoso JC (1994) Differences in the pattern of hippocampal neuronal loss in normal ageing and Alzheimer's disease. Lancet 344:769–772
9. Pasquier F, Bail L, Lebert F, et al (1994) Determination of medial temporal lobe atrophy in early Alzheimer's disease with computed tomography. Lancet 343:861–862

MRI and neuropsychological correlates in presumed vascular dementia

S. Bastianello[1], F. Giubilei[1], A. Paolillo[1], C. Gasperini[1], A. Bozzao[1], A. Gragnani[1], M. Antonelli[2], L. Bozzao[1]

[1] Department of Neurological Sciences, University of Rome "La Sapienza", Rome, Italy
[2] Istitutó Mediterrano Neuroscienze Pozzilli (IS), Rome, Italy

Abstract. We studied 34 patients with presumed vascular dementia (20 men and 14 women, average: 69.86) on a 0.2T MR system. T2-weighted on axial images and T1-weighted midsaggital images were obtained. The volumes of the subarachnoid and ventricular spaces, brain parenchyma and T2 signal-alteration areas were calculated using a semiautomated method. Volumes of supratentorial contents were normalised to relative values. We also calculated the ratio between the area of corpus callosum (CC) and the volume of supratentorial brain. Cognitive function was evaluated using a battery of neuropsychological tests. MRI showed an increase in size of the sulci and ventricle volumes correlated with parenchymal atrophy ($P<0.03$ and $P<0.001$, respectively); supratentorial T2 signal-alteration volumes were proportional to an increase in ventricle volumes ($P<0.001$) and to decrease in size of CC ($P<0.02$). A significant correlation was found between CC atrophy and deterioration of memory function ($P<0.002$) and ventricular enlargement also correlated with short-term memory impairment ($P<0.03$). A significant relationship between memory impairment and an increase of T2 signal-alteration volume was observed ($P<0.03$). Our methodological approach, which allowed us to obtain in vivo information and measurements of cerebral contents, suggests that CC atrophy might not be

Correspondence to: S. Bastianello, Department of Neurosciences, University of Rome "La Sapienza", Viale dell'Università 30, I-00185 Rome, Italy

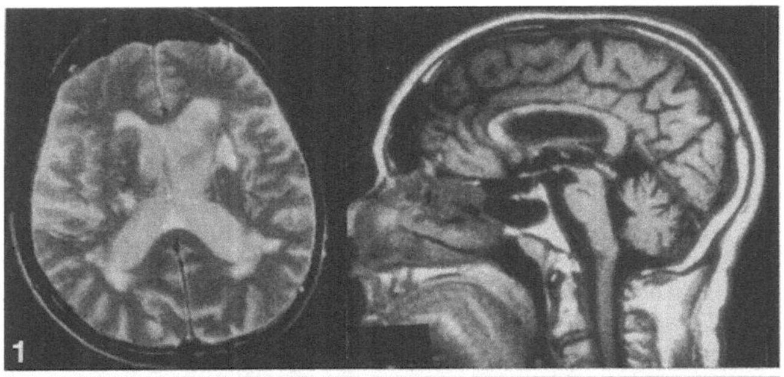

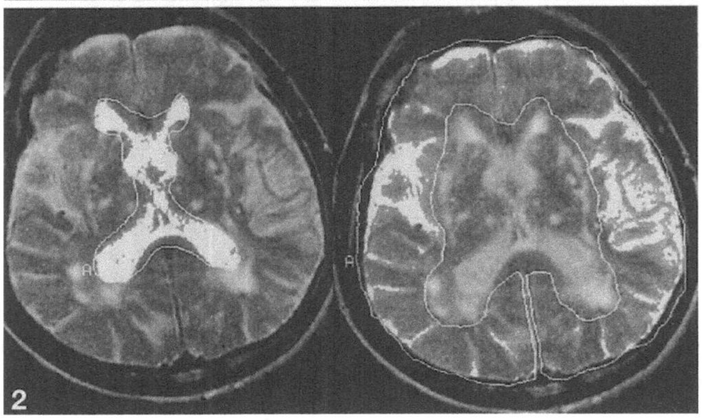

Fig. 1. MRI of patient with vascular dementia. Multiple areas of signal alteration, compatible with ischaemic foci, are well seen on axial T2-weighted images (*left*); cortical atrophy, corpus callosum and midbrain involvement are well documented on midsagittal T1-weighted image (*right*)

Fig. 2. Axial T2-weighted image in a patient with vascular dementia. Volume measurements of ventricles (*left*) and subarachnoid spaces (*right*), using a semiautomated technique based on different signal intensity values of each cerebral structure

simply an element of diffuse brain atrophy but an evident sign of the disease, and could be used as useful indicator in the assessment of specific cognitive disfunctions correlated with vascular dementia.

Key words: Vascular dementia – Magnetic resonance imaging – Neuropsychological test

Vascular dementia (VD) and Alzheimer's disease (AD) are the most common causes of dementia in older people, and are estimated to account for 70–85% of demented states [1–3]. The prevalence of VD is constantly increasing and proportional to advancing age [2–5]. The increase of VD and its various clinical pictures, requires more efficient diagnostic criteria. A great help in VD diagnosis are brain-imaging techniques, especially MRI [6].

MRI shows cerebral modifications in exceptional detail, but its potential role in differentiating specific causes of cognitive decline has not yet been determined (Fig. 1) [6]. Moreover, cortical atrophy, ventricle enlargement and pathological signal intensity areas are not well framed, depending on subjective criteria.

We performed quantitative MRI evaluation of supratentorial cerebral contents in patients with VD using a semiautomated technique.

Table 1. Absolute and normalised volumes of the supratentorial contens in VD patients, expressed in millimeters and as ratios between different structures

	Absolute data (SD)	Normalised data[a] (SD)
Sulci (CSF)	144.7 (29.3)	12.2 (1.9)
Ventricles	61.9 (24.4)	6.2 (2.1)
Total brain	943.2 (98.3)	81.8 (2.8)
T2 signal-alteration foci	14.4 (12.8)	1.2 (1.1)
Corpus callosum (cm^2)	5.05 (0.5)	-

[a] Normalised volumetric data: percentage of sulcal CSF volume = extraventricular CSF/total CSF + total brain; percentage of ventricular CSF volume = ventricular CSF/total CSF + total brain; percentage of relative brain volume = brain/total CSF + total brain; percentage of T2 signal-alterations volume = T2 signal-alterations volume/total CSF + total brain volume

Materials and methods

We studied 34 patients (20 men and 14 women, average age: 69.86 years) with VD diagnosed according to clinical (DSM-III) and radiological parameters [1, 7].

MR imaging. All patients were scanned on a 0.2T MRI system. Sequences of T2-weighted contiguous images, 7.5 mm thick with no gap (TR = 2500, TE = 30–110; 2 measures 256 × 192 matrix) on axial planes and T1 (TR = 400, TE = 25; 4 measures, 256 × 192 matrix on sagittal planes were obtained. T1 images were obtained to calculate the corpus callosum (CC) area.

Volumes of subarachnoid and ventricular cerebrospinal fluid (CSF), parenchymal brain tissue and T2 signal-alteration areas were calculated using a quantitative semiautomated method (Fig. 2). This technique involved intensity threshold segmentation in order first to isolate the brain from surrounding tissue, and then to identify T2 signal-alterations, ventricles and sulci CSF [8]; all volumes were measured in millilitres.

In order to compensate for variability in intracranial sizes, absolute volumetric measurements were normalised to relative values.

Based on limited methodological and subjective bias, we considered the values expressed by ratios between different structures (sulci, ventricles and parenchyma).

Neuropsychological assessment. The neuropsychological test battery consisted of measures of general intelligence, general cognitive abilities, language, memory, visuospatial abilities, and constructive apraxia and lasted approximately 2 h [9, 10].

Results

All VD patients showed cognitive impairment of various degrees in different tests. The absolute and normalised data of supratentorial contents are reported in Table 1. The correlation of normalised volumetric data was significant, showing an increase of CSF sulci and ventricle volumes correlated with parenchymal atrophy ($P < 0.03$ and $P < 0.001$ respectively). Moreover, supratentorial T2 signal-alteration volumes resulted proportional to an increase of ventricle volumes ($P < 0.001$) and to a decrease in size of CC ($P < 0.02$). Comparing supratentorial cerebral structure values with neuropsychological performances a significant correlation was found between CC atrophy and memory function deterioration ($P<0.002$) and between ventricular enlargement and short-term memory impairment ($P<0.03$). A memory impairment during a digit span test was also observed in correlation with an increase of T2 signal-alteration areas ($P<0.03$).

Discussion

Involvement of cortical functions can be indicative of dementia [1]. CT and particularly MRI can nowadays help clinicians in the diagnosis of VD, showing the presence of single or multiple ischaemic infarcts [6]. While CT appearances of ischaemic lesions are well known, the significance of signal-alterations on T2-weighted images, frequently disclosed on white matter, are often discussed but of unclear aetiology (ischaemic lesions, leucoaraiosis, apparently normal findings in elderly subjects) [1, 6, 11] and might lead to an overestimation of cerebral involvement. Notwithstanding these considerations, we assume that these findings could represent cerebral involvement probably due to ischaemic lesions, according to clinical data. Precise measurement of cerebral contents and pathological findings is not currently feasible, but there are methods, such as the one used in this study, by which the supratentorial contents of the ventricles, sulci, parenchymal and T2 signal alterations can be estimated [8, 12]. We did not observe a significant relationship between single cerebral contents and verbal fluency, visuospatial memory and long-term memory, which were the most severely impaired cognitive functions. Furthermore, we compared psychometric functions with total volumes of cerebral contents and not with those of specific structures or sites, such as frontal lobe, which is mainly involved when verbal fluency is compromised. A significant correlation was also found between ventricular enlargement and an increase of T2 signal-alteration volumes with short-term memory impairment, which could indicate a possible involvement of subcortical brain structures in the development of memory disfunction. These findings may ultimately support the ischaemic origin of the T2 signal-alteration areas seen at MRI in our VD patients. In our patients, the most significant finding was the atrophy of CC correlated with memory impairment. This structure, made up myelinated fibres, represents the most important medial structure linking the two cerebral hemispheres. Moreover, CC involvement could represent a secondary event generally due to corticosubcortical infarction with secondary Wallerian degeneration. The degree of CC involvement may parallel the extent of periventricular high-signal alterations [13–15]. The role of CC atrophy remains uncertain and speculative. We believe that CC atrophy might not be simply an element of diffuse brain atrophy but an evident sign of the disease process that it could be used as a useful indicator in the diagnosis of specific cognitive dysfunctions correlated with vascular dementia.

References

1. Chui HC, Victoroff JI, Margalin D, Jagus W, Shankle R, Katzman R (1992) Criteria for the diagnosis of ischemic vascular dementia proposed by the state of California. Alzheimer's disease. Neurobiol Aging 8:521–545
2. O'Brien HC (1989) Vascular dementia is underdiagnosed. Arch Neurol 45:797–798
3. Jorm AF, Korten AE, Henderson AS (1987) The prevalence of dementia: a quantitative integration of the literature. Acta Pschiatr Scand 76:465–479
4. Kase CS (1991) Epidemiology of multi-infarct dementia. Alzheimer Dis Assoc Disord 5:71–76
5. Rocca WA, Hofman A, Brayne C, et al (1991) The prevalence of vascular dementia in Europe: facts and fragments from 1980–1990 studies. Ann Neurol 30:817–824
6. Johnson KA, Davis KR, Buonanno FS, et al (1987) Comparison of magnetic resonance and roentgen ray computed tomography in dementia. Arch Neurol 44:1075–1080
7. American Psychiatric Association (1987) Diagnostic and statistical manual of mental disorders, 3rd edn, rev. American Psychiatric Association, Washington
8. Tanna NK, Koh MI, Horwich DN, et al (1991) Analysis of brain and cerebrospinal volumes with MR imaging: impact on PET data correction for atrophy. Radiology 178:123–130
9. Folstein MS, Folstein SE, McHugh PR (1975) Mini mental state. J Psychiatr Res 12:189–198
10. Lezak MD (1983) Neuropsychological assessment, 2nd ed. Oxford University Press, New York
11. Brust JCM (1988) Vascular dementia is overdiagnosed. Arch Neurol 45:799–801
12. Walser RL (1975) Automatic interpretation of reconstructed objects: Finding the volume of brain ventricle. Master's Thesis, Department of Information Engineering, University of Illinois at Chicago Circle
13. Habib M, Poncet M (1990) Callosal disconnection syndrome caused by left hemisphere infarction. Rev Neurol (Paris) 146:19–24
14. Risse GL, Gates J, Lund G, Maxwell R, Rubens A (1989) Interhemispheric transfer in patients with complete sections of the corpus callosum: anatomic verifications with magnetic resonance imaging. Arch Neurol 46:437–443
15. Laissy JP, Patraux B, Duchateau C, et al (1993) Midsagittal MR measurements of the corpus callosum in healthy subjects and diseased patients: a prospective survey. AJNR 14:145–154

Corticobasal degeneration: MRI and SPECT

K. Negoro, T. Fukusako, N. Tsuda, M. Morimatsu

Department of Neurology, Yamaguchi University School of Medicine, Yamaguchi, Japan

Abstract. We studied seven patients (4 men and 3 women, aged 64–82 years) diagnosed clinically as having corticobasal degeneration. MRI was performed on a 1.5 T MRI unit using a T2-weighted spin echo (SE) sequence (TR 3000, TE 80–90 ms), a T1-weighted SE sequence (TR 550–600, TE 15–20 ms) and a proton density-weighted SE sequence (TR 3000 ms, TE 12–22 ms). Brain perfusion SPECT studies were performed in six patients with ^{123}I-IMP and in one patient with ^{99m}Tc-HMPAO. MRI revealed diffuse brain atrophy in six patients and asymmetrical front parietal atrophy, especially in posterior central gyri and superior parietal lobules, in four contralateral to the most affected limbs. SPECT disclosed a decrease in cerebral blood flow in two patients in the thalamus or basal ganglia on the side opposite the affected limbs.

Key words: Corticobasal degeneration – Magnetic resonance imaging – Single photon emission computed tomography

Corticobasal degeneration is a slowly progressive disorder characterised by an asymmetrical akinetic-rigid syndrome and often accompanied by other involuntary movements and lateralised cortical signs such as alien limb and sensory impairment and apraxia [1, 2]. Cognitive decline usually develops late in the course of the disease, and language disturbance is absent or mild. Computed tomography (CT) or MRI may demonstrate asymmetrical frontparietal cortical atrophy in the later stages of the illness [1, 2]. Positron emission tomography shows a combination of parietal and frontal hypometabolism and an asymmetrical decrease of fluorodopa uptake in the striatum and medial frontal cortex [3, 4]. We report clinical and radiological findings in seven patients with clinical sign suggestive of corticobasal degeneration.

Patients and methods

We studied seven patients (4 men and 3 women, aged 64–82 years) with clinical findings compatible with corticovasal degeneration (Table 1). All presented with unilateral akinetic-rigid syndrome, which progressed to involve the other limbs within a few years. Some of the following lateralised cortical signs were present in the seven

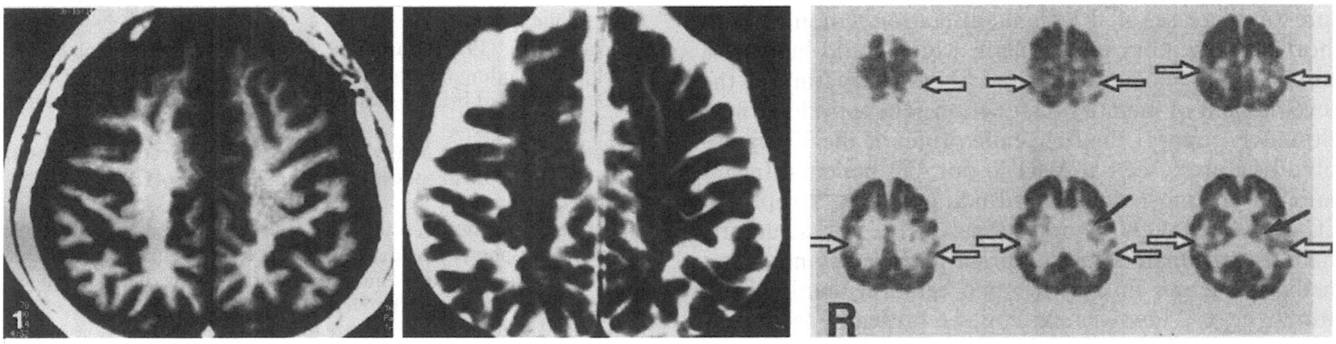

Fig. 1. Case 1. MRI showed severe fronto-parietal brain atrophy. SPECT revealed hypoperfusion in parieto-temporal cortex and left thalamus

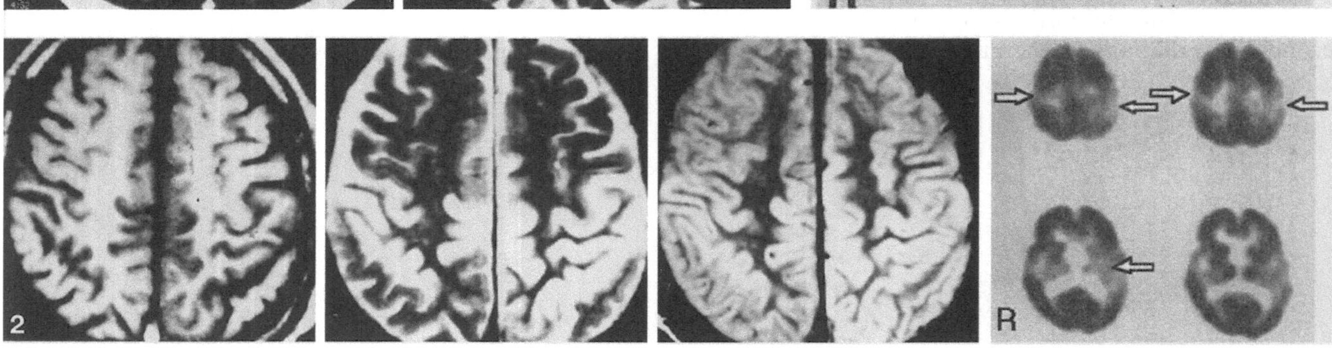

Fig. 2. Case 4. MRI showed diffuse brain atrophy and cortical high signal in parieto-temporal cortex on T-weighted and PD-weighted images. SPECT revealed hypoperfusion in parieto-temporal cortex and left basal ganglia

Correspondence to: K. Negoro

Table 1. Clinical features

Case	Age (years)	Sex	Side	Duration (years)	Akinetic-rigid	Grasp reflex	Alien limb	Limb dystonia	Pyramidal sign	Supranuclear gaze palsy	Limb-kinetic apraxia	Cortical sensory disturbance	Mini-Mental State score
1	65	F	L → both	5	+	+	+	+	–	+	+	–	27
2	72	M	R	4	+	+	+	+	–	–	+	–	28
3	82	M	R	2	+	+	–	+	+	+	+	–	28
4	65	M	R → both	0.5	+	+	+	–	–	+	+	+	24
5	70	M	L → both	2	+	–	–	–	+	+	+	–	28
6	66	F	R → both	2	+	+	–	–	+	+	+	–	24
7	64	F	L → both	3	+	+	+	+	–	+	+	+	26

Table 2. MRI and SPECT

Case	MRI	SPECT: reduced CBF
1	Severe fronto-parietal atrophy	Parieto-temporal (right > left): left thalamus
2	Diffuse brain atrophy: severe left parietal atrophy	Left parieto-temporal
3	Diffuse brain atrophy	Left parietal
4	Diffuse brain atrophy: abnormal signal in parieto-temporal area (right > left)	Parieto-temporal (right > left): left basal ganglia
5	Diffuse brain atrophy: parietal atrophy (right > left)	Left parieto-temporal
6	Diffuse brain atrophy: parietal atrophy (right > left)	Both parieto-temporal
7	Parietal atrophy (right > left): abnormal cortical signal	Right parieto-temporal

patients: grasp reflex, alien limb, limb-kinetic apraxia, pyramidal signs, and cortical sensory disturbance. Dementia was not evident in these patients, and motor symptoms were universally refractory to levodopa and dopamine agonists. Family histories were negative in all patients, and there was no history of drug exposure, head injury, encephalitis, or metabolic disease.

MRI was performed on 1.5 T unit using a T2-weighted spin echo (SE) sequence (TR 3000, TE 80–90 ms), a T1-weighted SE sequence (TR 550–600, TE 15–20 ms) and a proton density (PD)-weighted SE sequence (TR 3000, TE 12–22 ms).

Brain perfusion single photon emission computed tomography (SPECT) studies were performed in one patient with ^{123}I-IMP and in six patients with ^{99m}TC-HMPAO.

Results

MRI revealed diffuse brain atrophy in six cases and asymmetrical fronto-parietal atrophy, especially in posterior central gyri and superior parietal lobules, in four contralateral to the most badly affected limbs (Table 2). MRI in case 4 disclosed bilateral abnormal cortical high signals in the parieto-temporal cortex on T2- and PD-weighted images. In case 7, T2-weighted images revealed low signal in anterior and posterior central gyri bilaterally, and PD-weighted images revealed high signal in the left posterior central gyrus. SPECT showed a decrease in regional cerebral blood flow (CBF) in the posterior frontal and parieto-temporal regions bilaterally, which was more marked contralateral to the most affected limbs. SPECT disclosed a decrease CBF in the thalamus or basal ganglia in two cases.

Discussion

Corticobasal degeneration is an extrapyramidal syndrome that is often misdiagnosed, characterised by progressive unilateral akinesia and rigidity, associated with lateralised cortical signs such as alien limb, limb-kinetic apraxia, cortical sensory disturbance, and limb dystonia [1, 2]. The asymmetry of symptoms and signs is often striking. A clinical diagnosis of corticobasal degeneration should be considered if any of them occur together. Abnormalities demonstrated by MRI and SPECT contralateral to the most badly affected limbs strongly suggest the diagnosis of corticobasal degeneration.

References

1. Gibb WRG, Luthert PJ, Marsden CD (1989) Corticobasal degeneration. Brain 112:1171–1192
2. Eidelberg D, Dhawan V, Moeller JR, Sidtis JJ, Ginos JZ, Strother SC, Cederbaum J, Greene P, Fahn S, Powers JM, Rottenberg DA (1991) The metabolic landscape of cortico-basal ganglionic degeneration: regional asymmetries studied with positron emission tomography. J Neurol Neurosurg Psychiatry 54:856–862
3. Riley DE, Lang AE, Lewis A, Resch L, Ashby P, Hornykiewicz O, Black S (1990) Cortical-basal ganglionic degeneration. Neurology 40:1203–1212
4. Sawle GV, Brooks DJ, Marsden CD, Frackowiak RSJ (1991) Corticobasal degeneration. A unique pattern of regional cortical oxygen hypometabolism and striatal fluorodopa uptake demonstrated by positron emission tomography. Brain 114:541–556

Analysis of cerebrospinal fluid of patients with parkinsonism by proton nuclear magnetic resonance spectroscopy

Wu-Chung Shen[1], Chi-Chang Chen[1], San-Kan Lee[1], Hua-Jin Lin[2], Kuan Rong Lee[2]

[1] Department of Radiology, Veterans General Hospital, Taichung, Taiwan
[2] Institut of Life Science, National Tsing Hua University, Hsin-chu, Taiwan

Abstract. High-resolution proton magnetic resonance spectroscopy was used to study the concentrations of metabolites in the cerebrospinal fluid (CSF) of patients with parkinsonism. The results indicated that the glucose concentration was significantly lower than in that of a normal control group; the lactate-to-glucose ratio was higher for the parkinsonism group, as was the citrate concentration. Other metabolites detected by proton nuclear magnetic resonance (NMR), such as lactate, acetate, creatine, glutamine and alanine, did not show significant differences between the parkinsonism and normal group. Our findings suggest that glucose is used more in the brain of patients with parkinsonism and therefore results in a higher lactate-to-glucose ratio. The higher level of citrate possibly indicated a disorder of the TCA cycle or acetyl CoA transfer in the so-called citrate-pyruvate cycle during fatty acids synthesis in certain areas of brain.

Key words: Parkinsonism – Metabolism – Glucose – Lactate – Citrate – Magnetic resonance spectroscopy

High resolution magnetic resonance spectroscopy (MRS) has been used to study the cerebrospinal fluid (CSF) for the detection of tumours and disc herniations [1], bacterial meningitis [2], subarachnoid haemorrhage [3], mythelmalonic acid in vitamin B_{12} deficiency [4] and Alzheimer's disease [5]. MRS has proved to be valuable in analysing more than one chemical component at a time without tedious sample preparations [6].

The identification of biological molecules by MRS is based on several parameters. Chemical shift (in ppm) and coupling constant (in hertz) offer information about chemical formula, and the signal area reveals the relative concentration of each substance. MRS in combination with MRI may be useful for clinical diagnosis in the future [7]. A detailed review concerning an in vivo study of MRS has been reported [8]. In this study, we applied proton NMR to quantitative comparison of the concentrations of major water-soluble metabolites in the CSF of normal control and patients with parkinsonism. The results of amino acid analysis and creatinine analysis of the CSF samples are also described.

Correspondence to: Kuan Rong Lee, Institute of Life Science, National Tsing Hua University, Hsin-chu, Taiwan 300

Table 1. The average concentration (mmol/l) of major water-soluble metabolites in the CSF of 25 patients with parkinsonism and 12 normal controls measured by proton nuclear magnetic resonance

Metabolite	Parkinsonism	Normal control	*P*-value
Glucose	2.11 ± 0.79	3.11 ± 0.74	0.001
Lactate	1.22 ± 0.42	1.37 ± 0.21	0.179
Lactate/glucose ratio	0.60 ± 0.13	0.46 ± 0.11	0.002
Citrate	0.19 ± 0.07	0.12 ± 0.03	0.000
Creatine	0.08 ± 0.04	0.10 ± 0.02	0.070
Alanine	0.05 ± 0.02[a]	0.04 ± 0.01[a]	0.146
Glutamine	0.38 ± 0.14	0.39 ± 0.12	0.789
Acetate	0.13 ± 0.06	0.09 ± 0.04	0.083

[a] Only 8 patients and 9 normal controls had a measurable alanine signal

Materials and methods

We used deuterium oxide (both 99.8% and 99.99% D atom) and sodium 3-trimethylsilyl-propionate-2,2,3,3-d_4 (TSP); all reagents were of analytical grade.

The 25 patients with parkinsonism were aged between 45 and 81, with an average of 66; there were 18 men and 7 women. Parkinsonism was diagnosed on the basis of the clinical symptoms and signs. CSF was taken by lumbar puncture, and 2–3 ml of clear CSF was collected and poured through a microconcentrator to remove the high-molecular-weight content. One millilitre of this CSF was lyophilised and exchanged once with deuterium oxide (99.8% D atom) and resuspended TSP/D_2O (99.996% D atom).

The spectra were recorded on a spectrometer operating at 300.13 MHz. The parameters were as follows: transmitter pulsing angle 45°, repetition rate 3.0 s, number of signals averaging 512 or 1024, data size 16K. A line-broadening factor of 0.5 Hz was routinely applied to improve the signal-to-noise ratio. Some of the spectra were recorded with a presaturation pulse to suppress the residual water signal. The chemical shift of methyl protons of TSP was used as an internal reference and its signal area was normalised to 1.0 for quantitative comparison of the concentrations of metabolites.

Results

Figure 1 shows a typical proton NMR spectrum and the signal assignments of CSF of a patient with parkinsonism. Table 1 shows the average concentrations of major water-soluble metabolites in the CSF of the normal control group and the group with parkinsonism.

Discussion

In our study, the glucose concentration and lactate-to-glucose (L/G) ratio in the CSF of patients with parkinsonism seemed to be the most useful parameters for clinical

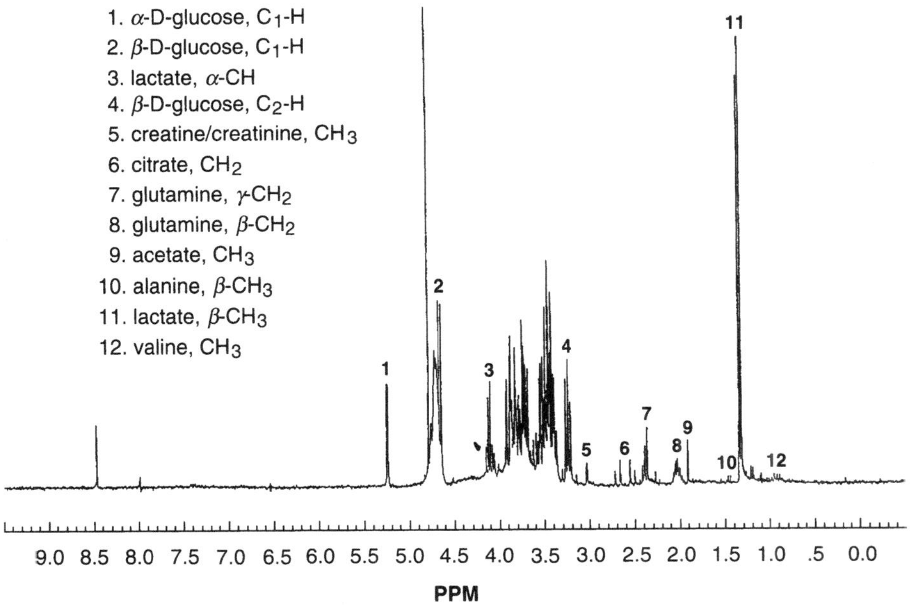

Fig. 1

reference. The glucose concentration was below 2.2 mmol/l in 13 patients (52%), which was definitely abnormal, while only 1 subject in the normal group showed a low glucose content. Therefore, the brain glucose is used more in patients with parkinsonism and results in a higher L/G ratio. In most patients with parkinsonism, the ratio is higher than 0.50 (20 of 25 patients; 80%), whereas only 3 cases (25%) in the normal control group showed a high L/G ratio. Since glucose and lactate signals are the largest two peaks in the proton NMR spectrum, the measurements of their concentrations are highly reliable, and accurate to within 5%. In a separate experiment, serial dilution of glucose and lactate at different concentrations also confirmed that our results were accurate to within 5%. Interestingly, the lactate concentration itself was not statistically significant. This was also observed in our malignant tissues, such as hepatocellular carcinoma and brain tumour (to be published), in which L/G ratio was significant and lactate concentration alone was not. Lactate participates in several biochemical routes, such as interconversion of lactate and pyruvate in glycolysis and gluconeogenesis. The reason why lactate is not statistically significant remains to be answered.

The reason for the higher citrate concentration in patients with parkinsonism is not clear. Citrate is involved primarily in the TCA cycle as an intermediate metabolite, and in the transfer of acetyl CoA from mitochondria to cytosol as an acetyl CoA carrier during fatty acid synthesis. Our observations imply a certain degree of disorder in the TCA cycle and/or in the acetyl CoA transfer between mitochondria and cytosol in the area of a brain lesion. Creatine and alanine are both involved in the energy consumption of brain cells, but our study did not reveal the importance of these two metabolites in parkinsonism. In a separate experiment performed by amino acid analyser, the contents of 20 free amino acids in the CSF did not show a statistically significant difference.

Acknowledgement. This study was supported by grant no. VGH-TC 835501 from the Veterans General Hospital.

References

1. Koschorek F, Gremmel H, Stelten J, Offermann W, Leibfritz D (1983) Cerebrospinal fluid: detection of tumors and disk herniations with MR spectroscopy. Neuroradiology 16:813–816
2. Bell JD, Brown JCC, Sadler PJ, Hughes RD, Williams R (1987) High-resolution proton nuclear magnetic resonance studies of human cerebrospinal fluid. Clin Sci 72:563–570
3. Koschorek F, Gremmel H, Stelten J, Offermann W, Kruger E, Leibfritz D (1989) Characterization of CNS lesions by using high-resolution ^{1}H MR spectroscopy of CSF: preliminary results. AJNR 10:523–527
4. Commodari F, Arnold DL, Sanctuary BC, Shoubridge EA (1991) ^{1}H NMR characterization of normal human cerebrospinal fluid and the detection of methylmalonic acid in a vitamin B_{12} deficient patient. NMR Biomed 4:192–200
5. Miller BL, Moats RA, Shonk T, Ernst T, Woolley S, Ross BD (1993) Alzheimer disease: depiction of increased cerebral myo-inositol with proton MR spectroscopy. Radiology 187:433–437
6. Nicholson JK, Wilson ID (1989) High resolution proton nuclear magnetic resonance spectroscopy of biological fluids. Prog NMR Spectr 21:449–501
7. Lundberg P, Harmsen E, Ho C, Vogel HJ (1990) Nuclear magnetic resonance studies of cellular metabolism. Anal Biochem 191:193–222
8. Howe FA, Maxwell RJ, Saunders DE, Brown MM, Griffiths JR (1993) Proton spectroscopy in vivo. Magn Reson Q 1:31–59

MRI in Minamata disease (organic mercury poisoning): correlation with visual field abnormalities

T. Okuda[1], Y. Korogi[1], M. Takahashi[1], Y. Sakamoto[1], T. Hirai[1], S. Hamatake[1], R. Murakami[1], T. Okajima[2]

[1] Department of Radiology, Kumamoto University School of Medicine, Kumamoto, Japan
[2] Jonan Hospital, Kumamoto, Japan

Abstract. The purpose of this study was to review MRI findings in Minamata disease (MD), and to correlate these with visual field abnormalities. MRI at 1.5T and visual field tests were performed in 20 patients with a mild type of MD, 8 patients with typical MD, and 10 control subjects. The atrophic portions of the calcarine areas were measured in the sagittal planes. In patients with constriction of the visual fields, the anterior portion of the calcarine fissure was significantly dilated, reflecting atrophy of the visual cortex. There was significant correlation between the degree of the temporal visual fields and the width of the calcarine sulci ($r = 0.753$, $P < 0.0001$). MRI has proved to be useful in studying abnormalities of the calcarine area due to methylmercury poisoning.

Key words: Minamata disease – Magnetic resonance imaging – Calcarine fissure – Visual cortex – Visual field abnormalities

Minamata disease (MD), a form of methylmercury poisoning, is a neurological illness caused by ingestion of contaminated seafood [1, 2]. It is characterised by cerebellar and cerebal atrophy, relatively localised in the occipital lobe [3]. Typical neurological findings in MD are sensory disturbance, concentric constriction of the visual fields, and ataxia. Concentric constriction of the visual fields, reflecting atrophy of the calcarine area, is one of the most important symptoms of MD. We have reported that MRI can demonstrate gross pathologic changes [4, 5]. In this study we evaluated MRI focusing on the atrophy of the calcarine area in MD, and correlated this with visual field abnormalities.

Materials and methods

MRI studies were correlated with visual fields in 20 patients with mild MD (mean age 80.6 ± 9.4 years), 8 patients with typical MD (mean age 5.2 ± 5.3 years), and 10 control subjects (mean age 65.2 ± 4.9 years). The visual fields have been followed periodically since the onset of disease, including within 1 month of the MRI study. In 2 patients with typical MD the visual fields were almost normal at the time of examination, although both had shown concentric constriction of the visual field at least until 1969. The remaining 6 patients showed no improvement of the visual field abnormalities. Therefore, the degree of the most severe constriction of the visual fields was adopted.

Correspondence to: T. Okuda, Department of Radiology, Kumamoto University School of Medicine, 1-1-1 Honjo, Kumamoto 860, Japan

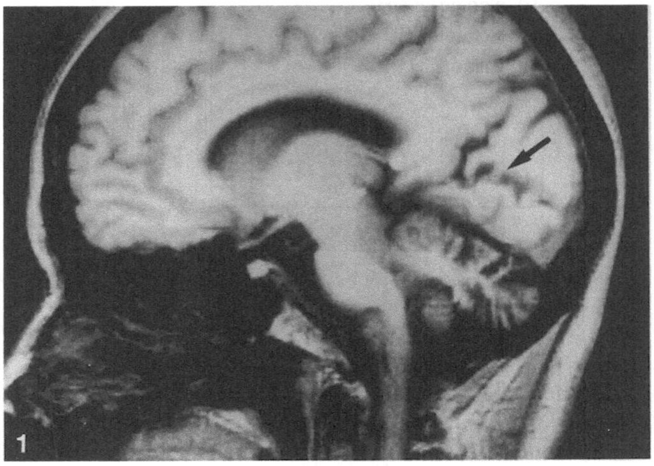

Fig. 1. A 52-year-old woman with typical MD. Sagittal T1-weighted image shows marked dilatation of the anterior portion of the calcarine fissure (*arrow*)

The MR unit used was a 1.5T superconductive type. T1-weighted images were obtained in sagittal sections using a spin-echo technique (TR 600/TE 13-20/2 NEX). The slice thickness was 4–6.5 mm with a 1.0–1.2 mm interslice gap. The field of view was 25 cm, and the matrix size was 192 × 256.

To estimate the degree of atrophy in the calcarine area, the width of the anterior calcarine fissure was measured. Line measurements were made in both the lateral sagittal planes with magnified images directly displayed on an imager console.

Results

The mean width of the calcarine fissure was 2.3 ± 0.4 mm in the mild MD group, 3.6 ± 1.0 mm in the typical MD group, and 1.8 ± 0.4 mm in the control group. The differences between the three groups were all statistically significant ($P < 0.0001$).

In cases with MD, the visual field tests revealed mild to severe concentric constriction of the visual fields (Fig. 1). The temporal visual fields ranged between 25° and 92° from the point of fixation in the mild MD group, and in the typical MD group between 5° and 80°. The visual fields of 10 healthy controls were all normal, with 80° or more.

The relationship between the degree of the unilateral temporal visual fields and the width of the contralateral calcarine fissure was evaluated. The degree of the temporal visual fields (y) and the width of the calcarine fissure (x) showed significant correlation. ($y = -23.27x + 125.6$, $r = -0.744$, $P < 0.0001$) (Fig. 2.)

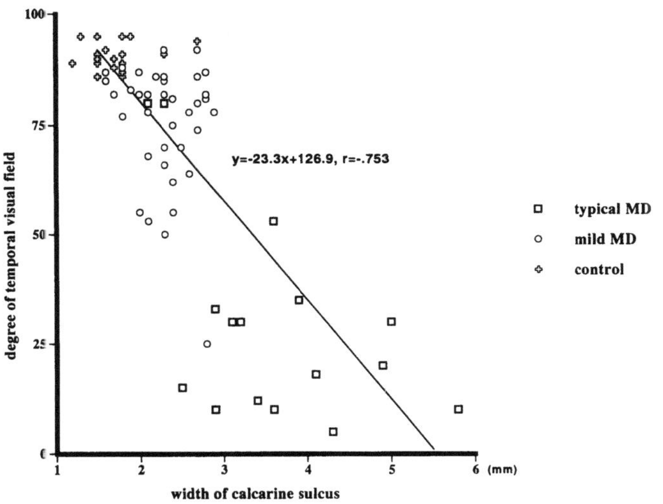

Fig. 2. Correlation between loss of the temporal visual field and the width of the calcarine fissure

Discussion

MD was caused by ingestion of methylmercury-contaminated seafood from Minamata Bay in Japan [1, 2]. The anterior regions of the visual cortex are the most severely disturbed. Since the central portion of the visual fields occupies the posterior area, while the periphery is represented anteriorly, this gives rise to concentric constriction of the visual fields, the most characteristic signs in MD. Pathologic changes in the cerebrum usually take the form of destruction of the normal cortical striation of Gennari. Disintegration and loss of neurons is a basic finding on microscopic examination, and, in moderate to severe cases, the neurons in calcarine areas almost always disappear entirely (status spongious) [1]. In recent years, MRI has become an important diagnostic tool for the demonstration of fine anatomical structures and pathologic changes in the brain. It clearly depicts the unique localisation of calcarine involvement [4, 5]. In this study we evaluated the correlation between MR findings in MD and visual field abnormalities quantitatively. There was significant correlation between the degree of the temporal visual fields and the width of the calcarine fissure, which has revealed that quantitative analysis of MRI is useful not only as a diagnostic aid, but also for providing insight into the pathological process of MD.

References

1. Takeuchi T, Morikawa N, Matsumoto H, Shiraishi Y (1962) A pathologic study of Minamata disease in Japan. Acta Neuropathol (Berl) 2:40–57
2. Tokuomi H, Okajima T, Kanai J, et al (1961) Minamata disease. World Neurol 2:536–545
3. Hunter D, Russell DS (1954) Focal cerebral and cerebellar atrophy in a human subject due to organic mercury compounds. J Neurol Neurosurg Psychiatry 17:235–241
4. Korogi Y, Takahashi M, Shinzato J, Okajima T (1994) MR findings among seven patients with organic mercury poisoning: Minamata disease. AJNR (in press)
5. Korogi Y, Takahashi M, Sumi M, et al (1994) MR imaging of Minamata disease: qualitative and quantitative analysis. Radiat Med (in press)

MRI in chronic toluene abuse

K. Ando[1], S. Tominaga[1], R. Ishikura[2], Y. Takayasu[1], K. Miura[1], N. Nakao[1], M. Yoshihara[3], A. Ueki[3], K. Miyoshi[3]

[1] Department of Radiology, Hyogo College of Medicine
[2] Department of Radiology, Takahazura City Hospital, Hyogo, Japan
[3] Department of Psychiatry, Hyogo College of Medicine, Hyogo, Japan

Abstract. We present two Japanese men with a more than 10-year history of toluene inhalation. In one patient with severe neurological impairments, T2-weighted MRI images showed symmetrical high-signal areas in the posterior limbs of the internal capsules, cerebral white matter, and cerebellar peduncles. There were bilateral reduced intensity areas in the thalami, basal ganglia, and cerebral cortex. Signal intensity changes of the other patient were mild; reduced intensity of the brain cortex has not been reported previously.

Correspondence to: K. Ando, Department of Radiology, Hyogo College of Medicine, 1-1 Mukogawa-cho, Nishinomiya, Hyogo, 650 Japan

Key words: Toluene – Brain – Magnetic resonance imaging – Iron

Chronic toluene abuse causes severe brain damage. MRI studies in two patients suggest that brain iron metabolism may be disturbed.

Case reports

Case 1: A 25-year-old Japanese man had a 15-year history of frequent toluene inhalation. He had noted tremor of the hands for 6 months. Neurological examination revealed cerebellar ataxia, tremor of the limbs, hyperactive tendon reflexes in both legs, bilateral visual disturbance, bilateral hearing loss, and dementia. His own past history and the family were unremarkable.

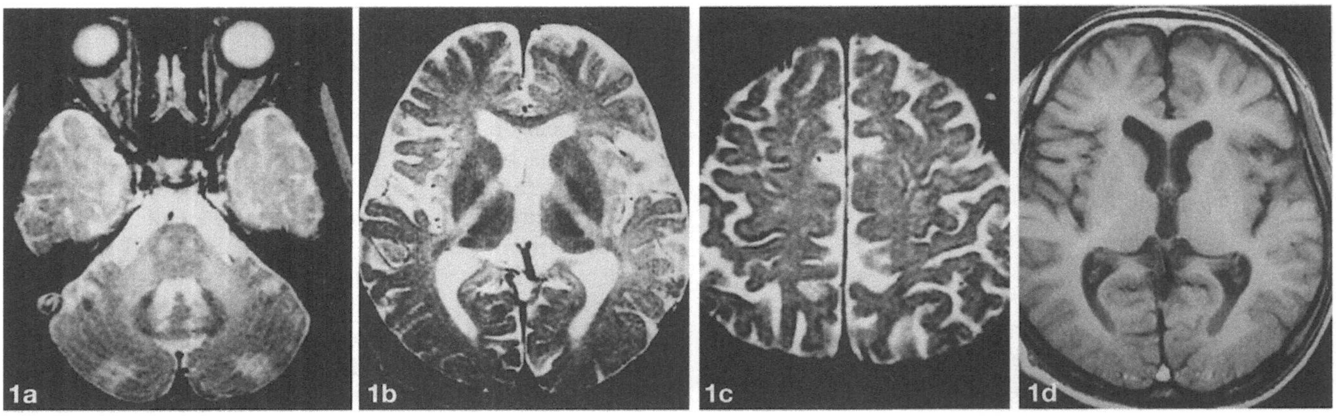

Fig. 1 a–d. Case 1. 25-year-old man with chronic toluene abuse. **a–c** Axial fast spin-echo (TR/TE = 4000/80, echo train = 8) images show symmetrical high signal in the periventricular and deep white matter, pyramidal tracts, including the posterior limb of the internal capsule, and middle cerebellar peduncles. The basal ganglia, thalami and cortical grey matter give low signal. **d** Axial T1-weighted conventional spin-echo (TR/TE = 600/13) image shows brain atrophy

T2-weighted MRI showed symmetrical high-signal areas in the periventricular and deep white matter, pyramidal tracts including the posterior limb of the internal capsule, and middle cerebellar peduncles (Figs. 1a, b). The basal ganglia and thalami bilaterally showed *reduced* intensity on T2-weighted images (Fig. 1b).

Cortical grey matter (especially in the occipital and parietal regions) also showed low-signal areas on T2-weighted images (Fig. 1c). T1-weighted images showed diffuse brain atrophy (Fig. 1d).

Case 2: A 27-year-old Japanese man had a 13-year history of toluene abuse. He frequently fell into hallucinatory confusion after sniffing glue, and his family took him to the hospital for further examination. His own past history and the family history were unremarkable. On neurological examination, visual disturbance and dementia were found. MR signal intensity changes were mild in this patient; T2-weighted images showed symmetrical high-signal areas in the posterior limb of the internal capsule, and low-signal areas bilateral in the thalami. The cortex retained its normal intensity. There were no abnormal intensity areas on T1-weighted images.

Discussion

Toluene is a neurotoxic organic solvent that mainly affects the central nervous system (CNS). Chronic toluene inhalation causes many progressive neurological impairments.

T1-weighted MRI shows diffuse brain atrophy. Findings from T2-weighted MRI in previous reports are as follows [1, 2]: symmetrical increased signal intensity in pyramidal tracts, cerebal white matter and cerebellar peduncles; symmetrically *reduced* signal intensity of the thalami and basal ganglia. In addition to these findings, the cerebral cortex of our case 1 gave reduced signal intensity on T2-weighted images.

Arai et al. [3] reported the neuropathological findings in a toluene intoxication subject, including diffuse demyelination and gliosis in the cerebral and cerebellar white matter. The cause of the areas of abnormally increased intensity in the cerebral white matter, pyramidal tracts, and middle cerebellar peduncles is suggested to be degeneration or demyelination.

Some authors suggest iron deposition as a cause of the decreased intensity areas in the thalami and basal ganglia [1, 2]. Abnormal low-signal areas in the cortex have been reported in amyotrophic lateral sclerosis, and Alzheimer's disease [4, 5]. Oba et al. [4] reported reduced signal intensity in the motor cortex of ALS and suggested that iron deposition, with the degenerative process of the pyramidal tract and of the motor cortex, could be the source of T2 shortening.

We speculate that diffuse demyelination following severe toluene intoxication may cause the iron deposition in the cerebral cortex, which results in the reduced intensity on T2 weighting.

References

1. Caldemeyer KS, Pascuzzi RM, Moran CC, Smith RR (1993) Toluene abuse causing reduced MR signal intensity in the brain. AJR 161:1259–1261
2. Xiong L, Matthes JD, Jinkins JR (1993) MR imaging of "spray heads": toluene abuse via aerosol paint inhalation. AJNR 14:1195–1199
3. Arai K, Tokumara S, Yagishita T, Hirayama K, Iwasaki I (1986) Chronic toluene intoxication and hyperkinésie volitionelle. Brain Nerve 38:1181–1186
4. Oba H, Araki T, Ohtomo K, Monzawa S, Uchiyama G, Koizumi K, Nogata Y, Kachi K, Shiozawa Z, Kobayashi M (1993) Amytrophic lateral sclerosis: T2 shortening in motor cortex at MR imaging. Radiology 189:843–846
5. Drayer BP (1988) Imaging of the aging brain. Pathologic conditions. Radiology 166:797–806

MRI and pathological changes in the brain of patients with chronic liver dysfunction

R. Ishikura[1], K. Ando[2], T. Okawa[2], K. Narasaki[2], T. Morikawa[2], S. Tominaga[2], K. Miura[2], Y. Takayasu[2], N. Nakao[2], J. Inoue[3]

[1] Department of Radiology, Takarazuka City Hospital, Hyogo Japan
[2] Department of Radiology, Hyogo College of Medicine, Hyogo, Japan
[3] Department of Radiology, Ashiya City Hospital, Hyogo, Japan

Abstract. Three patients with chronic liver dysfunction underwent cerebral magnetic resonance imaging and pathological studies of the brain at autopsy. All showed high-signal basal ganglia on T1-weighted images. Proliferation of astrocytes in the globus pallidus was observed in only one of the three brains. Increased amounts of paramagnetic trace metals (Fe, Mn, Zn, and Cu) were detected in the globus pallidus of two brains, but there was no increase in the third brain. These results suggest that an MR signal change in a patient with chronic liver dysfunction does not directly reflect astrocyte proliferation or deposition of paramagnetic trace metals.

Key words: Basal ganglia – Magnetic resonance imaging – Liver cirrhosis

We suggest that a hyperintense basal ganglia in patients with chronic liver dysfunction does not directly reflect the deposition of paramagnetic trace metals or the proliferation of astrocytes.

Materials and methods

Three patients with posthepatic cirrhosis (two men and one woman, ages 53–68 years) underwent cerebral MRI and pathological examinations of the brain at autopsy.

MRI was obtained with a 0.5T super-conducting system using a T1-weighted spin-echo sequence of 500/22 (TR/TE). Pathological examination included macroscopic and light microscopic studies of autopsy brain. Trace metal analysis in the globus pallidus (dried material) was performed by an induction-coupled plasma method. As controls, three autopsy brains from patients without liver dysfunction were also investigated.

Results

The Child-Turcotte classification and the portal-systemic shunts of the three patients at the time of the MRI examination are presented in Table 1. All had portal-systemic collateral vessels. The MRI findings of the three patients are summarised in Table 2. All three showed symmetrical increased intensity in the globus pallidus (GP) on T1-weighted images (Fig. 1a). Cases 2 and 3 also showed a mildly increased intensity in the surrounding structures.

Correspondence to: R. Ishikura, Department of Radiology, Hyogo College of Medicine, 1-1 Mukogawa-cho, Nishimo miya, Hyogo 650, Japan

Table 1. Clinical status and portal-systemic shunts

Case	Age (years)/ sex	Child-Turcotte classification	Types of collateral vessel
1	60/M	B	SMV-IMV; Oesophageal varix
2	68/M	B	Oesophageal varix
3	53/F	B	Paraumbilical; Oesophageal varix

Table 2. MRI findings

Case	High-signal areas on T1-weighted image				
	Globus pallidus	Putamen	Cerebral peduncles	Temporal white matter	Pituitary gland
1	+				
2	+			+	
3	+	+	+	+	+

Table 3. Trace metal analysis of globus pallidus

Case	Metal content (dried material) (ratio patient control)			
	Zn	Fe	Mn	Cu
1	1.80	1.24	1.56	2.18
2	0.96	0.75	0.96	1.09
3	1.27	2.14	2.82	3.48

At autopsy, the brains of these patients showed no macroscopic change in the GP. On microscopic study, type II Alzheimer astrocytes were numerous in the GP of case 3 (Fig. 1b), but were rare in the other two cases. The results of trace metal analysis in the GP are shown in Table 3. Increased amounts of manganese, iron, zinc, and copper were detected in cases 1 and 3, but no metal content was increased in case 2.

Discussion

Deposition of paramagnetic trace metals and/or an astrogliotic reaction have been suggested as the basis for an altered signal intensity of the basal ganglia in patients with chronic liver dysfunction [1] or other diseases [2, 3].

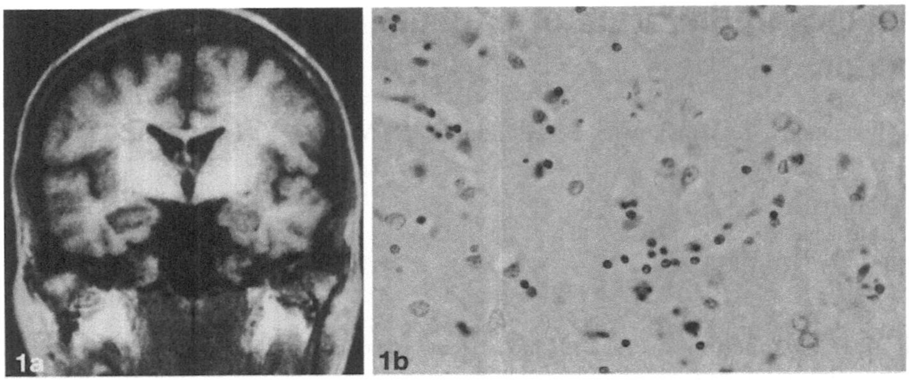

Fig. 1 a, b. Case 3. A 53-year-old woman with posthepatitic cirrhosis. **a** Coronal T1-weighted image (500/22) shows symmetrical increased intensity areas in globus pallidus, putamen, and temporal white matter. **b** Photomicrograph of histological specimen from globus pallidus shows proliferation of type II Alzheimer astrocytes

In this study, we report that the proliferation of astrocytes and an increased content of paramagnetic trace metals (zinc, manganese, iron, and copper) does not always exist in a hyperintense GP. These results lead to the suggestion that an MR signal change does not directly reflect astrocyte proliferation or deposition of paramagnetic trace metals. Uchino et al. [4] suggested that portal-systemic collaterals and cholestasis had a prominent role in the causation of cerebral abnormalities in T1-weighted images. Both present an abnormal metabolic status without normal hepatic clearance. Pujol et al. [5] reported a regression of abnormal signal intensity after liver transplantation.

We speculate that the deposition of unknown metabolites with T1-shortening effects (some kind of protein, for example,) bypassing the hepatic clearance may have some role in signal intensity alteration.

References

1. Inoue E, Hori S, Narumi Y, Fujita M, Kuriyama K, Kadota T, Kuroda C (1991) Portal-systemic encephalopathy: presence of basal ganglia lesions with high signal intensity on MR images. Radiology 179:551–555
2. Mirowitz SA, Westrich TJ, Hirsch JD (1991) Hyperintense basal ganglia on T1-weighted MR images in patients receiving parenteral nutrition. Radiology 191:117–120
3. Mirowitz SA, Sartor K, Gado M (1990) High-intensity basal ganglia lesions on T1-weighted MR images in neurofibromatosis. AJNR 10:1159–1163
4. Uchino A, Hasuo K, Matsumoto S, Masuda K (1993) Cerebral MR imaging in patients with primary biliary cirrhosis. Nippon Acta Radiol 53:145–149
5. Pujol A, Graus F, Peri J, Mercader JM, Rimalo A (1991) Hyperintensity in the globus pallidus on T1-weighted and inversion-recovery MRI: a possible marker of advanced liver disease. Neurology 41:1526–1527

Inflammation

Imaging of HTLV-1 neurological disease in a new endemic area

H. J. Robertson[1], **G. J. Parry**[2], **P. Correa**[3]

[1] Department of Radiology, Louisiana State University Medical Center, New Orleans, Louisiana, USA
[2] Department of Neurology, Louisiana State University Medical Center, New Orleans, Louisiana, USA
[3] Department of Pathology, Louisiana State University Medical Center, New Orleans, Louisiana, USA

Abstract. The extent of HTLV-1 myelopathy and encephalopathy can be shown by standard MRI techniques without intravenous contrast medium injections. CT myelography is less sensitive but can show advanced myelopathy.

Key words: HTLV-1 – Myelopathy – Brain – Magnetic resonance imaging – Computed tomography

The retrovirus, human T-cell lymphotropic virus type 1 (HTLV-1) is a cause of adult T-cell leukemia and lymphoma, myelopathy (HAM), polymyositis and lymphocytic meningitis [1, 5]. MRI facilitates diagnosis and demonstrates the extent of myelopathy and cerebral white matter disease. We illustrate the constitution of MRI in four cases.

Case reports

Case 1. A 34-year-old HTLV-1 seropositive man with a history of intravenous drug abuse had progressive spasticity of the legs with mild weakness for 5 years. There was urinary frequency. No sensory changes were found on examination. MRI showed atrophy of the cord (Fig. 1).

Case 2. A 55-year-old man seropositive for HTLV-1 had progressive stasticity of the legs with mild weakness. Spinal cord atrophy and brain lesions were shown by MRI (Fig. 2).

Case 3. A 54-year-old man HTLV-1 seropositive, had progressive paraparesis for several years. There was no history of intravenous drug abuse or other known factors of HTLV-1 spread. He also had an atrophic spinal cord (Fig. 3).

Case 4. A 42-year-old woman, HTLV-1 seropositive, had progressive leg spasticity and mild weakness and cerebellar ataxia. There was no history of known HTLV-1 modes of infection. There was a previous erroneous diagnosis of multiple sclerosis. MRI revealed not only an atrophic spinal cord, but a Chiari malformation (Fig. 4).

Discussion

HTLV-1 associated myelopathy (HAM) is a progressive spastic paraparesis affecting the legs with predominant motor tract involvement and typically sparing the arms [1]. HAM occurs in an estimated 10% seropositive individuals. It has a slow progressive course over many years. HTLV-1 disease is endemic in Jamaica and Martinique in the Caribbean region, in Columbia, South Africa, Ivory Coast in West Africa, Souther India, Okinawa and Southern Japan [1, 2]. New endemic areas have recently been found in the United States. The pathology is meningomyelitis with progressive demyelination within the spinal cord and mild focal inflammation and demyelination in the brain. Spinal cord disease results in total disability after several years while the commonly occurring brain white matter lesions are less symptomatic [2].

MRI shows atrophy occurring earliest in the lower half of the thoracic cord on T1-weighted sagittal and axial images. Progressive spinal cord atrophy subsequently involved the entire thoracic and cervical spinal cord and medulla oblongata. The anatomical cervical cord enlargement becomes less conspicuous with progressive atrophy. The conus medullaris cord enlargement is relatively preserved until spinal cord atrophy is severe. We have not detected abnormal signal intensity within the spinal cord on T1- or T2-weighted images nor have we seen abnormal enhancement of tissues after intravenous injection of gadolinium DTPA.

MRI usually also shows one or more small focal areas of cerebral white matter increased signal on T2-weighted images [3, 5]. CT myelography may detect intermediate and late spinal cord atrophy, but the subtle brain lesions are usually not detected by CT of the brain. Incidental spinal disease such as cervical sponylosis may mask the underlying HTLV-1 myelopathy [2]. Serological studies are indicated, particularly in endemic areas, where there is suspicion of spinal cord atrophy.

References

1. Osame M, Usuku K, Izumo S, et al (1986) HTLV-1 associated myelopathy: a new clinical entity. Lancet II:1031–1032
2. Cruickshank JK, Rudge P, Dalgleish AG, et al (1989) Tropical spastic paraparesis and human T-cell lymphotropic virus type 1 in the United Kingdom. Brain 112:1057–1090
3. Kira J, Minato S, Yasuto I, et al (1988) Leukoencephalopathy in HTLV-1 associated myelopathy: MRI and EEG data. J Neurol Sci 87:221–232
4. Furukawa Y, Osame M, Une F (1989) Magnetic resonance imaging (MRI) abnormalities in HTLV-1 associated myelopathy (HAM) In: HTLV-1 and the nervous system. Liss, New York, pp 393–396
5. Kira J, Fujihara K, Itoyama Y, et al (1991) Leukoencephalopathy in HTLV-1 associated myelopathy/tropical spastic paraparesis: MRI analysis and a two year follow-up study after corticosteroid therapy. J Neutrol Sci 106:41–49

Correspondence to: J. Robertson, Department of Radiology, LSU Medical Center, 1542 Tulane Avenue, New Orleans, LA TOIR, USA

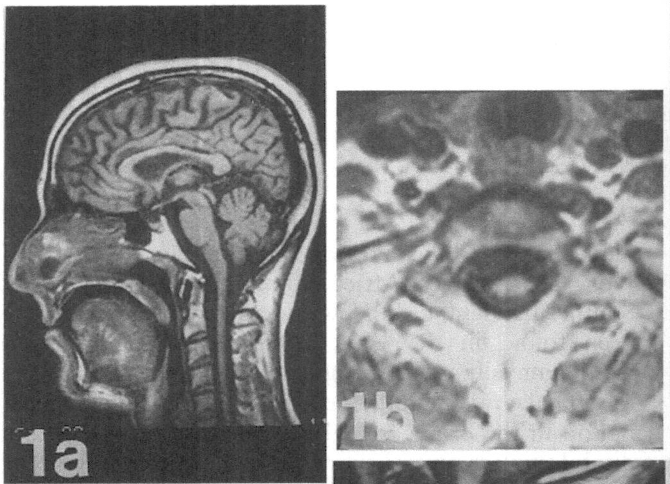

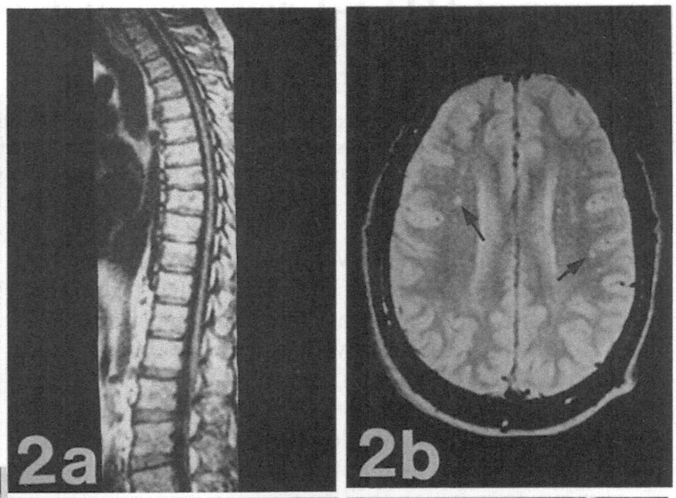

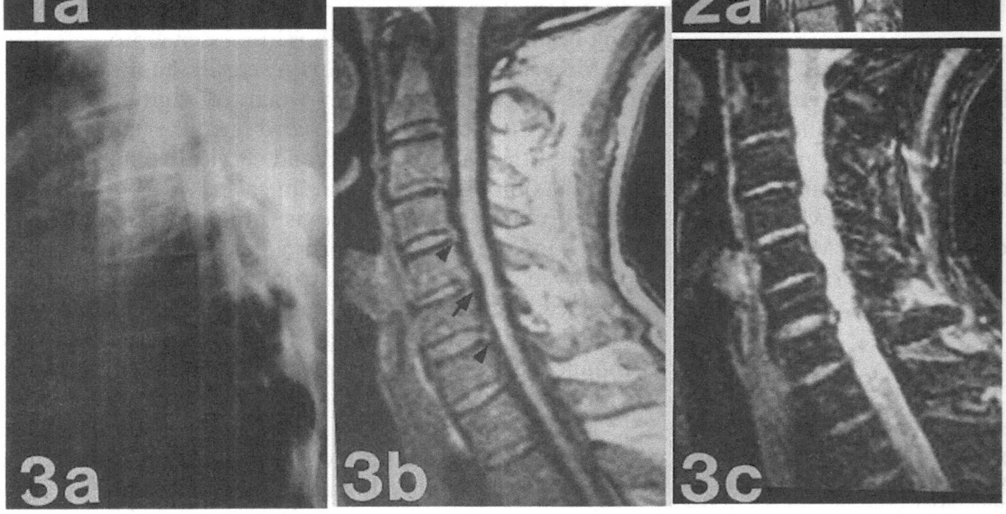

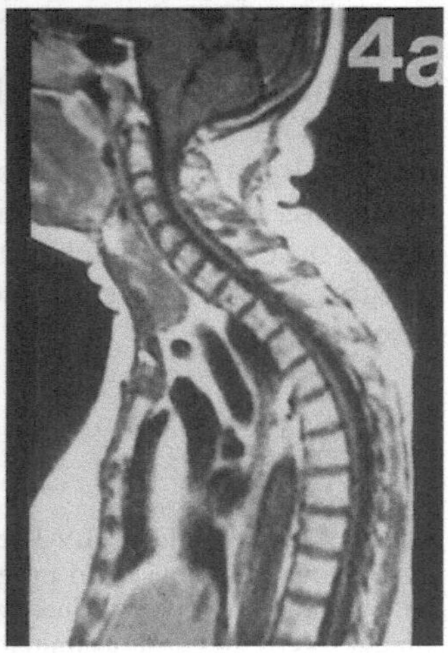

Fig. 1a, b. Case 1. **a** T1-weighted sagittal image shows moderately severe cervical spinal cord atrophy and probable medulla oblongata atrophy. **b** An axial image at the C7 level showing flattened oval atrophic cord

Fig. 2a, b. Case 2. **a** Moderate thoracic spinal cord atrophy on a T1-weighted sagittal image. **b** Multiple focal cerebral white matter lesions on a proton-density image

Fig. 3a–c. Case 3. **a** Lateral thoracic projection of myelogram showing moderate cord atrophy. **b** T1-weighted sagittal cervical spine images show moderate cervical spinal cord atrophy C5-6 spondylosis (*arrow*) C4-5 and C6-7 disc protrusion (*arrow heads*)

Fig. 4. Case 4. Moderate cervical and thoracic cord atrophy on T1-weighted sagittal spine image. Incidental Chiari malformation with cerebellar tonsillar ectopia

Gd-DTPA-enhanced MRI of intracranial tuberculomas

R. Kapur, S. K. Aggarwal, R. Gothi, S. S. Doda, R. Dutta

Diwan Chand Satya Pal Aggarwal Imaging Research Centre, 10-B, Kasturba Gandhi Marg, New Delhi, India

Abstract. Tuberculosis, a necrotising bacterial infection, is amongst the forerunners of health problems in the developing world. It is often not possible to differentiate tuberculomas from other inflammatory granulomas, small gliomas or metastasis on imaging.

Correspondence to: R. Kapur

Key words: Magnetic resonance imaging – Brain – Tuberculoma – Gadolinum-DTPA

The purpose of this study is to determine the diagnostic value of gadolinum (Gd)-DTPA-enhanced magnetic resonance imaging (MRI) in intracranial tuberculosis. The

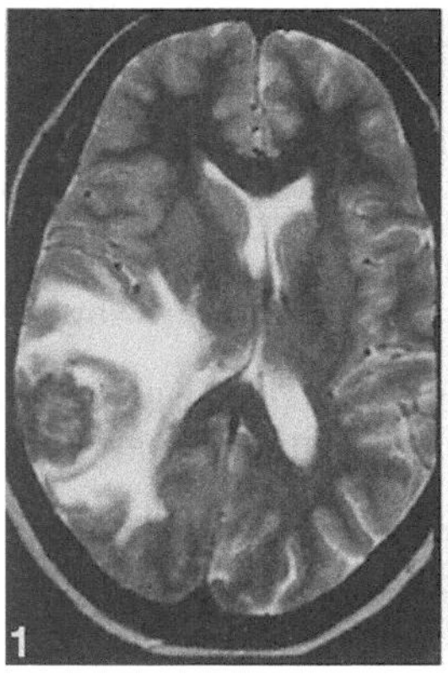

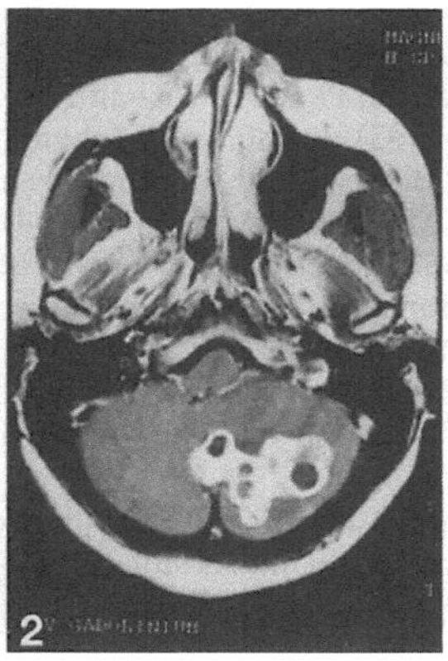

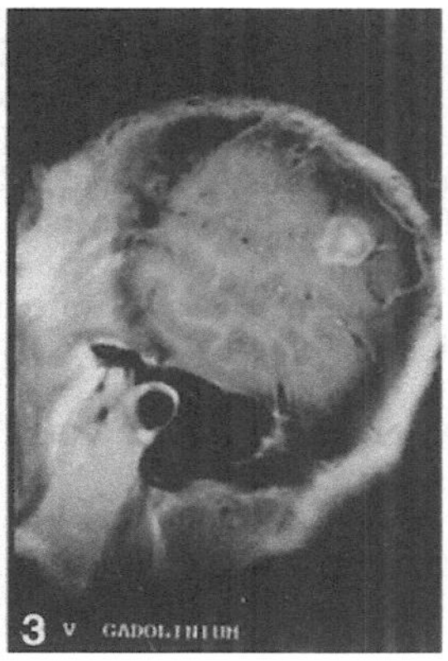

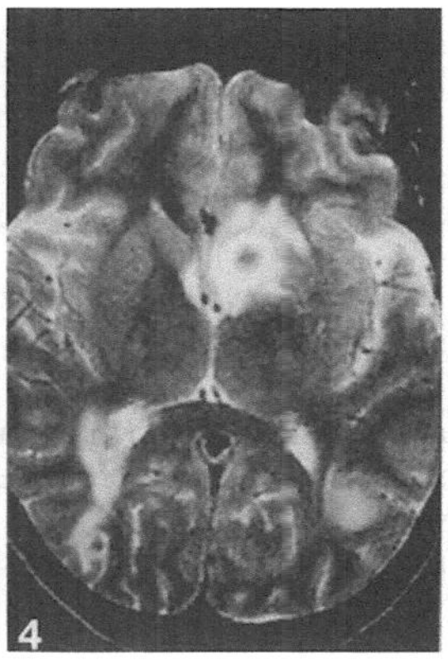

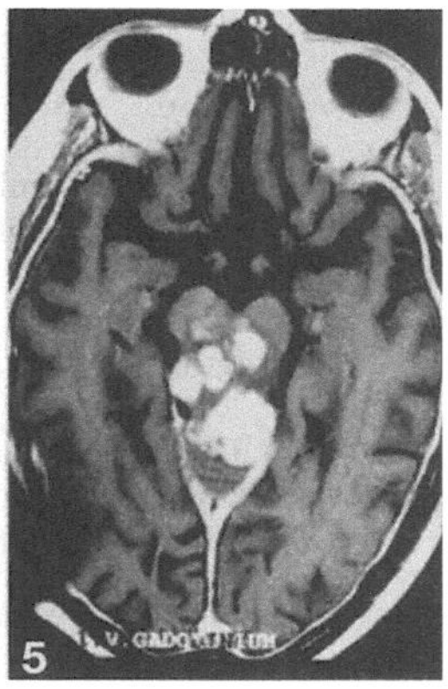

Fig. 1. Axial T2-weighted image shows a solid, well-defined, low signal intensity mass with multiple nubbins and surrounding oedema, causing ventricular compression

Fig. 2. Gd-DTPA-enhanced axial T1-weighted image. There are multiple small tubercles, some with caseating and liquified centres dispersed within an oedematous brain; there is a cluster of ring-enhancing lesions

Fig. 3. Contrast-enhanced T1-weighted sagittal image shows peripheral enhancing lesion with central pooling of contrast medium – the 'target sign'

Fig. 4. Multiple nodular lesions displaying crescentic rings of progressive bright signal intensity from centre outwards on T2-weighted imaging giving an "onion skin" appearance

Fig. 5. Axial Gd-DTPA-enhanced T1-weighted image shows multiple enhancing lesions in the midbrain and quadrigeminal cistern. Diffuse leptomeningeal enhancement is seen

special emphasis is on documenting the signs of tuberculomas on MRI, which would differentiate them from mitotic lesions and thus allow early institution of appropriate therapy.

Materials and methods

Thirty-five patients presumed to harbour intracranial tuberculomas were studied with Gd-DTPA on a 1.0 T system. In 4 patients the diagnosis was confirmed by biopsy and 10 showed improvement on antituberculous therapy (ATT). The age of the patients ranged from 3 to 60 years.

Results

Disc/ring-enhancing lesions were the most frequent morphological features observed. In 7 patients, a conglomerate, grape-like cluster was seen, along with enhancement of the adjacent leptomeninges. A central pooling of contrast medium within the granuloma was present in 2 patients, while a lamellated, "onion-skin" appearance was seen in 4.

Discussion

The typical tuberculoma is a solid, well-defined avascular mass with multiple nubbins extending to and compressing the surrounding brain. It has a firm collagenous capsule surrounding an often gritty, caseating central core. This is usually referred to as the mature form of tuberculoma [1].

Few reports have dealt with the MR appearances of tuberculomas [2–5]. The appearance of iso- to hypointense lesions on T1-weighted images, which become progressively hypointense on T2-weighted images, has been reported to be pathognomonic of tuberculomas [4]. Of 35 patients presumed to harbour cerebral tuberculomas (4 were confirmed by biopsy and 10 showed a therapeutic response to ATT), the lesions were found to be either homogenously hypointense or revealed a central hyperintense nidus within the hypointense lesion on T2-W images (Figs. 1, 2). The T2 hypointensity (T2 shortening) may be a reflection of the relative proportion of macrophages, cellular infiltrates and fibrosis within the granuloma [5, 6]. However, hypointensity on T2-weighted images has also been seen in fungal granulomas, haemorrhagic metastases and cysticeral granulomas. The target sign, supposedly a pathognomonic, albeit infrequent, sign [7, 8], was seen in 2 patients (Fig. 3). We observed a lamellated, "onion-skin" appearance (Fig. 4) in 4 patients, which we feel is specific to a benign aetiology and possibly exclusively indicates tuberculomas (3 of these patients had a surgically proven diagnosis in our series).

The MRI morphological features of tuberculomas can be classified into two categories:

1. Major criteria (cluster formation, onion-skin appearance, target sign on contrast enhancement)
2. Minor criteria (low signal intensity on T2-weighted images, enhancement of adjacent leptomeninges (Fig. 5), peripheral distribution, CSF biochemistry, positive chest radiographs, blood ELISA, Mantoux test)

Based on these criteria, one major and at least two minor criteria on patients may be considered sufficient evidence for tuberculosis, and the patient is put on ATT. This attains importance because specific therapy is most effective when instituted early on, and irreversible brain damage may result from waiting 6–8 weeks for culture proof of diagnosis.

References

1. Dastur HM (1975) Tuberculoma. In Vinken PJ, Bruyn GW (eds) Handbook of clinical neurology, 18. Elsevier, New York, pp 413–426
2. Chang KH, Han MH, Roh JK, et al (1990) Gd-DTPA-enhanced MR imaging in intracranial tuberculosis. Neuroradiology 32: 19–25
3. Gupta RK, Jena A, Sharma A, Guha DK, Khushru S, Gupta AK (1988) MR imaging of intracranial tuberculomas. J Comput Assist Tomogr 12:280–285
4. Desai SB, Shah VC, Tavri OJ, Rao P (1991) MRI: more specific than CT in cranial tuberculomas. Neuroradiology 33 [Suppl]: 216–218
5. Gupta RK, Pandey R, Khan EM, Mittal P, Gujral RB, Chhabra DK (1993) Intracranial tuberculomas: MRI signal intensity correlation with histopathology and localized proton spectroscopy. Magn Reson Imaging 11:443–449
6. Sze G, Zimmerman RD (1990) Magnetic resonance imaging of infections and inflammatory diseases. Radiol Clin North Am 26:839–858
7. Van Dyke A (1988) CT of intracranial tuberculomas with specific reference to the 'target sign'. Neuroradiology 30:329–336
8. Welchman JM (1979) Computerised tomography of intracranial tuberculoma. Clin Radiol 30:567–573

CT in intracranial tuberculosis in children: clinicoradiological correlations

S. Kataria[1], A. Kumari[1], N. Khandelwal[1], D. Takhtani[1], L. Kumar[2], S. Suri[1]

[1] Department of Radiodiagnosis, Postgraduate Institute of Medical Education and Research, Chandigarh, 160012 India
[2] Department of Paediatrics, Postgraduate Institute of Medical Education and Research, Chandigarh, 160012 India

Abstract. Clinicoradiological correlations in neurotuberculosis were studied in 30 children with the help of contrast-enhanced computed tomography (CT) carried out on admission, and after 2 months, 6 months and 1 year. Moderate to severe hydrocephalus with periventricular lucency was a bad prognostic sign. Fourteen of the 18 tuberculomas responded clinically to antituberculous treatment, but 50% showed radiological sequelae which included focal atrophy and calcification. Moderate to severe exudates, when seen on the initial CT scan, were associated with poor outcome. Newer lesions seen in 8 patients included six tuberculomas and four infarcts, which developed in patients having exudates on the initial scan, and 1 patient with a tuberculoma developed exudates later on. The appearance of newer lesions during antituberculous therapy was associated with a poor host response.

Key words: Tuberculosis – Intracranial computed tomography

Computed tomography (CT) offers a unique, rapid, sensitive and non-invasive tool for documenting the pathoanatomical changes seen in intracranial tuberculosis [1–3]. It is also an excellent modality for following up the patient while on treatment. There is plenty of literature describing the spectrum of intracranial tuberculosis, but very few studies have been done where follow-up CT studies are available while on treatment, especially in children. The aim of this study was to investigate and establish the clinicoradiological correlations in intracranial tuberculosis in a paediatric population, using CT.

Correspondence to: S. Kataria

Methods

Thirty consecutive paediatric patients with high clinical suspicion and laboratory parameters suggesting intracranial tuberculosis formed the study group. All patients had a detailed clinical examination and underwent contrast-enhanced CT (CECT) of the head and follow-up head CECT after 2 months, 6 months and 1 year. The status of the ventricular system, exudates (especially in the basal clisterns), focal parenchymal lesions, and associated oedema or infarcts were specially noted in the initial work-up, and subsequently correlated with the follow-up scan while the patients were on antituberculous treatment (ATT). Ten patients required shunt surgery.

Results

Clinically, the children presented with vomiting (66.2%), convulsions (56.6%), fever (53.3%), meningeal signs (40%) and headache (10%). Neurological examination revealed signs of meningeal irritation (40%), papilloedema (50%), altered sensorium (40%), cranial nerve palsy (33%), hemiparesis (10%), and decerebrate posture (10%). Thirteen patients (43.3%) had no neurological deficits.

Chest radiography was abnormal in 7 patients (23.3%). Cerebrospinal fluid (CSF) examinations in 16 cases showed raised protein levels (15), reduced sugar (12), and raised total cell count (15).

All the CT studies were done on a Schimadzu 2000 scanner, using a 10-mm slice thickness at 10-mm table steps after giving bolus contrast. CT findings at the time of admission are given in Table 1. Hydrocephalus was mild (ventricle-head ratio-VHR 30–39%) in 5, moderate (VHR 40–46%) in 5 and severe (VHR >47%) in 4 cases. Periventricular lucency was associated with severe hydrocephalus in 4 patients and with moderate hydrocephalus in 3. Exudates were noted in 12 patients, most com-

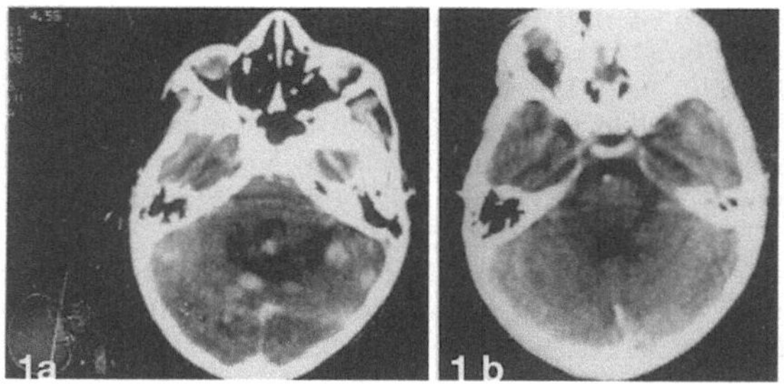

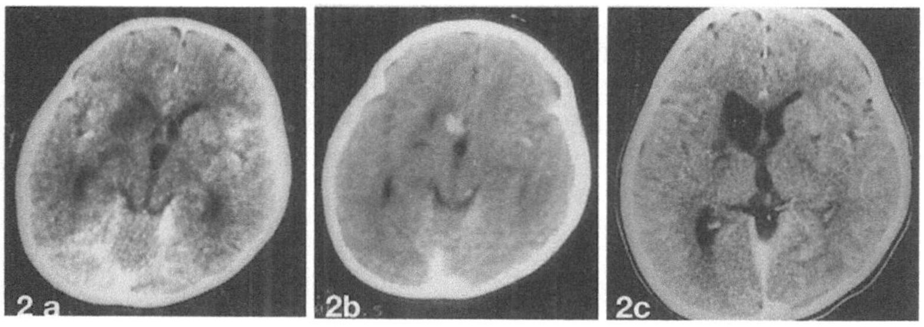

Fig. 1. a Contrast-enhanced CT on admission, showing multiple ring and disc lesions in posterior cranial fossa. **b** At 6 months the lesions have completely disappeared

Fig. 2. a Contrast-enhanced CT on admission: acute infarct in left middle cerebral artery territory and exudate in right sylvian fissure. **b** At 2 months a new parenchymal lesion has appeared. Note reduction in exudates in sylvian fissure. **c** At 6 months exudates have completely cleared, and chronic infarct is seen, with a dilated left frontal horn

monly in the suprasellar and ambien cisterns (100%), quadrigeminal cisterns (91.67%), and sylvian fissure (83.3%). Exudates were graded as mild, moderate and severe as suggested by Bhargava et al. [5]. Large ring lesions were the commonest focal parenchymal abnormalities (13/18), followed by disc lesion (3/18), and conglomerate lesion (2/18). Twelve of 18 focal lesions were situated supratentorially, 2 were infratentorial, and the remaining 4 had multiple lesions above and below the tentorium. Two patients had infarcts on the initial CT. The follow-up scan showed the appearance of new lesions during treatment in 8 patients. The nature of new lesions, their time of appearance and the initial lesions over which these developed are given in Table 1. The final clinical outcomes of patients with various CT findings at admission are summarised in Table 1. Four of the 8 patients developing new lesions on therapy had a clinical outcome consistent with group III, and 3 patients with group II of the classification suggested by Kingsley et al. [4]. One patient from this group, who had developed a bilateral middle cerebral artery infarct, succumbed to the disease in the 8th month.

Table 1. Final outcome and CT findings in clinical groups suggested by Kingsley et al. [4]

	Group I	Group II	Group III	Group IV
Hydrocephalus				
Mild	2	2	1	–
Moderate	–	3	2	–
Severe	–	2	2	–
Periventricular lucency	1	3	3	–
Focal parenchymal lesion				
Disc	2	–	1	–
Ring	11	1	–	
Conglomerate	1	–	1	–
Exudates				
Mild	1	–	–	–
Moderate	–	3	3	–
Severe	–	1	3	1
Infarcts	–	1	1	–

Discussion

In a proper clinical setting and supportive CSF findings, the head CT may suggest a diagnosis of neurotuberculosis. Periventricular lucency, which is present in moderate to severe hydrocephalus, was also associated with poor prognosis. The presence of exudates was also related to a poor final outcome of the disease, as 11 cases of moderate to severe exudates showed poor response to the treatment, probably due to lingering infeciton as they turn fibrous during treatment.

Eighteen patients showed focal parenchymal lesions on the initial CT. The commonest form of parenchymal involvement seen in our series was large ring lesions, either single or multiple (72.7%). Other patterns observed were disc lesions and conglomerate lesions. Two distinct patterns of resolution were observed. The commoner pattern was a decrease in size, perifocal oedema and contrast enhancement of the lesion initially, with focal atrophy and calcification later on (50%). In another pattern of resolution, ring lesions showed increased hypodensity in the centre before finally disappearing completely (16.6%). In 3 patients the first step in the resolution of these lesions was only the decrease and subsequent disappearance of the oedema before the focal lesion disappeared. The majoritiy of the parenchymal lesions in our study disappeared after 2–6 months of therapy (Fig. 1). Of the four focal lesions which did not respond to therapy, two were ring lesions, one a disc lesion and one a conglomerate lesion. In fact, surgery was performed in the patient with the latter lesion, as the size of the lesion increased in the follow-up CT, arousing suspicion of glioma. Contrary to earlier reports that the incidence of calcification is not common in treated neurotuberculosis [6], we observed calcification in 9 out of 18 patients treated with ATT, including calcification of exudates in 2 patients.

Cerebral infarcts, which have been well described [7], were also seen in 2 patients in our series on the first CT. Both these infarcts were situated in the middle cerebral (MCA) territory. Four patients developed infarcts during the course of treatment, and the MCA territory was the commonest involved in this group as well.

The development of new lesions in patients on ATT is well documented [8, 9], as was also observed in our series, in which 8 patients developed new lesions while on therapy. Exudates in the initial CT are more likely to be associated with the development of new lesions. Patients with new lesions developing during therapy showed varied clinical outcomes ranging from group II to group IV, thus showing mixed clinical results.

References

1. De Angelis LM (1981) Intracranial tuberculoma - case report and review of literature. Neurology 31:1133–1136
2. Enzmann DR, Norman D, Mani J, et al (1976) Computed tomography of granulomatous basal arachnoiditis. Radiology 120:341–344
3. Whelan MA, Stern J (1981) Intracranial tuberculoma. Radiology 138:75–81
4. Kingsley DP, Hendrickse WA, Kendall BE, Swash M, Singh V (1987) Tuberculous meningitis: role of CT in management and prognois. J Neurol Neurosurg Psychiatry 50:30–36
5. Bhargava S, Gupta AK, Tandon PN (1982) Tuberculous meningitis - CT study. Br J Radiol 55:189–196
6. Enzmann DR (1984) Imaging of infections and inflammations of central nervous system - computed tomography, ultrasound and nuclear magnetic resonance. Raven Press, New York
7. Hsieh FY, Chia LG, Shen WC (1992) Locations of cerebral infarctions in tuberculous meningitis. Neuroradiology 34:197–199
8. Lees AJ, Macleod AF, Marshall J (1980) Cerebral tuberculoma developing during the treatment of TBM. Lancet I:1208–1211
9. Malone JL, Paparello S, Rickman LS, et al (1990) Intracranial tuberculoma developing during therapy for tuberculous meningitis. West J Med 152:188–190

Dissemination of tuberculous granuloma after stereotactic needle brain biopsy

A. C. A. Magalhães, L. A. Bacheschi, S. C. Mathias

Department of Radiology, Section of Magnetic Resonance, Hospital das Clínicas, University of São Paulo, São Paulo, Brazil

Abstract. Two patients with dissemination of tuberculous granuloma after needle brain biopsy were seen. The first was a 42-year-old man with headache, dizziness and fever for 1 month. MRI revealed a right cerebellar and parietal abscess. A stereotactic needle brain biopsy of the cerebellar lesion was performed, with aspiration of suppurative material positive for *Mycobacterium tuberculosis.* MRI showed multiple variously sized lesions, with contrast enhancement at the right cerebellar lobe along the course of the needle biopsy. The second was a 17-year-old woman undergoing 3 months of unsuitable treatment for pulmonary tuberculosis, who developed fever, headache, and right hemiparesis. MRI revealed a left granulomatous thalamic lesion and hypertensive hydrocephalus. She was submitted to a ventricular shunt and stereotactic needle biopsy of the lesion. After 12 days, MRI showed multiple size-variegated lesions, with contrast enhancement in the left temporal region along the course of the needle.

Key words: Tuberculosis - Brain, infections - Brain, biopsy

We report two cases of brain tuberculosis, submitted to stereotactic needle biopsy for diagnostic purposes. In both cases, after 30 and 12 days MRI showed multiple variously sized lesion with contrast enhancement along the route of the stereotactile needle.

Correspondence to: L. A. Bacheschi, University São Paulo School of Medicine, 05444-010-Rua dos Tamanas 506, São Paulo, SP, Brazil

Case reports

Case 1

A 42-year-old man, previously healthy, had suffered from headache, dizziness and fever for 1 month. Neurological examination showed cerebellar ataxia. CT revealed a left cerebellar and right frontal abscess. Chest radiography revealed a pulmonary nodule. Anti-HIV ELISA and Western blot were positive. A stereotactic needle brain biopsy was performed with aspiration of supparative material positive for *Mycobacterium tuberculosis.* Antituberculosis therapy was initiated, with clinical improvement. The patient left the hospital after 20 days of treatment. Two weeks later he returned with fever and signs of intracranial hypertension. MRI showed multiple, variously sized lesions at the cerebellar lobe, along the course of the needle biopsy (Fig. 1). Antituberculous drugs were continued and dexamethasone was added, with progressive improvement and discharge within 40 days.

Case 2

A 17-year-old woman undergoing 3 months of unsuitable treatment for pulmonary tuberculosis developed fever, headache, and right cerebellar and pyramidal signs. Neurological examination showed bilateral papilloedema, right cerebellar ataxia and right hemiparesis. MRI revealed a granulomatous thalamic lesion with perifocal oedema and mass effect, and hypertensive hydrocephalus. Anti-HIV ELISA and Western blot were negative. The patient was submitted to a ventricular shunt and stereotactic needle biopsy. The material obtained was negative for *Mycobacterium tuberculosis*, *Toxoplasma gondii*, and other pyogenic agents. Nevertheless, the patient reinitiated antituberculosis treatment, with good outcome. Twelve days after the stereotactic needle biopsy, the clinical picture worsened, with seizures, fever and stupour. MRI showed multiple variously sized lesions in the left temporal region, along the course of the needle biopsy (Fig. 2). Another needle biopsy was performed, with the location of a Rickhan chamber to administer streptomycin inside the

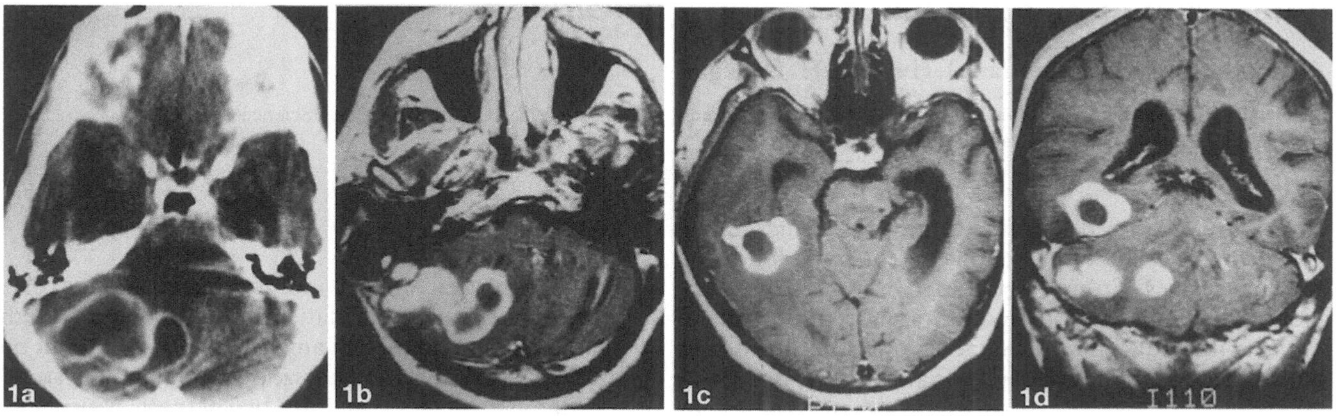

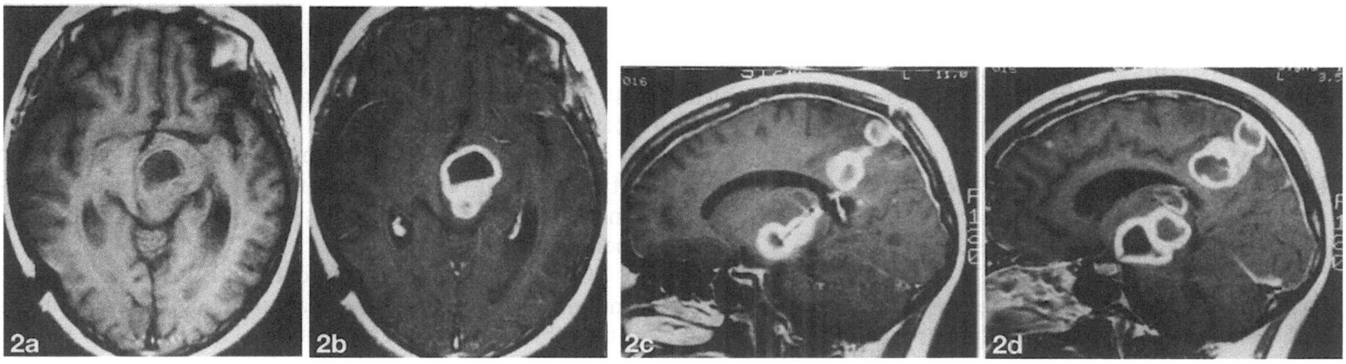

Fig. 1 a–d. A 42-year-old man with headache, dizziness and fever for 1 month. Neurological examination showed cerebellar ataxia. **a** CT revealed left cerebellar and right frontal abscesses. A stereotactic needle brain biopsy was performed, with aspiration of suppurative material positive for *M. tuberculosis*. **b–d** MRI 5 weeks after the biopsy (axial T1-weighted and coronal contrast-enhanced T1-weighted images) show multiple lesions on the cerebellum along the course of the needle biopsy

Fig. 2 a–d. A 17-year-old girl undergoing 3 months of unsuitable treatment for pulmonary tuberculosis developed fever, headache, and right cerebellar and pyramidal signs. **a, b** MRI (axial T1-weighted images before and after contrast medium) show a thalamic granuloma with perifocal oedema and mass effect, and hydrocephalus. **c, d** MRI (sagital contrast-enhanced T1-weighted images) show multiple and varied-size lesions in the left temporal region, along the course of the needle biopsy

lesion once a week for 5 weeks. The mental state and intracranial pressure improved and the seizures were under control, but the right motor deficit remained until she left hospital.

Discussion

In developing countries 5–8% of space-occupying lesions of the central nervous system are tuberculomae [1]. CT and MRI are equally sensitive to show deeply located tuberculomae [2]. Diagnosis can be difficult in the absence of extracranial tuberculosis, and in MRI studies other infections or neoplastic diseases may present similar findings [1, 2], although some distinctive features have been stressed [3]. Brain biopsy had to be considered in these cases [1, 4] until other noninvasive methods, like MR spectroscopy, had been developed [5]. These cases demonstrate the high sensibility of MRI to dissemination of infectious processes, either in the cerebrospinal fluid spaces or inside the cerebral paranchyma [1, 3].

Stereotactic biopsy allows diagnosis and permits abscess drainage. In this opened condition, the lesion becomes more susceptible to specific drug therapy [4, 5]. In these two cases, the dissemination of tuberculous granuloma did not lead to failure of specific treatment.

References

1. Bouchama A, al-Kawi MZ, Kanaan I, Coates R, Jallu A, Rahm B, Siqueira EB (1991) Brain biopsy in tuberculoma: the risk and benefits. Neurosurgery 29:405–409
2. Salgado P, Del Brutto OH, Talamas O, Zentero MA, Rodríguez-Carbajal J (1989) Intracranial tuberculoma: MR imaging. Neuroradiology 31:299–302
3. Gupta RK, Jena A, Sharma A, Guha DK, Khushu S, Gupta AK (1988) MR imaging of intracranial tuberculomas. J Comput Assist Tomogr 12:280–285
4. Gupta RK, Jena A, Singh AK, Sharma A, Puri V, Gupta M (1990) Role of Magnetic resonance (MR) in the diagnosis and management of intracranial tuberculomas. Clin Radiol 41:120–127
5. Gupta RK, Pandey R, Khan EM, Mittal P, Gujral RB, Chhabra DK (1993) Intracranial tuberculomas: MR signal intensity correlation with histopathology and localised proton spectroscopy. Magn Reson Imaging 11:443–449

Follow-up imaging in parenchymal cysticercosis

C. S. Zee, M. Terk, S. Destian, J. Huprich, H. D. Segall

University of Southern California School of Medicine, Department of Radiology, LAC + USC Imaging Science Center, 1744 Zonal Avenue, Los Angeles, CA 90033, USA

Abstract. We studied the natural history of intracranial parenchymal cysticercosis lesions by obtaining follow-up imaging studies. From 6 weeks to 4 years in 92 patients, along with their clinical findings and laboratory data. Patients treated with medical therapy were excluded. The natural history in the majority of patients with intracranial parenchymal cysticercosis cysts without medical or surgical intervention is self-limiting. Treatment is not warranted in these patients. However, a small group of patients with progression of the disease documented on follow-up imaging studies may require medical or surgical intervention.

Key words: Cysticercosis, parenchymal – Cysticercosis, natural history

---

Pathologists have identified a series of alterations occurring within and surrounding the parenchymal cysticercal larva from its earliest viable stage to its final stage. Escobar [1] identified four stages the parasite within the cerebral paranchyma undergoes. In the first (vesicular) stage, the larva is seen as a small marginal nodule projecting into a small cyst containing clear fluid; a very thin capsule surrounds the cyst. In the next (colloidal vesicular) stage, the larva begins to degenerate and mineralize, the cyst fluid becomes turbid and its capsule is thicker. By the granular nodular (third) stage, the cyst has undergone refraction, its coarsely granular contents have mineralized further, and its capsule is quick thick and collagenous. By the final (nodular calcified) stage, the lesion has shrunk to one half or even one quarter of its original size and its completely mineralized. On computed tomography (CT) this noncystic lesion is represented by a small, completely calcified nodule. This dormant, calcified, long-standing residue exhibits no imaging manifestations of surrounding active brain reaction [2–5].

Materials and methods

Ninety-two patients with appropriate, comparable studies and adequate clinical information were selected for study from a group of 320 patients with neurocysticercosis who had neuroimaging studies. Of the 92 patients, the majority (56 patients) had follow-up studies within 3–6 months (range: 4 weeks–4 years).

Correspondence to: C. S. Zee

Results

The patients were divided into four major groups.

Group 1 consists of patients whose imaging studies demonstrated evolution of any or all the cysts into the next stage(s), or a decrease in the size of any or all the cysts with or without a calcification. Fifty-two of the 92 patients with parenchymal cysts (57%) fell within this group (Fig. 1A–D, Fig. 2A, B, C).

Group 2 consists of patients who exhibited no change in any cyst on follow-up studies. Sixteen patients (17%) demonstrated no change.

Group 3 consists of patients whose follow-up imaging studies displayed the appearance of new cyst(s), or an increase in the size of the cyst(s). Eleven patients (12%) belonged to this group.

Group 4 consists of patients with mixed findings on imaging studies, i.e. some cysts showing group 1 findings and others showing progression. There were 13 patients (14%) in this group.

Discussion

Our experience indicates that the majority of the patients with parenchymal cysticercal cysts (68/92, 74%) who had no medical or surgical treatment directed at the cysts exhibited either evolution of any or all the cysts into subsequent stages, or a decrease in size of any or all of the cysts, or resolution of any or all of the cysts with or without calcification, or no change (i.e. groups, 1 or 2) on follow-up imaging studies. Since the majority of parenchymal cysticercal cysts frequently abate (some leaving only a small calcified residue on CT studies), a conservative follow-up study is advocated at our institution whenever urgent intervention can be avoided. It is desirable to perform a follow-up imaging within 3–6 months, to evaluate the natural course of the disease for each patient. In addition, when a single ring-like enhancing lesion is encountered, the differential diagnosis could include a glioma, an abcess and cysticercosis. An abcess can usually be excluded by evaluating clinical information such as fever, nuchal rigidity, etc. A glioma can be excluded by the absence of elevated cysticercosis titer in the blood and cerebrospinal fluid (CSF). An increase in the size of a ring-like enhancing lesion on imaging studies makes the lesion more likely to be a glioma. Of course, cases of cerebral abscesses and gliomas are excluded for the current study.

Acknowledgement. We wish to express our appreciation to Linda Needham and her colleague for their cooperation in the preparation of this manuscript.

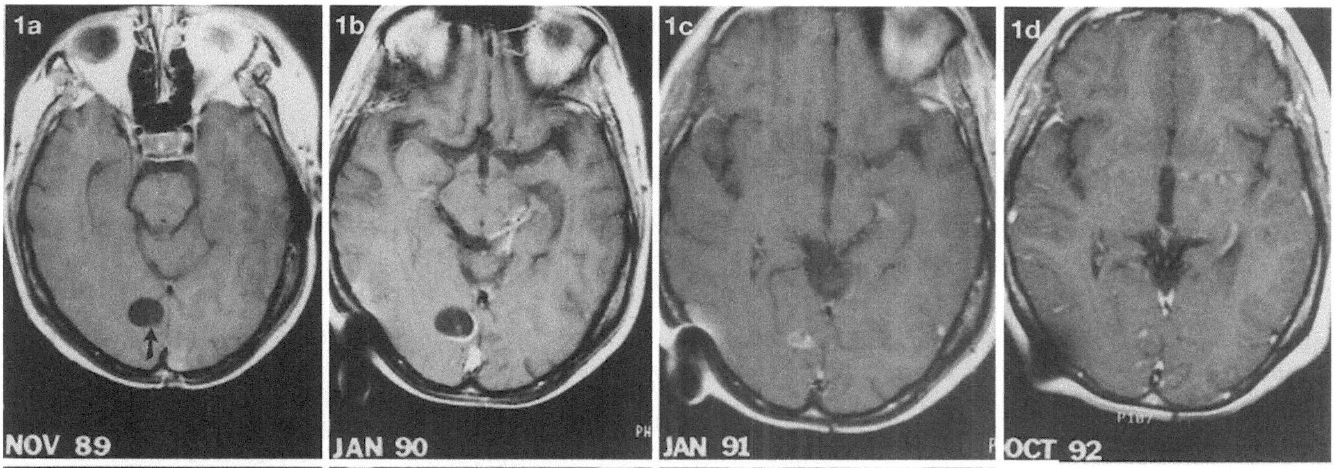

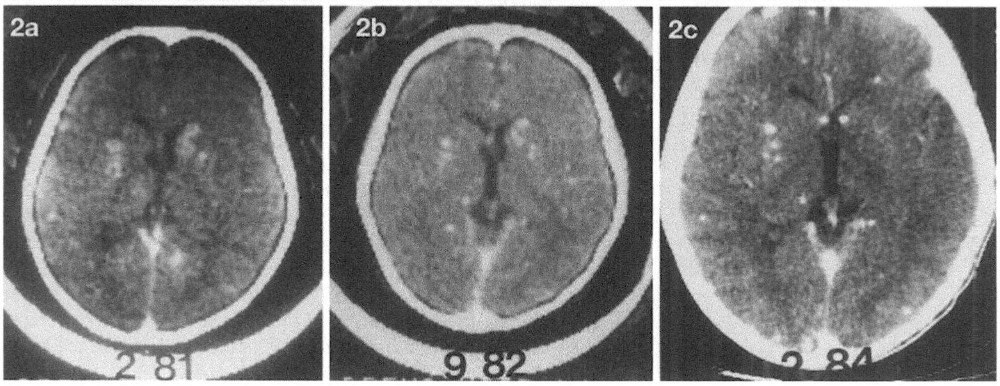

Fig. 1 a–d. Resolution of a parenchymal cysticercosis cyst, demonstrated by serial MRI over 3 years. **a** Axial Gd-enhanced T1-weighted image shows a low signal intensity cyst with an eccentric isointense area (*arrow*), consistent with a scolex. Minimal contrast enhancement of the cyst wall is seen posteriorly and medially. This corresponds to Escobar's vesicular stage. **b** Repeat study shows partial enhancement of the cyst wall posteriorly and medially, as well as enhancement of the scolex. **c** A year later there is a very small, residual ring-like enhancement. Compared to **b** there is a significant decrease in the size of the lesion; Escobar's granular nodular stage. **d** Last contrast-enhanced image shows no significant abnormality

Fig. 2 a–c. Evolution of cysts from colloidal vesicular stage to nodular calcified stage. **a** Contrast-enhanced CT demonstrates multiple ring and nodular enhancing lesions, consistent with colloidal vesicular and granular nodular stages of the disease. **b** CT 19 months later demonstrates nodular enhancing lesions, consistent with granular nodular stage. **c** CT 36 months later demonstrates multiple areas of calcification, consistent with nodular calcified stage. No enhancing lesion was identified

References

1. Escobar A (1983) The pathology of neurocysticercosis. In: Palacios E, Rodríguez-Carbajal J, Taveras J (eds) Cysticercosis of the central nervous system. Thomas, Springfield, pp 27–54
2. Zee CS, Segall HD, Miller C, et al (1980) Unusual neuroradiological features of intercranial cysticercosis. Radiology 137:397–407
3. Zee CS, Segall HD, Boswell WD, et al (1986) MR imaging of neurocysticercosis. J Comput Assist Tomogr 10:195–198
4. Martínez HR, Rangel-Guerra R, Elizondo G, et al (1989) MR imaging in neurocysticercosis: a study of 56 cases. AJNR 10:1011–1019
5. Chang KH, Lee JH, Han MH, et al (1991) The role of contrast-enhanced MR imaging in the diagnosis of neurocysticercosis. AJNR 12:509–512

Central nervous system involvement in progressive facial hemiatrophy: further evidence of chronic localised meningoencephalitis

K. Terstegge [1], **W. Küster** [2], **S. Felber** [3], **H. Henkes** [4], **R. Felix** [1]

[1] Department of Radiology, Universitätsklinikum Rudolf Virchow, Berlin, Germany
[2] Department of Dermatology, Klinikum der Phillips-Universität, Marburg, Germany
[3] Institute of Magnetic Resonance, Universitätsklinikum, Innsbruck, Austria
[4] Institute of Neuroradiology, Universitätskliniken, Homburg/Saar, Germany

Abstract. Progressive facial haemiatrophy is a sporadic disease that affects children and adolescents and leads to atrophy and derformity of one side of the face. It was recently suggested that a characteristic form of chronic localised meningoencephalitis may be the histological correlate of occasional central nervous system (CNS) involvement. We performed an analysed MRI CT and cerebrospinal fluid (CSF) examinations and ophthalmoscopy in 15 patients with CNS involvement, and present our preliminary data. The triad of corticomeningeal dysmorphia, white matter lesion and homolateral hemiatrophy represented a typical (but not always complete) morphological pattern. The cortical lesions were of variable size. Five patients had small areas of cortical calcification. In 2 patients MRI revealed regional parenchymal and meningeal contrast enhancement. Contrast enhancement, CSF findings and ophthalmoscopic findings support the hypothesis of an inflammatory disease of the CNS.

Key words: Progressive facial hemiatrophy – Central nervous system – Meningoencephalitis – Magnetic resonance imaging

Progressive facial haemiatrophy (PFH) is a sporadic disease most often occurring in the first decade. It leads to variable deformity of one side of the face [1–3]. The subcutaneous fat represents the site of the most substantial loss, but the process may extend to various other tissues [1, 4–7]. At least in some of the cases the atrophy is secondary to localised scleroderma. However, it has also been suggested that this morphologically inhomogenous dermatological disease occurs early in the course in all cases. It may have a relatively inconspicuous and insidious cutaneous aspect that does not necessarily lead to its diagnosis [1, 2]. Some patients with PFH have epilepsy of neurological symptoms of central nervous system (CNS) dysfunction [1, 4, 8–11]. Although rare, and as yet lacking histological confirmation, a pattern analysis supported evidence that the brain involvement is disease-related [8]. It has recently been suggested that in these patients the facial inflammation may transcranially invade and then lead to a distinct form of localised meningoencephalitis [8]. It was our aim to examine whether neuroimaging examinations and laboratory findings reveal signs of inflammatory CNS disease. We performed a highly selective multiregional investigation of CNS-symptomatic PFH, to look for data supporting the hypothesis of an inflammation of meninges and CNS in this group.

Correspondence to: K. Terstegge, Department of Radiology, Universitätsklinikum Rudolf Virchow, Augustenburger Platz 1, D-13353 Berlin, Germany

Patients and methods

The diagnosis of PFH with CNS involvement was restricted to patients who had reported unequivocally new onset after the 1st year of life, a progressive course of the disease, or a history of epilepsy or (central) neurological deficits. We undertook no efforts to discriminate between the two diagnoses of "primary" PFH (Romberg's disease) and "secondary" PFH complicating facial morphea (localised scleroderma). We studied 15 patients (13 females and 2 males). Age (11–67 years) and duration of the disease (3–47 years) were wide ranging. The onset of facial symptoms occurred between the age of 1 and 25 years, and all patients had a delayed onset of neurological symptoms (in 9/15, within 3 years). Thirteen of 15 patients had partial epilepsy, and 2 patients had bilateral facial involvement.

We reviewed routine MRI (13 patients) examinations for corticomeningeal dysmorphia, white matter lesions and ventricular enlargement; descriptional criteria that have been published earlier [8]. In 11 patients the study included injection gadiolinium dimeglumine. CT studies were reviewed for calcification (12 patients). In 7 patients with recent increase of seizures or deficits, CSF was analysed, and in 7 CSF findings from examinations during the initial stage of neurological symptoms were reviewed. Ten patients had a complete ophthalmological examination.

Results

Four patients had CSF pleocytosis between 50 and 350 lympocytes mm^3 in the initial phase of their neurological symptoms. One patient had positive oligoclonal bands in the micrelectrophoresis during this period. Two patients, one of whom also had early pleocytosis, had oligoclonal bands in follow-up CSF examinations. Five patients, four of whom also had CSF abnormalities, had severe inflammatory ophthalmological affection of the homolateral eye (i. e. posterior uveitis, retinitis, optic neuritis, vitriitis).

Corticomeningeal dysmorphia was the most frequent finding (13/15 patients) on MRI and CT. The extent of the lesions varied between areas of a few gyri (Fig. 1) and subtotal involvement of one whole hemisphere. The extent of the corticomeningeal dysmorphia correlated with the size of white matter lesions and ventricular enlargement. Cortical calcification in these areas was seen in five patients, and did not correlate with any other morphological criteria. Two patients had either a little focal enhancement in cortical zones and adjacent to the leptomeninges

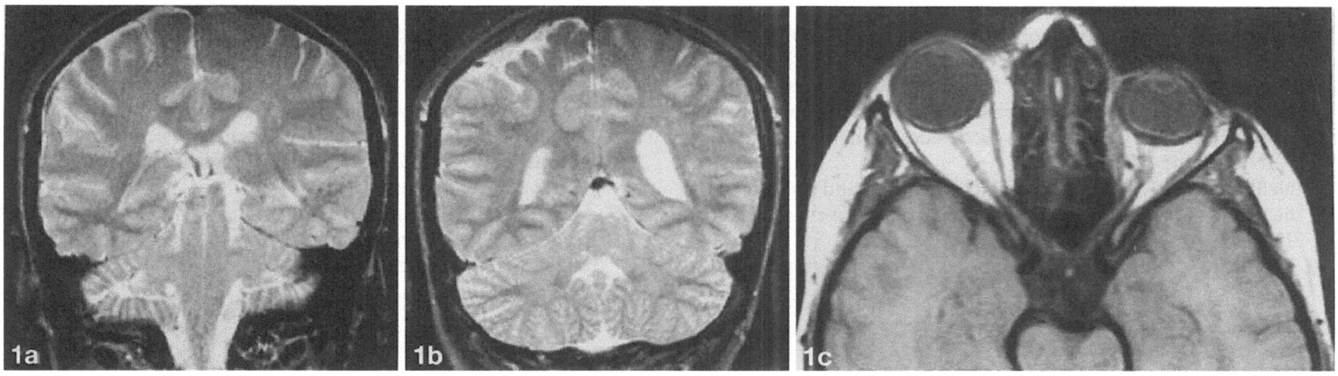

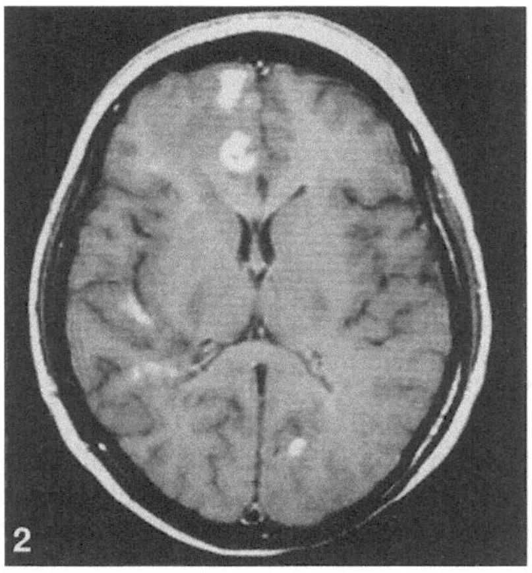

Fig. 1a–c. Woman aged 19 years. Onset of skin changes and alopecial areata in the left frontal region at 15 years. At 17 sudden onset of subtotal visual loss, optic neuritis, posterior uveitis and panophthalmitis. Repeated attacks of sensory Jacksonian seizures of the right arm, and repeated periods of hypoaesthesia of the right arm since the age of 18. **a, b** Control T2-weighted images. The left paramedian cortical surface was much closer to the bone and dura mater over an anteriorposterior distance of 10 cm in all coronal images. The gyri seem ill-formed, and the fluid signal in the sulci is reduced. There is reduction of corticomedullary contrast in this region. This was rated as a minimal form of corticomeningeal dysmorphia; the lesion also involved the region of the epileptigenic focus. **c** Axial T1-weighted image obtained 2 years after a documented episode of posterior uveitis, optic neuritis and panophthalmitis which led to phthisis bulbi. The globe is become much smaller, the signal from the vitreous humour is increased, the retrobulbar fat largely reduced and the extraocular muscles show structural changes. These findings represent a maximal degree of homolateral inflammatory eye involvement, seen in three patients

Fig. 2. Woman aged 30 years. Onset of facial changes at the age of 7 years, and onset of neurological deficits (left hemianopa and left partial seizures) at 28.. This patient has bilateral facial changes, more marked on the left. Contrast-enhanced T1-weighted image shows multifocal contrast enhancement, predominantly in the right cerebral hemisphere. Most foci are cortical, and seem to have direct contact with the subarachnoid space or leptomeninges. There is one small focus in the left occipital region. The high signal in the left frontoparietal diple was present on unenhanced mages. Loss of subcutaneous tissue is visible in the left occipital region

(Fig. 2), or focal meningeal enhancement. In patients with unilateral PFH, all these alterations were always seen on the side of the facial disease.

Discussion

Of 15 patients 6 showed signs of inflammation either in the CSF or on ophthalmoscopy, and in 2 patients with relatively new onset of neurological symptoms, focal contrast enhancement was observed on MRI. These data strongly support the hypothesis that CNS involvement in PFH represents an infrequent, clinically and morphologically distinct form of meningoencephalitis that requires further description. The inflammation may be related to autoimmune phenomena alone, but it is our impression that regularly continuous extension of the faciocranial inflammation with obvious lack of tissue preference, and a monophasic course of the clinical and CSF findings may be better explained by a causative yet unknown transmitted agent, as suggested earlier by some investigators [9, 12, 13].

Acknowledgements. This paper is dedicated to the IInd Department of Surgery of the Kumamoto University Medical School. The first author would like to take this opportunity of expressing his heartfelt thanks for all the kind support received, with personal admiration to K. Sakamoto, MD, PhD, to Dr. S. Tomiyasu, and to the nursing staff for untiring and personal care, and also to all those who were active behind the scenes, expecially Y. Korogi, MD, Mrs. J. Korogi and Ms. H. Usa.

References

1. Wartenberg R (1945) Progressive facial hemiatrophy. Arch Neurol Psychiatr 54:75–96
2. Rees TD (1976) Facial atrophy. Clin Plast Surg 3:637–646
3. Pensler JM, Murphy GF, Mulliken JB (1990) Clinical and ultrastructural studies of Romberg's hemifacial atrophy. Plast Reconstr Surg 85:669–674
4. Fry JA, Alvarellos A, Fink CW, Blaw ME, Roach ES (1992) Intracranial findings in progressive facial hemiatrophy. J Rheumatol 19:956–958
5. Goldenstein-Schainberg C, Rodrigues Pereira RM, Gusukama MC, Messina WC, Cossermeli W (1990) Childhood linear scleroderma "en coup de sabre" with uveitis. J Pediatr 117:581–584
6. Ong K, Billson FA, Pathirna DS, Clift-Bligh P (1991) A case of progressive facial hemiatrophy with uveitis and retinal vasculitis. Austr N Z J Ophthalmol 19:295–298
7. Goldhammer Y, Kronenberg J, Tadmor R, Braham J, Leventon

G (1981) Progressive hemifacial atrophy (Parry-Romberg's syndrome), principally involving bone. J Laryngol Otol 95:643–647
8. Terstegge K, Kunath B, Felber S, Speciali JG, Henkes H, Hosten N (1994) MR of brain involvement of progressive facial hemiatrophy (Romberg's disease): reconsideration of a syndrome. AJNR 15:145–150
9. Nellhaus G (1970) Aquired unilateral vitiligo and poliosis of the head and subacute encephalitis with partial recovery. Neurology 20:965–974
10. Merrit KK, Faber HK, Bruch H (1937) Progressive facial hemiatrophy: report of two cases with cerebral calcifications. J Pediatr 10:374–395
11. Asher SW, Berg BO (1982) Progressive facial hemiatrophy: report of three cases, including one observed over 43 years, and computed tomography findings. Arch Neurol 39:44–46
12. Möbius PJ (1895) Der umschriebene Gesichtsschwund. In: Nothnagel CWH (ed) Specielle Pathologie und Therapie, vol 11, part 2. Hölder, Vienna
13. Abele DC, Bedingfield RB, Chandler FW, Given KS (1990) Progressive facial hemiatrophy (Parry-Romberg syndrome) and borreliosis. J Am Acad Dermatol 22:531–533

The radiology of progressive multifocal leukoencephalopathy

S. Batnitzky[1], **H. I. Price**[1], **D. A. Eckard**[1], **P. L. O'Boynick**[2], **S. J. Rosenthal**[1]

[1] Department of Radiology, University of Kansas School of Medicine, Kansas City, Kansas, USA
[2] Department fo Neurosurgery, University of Kansas School of Medicine, Kansas City. Kansas, USA

Abstract. Progressive multifocal leukoencephalopathy (PML) is a progressive multifocal disease of the brain secondary to an opportunistic viral infection that primarily affects immunosuppressed patients. Fifty-five to 85% of PML cases are directly attributable to the acquired immunodeficiency syndrome. The neuroimaging findings of PML parallel the pathologic changes and have a variable appearance on CT and MRI. The features are nonspecific and can mimic a wide spectrum of pathologic states.

Key words: Progressive multifocal leukoencephalopathy – Acquired immunodeficiency syndrome – Demyelinating disease

Progressive multifocal leukoencephalopahty (PML) is a progressive demyelinating disease of the brain secondary to an opportunistic viral infection that primarily affects immunosuppressed patients, especially those with defective cell-mediated immunity [1]. The virus responsible for PML, known as the JC virus, is a polyomavirus, which is a subgroup of the papovavirus group. Pathologically the major target cell is the oligodendrocyte, which undergoes cytolytic destruction. The usual clinical course of the disease is one of the progression to coma leading to death in 3–6 months after the onset of symptoms [1], although there have been reports of survival up to 10 years [2]. Today AIDS is the most frequent predisposition to PML [1]. Fifty-five to 85% of PML cases are directly attributable to AIDS [3].

Correspondence to: S. Batnitzky, Department of Radiology, University of Kansas Medical Center, 3901 Rainbow Boulevard, Kansas City, KS 66160-7234, USA

Methods and materials

The CT and/or MRI studies of 14 patients with pathologically proven PML were reviewed. Eight patients had associated AIDS. Six patients had compromised immune systems secondary to a variety of chronic diseases such as lymphoma, leukemia, sarcoidosis, and post-renal transplant treatment with immunosuppressive drugs.

Results

On CT, PML lesions appear as focal, nonenhancing regions of low attenuation in the white matter that exhibit no mass effect. On MRI the lesions are hypointense on T1-weighted images and hyperintense on T2-weighted images. MRI is superior to CT in demonstrating the extent and involvement of the disease.

Although any part of the brain may be involved, there is a predilection for the parieto-occipital area (Fig. 1). This disease initially involves the peripheral white matter following the contours of the gray/white matter interface to give scalloped lateral margins. With progression, the disease spreads to the deep white matter. Initially the lesions are multifocal (Fig. 2), but with progression of the disease the lesions coalesce, forming single or multiple large areas of demyelination (Fig. 3). Asymmetric cerebral involvement is a characteristic feature. In non-AIDS PML cases the cortical gray matter is usually spared. Vascular territories and the corpus callosum can be crossed, resulting in butterfly distribution of the disease (Fig. 3).

The majority of PML cases do not demonstrate contrast enhancement either on CT or MRI. However, in some cases contrast enhancement may be seen both on CT and MRI (Fig. 1).

The imaging findings of PML in patients with AIDS have a variable appearance, and have many characteristics that differ from those seen in PML in non-AIDS patients. The parieto-occipital location is not as notable in AIDS patients. PML in AIDS patients tends to have a more

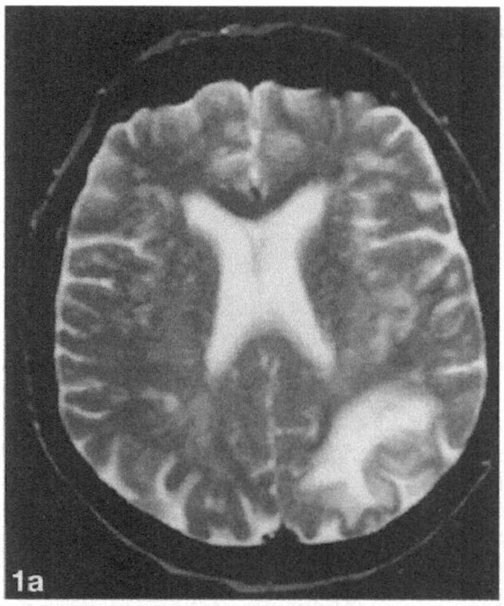

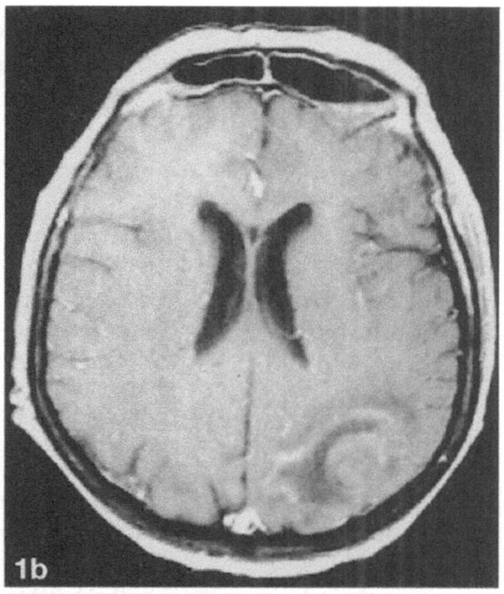

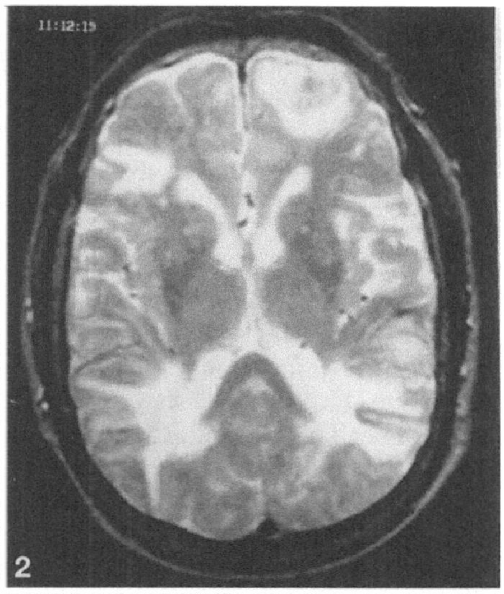

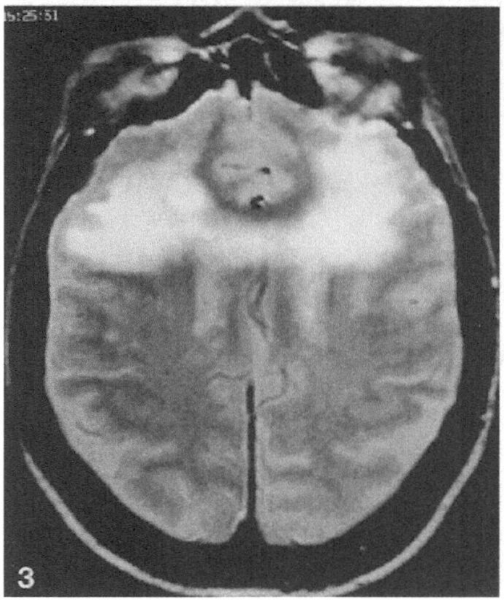

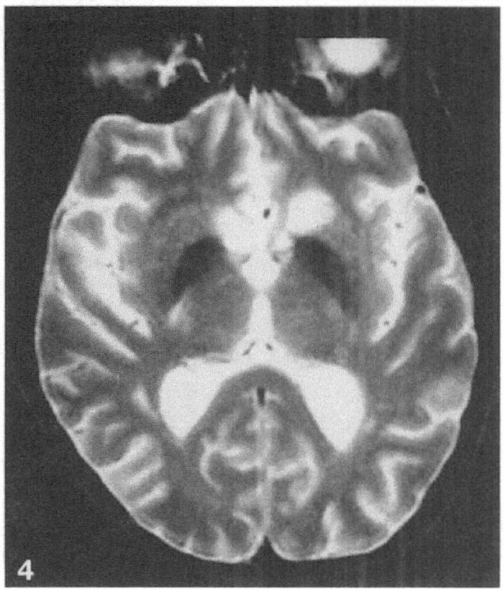

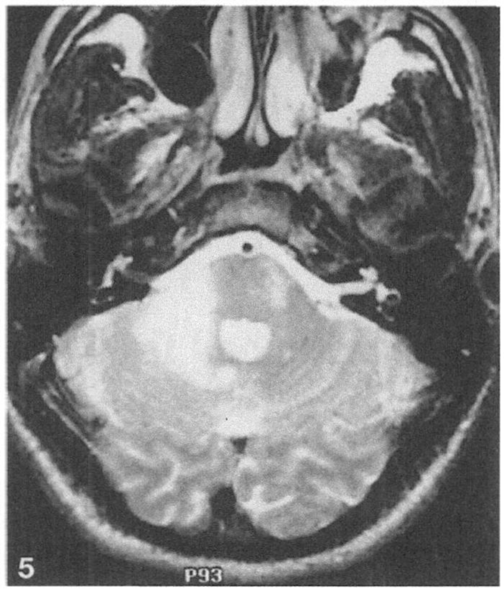

Fig. 1a, b. Progressive and multifocal leukoencephalopathy (PML) in 70-year-old woman with history of intra-abdominal lymphoma. T2-weighted image (**a**) demonstrates increased signal intensity in the left occipital subcortical white matter. Following IV gadolinium (**b**), the left occipital lesion enhances. Biopsy confirmed the diagnosis

Fig. 2. Pathologically proven PML in 63-year-old man with chronic lymphocytic leukemia. T2-weighted image demonstrates bilateral extensive white matter increased signal intensity. No contrast was demonstrated

Fig. 3. Pathologically proven PML in 54-year-old woman who had a renal transplant. T2-weighted image demonstrates bilateral frontal areas of increased signal intensity, which cross the midline. No contrast enhancement was demonstrated

Fig. 4. PML in a 40-year-old man with AIDS. T2-weighted axial image demonstrates abnormal increased signal intensity in both caudate nuclei. Postmortem confirmed the diagnosis

Fig. 5. A 36-year-old man with AIDS with pathologically proven PML in the right cerebellum and left pons. T2-weighted axial image demonstrates areas of increased signal intensity. No contrast enhancement was seen

atypical presentation. Although most lesions invovle the white matter, gray matter involvement occurs in 50% of patients (Fig. 4). Posterior fossa disease is common and is seen in approximately one-third of PML cases (Fig. 5). These are usually associated with supratentorial lesions as well. However, in 10% of cases involvement is solely infratentorial. Posterior fossa involvement can also occur in non-AIDS patients.

Discussion

PML was originally described in patients with chronic diseases associated with compromising immune response, such as lymphoma, leukemia, carcinomatosis, sarcoidosis, tuberculosis, systemic lupus erythematosus, nontropical sprue, Whipple' disease, as well as transplant recipients, especially renal transplants treated with immunosuppressive drugs [1]. Today AIDS is the most frequent predisposition to PML [1, 3]. A few patients with PML have no known underlying illness [1].

PML is characterized phatologically by focal or confluent areas of demyelination mainly distributed through the cerebral white matter. There is a predilection for the parieto-occipital area [4], although any area may be involved. The earliest lesions of PML are found in the subcortical white matter, spreading to the deeper white matter late in the course of the disease.

The neuroimaging findings of PML parallel the pathologic changes and have a variable appearance, as described above [1, 3–5].

The majority of cases of PML do not demonstrate contrast enhancement either on CT or MRI [4]. This may be due to the lack of an accompanying inflammatory component to the changes seen in the oligodendrocyte and astrocyte. However, cases of contrast enhancement may be seen both on CT and RMI. Thus, the demonstration of contrast enhancement does not exclude the diagnosis of PML.

The CT and MRI features of PML are nonspecific and can mimic a wide spectrum of pathologic states [1]. The differential diagnosis includes other opportunistic infections such as HIV encephalitis, cytomegalovirus encephalopathy, toxoplasmosis, lymphoma, primary and metastatic disease, and other causes of demyelination such as multiple sclerosis and also ischemic changes. Many of these diseases can be excluded on clinical and laboratory findings. The definitive diagnosis of PML can only be made by histologic examination following brain biopsy or necropsy.

References

1. Caldemyer KS, Edwards MK, Smith RR, Moran CC (1993) Neuroimaging Clin North Am 3:305–317
2. Kepes JJ, Chou SM, Price LW (1975) Progressive multifocal leukoencephalopathy with 10-year survival in a patient with nontypical sprue. Neurology 25:1006–1012
3. Berger JR, Kaszowitz B, Post MJD, Dickinson G (1987) Progressive multifocal leukoencephalopathy associated with human immunodeficiency virus infection. A review of the literature with a report of sixteen cases. Ann Intern Med 107:78–87
4. Guilleux MH, Steiner RE, Young IR (1986) MR imaging in progressive multifocal leukoencephalopathy. AJNR 7:1033–1035
5. Mark AS, Atlas SW (1989) Progressive multifocal leukoencephalopathy in patients with AIDS: appearance on MRI image. Radiology 173:517–520

Cerebral blood flow and metabolism in progressive multifocal leukoencephalopathy

K. Mineura [1], T. Sasajima [1], K. Nishino [1], M. Kowada [1], N. Tomura [2], T. Ogawa [3], J. Hatazawa [3], K. Uemura [3]

[1] Neurosurgical Service, Akita University Hospital, Akita, Japan
[2] Department fo Radiology, Akita University Hospital, Akita, Japan
[3] Department of Radiology and Nuclear Medicine, Research Institute for Brain and Blood Vessels, Akita, Japan

Abstract. We report a case of progressive multifocal leukoencephalopathy (PML) studied by positron emission tomography. Regional cerebral circulation increased greatly in the white matter lesion, whereas oxygen metabolism was reduced to a considerable extent. Increased circulation reflected angiographic findings of vascular blush and early venous filling. There was less accumulation of ^{11}C-methyl-L-methionine in PML lesions, than in brain tumours.

Key words: Positron emission tomography – Progressive multifocal leukoencephalopathy – Cerebral blood flow – ^{11}C-methyl-L-methionine

Progressive multifocal leukoencephalopathy (PML) is a rare, slowly progressing demyelinating disease, occurring predominantly in patients with impaired cell-mediated immunity. Neuroradiological findings of this entity have been well described, with the recent introduction of MRI showing better resolution of white matter lesions [1–3]. Knowledge of blood flow and metabolism of this entity has been scarce [4]. In the current study, cerebral blood flow and metabolism were measured by positron emission tomography (PET) in a patient with PML who had presented with mild right-sided weakness.

Correspondence to: K. Mineura

Case report

A 51-year-old woman presented with mild right-sided weakness. She was clear and alert. No neurological deficit except for right hemiparesis was noted. CT showed relatively well-bordered low density areas in the white matter of the left parietal and frontal lobes (Fig. 1a). T2-weighted MRI revealed more precisely the location and shape of high-intensity signal lesions scattered in the white matter, where neither mass effect nor enhancement effect was present (Fig. 1b, c). Cerebral angiography showed vascular staining in the left parietal region, and early filling and dilatation of medullary veins which converged onto the wall of the lateral ventricle [5].

Cerebral circulation and metabolism were examined using PET with $C^{15}O_2$, $C^{15}O$, $^{15}O_2$, and ^{11}C-methyl-L-methionine (^{11}C-Met). Regional cerebral blood flow (rCBF) and blood volume (rCBV) increased in the left parietal lesions as compared with the contralateral region, whereas the oxygen extraction fraction (rOEF) and

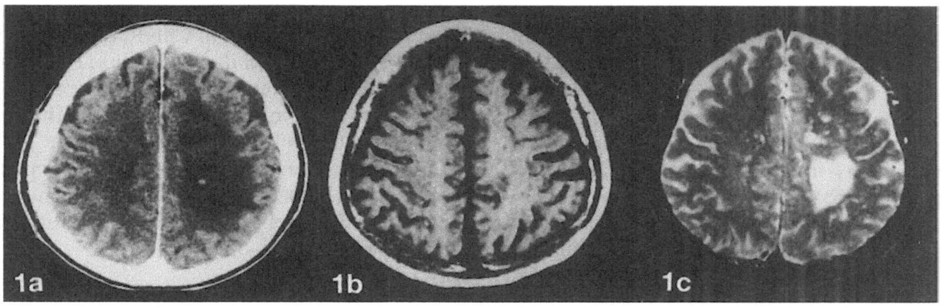

Fig. 1. Contrast-enhanced CT (**a**), Gd-DTPA-enhanced T1-(**b**), and T2-weighted (**c**) images. Relatively well-bordered low density and high signal intensity areas were detected in the left parietal white matter on CT and T2-weighted. The lesion did not show contrast enhancement

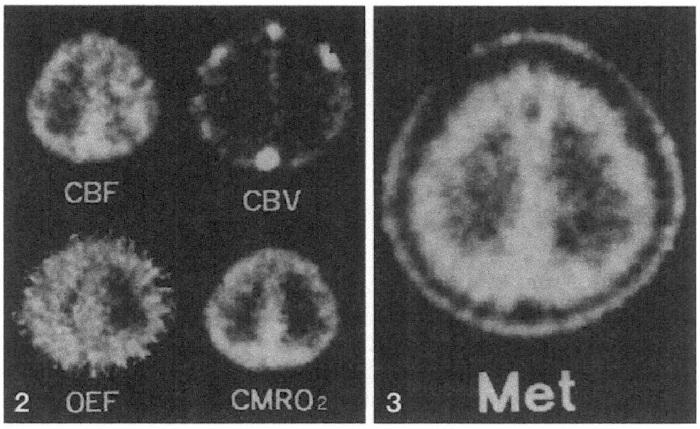

Fig. 2. All parameters ecxept for rCBF were reduced in the left parietal lesion. rCBF increased markedly and corresponded to angiographic findings of vascular blush and early venous filling. *CBF*,Cerebral blood flow; *CBV*, blood volume; *OEF*, oxygen extraction fraction; *CMRO*$_2$, metabolic rate of oxygen

Fig. 3. ^{11}C-methyl-L-methionine PET showed no accumulation of tracers in the left parietal lesion

oxygen consumption (rCMRO$_2$) were reduced to a considerable extent (Fig. 2). No accumulation of ^{11}C-Met was noted in the lesions (Fig. 3).

The patient underwent CT-guided stereotactic biopsy to obtain a definite diagnosis and to achieve differentiation from brain tumours. The histological findings of biopsy specimens were those of PML, since immunohistochemical methods revealed oligodendrocytes infected with the JC virus, a human papovavirus. Her neurological signs deteriorated gradually, resulting in tetraparesis and akinetic mutism.

Discussion

The diagnosis of PML is hardly differentiated from multiple sclerosis and other white matter diseases. The present case suffered from PML without underlying diseases. The different diagnosis included common CNS diseases such as cerebral infarction or low-grade gliomas and other demyelinating diseases. The pathology of biopsy specimens identified cells containing viral particles.

Neuroradiological interventions are expected to faciliate the diagnosis of this entity in a non-invasive manner. MRI is the best method for revealing topographic abnormalities in PML. High signal intensity on both T1- and T2-weighted images spreads asymmetrically without mass effect, and is confined to the white matter, distant from the periventricular region [2].

Reports on PET findings of PML have been few. Our results showed increased rCBF and rCBV in the white matter lesion, corresponding to the hyperperfused and hypervascular area revealed by cerebral angiography. The rCBF increased in the leson, as compared with the contralateral region, reflecting angiographic findings such as vascular blush and early venous fillings. As with oxygen metabolism, rCMRO$_2$ fell widely in the vicinity of the lesion, including the adjacent grey matter. Because of low rOEF, the lesion received an excessive blood supply beyond oxygen demand. In ^{11}C-Met images obtained 45 min after an intravenous injection, the tracer did not accumulate in the lesion corresponding to the low density area on CT. Because gliomas had a high accumulation of ^{11}C-Met [6, 7], no uptake of ^{11}C-Met in the PML lesion was an important landmark in the differential diagnosis. These PET findings proved the lesion to be hyperdynamic, but to be hypometabolic related to amino acids and oxygen.

Kiyosawa et al. [4] have described the glucose metabolism of a patient with PML using ^{18}F-fluorodeoxyglucose. Cortical glucose metabolism was decreased due to the white matter disease. This metabolic depression may be caused by a retrograde effect of axonal destruction in the white matter or by deafferentation. In contrast, the mostly deep white matter lesions showed a relatively increased glucose metabolism, which resembled metabolic changes in areas with inflammatory cellular infiltration [4]. Since a regional cerebral metabolic rate of glucose (rCMRGl) value depends not only on phosphorylatin but also on diffusion through the blood-tissue barrier, increased rCMRGl may be due in part to hyperperfusion, as implicated by our results. The circulation and metabolism of PML may vary from stage to stage of disease progression in PML. Further PET studies will provide knowledge on blood flow and metabolism in PML, and may result in an early diagnosis different from that of other white matter lesions.

References

1. Levy JD, Cottingham, KL, Campbell RJ, Moore GK, Gyorkey F, Ashizawa T, Goldman AM (1986) Progressive multifocal leukoencephalopathy and magnetic resonance imaging. Ann Neurol 19:399–401
2. Guilleux MH, Steiner RE, Young IR (1986) MR imaging in progressive multifocal leukoencephalopathy. AJNR 7:1033–1035

3. Tashiro K, Doi S, Morikawa F, Maruo Y, Nomura M (1987) Progressive multifocal leucoencephalopathy with magnetic resonance imaging verification and therapeutic trials with interferon. J Neurol 234:427–429
4. Kiyosawa M, Bosley TM, Alavi A, Gupta N, Rhodes CH, Chawluk J, Kushner M, Savino PJ, Sergott RC, Schatz NJ, Reivich M (1988) Positron emission tomography in a patient with progressive multifocal leukoencephalopathy. Neurology 38:1864–1867
5. Tomura N, Watanabe M, Kato T, Nishino K, Kowada M (1994) Case report: progressive multifocal leukoencephalopahty with prominent medullary veins on angiogram. Clin Radiol 49:66–68
6. Mineura K, Sasajima T, Suda Y, Kowada M, Shishido F, Uemura K (1990) Amino acid study of cerebral gliomas using positron emission tomography: analysis of (^{11}C-metyhl-)L-methionine uptake index. Neurol Med Chir (Tokyo) 30:997–1002
7. Ogawa T, Shishido F, Kanno I, Inugami A, Fujita H, Murakami M, Shimosegawa E, Ito H, Hatazawa J, Okudera T, Uemura K, Yasui N, Mineura K (1993) Cerebral glioma: evaluation with methionine PET. Radiology 186:45–53

Subacute sclerosing panencephalitis: MRI and neuropathology

T. Kryst, G. Szpak, J. Kulczycki, E. Lewandowska

Institute of Psychiatry and Neurology, Warsaw, Poland

Abstract. Substrate sclerosing panencephalitis (SSPE) is a late complication of measles, occurring 6–8 years after infection and leading to progressive impairment of brain function and death. MRI is not specific, but in every stage abnormal diffuse high intensity areas are seen in the periventricular white matter regions. Of 32 cases under observation, 2 patients died in the subacute and chronic clinical stages, and a morphological assessment was carried out. In the subacute clinical case, inflammatory infiltration, diffuse proliferation of glial cells, degeneration of myelin, and intranuclear inclusion bodies were found in the patomorphological examination and in the chronic case neurofibrillary tangles were found. Typical nucleocapsids of paramyxoviruses, nuclear bodies and demyelinating changes have been observed by electron microscopy.

Key words: Substrate sclerosing panencephalitis – Magnetic resonance imaging – White matter disease – Nucleocapsid-Neurofibrillary tangles

Subacute sclerosing panencephalitis (SSPE) is a slow, progressive infection by the measles virus, which causes an often fatal condition and typically affects children aged between 5 and 12 years who had clinical measles usually before the age of 3. Diagnosis is established by the presence of elevated titres of measles antibodies in the cerebrospinal fluid (CSF) and serum, abnormal complexes in the EEG, and clinical manifestations. The most significant hypodense areas in the posterior parietal regions and generalised brain atrophy were found on CT [1]. MRI in all stages reveals diffuse periventricular white matter hyperintensity [2].

Correspondence to: T. Kryst, Magnetic Resonance, Institute of Psychiatry and Neurology, Al. Sobieskiego 1/9, 02-957 Warsaw, Poland

Materials and methods

Our material consists of MRI examinations of 32 patients with SSPE. Two of them died in the III/IV stage, one in the subacute clinical stage, the second in the chronic clinical stage. MRI examinations were done on a 0.4 T resistive system, using standard protocol SE sequences and T1- and T2-weighted images. Neuropathological examinations were carried out by the PTAH, H & E and Klüver-Barrera methods. For electron microscopy, the autopsy material was fixed in glutaraldehyde and postfixed in osmium tetroxide. After dehydration, the material was embedded in epon. Ultrathin sections were stained with uranyl acetate and lead citrate.

Results

MRI examinations revealed, in the T2 sequences, diffuse bilateral periventricula hyperintensity in the white matter of the parietal, occipital, frontal and temporal lobes, with involvement of the frontal and occipital cortex (Figs. 1, 2). Neuropathological examinations revealed diffuse proliferation of the glial cells, degeneration of myelin, intranuclear inclusion bodies, inflammatory infiltration and in the chronic case, neurofibrillary tangles (Figs. 3, 4). By electron microscopy, the typical nucleocapsids of the measles virus were found in the nuclei of the glial cells (Figs. 5 and 6). In both cases, numerous nuclear bodies were observed in the glial cells, as well as the nuclei of glial cells with changes in the ultrastructural image. Reactive astrocytes containing abundant intracytoplasmatic glial filaments were numerous. Degenerated axons and demyelinic changes were seen in both cases.

Discussion

MRI demonstrated periventricular white matter lesions with abnormal signal intensity, due to prolonged relaxation times and increased water content without mass effect. Frontal and parieto-occipital white matter involvement was extensive in both cases. Diffuse brain atrophy and prominent lateral ventricles are thought to represent

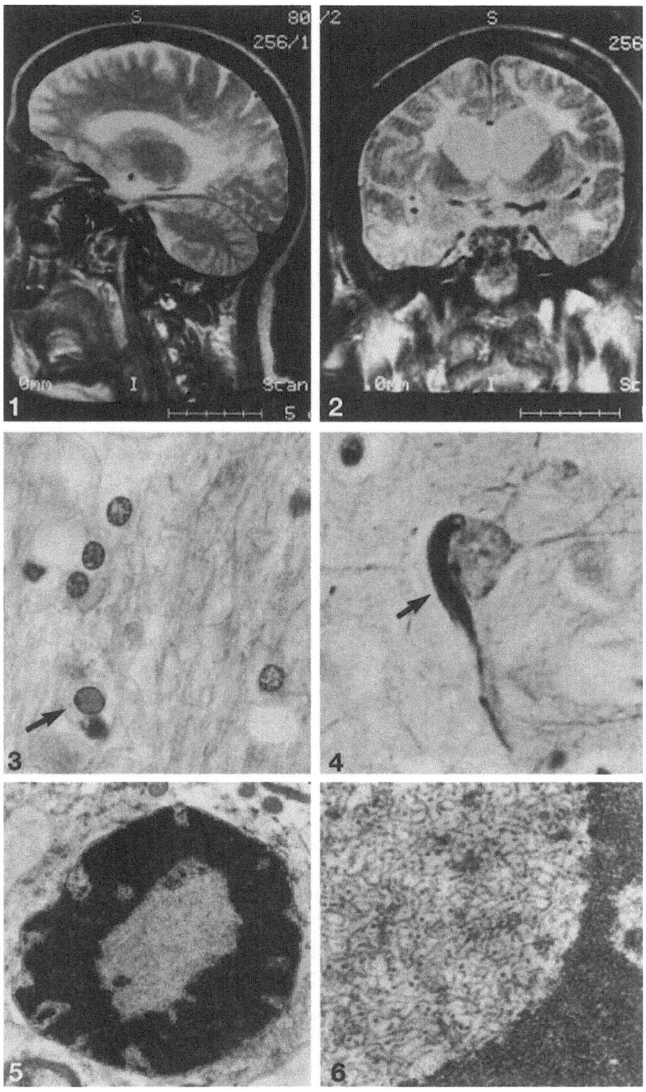

Fig. 1. Sagittal T2-weighted SE image. Pathological signal increase in the parieto-occipital region, in the periventricular white matter, and cortex. Subacute clinical stage

Fig. 2. Coronal image: diffuse bilateral periventricular white matter pathological changes are seen in the temporal and frontal lobes, on the left side of the affected cortex. Prominent lateral ventricles. Chronic clinical stage

Fig. 3. Intranuclear inclusion body, oligodendrocyte (*arrow*). Haemotoxylin and eosin stain. Subacute clinical stage

Fig. 4. Neurofibrillary tangles in the cerebral cortex (*arrow*). Bielschowsky stain. Clinical chronic stage

Fig. 5. Glial cell, presumably oligodendrocyte: dense aggregate of chromatin at the periphery of the nucleus. In the clear central area multiple nucleocapside are seen. × 17000

Fig. 6. Part of the nucleus of the oligodendrocyte with smooth nucleocapsids of paramyxovirus. Higher magnification. × 70000

demyelination and gliosis primarily, but may also be due to inflammation. No difference between the subacute and chronic clinical stages was observed on MRI. Microscopic analysis permitted us to follow up the pathological process from the subacute stage of inflammatory infiltration, throughout the increasing reaction of neuroglia and demyelination, up to the late changes of encephalopathic type with the appearance of Alzheimer's neurofibrillary degeneration [3]. The intranuclear inclusion bodies were found in all stages of the disease in the neurons, oligodendroglia and in the astroglial cells. In the intranuclear inclusion bodies, the typical nucleocapsids of paramyxoviruses were observed by electron microscopy.

References

1. Kryst-Widzgowska T, Sobczyk W, Kulczycki J, Kozlowski L (1991) Subacute sclerosing panencephalitis: CT findings in acute and chronic. Neuroradiology 33 [Suppl]:612–613
2. Case records of the Massachusetts General Hospital (case 25-1986). (1986) N Engl J Med 314:1686–1700
3. Wiśniewski HM, Dymecki J, Węgiel J, Kulczycki J, Schmidt-Sidor B, Grundke-Iqbal I, Strojny P (1991) Neurofibrillary pathology in subacute sclerosing panencephalitis. Dementia 2:133–141

MRI in intracranial paracoccidioidomycosis

A. C. A. Magalhães, P. Caramelli, J. R. Menezes, L. S. Lo, M. H. Chen, L. A. Bacheschi, S. C. Mathias, A. Magalhães

Department of Radiology, Section of Magnetic Resonance, Hospital das Clínicas, University of São Paulo, São Paulo, Brazil

Abstract. Five male patients, aged between 10 and 55 years, with diagnosed central nervous system paracoccidioidomycosis were examined with a 1.5 TMR system. T1- and T2-weighted spin-echo sequences were obtained before and after contrast medium MRI findings ranged from a single lesion in one patient to multiple rounded lesions in four. The lesions were iso- to hypointense on T1-weighted images and hypo or hyperintense on T2-weighted images. After contrast injection, there was ring and/or nodular enhancement. The lesions had a slight preference for the posterior cranial fossa, but were also found in many other

Correspondence to: A. C. A. Magalhães, University of São Paulo, School of Medicine, 01415-000, Rua Bela Cintra, 1600, São Paulo, SP, Brazil

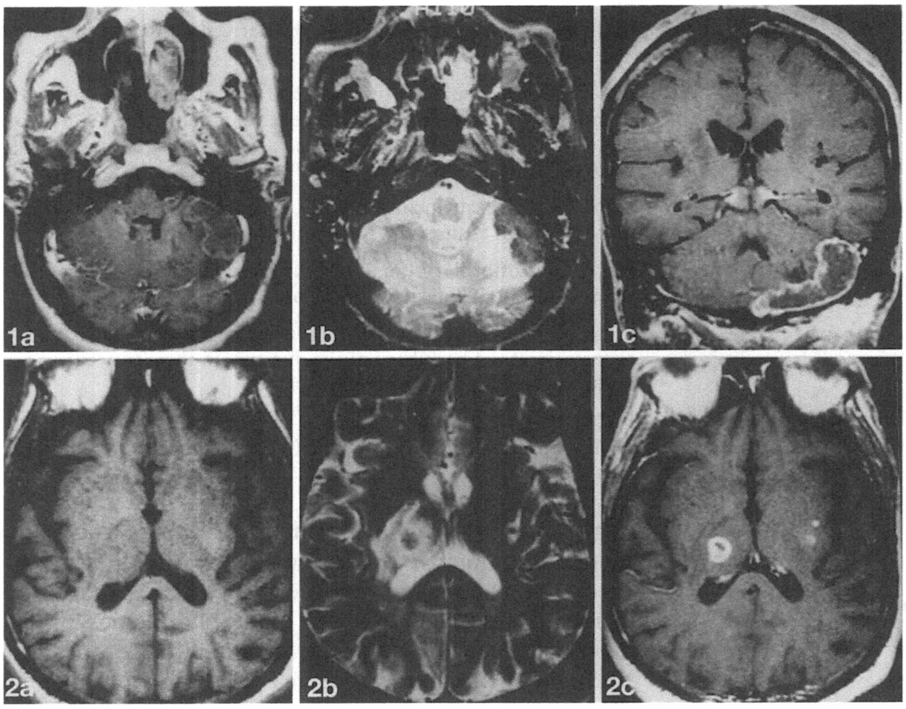

Fig. 1a–c. Paracoccidioidomycosis. **a, b** Axial T1- and T2-weighted and coronal contrast-enhanced T1-weighted images show large lesion in the left cerebell for hemisphere, isointense in **a**, low intensy in **b**, and showing peripheral contrast enhancement

Fig. 2a–c. Paracoccidioidomycosis. **a–c** Images weighted as in Fig. 1 show multiple lesions in the thalamus, iso- or hyperintense in **a**, hypointense in **b**, with ring or nodular contrast enhancement

supratentorial areas. MRI proved to be a good method for the demonstration of paracoccidioidomycosis brain involvement, especially with the use of contrast medium.

Key words Paracoccidioidomycosis – Blastomycosis – Brain, infections – Brain, magnetic resonance imaging

Paracoccidioidomycosis, also called South American blastomycosis, is a systemic mycosis caused by *Paracoccidioides brasilliensis,* endemic mainly in the countries of South and Central America. The disease involves many organs, including the central nervous system (CNS), which may be affected in almost 10% of cases. CNS involvedment is characterized by a meningeal form with inflammation of the leptomeninges, predominantly at the skull base, and a pseudotumoral or granulomatous form [1, 2]. Neuroradiological methods are essential to demonstrate neurological involvement by the disease, mainly in the granulomatous form [3, 4]. The purpose of this study is to describe the MRI findings in a group of patients with intracranial paracoccidioidomycosis.

Patients and methods

Five men, aged 31–55 years, with neurological complaints underwent biopsy, which proved they were suffering from systemic paracoccidioidomycosis. They underwent MRI on a 1.5 T system; T1- and T2-weighted sequences (TR 400/TE 15; TR 2000/TE 30–90) were obtained before and after the administration of gadolinium-diethylenetriamine pentaacetic acid (DTPA), with multiplaner acquisitions.

Results

All patients had multiple, round or lobulated lesions. On precontrast T1-weighted images relative to the surrounding brain the lesions were isointense in four patients and hyperintense in two. On postcontrast T1-weighted images, there was ring enhancement of the lesions in all patients, with concomitance of multiple nodular enhancing lesions in one patient. On T2-weighted images hypointense lesions were seen in all patients, with central hyperintensity in two and perilesional oedema in four. One patient also had homogeneous multiple hyperintense lesions on T2-weighted images (Figs. 1, 2).

Discussion

Paracoccidioidomycosis is acquired by fungus inhalation, involving primarily the lungs and the superior air tract. After haematogenous dissemination, other organs can be affected: lymph nodes, adrenal glands, CNS, spleen, liver, bones and gastrointestinal tract. CNS involvement occurs in almost 10% of patients with this disease, including a meningeal form leading to leptomeningitis of the skull base, similar to tuberculous meningitis, and a pseudotumoral or granulomatous form with single or multiple intraparenchymatous granulomata, mostly supratentorial [1, 2]. Posterior fossa and spinal cord lesions are also observed [5–9]. The granulomatous form is more common and may give rise to different signs and symptoms, mainly intracranial hypertension, seizures, motor and sensory deficits, cerebellar ataxia, and aphasia [2].

In the present study, MRI was able to identify lesions throughout the brain, including the posterior fossa, characterized by isointensity or hyperintensity on precontrast T1-weighted images, hypointensity on T2-weighted images with or without peripheral oedema, and ring or nodular enhancement on postcontrast T1-weighted images.

The hyperintensity on precontrast T1-weighted images, observed in two patients, could be due to the presence of fat in macrophages, usually seen in granulomatous lesions, or the presence of methaemoglobin. Hypointense lesions on T2-weighted images observed in all patients, could relate to the chronic granulomatous inflammation or haemosiderin deposits, but the exact explanation awaits pathological correlations. The hyperintensity observed on T2-weighted images in patient 2 is probably due to the acute phase of the same process. In patients 2 and 4, hypointense lesions on T2-weighted images had a central area of hyperintensity, which was most likely related to necrosis with cyst formation.

In the present series, supratentorial lesions were more frequent than infratentorial lesions, which were observed in three of the five patients. Therefore, due to its high sensitivity to posterior fossa lesions, MRI, especially postcontrast T1-weighted sequences, is superior to CT in these circumstances.

In conclusion, MRI is a sensitive method for the detection of intracranial granulomata of paracoccidioidomycosis, and may be more specific than CT in establishing this diagnosis. Pathological correlation studies will be necessary in order to understand better the varied signal intensity of lesions observed on T1- and T2-weighted images.

References

1. Pereira WC, Raphael A, Sallum J (1965) Lesões neurológicas na blastomicose sul-americana: estudo anátomo-patológico de 14 casos. Arq Neuropsiquiatr 23:95–112
2. Nóbrega JPS (1982) Micoses do sistema nervoso central. Arq Bras Neurocirurg 1:157–171
3. Hutzler RU, Brussi MLP, Capitani CM, Lima SS (1985) Acometimento neurológico da paracoccidioidomicose, avaliado pela tomografia computadorizada de crânio. Rev Paul Med 103:243–244
4. Minguetti G, Madalozzo LE (1983) Paracoccidioidal granulomatosis of the brain. Arch Neurol 40:100–102
5. Teive HAG, Arruda WO, Ramina R et al (1991) Paracoccidioidomycosis granuloma simulating posterior fossa tumor. J R Soc Med 84:562–563
6. Morato-Fernández RN, Beraldo PSS, Masini M, Costa PHC (1991) Paracoccidioidomicose de localização intramedular e cerebral. Arq Neuropsiquiatr 49:192–197
7. Guerreiro CAM, Chuluc SSD, Branchini MLN (1987) A new treatment for large cerebral paracoccidioidomycosis. Arq Neuropsiquiatr 45:419–423
8. Araujo JC, Werneck L, Cravo MA (1978) South American blastomycosis presenting as a posterior fossa tumor. J Neurosurg 49:425–428
9. Aun RA (1957) Blastomicose do cerebelo: forma tumoral. Arq Hosp Santa Casa S Paulo 3:31–38

White matter, trauma, epilepsy

Demonstration of multiple sclerosis brain lesions with rapid inversion-recovery fluid-attenuated MRI

I. Berry [1,3], J. M. Franconi [4], M. Clanet [2], C. Manelfe [1]

[1] Department of Neuroradiology, University Hospital Purpan, F-31059 Toulouse, France
[2] Department of Neurology, University Hospital Purpan, Toulouse, France
[3] Biophysics, University Hospital Rangueil, Toulouse, France
[4] Siemens, Saint-Denis, France

Abstract. Turbo-FLAIR seems to be a reliable and practical method, more sensitive than T2-weighted spin-echo, for detection of multiple sclerosis. It offers an excellent compromise, allowing multisclice acquisition in a reasonable time without the disadvantages of limited resolution and edge artefacts of single shot techniques like echo-planar imaging. The results on 20 patients suspected of having multiple sclerosis are presented.

Key words: Multiple sclerosis - Magnetic resonance imaging - Demyelinating diseases

Multiple sclerosis brain lesions are detected on MRI with high sensitivity in white matter because they produce bright signal intensity on T2-weighted sequences, although the periventricular plaques may be difficult to separate from the signal of the cerebrospinal fluid. Several techniques have been used to solve this problem, i.e. dual spin-echo and fluid-attenuated inversion recovery (FLAIR).

The FLAIR sequence is highly beneficial to study of the periventricular region but requires long acquisition times. The data collection may be significantly shortened if several echoes are obtained and rearranged in the Fourier space. This has been applied to inversion recovery and names turbo-inversion recovery on our MRI system.

We optimised the turbo-inversion recovery for fluid attenuation and evaluated the visualisation of multiple sclerosis plaques in the periventricular and subcortical white matter.

Patients and methods

Brain imaging was performed in 20 patients suspected of having multiple sclerosis. MRI was obtained at 1.5 T, comparing during the same examination:

1. Turbo-fluid-attenuated inversion recovery (turbo-FLAIR) with the following parameters: TR 8000 ms, TE 119 ms, TI 2100 ms, 1 excitation, acquisition time 4.24 min, 15 slices 4 mm thick, interslice gap 20%, rectangular field of view and matrix (224×256)
2. T2-weighted sequence taken as reference with the turbo-dual spin-echo technique with the following contrast parameters: TR 3800, TE 16/98 ms, 1 excitation, acquisition time 2.56 min and the same slice parameters as above.

Correspondence to: I. Berry

Results

Turbo-FLAIR results in better visibility of multiple sclerosis lesions when compared with spin-echo: clear demonstration of periventricular multiple sclerosis lesions (Fig. 1); improved visibility of supratentorial subcortical multiple sclerosis lesions, related to better separation between deep sulci and gyri; improved confidence to exclude false positive lesions on T2-weighted images due to volume averaging of the cerebrospinal fluid and cortex, or dilated Virchow-Robin spaces (Fig. 2).

With FLAIR we noted a conspicuous thin bright rim at the interface between the ventricles and the brain, occurring also in normal individuals and a less conspicuous but usually visible bright rim at the interface of the subarachnoid space and the brain.

Discussion

Cerebrospinal fluid signal may be suppressed by inversion recovery while maintaining good T2 weighting of the other tissues. This method (FLAIR) relies on the differential values of T1 relaxation time of the brain and the cerebrospinal fluid which has a longer T1 than all the others including brain parenchymal lesion (i.e. multiple sclerosis plaques). The combination of a long inversion time (i.e. 1–3 s) and a long repetition time (typically 8 s) gives a differential nulling of the cerebrospinal fluid signal on inversion recovery. Drawbacks are the long acquisition time (over 17 min) and the single slice character of this method. In some more recent versions, FLAIR has been developed for multislice capabilities [1], although remaining with a limited number of slices. Poor image quality is one of the major problems, related to a lower signal to noise ratio as compared with conventional techniques.

Nevertheless the initial clinical report describes improvement in delineation of pathological findings in infarction, low-grade astrocytoma and diplegia [2]. It also shows excellent anatomical details in the brain stem. Subsequent clinical series confirmed improved lesion delineation in a series of FLAIR versus spin-echo, examined by two radiologists for lesion number, visibility and extent (48 lesions: 22 FLAIR > spin-echo, 26 FLAIR = spin-echo) [3].

One of the initial findings was that normally appearing white matter is brighter in the centrum semiovale, posterior internal capsule, parietopontine tract, occipitothalamic radiation and brain stem than the surrounding white

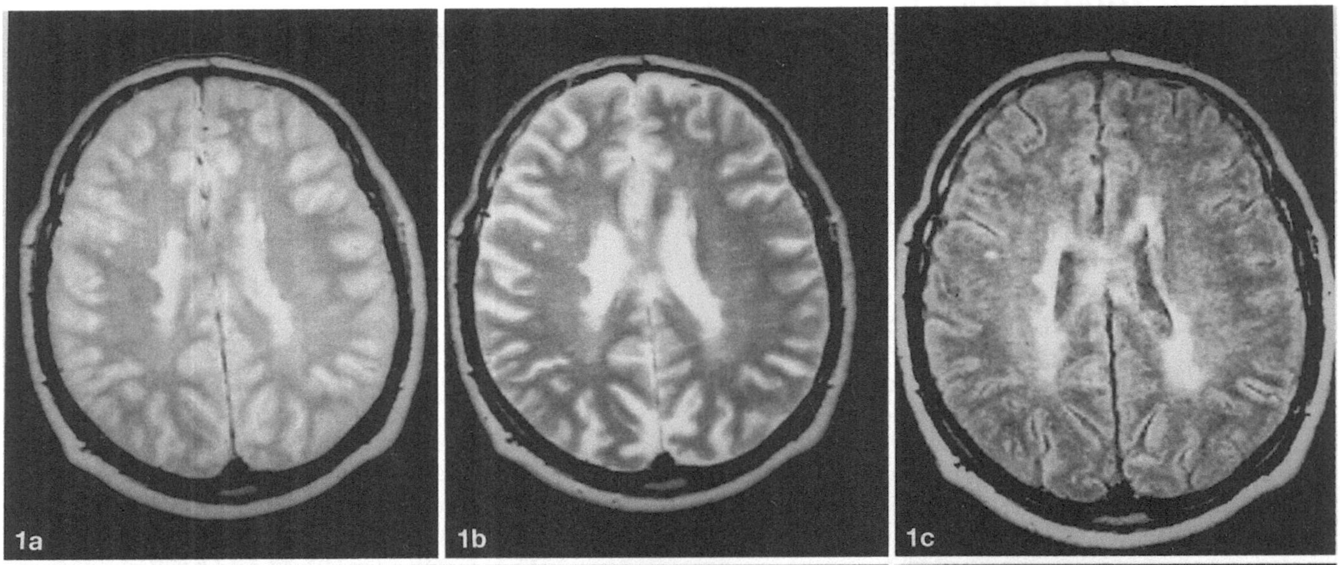

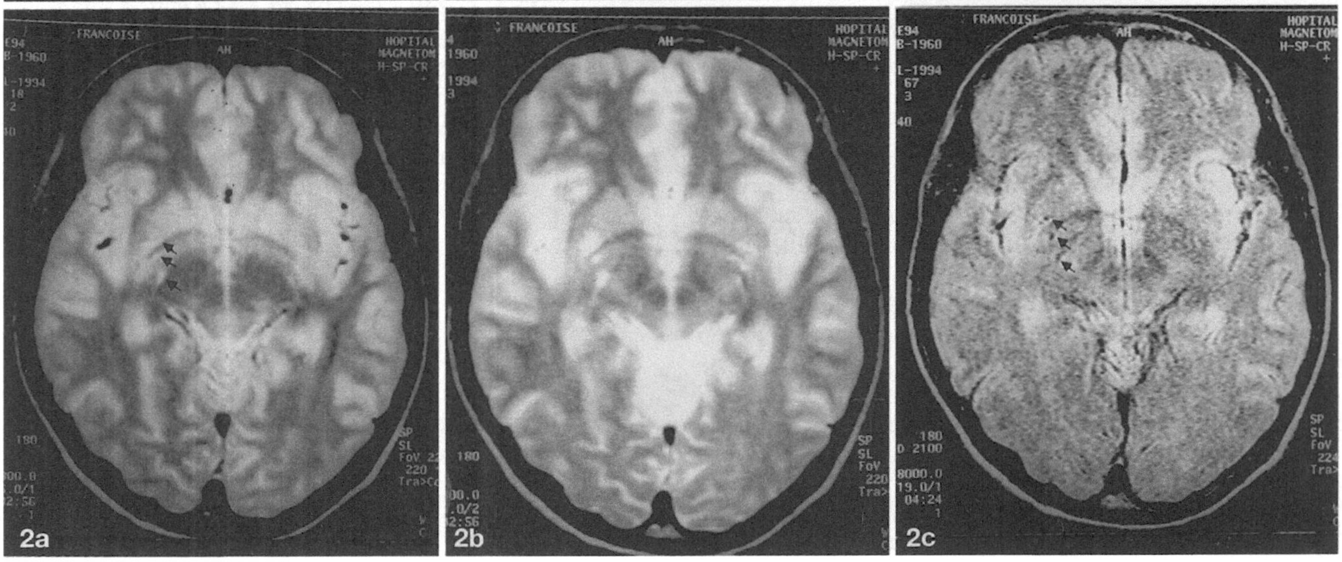

Fig. 1a–c. Improved demonstration of periventricular lesions on turbo-FLAIR. Dual turbo-spin-echo: first **(a)** and second **(b)** echoes; **c** turbo-FLAIR. The bright intensity signal of the periventricular plaques is well differentiated from the nulled signal of cerebrospinal fluid on FLAIR

Fig. 2. Dual turbo-spin-echo: first **(a)** and second **(b)** echoes; **c** turbo-FLAIR. Plaques are excluded on turbo-FLAIR, which shows high-signal areas (**a** *arrows*) dilated to be Virchow-Robin spaces (**c** *arrows*) because the signal is attenuated as cerebrospinal fluid

matter. One possible explanation is the influence of anisotropic differences in magnetic susceptibility [1].

Turbo-FLAIR was proposed by den Boer, who used a turbo-spin-echo preceded by an inversion delay sufficient to suppress the cerebrospinal fluid signal. Therefore multiple echoes are acquired and rearranged in the *k* space according to the RARE technique [4]. In the initial publication, 16–20 echoes were used, leading to an echo train of about 200 ms thereby reducing acquisition time by a factor of 16–20. The sequence can be made multislice, taking advantage of the long inversion times to interleave inversion pulses and echo trains of subsequent slices within one repetition time. Some flow artefacts, however, appear related to the inflow of cerebrospinal fluid during the inversion time. Slice rearrangement is a way of partially alleviating this problem. The interesting diagnostic capacities we have reported here are consistent with other authors' findings in recent preliminary reports. Unlike FLAIR, brighter deep white matter tracts did not occur in our experience, probably because of relatively shorter effective echo time (119 ms), allowing less expression of diffusion effects.

Further development may involve the use of echo-planar imaging (EPI). Image acquisition of a single slice (matrix 256 × 128) is as short as 46 s. The results tested for multiple sclerosis plaques remain, although limited in terms of image quality, lesion delineation and diagnostic confidence. A blinded review by six specialists compared spin-echo T2-weighted images and EPI-FLAIR and concluded that a T2-weighted spin-echo was of superior diagnostic value, except in one case where motion artefact was a concern. The magnetic susceptibility artefacts at the skull base and sinus interfaces are also a limitation. Again, it is only for periventricular lesions or lesions adjacent to cortical sulci that EPI-FLAIR was superior to T2-weighted spin-echo (10.4%).

References

1. Hajnal JV, de Coene B, Lewis PD et al. (1992) High signal regions in normal white matter shown by heavily T2-weighted CSF nulled IR sequences. J Comput Assist Tomogr 16:506–513
2. Hajnal JV, Bryant DJ, Kasuboski L et al. (1992) Use of fluid attenuated inversion recovery (FLAIR) pulse sequences in MRI of the brain. J Comput Assist Tomogr 16:841–844
3. de Coene B, Hajnal JV, Gatehouse P et al. (1992) MR of the brain using fluid-attenuated inversion recovery (FLAIR) pulse sequences. AJNR 13:1555–1564
4. Hennig J, Naureth A, Friedburg H (1986) RARE imaging: a fast imaging method for clinical MR. Magn Reson Med 3:823–833

Large focal cerebral demyelinating lesions mimicking intracranial neoplasms: imaging features

S. Batnitzky [1], D. A. Eckard [1], J. J. Kepes [2], H. J. Robertson [3]

[1] Department of Radiology, University of Kansas School of Medicine, Kansas City, KS 66160 - 7234, USA
[2] Department of Pathology and Laboratory Medicine, University of Kansas School of Medicine, Kansas City, Kansas, USA
[3] Department of Radiology, Louisiana State University, New Orleans, Louisiana, USA

Abstract. The CT and MRI features of 41 patients with histologically proven demyelinating lesions that mimicked intracranial neoplasms, both clinically and radiologically, were studied retrospectively. There were 32 patients with single and 9 with multiple lesions. In 40 cases the lesions characteristically involved the hemisphere white matter with no predilection for the periventricular areas, optic pathways or brain stem. The CT and MRI features are nonspecific and the true nature of the lesion was demonstrated by histology. All patients showed marked improvement following steroid therapy.

Key words: Demyelinating lesion – Neoplasm – Metastases

Demyelinating diseases of the central nervous system (CNS) are numerous, with multiple sclerosis (MS) being the most common and best known. In MS multiple demyelinating lesions, separated from each other in space and time, involve the CNS with certain areas of preference, such as periventricular white matter, the optic pathways, cerebellum, brain stem and spinal cord. While MS is nosologically well delineated, diseases in which large confluent territories of cerebral white matter become demyelinated comprise a less well understood group. These lesions can mimic intracranial tumors both clinically and radiologically [1–4].

Correspondence to: S. Batnitzky

Patients and methods

We reviewed the imaging findings of 41 patients with proven demyelination following open biopsy. Prior to biopsy, these patients were diagnosed as having a brain tumor, multiple abscesses, parasitic cysts, or metastases.

CT before and after contrast medium was obtained in 18 patients; 26 underwent MRI, with postgadolinium examinations in 22. Both CT and MRI were performed in 3 patients.

Follow-up CT or MRI examinations were obtained in 36 patients following open biopsy and treatment with corticosteroids, periods ranging from 1 month to 1 year after the initial study. Of these patients 27 had several imaging examinations up to 12 years following initial diagnosis.

Results

The patients were divided into two groups. Group A consistedof 32 patients, each of which had a single large lesion, and Group B of 9 patients with multiple lesions. Group A consisted of 23 females and 9 males; in group B there were 6 females and 3 males. The age of the patients at onset of symptoms was 5–77 years.

One patient presented with a solitary lesion in the cerebellar white matter (Fig. 1). All the other lesions characteristically involved hemisphere white matter, with no predilection for the periventricular areas, optic pathways or brain stem. Shift of midline structures was not commensurate with the size of the mass. Despite the fact that the diameter of most of the lesions in group A was more than 2.5 cm, the largest lesion measuring 9 cm, only minimal shift was noted. In group B, the lesions ranged from 0.5 cm to 4 cm in diameter.

The CT and MRI features were variable and not specific. On CT the lesions appeared as low-density areas

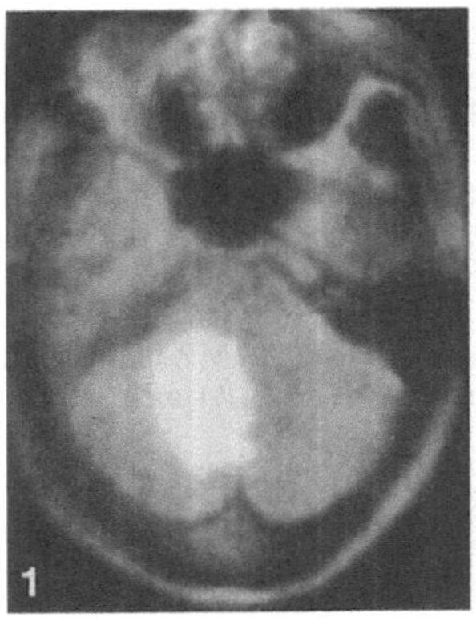
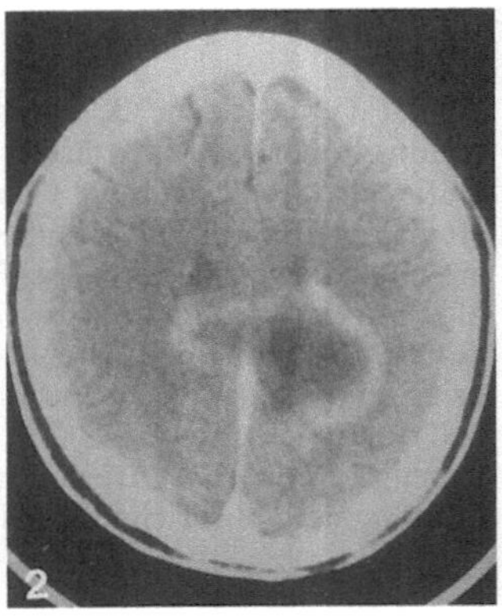
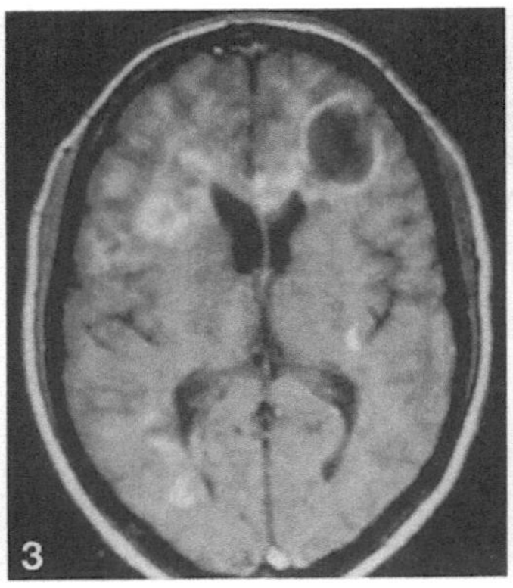
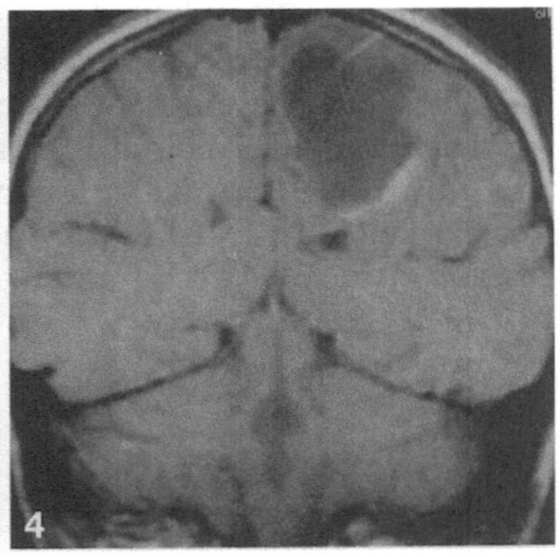
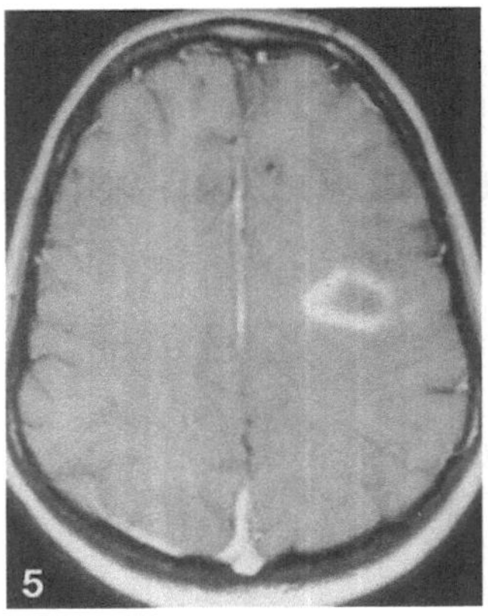
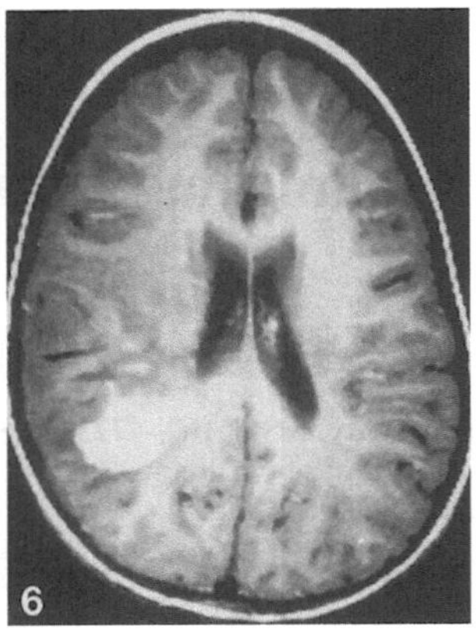

Fig. 1. Demyelination mimicking cerebellar tumor. T2-weighted axial MRI in a 37-year-old man demonstrates a large area of increased signal intensity in the right cerebellum

Fig. 2. Demyelination mimicking "butterfly" metastasis. Contrast-enhanced axial CT in a 41-year-old man with a retroperitoneal seminoma demonstrates a large irregular ring enhancing lesion in the posterior corpus callosum, believed to be a metastasis. Biopsy showed an area of demyelination

Fig. 3. Multiple demyelinating mass lesions. Contrast-enhanced axial T1-weighted MRI of a 24-year-old woman demonstrates multiple, ring enhancing masses of varying size in both hemispheres. Biopsy of a lesion in the right frontal lobe demonstrated an area of demyelination

Fig. 4. Contrast-enhanced coronal T1-weighted MRI at a 10-year-old boy suspected clinically of having a brain tumor demonstrates a large low-signal mass in the left parietal region. Peripheral ring enhancement is most marked on its inferiolateral aspect. The histological diagnosis was demyelination

Fig. 5. A 31-year-old woman was diagnosed as having a left parietal glioma; she had an influenza vaccination 10 days prior to admission. Contrast-enhanced axial T1-weighted MRI demonstrates ring enhancement in the left parietal region. Biopsy show an area of demyelination

Fig. 6. Focal demyelination mimicking intracranial neoplasm in 5-year-old girl. Contrast-enhanced axial T1-weighted MRI demonstrates an area of intense enhancement in the right parietal lobe with slight shift of the midline structures to the left. The trigone of the right lateral ventricle is effaced. The pre-operative and operative diagnosis was that of a glioma, but histology revealed an area of demyelination

with ill-defined margins. In 20% of the solitary lesions and 80% of the multiple lesions, a peripheral rim of increased density was present on unenhanced CT. Contrast enhancement was seen in 96% of cases. This varied from peripheral ring enhancement in 80% (Fig. 2) to dense homogeneous or heterogeneous enhancement in the remaining 20%. Calcification was not seen in any lesions.

On MRI, the lesions gave low signal on T1-weighted images and high signal on proton density and T2-weighted images. Contrast enhancement with intravenous gadolinium injection was present in 98% of cases. As with CT, this was peripheral in 80% (Figs. 3–5) and homogeneous (Fig. 6) or heterogeneous in 20%. In all cases the area of enhancement was smaller than the lesion seen on the T2- and proton-density-weighted images, suggesting perilesional edema.

The histological picture was essentially identical in each patient. In the subcortical white matter, large numbers of foamy macrophages were seen intermingled with large-bodied reactive astrocytes. In some areas, perivascular lymphocytic infiltrates were identified. On myelin stain, near total or total loss of myelin was observed. However, there was always relative preservation of a moderate to large number of axons in these areas.

All patients showed marked improvement following corticosteroid therapy. In 36, no additional lesions were documented clinically or radiologically during follow-up ranging from 9 months to 12 years, with complete resolution of the lesions on follow-up imaging. One patient remained hemiparetic although no additional lesions were documented clinically or radiologically during a 3-year period. Her initial lesion showed incomplete resolution on follow-up MRI. Four patients developed additional lesions following the pattern of MS both clinically and radiologically over a 1–4 year period after the initial diagnosis.

Discussion

These cases underline the diagnostic difficulties the clinician and radiologist may encounter when dealing with demyelinating disease presenting as and operated upon as presumed CNS tumors. In our series, the great majority of cases (37) behaved as a "single event" disease with no relapses and exacerbations, both clinically and on imaging studies in follow-up periods ranging from 1 to 14 years. Even the pathologist may encounter difficulties if special stains for myelin and axons are not used. In 14 patients in this series, the initial histopathological findings were misleading, suggesting the presence of a neoplasm. Special stains for myelin and axons revealed the total to near total loss of myelin with relative preservation of axons, which revealed the true nature of the lesion.

One of us [5] reported on the pathological features of single event demyelination in 31 of these cases. While histologically these lesions resemble MS, they differ from it in a number of ways. It was suggested that most large focal demyelinating lesions of the brain that mimicked intracranial neoplasms represent an entity intermediate between classical MS and postinfectious and postvaccination encephalomyelitis.

Neither CT nor MRI is specific. Demyelinating lesions should be considered in the differential diagnosis of both single and multiple space-occupying lesions. On imaging features alone, it is not possible to differentiate these lesions from other mass lesions such as gliomas, abscesses, and metastases. The true nature of these lesions is usually established only through biopsy.

References

1. Van der Velden M, Bots GTAM, Endtz LJ (1979) Cranial CT in multiple sclerosis showing a mass effect. Surg Neurol 12:307–310
2. Rieth KG, Di Chiro G, Cromwell LD et al. (1981) Primary demyelinating disease simulating glioma of the corpus callosum. J Neurosurg 55:620–624
3. Sagar HJ, Warlow CP, Sheldon PWE et al. (1982) Multiple sclerosis with clinical and radiological features of cerebral tumour. J Neurol Neurosurg Psychiatry 45:802–808
4. Ishihara O, Yamaguchi Y, Matsuishi T et al. (1984) Multiple ring enhancement in a case of acute reversible demyelinating disease in childhood suggestive of acute multiple sclerosis. Brain Dev 6:401–406
5. Kepes JJ (1993) Large focal tumor-like demyelinating lesions of the brain: Intermediate entity between multiple sclerosis and acute disseminated encephalomyelitis? A study of 31 patients. Ann Neurol 33:18–27

Central pontine myelinolysis: magnetic resonance imaging

L. A. Bacheschi, S. C. Mathias, A. C. A. Magalhães

Department of Radiology, Section of Magnetic Resonance, Hospital das Clinicas, University of São Paulo, São Paulo, Brazil

Abstract. Three patients with central pontine myelinolysis underwent MRI study. The first case, with a good outcome, had small pontine lesions. The second, with incomplete recovery, showed large pontine lesions; and the third, who died showed severe brain-stem involvement. MRI showed central pontine myelinolysis as lesions with low signal on T1-weighted images and high signal on T2 weighting without contrast enhancement. The severity of the clinical picture was proportional to the extension of the lesions.

Key words: Central pontine myelinolysis – Brain-Magnetic resonance imaging – Demyelinating disease

Central pontine myelinolysis (CPM) is a rare disorder caused by essentially demyelinating lesions which affect mainly the middle portion of the basis pontis. Initially, the majority of the cases had been related to late stages of chronic alcoholism. Recently it was observed that even in alcoholic patients the development of CPM was associated with rapid correction of severe hyponatraemia [1–5].

Correspondence to: L. A. Bacheschi, University of São Paulo, School of Medicine, 05444-010 - Rua dos Tamanas 506, Sao Paulo, SP, Brazil

Case reports

Three adult patients who developed disturbed consciousness and quadriparesis after rapid metabolic control are presented. In these patients, MRI studies were performed with a 1.5 T imager.

Case 1

A 39-year-old woman with renal failure following childbearing and severe hyponatraemia developed stupor and spastic tetraparesis after a rapid metabolic correction. MRI showed central pontine lesion with low signal on T1-weighted and high signal on T2-weighted images without mass effect or contrast enhancement (Fig. 1). This patient made a good recovery.

Case 2

A 28-year-old chronic alcoholic man was admitted because of disturbed consciousness due to septicaemia, rhabdomyolysis and acute renal failure. After metabolic control he developed a tetraparesis. MRI showed central pontine lesion with the same characteristics as in case 1 (Fig. 2). This patient made an incomplete neurological recovery.

Case 3

A 28-year-old man with recurrent otitis media developed an acute bacterial meningoencephalitis. After the introduction of antimicrobial drugs and metabolic control, he developed coma and spastic

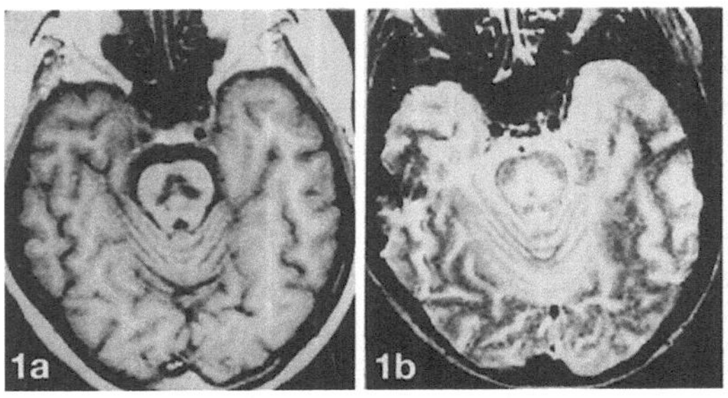

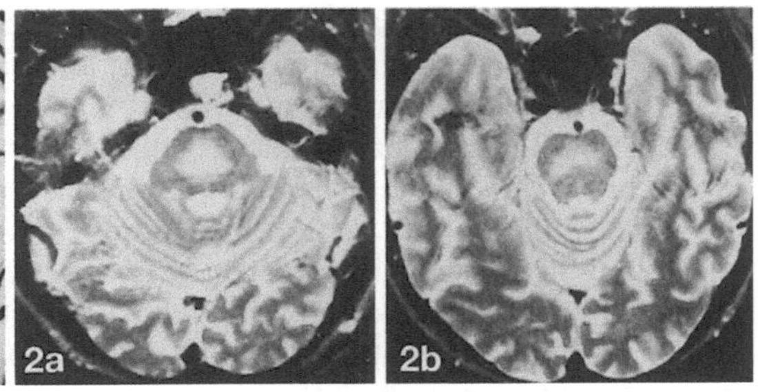

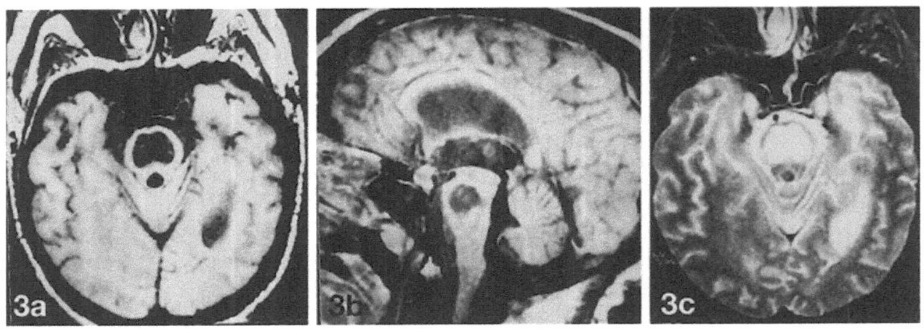

Fig. 1 a–c. Case 1. MRI (**a** axial T1-weighted, **b** axial T2-weighted, **c** sagittal contrast-enhanced T1-weighted) show a large lesion with low signal on T1 weighting and high signal on T2 weighting in the middle of the pons, without mass effect or contrast enhancement

Fig. 2 a, b. Case 2. Axial T2-weighted images show a large round lesion with high signal in the middle of the pons

Fig. 3 a–c. Case 3. Axial T1- **(a)** and T2-weighted **(b)** and sagittal T1-weighed images **(c)** show ventricular enlargement and a large round lesion in the middle of the pons

tetraparesis. MRI showed ventricular enlargement and a large round lesion in the middle of the pons and brain-stem isthmus (Fig. 3). This patient died, and at autopsy the pontine lesion seen on MRI had the same shape, corresponding to a complete necrotic cavity.

Discussion

The clinical features of CPM include spastic tetraparesis, pseudobulbar palsy and consciousness level alterations which can deteriorate to coma. The pontine lesions can be associated with points of myelinolysis in other areas symmetrically distributed in thalamus, subthalamic nucleus, striatum, internal capsule, cerebellar white matter, internal layer of cerebral cortex and adjacent white matter [2, 3, 6].

The pathological features consist of myelin sheath destruction with partial sparing of axons and pontine nuclei. These alterations begin inside the lesion in an intense manner leading to frank tissue necrosis. Signs of inflammatory activity are generally absent [7].

The causes of CPM are not well understood. The most important pathogenic factor is the rapid correction of severe states of hyponatraemia to normal or higher serum sodium levels. Other correlated features include nutritional disturbances, severe serum hyperosmolarity, hypernatraemia, hyperglycaemia and azotaemia.

The demyelination lesions appear as low signal areas on T1-weighted images and high signal areas on T2 weighting. With contrast media there is no pathological enhancement. The specific feature is the preferential localisation of the demyelination lesions in the central pontine area. Associated extrapontine lesions must be differentiated from other white matter alterations like infarcts, multiple sclerosis, brain-stem gliomas and radiotherapy-related lesions [2]. In the present cases, the severity of the clinical picture was proportional to the extent of the lesions, but sometimes clinical symptoms were mild despite extensive pontine lesions [8].

References

1. Brunner JE, Redmond JM, Haggar AM, Elias SB (1988) Central pontine myelinolysis after rapid correction of hyponatremia: a magnetic resonance imaging study. Ann Neurol 23:389–391
2. Miller GM, Baker HL Jr, Okazaki H, Whisnant JP (1988) Central pontine myelinolysis and its imitators: MR findings. Radiology 168:795–802
3. Estol CJ, Faris AA, Martínez AJ, Ahdab-Barmada M (1989) Central pontine myelinolysis after liver transplantation. Neurology 39:493–498
4. Ragland RL, Duffis AW, Gendelman S, Som PM, Rabinowitz JG (1989) Central pontine myelinolysis with clinical recovery. MR documentation. J Comput Assist Tomogr 13:316–318
5. Castillo RA, Ray RA, Yagmai F (1989) Central pontine myelinolysis and pregnancy. Obstet Gynecol 73:459–461
6. Ho VB, Fitz CR, Yoder CC, Geyer CA (1993) Resolving MR features in osmotic myelinolysis (central pontine and extrapontine myelinolysis). AJNR 14:163–167
7. Thompson AJ, Brown MM, Swash M, Thakkar C, Scholtz C (1988) Autopsy validation of MRI in central pontine myelinolysis. Neuroradiology 30:175–177
8. Korogi Y, Takahashi M, Shinzato J, Sakamoto Y, Mitsuzaki K, Hirai T, Yoshizumi K (1993) MR findings in two presumed cases of mild central pontine myelinolysis. AJNR 14:651–654

MRI in neuro-Behçet's disease: clinical correlation

Young Kuk Cho [1], Dong Ik Kim [1], Eun Young Kim [1], Tae Sub Chung [1], Jung Ho Suh [2], Il Nam Sunwood [3]

[1] Department of Diagnostic Radiology, Yonsei University College of Medicine, Seoul, Korea
[2] Department of Neurology, Yonsei University College of Medicine, Seoul, Korea
[3] Department of Diagnosic Radiology, College of Medicine, Ajou University, Suwon, Korea

Abstract. We reviewed brain MRI patterns of 4 patients with neuro-Behçet's disease and correlated them with the patients' clinical status. The frequent neurological symptoms at the time of MRI were dysarthria, headache, motor weakness, diplopia, and ataxia (in order of frequency). T2-weighted axial images showed multiple, discrete or patchy high signal intensities in the brain stem (medulla, pons, midbrain), deep cerebral nuclei (thalamus, basal ganglia), centrum semiovale, corpus callosum, and other supratentorial grey and white matter. The frequently affected regions were pons ($n=11$) and lentiform nuclei ($n=11$). During the initial neurological attack, anatomical regions of high-signal intensities were more widely distributed. The more the previous neurological insults, the less was the number of affected anatomical regions. The predominance of high signal intensities in the brain stem and deep cerebral nuclei with relatively scarce lesions in the cerebral hemisphere may suggest the possibility of central nervous system involvement in Behçet's disease patients. As well as the clinical settings such as severe headache, dysarthria and motor weakness, brain MRI may be a helpful aid in the diagnosis of neuro-Behçet's disease.

Key words: Neuro-Behçet's disease – Behçet's disease – Magnetic resonance imaging

Behçet's disease is characterised clinically by the presence of a diagnostic triad of stomatitis, genital ulceration and uveitis [1]. Other multiple organ systems may be involved. As in other rheumatological diseases and vasculitis, central nervous system (CNS) findings can be present without any peripheral evidence of underlying processes [2]. The purpose of this study was to categorise the MRI manifestations of neuro-Behçet's disease and to correlate the clinical findings with the images.

Patients and methods

We reviewed the records and brain MRI findings of 14 patients (8 men, 6 women, aged 27–55 years, median 32 years) with neuro-Behçet's disease. We adopted diagnostic criteria of Behçet's disease suggested by the Behçet's Disease Research Committee of Japan [3].

MRI was performed in 12 patients with a 1.5 T superconducting system, in 1 at 0.5 T, and in another at 1.0 T. All had 5- or 10-mm axial, coronal, and sagittal contiguous sections using spin-echo (SE) sequences (SE200/20–SE500/30, SE2500/80–SE3000/100).

Correspondence to: Y. K. Cho, Department of Diagnostic Radiology, Yonsei University College of Medicine 134, Shinchon-dong, Seodaemunku, Seoul, 120-752 Korea

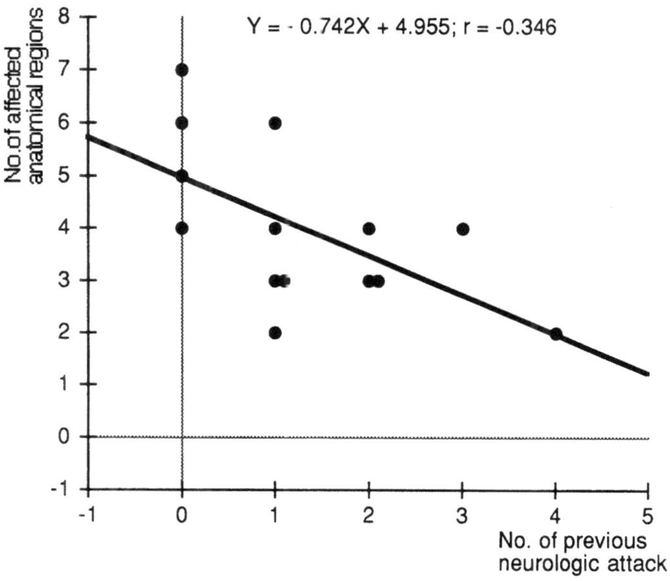

Fig. 1. Significant ($P<0.05$), negative correlation ($Y=0.742X+4.955$; $r=0.346$) between the number of affected anatomical regions and the number of previous neurological attacks

The brain MRI findings were reviewed, paying special attention to the distribution of high signal intensities in proton density and T2-weighted axial images. Anatomical regions which showed high signal intensities were arbitrarily divided into ten regions: medulla, pons, midbrain, thalami, caudate nuclei, lentiform nuclei, corpus callosum, centrum semiovale and other supratentorial grey and white matter.

The numbers of affected anatomical regions in each patient that showed high signal intensities were correlated with each patient's clinical information, such as the number of previous neurological attacks, the interval between the first neurological attack and the present attack, that between the onset of recent neurological symptoms and the day on which MRI was performed, and that between the day on which Behçet's disease was diagnosed and the onset of neuro-Behçet's disease. To assess the correlation, linear regression analysis was performed on all occasions.

Results

Both clinical and MRI findings in the 14 patients are summarized in Tables 1 and 2. The pons and the lentiform nuclei were the most frequently affected regions. The medulla oblongata, midbrain, and supratentorial white matter except the centrum semiovale were the second most common regions. The caudate nuclei, thalamus, other supratentorial grey matter, centrum semiovale and corpus callosum were less commonly affected. Brain-stem atrophy was seen in two patients.

Table 1. Clinical features of 14 patients with neuro-Behçet's disease

No/age (years)/sex	No. of previous neurological attacks	Interval between previous attack and present (years)	Interval between onset of Behçet's disease and neurological involvement (years)	Interval between recent neuro-logical attack and MRI (days)	Major neurological findings
1/27/F	0	0	6	25	Confusion, weakness
2/30/F	0	0	4	8	Headache, dysarthria
3/30/F	0	0	4	150	Weakness
4/53/M	0	0	1	15	Headache, dysarthria
5/27/M	1	1	3	24	Headache, blurred vision
6/29/F	1	0.67	1	7	Severe headache
7/30/M	1	0.25	0.75	5	Dysarthria, weakness
8/34/M	1	2	8	2	Diplopia, dizziness
9/36/M	1	1.25	2	7	Seizure
10/32/M	2	3	5	1	Severe headache
11/33/F	2	9	5	4	Confusion, dysarthria, weakness
12/55/F	2	5	3	8	Dysarthria, weakness
13/32/M	3	3	2	10	Diplopia
14/32/M	4	8	5	3	Dysarthria, ataxia

Table 2. Distribution of high signal intensity on T2-weighted images of 14 patients with neuro-Behçet's disease

Case	Medulla	Pons	Mid-brain	Caudate nucleus	Lenti-form nucleus	Thalami	Corpus callosum	Centrum semi-ovale	Other STGM	Other STWM	Total
1	−	−	−	+	+	−	+	+	−	+	5/10
2	−	+	+	+	+	+	−	−	+	+	7/10
3	+	+	+	−	+	−	−	−	−	−	4/10
4	−	+	+	−	+	+	−	+	−	+	6/10
5	+	−	+	+	+	−	−	−	−	−	4/10
6	−	+	+	−	+	−	−	−	−	−	3/10
7	+	+	−	−	−	−	−	−	−	−	2/10
8	+	+	+	−	+	+	−	−	−	+	6/10
9	−	−	−	+	+	−	−	−	−	+	3/10
10[a]	+	+	+	−	−	−	−	−	−	−	3/10
11[b]	+	+	−	−	−	−	−	−	+	+	4/10
12	+	+	−	−	+	−	−	−	−	−	3/10
13	−	+	−	−	+	+	−	−	−	+	4/10
14	−	+	−	−	+	−	−	−	−	−	2/10
Total	7/14	11/14	7/14	4/14	11/14	4/14	1/14	2/14	2/14	7/14	56/140

STGM Supratentorial grey matter; STWM supratentorial white matter other than corpus callosum, and centrum semiovale
[a] These two patients showed brain stem atrophy

The number of previous neurological attacks was significantly correlated to the number of affected anatomical regions ($Y = -0.742\times + 4.955$; $r = -0.346$) ($P < 0.05$) (Fig. 1). The interval between the onset of recent neurological symptoms and the day on which MRI was performed and the interval between the day on which Behçet's disease was diagnosed and the onset of neuro-Behçet's disease was not significantly correlated with the number of anatomical regions affected.

Discussion

Behçet's disease, a rare multisystem immune-related vasculitis, is prevalent in Korea, Japan, the Middle East, and many Mediterranean countries. CNS manifestations are frequently seen in association with vasculitic disorders. Behçet's disease in particular often has associated neurological features. The frequency of CNS involvement in Behçet's disease is 8–10% [4, 5].

MRI findings in neuro-Behçet's disease consist of small foci of high signal intensity on T2-weighted images, which are iso- or hypointense, relative to brain, on T1-weighted images. The lesions may be circular, linear, crescentic, or irregular, and occur most frequently within the brain stem, especially around the cerebral peduncles and in the pons. The thalamus and basal ganglia are second in frequency and similar foci may be seen in the cerebral hemispheres, spinal cord, or the cerebellum.

Histological findings in nervous system involvement in Behçet's syndrome include infiltrations rich in lymphocytes in the meninges, scattered small necrotic or softened

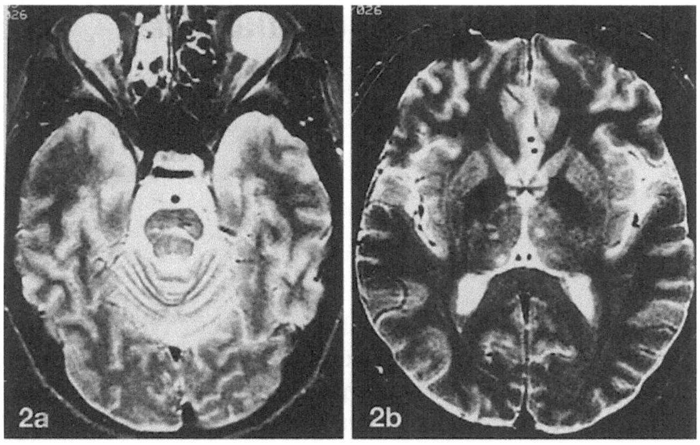

Fig. 2. T2-weighted MRI of case 13. This patient had three neurological attacks within 3 years. Multiple high signal intensity areas are noted in the pons and thalamus

foci in the white matter, perivascular lymphocytic cuffing, especially around venules, and diffuse demyelination and axonal degeneration. These changes are most prominent in the brain stem (midbrain, pons, medulla oblongata, and crus cerebri) [3].

In our study, there was a tendency for the patient to experience other previous neurological attacks, each of which had a smaller number of affected anatomical regions (Fig. 2). A possible explanation of our result is a reversibility of neuro-Behçet's lesions, and a better result after previous treatments with steroids, or a combination of steroid and immunosuppressive drugs. Other articles reported the reversibility of the brain stem lesions in neuro-Behçet's disease [6, 7].

Previous case reports of sequential brain CT and MRI in brain-stem typeneuro-Behçet's syndrome may provide another explanation. The most frequently affected structures in these cases were distributed over the pontine base, pontine tegmentum, cerebral peduncle and posterior limb of the internal capsule. This rostrocaudal distribution of lesions can be explained not by arterial occlusion but by a disturbance of the venous outflow from the brain stem [8].

In a very interesting report, the authors hypothesized that small cortical vein thromboses were the underlying causes of transient cortical lesions affecting both grey and white matters. These are frequently located in the occipital and posterior parietal areas, although in cases of malignancy, aplastic anaemia, and AIDS [9] they are located in the cerebral hemispheres. We believe that there may be many diseases showing similar changes, as in neuro-Behçet's disease.

In a report of MRI in six neuro-Behçet's patients, the authors suggested three different stages of imaging appearance. There were scattered areas of high signal intensity on T2-weighted images with predilection to the central structures of the cerebrum, the cerebral peduncles, and basis pontis in the acute stage. During the recovery phase, most of these findings improved, but some white matter high signal areas persisted in the upper brain stem and peripheral subcortical white matter. Occasionally, findings suggest microhaematoma. In the chronic phase, atrophy of posterior fossa structures became evident with decreased signal intensity suggestive of haemosiderin deposits [10].

In conclusion, diagnostic sensitivity of T2-weighted images for neuro-Behçet's disease seems to be high, and MRI is useful for studying CNS lesions in Behçet's disease.

The predominance of high signal intensities at the brain stem, basal ganglia, and thalamus with relatively scarce abnormalities in the cerebral hemispheres may suggest the high possibility of neuro-Behçet's disease in Behçet's disease patients. As well as the clinical setting such as severe headache, dysarthria and motor weakness, brain MRI may be helpful in the diagnosis of neuro-Behçet's disease.

References

1. Katoh K et al. (1985) Pathologically defined neuro-, vasculo-, entero-Behçet's disease. J Rheumatol 12:1186–1190
2. Sigal LH (1987) The neurologic presentation of vasculitic and rheumatologic syndromes. A review. Medicine (Baltimore) 66:157–180
3. Shimizu T, Ehrlich GE, Inaba G, Hayashi K (1979) Behçet's disease (Behçet's syndrome). Semin Arthritis Rheum 8:223–260
4. Chajek T, Fainaru M (1975) Behçet's disease. Report of 41 cases and review of the literature. Medicine (Baltimore) 54:179–196
5. Alema G (1978) Behçet's disease. In: Vinken PJ, Bruyn GW (eds) Handbook of clinical neurology, vol 34. Infections of the nervous system, part 2. North-Holland, Amsterdam, pp 475–512
6. Mizukami K et al. (1992) CNS changes in neuro-Behçet's disease: CT, MR, and SPECT findings. Comput Med Imaging Graph 16:401–406
7. Patel DV, Neuman MJ, Hier DB (1989) Reversibility of CT and MR findings in neuro-Behçet's disease. J Comput Assist Tomogr 13:669–673
8. Kataoka S, Hirose G, Tsukada K (1989) Brain stem type neuro-Behçet's syndrome. Correlation of enhanced CT scans and MRI during the acute and chronic stage of illness. Neuroradiology 31:258–262
9. Patronas NJ, Argyropoulou M (1992) Intravascular thrombosis as a possible cause of transient brain lesion: CT and MRI. J Comput Assist Tomogr 16:849–855
10. Al Kawi MZ, Bohlega S, Banna M (1991) MRI findings in neuro-Behçet's disease. Neurology 41:405–408

Brain and spinal MRI in patients with systemic lupus erythematosus

S. Kan [1], T. Ikeda [1], S. Katagiri [1], S. Nishiyama [1], T. Matsubayashi [1], J. Okada [2]

[1] Department of Radiology, Kitasato University, Kanagawa, Japan
[2] Department of Internal Medicine, Kitasato University, Kanagawa, Japan

Abstract. We have examined 80 patients with systemic lupus erythematosus. Of 127 head MRI studies 75 showed parenchymal changes. Brain MRI findings were classified roughly into six groups: multiple high-intensity spots on T2-weighted images, 28 studies; infarction, 33 studies; transient high-intensity lesions on T2-weighted images, 8 studies; sinus thrombosis, 3 studies (1 patient); diffuse intracranial calcification, 2 studies; inflammation, 1 study. Significant differences were noted between MRI positive and MRI negative patients with regard to age and duration of the disease. Patients with MRI lesions were significantly older than MRI negative patients, and had a longer duration of the disease. There was no significant difference in the two groups with regard to lupus anticoagulant and the level of anticardiolipin antibody.

Key words: Magnetic resonance imaging – Systemic lupus erythematosus

Involvement of the central nervous system (CNS) by systemic lupus erythematosus (SLE) is relatively common. A frequency (70%) of central nervous system (CNS) involvement is reported, according to Small et al. [1]. MRI is known to be useful in displaying brain lesions with neuropsychiatric SLE. Several studies of neuropsychiatric SLE with MRI have been made [2–5]. The purpose of this study is to determine the correlation between MRI findings and clinical variables, including data, and to analyse MRI findings in patients with SLE.

Patients and methods

We examined 80 patients with SLE. The group consisted of 76 females and 3 males who ranged in age from 13 to 68 years (mean, 33 years). MRI was performed on a 0.5 T MR unit. Brain MRI included T1-weighted, T2-weighted and proton density images. The slice thickness was 7 mm. Most of the head MRI studies were acquired in the axial plane. Contrast media was given in a few cases. Spinal MRI was carried out in 3 cases. Spinal MRI included T1-weighted, proton density and T2-weighted images. The slice thickness was 5 mm. A total of 130 head and spinal MRI examinations were performed. The following clinical parameters are reviewed: patient age, duration of the disease, activity of the disease, facial butterfly, renal involvement and type of CNS manifestation. Lupus anticoagulant and anticardiolipin antibodies were measured in most cases.

Correspondence to: S. Kan

Results

Seventy-five of 127 (59%) showed parenchymal changes. Atrophic change and extracerebral haemorrhage were not considered brain parenchymatous change. One of 3 spinal MRI studies showed abnormal findings. Brain MRI findings were classified roughly into six groups: (1) multiple high-intensity spots on T2-weighted images (migraine-like type), 28 studies; (2) infarction which had low intensity on T1-weighted images or low density on CT, 33 studies; (3) transient high-intensity lesion on T2-weighted images (eclampsia-like, encephalitis-like type), 8 studies; (4) sinus thrombosis, 3 studies (1 patient); (5) diffuse intracranial calcification, 2 studies; (6) inflammation, 1 study.

Spinal MRI did not detect any abnormality in the two cases of transverse myelitis.

First, we compared the number of patients with positive versus negative MR findings with regard to multiple clinical variables and laboratory data. Significant differences were noted in two groups (MR-positive versus MR-negative patients) with regard to age and duration of the disease ($P < 0.05$). Patients with MRI-positive lesions were significantly older than MRI-negative patients, and had longer duration of the disease than MRI-negative patients.

Secondly, we compared a number of patients between a subtype of MRI findings (normal and above-mentioned six types of positive MRI findings) with regard to multiple clinical variables and laboratory data. Significant differences were noted within a subtype of MRI findings with regard to renal involvement, duration of the disease, patient's age, facial butterfly and activity of the disease. Patients with types 1 and 2 were older than MRI-negative patients. Patients with eclampsia-like pattern (type 3) were younger than patients with types 1 and 2. The activity of the disease was highest in the type 3 group of patients. All patients with types 4–6 had renal involvement. Patients with type 2 had significantly longer duration of the disease than patients with normal MRI. Facial butterfly flush was frequently seen in the type 3 patients.

Discussion

Aisen et al. [5] analyse MRI of SLE involving the brain, and three patterns of findings were reported: cerebral infarction (type 1 of our study), multiple small areas of increased intensity (type 2), and focal areas of increased intensity, predominantly in the cerebral grey matter (type 3). Because of the similarity of MRI findings, we named type 1 migraine-like, type 2 frank infarction, and type 3 eclampsia-like, encephalitis-like. We have encountered types other than those in Aisen's study, i.e. type 4 sinus

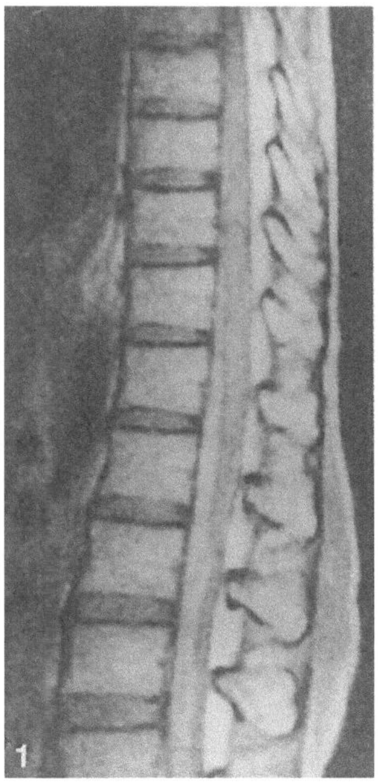

Fig. 1. Spinal subdural haematoma in a patient with severe back pain. T1-weighted image: diffuse high intensity in thorac-lumbar spinal canal subcutaneous haematoma is seen as an isointense mass

thrombosis, type 5 diffuse calcification and type 6 inflammation. Those types of MRI findings are not frequent in our series.

The exact cause of neuropsychiatric manifestation is not known. From pathological studies, typical findings are as follows: microvascular abnormalities (endothelial proliferation, perivascular gliosis, hyalinization), microinfarcts in the cortex, perivascular "cuffing" of small arteries, infrequent arteritis and arterial thrombosis. True vasculitis is not common in the nervous system. From an immunopathological point of view, two causes are postulated: immune-complex-mediated vascular damage and the direct interaction of autoantibody with membrane molecules of neurons [6].

The MRI findings of our study indicate that type 1 might be due to micro-infarction and type 2 is infarction due to arterial disease. MR angiography may play an important role in type 2. In some cases of type 3 MRI findings, the cause is probably the same as that of eclampsia. All such cases had renal involvement and distribution of multiple high-intensity lesions, which is quite similar to typical MRI of eclampsia. However, there are cases of type 3 whose MRI showed high-intensity lesions in the insular cortex and temporal lobes. This finding is similar to herpes encephalitis, but no definite evidence of herpes encephalitis was noted, so the exact cause is unknown.

Spinal subarachnoid haemorrhage associated with SLE is quite rare [7]. In our series, one case of spinal subdural haematoma was encountered (Fig. 1). MRI findings of transverse myelitis have been reported [8].

Significant clinical variables between subtypes of MRI findings are the patient's age, duration of the disease, facial butterfly, renal involvement and activity of the disease. In McCune's study of neuropsychiatric SLE [2], the most significant parameter associated with MRI findings by multivariate analysis was age. This result was the same as our study. In contrast to McCune's study, half of the patients without CNS manifestation showed abnormal MRI findings.

References

1. Small P, Mass MF, Kohler PF, Haarbech RJ (1977) Central nervous system involvement in SLE: diagnostic profile and clinical features. Arthritis Rheum 20:869–878
2. McCune WJ, MacGuire A, Aisen A, Gebarski S (1988) Identification of brain lesions in neuropsychiatric systemic lupus erythematosus by magnetic resonance scanning. Arthritis Rheum 31:159–166
3. Jacob L, Kinkel PR, Costello PB, Alukal MK, Kinkel WR, Green FA (1988) Central nervous system lupus erythematosus: the value of magnetic resonance imaging. J Rheumatol 15:601–606
4. Lim L, Ron MA, Ormerod IEC, Miller DH, Logsdail SJ, Walport MJ, Harding AE (1988) Psychiatric and neurological manifestations in systemic lupus erythematosus. Q J Med 249:27–38
5. Aisen AM, Gabrielsen TC, McCune WJ (1985) MR imaging of systemic lupus erythematosus involving the brain. AJNR 6:197–201
6. Bluestein HG (1992) The central nervous system in systemic lupus erythematosus. In: Lahita RG (ed) Systemic lupus erythematosus. Churchill Livingstone, Edinburgh, pp 639–655
7. Fody EP, Netsky MG, Mrak RE (1980) Subarachnoid spinal hemorrhage in a case of systemic lupus erythematosus. Arch Neurol 37:173–174
8. Boummpas DT, Patronas MJ, Dalakas MC, Hakim CA, Klippel JH, Balow JE (1990) Acute transverse myelitis in systemic lupus erythematosus: magnetic resonance imaging and review of the literature. J Rheumatol 17:89–92

Multiple cystic lesions in white matter without clinical manifestations (unidentified black holes)

L. A. Bacheschi, A. C. A. Magalhães, S. C. Mathias

Department of Radiology, Section of Magnetic Resonance, Hospital das Clínicas, University of São Paulo, São Paulo, Brazil

Abstract. We report three patients with normal daily life and normal professional or school activities who were submitted for cerebral MRI studies owing to minor symptoms. MRI showed multiple and wide lesions in one or both hemispheres which were iso-intense relative to cerebrospinal fluid on all pulse sequences. No convincing clinical or laboratory evidence was found to explain the exact nature of these lesions. The possibility of dilated Virchow-Robin spaces (VRS) seems too simplistic because of the size and shape, specifically of the unilateral lesions, which are not usual characteristics of VRS.

Key words: Virchow-Robin spaces – Brain abnormalities – Magnetic resonance imaging

Multiple cerebral white matter lesions, seen in cranial MRI studies and which are iso-intense relative to cerebrospinal fluid (CSF) on all pulse sequences, may have different origins. More often they represent idiopathic dilated Virchow-Robin spaces (VRS). These enlarged perivascular spaces may also be seen in brain storage disorders like mucopolysaccharidoses [1] and brain infections like cryptococcosis [2]. These lesions, seen like brain black holes on T1-weighted sequences, may also represent desctructive lesions of multiple causes, which underwent cystic transformation [3].

Fig. 1 a, b. Case 1. Axial T1 **(a)** and T2-weighted **(b)** images show multiple cystic areas in the left cerebral hemisphere

Fig. 2 a, b. Case 2. Coronal T1 **(a)** and T2-weighted **(b)** images show multiple cystic areas in the left cerebral hemisphere

Fig. 3 a–c. Sagittal, axial and coronal T1-weighted images **(a–c)** show multiple cystic areas in both hemispheres

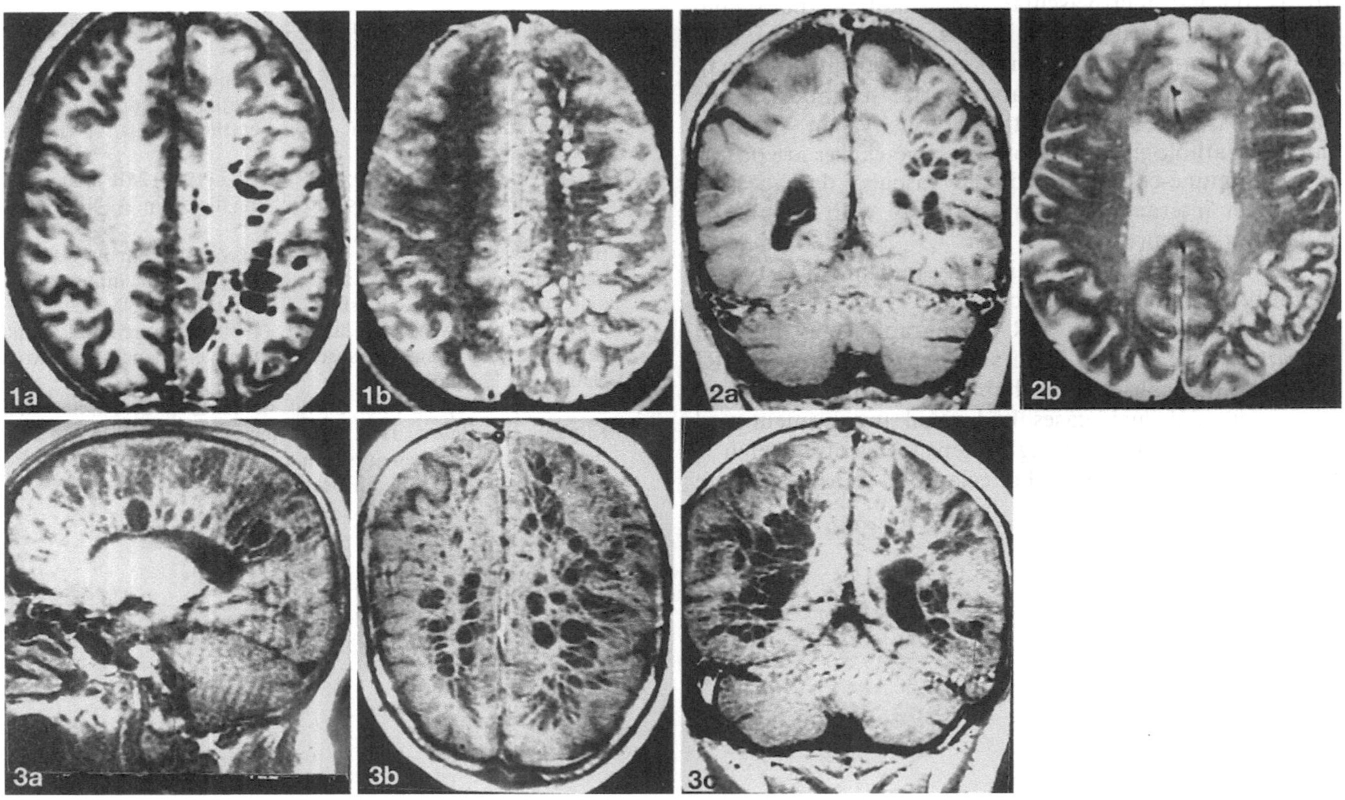

Correspondence to: L. A. Bacheschi, University of São Paulo, School of Medicine, 05444-010 – Rua dos Tamanas 506, São Paulo, SP, Brazil

Patients and methods

Three patients with normal daily life and normal professional or school activities were submitted to CT scans, for investigation of minor symptoms. White matter lesions were described in all three cases. Subsequently, MRI studies were performed with a 1.5 T imager.

Results

Case 1 was a 21-year-old man, a university student with essential tremor of the right hand. MRI showed cystic areas, iso-intense to CSF, in the right hemisphere (Fig. 1). Case 2 was a 57-year-old man, an engineer with sporadic migraine-like headaches for ten years. MRI study showed lesions similar to case 1, in the left hemisphere (Fig. 2). Case 3 was a 58-year-old man, a civil servant who received treatment for bipolar depression for 22 years but carried out normal activities. MR showed multiple and wide cystic areas in both hemispheres (Fig. 3). No other disturbances were found in mental or neurological examinations of the three patients. Routine laboratory investigation was also normal and all the patients refused to be submitted to invasive examination.

Discussion

The significance of iso-intense lesions relative to CSF in white matter has been studied in recent years, specifically to differentiate idiopathic dilated VRS of ischaemic or demyelinating lesions [3–7]. Enlarged VRS were associated with increased age [5], but they can also be seen in children [1]. Recently Rollins et al. [1] reported the association of dilated VRS with the incidence of functional neuropsychiatric disorders in children.

In our cases, it is very difficult to explain the relationship between the minor symptoms and the MRI findings. In case 1, the essential tremor was ipsolateral to the hemispheric lesions. The sporadic headaches of case 2 may be poorly related to the cerebral lesions and in case 3, it remains unclear to what extent the bilateral hemispheric lesions can be correlated with the patient's bipolar depressive state.

It would be helpful to study the occurrence of similar cases and their correlation with clinical findings.

References

1. Rollins NK, Deline C, Morriss MC (1993) Prevalence and clinical significance of dilated Virchow-Robin spaces in childhood. Radiology 189:53–75
2. When SM, Heins ER, Burgen PC, Boyko OB (1989) Dilated Virchow-Robin spaces in cryptococcal meningitis associated with AIDS: CT and MR findings: J Comput Assist Tomogr 13:756–762
3. Braffman BH, Zimmerman RA, Trojanowiski JQ, Gonatas NK, Hickey WS, Schlaepfer WW (1988) Brain MR: pathologic correlation with gross and histopathology. 1. Lacunar infarction and Virchow-Robin spaces. AJR 151:551–558
4. Jungreis CA, Kanal E, Hirsch WL, Martinez AJ, Moossy J (1988) Normal perivascular spaces mimicking lacunar infarction: MR imaging. Radiology 169:101–104
5. Heir LA, Bauer CJ, Schwartz L, Zimmerman RT, Morgello S, Deck MD (1989) Large Virchow-Robin spaces: MR-clinical correlation. AJNR 10:929–936
6. Esiri MM, Gay D (1990) Immunological and neuropathological significance of the Virchow-Robin space. J Neurol Sci 100:3–8
7. Yetkin FZ, Haughton VM, Fischer ME, Papke RA, Daniels DL, Mark LP, Hendrix LE, Asleson RJ, Johansen J (1992) High-signal foci on MR images of the brain: observer variability in their quantification. AJR 159:185–188

MRI of diffuse axonal injury

K. Ishii[1], T. Onuma[2], T. Kinoshita[1], G. Shiina[2], Y. Shimosegawa[2], H. Naganuma[3]

[1] Department of Radiology, Sendai Municipal Hospital, Sendai, Japan
[2] Department of Neurosurery, Sendai Municipal Hospital, Sendai, Japan
[3] Department of Pathology, Sendai Municipal Hospital, Sendai, Japan

Abstract. We reviewed spin-echo MRI of 53 patients with diffuse axonal injury (DAI). Initial MRI was obtained with 0.5–1.5 T systems within 7 days of injury. T2-hyperintense areas with or without haemorrhagic foci were found in 51 patients. The sites of lesions demonstrated on MRI were as follows: corpus callosum in 48 patients (mostly in body and splenium), subcortical cerebral white matter in 23, cerebral cortex in 20, midbrain in 19, parahippocampal gyrus in 14, central grey matter in 14, pons in 6, and cerebellum in 3. Two corpus callosum lesions were missed on MRI within 6 h of injury which appeared obvious 6 days later. In one autopsy case, MRI missed some axonal lesions which were appreciated microscopically.

Key words: Brain injury – Diffuse axonal injury – Magnetic resonance imaging

Correspondence to: K. Ishii, Department of Radiology, Sendai Municipal Hospital, 3-1, Shimizu Koji, Wakabayashiku, Sendai, 980 Japan

Table 1. Conscious level of 53 patients on hospitalisation

Glasgow Coma Scale	Patients
3–4	6
5–6	17
7–8	30

Table 2. Outcome in 53 patients

Glasgow outcome scale	Patients
Good recovery	20
Moderate recovery	17
Severely disabled	13
Persistent vegetative state	1
Dead	2

Table 3. Lesions demonstrated on MRI in 53 patients

Site	Lesions
Corpus callosum	48
body	39
splenium	28
genu	10
Subcortical white matter	23
gliding contusion	12
Cerebral cortex	20
Midbrain	19
dorsal	12
ventral	7
Parahippocampal gyrus	14
Central grey matter	14
Pons	6
Cerebellum	3

Diffuse axonal injury (DAI) occurs as a result of shear and tensile strains affecting axons induced by sudden acceleration/deceleration or rotational forces on the brain and is identified as the most important cause of significant morbidity in traumatic brain injuries [1, 2]. Few prior papers have documented MRI findings of the acute phase of DAI [3]. The purpose of this study was to evaluate MRI of DAI in the acute phase and to correlate it with previously described neuropathological and MRI findings on this disorder.

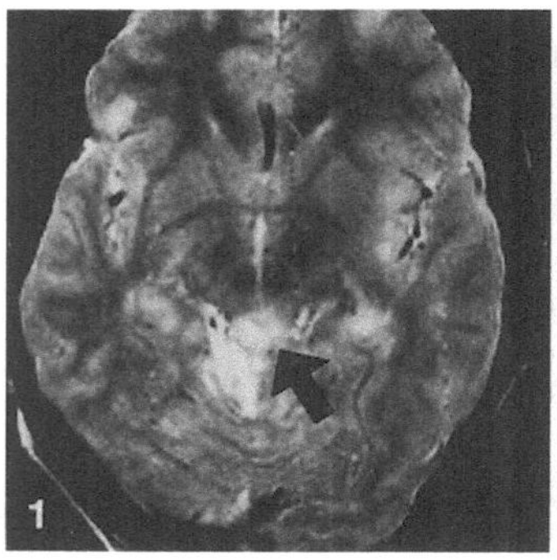

Fig. 1. A 22-year-old man [Glasgow Coma Scale (GCS): 4; Glasgow Outcome Scale (GOS): persistent vegetative state]. T2-weighted axial image (3000/90) 7 days after injury shows hyperintense areas in dorsal midbrain *(arrow)*, cerebellar vermis, subcortical white matter and left insular cortex

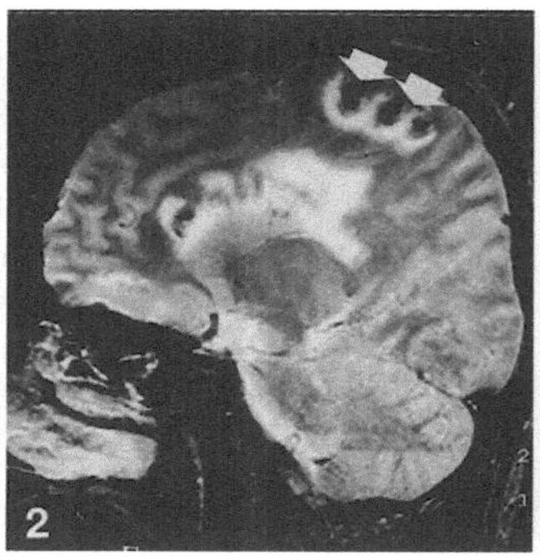

Fig. 2. A 28-year-old man (GCS: 6; GOS: severely disabled). T2-weighted sagittal image (2000/80) 7 days after injury shows hypointense areas with peripheral hyperintense areas representing haemorrhagic contusion in the right parasagittal region (gliding contusion; *arrows*). Hyperintense areas are also noted in the cingulate gyrus

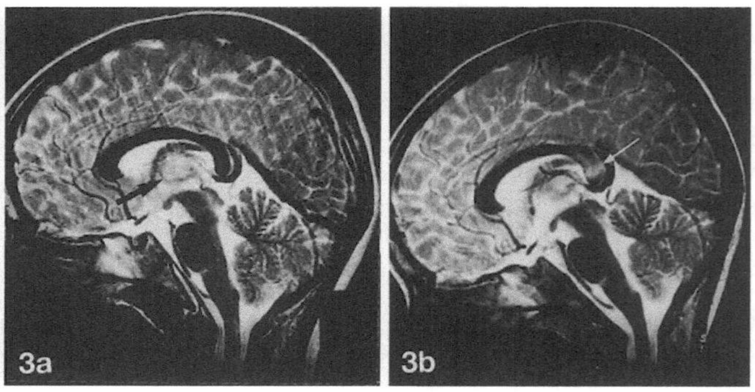

Fig. 3 a, b. A 9-year-old girl (GCS: 7; GOS: good recovery). T2-weighted sagittal images (400/90) obtained 2 h (**a**) and 6 days (**b**) after head injury. **a** A hyperintense area is found in the thalamus *(arrow)*; however, the corpus callosum is spared. **b** A hyperintense area appears in the splenium of the corpus callosum *(arrow)*

Patients and methods

We reviewed MRI of 53 patients with DAI (44 men, 9 women; age range, 2–79 years; mean, 25.7 years). Diagnosis was made based on Gennarelli's criteria, i.e. traumatic coma (Glasgow Coma Scale and was below 8) lasting more than 6 h without discernible intracranial space occupying lesions, or considerable brain-stem lesions responsible for loss of consciousness [2]. All patients had MRI within 7 days of injury (5 of them within 24 h). MRI was performed at 0.5 T in 12 cases, 1.0 T in 26, and 1.5 T in 15. Axial T1-weighted spin-echo (SE) images (0.4–0.5 s/15–20 ms; repetition time/echo time) and axial, coronal and sagittal T2-weighted images (2–3 s/80–90 ms, or fast SE: 3.7 s/85 ms) were obtained with 5–10 mm slice thickness and 2–3 mm interslice gap. Follow-up MRI was performed in 21 patients 2 months after injury. Autopsy was done in one patient. MRI findings were correlated with patients' clinical outcome estimated by the Glasgow outcome scale, 3 months or more after injury.

Results

Conscious level on hospitalisation and clinical outcome of 53 patients are shown in Tables 1 and 2. Traumatic lesions appeared hyperintense on T2-weighted images with or without hypo-intense areas reprsenting haemorrhage in 51 patients. Locations of lesions demonstrated on MRI are shown in Table 3. Cerebral subcortical white matter included 12 cases of gliding contusion (haemorrhagic lesions in parasagittal white matter [4]), (Figs. 1–4). Callosal lesions frequently involved the posterior half of the trunk followed by the splenium, mostly slightly

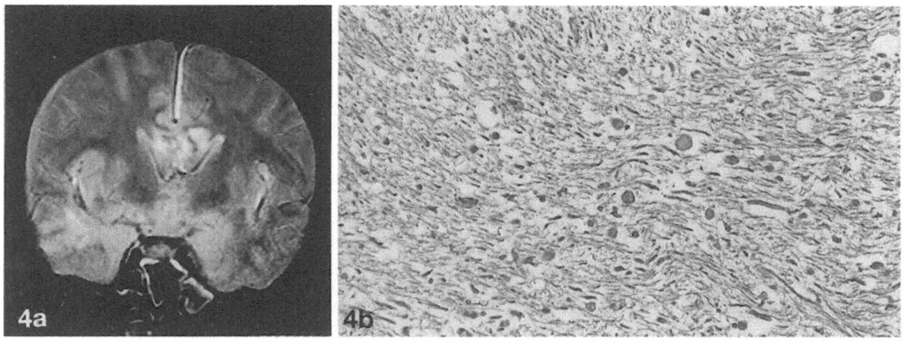

Fig. 4 a, b. A 19-year-old man (GCS: 6; GOS: dead). **a** T2-weighted coronal image (2000/80) obtained 6 days after injury shows hyperintense areas with irregular hypo-intense areas in the trunk of the corpus callosum and hyperintense areas in the insular cortex, basal ganglia, parahippocampal gyri bilaterally and right temporal and parietal lobes. **b** Microscopic specimen of centrum semiovale with Bodian's stain (×100) shows multiple axonal retraction balls. Similar findings were also found in internal capsule, cerebellar white matter, and tegmentum of pons

eccentric to the midline. MRI of 5 patients obtained within 24 h of trauma disclosed most of the lesions; however, two callosal lesions were missed on MRI within 6 h of injury, which appeared obvious 6 days later (Fig. 3). Follow-up MRI obtained 2 months after trauma showed diffuse cerebral atrophy in 16 of 21 patients. In one autopsy case, several hyperintense areas were found on T2-weighted MRI; however, histopathological examination showed multiple scattered foci of axonal retraction balls, representing axonal disruption in the centrum semiovale, internal capsule, cerebellar white matter, and tegmentum of the pons, which were not demonstrated on MRI (Fig. 4). No definite correlation was found between patients' clinical outcome and MRI findings, including the number of lesions and brain-stem lesions.

Discussion

DAI was first described by Adams et al. [1] based on neuropathological analysis of 45 patients, which was characterised by focal lesions in the corpus callosum and in the dorsolateral quadrant of the rostral brain stem, and diffuse damage to the axons. Clinically, Gennarelli classified diffuse brain injury into three categories based on the severity of disturbance of consciousness [2]. DAI is the most severe form of diffuse brain injury.

MRI is regarded as valuable for evaluating unexplained neurological findings and determining the full extent of lesions in head injury. Gentry et al. [3] first described MRI findings of DAI, in which the majority (67%) of lesions were located in the peripheral lobar white matter (most common in the frontal parasagittal regions), followed by the corpus callosum (21%, frequent in the posterior trunk and splenium and slightly eccentric to the midline) and brain stem [3]. Our results were different from those, i.e. the corpus callosum was by far the most frequent site (91%) followed by the cerebral subcortical white matter (43%).

The posterior part of corpus callosum is thought to be the most vulnerable to shearing injury, because tensile and shear strains develop at the connecting point of the two hemispheres (corpus callosum), and posterior falx is larger, which prevents displacement of the brain across the midline. In one autopsy case, microscopic examination disclosed much more axonal damage than was demonstrated on MRI. It also disclosed macroscopic lesions. MRI is sensitive to detect brain lesions in the acute phase of DAI; however, many microscopic lesions seem to be missed on SE images. We suggest newer techniques of MRI might be able to detect more lesions in patients with DAI.

References

1. Adams JH, Doyle D, Murray LS et al. (1982) Diffuse axonal injury due to nonmissile head injury in humans: an analysis of 45 cases. Ann Neurol 12:557–563
2. Gennarelli TA (1987) Cerebral concussion and diffuse brain injuries. In: Cooper PR (ed) Head injury, 2nd edn. Williams & Wilkins, Baltimore, pp 108–124
3. Gentry LR, Godersky JC, Thompson BH (1988) MR imaging of head trauma: review of the distribution and radiopathologic features of traumatic lesions. AJR 150:663–672
4. Adams JH, Doyle D, Graham DI et al. (1986) Gliding contusions in nonmissile head injury in humans. Arch Pathol Lab Med 110:485–488

Oedema fluid clearance within cerebral contusion studied by MRI

H. Kushi, M. Fujii, T. Shibuya, Y. Katayama, T. Tsubokawa

Department of Neurological Surgery, Nihon University School of Medicine, Tokyo, Japan

Abstract. Peripheral oedema associated with cerebral contusion is life-threatening in severe head injury. The present study was conducted to make clear the time sequence of development of post-traumatic vascular permeability using gadolinium (Cd)-DTPA-enhanced MRI. We examined 10 patients with traumatic cerebral contusion (mean age 38 years; 8 men and 2 women) with Gd-DTPA-enhanced MRI 1–3 days after head trauma. Gadolium-DTPA (0.3 mmol/Kg) was administered by intravenous drip infusion for 30 min. MRI was performed before, and 2 and 4 h after infusion. The contusional oedema area frequently enhanced with Gd-DTPA 2 h after infusion. After 4 h, the enhancement had already begun to decrease. These findings suggest that increased vascular permeability in the very acute phase of head injury may contribute in part to the formation of contusional oedema and that the oedema fluid clearance within cerebral contusion is more rapid than previously thought.

Key words: Cerebral contusion – Vasogenic oedema – Magnetic resonance imaging – Gadolinium-DTPA enhancement

Cerebral contusion in head trauma causes progressive contusional oedema, sometimes leading to clinical deterioration during the first 1–3 days after trauma [1], but the factors related to formation and development of contusional oedema are not clear. An experimental study showed no leakage of Evans blue in the early stage of cortical contusion [2]. In addition, post-mortem plasma protein staining in patients revealed no positive staining early after contusion [3]. These findings seem to indicate that, in the early phase of cerebral contusion, the formation of contusional oedema is not related to an increase in vascular permeability. However, it seems possible that these findings might have resulted from inadequate detection of increased vascular permeability. Therefore we evaluated a method by which an increase in blood-brain barrier (BBB) permeability can be detected in the early stage of cerebral contusion [4] to clarify the time-sequence of the development of post-traumatic vascular permeability by gadolinium-DTPA-enhanced MRI.

Patients and methods

A total of 10 patients with acute cerebral contusion were included in this study (Table 1). They were 8 men and 2 women whose mean age was 38 years (range 17–60 years). Six patients were injured in traffic accidents and 4 in falls. On admission, 4 patients had a conscious level lower than Glasgow Coma Scale (GCS) 8, and 6 of 9–14. Plain skull films revealed fracture lines in the skull vault in 8 patients; no fracture line was observed in the remaining 2 patients. CT at the time of admission showed cerebral contusion in 9 patients (frontal lobe in 4, temporal lobe in 5). In the other patient, contusional haemorrhage occurred in the left temporal lobe after the removal of a right acute extradural haematoma. The cerebral contusion was never restricted to the cortex but extended to the white matter. CT and MRI at 1.5 or 0.5 T were performed on all patients. CT was carried on three occasions: within 24 h at 36–48 h and about 1 week after the trauma. Axial and coronal MRI was performed within 24 h of the trauma, and Gd-DTPA-enhanced MRI after 36–48 h. The dose of Gd-DTPA was 0.3 mmol/kg and the infusion lasted 30 min. MRI was performed 2 and 4 h after Gd-DTPA administration.

Table 1. Clinical data and radiological findings in 10 patients

Patient	Sex	Age	GCS	Skull fracture	CT findings	Diagnosis
1	M	44	12	Parietotemporal	Temporal contusion	Focal contusion
2	M	17	6	None	Temporal contusion	Diffuse brain injury, multiple contusions
3	F	58	14	Occipital	Bifrontal contusion	Bifrontal contusion
4	M	20	6	Occipital	Temporal contusion	Multiple contusions
5	M	25	9	Frontal	Frontal contusion	Focal contusion
6	M	60	10	Temporal	Temporal contusion	Focal contusion
7	F	19	6	None	Frontal contusion	Focal contusion
8	M	51	14	Parietal	Frontotemporal contusion	Focal contusion
9	M	29	12	Temporal	Temporal contusion	Multiple contusions
10	M	57	7	Parietotemporal	Extradural haematoma, temporal contusion	Focal contusion

GCS, Glasgow Coma Scale

Correspondence to: H. Kushi

Table 2. MRI findings

Patient	Lesion on first MRI			Lesion enhancement after Gd-DTPA			
	Cortical subcortical	Deep white matter	Extradural haematoma	At 2 h		At 4 h	
				Contusional necrosis	Contusional infarct	Contusional necrosis	Contusional infarct
1	+	–	–	++	–	+	–
2	+	+	–	++	±	+	–
3	+	–	–	+	–	±	–
4	+	+	–	++	±	+	–
5	+	–	–	++	++	+	–
6	+	–	–	+	±	–	–
7	+	+–	+	+	–	–	
8	+	–	–	+	+	–	–
9	+	–	–	++	++	+	–
10	+	+	+	+	–	–	–

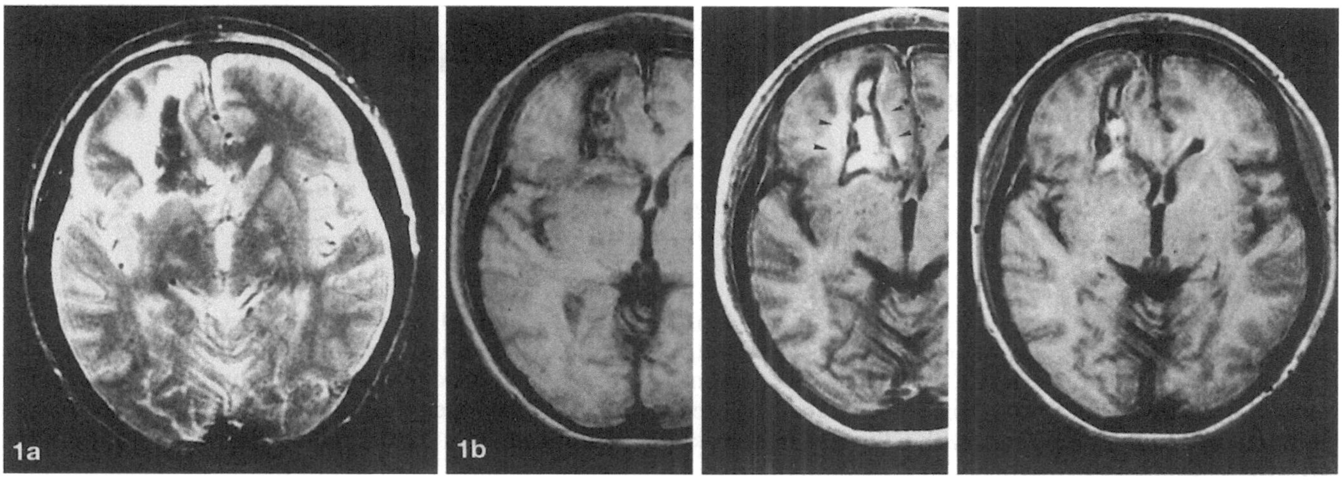

Fig. 1 a, b. MRI of a 25-year-old man (48 h after injury in a fall). His GCS on admission was 9. CT showed haemorrhagie contusion in the left frontal lobe. **a** T2-weighted images show the contusional oedema extending along the white matter tracts. **b** T1-weighted image left without enhancement. *Middle*, 2 h after Gd-DTPA administration: note enhancement of the contusional oedema area in the white matter surrounding the cerebral contusion (*arrow*). *Right*, 4 h after Gd-DTPA the enhancement had diminished

Results

Cerebral contusions enhanced with Gd-DTPA as early as 1–2 days after head injury. Gd-DTPA enhancement on MRI was recognised as falling into two categories: contusional necrosis and contusional oedema. MRI showed enhancement in both types 2 h after Gd-DTPA infusion, but enhancement in the contusional oedema area was markedly decreased 4 h after infusion (Table 2).Figure 1 shows a representative case.

Discussion

Because Gd-DTPA cannot pass through the BBB, like plasma proteins, contrast enhancement on MRI implies an increase in BBB permeability. Thus, we examined the time at which vascular permeability increase occurs in cerebral contusion using Gd-DTPA-ehanced MRI. Previously, Gd-DTPA (0.2 mmol/kg) was administered by bolus in i.v. and MRI was begun immediately after; enhancement was noted 6 days after trauma when early and 9 days when late [5]. This was markedly different in time from the BBB permeability increase in experimental animals. The compliance of brain tissue is essentially small at the early stage of vasogenic oedema development, and the progression and extension of oedema require increased capillary perfusion pressure [6]. However, once the extracellular space has been enlarged, and the compliance of brain tissue has thereby been increased, even a slight elevation in capillary perfusion pressure causes vasogenic oedema. To detect this vasogenic oedema early by Gd-DTPA-MRI, it is necessary to maintain an adequate blood Gd-DTPA concentration and to consider the time required for the passage of Gd-DTPA through the BBB. Our Gd-DTPA administration method enables compensation for the gap between animal and clinical studies. These findings show that vasogenic oedema plays a part in contusional oedema from an early stage and that oedema fluid clearance in cerebral contusion is more rapid than previously thought.

References

1. Katayama Y, Tsubokawa T, Miyazaki S, et al (1990) Oedema fluid formation within contused brain tissue as a cause of medically uncontrollable elevation of intracranial pressure in head trauma patients. Acta Neurochir (Wien) [Suppl] 51:308–310
Tornheim PA, Prioleau GR, McLaurin RA, et al (1984) Acute responses to experimental blunt head trauma topography of cerebral cortical edema. J Neurosurg 60:473–480
2. Lang DA, Hadley DM, Teasdale GT, et al (1991) Gadolinium DTPA enhanced magnetic resonance imaging in acute head injury. Acta Neurochir 109:5–11
3. Kushi H, Katayama Y, Shibuya T, et al (1994) Gadolinium DTPA-enhanced magnetic resonance imaging of cerebral contusion. Acta Neurochir (Wien) [Suppl] 60:472–474
4. Niendorf HP, Haustein J, Louton T, et al (1991) Safety and tolerance after intravenous administration of 0.3 mmol/kg Gd-DTPA. Results of randomized, controlled clinical trial. Invest Radiol [Suppl] 26:221–223
5. Maramrou A, Takagi H, Shulman K (1980) Biomechanics of brain edema and effects on local cerebral blood flow. (Advances in neurology, vol 28) Raven, New York, pp 345–358
6. Reulen HJ, Graham R, Spatz M, et al (1977) Role of pressure gradients and bulk flow in dynamics of vasogenic brain edema. J Neurosurg 46:24–35

The significance of MRI changes in the hippocampal formation in patients with extrahippocampal epilepsy

D. I. Kim[1], J. I. Chung[1], B. I. Lee[2]

[1] Department of Diagnostic Radiology, Yonsei University, College of Medicine, Seoul, Kòrea
[2] Department of Neurology, Yonsei Univerity, College of Medicine, Seoul, Korea

Abstract. Our purpose was to investigate abnormalities on MRI in the hippocampal formation (HF) in patients with complex partial seizure (CPS) whose MRI studies demonstrated an extrahippocampal epileptogenic focus. Three hundred and forty-one patients with CPS were retrospektively reviewed and 107 patients with extrahippocampal epileptogenic foci were investigated. Seventeen patients had an extrahippocampal temporal lobe lesion, and the remaining 90 had an extratemporal lesion on MRI. Overall 21 (19.6%) patients with extrahippocampal epilepsy (EHE) showed decreased HF volume and 11 of these had associated high signal changes of HF. In addition, 5 of 17 (29.4%) patients with an extrahippocampal temporal lobe lesion had a decreased HF volume, and 3 of them had high signal changes of HF. These 5 patients showed 4 unilateral HF abnormalities and 1 contralateral HF lesion. There were 2 tumours (1 ganglioglioma and 1 astrocytoma), 1 temporal lobe atrophy, 1 postsurgical status of temporal lobe and 1 inflammatory granuloma. The remaining 16 of 90 (17.8%) cases of extratemporal lesions were 7 of encephalomalacia, 4 of hemiatrophy, 2 of cortical atrophy, 1 of cortical dysplasia, 1 of heterotopia and 1 of glial tumour.

Key words: Extrahippocampal epilepsy – Hippocampus – Magnetic resonance imaging – Complex partial seizures

Correspondence to: S. I. Kim, D. M., Department of Diagnostic Radiology, College of Medicine, Yonsei University, 134 Shinchon-dong, Seodaemoonn-ku, Seoul, 120-752 Korea

Mesial temporal sclerosis is one of the most important pathologic entities of complex partial seizure. However, the presence of additional lesions confounds the definition of the epileptogenic focus in some cases. The effects of repetitive partial seizures and the presence of extrahippocampal lesions in relation to the development of hippocampal sclerosis are still controversial [1]. We evaluated the structural abnormalities of the hippocampal formation in patients with complex partial seizure whose MRI demonstrated extrahippocampal epileptogenic foci.

Materials and methods

We carried out a retrospective study of 341 patients with clinically diagnosed complex partial seizures (CPS), and symptoms of typical aura and significant EEG findings. Among them, 107 patients had a structural abnormality on MRI, consisting of 90 extratemporal lesions and 17 extrahippocampal temporal lesions. 1.5 T and 1.0 T images were used to obtain 3 mm inclined axial and coronal short TR/TE and long TR/TE images of the hippocampus. The criteria for abnormality of the hippocampus included visual detection of significant volume loss and/or high signal changes on T2-weighted images.

Results

Overall, 21 of 107 (19.6%) patients with extrahippocampal epilepsy (EHE) had structural changes in the hippocampus including a decrease in its volume, and 11 had high signal changes on T2-weighted images. Five out of 17 (29.4%) patients with an extrahippocampal temporal

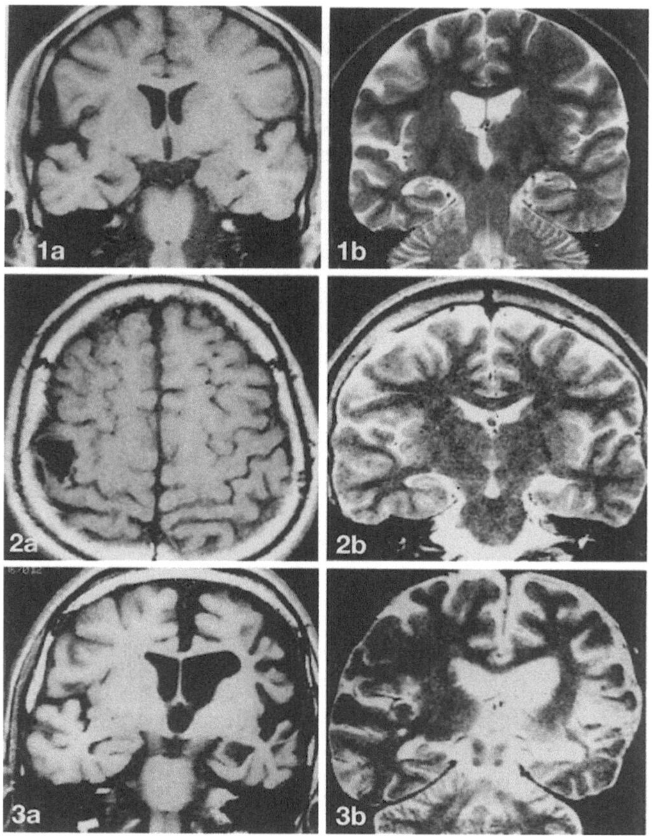

Fig. 1 a, b. A woman with an extrahippocampal temporal lesion and atrophy of right parietotemporal lobe. EEG showed a now amplitude spike from the left anterior or mesial temporal region. **a** T1-weighted coronal image shows sulcal widening and cortical atrophy of right parietotemporal region. **b** T2-weighted coronal image demonstrates volume loss of right hippocampus with dilatation of temporal horn. High signal change in the hippocampus is also noted

Fig. 2 a, b. A 15-year-old boy with a history of complex partial seizures. **a** T1-weighted axial image shows focal encephalomalacia in right anterior parietal lobe. **b** T2-weighted coronal image shows volume loss and high signal in left hippocampus. EEG findings were focal sharp waves in the right central and temporal regions

Fig. 3 a, b. A 37-year-old man with an extratemporal lesion. **a** diffuse gyral thinning with sulcal widening is seen in the left hemisphere, with secondary dilatation of the lateral ventricle and atrophy of the hippocampus on a T1-weighted coronal image. **b** T2-weighted coronal image shows increased signal intensity, suggesting marked hippocampal neuronal loss and sclerosis

lesion had a decreased HF volume, and 3 had associated high signal changes: 4 of them had an ipsilateral hippocampal abnormality whereas the other 1 had a contralateral hippocampal abnormality. These extrahippocampal temporal lesions were 2 tumours (1 ganglioglioma, 1 astrocytoma), 1 temporal lobe atrophy (Fig. 1), 1 postsurgical state of temporal lobe, and 1 inflammatory granuloma. Among the 90 patients with extratemporal lesions 16 (17.8%) had encephalomalacias (7 patients; Fig. 2), hemiatrophy (4; Fig. 3), cortical atrophy (2), nonlissencephalic cortical dysplasia (1), heterotopia (1) of glial tumour (1).

Discussion

We demonstrated that extrahippocampal lesions in patients with CPS were associated with relatively frequent hippocampal abnormalities, including decreased volume or signal alterations. In patients with extrahippocampal epilepsy, MRI should be compatible with clinical, EEG and other relevant clinical data for the precise evaluation of epileptogenic focus. Recent developments of neuroimaging techniques, including MRI, PET and SPECT provide proper localisation and detection of epileptogenic foci including hippocampal sclerosis and extrahippocampal lesions [2, 3]. Furthermore, dual pathology definition was reported when extrahippocampal lesions were found in association with hippocampal sclerosis during surgery for partial epilepsy [4]. However, significant neuronal loss of the hippocampus during recurrent partial seizures is still controversial. Different clinical and experimental results have been demonstrated as either non-progressive hippocampal neuronal loss [5] or progressive hippocampal neuronal loss induced by cumulative damage of recurrent seizures or by kindling [6, 7]. If kindling or successive partial epilepsy should play a role in the loss of hippocampal neurons, the latter mechanism of repetitive seizure causes the neuronal loss of hippocampus.

These dural abnormalities are found in 8–22%, consisting of hippocampal sclerosis in combination with either glioma, hamartoma or heterotopia [8]. In our cases, diffuse cerebral morphological changes such as cortical atrophy, encephalomalacia and hemiatrophy that had resulted from previous episodic insults of trauma, hypoxia and febrile convulsions were included as an EHE group. Levesque et al. [4] also described how prior severe head injury was associated with severe hippocampal cell loss. These findings may suggest the possibility of more frequent loss of hippocampal neurons other than tumorous conditions, including glioma, hamartoma or migrational anomaly. Findings with contralateral side hippocampal sclerosis were seen in some cases; either extrahippocampal temporal lesion or extratemporal lesion (Fig. 2). This illustrated case shows that an EHE focus may play a role in the formation of hippocampal sclerosis under the hypothesis of neuronal loss by recurrent seizures [6]. However, focus of mesial temporal sclerosis with incidentally found extrahippocampal lesions cannot be excluded according to the EEG criteria of temporal lobe epilepsy. The mechanism of contralateral involvement of hippocampal formation is not yet known. However, previous surgical trauma may be partly responsible since another of our cases demonstrated the contralateral hippocampal neuronal loss on follow-up MRI and EEG findings, following previous temporal lobectomy. A good anatomoclinical correlation of EHE focus was found between the temporal, occipital and frontal lesions but not with parietal lesions [9]. Parietal lobe involvement by an EHE focus may obscure the epileptogenic foci on the clinical basis of EEG criteria (Fig. 1). Since our cases were selected by exclusive criteria of MRI on HF with or without concordance with clinically available data such as EEG, SPECT or neuropsychological tests. Therefore, distant lesions found incidentally or clinically undetermined epileptogenic foci may not predict the degree of significant hippocampal neuronal loss secondary to the partial seizures.

Our results suggest that one should always evaluate the hippocampus in patients with partial epilepsy regardless of distant lesion. These findings must also correlate with other clinically available data according to the institution's policy of management of intractable seizures.

References

1. Sagar HJ, Oxbury JM (1987) Hippocampal neuron loss in temporal lobe epilepsy: correlation with early childhood convulsions. Ann Neurol 22:334–340
2. Jabbari B, Nostrand DV, Gunderson CH, Bartoszek D, Mitchell MH, Lombardo M, Citrin C, Sherman J (1991) EEG and neuroimaging localization in partial epilepsy. Electroencephalogr Clin Neurophysiol 79:108–113
3. Bronen RA (1992) Epilepsy: the role of MR imaging. AJR 159:1165–1174
4. Levesque MF, Nakasato N, Vinters HV, Babb TL (1991) Surgical treatment of limbic epilepsy associated with extrahippocampal lesions: the problem of dual pathology. J Neurosurg 75:364–370
5. Bertram EH, Lothman EW, Lenn NJ (1990) The hippocampus in experimental chronic epilepsy: a morphometric analysis. Ann Neurol 27:43–48
6. Dam AM (1980) Epilepsy and neuron loss in the hippocampus. Epilepsia 21:617–629
7. Cavazos JE, Sutula TP (1990) Progressive neuronal induced by kindling: a possible mechanism for mossy fiber synaptic reorganization and hippocampal sclerosis. Brain Res 527:1–6
8. Babb TL, Brown WJ (1987) Pathological findings in epilepsy. In: Engel JJ, ed. Surgical treatment of the epilepsie. Rafen Press, New York, pp. 511–540
9. Boon PA, Williamson PD, Fried I, Spencer DD, Novelly RA, Spencer SS; Mattson RH (1991) Intracranial, intraaxial, space-occupying lesions in patients with intractable partial seizures: an anatomical, neuropsychological, and surgical correlation. Epilepsia 32:467–476

The role of MRI in epilepsy surgery

K. Moritake, A. Fukuma, M. Takaya, T. Yamasaki, J. Ohta

Department of Neurosurgery, Shimane Medical University, 89-1, Enya-cho, Izumo, 693 Japan

Abstract. MRI has made it possible to identify anatomical brain lesions that are responsible for refractory epilepsy, which previously had not been diagnosable. We have developed a protocol for the surgical treatment of epilepsy, which uses MRI as the primary diagnostic tool for identifying the lesion to be resected. MRI enabled identification of a cerebral lesion in 42 patients with intractable epilepsy. Preoperative and intraoperative examinations, including ictal EEG, confirmed that the lesion identified by MRI was the source of the seizures. The lesion was resected as completely as possible in all cases. The outcome was excellent in 60% and good in 30% of cases.

Key words: MRI – Intractable epilepsy, surgical treatment

Technological advances have made it possible to locate epileptogenic lesions of the brain in patients with refractory epilepsy, which previously had not been identifiable. MRI has been especially useful in showing lesions amenable to surgical intervention [1–4]. Soon after its introduction, we developed a protocol for use of MRI to diagnose epileptogenic lesions amenable to surgical treatment [5]. This paper discusses the role of MRI in the surgical treatment of epilepsy based on our clinical experience.

Correspondence to: K. Moritake

Table 1. Pathology of epileptogenic lesions identified by MRI

Neuronal loss and Gliosis	15	4 porencephaly 4 arachnoid cysts 4 post-traumatic scars 3 nonspecific (infarct)
Hamartomatous lesions	10	1 hamartoma 8 tuberous sclerosis 1 dysgenesis of cerebral gyrus
Neoplasms	8	3 ganglioglioma 1 dysembryoplastic neuroepithelial tumour 2 astrocytoma (low-grade) 1 oligodendroglioma 1 epidermoid
Vascular anomaly	3	1 arteriovenous malformation 1 cavernoma 1 venous angioma

Methods

From December 1985 through April 1992, 42 patients underwent surgical resection for intractable epilepsy. Their age at the time of surgery ranged from 2 to 51 years, with a mean age of 18 years. The duration of the seizure disorder was from 1 to 41 years; the mean was 10 years. Lesions identified by MRI were resected as completely as possible. The pathology of the surgical specimens is shown in Table 1.

As illustrated in Fig. 1 whether or not a lesion identified by MRI is an epileptogenic focus is determined by noninvasive methods, including ictal EEG analysis using video-monitor and/or ambulatory EEG and regional cerebral blood flow studies by single photon

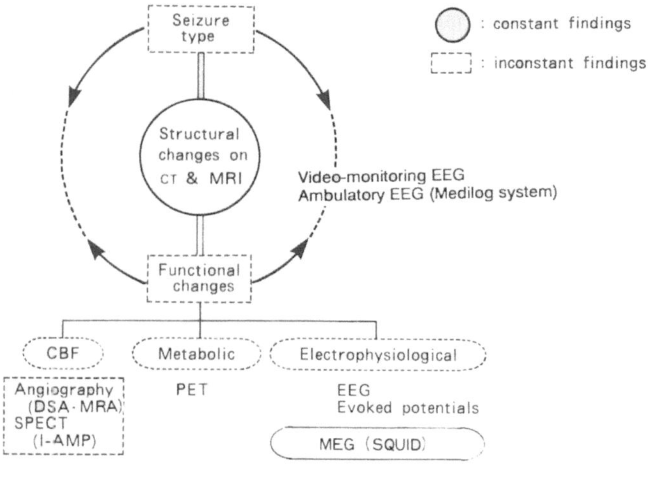

Fig. 1. Preoperative identification of an epileptogenic lesion by MRI

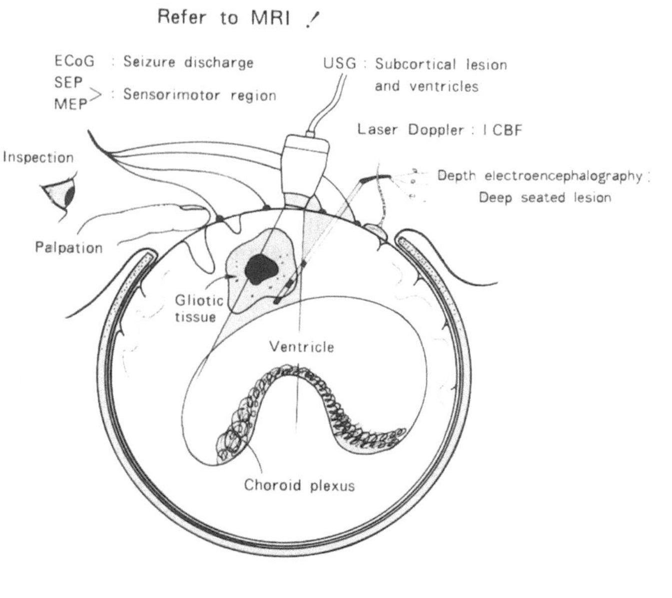

Fig. 2. Intraoperative identification of an epileptogenic lesion

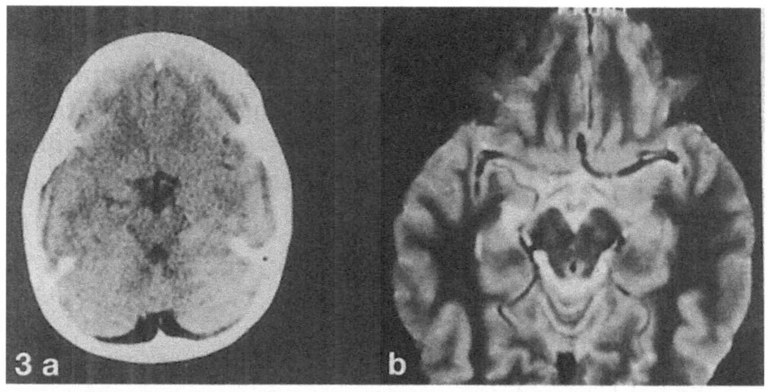

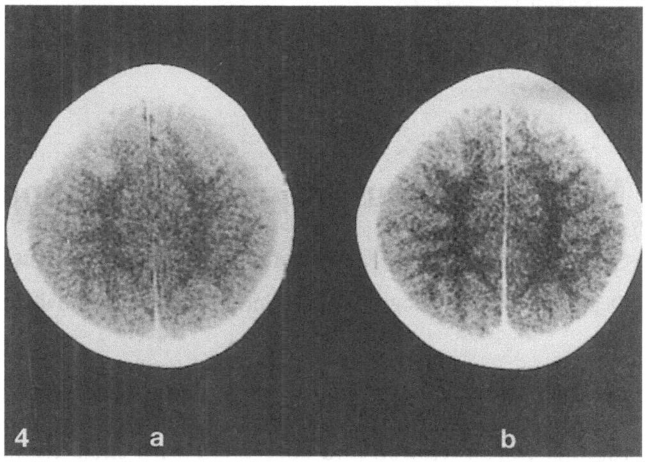

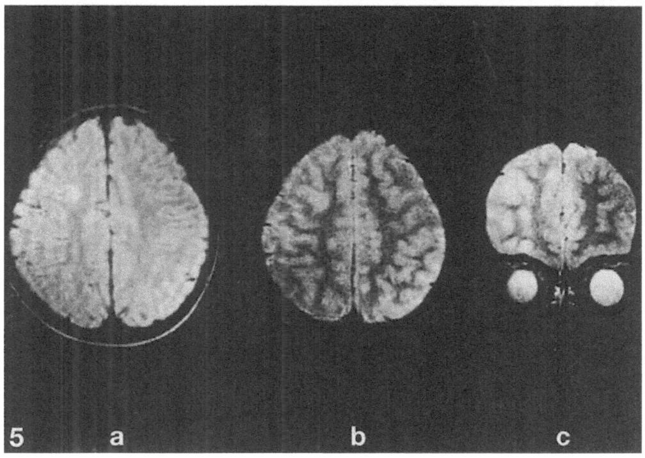

emission computed tomography. If epileptogenicity is confirmed, we proceed to craniotomy. As shown in Fig. 2, we localise the lesion intraoperatively and use electrophysiological and haemodynamic studies to confirm that we have found the true source of the seizures.

Results

Figure 3 shows CT and MRI in a patient with a medial temporal lobe lesion; Fig. 4 shows CT and Fig. 5 MRI of an extratemporal lesion in a patient with medically refractory epilepsy; both lesions are clearly depicted on MRI. On both proton-density and T2-weighted MRI, most epileptogenic lesions appear as a high-intensity area with a clear margin.

Fig. 3. CT (**a**) and T2-weighted MRI (**b**) of an 8-year-old girl with intractable epilepsy. A focal lesion in the right medial temporal lobe, which does not appear on CT, is clearly shown by MRI

Fig. 4a, b. CT before (**a**) and after (**b**) contrast medium in a 6-year-old boy with intractable epilepsy. An area of slightly low density with an ambiguous border is seen in the subcortex of the right frontal lobe. This area did not enhance with contrast medium

Fig. 5. Proton density- (**a**) and T2-weighted (**b, c**) MRI in the patient shown in Fig. 4. The abnormal area seen on CT is clearly visible as a high signal area, especially on T2-weighted images

Discussion

The common pathological feature among these lesions was the proliferation of abnormal glial cells, which are clearly visualised on MRI, expecially on T2-weighted images [5]. For both temporal and extratemporal lesions, seizure resolved completely or almost completely in about 60% of patients and clearly improved in about 30%. No patient suffered permanent neurological injury. In conclusion, MRI is a sensitive technique for identifying epileptogenic lesions in patients with medically intractable epilepsy. MRI is also useful in planning of the surgical approach.

References

1. Gerard G, Shabas D, Rossi D (1987) MRI in epilepsy. Comput Radiol 11:223–227
2. McLachlan RS, Nicholson RL, Black S, Carr T, Blume WT (1985) Nuclear magnetic resonance imaging, a new approach to the investigation of refractory temporal lobe epilepsy. Epilepsia 26:555–562
3. Oldendorf WH (1984) The use and promise of nuclear magnetic resonance imaging in epilepsy. Epilepsia 25:S105–S117
4. Schoerner W, Meencke HJ, Felix R (1987) Temporal-lobe epilepsy: comparison of CT and MR imaging. AJNR 8:773–781
5. Moritake K, Kikuchi H, Minamikawa J, Yamamura K, Takaya M, Yamasaki T, Fujisawa I, Asato R, Nishizawa S, Okuno T (1990) MRI and pathological findings of epileptogenic lesions removed surgically. Prog CT 12:167–173

MRI of obvious lesions in the hippocampus and/or juxtahippocampal region

S. Takahashi, K. Ishii, K. Matsumoto, S. Higano, N. Kurihara, K. Sakamoto

Department of Radiology, Tohoku University School of Medicine, 1-1 Seiryomachi, Aoba-ku, Sendai, 980, Japan

Abstract. The MR images of 38 patients with obvious lesions in the hippocampal and/or juxtahippocampal regions were reviewed and correlated with their clinical features. Based on the MRI and clinical findings, the patients were divided into 4 groups: (1) 10 patients with massive lesions causing symptomatic temporal epilepsy; (2) 14 patients with hippocampal infarcts, those on the left causing amnesia; (3) 10 patients with encephalitis, generally accompanied by both amnesia and epilepsy; (4) 4 patients with localised temporal atrophy and presenile dementia of subacute onset. MRI allowed precise localisation and clinical correaltion of hippocampal and juxtahippocampal lesions.

Key words: Magnetic resonance imaging – Hippocampus – Amnesia

The hippocampus has attracted attention with respect to both temporal lobe epilepsy and memory function [1]. This study compares the MRI appearances of obvious hippocampal and juxtahippocampal lesions with the clinical features.

Materials and methods

MRI studies of 38 patients (14 female and 24 male) aged 2–83 years (mean 53.2 years) and with obvious abnormalities of the hippocampus and/or juxtahippocampal region were reviewed. Patients who had mesial temporal sclerosis only or Alzheimer's disease were excluded. Patients with herpes simplex encephalitis primarily localised in the temporal lobe were included.

Using a 1.5 T or 0.5 T imager, spin-echo T1-weighted (TR/TE/excitations = 600–800 ms/11–30 ms/1–2) and double-echo long TR (2500–3500/18–25) images were obtained in the axial and basiparallel coronal planes.

We also reviewed the medical records to determine whether significant clinical symptoms or signs attributable to the hippocampal lesion were present or not.

Results

The patients were classified into four groups on the basis of imaging findings and clinical data: symptomatic temporal epilepsy; infarcts involving the hippocampus and adjacent structures; encephalitis; and progressive dementia.

Symptomatic temporal epilepsy

Ten patients were allocated to this group on the basis of MRI findings indicating a unilateral massive hippocampal lesion. Histological confirmation was obtained in 2 patients with astrocytoma and 1 patient with toxoplasmosis. Among the rest, the MRI diagnosis was cavernous angioma in 4, arachnoid or epidermoid cyst in 2, and other lesions in 2. Clinically, all presented with psychomotor seizures and epileptic discharges were seen on electroencephalography in 9. An amnesic syndrome was found in 2 patients.

Infarcts of medial temporal region, including the hippocampus

This group comprised 14 patients with 16 juxtahippocampal lesions. The hippocampus is supplied mainly by hippocampal arteries from the posterior cerebral artery.

Correspondence to: S. Takahashi

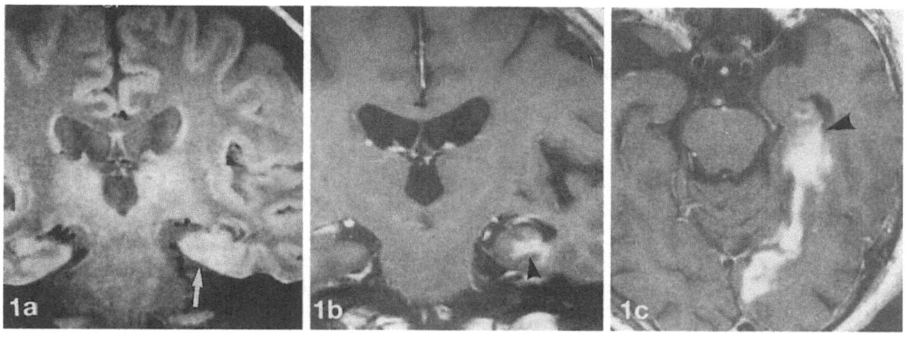

Fig. 1a–c. MRI of a 70-year-old man with a left hippocampal infarct, who suddenly developed memory disturbance and right hemianopia. **a** Coronal proton-density-weighted image obtained on day 24 shows a hyperintense lesion in left hyppocampus (↖). **b, c** Coronal and axial contrast-enhanced T1-weighted images show contrast enhancement in this hippocampus-subiculum (▲) and medial occipital region

The pattern of hippocampal infarcts in our patients corresponded with the distribution of these arteries (Fig. 1).

Clinically, 8 of the 9 patients with left or bilateral hippocampal infarcts presented with an amnesic syndrome: 4 had isolated disturbance of recent memory, and 4 had disturbance of both recent and remote memory. Amnesia was present in 5 of 6 patients with no infarct in the anterior/medial thalamus, which can also cause amnesia. In contrast, 4 of the 5 patients with right hippocampal infarcts had no amnesia. Epilepsy was not observed in any of these patients.

Encephalitis

There were 10 patients in this group, 7 with bilateral and 3 with unilateral juxtahippocampal involvement. In 4 patients, the diagnosis was *Herpes simplex* encephalitis, while the aetiology was not identified in the other 6. On neurological examination in the chronic stage, all 8 patients with bilateral or left hippocampal involvement showed marked memory disturbance, while 2 patients with right-sided involvement showed good recovery. In 7 patients, temporal lobe epilepsy was noted.

Presenile dementia

All 4 patients with presenile dementia had an insidious onset of forgetfulness in their fifties and gradual dementia. MRI revealed atrophy of the left temporal lobe with high signal on T2-weighted images. We suspect that the 4 patients with both left temporal atrophy and progressive dementia had a temporal form of Pick's disease [2].

Discussion

Patients with obvious lesions of the juxtahippocampal region thus feel into four groups. Infarction or encephalitis involving the left or both hippocampal regions was confirmed as causing an amnesic syndrome as a deficiency symptom, being consistent with the previous observation of memory impairment following its surgical ablation [3]. MRI particularly including coronal imaging, enabled precise anatomical assessment and correlation with clinical features of juxtahippocampal lesions.

References

1. Watson C, Anderman F, Gloor P, Jones-Gotman M, Peters T, Evans A, Olivier A, Melanson D, Ledroux G (1992) Anatomic basic of amygdaloid and hippocampal volume measurement by magnetic resonance imaging. Neurology 42:1743–1750
2. Cummings JL, Duchen LW (1981) Klüver-Bucy syndrome in Pick disease: clinical and pathological correlations. Neurology 31:1415–1422
3. Scoville WB, Milner B (1957) Loss of recent memory after bilateral hippocampal lesions. J Neurol Neurosurg Psychiatry 20:11–21

A study of epileptogenic foci with ^{31}P-chemical shift imaging

K. Nakamura [1], T. Asakura [1], M. Sasahira [1], W. Hirakawa [1], A. Haruzono [2], T. Fujimoto [3]

[1] Department of Neurosurgery, Faculty of Medicine, University of Kagoshima, 8-35-1 Sakuragaoka, Kagoshima 890, Japan
[2] Department of Neurosurgery, Fujimoto Hospital, Miyakonjo 885, Japan
[3] Department of Psychiatry, Fujimoto Hospital, Miyakonjo 885, Japan

Abstract. The subjects of this study were 36 epilepsy patients aged 8–62 years, who were examined 45 times; 25 had partial and 11, generalised seizures. ^{31}P-chemical shift imaging (CSI) was acquired with three-dimensional Fourier transformation (3DFT) multivoxel spectroscopy. The ^{31}P-CSI method detected abnormalities in 30 of the 36 patients (83.3%), 25 of whom had partial seizures. In patients with no apparent organic lesion, an elevation in organic phosphate (Pi) levels was observed in the peri-ictal stage. Twenty-two patients also underwent ^{123}I-IMP and ^{99m}HM-PAO single photon emission CT (SPECT), and 19 of them were found to have hypoperfusion in the regions identical to those appearing abnormal on CSI. One patient in whom no abnormalities had previously been observed was found to have abnormalities on CSI. In patients with apparent organic lesions, the signals of phosphocreatine (PCr), ATP and Pi were lower in the pathological hemisphere than in the contralateral hemisphere. These changes in phosphate levels seem to suggest that energy metabolism was reduced in the brain regions around the seizure foci in the interictal stage. Imaging diagnosis plays an important role in identifying seizure foci. ^{31}P-CSI appeared to be effective for diagnosing the disease foci in patients with refractory epilepsy.

Key words: ^{31}P-chemical shift imaging – ^{31}P-magnetic resonance spectroscopy – Epilepsy

We investigated the efficacy of MRI for identifying foci in patients with refractory epilepsy and evaluating candidates for surgical treatment [1]. Recently, in vivo ^{31}P-MR spectroscopy has been adopted to test for metabolism disorders in epileptic brains. We investigated cerebral metabolism, localisation and pathophysiology in epileptic patients with ^{31}P magnetic resonance spectroscopy (MRS) in addition to conventional MRI. ^{31}P-CSI was acquired with spectroscopy imaging performed with three-dimensional Fourier transformation (3DFT) multivoxel spectroscopy.

Subjects and methods

The distribution of various phosphides can be shown in separate slices by CSI. We compared the distribution of total phosphate, phosphocreatine (PCr), inorganic phosphate (Pi), ATP, phosphodiesters (PDE) and phosphomonoesters (PME) between the cerebral hemisphere with lesions and the contralateral hemispheres. An MRI apparatus with a magnetic field strength of 2.0 T was employed. The introduction of 3DFT multivoxel spectroscopy has made it possible to produce clear spectra and acquire coronal images. This method facilitates the diagnosis of temporal lobe epilepsy. ^{31}P-CSI was performed by three-dimensional CST method. Voxel size was $3 \times 3 \times 4$ cm. Tr was 2 s. Metabolic images such as total ^{31}P, PME, Pi, PDE, PCr and ATP were generated and overlaid on the corresponding proton image. The subjects comprised 36 patients and they were examined 45 times. A total of 36 patients including 23 males and 13 females whose ages ranged from 8 years to 62 years were studied. Out of 25 patients with partial seizure and 11 with generalized seizure, 15 patients suffered from intractable epilepsy which was difficult to control by medication and frequently recurred. Abnormal foci were identified on EEG in 27 patients out of the 36. The epileptic focus was apparently localized on the frontal and lateral lobes in 26 patients. Abnormalities were demonstrated by conventional MRI but not by CT in 7 patients, of whom 5 were demonstrated to have a high-signal lesion on T2 weighted imaging in accordance with the abnormality seen on EEG.

Correspondence to: K. Nakamura

Results

CSI studies were abnormal in 30 of 36 patients: 25 of 25 patients with partial seizure and 5 of 11 with generalized seizures. In addition, images of the focal side were abnormal in all the patients with partial seizures.

Signals for Pi increased and those for PCr were decreased in peri-ictal patients. Signals for ATP as well as those for Pi and PCr decreased in the affected side in patients with an apparent organic lesion. Nineteen patients out of 22 had abnormal findings on SPECT. One patient who was not seen to be abnormal on SPECT was identified as being abnormal on CSI. These alterations in phosphate compounds during remission may account for a decrease in energy metabolism around an epileptic focus. Thus, these findings provide accurate information on remission or relapse, status of disease focus, and alteration associated with organic disease. However, in patients with epilepsy, the results may be altered by relapse and antiepilepsy drugs.

Discussion

We studied phosphate metabolism for cerebral infarction by ^{31}P-CSI. The signals for Pi increased in the acute phase of cerebral infarction, and those for PCr and ATP decreased in an area of hypoperfusion. In the chronic phase, signals for all these substances apparently decreased. Ischaemia may increase Pi, which may be gradually washed out into the blood stream, eventuating in a decrease of cellular activities due to ischaemia in the chronic phase. During remission, metabolism around the epileptic focus decreased, while Pi increased during re-

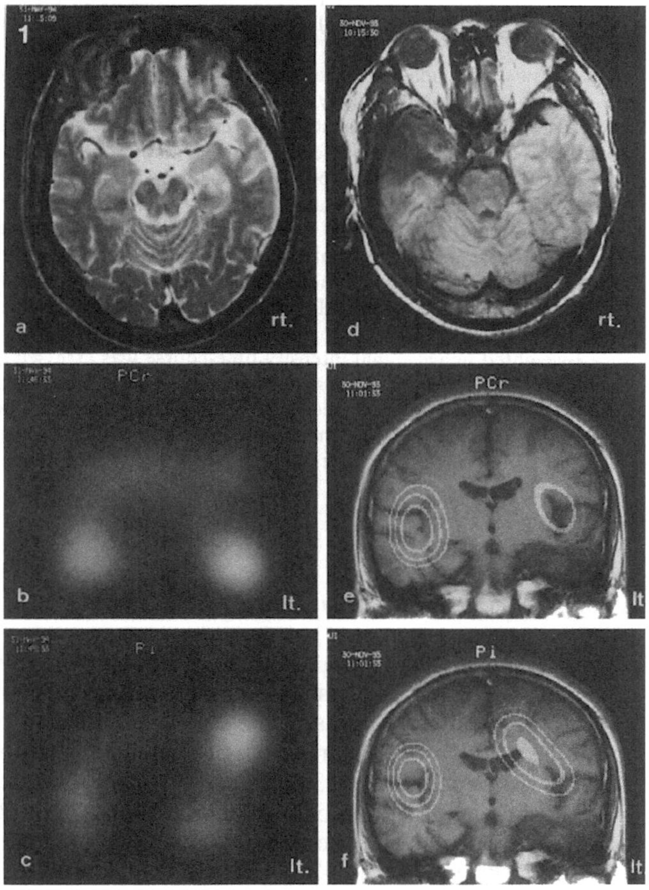

Fig. 1 a–f. A 43-year-old patient with right temporal lobe epilepsy. **a** T2-weighted image shows high signal in right hippocampus. **b** CPCr and Pi images show decrease in right temporal region. **c–f** A 41-year-old patient following a left lobectomy. **d** Proton density-weighted image shows temporal lobectomy. **e** PCr contour map shows decrease, while **f** Pi image shows increase on the left

lapse. However, specific changes in each case may be involved in the pathogenesis of epilepsy, with epilepsy being a reversible phenomenon which relapses, in contrast to cerebral infarction. Simple measurement of phosphate metabolism during relapse and remission may be useful; therefore, CSI is a useful method for clarifying the biochemical mechanism of epileptic seizures. PDE is said to be involved in phosphate metabolism of the membrane. However, as shown in the figure, PME as well as PDE share similar signals with PDE and other substances. Further study on this subject is warranted.

Reference

1. Asakura T, Sasahira M, Uchimura K (1989) Chemical shift imaging. J Med Imaging Jpn 9:942–952

Apparent diffusion coefficient alterations associated with experimental complex partial status epilepticus

A. Righini[1], **C. Pierpaoli**[2], **J. R. Alger**[2], **M. Leonardi**[1], **G. Di Chiro**[2]

[1] Neuroradiology Department, Ospedale Maggiore, Milan, Italy
[2] Neuroimaging Branch, NINDS, NIH, Bethesda, Md., USA

Abstract. The objective of this study was to evaluate whether water apparent diffusion coefficient (ADC) measurements provide more specific information than T2-weighted MRI about brain parenchyma lesions secondary to prolonged complex partial seizure. We measured the ADC in the brain of rats exhibiting prolonged complex partial seizures induced by an intraperitoneal injection of kainic acid (KA). The animals were imaged with diffusion and T2-weighted MRI at 2 T from 3 h to 9 days after the KA injection. In the piriform cortex and amygdala, the T2-weighted MRI signal intensity appeared to be uniformly increased from 24 to 72 h after KA injection, and to return to normal by 9 days after. In the same regions between 24 and 72 h, the ADC first decreased and then increased. The ADC changes were consistent with the known histopathological alterations. In this complex partial seizure model, the ADC measurement provides

Correspondence to: A. Righini, Servizio di Neuroradiologia Ospedale Maggiore-Policlinico, Via F. Sforza 35. I-20122 Milan, Italy

more specific information than T2-weighted MRI about the histopathological evolution of the lesions.

Key words: Magnetic resonance imaging – Epilepsy – Diffusion imaging – Rat brain

An MRI procedure for identifying histopathological alterations (cytotoxic edema, cellular death, etc.) consequent on prolonged seizures would be clinically valuable, because the extent to which seizures result in brain parenchyma alterations cannot be easily assessed. In fact, the oportunity to perform neuropathology studies soon after an ictal event is rare. However, conventional MRI appears to be relatively insensitive to the alterations associated with acute seizure activity. Diffusion MRI is a recently developed imaging technique that is sensitive to the rate of Brownian motion of water molecules. With this technique it is possible to measure the water apparent diffusion coefficient (ADC) in living tissues [1]. Diffusion MRI has proven valuable for detecting early or transient ADC changes associated with cerebral ischemia in experimental [2, 3] and clinical [4] settings. It also appears to provide more information on the histopathological features of evolving stroke than conventional MRI [5]. The studies noted above lead to the hypothesis that diffusion MRI may provide a noninvasive means of monitoring the histopathological sequelae of prolonged and multiple seizures.

We have measured the ADC in rats exhibiting prolonged complex partial seizures induced by systemic administration of kainic acid (KA), an agonist for a glutamate receptor subtype. KA acts as a potent neuroexcitant and neurotoxic agent [6].

Methods

Seizure induction. Adult male Sprague Dawley rats (260–310 g) were allowed free access to food and water until KA injection. KA, 8 mg/kg i.p. dissolved in saline, was injected into unanesthetized animals.

Magnetic resonance imaging. Diffusion and T2-weighted spin-echo images were acquired from a group of 5 rats at 3–5, 24, 48 and 72 h and 9 days after KA injection. One animal died between the 72-h and 9-day examinations, so that only 4 animals were included in the 9-day analysis. During imaging the animals were positioned prone in the magnet with the head in a plexiglas tube into which an anesthetic mixture of 85% O_2, 14% N_2O and 1% isoflurane was delivered. Rectal temperature was monitored with an optic fiber thermometer and kept constant at 37 ± 1 °C by a water-heated pad.

All MRI procedures were conducted with a 2 T chemical shift imaging system equipped with a horizontal 35-cm clear bore and self-shielded gradients coils. A home-built, saddle-shaped radio frequency coil (diameter = 40 mm) was used as transmitter and receiver. Four contiguous 2-mm-thick coronal diffusion-weighted and T2-weighted images were collected, with offsets chosen to correspond approximately to section at −5.80, −3.80, −1.80, +0,20 mm to the bregma, as shown by Paxinos and Watson [7]. T2-weighted images had the following parameters: TR 2600, TE 80 ms, 2 exitations, matrix 256, field of view 64 mm. Diffusion-weighted images were obtained using a modified Steijskal and Tanner spin-echo sequence [8]. The parameters of diffusion-weighted and T2-weighted images were the same, but a diffusion sensitizing gradient (3.25 G/cm) was applied in the phase-encoding (ventrodorsal) direction before and after the 180° pulse, leading to b-factor values (as defined by LeBihan [1]) as high as 890 s/mm^2.

Data analysis. ADC maps were calculated by a two-point linear fit of the logarithm of signal intensity versus the b-factor on a pixel-by-pixel basis [9]. Regions of interest (ROI) were traced on T2-weighted images and automatically transferred to ADC maps. The following ROI were selected form the four MRI sections: parietal cortex, hippocampus, thalamus, cingulate cortex, amygdala and piriform cortex. To obtain baseline ADC values, 5 rats that had not received ions of KA were imaged as controls. Student's *t*-test for unpaired samples was used to assess differences between ADC values in KA-treated animals and in controls. P-values lower than 0.05 were taken as significant.

T2-weighted image signal intensity time-course was assessed by calculation of the ratio between signal intensity in the different ROI and the signal intensity of one ROI (parietal cortex) that had displayed no significant ADC changes. Statistical methods equivalent to those described above were used for the T2-weighted images.

Results

Behavioral effect of KA treatment

After KA injection, all animals exhibited similar behavioral changes. During the first few minutes after injection exploratory activity decreased and the rats tended to be motionless with a fixed stare for many seconds. Wet-dog shakes were apparent by 30–50 min. At 40–70 min the animals showed clear signs of limbic convulsions (multiple episodes of orofacial automatism, head bobbing and forelimb clonus). At 1.5–2 h after KA injection they started having consecutive seizures characterized by intense forelimb clonus, profuse salivation, rearing, and loss of postural control. The seizures went on until the anesthesia for the first imaging procedure was administered (3–5 h after KA injection). No seizures were noted during the 1-h-long MRI session. After recovery from anesthesia, the rats exhibited spontaneous or noise-induced wet-dog shakes, and episodes of orofacial automatism and forelimb clonus. The frequency of these episodes decreased and, beyond 12 h after KA injection, only occasional wet-dog shakes and forelimb clonus were observed.

Imaging

In all animals, the T2-weighted images signal intensity (assessed by visual inspection) in the piriform cortex and amygdala was increased at 24 h after KA injection. The signal remained hyperintense at 72 h, but it appeared to be normal at 9 days; at this time some animals showed moderate brain atrophy. The T2-weighted image signal intensity ratios for the amygdala (amygdala ROI/parietal cortex ROI) and for the piriform cortex (piriform cortex ROI/parietal cortex ROI) confirmed this observation. In the two piriform cortex ROI, at 3 h there were no significant signal differences from the control values. From 24 h to 72 h an increase of about 30% in signal was noted with respect to the control value, but there was no statistically significant difference between the amount of signal increase at 24, 48, and 72 h. At 9 days the signal decreased to values no different from those of the controls. In the amygdala ROI the T2-weighted image signal intensity evolved in a similar way; no significant differences were noted between the measurements at 24, 48, and 72 h.

In the two piriform cortex ROI, The ADC values at 3 h [$0.678 \pm 0.074 \times 10^{-3}$ and $0.487 \pm 0.065 \times 10^{-3}$ mm^2/s (means ± standard deviations)] were reduced by 9% and 19% with respect to controls ($0{,}747 \pm 0.094 \times 10^{-3}$ and $0.604 \pm 0.151 \times 10^{-3}$ mm^2/s). However, this reduction was not statistically significant. A significant ($0.376 \pm 0.027 \times 10^{-3}$ and $0.277 \pm 0.133 \times 10^{-3}$ mm^2/s) and substantial decrease was apparent at 24 h (−49% and −54%). From 48 h onwards the ADC rose to values significantly different from the 24 h values and close to control values. In the amygdala ROI the ADC (controls = $0.661 \pm 0.142 \times 10^{-3}$ mm^2/s) exhibited a 20% reduction at 3 h ($0.525 \pm 0.067 \times 10^{-3}$ mm^2/s), which became significant ($0.424 \pm 0.147 \times 10^{-3}$ mm^2/s) at 24 h (−36%), followed by a course similar to that noted in piriform cortex ROI. In the parietal cortex, hippocampus, thalamus, and cingulate cortex ROI, the ADC did not show any significant change relative to the ADC in the corresponding ROI of control animals.

Discussion

The most relevant result is that from 24 to 72 h after KA injection, the ADC decreased and subsequently increased in the lesions, while in the same period the T2-weighted image signal remained uniformly hyperintense.

The T2-weighted high signal in the amygdala and piriform cortex regions is consistent with an increase in the total amount of water in the tissue (vasogenic edema) secondary to the increased blood–brain barrier permeability reported in this model [10].

The ADC changes can be discussed in the light of the several reports on the histopathological changes noted previously in this model [11–14]. In the piriform cortex and amygdala, between 2 and 24 h after systemic injection of medium to high doses of KA (7–12 mg/kg) the following histological abnormalities have been reported: vacuolated neuropil, swollen astrocytes (especially perineuronal and perivascular processes), dark and shrunken neurons, endoplasmic reticulum swelling and vacuolation of the mitochondria. After 24 h, electron microscopy revealed fragmentation of the neuropil and light microscopy revealed that most of the neuronal somata had disappeared. Based on these data we propose that, in this model, the initial ADC decrease is associated with the neuropil swelling and that the subsequent increase in ADC results from the neuropil fragmentation and the consequent loss of diffusion barriers.

The ADC and histological changes described in this model have many features in common with the alterations observed in a rat model of focal irreversible ischemia [5]. These similarities are in line with the observations from human neuropathology that, at the cellular level, ischemic lesions are not easily distinguished from those produced by prolonged seizures [15]. Our observations are also consistent with the propos hypoxic-ischemic pathogenesis of seizure-induced lesions [15]. Moreover, the excitotoxic effect of the massive release of excitatory aminoacids seems to play an important part in both the ischemic damage and the epilepsy-related damage. In our model the lesions in the piriform cortex and amygdala are believed to be due mostly to the prolonged epileptic discharge of the neurons in these areas and to the associated hypoxic-ischemic damage [11].

In this complex partial seizure model, the ADC measurement provides more specific information than the T2-weighted images on the evolution of the lesions. This supports the proposal that diffusion MRI may be valuable for the study of the neuropathological sequelae in patients with multiple or prolonged seizures.

References

1. LeBihan D, Breton E, Lallemand D, Grenier P, Cabanis E, Laval-Jeantet M (1986) MR imaging of intravoxel incoherent motions: application to diffusion and perfusion in neurologic disorders. Radiology 161:401–407
2. Moseley ME, Kucharczyk J, Mintorovitch J, et al (1990) Diffusion-weighted MR imaging of acute stroke: correlation with T2-weighted and magnetic susceptibility-enhanced MR imaging in cats. AJNR 11:423–429
3. Mintorovitch J, Moseley ME, Chileuitt L, Shimizu H, Cohen Y, Weinstein PR (1991) Comparison of diffusion- and T2-weighted MRI for the early detection of cerebral ischemia and reperfusion in rats. Magn Reson Med 18:39–50
4. Warach S, Chien D, Li W, Ronthal M, Edelman RR (1992) Fast magnetic resonance diffusion-weighted imaging of acute human stroke. Neurology 42:1717–1723
5. Pierpaoli C, Righimi A, Linfante I, Cheng JHT, Alger JR, Di Chiro G (1993) Histopathological correlates of abnormal water diffusion in cerebral ischemia: a diffusion-weighted MRI, light and electron microscopy study. Radiology 189:439–448
6. Cooper JR, Bloom FE, Roth RH (1991) The biochemical basis of Neuropharmacology, 6th edn. Oxford University Press, New York, pp 133–189
7. Paxinos G, Watson C (1986) The rat brain in stereotaxic coordinates, 2nd edn. Academic Press, San Diego, Calif
8. Steijskal EO, Tanner JE (1963) Spin diffusion measurement: spin echoes in the presence of a time-dependent field gradient. J Chem Phys 41:288–292
9. Goldberg R, LeBihan D (1992) Interactive data processing for magnetic resonance imaging: application to diffusion and perfusion imaging. In: Brody WR, Johnston GS (eds) Computer application to assist radiology. Symposia Foundation, Carlsbad, Calif, pp 384–386
10. Lothman EW, Collins RC (1981) Kainic acid induced limbic seizures: metabolic, behavioral, electroencephalographic and neuropathological correlates. BrainRes 218:299–318
11. Lothman EW, Collins RC, Ferrendelli JA (1981) Kainic acid-induced limbic seizures: electrophysiologic studies. Neurology 31:806–812
12. Nadler JW (1981) Kainic acid as a tool for the study of temporal lobe epilepsy. Life Sci 29:2031–2042
13. Schwob JE, Fuller T, Price JL, Olney JW (1980) Widespread patterns of neuronal damage following systemic or intracerebral injections of kainic acid a histological study. Neuroscience 5:991–1014
14. Lassmann H, Petsche U, Kitz K, et al (1984) The role of brain edema in epileptic brain damage induced by systemic kainic acid injection. Neuroscience 13:691–704
15. Meldrum BS, Bruton JC (1992) Epilepsy, In: Adams JH, Duchen LW (eds) Greenfield's neuropathology, 5th edn. Oxford University Press, New York, pp 1246–1283

Comparison of positron emission tomography, xenon CT and single photon emission CT in infants with intractable seizures

M. Mosskin [1], K. J. Poskitt [2], M. Connolly [2], K. Farrell [2], H. Nadel [2]

[1] Department of Radiology, Karolinska Hospital, S-17/76 Stockholm, Sweden
[2] British Columbia's Children's Hospital, Vancouver, B. C., Canada

Abstract. Ten infants with intractable seizures were examined with fluorodeoxyglucose positron emission tomography, xenon CT and HMPAO single photon emission computed tomography and with anatomical CT and MRI. Three were abnormal anatomically. In these three cases and in one anatomically normal case all the functional studies were abnormal. Functional imaging was expected to yield more information in the anatomically normal child.

Key words: Infantile spasus – Seizures – Positron emission tomography – Xenon computed tomography – Single-photon emission computed tomography

Infantile spasms are a unique type of seizure that occur mainly in the first year of life and have a poor prognosis: the Mortality rate is 5–15% [1]; cerebral palsy arises in 33–50% [2–4] and mental retardation in 71–85% of the infants affected [2]. Chugani et al. [5] reported the positron emission tomography (PET) findings of diminished focal cortical fluorodeoxyglucose (FDG) uptake in 13 children with cryptogenic infantile spasms. Four of these children underwent surgical excision of regions of "dysfunctional cortex" and have remained seizure-free with a significant improvement in neurological development. Neurohistopathological examination of surgical specimens showed cortical dysplasia, in keeping with pathological findings described at autopsy.

Measuring regional glucose metabolism with 18F-FDG PET has usually involved adult patients with epilepsy, demonstrating areas of interictal hypometabolism that correlate to EEG and pathological changes at surgery [6–9]. Thus, FDG-PET is considered the functional imaging gold standard for seizure localization in patients with intractable seizures. Unfortunately, PET is expensive and not widely available for paediatric use.

Our goal was to determine whether other available methods of measuring brain functions are as efficacious as PET in demonstrating focal abnormalities in a population similar to that of Chugani et al. [5]. We chose to evaluate the utility of regional blood flow as imaged with stable xenon-enhanced CT (XE-CT) and HMPAO single photon emission CT (SPECT) and compare results with those of FDG-PET. We regard this work as hypothesis-generating: our initial premise was that there is no significant difference between the ability of FDG-PET, Xe-CT or HMPAO-SPECT to localise seizure foci in young children with intractable seizures.

Correspondence to: M. Mosskin

Materials and methods

Eligibility criteria for patients included intractable infantile spasms or partial seizures within the first year of life that had proved resistant to standard treatment for at least 3 months. Patients with isolated focal partial seizures and a focal structural abnormality on anatomical imaging were excluded. During the study the inclusion criteria were modified to include patients with focal structural lesions if clinical seizure localisation remained unclear. These patients were part of a larger prospective series of 60 children with intractable seizures.

Ten patients, five of each sex with a median age of 4 months (range 0–10 months), comprised the study population. Eight had infantile spasms, while two suffered from intractable partial seizures arising from an incertain focus. At the time of functional imaging the patient population had an average of 26 months (range 5–63 months). The clinical data on each patient included seizure classification, neurological development, EEG and video EEG localization. Each patient had an average of seven EEG examinations to determine seizure localization, and clinical follow-up ranged from 8 month to 5 years. Only one patient has underogne surgical resection.

Each patient had a standard CT and MRI scan of the head. If the patient remained eligible for study, then FDG-PET, Xe-CT and HMPAO-SPECT studies were performed in random order within 3 months of any anatomical imaging. All examinations were evaluated in a blinded fashion by at least two investigators. When any imaging study was performed or interpreted such information as seizure type, EEG findings, suspected clinical focus or previous imaging findings, which might have permitted identification, was withheld.

All CT examinations consisted of axial 5-mm-thick slices. Additional contrast-enhanced coronal images were acquired if clinically indicated. The MRI examinations were performed using 1.5 T systems. All MRI examinations consisted of axial and coronal 5-mm T1 (600/20/2)- and T2 (2500/30/90/1)-weighted images as well as selected coronal images from an IR sequence (5 mm, gap 1.5 mm) or a selective 3D T1-weighted sequence (2 mm). CT and MRI were interpreted independently by two neuroradiologists (M.M., KJP) and any differences settled by consensus.

Xe-CT for estimation of regional cerebral blood flow were performed in the interictal state following the intravenous administration of 3–6 mg/kg Nembutal. A single Xe-CT study sampling 5 axial levels with the slices selected to cover the basal ganglia, temporal, frontal, partial and occipital lobes was performed. Each Xe-CT study consisted of an inhalation of a mixture of 28% xenon, 30% oxygen and 42% nitrogen over 5 min using a xenon rebreathing inhaler. Each level was sampled to create a combined wash-in, plateau and wash-out study.

Nuclear medicine imaging comprised HMPAO-SPECT using a single-headed camera. The infants each received 27 MBq/kg Tc-HMPAO by injection in the EEG department following monitoring for at least 10 min, continued for at least 10 min after injection. Image acquisition parallel with the cantomeatal line was performed 1–2 h after injection of the pharmaceutical preparation. If necessary the patient was sedated. The data were reconstructed in the axial, sagittal and coronal planes using a modified Butterworth algorithm.

The FDG-PET studies were carried out in the interictal state. During the procedure each infant was sedated with 50–100 mg/kg chloral hydrate. A venous catheter was inserted in either a hand or a foot and the limb heated to 44°C to allow "arterialization" of venous blood for sampling purposes [10]. In another venous catheter remote from the "arterialized" one, 0.143 mCi/kg 18-FDG was injected. Periodic blood samples were acquired to determine plasma FDG and glucose concentrations. The infants were imaged 40 min after the FDG administration, and 31 axial images of relative FDG activity were reconstructed.

Xe-CT regional cerebral blood flow maps were generated by the provided software, creating a pixel-by-pixel map of flows measured in ml/100 g tissue/min with an associated confidence interval. The assessment of the XE cerebral blood flow maps included freehand irregular anatomical regions of interest (ROI) involving grey or white matter, ranging in area from 1–5 cm^2. The procedure was repeated with circular ROI measuring 2 cm^2 in area placed over the sampled cortex. A comparison of side-to-side variability was carried out by one researcher (KJP) using visual inspection and direct comparison of both sets of ROI. For this study a significant difference of regional cerebral blood flow was defined as a greater than 20% side-to-side variability in comparable ROI or a difference in flow values of greater than 10 ml/100 g tissue/min, provided the confidence limits of measurement did not exceed the calculated difference.

For HMPAO-SPECT image interpretation the EEG status at the time of pharmaceutical injection and a baseline anatomical map, either CT or MRI, was available. The anatomical map was used for anatomical/functional correlation. The HMPAO-SPECT data were visually assessed independently by a nuclear medicine specialist (H.N.) and a neuroradiologist (KJP) and any disagreements were settled by consensus.

PET image interpretation was approached in a similar fashion. The images were visually assessed independently by two neuroradiologists (M.M., KJP), and any disagreements were settled by consensus. Symmetrical ROI of grey and white matter analogous to those used in evaluating Xe-CT were also used by one observer (M.M.). Specific comments were made regarding the overall uptake of the tracer and any dominant focal abnormalities observed.

Results

The 19 CT and 14 MRI studies available for study documented diffuse cerebral volume loss in seven of the ten patients during treatment and demonstrated that three patients had structural abnormalities: a suprasellar mass; hemimegalencephaly; and Aicardi's syndrome, with cortical abnormalities and dysgenesis of the corpus callosum. The suprasellar mass had imaging characteristics of a hamartoma and was the only lesion detected in the two patients who had intractable partial seizures without infantile spasms.

Among the functional imaging studies there were 10 XeCT, 10 FDG-PEWT and 13 HMPAO-SPECT studies, the latter including 2 ictal examinations, for assessment. FDG-PET studies were abnormal in all three patients with structural abnormalities seen on standard imaging. XeCT imaging demonstrated complete congruence with PET localization. HMPAO-SPECT imaging was positive in all patients with structural abnormalities but agreed with PET data in only five of seven patients with normal anatomic imaging. In both cases of disagreement, the SPECT studies suggested possible foci not detected by FDG-PET and not supported by clinical or EEG localization. When comparing PET and XeCT localization of seizure foci with all available clinical data, there was congruence of data in seven of ten cases. SPECT imaging and clinical data were in agreement in five of ten cases.

Discussion

Based on the work of Chugani et al. [5], we had expected to find a higher prevalence of abnomal FDG uptake on PET studies in young children with infantile spasms and normal anatomical imaging. A high percentage of those studied by Chugani et al. demonstrated focal, central or hemispheric alterations in FDG uptake while only one of six in our series was abnormal. This one patient (case 9) suffered from partial seizures as well as infantile spasms. This combination is common in the cases reported by Chugani et al. and may reflect an important selection criterion. The only other patient with infantile spasms and partial seizures was case 5, who also had dysgenesis of the corpus callosum as part of Aicardi's syndrome.

Our difficulties in finding infants meeting the inclusion criteria led us to include two additional patients in whom we were uncertain of their seizure focus on clinical grounds and one patient with infantile spasms and hemimegalencephaly. In all three cases FDG-PET, XeCT and HMPAO-SPECT were congruent in documenting abnormal uptake and blood flow, respectively, in the structural abnormalities. To date only the patient with the suprasellar mass has undergone surgery. The initial needle biopsy suggested the lesion was a hamartoma, but at histopathology after resection the mass was found to be a ganglioglioma. Thus, in infants with intractable seizures, an anatomical abnormality and partial seizures we were unable to detect any difference in the efficacy of FDG-PET, XeCT or HMPAO-SPECT.

In patients with intractable infantile spasms and normal anatomical imaging there was complete congruence of data between PET and XeCT, while HMPAO-SPECT yielded two "false-positions". The HMPAO data are regarded as suspect, since no clinical data supported the suggested localization and we had defined FDG-PET as our gold standard. We do not have a good explanation for the discrepancy and remain surprised at this observation, since in a larger series of 60 children with seizures there was excellent agreement between the Xe-CT and HMPAO studies performed.

Our study was designed to compare FDG-PET, XeCT and HMPAO-SPECT in localizing seizure foci in infants with intractable seizures. We did not find any difference in the results derived from PET and XeCT, while HMPAO-SPECT data was mildly discordant. These results suggest that if there is a significant difference among the functional modalities, it is likely to be modest, and a large series of patients would be necessary to ascertain this. The data suggest that partial seizures in infants with infantile spasms in combination with normal anatomical imaging may be an important selection criterion that should be fulfilled before embarking on functional imaging in these challenging patients. In infants with partial seizures with or without infantile spasms, PET, XeCT and HMPAO-SPECT are likely to be comparable in value for localizing altered regions of glucose metabolism or regional cerebral blood flow.

Acknowledgements. This work was supported by the Wenner-Gren Foundation, the Maj Lalander Fondation, the Swedish Society of Medicine, the Swedish Medical Research Council, and British Columbia's Health Care Research Foundation.

References

1. Glaze DG, Hrachovy RA, Frost JD, Kellaway P, Zion TE (1988) Prospective study of outcome of infants with infantile spasms treated during controlled studies of ACTH and Prednisolone. J Pediatrics 11:389–396
2. Aicardi J, Chevrie JJ (1978) Les spasmes infantiles. Arch Fr Pédiatr 35:1015–1023
3. Pollack MA, Zion TE, Kellaway P (1979) Long-term prognosis of patients with infantile spasms following ACTH therapy. Epilepsia 20:255–260
4. Seki T, Kawahara Y, Hirose M (1977) The longterm prognosis of minor seizures in childhood epilepsy. Fol Psychiatr Neurol Jpn 31:315–326
5. Chugani HT, Shields WD, Shewmon DA, Olson DM, Phelps ME, Peacock WT (1990) Infantile spasms: I. PET identifies focal cortical dysgenesis in cryptogenic cases for surgical treatment. Ann Neurol 27:406–413
6. Engel J, Kuhl DE, Phelps ME, Maziotta JC (1982) Interictal cerebral glucose metabolism in partial epilepsy and its relation to EEG changes. Ann Neurol 12:510–517
7. Engel J, Kuhl DE, Phelps ME, Sato S, et al (1983) Local cerebral metabolism during partial seizures. Neurology 33:400–413
8. Theodore WH, Newmark ME, Sato S, et al (1983) [^{18}F] Fluorodeoxyglucose positron emission tomography in refractory complex partial seizures. Ann Neurol 14:429–437
9. Aboul-Khalil BW, Siegel GJ, Sackellares JC, Gilman S, Hichawa R, Marshall R (1987) Positron emission tomography studies of cerebral glucose metabolism in chronic partial epilepsy. Ann Neurol 22:480–486
10. Phelps ME, Huang SC, Hoffman EJ, et al (1979) Tomographic measurement of local cerebral glucose metabolic rate in humans with (F-18)2-fluoro-2-deoxy-D-glucose: validation of method. Ann Neurol 6:371–388

Paediatrics

Magnetization transfer suppression in gadolinium enhancement of the child's brain

R. A. Zimmerman, J. C. Haselgrove, L. T. Bilaniuk, J. V. Hunter

Department of Radiology, The Children's Hospital of Philadelphia, Philadelphia, Pennsylvania, USA

Abstract. Magnetization transfer suppression (MTS) pulse was applied to a T1-weighted sequence and compared to the same sequence without MTS in order to detect its effect on gadolinium-enhancing intracranial pathology in children.

We examined 71 patients, 43 girls and 28 boys, ages 6 months to 18 years. There were 7 (8%) seen only with MTS, 42% were better defined with MTS than without, and 50% in which the two examinations were equal. In conclusion, gadolinium-enhanced T1-weighted MTS pulse sequences provided improved detection and delineation of contrast-enhancing brain lesions.

Key words: Magnetic resonance imaging – Magnetization transfer – Brain, children

Improvement in conspicuity of contrast enhancement in abnormal cerebral tissue that results from a disruption in the blood brain barrier (BBB) has been achieved in the past with the transition from the use of iodinated contrast media with CT to the use of gadolinium contrast media with magnetic resonance imaging (MRI). Given the high sensitivity of gadolinium-enhanced MRI, the question is whether there is still the possibility of further improvement.

Recently, triple-dose (0.3 mmol) gadolinium contrast medium has been compared to single dose (0.1 mmol) in adults in the detection of metastatic disease and found to be more sensitive [1]. We have also used triple-dose in comparison to single-dose in childhood CNS diseases and found that the triple-dose showed an improved diagnostic yield. However, triple-dose costs three times as much as single-dose, which is already a significant expense. More recent work, utilizing magnetization transfer suppression (MTS) pulse sequences in adult patients, have also shown an improvement in the conspicuity of contrast-enhancing lesions that approaches the results achieved with the higher doses of gadolinium [2]. The advantage of the MTS study is that it utilizes only the single dose of contrast medium. This study was undertaken in order to see if results could be improved in children with their pathological processes, which, unlike adults, does not include hematogenously disseminated brain metastatic disease as a common occurrence.

Correspondence to: R. A. Zimmerman

Table 1. Findings on contrast-enhanced images

Category	Lesions (%)
Seen only with MTS	7 (8)
Seen better with MTS	37 (42)
Seen equally with and without MTS	45 (50)
Seen better without MTS	0 (0)
Seen only without MTS	0 (0)
Total	89 (100)

Table 2. Effect of type of disease on improvement in visualization with MTS on contrast-enhanced images

Disease	Patients	Lesions	Improvement with MTS
Brain Tumor	51	58	
Primary, residual or recurrent			35%
CSF tumor dissemination			78%
Infarction (acute or subacute)	7	11	82%
Infection	5	7	86%
Inflammatory disease	4	5	20%

Materials and methods

Over a 2-month period, all patients requiring the injection of intravenous gadolinium for a question of brain pathology were examined utilizing the same pulse sequence (TR 600 TE 22 ms) with and without the additional use of an MTS pulse. In half the patients, the pulse sequence with MTS preceded the non-MTS sequence, and in half it did not. This was done in order to remove a time delay variable in enhancement from consideration. Both imaging sequences were obtained in axial plane, and both utilized similar slice thicknesses and similar slice locations. Only the patients with contrast-enhancing pathology have been included in the subsequent data: 71 patients, 43 girls and 28 boys, ranging in age from 6 months to 18 years.

Examinations were performed at 1.5 T.

Patients between 6 months and 6 years of age were routinely sedated with intravenous Nembutal, in a dose between 1–6 mg/kg. Patients over age 6 were usually not sedated.

Results

There were 89 contrast-enhancing lesions or areas in the 71 patients. These were divided into 5 categories (Table 1). The results are that 8% of lesions were seen only with MTS enhanced gadolinium study (Fig. 1), 42% were better defined with MTS than without (Figs. 2, 3), and 50% showed no difference between gadolinium enhancement with or without MTS. The usefulness of the MTS gadolin-

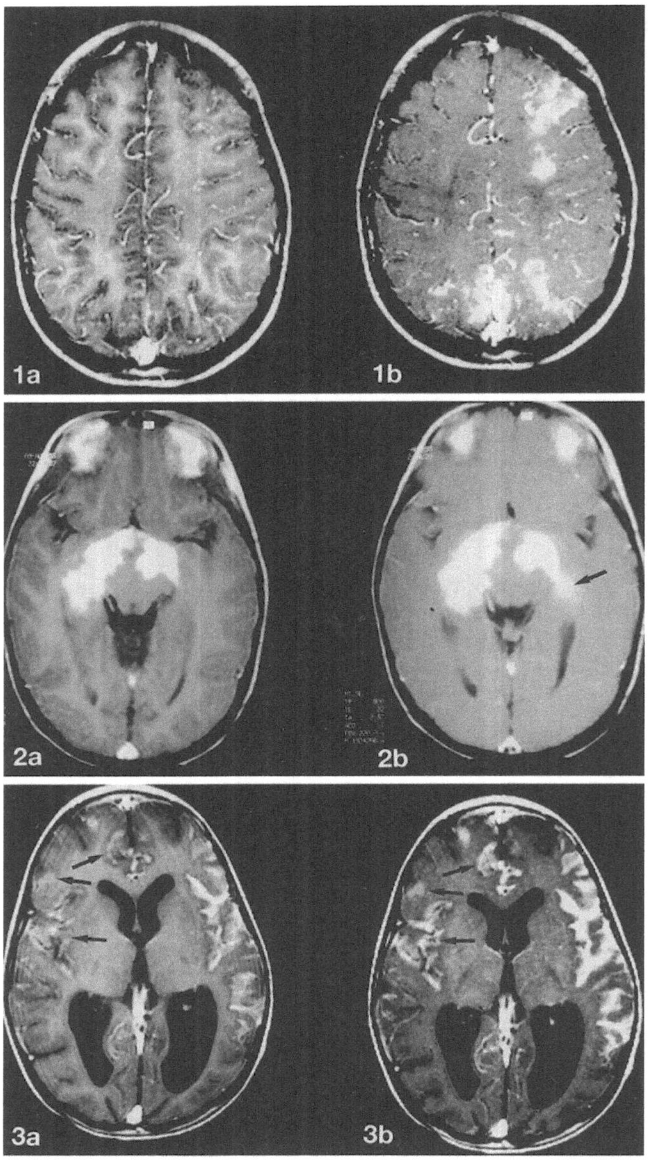

Fig. 1 a, b. Acute watershed infarcts. **a** Axial image after gadolinium injection shows no abnormal contrast enhancement. **b** With MTS extensive contrast enhancement is seen in a watershed distribution between the left anterior and middle cerebral arteries and between the middle and posterior cerebral arteries on both sides. There is deeper enhancement on the right, extending into the vascular territory of the posterior cerebral artery

Fig. 2 a, b. Visual pathway glioma. **a** Gadolinium-enhanced image shows involvement of the optic chiasm and both optic tracts, extending to the right lateral geniculate body, but not the left. **b** With MTS the more posterior extent of tumor on the left *(arrow)* is evident

Fig. 3 a, b. Subarachnoid dissemination of primitive neuroectodermal tumor of the posterior cranial fossa. **a** Gadolinium-enhanced image shows bilateral subarachnoid dissemination of contrast-enhancing tumor. **b** MTS image demonstrates a greater degree of enhancement, making some of the ill-defined areas *(arrows)* clear-cut

ium-enhanced sequence varied according to the pathological process (Table 2). Improvement in the recognition of primary, residual or recurrent brain tumors was only 35%, whereas the improvement in the detection of tumor dissemination within the intracranial subarachnoid space and ventricles was 78%. Both infarction and infection showed an improvement in the 80%+ range, while the improvement in inflammatory disease was only in the order of 20%.

Discussion

Prior studies have shown a positive relationship between the concentration of paramagnetic contrast agents and the detection of contrast-enhancing CNS pathology [1]. This was demonstrated in the triple-dose gadolinium studies using gadopentetate dimeglumine or gadoteridol [1]. Our own experience in eight patients showed a similar improvement in diagnosis. However, the cost of triple-dose gadolinium is a consideration and raises issues that relate to cost effectiveness.

Within the tissue being examined there appear to be two pools of protons. The pool of protons that are routinely imaged are those that are "free". These respond to the on-resonant radio-frequency (RF) pulse that is used to energize them, with tissue relaxation giving rise to the signal intensity that produces the MR image. There is a second pool of "bound" protons that are associated with the macromolecules such as the proteins and cell membrane constituents. These are the so-called invisible protons that contribute to the background's signal intensity by cross-relaxation with the "free" bulk water protons. MTS is produced when an off-resonant RF energy pulse saturates the bound protons, suppressing their contribution to the background signal intensity. This is presumably by means of dipolar cross-coupling and by chemical-exchange interactions [3–5].

Finelli et al. [2], in 110 consecutive adult patients, 88 of whom had positive MRI findings with 201 enhancing lesions, found that the contrast-to-noise (C/N) ratio of the enhancing lesions was more than doubled by utilizing an MTS T1-weighted spin echo (SE) sequence technique. However, their results did not indicate the percentage of patients in whom this improvement in C/N achieved with MTS and gadolinium-detected lesions not seen without MTS, or in what proportion there was or was not an improvement in detecting the size and extent of disease with the MTS sequence that was already shown on the non-MTS sequence.

In this series of children (Table 2), the improvement lesion(s) conspicuity was 50%, in 8% the diagnosis only being made on the MTS sequence, and in 42% the size and extent of disease being more obvious on the MTS sequence. In 50%, primarily those patients with large, densely enhancing intracranial masses, the improvement in C/N with MTS did not result in observable improvement in lesion evaluation, as the non-MTS already showed the full extent of the lesion. It is important to note that in no instance did the MTS study fail to show information equal to the non-MTS study.

References

1. Yuh WTC, Engelken JD, Muhonen MG, Mayr NA, Fisher DJ, Ehrhardt JC (1992) Experience with high-dose gadolinium MR imaging in the evaluation of brain metastases. AINR 13:335–345
2. Finelli DA, Hurst GC, Gullapali RP, Bellon EM (1994) Improved contrast of enhancing brain lesions on postgadolinium, T1-weighted spin-echo images with use of magnetization transfer. Radiology 190:553–559
3. Forsen S, Hoffman RA (1963) Study of moderately rapid chemical exchange reactions by means of nuclear magnetic double resonance. J Chem Phys 39:2892–2901
4. Koenig SH, Bryant RG, Halenga K, Jacob GS (1978) Magnetic cross relaxation among protons in protein solution. Biochemistry 17:4348–4358
5. Edzes HT, Samulski ET (1977) Cross relaxation and spin diffusion in the proton NMR of hydrated collagen. Nature 265:521–523

Correlation between brain stem dysfunction and morphological abnormalities in Chiari II malformation

T. Nishimura[1], **K. Mori**[2]

[1] Department of Neurosurgery, Kaisei Hospital, Kagawa, Japan
[2] Department of Neurosurgery, Kochi Medical School, Kochi, Japan

Abstract. To assess any changes in the anatomical relationships in Chiari II malformation, we reviewed serial MRI studies in 20 patients with myelomeningocele (MMC). A ratio (distance C / diameter F, distance M / diameter F) was established between the distance from the foramen magnum to the caudal tip of the herniated vermian peg of the cerebellum (distance C) or to the caudal tip of the kinked medulla (distance M) and the anteroposterior diameter of the foramen magnum (diameter F). Both the ratio of distance C / diameter F and distance M /diameter F tended to increase with increasing age. This indicates the continuous anatomical change of the Chiari II malformation and the skull base occurs during growth. A combination of compression and traction forces due to this change may be applied to the anomalous hindbrain and its connections. Electrophysiological studies, using brainstem auditory evoked potential (BAEP) and somatosensory evoked potential (SEP), indicated gradual latent prolongation of the peripheral components and latent shortening of the brainstem components. Thus, while the primary brainstem dysfunction may gradually improve during growth, the secondary dysfunction due to the compression and traction of the lower cranial nerves and cervical nerve roots may intensify. The natural course of Chiari II malformation involves these opposite phenomena in the hindbrain and its connections, despite the anatomical progression.

Key words: Chiari II malformation – Myelomeningocele – Magnetic resonance imaging – Brainstem auditory evoked potential – Somatosensory evoked potential

Brainstem dysfunction because of Chiari II malformation in patients with myelomeningocele is well known [1]. Hindbrain dysfunction has been reported to be responsible for 73% of all deaths of children with myelomeningocele [2]. Those types that present clinical symptoms of hindbrain involvement are currently unclear. The natural course of this anomaly is unknown. We are not sure if morphological abnormalities in the hindbrain correlate with functional disorder.

In this study, we investigated MRI, brain stem auditory and somatosensory evoked potentials (BAEP, SEP) serially in patients with myelomeningocele and a Chiari II malformation to elucidate what is occurring in the hindbrain and its connections during growth, and how the brainstem dysfunction correlates with the morphological abnormality of this anomaly.

Correspondence to: T. Nishimura, Department of Neurosurgery, Kaishei Hospital, Muromachi Chyo 3-5-28, Sakaide City, Kagawa Pref, Japan

Materials and methods

As functional aspects, the I–III interpeak latency (IPL) of the BAEP and EP-N13(formel) IPL of the SEP tended to become gradually prolonged from the normal range during growth. These findings may indicate that cochlear nerves and lower cervical nerve roots become stretched and the cervical spinal cord strangled during growth. Stretching of the cochlear nerve may coexist in most cases with elongation and stretching of other lower cranial nerves and of the hindbrain [3]. Functional deterioration, reflected in I–III IPL on BAEP and EP-N_{13} IPL on SEP, may result from the anatomical progression of this anomaly, described above.

On the other hand, the III–V IPL of the BAEP and N_{13}–N_{20} IPL of the SEP were initially prolonged and deceased progressively to the normal range (Figs. 1, 2). As morphological aspects, both the ratio of distance C /diameter F, and that of distance M /diameter F tended to increase gradually during growth (Figs. 3, 4).

Results and discussion

The MRI findings indicate that a combination of compression and traction forces, due to this change, continues to be added on the anomalous hindbrain and its connections. The neurophysiological findings may indicate that there are primary intrinsic functional disorders in the

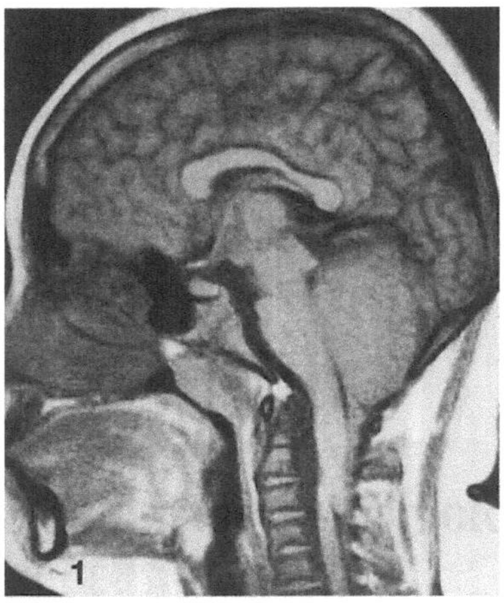

Fig. 1. Midsagittal MRI demonstrating Chiari II malformation, consisting of protrusion of the vermis of the cerebellum and brain stem through the foramen magnum, together with elongation of the fourth ventricle into the cervical spinal canal

brainstem and that the functional disorders gradually improve during growth [3] despite the progression of the compression and traction forces added on the anomalous hindbrain.

The degree of electrophysiological abnormalities did not always correlate with the amount of caudal displacement of the brainstem in patients with a Chiari malformation. This suggests that a functional disorder in the myelomeningocele brainstem, regardless of the existence of a Chiari malformation, may be present [3, 4]. Therefore, in patients with a Chiari malformation, functional disorders due to compression and traction forces compatible with the degree of morphological abnormality may be added to an intrinsic dysfunction or pathological changes within the brainstem.

Continuous anatomical changes between the Chiari II malformation and the skull base occur during growth [5]. Compression and traction forces due to this change strangle the cervical spinal cord and the kinked medulla, or stretch the cervical nerve roots and lower cranial nerves. On the other hand, primary intrinsic functional disorders in the brainstem gradually improve during growth. The natural history of Chiari II malformations involves these opposite dynamic phenomena in the hindbrain and its connections, despite the anatomical progression.

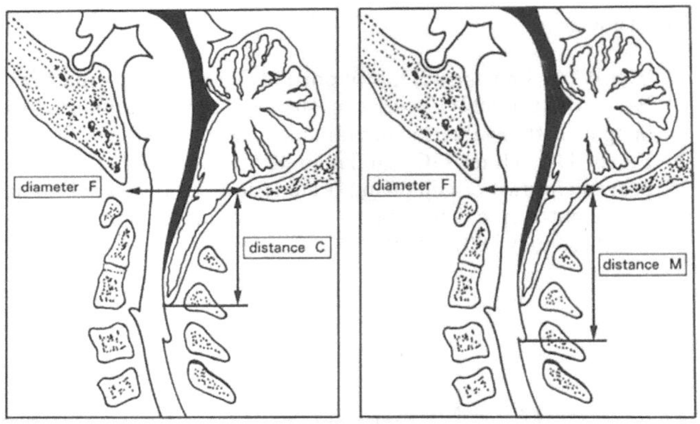

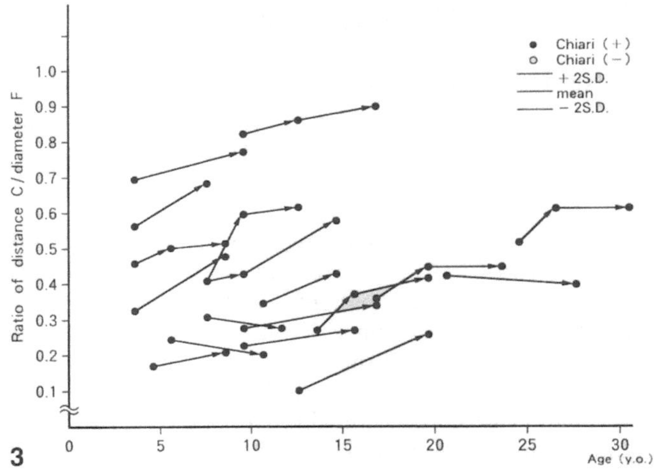

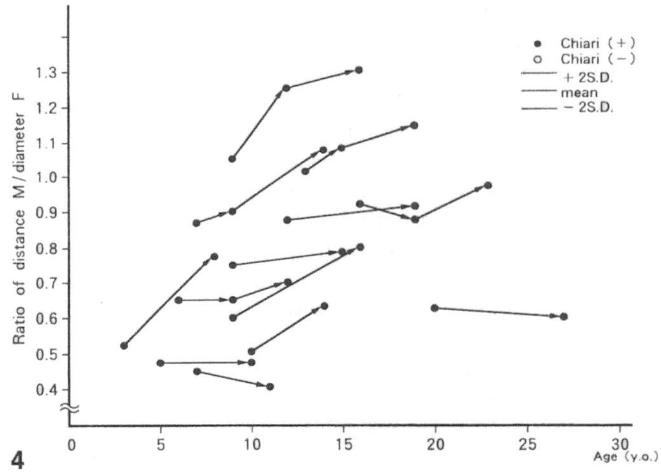

Fig. 2. We measured the distance from the foramen magnum to the caudal tip of the herniated vermias (*distance C*) and from the foramen magnum to the caudal tip of the kinked medulla (*distance M*) and the anteroposterior diameter of the foramen magnum (*diameter F*). The ratios of distance C / diameter F and distance M / diameter F were calculated and compared on serial MRI studies

Fig. 3. Chronological changes of the ratio distance C / diameter F

Fig. 4. Chronological changes of the ratio distance M / diameter F

References

1. Mori K (1985) Anomalies of the central nervous system. Thieme-Stratton, New York, pp 97–109
2. McLone DG, Naidich TP (1989) Myelomenigocele: outcome and late complications. In: McLaurin R, Schut L, Venes J, Epstein F (eds) Pediatric neurosurgery, 2nd edn. Saunders, Philadelphia, pp 53–70
3. Nishimura T, Mori K, Uchida Y, Ohira T, Tamura K (1991) Brainstem auditory evoked potentials in meningomyelocele. Natural history of Chiari II malformation. Child's Nerv Syst 7:316–326
4. Nishimura T, Mori K (1994) Blink reflex in myelomeningocele, with special reference to its usefulness in the evaluation of brainstem dysfunction. Child's Nerv Syst (in press)
5. Ruge JR, Masciopinto J, Storrs BB, McLone DG (1992) Anatomical progression of the Chiari II malformation. Child's Nerv Syst 8:86–91

Imaging of frontoethmoidal encephalomeningoceles

N. Suwanwela[1], **C. Suwanwela**[2]

[1] Department of Radiology, Chulalongkorn University, Bangkok, Thailand
[2] Department of Surgery, Chulalongkorn University, Bangkok, Thailand

Abstract. An exceptionally high incidence of frontoethmoidal encephalomeningocele is found in Southeast Asia. Diagnosis, with details of the bones and intracranial abnormalities, must be studied for treatment. Bone defects in 120 patients were assessed on plain radiograms. CT in 110 patients was found to be useful for confirming the diagnosis, classifying the lesions and demonstrating more details of facial abnormalities. The content of the sac and intracranial abnormalities can be assessed by CT, but MRI is more useful in demonstrating the details in multiple planes. MRI and MRA are non-invasive studies of the blood vessels at the base of the brain. These also help in the planning and selection of an operative approach.

Key words: Frontoethmoidal encephalomeningocele – Computed tomography – Magnetic resonance imaging – Magnetic resonance angiography

An exceptionally high incidence of frontoenthmoidal encephalomeningocele is found in Southeast Asia [1–5]. Imaging has been proved to be essential in the preoperative investigation of patients. Plain radiography of the skull is of limited use, because the superimposition of bony structures obscures essential details. Before the availability of CT and MRI, pneumoencephalography and cerebral angiography were known to provide important information [6]; however, these studies were invasive and their applications in young children limited. Isotope cisternography and ventriculography have also been used [7]. This new report describes the findings of different imaging modalities, including CT, MRI and MR angiography in patients with frontoenthmoidal encephalomeningoceles.

Materials and methods

We reviewed the CT studies of 110 children with frontoethmoidal encephalomeningocele and MRI investigations of a further 8 patients. We assessed the utility of each technique as regards preoperative data.

Correspondence to: N. Suwanwela, Department of Radiology, Faculty of Medicine, Chulalongkorn University, Bangkok 10330, Thailand

Table 1. Morphological classification of encephalomeningocele

1. Occipital encephalomeningocele
2. Encephalomeningocele of the cranial vault
   A. Interfrontal
   B. Anterior fontanelle
   C. Interparietal
   D. Posterior fontanelle
   E. Temporal
3. Frontoethmoidal encephalomeningocele
   A. Nasofrontal
   B. Nasoethmoidal
   C. Naso-orbital
4. Basal encephalomeningocele
   A. Transethmoidal
   B. Sphenoethmoidal
   C. Trans-sphenoidal
   D. Frontosphenoidal or spheno-orbital
5. Cranioschisis
   A. Cranial-upper facial cleft
   B. Basal-lower facial cleft
   C. Occipitocervical cleft
   D. Acrania and anencephaly

Results

Visualisation of bones

CT in axial and coronal planes with bone windows was very helpful for demonstrating the bony details and their relationships. Sagittal reconstructions also helped in visualisation of the displaced frontal and nasal bones. Three-dimensional reconstruction of craniofacial deformities, in particular using spiral CT, is an excellent modality for showing the bony defects and related bone deformities [8, 9].

MRI is an appropriate method for studying children because it does not use ionising radiation [10, 11]. Imaging in multiple planes, especially the sagittal plane, is particularly helpful in this disease, which has a mass in the frontal midline.

Visualisation of bony structures was used:

1. To demonstrate the existence of bone defect. In a small number of patients with masses in the glabellar or nasal regions, no bony defect was present. The lesion was exclusively extracranial, being a nasal glioma or a congenital cyst. CT demonstration of the absence of a bony defect led to the correct diagnosis, and intracranial surgical intervention could be avoided.
2. To classify the subtypes of frontoethmoidal encephalomeningocele. Based upon bony defects found at postmortem, a morphologic classification (Table 1) has been proposed [12] and adopted or modified for subsequent use [13]. Such a classification is helpful in the selection of the

operative approach. Cranial CT is very helpful for outlining the defect and position of nasal and ethmoidal bones, upon which the classification is based.
3. To assess the deformity of the bones of the face. Deformities of the facial bones vary greatly, depending on the size of the defect and the compressing mass. For plastic reconstruction of the facial structures, CT – especially three-dimensional reconstruction – is very helpful in planning surgery.

A large nasofrontal lesion is associated with a deep anterior cranial fossa, low position of the nasal bones below the defect, and lateral displacement of the medial orbital walls. Facial deformity is more severe in patients with large nasoethmoidal lesions. The nasal bones and the free frontal processes of the maxillary bones are displaced markedly upwards and located above the mass. The nasal bridge, which consists of nasal cartilage and adjoining maxillary bones, is below the mass, resulting in a long nose after repair. The medial orbital walls are displaced and become convex laterally, leading to wide interorbital distance. The naso-orbital lesion is associated with deformed orbits, while the frontal and nasal bones and the nasal cartilage are in normal relationship.

Visualisation of the brain

CT and MRI have completely replaced air studies. They can demonstrate brain structures both in the sac and intracranially.

1. *The amount of herniated brain.* Some patients had a large mass, which mainly consisted of CSF, and the herniated brain was small, while in others the whole sac was filled with brain tissue. As much as half of the cerebrum was herniated into the sac. The size of the mass does not usually reflect the extent of brain herniation. CT, and particularly sagittal MRI, can clearly demonstrate the brain inside the sac.
2. *Distortion of brain structures.* When a large amount of the frontal lobes are herniated, intracranial structures are pulled forward. The cerebrum, basal ganglia, and brain stem are more anterior in position than normal. Angulation of the brain stem is occasionally seen. The hypothalamus and optic chiasm are displaced anteriorly. The foramen of Monro can be displaced and at times obstructed, resulting in unilateral or bilateral hydrocephalus. Since the abnormalities occur early in life, the falx cerebri is laterally displaced in cases of unilateral hydrocephalus, leading to an asymmetrical head.
3. *Associated anomalies of the brain.* Porencephalic cysts, agenesis of corpus callosum, polymicrogyria, agyria, macrogyria and cortical scans can be clearly seen on CT or MRI.
4. *Blood vessels of the brain.* Distortion of the intracranial blood vessels follows brain abnormalities. Forward displacement of the anterior cerebral arteries was seen to be as far as the bony defect. This demonstration would assist the surgeon in preventing damage to them during amputation of the brain at the intracranial end of the defect. MRA is therefore useful in selected cases [14, 15]. Abnormal position of dural venous sinuses can also be demonstrated.
5. *Cranial nerves.* Distortion and anomalies of cranial nerves can be identified on MRI. A number of patients were blind, and in some blindness followed surgical repair. Anteriorly, displaced optic nerve and optic chiasm are believed to be responsible for the blindness.
6. *CSF flow.* In some patients, CT was obtained after intrathecal water-soluble instillation of contrast medium. CSF flow can be assessed; a subarachnoid block at the basal cisterns has been demonstrated. Retrograde flow of the contrast medium into the fourth and third ventricles was also encountered.

Discussion

CT and MRI have been found to be very useful in the assessment of patients with frontoethmoidal encephalomeningocele. The tomographic nature of bony CT renders it very useful in the detail evaluation of bony structures. Coronal CT contributes to the recognition of each bone of face. Three-dimensional spiral CT is very helpful in planning surgical treatment. MRI is better than CT in providing multiplanar images, especially the sagittal view. This modality also demonstrates the brain and other intracranial structures in great detail. Both CT scan and MRI show contents in the sac, including herniated brain tissue. On T2-weighted MRI, the herniated brain invariably appears with high signal intensity similar to gliotic or sclerotic cerebral tissue. Sclerotic change of the herniated brain has been proven histologically in the study of surgically removed tissue.

Our colleagues have demonstrated the extension of brain tissue into the sac of frontoethmoidal encephalomeningocele by using Technitium 99-m hexamethyl prophyleneamine oxim radionuclicle imaging [15]. The deposition in the brain is believed to be proportional to cerebral blood flow. The presence of blood flow in the herniated brain can thus be demonstrated.

References

1. Suwanwela C, Hongsaprabhas C (1966) Frontoethmoidal encephalomeningocele. J Neurosurg 25:172–182
2. Suwanwela C, Suwanwela N (1971) Frontoethmoidal encephalomeningocele. Surgery 69:617–625
3. Suwanwela C (1972) Geographical distribution of frontoethmoidal encephalomeningocele. Br J Prev Soc Med 26:193–198
4. Suwanwela C (1976) Craniomeningocele and encephalomeningocele. In: Sano K et al (eds) Recent progress in neurological surgery. Elsevier, New York, pp 49–55
5. Suwanwela C, Suwanwela N (1979) Congenital malformations of the nervous system as a regional problem. In: Isler H (ed) Neurological sciences in developing countries. University of Malaya Press, Malaya, pp 444–445
6. Suwanwela C, Suwanwela N (1972) Air study in infants and children with frontoethmoidal encephalomeningocele. Neuroradiology 4:190–194
7. Suwanwela C, Poshyachinda V, Poshyachinda M (1973) Isotope cisternography and ventriculography in frontoethmoidal encephalomeningocele. Acta Radiol 14:5–8

8. Hemmy DC, David DJ, Herman GT (1983) Three-dimensional reconstruction of craniofacial deformity using computed tomography. Neurosurgery 13:534–541
9. Coleman LT, Zimmerman RA (1994) Pediatric craniospinal spiral CT: current applications and future potential. Semin Ultrasound CT MR 15:148–155
10. Naidich TP, Zimmerman RA (1987) Common congenital malformations of the brain. In: Brant - Zawadzki M, Norman D (eds) Magnetic resonance imaging of the central nervous system. Raven Press, New York, pp 131–150
11. Bayer RS (1988) Editorial. Semin Ultrasound CT MR 9:183–185
12. Suwanwela C, Suwanwela N (1972) A morphological classification of sincipital encephalomeningoceles. J Neurosurg 36: 201–211
13. Naidich TP, Osborn RE, Bauer BS, Mc Lone DG, Kernahan DA, Zaparackas ZG (1991) Embryology and congenital lesions of the midface. In: Som PM, Bergeron RT (eds) Head and neck imaging. Mosby Year Book, St. Louis, pp 1–50
14. Edelman RR, Ahn SS, Chien D, Li W, Goldman A, Mantello M, Kramer J, Kleefield J (1992) Improved time-of-flight MR angiography of the brain with magnetization transfer contrast. Radiology 184:395–399
15. Poshyachinda M, Boonvisut S (1989) Cerebral blood flow imaging with 99 Tc m HMPAO. In: Dynamic functional studies in nuclear medicine in developing countries. IAEA, Vienna, pp 281–288

Normal CT anatomy of the lateral fontanelles

R. Silbergleit, E. M. Spickler

Department of Diagnostic Radiology, Henry Ford Hospital, 2799 West Grand Boulevard, Detroit, MI 48202, USA

Abstract. One hundred and thirteen CT studies of 107 patients ranging in age from several hours to 6 months were reviewed to study the anterolateral and posterolateral fontanelles. The lateral fontanelles were always patent in the first month of life and were almost always closed by 6 months of age. The appearance of the fontanelles before closure is variable. The membrane may be thick and nodular, thick and smooth, or thin. The membrane may show foci of ossification. There is generally uniform enhancement of the membrane. The presence of irregular nodularity and enhancement of the membrane should be recognized as a normal variant.

Key words: Fontanelles – Computed tomography – Normal development

The membranous bones of the cranial vault are separated by fibrous sutures and fontanelles [1–3]. Sutures are fibrous conections or joints with the opposing bones closely united. Fontanelles are fibrous connections in which the opposing surfaces are separated causing a soft spot. There are six constant fontanelles; the anterior, posterior, and the paired anterolateral (sphenoidal) and posterolateral (mastoidal) fontanelles [4]. The anterior fontanelle is often called the major fontanelle and the posterior fontanelle is called the minor fontanelle. The CT appearance of the anterolateral and posterolateral fontanelles is highly variable, and at times the normal fontanelle can mimic an aggressive process.

Correspondence to: R. Silbergleit

Patients and methods

One hundred and thirteen CT scans in 107 patients ranging in age from several hours to 6 months were reviewed. Patients with a history of trauma, neoplasm, or congenital CNS anomaly were excluded. Premature infants were also excluded. There were 63 boys and 44 girls. Seventy-nine CT scans were performed without injection iodinated contrast medium, 12 both before and after and 21 only after injection. We obtained E-mm-thick axial scans in most patients. In 8 patients 3 mm and in one patient 1.5 mm-thick axial scans were obtained through the orbits. In 2 patients 3-mm-thick coronal images of the orbits were performed. Each scan was studied to determine which fontanelles were open and to identify unusual appearances of the fontanelles. The interpretation was performed blinded to the patient's age. All patients had at least 6 months clinical follow-up to exclude neoplasm or systemic illness.

Results

At birth and through the first month of life, both anterolateral and posterolateral fontanelles were patent in all patients. There is a gradual decrease in sutural patency from the second through sixth month of life (Table 1, Fig. 1). During the sixth month of life only 9.1% of anterolateral fontanelles were open and all posterolateral fontanelles were closed. Up to 3 months of age more anterolateral fontanelles were closed than posterolateral fontanelles. From 3 to 6 months a larger percentage of posterolateral fontanelles were closed. In every case, if one posterolateral fontanelle was closed, the contralateral posterolateral fontanelle was closed. This was also the case for the anterolateral fontanelles, except for one case in which the right anterolateral fontanelle was open but the left anterolateral fontanelle was closed. There were cases in which both anterolateral fontanelles were open and both posterolateral fontanelles were closed, as well as cases in which both posterolateral fontanelles were open but both anterolateral fontanelles were closed. Contrast

Table 1. Sutural patency

	Age (months)					
	0–1	1–2	2–3	3–4	4–5	5–6
Anterolateral fontanelle open	48/48 (100%)	16.5/27 (61.1%)	5/9 (55.6%)	3/9 (33.3%)	4/10 (40%)	1/11 (9.1%)
Anterolateral fontanelle closed	0/48 (0%)	10.5/27 (38.9%)	4/9 (44.4%)	6/9 (66.7%)	6/10 (60%)	10/11 (90.9%)
Posterolateral fontanelle open	48/48 (100%)	21 /27 (77.8%)	6/9 (66.7%)	2/9 (22.2%)	4/10 (40%)	0/11 (0%)
Posterolateral fontanelle closed	0/48 (0%)	6 /27 (22.2%)	3/9 (33.3%)	7/9 (77.8%)	6/10 (60%)	11/11 (100%)

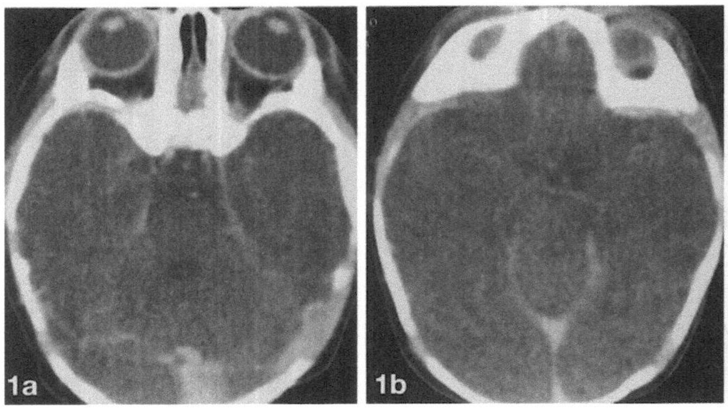
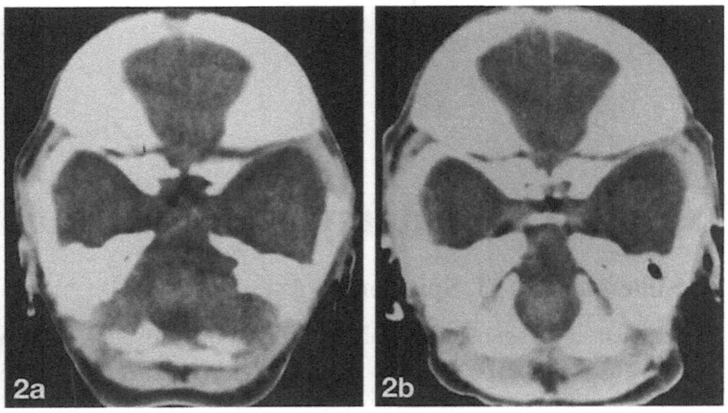
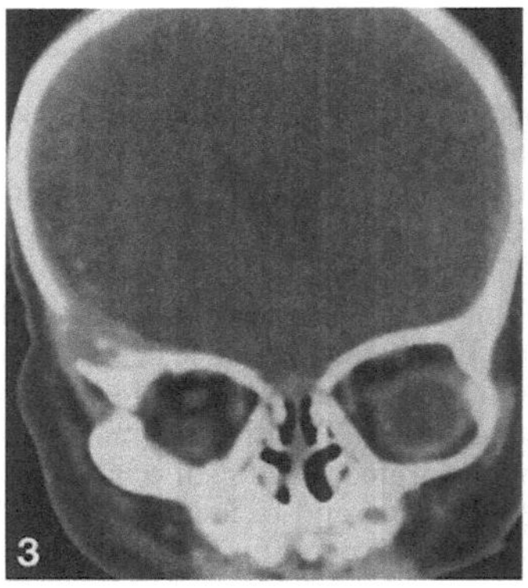
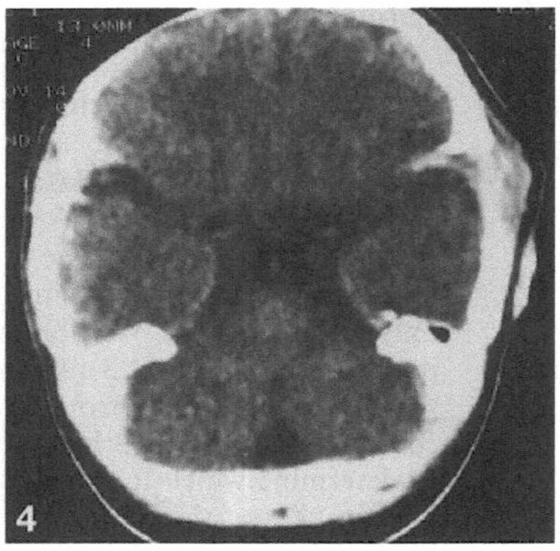

Fig. 1. A 3-day-old girl. Contrast-enhanced CT (3-mm sections) demonstrates normal appearance and enhancement of the anterolateral and posterolateral fontanelles

Fig. 2. A 4-day-old boy. CT (5-mm sections). **a** Before, **b** after enhancement. There is mild, homogeneous enhancement of the left anterolateral fontanelle

Fig. 3. A 4-day-old boy. Coronal contrast-enhanced CT (3-mm section). There is prominent enhancement of the right anterolateral fontanelle and partial ossification of the membrane

Fig. 4. A 13-day-old girl. Axial CT (5-mm sections) demonstrates a nodular left anterolateral fontanelle

enhancement of the membranes was usually uniform (Fig. 2). In four patients absence of bone and enhancement and irregularity of adjacent membranes suggested an aggressive process (Fig. 3). In four additional cases, nodularity of the membranes and irregularity of the osseous margin also suggested an aggressive process (Fig. 4).

Discussion

The anterolateral and posterolateral fontanelles are widely patent at birth. There is a gradual decrease in sutural patency over the first 6 months of life. By 6 months of age both the anterolateral and posterolateral fontanelles are usually closed. The appearance of the fontanelles before closure is variable. The membrane may be thick and nodular, thick and smooth, or thin. The membrane may show foci of ossification. There is generally uniform enhancement of the membrane. The presence of irregular nodularity and enhancement of the membrane should be recognized as a normal variant.

References

1. Gooding CA (1971) Cranial sutures and fontanelles. In: Newton TH, Potts DG (eds) Radiology of the skull and brain, book 1. Medibooks, Great Neck, NY, pp 216–237
2. Seagall HD, Mikity VG, Rumbaugh CL et al (1973) The radiology of the normal anterior fontanelle. Radiology 107:105–107
3. Acheson RM, Jefferson E (1954) Some observations on the closure of the anterior fontanelle. Arch Dis Child 29:196–198
4. Shapiro R (1981) Radiology of the normal skull. Year Book Medical Publishers, Chicago, pp 20–39

Development of the pineal gland: measurement with MR imaging

M. Sumida, A. J. Barkovich, T. H. Newton

Department of Radiology, University of California, San Francisco, California USA

Abstract. Our object was to analyze the size of the pineal gland in infants, children and adolescents using MRI. We retrospectively studied 249 patients aged 0–20 years. Their pineal glands were measured for maximum length (L) and height (H) on T1-weighted sagittal imaging and for width (W) on coronal or axial imaging. The volume was calculated with $1/2 \times L \times H \times W$. In patients 0–1 year of age, the gland was significantly smaller. It grew in size and remained stationary from 2 to 20 years old. There was a big variation in size in all age groups. There was no difference in size between males and females.

Key words: Pineal gland – Magnetic resonance imaging

The function of the pineal gland is not clear. For a long time pineal gland calcification has been focused upon in radiology. In a large review, physiological calcification on CT was not noted in patients younger than 5 years old but increased in prevalence dramatically and almost logarithmically with age [1]. However, because of various limitations, the growth process of the midline structures could not be fully analyzed with CT. In this study, we analyzed the size of the pineal gland in infants, children and adolescents, using MRI.

Patients and methods

We retrospectively studied 249 patients (129 males and 120 females) aged 0–20 years who had been examined by MRI. We excluded patients with any malignant tumor, glioma, radiation or chemotherapy.

A 1.5 T imager was used. T1-weighted spin echo 600/minimum/2 (TR/TEexcitations) images were obtained with a 256 × 192 matrix, a field of view of 20 cm, a 5-mm slice thickness and 1-mm gap. These patients were measured for maximum length (L) and height (H) on T1-weighted sagittal imaging and for width (W) on coronal or axial imaging. The volume was calculated with $1/2\ L \times H \times W$ [2].

Results

In patients 0–1 year of age, the gland was smaller (mean ± standard deviation L 4.8 mm ± 0.9, H 2.9 mm ± 0.6, W 3.7 mm ± 0.9, volume 26.9 mm^3 ± 12.4). It grew in size and remained stationary from 2 to 20 years old (average L 6.1 mm ± 1.2, H 3.7 mm ± 0.8, W 4.8 mm ± 1.1, volume 56.6 mm^3 ± 27.6) (Fig. 1). There was a big variation in size in all age groups. There was no significant difference in size between males and females. The gland in patients 0–1 year of age was significantly (P = .0001) smaller than the patients of 2–20 years of age.

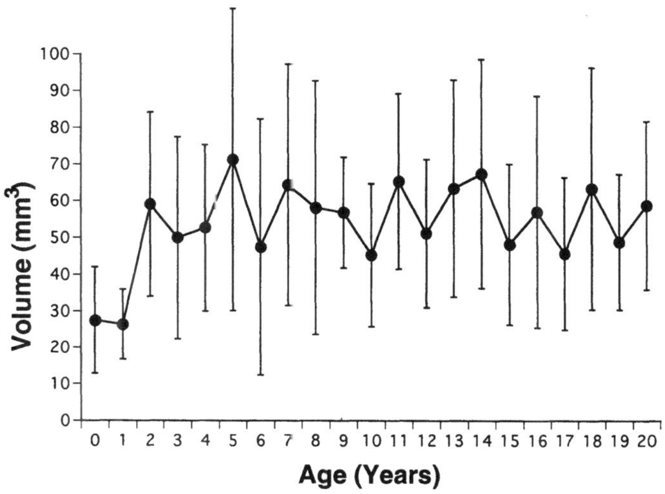

Fig. 1. Volume of the pituitary gland from birht to 20 years of age

Discussion

The pineal gland develops from the most caudal portion of the roof of the third ventricle, from an area of ependymal thickening that evaginates during the 7th week of gestation [3]. Initially, there is a patent cavity within the gland that connects to the third ventricle and is lined by ependyma. By the middle of first decade the structure of the pineal gland approaches that of a mature gland, consisting of pineocytes arranged into lobules separated by delicate connective tissue septa and thin-walled blood vessels.

In many lower vertebrates, the pineal gland is superficial and has a direct photoreceptor function. Even in humans, the regulation of biologic rhythms by the pineal gland responds to photoperiodic cues. The pineal gland receives this light or dark information via an accessory optic pathway that begins as the retinohypothalamic tract and passes through both sympathetic and parasympathetic innervation [4].

Most of the research concerned with the biological behavior of the pineal gland has been performed on animals, with most attention directed toward melatonin [5]. Melatonin in animals is essential in regulating circadation rhythms in endocrine activity and producing an antigonadal effect primarily through the hypothalamic-adenohypophyseal axis. Light inhibits melatonin production in animals and humans [6]. In humans the importance of melatonin is less well defined [7].

Correspondence to: M. Sumida, Department of Neurosurgery, Hiroshima University School of Medicine, 1-2-3 Kasumi, Minami-ku, Hiroshima, 734, Japan

In autopsy cases the average size of the pineal gland was 7.4 mm long, 6.9 mm wide and 2.5 mm high [8]. The weight of the pineal gland increased gradually from puberty to old age [9, 10]. The percentage of calcification showed no change after 30 years. However there are no reports about the development of the pineal gland concerning autopsy.

After the first report of pineal calcification on skull radiographs [11], the identification of pineal calcification has been of interest to the radiologist. CT is much more sensitive to calcification than skull radiographs [12]. In a large review of healthy patients, the youngest patient with a normally calcified pineal gland on CT was 61 years old. The incidence of pineal calcification as detected by CT shows an increase that coincides with the onset of puberty. The reason for pineal calcification has not been understood until now.

MRI has provided a marked improvement in the localization and characterization of tissue, as a result of facile multiplanar imaging and superior tissue contrast and resolution. Using MRI small soft structures which cannot be detected with CT are clearly shown especially in the midline with sagittal section [13].

In this study, the size of the pineal gland increased from 0 to 1 year of age and remained stationary from 2 to 20 years. The reason for this result has not been proved. It is well known that the size of the pituitary gland, one of the neuroendocrinological organs, well reflects the function of hormonal secretion. An understanding of the neuroendocrinologic function of the pineal gland may provide an answer in the near future. We believe that these data reflect the development and function of the pineal gland.

References

1. Zimmerman RA, Bilaniuk LT (1982) Age-related incidence of pineal calcification detected by computed tomography. Radiology 142:659–662
2. Lundin P, Pedersen F (1992) Volume of pituitary macroadenomas: assessment by MRI. J Comput Assist Tomogr 16:519–528
3. Langman J (1975) Medical embryology, 3th edn. William & Wilkins, Baltimore, pp 175–178, 318–364
4. Preslock JP (1984) The pineal gland: basic implication and clinical correlations. Endocr Rev 5:282–308
5. Lerner AB, Case JD, Takahashi Y et al (1958) Isolation of melatonin, the pineal gland factor that lightens melanocytos. J Am Chem Soc 80:2587
6. Lewy AJ et al (1980) Light suppresses melatonin secretion in humans. Science 210:1268
7. Reppert SM et al (1988) Putative melatonin receptors in a human biological clock. Science 242:78
8. Yamamoto Y, Kageyama N (1980) Microsurgical anatomy of the pineal region. J Neurosurg 53:205–221
9. Tapp E, Huxley M (1971) The weight and degree of calcification of the pineal gland. J Pathol 105:31–39
10. Tapp E, Huxley M (1972) The histological appearance of the human pineal gland from puberty to old age. J Pathol 108:137–144
11. Schüler A (1918) Roentgen diagnosis of diseases of the head. Mosby, St. Louis, p 156
12. Norman D, Diamond C, Boyd D (1978) Relative detectability of intracranial calcifications on computed tomography and skull radiography. J Comput Assist Tomogr 2:61–64
13. Hayakawa K, Konishi Y, Matsuda T et al (1989) Development and aging of brain midline structures: assessment with MR imaging. Radiology 172:171–177

Di- and Hemiplegic infants: clinical-MRI correlation and pathogenetic considerations

M. Sintini [1], E. Della Giustina [2], L. Mavilla [1]

[1] Section of Neuroradiology, University of Modena, I-44100 Modena, Italy
[2] Institute of Paediatrics, University of Modena, I-44100 Modena, Italy

Abstract. We studied 48 infants with cerebral palsy (24 diplegic and 24 hemiplegic) by MRI and correlated the findings with clinical status, pregnancy and delivery events. All hemiplegic infants were born at term, 18 diplegic were premature. MRI proved useful, showing that hemiplegia is often due to a malformation, mainly schizencephaly and cortical dysplasia, making it possible to demonstrate its prenatal origin. Only children with congenital defects developed late epilepsy. White and grey matter infarcts are the most frequent MRI findings, as on CT, and their extent does not correlate with the severity of the neurological deficit; there is no proof of a prenatal origin. Diplegic infants showed the typical periventricular white matter lesions which, when asymmetrical, did not correlate with the predominant side of plegic motor signs.

Key words: Cerebral palsy – Hemiplegia – Diplegia – Magnetic resonance imaging

According to Kotlarek et al. [1] congenital hemiplegia is a "nonprogressive spastic hemiplegia discovered in the first year of life without any history of brain accident postnatally". It has also been emphasized that this form of cerebral palsy has maintained the same incidence over recent years, while other forms such as spastic diplegia have decreased along with the improvement of perinatal

Correspondence to: M. Sintini

Table 1. Clinical and MRI correlations

Birth date	24 Hemiplegic children (9F, 15M), all born at term	24 Diplegic children (10F, 14M); 18 premature
Pregnancy	23 normal, 1 maternal diabetes mellitus	18 normal, 1 intrauterine death, 4 eclampsia 1 late haemorrhage
Delivery events	19 none, 1 CFB deceleration, 1 placental abruptio, 3 primary asphyxia	11 none, 5 primary asphyxia, 4 dystocia, 2 secondary asphyxia, 2 placental abruptio
Post natal pathology	20 none, 2 neonatal seizures (with primary asphyxia), 1 meningeal haemorrhage, 1 hypoglycaemia	4 none, 14 respiratory distress syndrome, 6 intracranial haemorrhage, 4 seizures
Late epilepsy	4 (all associated with cortical dysplasia)	13
MRI findings	7 congenital defects (1 hemimegalencephaly, 1 isolated cortical dysplasia, 2 grey matter dysplasia with associated schizencephaly, 3 bilateral schizencephaly) 12 ischaemic lesions along corticospinal tracts 5 bilateral periventricular white matter lesions with unilateral predomiance (3 with delivery asphyxia)	All with periventricular leukomalacia without grey matter abnormalities, with variable central atrophy (ventricular dilatation), asymmetrical in 8 cases

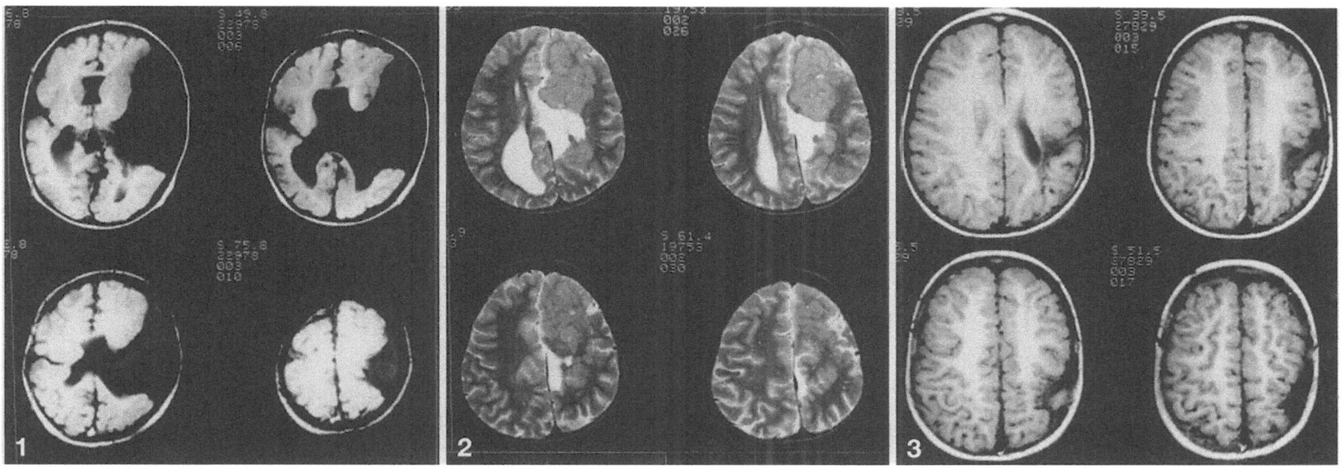

Abb. 1. Right hemiparesis in a 6-month-old boy. T1-weighted gradient-echo images showing bilateral schizencephaly, open on the left

Fig. 2. Right hemiparesis in a 12-year-old boy. T2-weighted spin-echo images. Large left frontal heterotopia associated with extensive cortical dysplasia and closed-lip parietal schizencephaly

Fig. 3. Right hemiparesis in a 4-year-old boy. T1-weighted gradient-echo images. Left Rolandic infarct

care [2]. The purpose of this study was to describe 48 cases of cerebral palsy (24 spastic diplegia and 24 spastic hemiplegia) in order to correlate them with clinical findings, as well as pregnancy and delivery events.

Materials and methods

We reviewed the MRI of 48 infants with cerebral palsy, 24 spastic hemiplegias and 24 spastic diplegias, all performed at 1.5 T, employing the usual T1 and T2-weighted spin-echo and gradient-echo sequences. In no case was Gd-DTPA administered. One of us (EDG) examined all the patients at the time of MRI and reconstructed clinical, pregnancy and delivery histories from parents and previous hospital admissions. We considered hemiplegia and hemiparesis together, as well as all the grading of spastic diplegias in order to correlate MRI with the severity of motor impairment. Mental development was not considered, late epilepsy being the only aspect of clinical outcome we annotated.

Results

See Table 1.

Discussion

MRI findings in our cases are in accord with those recently reported [3–7], except for the absence in our hemiplegic series of a normal picture. Above all we emphasize the incidence of congenital defects (about 30% in our group), namely cortical dysplasia, in hemiplegic infants providing a certain prenatal origin of motor impairment, regardless of the timing of cerebral insult. Of all 24 hemiplegic infants, only those affected by the above-mentioned brain malformations developed late partial epilepsy. Also, in hemiplegic children, ischaemic lesions were present in 50% of cases along the corticospinal tracts; the first year of life was clinically uneventful, except for the obvious discovery of spastic motor deficit, and one may suppose its prenatal origin even if, especially for mild hemiparesis, an inschaemic event with only motor impairment may pass unnoticed during the first months of life.

Finally, we found no correlation between the severity of hemiplegia and infarct extension. The diplegic group was more homogeneous at MRI, showing the typical periventricular findings whose side prevalence, when present, did not always agree with spastic motor signs. Few cases showed the MRI pattern of wallerian degeneration [6] of fibres in the internal capsule that, when present only in the posterior half of the internal capsule's posterior arm, they disagreed with the classical anatomical descriptions and supported the hypothesis that motor fibres also run there. Therefore, MRI proved very useful to demonstrate hemiplegic and diplegic syndromes as different entities in the pediatric population, the former showing excellent clinical-MRI correlations.

References

1. Kotlarek F, Rodewig R, Brull D (1981) Computed tomographic findings in congenital hemiparesis in childhood and their relation to etiology and prognosis. Neuropediatrics 12:101–108
2. Molteni B, Oleari G, Fedrizzi E et al (1987) Relation between CT patterns, clinical findings and etiological factors in children born at term, affected by congenital hemiparesis. Neuropediatrics 18:75–80
3. Steinlin M, Good M, Martin E et al (1993) Congenital hemiplegia: morphology of cerebral lesions and pathogenetic aspects from MRI. Neuropediatrics 24:224–229
4. Wiklund LM, Uvebrant P, Flodmark O (1990) Morphology of cerebral lesions in children with congenital hemiplegia. A study with computed tomography. Neuroradiology 32:179–186
5. Truwit CL, Barkovich AJ, Koch TK et al (1992) Cerebral palsy: MR findings in 40 patients. AJNR Am J Neuroradiol 13:67–78
6. Bouza H, Dubowitz LMS, Rutheford M et al (1994) Prediction of outcome in children with congenital hemiplegia: an MRI study. Neuropediatrics 25:60–66
7. Krageloh-Mann I, Hagberg B, Petersen D et al (1992) Bilateral spastic cerebral palsy – pathogenetic aspects from MRI. Neuropediatrics 23:46–48

Assessment of visuoperceptual disturbance in spastic diplegic children using measurements of the lateral ventricles on cerebral MRI

J. Ito[1], H. Tanaka[1], T. Tasaki[1], K. Cho[1], A. Miyamoto[2]

[1] Department of Paediatrics, Asahikawa Habilitation Center for Disabled Children, Asahikawa, Japan
[2] Institute of Paediatrics, Asahikawa Medical College, Asahikawa, Japan

Abstract. We assessed visuoperceptual disturbance in spastic diplegic children from the characteristics of the lateral ventricles on cerebral MRI. The ratio of the areas of the posterior horns to the anterior horns (P/A) had a high correlation with the degree of perceptual disturbance. This ratio could be used as an index to estimate perceptual disturbance in spastic diplegic children at an early age.

Key words: Spastic diplegia – Visuoperceptual disturbance – Cerebral magnetic resonance imaging

One of the main problems of children with cerebral palsy is visuoperceptual disturbance. Because of this, some of their performance abilities may be retarded compared with verbal ability [1–3]. There are few reports on the causes of visuoperceptual disturbances in these children [3–6], so we attempted to assess the morphological basis of this disorder from measurements of the lateral ventricles on cerebral MRI.

Correspondence to: J. Ito, Department of Pediatrics, Asahikawa Habilitation Center for Disabled Children, Shunkodai 1-1, Asahikawa City, Hokkaido 071, Japan

Patients and methods

We studied 27 children with spastic diplegia without involuntary movements. They had mild or no motor disturbance of the upper extremities, no disturbance of eye movements or visual fields, and could be assessed with both verbal and performance intellectual quotients (VIQ and PIQ) by the Wechsler intelligence test. Their VIQ was above 70. The presumed causes were premature birth (23 children), asphyxia (1 child), neonatal infection (1 child) and unknown (2 children).

Because our previous study showed that the point differential between PIQ and VIQ was an indicator of perceptual disturbance [2], we divided the children into two groups, SD(NR) and SD(R), based on the IQ difference (Table 1). Eleven children, whose IQ difference was within 14 points, were considered to have normal perceptual ability for their age [SD(N)]. Sixteen other children, whose IQ difference was more than 15 points, were considered to have retarded perceptual ability [SD(R)].

Table 1. Children studied. Subjects of our study

	Children	Age (mean)	IQ difference
SD (N)	12	8 years, 4 months	VIQ–PIQ≦14
SD (R)	15	8 years, 8 months	VIQ–PIQ>15
Controls	12	9 years, 2 months	VIQ–PIQ≦14

SD (N), Diplegic children considered to have normal perceptual ability for their age; SD (R), diplegic children considered to have retarded perceptual ability; VIQ PIQ, verbal and performance IQ

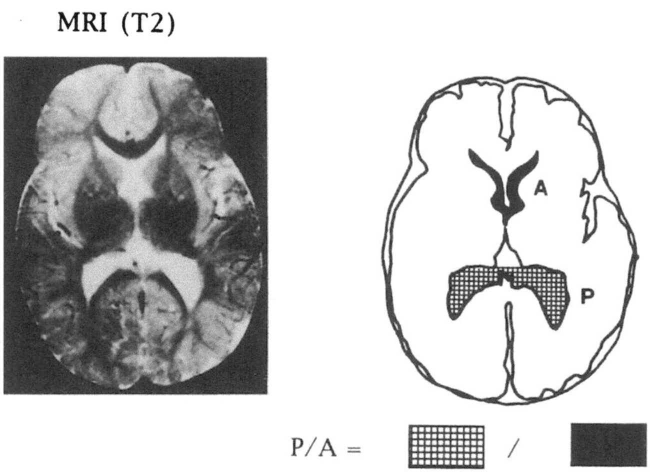

Fig. 1. Cerebral MRI of a child whose verbal and performance IQs were 111 and 76. Widening of posterior horns of the lateral ventricle was noted; P/A was 2.2

We defined P/A (Fig. 1) as the ratio of the areas of posterior horns to the anterior horns, using a computer-assisted image analyser and compared the results in the two groups. We also examined the correlation between their P/A and perceptual disability.

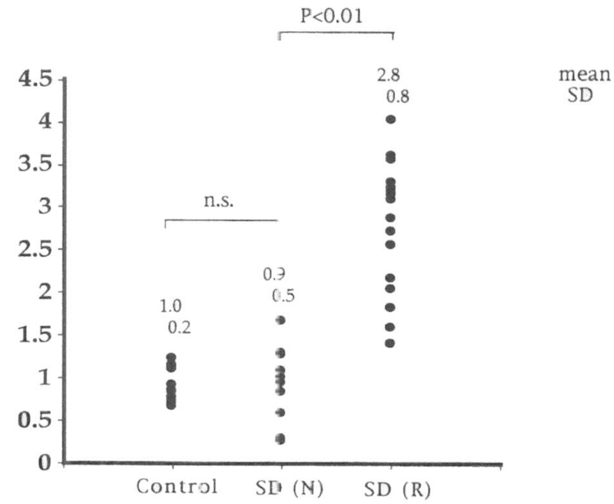

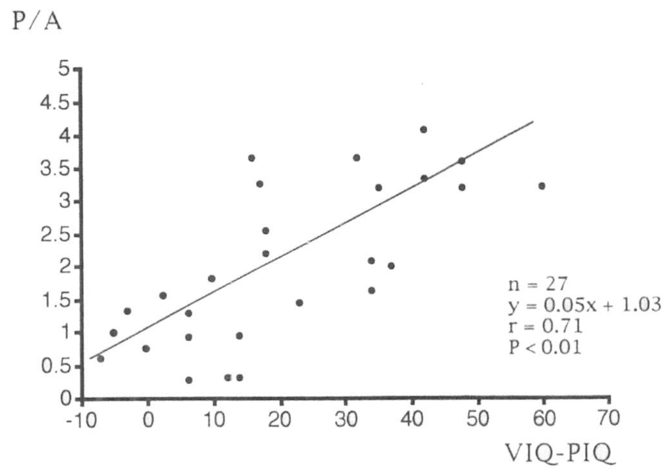

Fig. 3. Correlation between the degree of perceptual disturbance and P/A was highly significant

Results

As for the P/A, there was no difference between SD(N) and the control group, but SD(R) was significantly higher (Fig. 2). The correlation between P/A in spastic diplegic children and the degree of perceptual disturbance was highly significant ($r = 0.71$, $P < 0.01$) (Fig. 3).

Discussion

The visuoperceptual disturbance in spastic diplegic children is now suspected to be caused by damage to the visual pathway and/or occipital lobes [3–6]. Periventricular leukomalacia has recently come to be regarded as the underlying pathogenesis, especially in premature children. It was shown in this study that the widening of posterior horns of the lateral ventricles correlates with the visuoperceptual disturbance in spastic diplegic children. Our findings indicated atrophy of the optic radiation running at the posterior horn of the lateral ventricles and/or occipital lobes.

We also found that P/A, which could be easily assessed by eye, is an index of visuoperceptual disturbance in spastic diplegic children. Thus, a decision can be made to start occupational therapy for children with verbal and performance developmental discrepancies, as assessed by the P/A ratio on cerebral CT or MRI findings.

References

1. Abercrombie MLJ (1964) Visual, perceptual and visuo-motor impairments in physically handicapped children. Percept Mot Skills 18:583–594
2. Ito J, Kazuhiko C (1994) Relationship between intellectual status and disorders of visual perception in spastic diplegia (in Japanese). Shoni Hoken Kenkyu (Tokyo) 53:26–31
3. Koeda T, Takeshita K (1992) Visuo-perceptual impairment and cerebral lesions in spastic diplegia with preterm birth. Brain Dev 14:239–244

4. Van Nieuwenhuizen O, Willemse J (1984) CT-scanning in children with visual disturbance and its possible relation to hypoxia and ischemia. Brain Behav Res 14:143–145
5. Flodmark O, Jan JE, Wong PKH (1990) Computed tomography of the brains of children with cortical visual impairment. Dev Med Child Neurol 32:611–620
6. Scher MS, Dobson V, Carpenter NA et al (1989) Visual and neurological outcome of infants with periventricular leukomalacia. Dev Med Child Neurol 31:353–365

Neuroradiological follow-up in seven patients with idiopathic bilateral striatal necrosis

M. Gallucci[1], **A. Bozzao**[1], **V. Leuzzi**[2], **F. Cardona**[2], **B. Orlandi**[1], **A. Bottone**[1], **M. G. Alagia**[1]

[1] Department of Radiology, University of L'Aquila, L'Aquila, Italy
[2] Department of Child Neurology, University of Rome "La Sapienza", Rome, Italy

Abstract. Idiopathic bilateral striatal necrosis (IBSN) is a heterogeneous neuroradiological pathological group of unknown aetiology. We followed seven patients for a period ranging from 3 to 13 years. In all patients, other metabolic or other pathologies were excluded. CT and MRI demonstrated selective necrosis in the early phase of the disease (in 1 case the dentate nucleus was also involved). Follow-up showed progression of the disease, with involvement of the caudate nuclei in all patients except one, in whom cerebellar cortical necrosis was detected. All these findings preceded by months or years the clinical worsening of the disease.

Key words: Idiopathic bilateral striatal necrosis – Magnetic resonance imaging – Follow-up study

Idiopathic bilateral striatal necrosis (IBSN) is heterogeneous group of pathology manifesting as progressive dystonia in children [1]. The aim of this study was to follow seven children affected by the condition, taking particular account of the clinical and neuroradiological aspects as well as the differential diagnosis.

Patients and methods

Seven children (4 boys, 3 girls), age ranging from 3 to 13 years at first examination, were followed clinically and neuroradiologically for a period ranging from 3 to 13 years. At the onset, five patients had focal dystonia, associated with visual acuity defect in two (siblings). All these patients showed progressive worsening. The remaining two were affected by rigidity more than abnormal movements, with very slow progression. One also had seizures. Each had undergone repeated neurometabolic studies in order to identify known metabolic defects (in particular mitochondrial defects, organic aciduria and lysosomal diseases). All were negative. Neuroradiological examination was by CT and MRI (0.5 T, standard SE sequences).

Correspondence to: M. Galucci

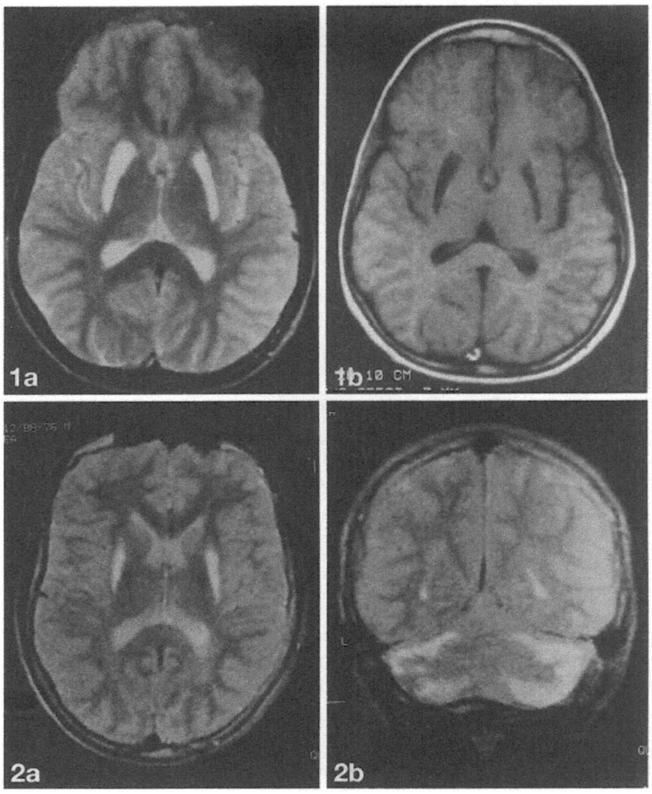

Fig. 1. Selective putaminal involvement in IBSN on T2-weighted (**a**) and T1-weighted (**b**) images

Fig. 2. Typical putaminal involvement (**a**) with cortical cerebellar changes on follow-up (**b**)

Results

CT and/or MRI showed in all cases selective putaminal necrosis, not necessarily symmetrical (Fig. 1). In one case, caudate necrosis was associated; in another the dentate nuclei were also involved. Neuroradiological follow-up invariably showed worsening of the illness: symmetrical extension to the whole neostriatum in all cases but one.

The latter showed bilateral neocerebellar cortical necrosis after 1 year (Fig. 2). Neuroradiological worsening always preceded the clinical progression by weeks or months. No strict relationship between the sites involved and the corresponding clinical syndrome was found.

Discussion

IBSN is very similar to some mitochondrial cytopathies (MC) from the clinical and neuroradiological points of view [1, 2]. Despite this, until now no enzyme deficiency has been detected and the clinical progression was usually milder. Our study led us to some conclusions. Radiological findings are usually those of neostriatal involvement [3–5].

As in MC and in particular in Leigh disease, selective neostriatal involvement is constant in IBSN. It was observed as soon as the clinical symptoms began. On the other hand, unlike MC, we never found atrophic changes or calcium deposits. Progression of the disease was always evident, even if slower than in MC. Extrastriatal extension is possible, even if the brainstem, white matter or cerebral cortex were always spared.

The differential diagnostic criteria between IBSN and MC may thus be easier in the early phases of the diseases, when only the putamen is involved in IBSN. In the later phases, because of progressive involvement on dentate nuclei and cerebellar cortex, the differential diagnosis might be much more difficult. The sparing of the brain stem, cerebral cortex and white matter may help since it was never observed in IBSN.

The neuroradiological findings always preceded the clinical ones by months or years, thus allowing prognostic consideration of the disease.

References

1. Roytta M, Olsson I, Sourander P et al (1981) IBSN. Clinical and morphological report of a case and review of the literature. Acta Neuropathol 55:97–103
2. Becker LE (1992) Lysosomes, peroxisomes and mitochondria: function and disorder. AJNR 13:609–620
3. Barkovich AJ (1990) Pediatric neuropathology. Raven Press, New York
4. Osborn AG (1994) Diagnostic neuroradiology. Mosby, St. Louis
5. Kendall BE (1992) Disorders of lysosomes, peroxisomes and mitochondria. AJNR 13:621–653

MRI of kernicterus

Wu-Chung Shen [1], Chi-Chan Chen [1], San-Kan Lee [1], Jeun-Horng Chen [2]

[1] Department of Radiology, Taichung Veterans General Hospital, Taichung, Taiwan
[2] Department of Pediatrics, Chung Shan Medical and Dental College Hospital, Taichung, Taiwan

Abstract. We report six cases of kernicterus examined by MRI. All showed symmetrical high-signal lesions in the globus pallidus bilaterally on long TR images. Two showed high-signal lesions in the subthalamic nuclei and in the corticospinal tracts of the midbrain. Three revealed dilatation of both lateral ventricles, reflecting atrophy of the hippocampus. The lesions described correspond to the pathological reports of kernicterus, that is, icteric discoloration, atrophy with loss of nerve cells and glial scarring in the globus pallidus, subthalamic nuclei and Ammon's horn of the hippocampus.

Key words: Kernicterus – Bilirubin encephalopathy – Magnetic resonance imaging

Kernicterus (bilirubin encephalopathy) is classically associated with icterus gravis in newborns and severe neurological damage in infants who survive [1, 2]. With the advent of neonatal exchange transfusion, phototherapy, and other techniques used to control serum bilirubin levels, both the incidence of kernicterus and the classical sequelae of neonatal hyperbilirubinaemia have been greatly reduced [1, 3]. The pathology of kernicterus has been well documented, and includes icterid discoloration, atrophy with loss of nerve cells and glial scarring in the pallidum, subthalamic nuclei, Ammon's horn, and substantia nigra [1, 4–6]. However, to the best of our knowledge, there are no published medical imaging reports concerning kernicterus. Here we report six children with kernicterus examined by MRI.

Correspondence to: Wu-Chung Shen, Department of Radiology, Taichung Veterans General Hospital, Taichung 407, Taiwan

Materials and methods

In the past 2 years (July 1992–July 1994), we have examined six cases of kernicterus by MRI. The diagnosis of kernicterus was based on a neonatal history of definite hyperbilirubinaemia (over 25 mg/dl) with later neurological deficits. The age range of the patients was 6 months to 5 years, with a mean age of 2 years. The patients were examined on a 1.0 T MRI machine in four cases, and on a 0.2 T MRI machine in two cases. The pulse sequences were spin echos of T1-weighted images and dual echoes of long TR images.

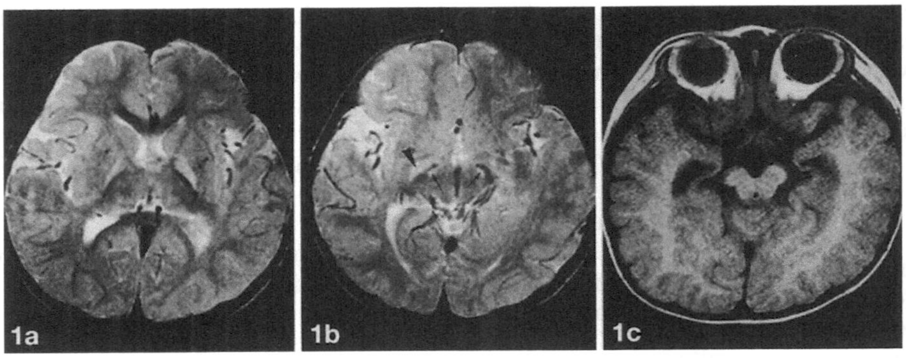

Fig. 1 a–c. Kernicterus in girl aged 2 years 9 months; presentation as cerebral palsy, extrapyramidal mixed with pyramidal type. **a, b** T2 WI (TR/TE 3500/80 ms). **a** Symmetrical high-signal areas bilaterally in globus pallidus. **b** Symmetrical high-signal lesions in the bilateral corticospinal tracts (*small arrows*) of the midbrain. Hypertense lesion in the subthalamic nucleus (*arrowhead*). **c** T1WI (TR/TE 750/20 ms). Dilatation of the temporal horns of bilateral lateral ventricles, reflecting atrophy of the hippocampus

Results

All six cases showed symmetrical high-signal lesions bilaterally in the globus pallidus long TR images (Fig. 1a). Two also showed high-signal lesions in the subthalamic nuclei and the corticospinal tracts of the midbrain (Fig. 1b). The temporal horns of both lateral ventricles were dilated in three cases (Fig. 1c), reflecting atrophy of the hippocampus.

All the children had cerebral palsy of extrapyramidal type and two who had lesions in the corticospinal tracts of the midbrain also had a pyramidal syndrome. Squint and hearing impairment were noted in one case.

Discussion

The classical diagnosis of kernicterus is based on the clinical findings of severe neonatal hyperbilirubinaemia and characteristic neurological symptomatology [1, 2]. In the early 1950s, survivors of primarily full-term gestations complicated by marked hyperbilirubinaemia accounted for approximately 6% of all cases of cerebral palsy seen in large clinics [7]. With improved control of the serum bilirubin level and the prevention of hyperbilirubinaemia, the classic clinical syndrome of kernicterus has decreased markedly [1, 3]. Furthermore, some workers consider that neonatal hyperbilirubinaemia in a healthy full-term infant does not necessarily cause brain damage [8]. However, the incidence of kernicterus is still high in Chinese term infants [9].

The gross features of kernicterus consist of icteric discoloration of nuclear groups in a symmetrical pattern. The most common sites are the pallidum, subthalamic nucleus and Ammon's horn; staining of the thalamus and the striatum is less common. Icteric staining in the brain stem involves mainly the cranial nerve nuclei of the tegmentum, particularly the oculomotor and dentate nuclei, and the cerebellar flocculi. Microscopically, the lesions are characterised by atrophy with loss of nerve cells and glial scarring [1, 4–6]. In all our cases the symmetrical high-signal lesions in the globus pallidus were very clear on long TR images (Fig. 1a). However, only two showed high-signal lesions in the subthalamic nuclei and midbrain (Fig. 1b). Three cases demonstrated dilatation of the temporal horns of the bilateral lateral ventricle, which possibly reflected atrophy of the hippocampus (Fig. 1c), due to involvement of Ammon's horn.

Neonatal hyperbilirubinaemia does not directly cause damage to the brain, except in association with brain hypoxia, prematurity, acidosis, or sepsis [4, 5, 8]. Perinatal asphyxia and kernicerus often coexist. Chen [5] observed amniotic aspiration in 84% of infants with kernicterus. Indeed, anoxia may increase the permeability of the blood-brain barrier in the damaged regions and trigger kernicterus [6–8, 10]. Hence, posticretic encephalopathy may coexist with lesions characteristic of perinatal asphyxia. However, in our study, only one child had a history of perinatal asphyxia and prematurity. In addition to the characteristic lesions of the globus pallidus, this patient also showed typical periventricular leucomalacia.

Acknowledgement. This study was supported by grant NSC 82-0412-B075A-029.

References

1. Turkel SB, Miller CA, Guttenberg ME, Moynes DR, Hodgman JE (1982) A clinical pathologic reappraisal of kernicterus. Pediatrics 69:267–272
2. Gerrard J (1952) Kernicterus. Brain 75:526–532
3. Brodersen R (1980) Bilirubin transport in the newborn infant, reviewed with relation to kernicterus. J Pediatr 96:349–355
4. Ahdab-Barnada M, Moosy J (1984) The neuropathology of kernicterus in the premature neonate: diagnostic problems. J Neuropathol Exp Neurol 43:45–56
5. Chen HC (1964) Kernicterus in the Chinese newborn. A morphological and spectrophotometric study. J Neuropathol Exp Neurol 23:527–549
6. Friede RL (1989) Kernicterus (bilirubin encephalopathy). In: Friede RL (ed) Develomental neuropathology. Springer, Berlin Heidelberg New York, pp 115–124
7. Byres RK, Paine RS, Crothers B (1955) Extrapyramidal cerebral palsy with hearing loss following erythroblastosis. Pediatrics 15:248–256
8. Newman TB, Maisels MJ (1990) Does hyperbilirubinemia damage the brain of healthy full-term infants? Clin Perinatal 17:331–358
9. Yeung CY (1985) Kernicterus in term infants. Aust Paediatr J 21:273–274
10. Levine RL, Fredericks WR, Rapoport SI (1982) Entry of bilirubin into the brain due to opening of the blood-brain barrier. Pediatrics 69:255–259

Neuroradiology of Pelizaeus-Merzbacher disease: a long-term follow-up study

A. Bozzao [1], M. Gallucci [1], F. Cardona [2], R. Manetta [1], E. Bielli [1], F. Navarra [1]

[1] Department of Radiology, University of L'Aquila, L'Aquila, Italy
[2] Department of Child Neurology, University of Rome "La Sapienza", Rome, Italy

Abstract. Pelizaeus-Merzbacher disease (PMD) is a leukodystrophy linked to an arrest of myelin formation of unknown aetiology. We report a longitudinal study (1–6 years) of seven affected patients. In all patients, MRI showed diffuse alteration of the supratentorial white matter. The infratentorial white matter was involved in the conatal form as well. Intermediate appearences were seen in the classical and non-X-linked forms. Except for the conatal case, little or no neuroradiological progression was seen in contrast with the slow progressive clinical worsening.

Key words: Palizaeus-Merzbacher disease – Magnetic resonance imaging – Follow-up

Pelizaeus-Merzbacher disease (PMD) is a rare leukodystrophy whose diagnostic classification is difficult [1, 2]. Until now, only sporadic case reports have been published [3–6]. We performed a long-term clinical neuroradiological follow-up of seven patients affected by the disease.

Patients and methods

We followed seven (six boys, one girl) affected by PMD (age at the first examination 1.5–6 years) for a period ranging from 5 to 8 years. The six boys (typical X-linked) were affected by classical (4 case) and conatal (1 case) type. The girl was affected by the classical form. MRI performed at 0.5 and 0.2 T using standard spin-echo sequences. Each patient underwent 2–4 MRI studies.

Results

The Seitelberger conatal form showed no myelin at all in any examination performed, without sparing of the brain stem or cerebellum (Fig. 1). All the other cases, including the autosomal type, showed total involvement of the supratentorial white matter without sparing the U fibres (Fig. 2). In 2 cases, the cerebellar white matter was

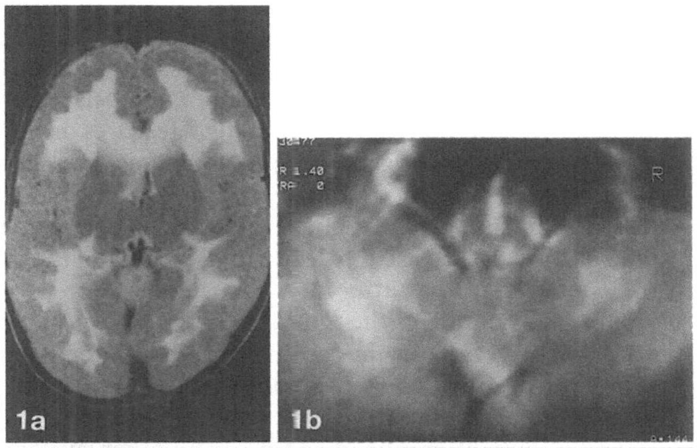

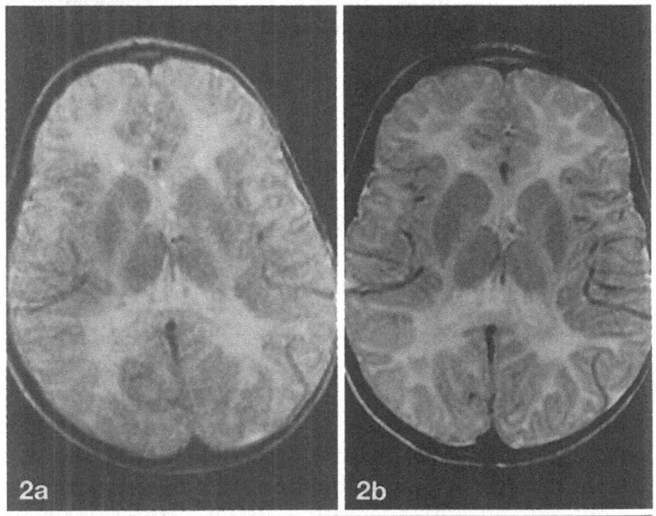

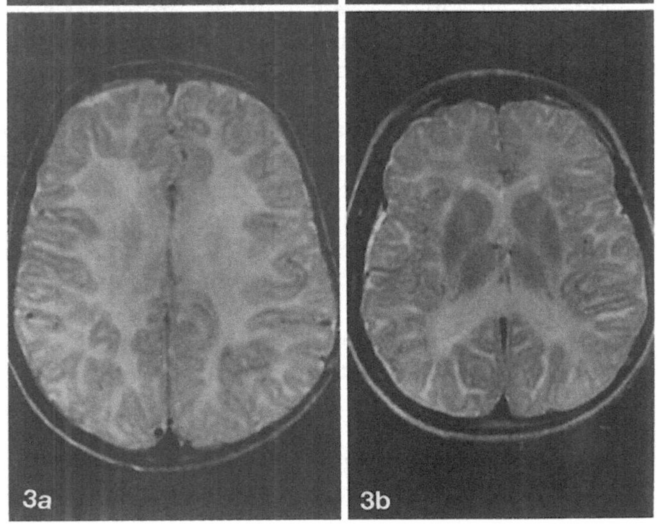

Fig. 1. Conatal form. Complete absence of myelin, both above (**a**) and below (**b**) the tentorium

Fig. 2. Transitional form. No changes in follow-up MRI (**b**) 4 years after the first (**a**)

Fig. 3 a, b. Affected girl. MRI findings are the same as in the X-linked form

Correspondence to: A. Bozzao

affected. The X-linked form showed no difference in the MRI findings (Fig. 3). Follow-up studies showed no extension of the disease, although clinical worsening was always present (Fig. 2).

Discussion

PMD is a rare X-linked leukodystrophy. Sporadic cases are described and autosomal-recessive transmission is reported [1, 2]. The disease manifests itself by wandering eye movements, failure to develop normal head control, tremor or shaking of the head, choreoathetosis, ataxic, spasticity and optic atrophy. The clinical features progress very slowly. The pathogenesis is unknown: recent findings suggest a defect of DND repair. Neuropathological studies show diffuse myelin damage with patchy demyelinate and sparing of perivascular white matter with a "tigroid" or "leopard-skin" pattern.

Our study confirms the typical neuroradiological pattern [3–6] absence of the normal white matter in the supratentorial regions with involvement of subcorcial U fibres, mild or absent atrophy.

This allows differential diagnosis from other leukodystrophies, e.g., Cockayne's disease. Our findings are in accordance with the hypothesis of a very slow breakdown of myelin, without demyelination. The MRI follow-up did not show changes in signal intensity or progressive atrophy. The neuroradiological patterns were in agreement with age of onset (no myelination in the infantile form). The X-linked form has shown to be clinically and neuroradiologically similar to the other forms.

References

1. Friede RL (1989) Patchy myelinopathies: Pelizaeus-Mezbacher disease, Cockayne syndrome, and others, also including a review of primary cerebral mineralizations. Dev Neuropathol 42:534–545
2. Becker LE (1992) Lysosomes, peroxisomes and mitochondria: function and disorder. AJ Neuroradiol 13:609–620
3. Barkovich AJ (1990) Metabolic and destructive brain disorders. Ped Neuroimaging 1:35–75
4. Caranci F, Cirillo S, Briganti F, Simonetti L, Del Basso de Caro ML, Gallucci M (1993) Malattia di Pelizaeus-Merzbacher. In: Elefante R (ed) Leucodistrofie, Col die Neurorad Liviana Medicina/Idelson, pp 33–39
5. Osborn AG (1994) Diagnostic neuroradiology. Mosby-Year Book, St. Louis, pp 716–747
6. Valk J, Knaap MS van der (1989) Magnetic resonance myelin, myelination, and myelin disorders. Springer, Berlin Heidelberg New York, pp 155–164

Abnormalities of the claustrum

R. N. Sener

Department of Radiology, Ege University Hospital, Bornova, Izmir, 35100-TR, Turkey

Abstract. The claustrum is a relatively thin anatomical structure. MRI is a sensitive modality showing the claustrum in a way not possible on CT. This paper presents eight patients with a variety of disease processes demonstrating claustral involvement. Seven were studied by MRI and one patient by CT. These included three patients with Wilson's disease, twins with cytoplasmically inherited strial degeneration, two patients with claustral infarctions associated with chronic meningitis and encephalomalacia (on CT), and a patient with a brain tumour and contralateral claustral haemorrhage. Claustral involvement was bilateral in most of the patients. In all the patients, accompanying lesions were evident in the brain.

Key words: Magnetic resonance imaging – Brain diseases – Brain anatomy – Computed tomography

Magnetic resonance imaging (MRI) is a sensitive method of detailing the normal anatomy and pathological changes of the brain parenchyma. Relatively thin anatomical structures such as the claustrum, which could have not been shown by CT, can be demonstrated by MRI. MRI of claustral involvement in Wilson's disease has recently been detailed [1, 2]. The current study investigated claustral involvement in a variety of disorders.

Correspondence to: R. N. Sener

Subjects and methods

1000 cranial MRI examinations during a period of 1 year, seven patients were found with claustral involvement. One patient with a claustral lesion seen on CT, who did not have an MRI study, is also included in this series. The ages of these eight subjects ranged from 1 to 47 years (average approximately 14 years). Five were female and three were male. The MRI studies were obtained on a 0.5 T unit.

Results

In five patients the claustrum gave apparently high signal on T2-weighted images. These included three patients with proven Wilson's disease (Fig. 1) and two siblings (twins) with a progressive neurological disorder presumed

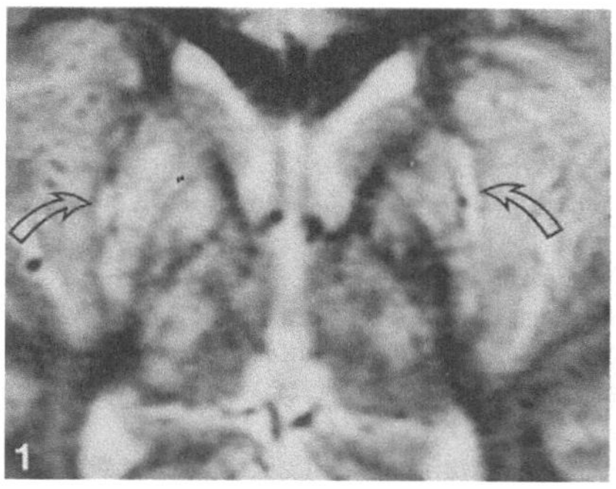
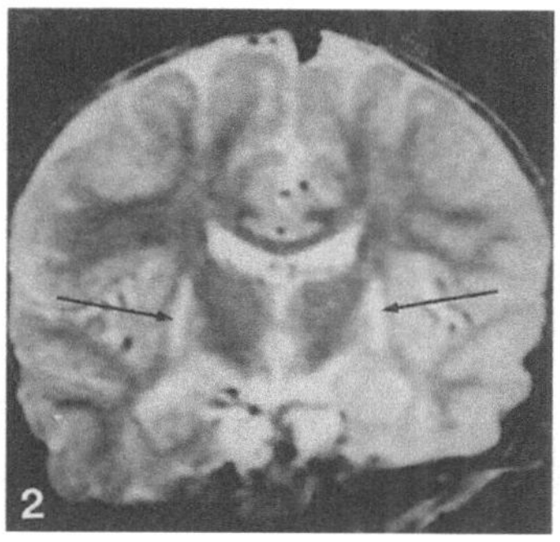
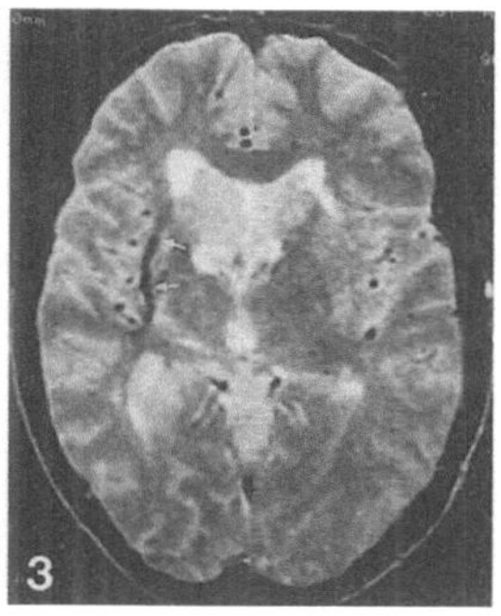
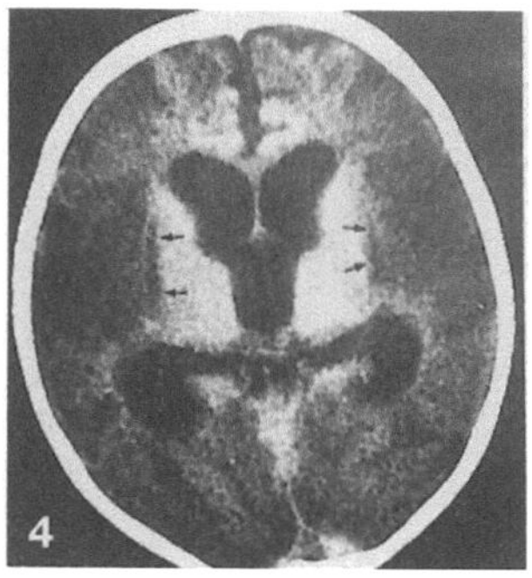

Fig. 1. T2-weighted image of a 12-year-old boy with Wilson's disease shows a high-signal, thickened claustrum on both sides (*arrows*). The lentiform nuclei and thalamus are affected

Fig. 2. T2-weighted image of one female twin with cytoplasmicaly inherited strial degeneration shows predominantly claustral involvement (*arrows*). Note also lesions in the heads of the caudate nuclei

Fig. 3. A 47-year-old man with a glial tumour in the left hemisphere and apparent shift of the midline structures. T2-weighted image shows the right claustrum to give low signal (*arrows*), suggesting chronic haemorrhage

Fig. 4. CT in a 1-year-old boy with multicystic encephalomalacia and the so-called reversal sign (high density of the basal ganglia) secondary to hypoxia. Note bilateral claustral infarcts (*arrows*)

to be "cytoplasmically inherited striatal degeneration" (Fig. 2). One patient had bilateral claustral infarctions. One patient showed unilateral claustral haemorrhage, contralateral to a brain tumour (Fig. 3). Another, studied only by CT, had bilateral claustral infarct (Fig. 4). In all patients, accompanying lesions were evident in the brain, i.e. no isolated claustral pathology was seen.

Discussion

The claustrum is a thin sheet of grey matter between the insula and utamen. It is separated from the putamen by the external capsule and from the insula by the extreme capsule. It is regarded by some as belonging to the corpus striatum. Animal studies suggest that the claustrum has corticoclastral and claustrocortical connections with many regions of the neocortex. In the human brain, however, the connections and functional significance of the claustrum are unknown [3].

The author recent reported the appearance of the normal claustrum on MRI as well as its brightness on T2-weighted MRI (Fig. 1) in Wilson's disease [1]. This finding is probably a consequence of involvement of the claustrum with one or more histopathological changes of Wilson's disease, because similar MRI findings have previously been reported in the basal ganglia and other cerebral locations in Wilson's disease [4–7].

The causes of bilateral basal ganglion lesions cover a wide variety of disorders, including Wilson's disease, Leigh's disease, mitochondrial encephalomyopathies, Hallervorden-Spatz disease, striatonigral degeneration, cytoplasmically inherited strial degeneration, barbiturate intoxication, hypoglycaemia, and carbon monoxide, cyanide, and hydrogen sulphide poisoning [8]. In our two patients, who were siblings, most of these could be excluded clinically and by laboratory studies, and the final presumed diagnosis was cytoplasmicaly inherited strial degeneration (Fig. 2).

The claustrum is supplied by the carotid system by medullary arteries, which are branches of the insular pial arteries of the middle cerebral artery [9]. On the other hand, the thalamic vascular territories are supplied by either the vertebrobasilar system or the carotid system [10, 11], and the amygdala by the middle cerebral artery [3]. These are usually end-arteries. In a patient with meningitis, bilateral infarcts in the thalamus, claustrum, and amygdala suggested arteriolopathic changes of these small end-arteries. In the other patient who developed the so-called reversal sign [12, 13] as a result of hypoxia during general anaesthesia, bilateral infarcts of the claustrum were evident on CT besides the major pathology, and peripheral encephalomalacia with hyperdensity of the centrally located structures (thalamus, basal ganglia, corona radiata, and brain stem) (Fig. 4).

In the patient with a brain tumour and contralateral shift of the midline structures, chronic haemorrhage was evident in the contralateral claustrum. On MRI the claustrum gave low signal on all sequences (more so on T2-weighting), suggesting the presence of haemosiderin (Fig. 3). These findings suggested a haemorrhagic infarct exclusively in the claustrum, probably due to compression of the small end-arteries supplying this region, secondary to the shift of the midline structures.

With respect to the bilateral claustral involvement by different pathologies in the current series, no definitive clinical signs and symptoms were noted that were attributable exclusively to the claustrum. The reason for this was possibly that the accompanying major lesions dominated the clinical presentation.

References

1. Sener RN (1993) The claustrum on MRI: normal anatomy, and the bright claustrum as a new sign in Wilson's disease. Pediatr Radiol 23:594–596
2. Sener RN (1993) Wilson's disease: MRI demonstration of caviations in basal ganglia and thalami. Pediatr Radiol 23:157
3. Williams PL, Warwick R, Dyson M, Bannister LH (1989) Gray's anatomy, 37th edn Churchill Livingstone, Edinburgh pp 748, 1034, 1080

4. Starosta-Rubinstein S, Young AB, Kluin K, Hill G, Aisen AM, Gabrielsen T, Brewer GJ (1987) Clinical assessment of 31 patients with Wilson's disease. Correlations with structural changes on magnetic resonance imaging. Arch Neurol 44:365–370
5. Aisen AM, Martel W, Gabrielsen TO, Glazer GM, Brewer G, Young AB, Hill G (1985) Wilson disease of the brain: MR imaging. Radiology 157:137–141
6. Lawler GA, Pennock JM, Steiner RE, Jenkins WJ, Sherlock S, Young IR (1983) Nuclear magnetic resonance (NMR) imaging in Wilson disease. J Comput Assist Tomogr 7:1–8
7. Prayer L, Wimberger D, Kramer J, Grimm G, Oder W, Imhof H (1990) Cranial MRI in Wilson's disease. Neuroradiology 32:211–214
8. Barkovich AJ (1990) Pediatric neuroimaging. Raven Press, New York, p 48
9. Takahashi S, Goto K, Fukasawa H, Kawata Y, Uemura K, Suzuki K (1985) Computed tomography of cerebral infarction along the distribution of the basal perforating arteries. Radiology 155:107–118
10. Bogousslavsky J, Regli F, Uske A (1988) Thalamic infarcts: clinical syndromes, etiology, and prognosis. Neurology 38:837–848
11. Sener RN, Alper H, Yunten N, Dundar C (1993) Bilateral acute thalamic infarcts causing thalamic dementia. AJR 161:678–679
12. Han BK, Towbin RB, De Courten-Myers G, McLaurin RL, Ball WS (1989) Reversal sign on CT: effect of anoxic/ischemic cerebral injury in children. AJNR 10:1191–1198
13. Vergote G, Vandeperre H, DeMan R (1992) The reversal sign. Neuroradiology 34:215–216

MRI of Hallervorden-Spatz disease

A. C. A. Magalhães, R. P. Maciel, L. A. Bacheschi, S. C. Mathias, J. R. Menezes, A. Magalhães[1]

Department of Radiology, Section of Magnetic Resonance, Hospital das Clínicas, University of São Paulo, Sáo Paulo, Brazil

Abstract. Two male and two female patients, aged between 10 and 28 years (mean = 16 years) with clinical features of Hallervorden-Spatz disease (HSD) were submitted to MRI examination with a 1.5 T system. T1- and T2-weighted spin-echo sequences were obtained. Two patients received paramagnetic contrast medium. All four cases had low signal in the globus pallidus. Three also had central high signal (target configuration). In one there was also low signal in the substantia nigra. There was no enhancement with contrast medium. The diagnosis of HSD was supported by the MRI study in all four cases. This method proved to be useful for an "in vivo" diagnosis of HSD, making MRI the procedure of choice for confirmation in patients with clinical findings of Hallervorden-Spatz disease.

Key words: Hallervorden-Spatz disease – Basal ganglia disease – Brain magnetic resonance imaging

Hallervorden-Spatz disease (HSD) was first described in 1922 as an uncommon autosomic recessive metabolic disorder, characterized by iron deposits in the globus pallidus, substantia nigra and red nucleus [1–3]. These iron deposits in the basal ganglia have not been associated with demonstrable abnormality of serum iron or iron metabolism. Before the advent of magnetic resonance imaging (MRI), diagnostic confirmation "in vivo" was not possible. The presumptive diagnosis was based only on the clinical picture, which begins in late childhood or adolescence as progressive pyraidal (spasciticity, hyperreflexia) and extrapyramidal (rigidity, tremor and choreoathetosis) disturbances and mental deterioration. Now MRI may confirm the diagnosis, demonstrating iron deposits in specific areas of the brain [4–7].

Case reports

We examined four patients (two males, and two females) aged 10–28 years on a 1.5 Tesla system, using spin-echo sequences weighted for T1 (TR 400 TE 16 ms) and T2 (TR 2100 TE 30–90 ms) with multiplanar acquisition with 5-mm thickness. Gadolinium DTPA was used in two cases; neither showed pathological contrast enhancement.

Case 1

A boy, 15 years old, had 2 years of progressive left arm dystonia, dysarthria and depression of the tendon reflexes. MRI showed bilateral, symmetrical intense low signal in the globus pallidus with a central area of high signal on T2 weighting (Fig. 1).

Case 2

A 12-year-old girl had 5 years of progressive urinary incontinence, a spastic tetraparesis with hyperreflexia and bilateral Babinski signs, gait ataxia and nistagmus. MRI showed intense low signal on T2 weighting in the globus pallidus and pars reticulata of the substantia nigra.

Case 3

A girl 10 years old, had 4 years of progressive gait and speech disturbances, and global dystonia. MRI showed symmetrical low signal in the globus pallidus with central high signal on T2-weighted images.

Correspondence to: A. C. A. Magalhães, University of São Paulo School of Medicine, 01415-000, Rua Bela Cintra, 1600, São Paulo, SP, Brazil

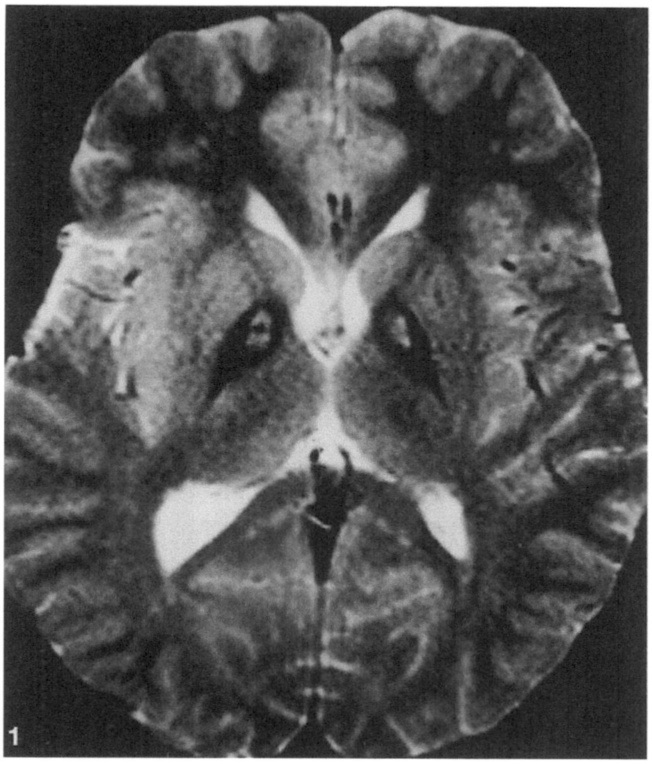

Fig. 1. Case 1. Coronal and axial T2-weighted images show bilateral, symmetrical low signal in the globus pallidus with a central area of high signal, the "eye of the tiger"

Case 4

A man, 28 years old, had 14 years of progressive gait disturbances, global dystonia and tremor; two sisters were similarly affected. MRI showed enlarged cortical sulci and basal cisterns. There was marked low signal in the globus pallidus, with central areas of high signal on T2 weighting.

Discussion

Iron pigmentation of the extrapyramidal system is physiological and occurs from progressive deposits of this metal in the basal ganglia throughout life. Iron depositions are abnormal before the age of 15 years and in these cases their detection by MRI is the basis of the diagnosis of HSD [1, 2].

The neuropathological features include bilateral, symmetrical damage to the globus pallidus, pars reticulata of the substantia nigra and red nucleus, with disseminated axonal spheroids (neuroaxonal dystrophy), demyelination, axonal lesions, and deposits of iron pigments in affected areas. The pathophysiological basis of this disease is pallidal degeneration [3, 4].

The literature includes a case with initial pallidal high signal on T2-weighted images, indicative of degeneration. This later changed to a peripheral low signal with a central area of high signal caused by iron deposition ("the eye-of the-tiger" sign) [5].

In our study, cases 1, 3 and 4 were characterised by symmetrical lesions of the globus pallidus with the "eye-of-the-tiger" sign formed by peripheral low signal with a central high signal on T2 weighting. Only case 2 showed substantia nigra involvement associated with the pallidal lesions without the high signal indicative of axonal lesions. There was no abnormal contrast enhancement in any case.

Pallidal low signal with central high signal on T2 weighting strongly suggests the diagnosis of Hallervorden-Spatz disease.

References

1. Atlas WS (1991) Magnetic resonance imaging of the brain and spine. Raven Press, New York, pp 594–597
2. Dooling EC, Schoene WC et al (1974) Hallervorden-Spatz syndrome. Arch Neurol 30:70–83
3. Galluci M, Cardona F, Arachi M et al (1990) Follow-up MR studies in Hallervorden-Spatz disease. J Comput Assist Tomogr 14:118–120
4. Savoiardo M, Halliday WC, Nardocci N, Strada L, D'Incerti L, Angelini L, Rumi V, Tesoro-Tess JD (1993) Hallervorden-Spatz disease: MR and pathologic findings. AJNR 14:155–162
5. Sethi KD, Adams RJ, Loring DW, el Gammal T (1988) Hallervorden-Spatz syndrome: clinical and magnetic resonance imaging correlations. Ann Neurol 24:692–694
6. Tanfani G, Mascalchi M, DalPozzo GC et al (1987) MRI in a case of Hallervorden-Spatz disease. J Comput Assist Tomogr 11:1057–1058
7. Trussart V, Leboucq N, Carlander B, Billiard M, Castan P (1993) Hallervorden-Spatz syndrome and MRI: "tiger's eye". One case. J Neuroradiol 20:70–75

Single-photon emission computed tomographic investigation of patients with school refusal

A. Tomoda[1], Y. Kai[1], T. Honda[1], K. Fukuda[1], T. Miike[1], M. Nabeshima[2], M. Takahashi[2]

[1] Department of Child Development, Kumamoto University School of Medicine, Kumamoto, Japan
[2] Department of Radiology, Kumamoto University School of Medicine, Kumamoto, Japan

Abstract. We studied 55 patients with school refusal by single-photon emission computed tomography to investigate the correlation between abnormalities of regional cerebral blood flow and clinical psychosomatic symptoms. Blood flow in the frontal, temporal and occipital lobes was significantly lower in patients with general fatigue, headache and memory disturbance than in those without these symptoms. These findings suggest that brain dysfunction followed by abnormal cerebral blood flow may be associated with the clinical psychosomatic symptoms in school refusal.

Key words: School refusal – Single-photon emission computed tomography – Brain dysfunction

It is well known that many school refusers show a sleep disturbance of defined onset, which is generally reported to follow a reversal of the daily rhythm of activity, with severe psychosomatic symptoms, such as headache, generalized fatigue, nausea, abdominal pain and anorexia [1–3]. In addition, although almost all school refusers have central nervous system involvement, that interferes significantly with normal school function, such as moderate to severe depression, memory disturbance, confusion and poor concentration, the regional cerebral blood flow has not previously been studied. We report here a single-photon emission CT (SPECT) study performed to measure regional cerebral blood flow semiquantitatively in school refusers.

Patients and methods

The subjects included 18 boys and 37 girls, aged 8–18 years (mean age, 14.5 years), refusing school for more than 2 months. All the following criteria had to be fulfilled for inclusion [1]: generalized fatigue; a report of memory disturbance; one of the following symptoms: headache, nausea, abdominal pain or anorexia; symptoms of sufficient severity to interfere significantly with normal school function; and a lack of detectable organic pathology accounting for the symptoms after appropriate investigation and consideration of the history by a paediatrician. Children who had recently started antidepressants or antianxiety drugs were excluded, as were patients with a neurological illness, migraine, mental retardation or serious psychopathology.

SPECT images were obtained with a ring-type multidetector scanner in the awake state, 30 min after intravenous injection of

Correspondence to: A. Tomoda, Department of Child Development, Kumamoto University School of Medicine, 1-1-1 Honjo, Kumamoto 860, Japan

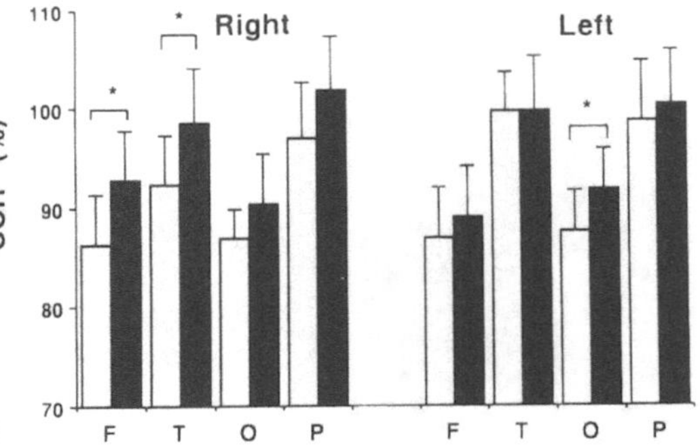

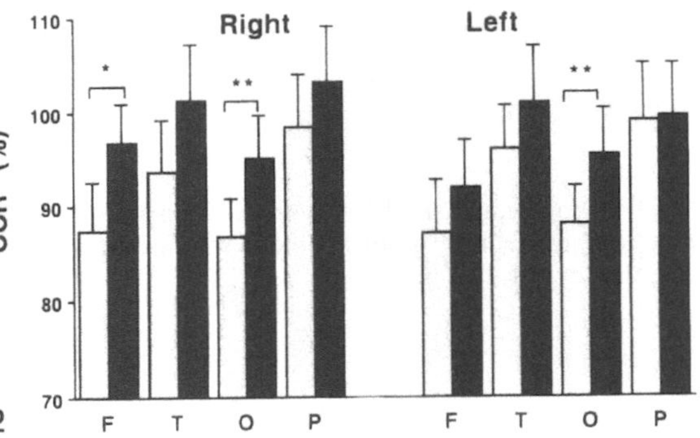

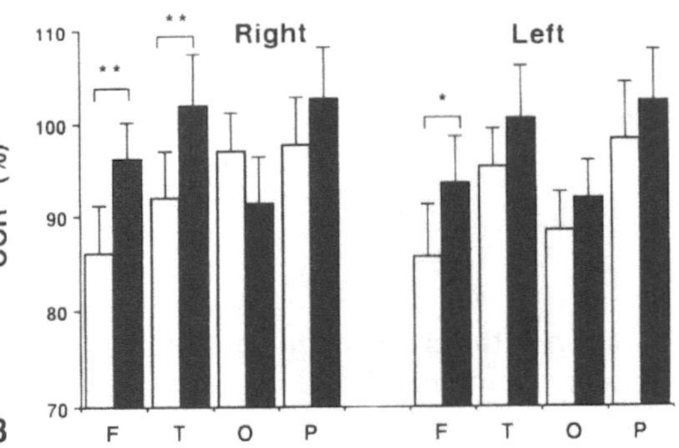

Fig. 1. Regional corticocerebellar ratio (CCR) and general fatigue. Blood flow in right frontal and both occipital lobes was significantly lower in patients with fatigue than in those without this symptom. All figures: $*P<0.05$, $**P<0.01$; F, frontal; T, temporal; O, occipital; P, parietal

Fig. 2. Regional corticocerebellar ratio (CCR) and headache. Blood flow in right frontal and both occipital lobes was significantly lower in patients with headache than in those without this symptom

Fig. 3. Regional corticocerebellar ratio (CCR) and memory disturbance. Blood flow in right frontal and both occipital lobes was significantly lower in patients with memory disturbance than in those without this symptom

111 MBq [^{123}I]-iodoamphetamine (^{123}I-IMP). After standard reconstruction of the images, an automated region of interest (ROI) computer program was applied to each tomographic brain image. The ratio of the mean activity per pixel in the ROI to that of the cerebellum (regional corticocerebellar ratio) was determined. To compare measures between the patients with and without variable complaints, the data were analysed statistically using an unpaired *t*-test, with the level of significance set at $P < 0.05$.

Results

The blood flow in the frontal, temporal and occipital lobes was significantly lower in patients with general fatigue, headache and memory disturbance than in those without these symptoms (Figs. 1–3). No patient had evidence of focal structural abnormalities on MRI.

Discussion

We have demonstrated abnormal cerebral blood flow in patients with school refusal. Furthermore, patients with memory disturbance, headache or general fatigue have a tendency to lower cerebral blood flow than those who have no symptoms. These findings suggest that brain dysfunction, followed by abnormal cerebral blood flow, may be associated with the clinical psychosomatic symptoms in school refusal even when MRI is normal.

References

1. Tomoda A, Miike T, Uezono K, Kawasaki T (1994) A school refusal case with biological rhythm disturbance and melatonin therapy. Brain Dev (Tokyo) 16:71–76
2. Ohta T, Iwata T, Kayukawa Y, Okada T (1992) Daily activity and persistent sleep-wake schedule disorders. Prog Neuropsychopharmacol Biol Pschiatry 16:529–537
3. Last CG, Strauss CC (1990) School refusal in anxiety-disordered children and adolescents. Adolesc Psychiatry 29:31–35

Superior sagittal sinus size as an indicator of cerebral perfusion in infants and children with hydrocephalus

I. Weitzner, Jr[1], D. Leslie[1], S. Rifkinson-Mann[2]

[1] Department of Radiology, New York Medical College, Valhalla, NY 10595, USA
[2] Department of Neurosurgery, New York Medical College, Valhalla, NY 10595, USA

Abstract. Nineteen infants and children with obstructive hydrocephalus were studied before and after shunting procedures. We compared ventricular size and superior sagittal sinus (SSS) size on CT. Clinical findings and transcranial Doppler resistivity index were correlated. Ventricular size and SSS were inversely related in 18 cases. In 2 cases the SSS correlated better than ventricular size with the clinical status. Resistivity index changes, when present, were useful. We felt that a qualitative guide to cerebral perfusion is available by inspecting the size and contour of the SSS on CT. This parameter may prove useful in decision-making in some cases.

Key words: Superior sagittal sinus – Cerebral blood flow – Hydrocephalus

Materials and methods

We retrospectively studied 19 consecutive patients who had undergone shunt procedures over a 12-month period. Their ages ranged from newborn to 14 years. Four variables were studied:

1. The size of the superior sagittal sinus (SSS) on axial CT was compared before and after shunt procedures. The comparisons were made at approximately the same place on the two studies, taking care to avoid the sinus confluence and higher slices that could be oblique to the sinus. Comparisons were visual and rated as smaller, larger, or no change. Contour differences were also assessed.
2. Ventricular size changes were noted.
3. Transcranial Doppler sonography (TCD) was correlated when available and when in a reasonable time span, i.e. when there was no change in clinical status between the time of the TCD and CT. The resistivity index (RI) = (systolic velocity – diastolic velocity)/systolic velocity was the value compared. Measurements were averaged at various points along the two middle cerebral arteries and compared on successive examinations, as well as with age-related normal values.
4. Clinical findings.

Results

An inverse relationship between ventricular size and SSS size held true in 18 of the 19 cases studied. In 6 cases the ventricles were judged more responsive to changes in pressure than the SSS. In 2 cases the SSS was more responsive than the venticles. In 1 case there was discordance, namely, when the SSS decreased in size, the ventricles were also smaller.

Correspondence to: I. Weitzner

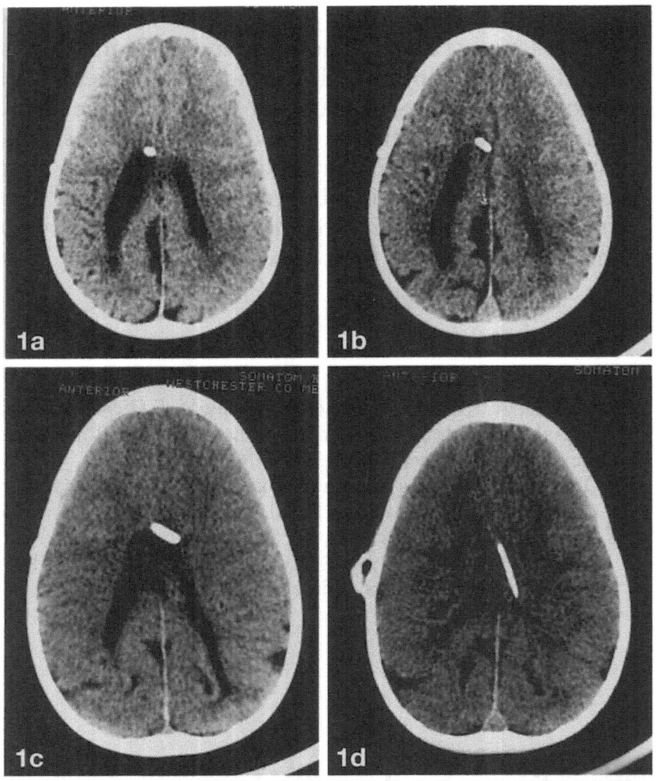

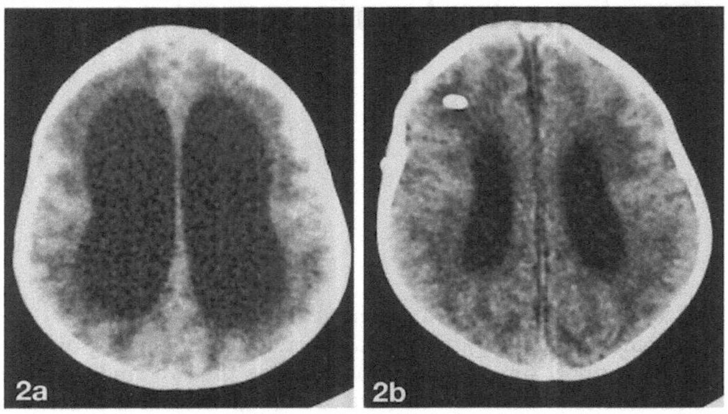

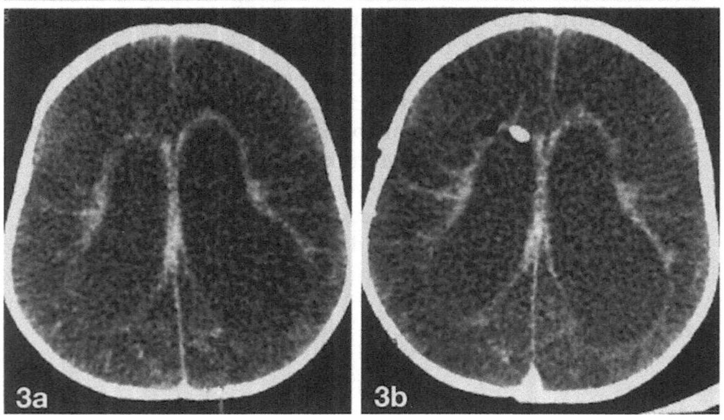

Twelve patients had TCD examinations. The RI had a positive correlation in 4 cases: as SSS size increased and ventricular size decreased, RI decreased; as SSS size decreased and ventricular size increased, RI increased. In 8 cases where there were changes of ventricular and SSS size, the RI was normal.

In every case where there were changes in SSS or ventricular size, there was positive correlation with the clinical findings.

Case reports

Case 1

A 1-year-old boy was shunted at the age of 3 months for hydrocephalus. Four days prior to admission he started vomiting after eating and became less active. CT (Fig. 1a) showed increase in the size of the posterior lateral ventricles. The SSS was virtually invisible. Shunt revision resulted in a decrease in ventricular size and a marked increase in the size of the SSS (Fig. 1b). RI at this time was normal. Clinical improvement coincided. The same sequence of events was repeated 9 months later (Fig. 1c, d). Although there was a decrease in ventricular size following shunt revision, there was a marked increase in SSS size. RI at the time of Fig. 1c was normal (0.56) and showed a decrease (0.50) following shunt revision.

Case 2

This patient was delivered by cesarean section. On the day of admission, aged 3 weeks, he became irritable. Head circumference was >98th centile with a tense anterior fontanelle. CT (Fig. 2a) showed marked hydrocephalus and a diminutive SSS. TCD on the following day revealed a high RI of 0.88 (normal 0.630). Aqueduct stenosis appeared to be the cause. A ventriculoperitoneal shunt was performed, and CT 3 days later (Fig. 2b) showed decreased ventricular size and an increase in the size of the SSS. TCD on the same day revealed a normal RI of 0.65.

Case 3

This 6-month-old was a "shaken baby" syndrome, with multiple brain hemorrhages, subdural hematoma, retinal hemorrhage and a skull fracture. On a later admission he presented with spastic quadriplegia and opisthotonus. CT (Fig. 3a) showed hydrocephalus, a very small SSS and a diffusely encephalomalacic brain. There was a markedly elevated RI with no diastolic velocity visible at times. At operation the CSF was under "significant pressure". CT following a shunt (Fig. 3b) showed no change in ventricular size, but a definite increase in SSS size. There was no change in the RI. Clinically there was slightly decreased spasticity and mild improvement of the opisthotonus.

Fig. 1a–d. A 1-year-old boy shunted at 3 months for hydrocephalus of unknown etiology. **a** increased ventricular size and invisible SSS due to shunt malfunction. **b** After shunt revision, decrease in ventricular size and marked increase in SSS size. **c, d** Same clinical and CT sequence 9 months later

Fig. 2a, b. A 3-week-old boy with aqueduct stenosis. **a** CT shows hydrocephalus and small SSS. **b** 3 days after shunting ventricular size has decreased and SSS size increased, indicating improved cerebral perfusion

Fig. 3a, b. A 6-month-old boy with a history of abuse. **a** Hydrocephalus, diminutive SSS, and encephalomalacia. **b** After shunting: definitive increase in SSS size suggests decresed pressure, although there is no change in ventricular size. Mild clinical improvement

Discussion

Increased intracranial pressure may cause functional changes by decreasing cerebral perfusion. Hypoxia at the cellular level is ultimately responsible for the clinical disturbances. The brain capillaries are most susceptible to increased intracranial pressure [1]. As pressure increases, arterial flow is reduced, although autoregulation may temporarily increase it. Veins, which may initially be engorged by mechanical compression, eventually collapse. Increased pressure may eventually collapse the SSS [1, 2].

The dural sinuses are the final pathway in cerebral blood flow. Although the dura mater has been thought of as rigid, the sinuses may passively change in size in response to alteration in cerebral perfusion. This may happen even in the absence of compression from contiguous brain (case 1). The SSS collects blood over the superior and mid-convexity. Pressure changes involving these areas will directly affect flow in the SSS. Blood collected from the infratentorial structures and the deep venous system enters sinuses inferior to the SSS. Changes in blood flow there can indirectly affect the SSS.

Imaging has classically focused on morphologic changes in ventricular and sulcal size in assessing the dynamics of hydrocephalus [3]. TCD has proved useful in management of hydrocephalus, but studies arterial flow uniquely. Stable xenon CT, while a promising tool, has not gained wide acceptance.

CT provides not only images of ventricles and other CSF spaces, but of the SSS. A qualitative assessment of cerebral perfusion may thus be obtained.

References

1. Hekmatpanah J (1970) Cerebral circulation and perfusion in experimental increased intracranial pressure. J Neurosurg 32:21–29
2. Cushing H (1902) Some experimental and clinical observations concerning states of increased intracranial tension. Am J Med Sci 124:375–400
3. Barkovich AJ (1990) Pediatric neuro-imaging: hydrocephalus. In: Contemporary neuro-imaging, vol 1. Raven Press, New York, pp 205–211

Hyperventilation in childhood head injuries causes unpredictable changes in cerebral blood flow

K. J. Poskitt, P. W. Skippen, J. Kestle, M. Mosskin, G. Annich

British Columbia's Children's Hospital, 4480 Oak Street, Vancouver, B. C. Canada

Abstract. Our purpose was to determine if changes in ventilation (P_aCO_2) cause predictable changes in regional cerebral blood flow (rCBF) in closed head injuries in children, and if ischaemic rCBF (< 20 ml/100 gm/min) occurs with hyperventilation. Eleven children with a Glascow Coma Scale < 8 were prospectively studied with xenon CT (XeCT) for measurements of rCBF. All underwent insertion of monitoring equipment, permitting measurement of P_aCO_2 cerebral perfusion pressure (CPP) and cerebral oxygen extraction (CEO_2) with rCBF derived from XeCT. Patients were studied with a three-level XeCT for estimation of rCBF at three random P_aCO_2 levels, determined clinically. The XeCT study was performed at early (< 24 h), intermediate (24–72 h) and late post-injury periods (> 72 h), if possible. Changes in rCBF from standard alterations in P_aCO_2 were unpredictable at all levels of P_aCO_2, but hyperventilation with P_aCO_2 values < 25 mmHg caused significantly more areas of regional ischemia than normocapnea ($P = 0.007$). There was no correlation between rCBF and CPP or CEO_2, although a $CEO_2 > 30\%$ ($P = 0.003$) was predictive of ischemia. Hyperventilation in pediatric head injuries caused variable changes in cerebral blood flow and increased the risk of regional ischemia.

Key words: Head injury – Hyperventilation – Cerebral blood flow – Children

Correspondence to: K. J. Poskitt

Severe head injury with a Glascow coma scale of less than 8 is associated with significant morbidity and mortality. Whether the poor outcome is due to the primary injury or is also influenced by treatment is unclear. Autopsies have shown that ischemia is common, suggesting that abnormalities of cerebral blood flow (CBF) may be important [1–3]. Elevated intracranial pressure (ICP) has been thought to be important in secondary brain injury, and controlling ICP with paralysis and hyperventilation has been thought to improve outcome [3, 4]. However, hyperventilation has not been shown to influence the mean hourly ICP or neurological outcome [5–7]. Hyperventilation is believed to cause a predictable decrease in CBF, but use of cerebral venous oxygen monitoring indicates that global ischemia is common [8–10], and recent adult studies with xenon CT (XeCT) have shown regional hypoperfusion [11, 12]. The pediatric literature continues to advocate the use of aggressive hyperventilation [13, 14], and we were concerned with the potential harmful effects of this approach. Thus, the purpose of this study was to test the null hypothesis that hyperventilation of childhood head injuries does not cause regional or global cerebral ischemia.

Materials and methods

We prospectively studied 11 patients with a Glascow Coma Scale < 8 who arrived at our institution within 12 h of head injury. All were managed with early intubation, controlled ventilation, CT, and urgent evacuation of any intracranial hematoma, if necessary. External ventricular drains and jugular venous bulb catheters were inserted into each patient before the XeCT study. Additional lines were inserted so that ICP, mean systemic arterial pressure, S_aO_2, and jugular venous co-oximetric oxygen saturation could be measured.

Estimates of regional CBF (rCBF) using XeCT were carried out after the patient was stabilized. A baseline CT was performed and a multilevel XeCT, for estimation of rCBF at three random P_aCO_2 levels, was carried out. Three axial 5-mm levels were selected that best sampled the brain stem, basal ganglia, frontal, temporal and occipital lobes and any obviously injured cerebral tissue. For each XeCT rCBF measurement, 28% xenon was administered over 5 min using an Anzai xenon rebreathing inhalator. Each level was sampled to create a combined wash-in, plateau, and wash-out study. All CBF measurements were performed with the patient paralyzed and sedated, and P_aCO_2 controlled by a real-time digital read-out. We attempted to perform XeCT studies, within 24 h, between 24 and 72 h and more than 72 h after cerebral injury, if clinically possible.

XeCT rCBF maps were generated by the provided software, creating a pixel-by-pixel map of flows, measured in ml/100 g of tissue/min with an associated confidence interval. The evaluation of the xenon cerebral blood-flow maps included estimates of global, hemispheric, and cortical rCBF, obtained with the placement of circular regions of interest (ROIs) measuring at least 2 cm^2. The procedure was repeated with free-hand irregular ROIs drawn to match the basal ganglia, cortex, or hemisphere.

Simultaneous clinical measurements from the inserted monitoring lines allowed calculation of cerebral perfusion pressure (CPP), cerebral oxygen extraction ratio (CEO_2) and CO_2 vasoresponsitivity, for each XeCT study performed. This communication primarily deals with CO_2 reactivity, which was defined as:

$$\frac{\%\text{change CBF}}{\text{mmHg } P_aCO_2} = \frac{([CBF_i\text{-}CBF_f]/CBF_i)*100}{P_aCO_2i\text{-}P_aCO_2f}$$

where CBF_i = initial CBF; CBF_f = final; P_aCO_{2i} = initial and P_aCO_{2f} = final.

For data analysis, oligemia was considered present in any ROI with a calculated flow of < 20 ml/100 g tissue/min. In order to test the hypothesis that hyperventilation does not result in ischemia, we required matched data sets from each study with P_aCO_2 values > 35 and between 25-35 mmHg. The data were analyzed with the McNemar chi-square test.

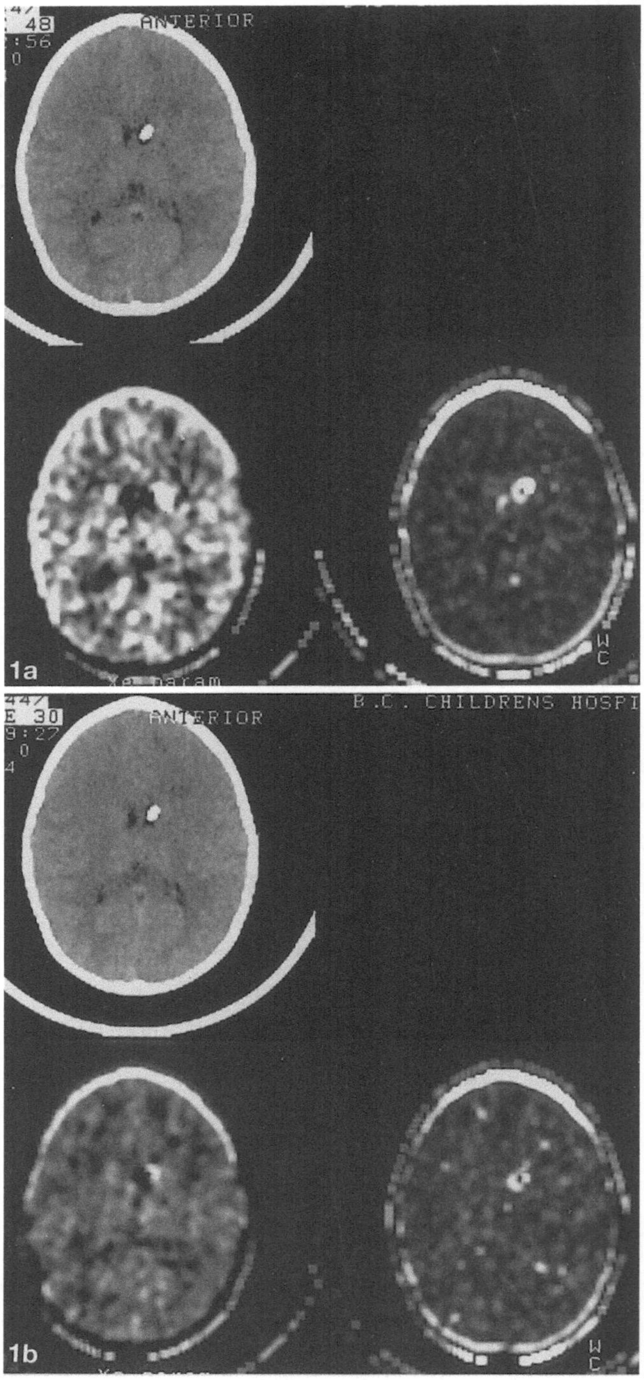

Fig. 1. Parameter images showing axial CT, CBF map and confidence map at P_aCO_2 values of 39 and 30 mmHg. Note the marked reduction in global CBF from 69 ml (**a**) to 15 ml/100 g tissue/min (**b**) with mild hyperventilation

Results

We studied 11 patients ranging in age from 2 to 15 years (6 girls/5 boys). Twenty-six XeCT studies were acquired, including 8 early studies (6–24 h after injury), 10 intermediate (24–72 h), and 8 late investigations (> 72 h). All patients had a Glascow Coma scale of < 8 and three required evacuation of intracranial bleeds. Ten patients were victims of trauma, (9 car accidents, 1 abuse) and one patient suffered from a ruptured arteriovenous malformation.

From these XeCT studies there were 52 alterations of P_aCO_2 with corresponding rCBF values of which 18 sets of paired data satisfied the inclusion criteria for statistical analysis of vasoreactivity. There was a statistically significant increase in the number of ischemic ROIs with hyperventilation (P = 0.007). Both global and regional ischemia occurred with moderate hyperventilation

($P_aCO_2 > 30$ mm Hg (Fig. 1) and the degree of vasoreactivity within individual patients ranged from −6% to +10%. Thus, in a given patient, the effect of standard change in P_aCO_2 was unpredictable. Similar trends were evident when the data over time were analysed, but the samples are too small to be significant. Finally, rCBF values for any given ROI at a common P_aCO_2 level also varied over time.

We were unable to demonstrate a consistent relationship between CPP and global CBF or rCBF. There was a statistical and clinically significant increase in the likelihood or regional oligemia with decreasing P_aCO_2 and $CEO_2 > 30\%$ ($P = 0.003$). The CEO_2 tended to increase predictability with reduction of P_aCO_2, but cases of regional and global oligemia did occur with CEO_2 values $< 30\%$.

Discussion

This study explored the effect of different levels of P_aCO_2 on cerebral blood flow using XeCT in head-injured children. Although in any patient the effect of hyperventilation was unpredictable with vasoreactivity ranging from −6% to +10%, the net effect was a significant increase in the number of regions of the brain rendered ishemic. This result agrees with the findings of others in adults [11, 12]. Of additional concern is that oligemic changes of both rCBF and global CBF occurred in some patients with P_aCO_2 values over 30 and 35 mm Hg, that up to now have been regarded as only mild hyperventilation.

Insufficient data are available from the CEO_2 extraction values to draw any conclusions, but the trend indicates that a $CEO_2 > 30\%$ may be a useful bedside indicator of oligemia. If hyperventilation is to continue to be used to decrease ICP in childhood head injuries, it is important to establish its efficacy and effects, as judged by patient outcome, and it will be necessary to develop a reliable bedside measure of cerebral oxygenation and/or perfusion.

Our preliminary work indicates that routine hyperventilation of head-injured patients results in an increased number of regions of CBF less than 20 ml/100 g per min and that this can occur even with mild hyperventilation. We believe that routine hyperventilation in all patients with raised ICP should be reevaluated.

References

1. Macpherson P, et al (1978) Correlation between angiographic findings and the ischemia of head injury. J Neurol Neurosurg Psychiatry 41:122–127
2. Graham DI, et al (1978) Ischemic brain damage in fatal nonmissile head injuries. J Neurol Sci 39:213–234
3. Graham DI, Ford I, Hume-Adams J, et al (1989) Ischemic brain damage is still common in fatal non-missile head injury. J Neurol Neurosurg Psychiatry 52:346–350
4. Marshall LF, Randall WS, Shapiro HM (1992) The outcome with aggressive treatment in severe head injuries. 1. The significance of intracranial monitoring. J Neurosurg 76:212–217
5. Muizelaar JP, Marmarou A, Ward JA, et al (1991) Adverse effects of prolonged hyperventilation in patients with severe head injury: a randomized clinical trial. J Neurosurg 75:731:739
6. Ward JD, Choi S, Marmarou A, et al (1989) Effect of prophylactic hyperventilation on outcome in patients with severe head injury. In Hoff JT, Betz AL (eds) ICP VII. Springer, Berlin, pp 630–634
7. Bruce DA, et al (1973) Regional cerebral blood flow, intracranial pressure, and brain metabolism in comatose patients. J Neurosurg 38:131–144
8. Sutton LN, et al (1990) Cerebral venous oxygen content as a measure of brain energy metabolism with increased intracranial pressure and hyperventilation. J Neurosurg 73:927–932
9. Sheinberg M, et al (1992) Continuous monitoring of jugular venous oxygen saturation in head-injured patients. J Neurosurg 76:212–217
10. De Deyne C, et al (1993) Jugular bulb metabolic monitoring during hyperventilation in severe head trauma patients. Crit Care Med 21 [Suppl]:S234
11. Marion DW, et al (1991) The use of stable xenon-enhanced CT studies of cerebral blood flow to define changes in cerebral carbon dioxide vasoreactivity caused by severe head injury. Neurosurgery 29:869–873
12. Stringer WA, et al (1993) Hyperventilation induced cerebral ischemia in patients with acute brain lesions: demonstrated by xenon CT. AJNR Am J Neuroradiol 14:475–484
13. Hammer G, Lindsay JN (1993) The neurosurgical pediatric patient. In: Andrews BT (ed) Neurosurgical intensive care. McGraw-Hill, New York
14. Davis RJ, Dean JM, Debrun GM, Carson BS, Rogers MC (1992) Head and spinal cord injury. In: Rogers NC (ed) Textbook of pediatric intensive care, 2nd edn. Williams and Wilkins, Baltimore

MRI in medulloblastomas and the significance of contrast-enhanced MRI of brain and spine for staging

Jae Joon Chung[1], **Dong Ik Kim**[1], **Jung Ho Suh**[2], **Tae Sub Chung**[1]

[1] Department of Diagnostic Radiology, College of Medicine, Yonsei University, Seoul, Korea
[2] Department of Diagnostic Radiology, College of Medicine, Ajou University, Suwon, Korea

Abstract. MRI of the brain in 18 patients (9 boys, 9 girls, mean age 9.4 years) with medulloblastomas were reviewed for signal intensity, contrast enhancement, presence of cyst and necrosis, and subarachnoid dissemination. In 14 patients, post-operative spinal MRI was reviewed for staging and therapeutic planning. Medulloblastomas showed low-to-intermediate signal intensity on T1-weighted images and moderately high signal intensity on T2-weighted images, compared to cerebellar white matter. Inhomogenous contrast enhancement was noted in 13 patients (72.2%). Cyst and necrosis within tumours were seen in 15 patients (83.3%). Subarachnoid dissemination was noted in 11 patients (61.1%), 6 demonstrated intracranial and 2 intraspinal disseminations. Three had both intracranial and intraspinal disseminations. Other associated findings included intratumoral haemorrhage (11.1%), peritumoral oedema (44.4%), tonsillar herniation (44.4%), hydrocephalus (88.9%) anc calcification (44.4%). Gd-DTPA-enhanced MRI of brain and spine was a useful diagnostic modality in pre-operative diagnosis and in post-operative staging of medulloblastomas.

Key words: Magnetic resonance imaging – Brain neoplasms – Posterior fossa – Spine

Medulloblastoma is one of the most common malignant tumours arising in the posterior cranial fossa of children and is a fairly demarcated and moderately enhanced solid tumour with frequent hydrocephalus, peritumoral oedema, subarachnoid dissemination and regional recurrence [1–3]. We analysed the MRI findings of the medulloblastomas and evaluated the significance of contrast-enhanced MRI of the brain and spine for staging.

Patients and methods

Brain MRI studies of 18 patients with surgically proven medulloblastoma were performed in addition to brain CT in all cases. There were 9 males and 9 females with ages ranging from 6 months to 22 years (mean age 9.4 years). T1-, T2- and proton density-weighted axial images, and sagittal T1-weighted images were obtained. Axial, sagittal and coronal T1-weighted images were also obtained after Gd-DTPA enhancement. About 2 weeks after operation, whole spine MRI studies, using surface coils, were performed in 14 patients to obtain sagittal images T1- and T2-weighted images and axial and sagittal images T1-weighted images after contrast enhancement.

Correspondence to: J. J. Chung, Department of Diagnostic Radiology, Yonsei University College of Medicine 134, Shinchon-dong, Seodaemun-ku, Seoul, 120-752 Korea

MRI findings were reviewed according to anatomical location, tumour size, MR signal intensity, appearance after contrast enhancement, presence of cyst and necrosis, degree of hydrocephalus, peritumoral oedema, intratumoral haemorrhage and subarachnoid dissemination. The location, shape and numbers of the disseminated lesions were analysed to investigate the characteristics of cerebrospinal fluid (CSF) seeding.

Results

The mean size of the tumour masses was 4.1 × 3.6 × 3.9 cm. Seventeen were located in the cerebellar vermis (inferior: 14, superior: 3) and 1 case was seen in the right cerebellopontine angle. Three cases of 17 vermian tumours invaded the right middle cerebellar peduncle. Seventeen cases (94.4%) showed well demarcated margins, and 1 case was ill-demarcated, which was pathologically proven to be the desmoplastic type.

Medulloblastomas showed low (17 cases, 94.4%) to intermediate (1 case, 5.6%) signal intensity on T1-weighted images, minimally high (11 cases, 61.1%) to intermediate (7 cases, 38.9%) signal intensity on T1-weighted images, minimally high (11 cases, 61.1%) to intermediate (7 cases, 38.9%) signal intensity on proton density images, and moderately high (15 cases, 83.3%) to intermediate (3 cases, 16.7%) signal intensity on T2-weighting, compared to cerebellar white matter (Fig. 1). Among them, one desmoplastic type showed intermediate signal intensity on all sequences, compared to the cerebellar hemispheres (Fig. 2). After Gd-DTPA enhancement, 13 cases (72.2%) showed inhomogenous enhancement, whereas 5 cases (27.8%) manifested homogenous and strong enhancement. Cyst and necrosis within tumours were seen in 15 patients (83.3%), and of these 10 cases were peripherally located. Intratumoral haemorrhage was seen in 2 cases (11.1%) with less than 1 cm in diameter, and calcifications with multiple nodular shapes within tumours were noted in 8 cases (44.4%). A mild degree of peritumoral oedema was seen in 8 cases (44.4%) and 8 cases (44.4%) showed herniation of the cerebellar tonsils. Non-communicating hydrocephalus was demonstrated in 16 cases (88.9%). A peritumoral crescent-shaped low-signal intensity area, having the same signal intensity as CSF, was noted in 12 cases (66.7%). Subarachnoid disseminations of medulloblastomas were noted in 11 patients (61.1%), and 6 intracranial and 2 intraspinal disseminations were demonstrated. Three had both intracranial and intraspinal dissemination. In 9 cases with intracranial lesions, there were intraparenchymal mass formations (7 cases), subarachnoid nodules (5 cases), infundibular lesions (2 cases) and diffuse gyral enhancement (1 case) (Fig. 3). In five cases with intraspinal lesions, there were extramedullary

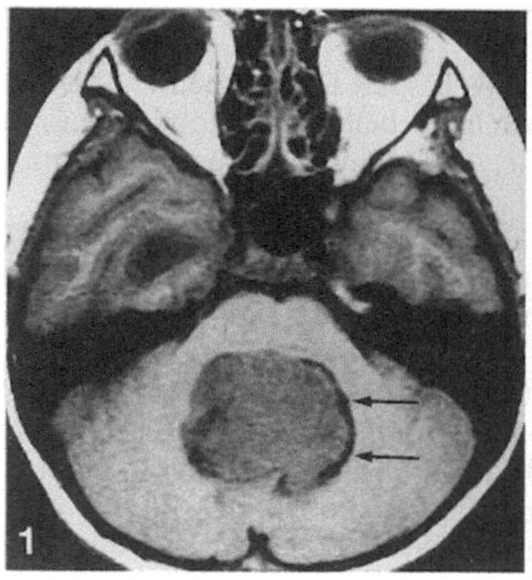

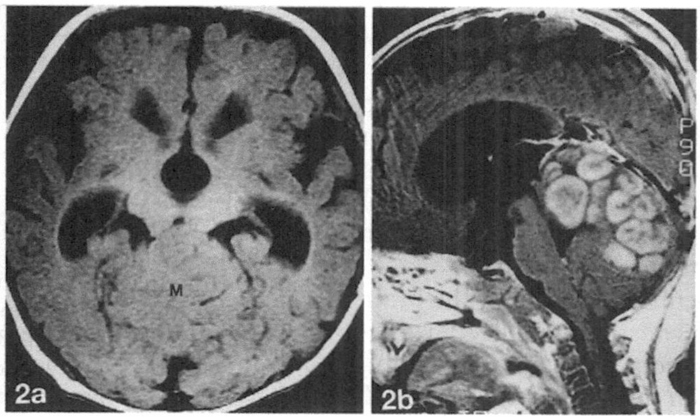

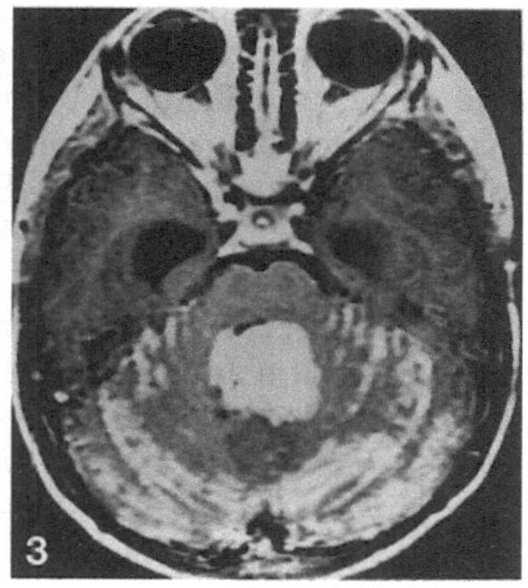

Fig. 1. Classical medulloblastoma (10-year-old girl). T1-weighted axial image shows solid mass of low-signal intensity in the vermis with a crescent low-signal intensity similar to that of CSF at its periphery (*arrows*)

Fig. 2a, b. Desmoplastic medulloblastoma (6-month-old boy). **a** Axial T1-weighted image demonstrates an ill-defined vermian mass (*M*) with giving signal similar to that of cerebellar parenchyma. **b** Contrast-enhanced sagittal image shows a lobulated mass with multiple ring enhancement

Fig. 3. Diffuse gyral dissemination (4-year-old boy). Contrast-enhanced axial image reveals strongly enhancing vermian mass and diffuse whirl-like gyral enhancement, not seen on unenhanced image

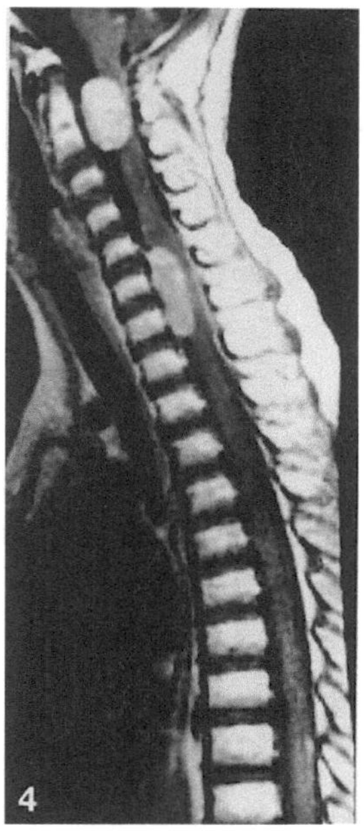

Fig. 4. Intradural masses (7-year-old girl). Contrast-enhanced sagittal image shows large enhancing intradural masses at the C1–2 and C6–7 levels

intradural small nodules (3 cases), central canal nodules (2 cases), intradural masses (1 case) (Fig. 4) and fine, nodular, and sheetlike leptomeningeal enhancement (1 case).

Discussion

Medulloblastoma is a primitive neuro-ectodermal tumour, arising from the inferior medullary velum or roof of the fourth ventricle, which is 33% of all posterior fossa tumours and about 25% of all intracranial tumours in children [1–3].

Meyers et al. [1] reported that there was no difference between pathologically classical and desmoplastic types, but one case of desmoplastic type with ill-demarcation in our study showed intermediate signal intensity on all sequences, compared to cerebellar white matter. Desmoplastic type displayed multilobulated, cobble-stone appearances and ringlike peripheral enhancement after contrast enhancement. These multilobulated masses were removed individually. Desmoplastic medulloblastomas with abundant reticulin fibres are generally rare, but occur frequently in the cerebellar hemispheres of older ages [4], having a better prognosis and poor contrast enhancement due to reticulin fibres than classical tumours [5].

It is well known that medulloblastomas have a relatively high cellularity and few cystic necroses [5], but in our study 15 cases (83.3%) showed cysts and necrosis in mostly peripheral locations. Other reports [6, 7] have cited an incidence of cystic necrosis in 16.7% to 45% of cases through analysis of CT, suggesting that a higher resolution of MRI, especially high-signal intensity on T2-weighting might be better in detecting small cysts than CT. Peritumoral oedema of variable incidence has been reported in the literature [1, 8], but in our study 8 cases (44.4%) manifested high-signal intensity with an irregularly spiculate, thin rim on T2-weighted images.

Meyers et al. [1] suggested that a peritumoral crescent-shaped space with a signal intensity identical to CSF might be peripheral necrosis, peritumoral oedema or entrapped CSF in the peritumoral space. However, because peripheral necrosis or peritumoral oedema showed more increased signal intensity on T1-weighting compared to CSF, we thought that it was CSF space surrounding the tumour mass in the dilated fourth ventricle.

Intracranial structures normally enhanced after Gd-DTPA injection are a part of the leptomeninges, pituitary gland, infundibulum, choroid plexus and small vessels on the cerebral cortical surface [9, 10]. Subarachnoid dissemination of medulloblastomas is manifested as intracranial of intraspinal parenchymal mass, leptomeningeal nodule, and linear or irregular gyral enhancement. It is known that a parenchymal mass develops by the tumour cells in CSF, entering through Virchow-Robin spaces on perivascular spaces. Recurrence or metastasis of the tumour should be considered if contrast-enhancing nodular masses are noted in the leptomeninges, ventricular wall, cisternal space, intradural space or central canal of the spine, and if linear or irregular leptomeningeal enhancement is seen on the follow-up MRI. It is important to decide when the follow-up MRI should be performed after operation because medulloblastomas had about 30% of subarachnoid dissemination in the early follow-up MRI [11], and a recurrence rate of 30–50% was reported even after radiation and chemotherapy.

In conclusion, Gd-DTPA-enhanced MRI of the brain and spine was a useful diagnostic modality in pre-operative diagnosis and post-operative staging of medulloblastomas, which was superior to contrast-enhanced CT or MRI without contrast medium.

References

1. Meyers SP, Kemp SS, Tarr RW (1992) MR imaging features of medulloblastomas. AJR 158:859–865
2. Rollins N, Mendelsohn D, Mulne A, et al (1990) Recurrent medulloblastoma: frequency of tumor enhancement on GD-DTPA MR imaging. AJNR 11:583–587
3. Gusnard DA (1990) Cerebellar neoplasms in children. Semin Roentgenol 25:263–278
4. Hubbard JL, Scheithauer BW, Kispert DB, Carpenter SM, Wick MR, Laws ER Jr (1989) Adult cerebellar medulloblastomas: the pathological, radiographic, and clinical disease spectrum. J Neurosurg 70:536–544
5. Bourgouin PM, Tampieri D, Grahovac SZ, Leger C, Carpio RD, Melancom D (1992) CT and MR imaging findings in adults with cerebellar medulloblastomas: comparison with findings in children. AJR 159:609–612
6. Zee CS, Segall HD, Miller C, et al (1982) Less common CT features of medulloblastoma. Radiology 144:97–102
7. Kingsley DPE, Kendall BE (1979) The CT scanner in posterior fossa tumours of childhood. Br J Radiol 52:769–776
8. Nelson M, Diebler C, Forbes WSC (1991) Paediatric medulloblastoma: atypical CT features at presentation in the SIOP II trial. Neuroradiology 33:140–142
9. Sze G, Soletsky S, Bronen R, Krol G (1989) MR imaging of the cranial meninges with emphasis on contrast enhancement and meningeal carcinomatosis. AJNR 10:965–975
10. Burke JW, Podrasky AE, Bradley WG Jr (1990) Meninges: benign postoperative enhancement on MR images. Radiology 174:99–102
11. North C, Segall HD, Stanley P, Zee CS, Ahmadi J, McComb JG (1985) Early CT detection of intracranial seeding from medulloblastoma. AJNR 6:11–13

CT and MRI of supratentorial intra-axial tumours in children

S. Higano[1], S. Takahashi[1], N. Kurihara[1], K. Matsumoto[3], T. Kayama[2], R. Katakura[4]

[1] Department of Radiology, Tohoku University School of Medicine, 1-1 Seiryo-machi Aobaku Sendai, Miyagi, 980, Japan
[2] Department of Neurosurgery, Tohoku University School of Medicine, Miyagi, Japan
[3] Department of Radiology, Miyagi Cancer Center, Miyagi, Japan
[4] Department of Neurosurgery, Miyagi Cancer Center, Miyagi, Japan

Abstract. MRI and CT of 32 children with pathologically proven supratentorial "intra-axial" tumours were retrospectively reviewed. Twelve histological types were included. The location of tumours is helpful for diagnosis. Cysts, calcification, and haemorrhage were found in 69%, 44% and 22%, respectively. Perifocal haemosiderin deposits were typical of cavernous angioma. An unenhanced CT high density was characteristic in some tumours, especially germinoma. Strong mass effect with marked perifocal oedema was suggestive of a malignant tumour. Although final diagnosis requires pathological study, these findings give some information for initial planning of treatment.

Key words: Supratentorial tumour – Paediatric brain tumour – Magnetic resonance imaging

Correspondence to: S. Higano, Department of Radiology, Tohoku University School of Medicine, 1-1 Seiryo-machi, Aobaku Sendai, Miyagi, 980, Japan

Supratentorial "intra-axial" tumours are not common in children, and their neuroradiological investigations are also limited. We aimed to review CT and MRI features of these lesions.

Patients and methods

MRI and CT of 32 children, 20 boys and 12 girls, aged 2 months–18 years (mean, 10 years) with pathologically proven supratentorial "intra-axial" tumours encountered in the last 5 years were reviewed retrospectively. Histological diagnosis was obtained by biopsy specimen in 9 cases, after partial/subtotal removal in 7 and after total removal in 16.

Twelve histological types were included (Table 1). A neurinoma in this series was a very rare case originating in brain parenchymy [1]. Although craniopharyngioma is extra-axial, we included one case with intra-axial extension in this study.

MRI studies were carried out in 31 cases (28 cases by 1.5 T unit; 3 by 0.5 T), and T1- and T2-weighted images and contrast-enhanced T1-weighted images with i.v. administration of Gd-DTPA were obtained, using conventional spin-echo or fast spin-echo sequences. CT was performed in 31 cases.

Table 1. Histological types

Histological type	Number
Malignant group	[11]
High-grade astrocytoma	5
Anaplastic ependymoma	2
Primitive neuroectodermal tumour	3
Choroid plexus carcinoma	1
Benign group	[21]
Low-grade astrocytoma	7
Germinoma	7
Cavernous angioma	2
Others	5 (1 each)
Oligodendroglioma, ganglioglioma giant cell astrocytoma neuroma, craniopharyngioma	

Table 2. Location of tumours

Location	Number	(%)
Frontal	9	(28)
Temporal	2	(6)
Parietal	1	(3)
Occipital	1	(3)
Basalganlia	7	(22)
Diencephalon	8	(25)
Foramen of monro	1	(3)
Cerebral hemisphere	3	(9)

Table 3. Comparison between 11 malignant and 2 benign tumours

Feature	Malignant		Benign		Significance
	Number	(%)	Number	(%)	
Contrast enhancement	8	(73)	17	(80)	
Calcification	4	(36)	11	(52)	
Cyst	7	(64)	15	(71)	
Haemorrhage	3	(27)	4	(19)	
Oedema					$P<0.01$
mild	3	(27)	16	(76)	
severe	8	(73)	5	(24)	
Mass effect					$P<0.001$
mild	0	(0)	16	(76)	
severe	11	(100)	5	(24)	

Results

All tumours were clearly depicted on MRI, while CT failed to detect two low-grade astrocytomas. In one case of craniopharyngioma with intra-axial extension, sagittal MRI revealed its continuity to the sellar region, although the lesion looked intra-axial on CT. MRI is superior to CT in detecting intratumoural haemorrhage, and CT in calcification. Apart from haemorrhage, MRI intensity patterns were relatively non-specific, while in some tumours, high density on unenhanced CT was characteristically found; especially germinomas (7 of 7) and cavernous angiomas (2 of 2).

The location of tumours is summarised in Table 2. Frontal lobe, basal ganglia and diencephalon were the most common sites. Around the foramen of Monro a giant cell astrocytoma occurred. Various kinds of tumours occurred in the frontal lobe. While 6 of 7 germinomas arose in basal ganglia and/or thalamus, 6 of 8 lesions of the diencephalon were astrocytomas, and half of the astrocytomas were located in the diencephalon.

Cysts, calcification and a haemorrhage were noted in 22 (69%), 14 (44%) and 7 cases (22%) respectively. Cysts were found to be various, with 11 kinds of tumours. Some tumours tend to have a high incidence of cystic components, such as germinomas. Primitive neuroectodermal tumours (PNET), and anaplastic ependymomas. With reference to the contrast enhancement pattern of the cyst wall, irregular enhancement was mostly found in malignant lesions such as PNET, anaplastic ependymomas and high-grade astrocytomas. Intratumoural haemorrhage was noted in 7 cases with five entities such as cavernous angiomas, high-grade astrocytomas, choroid plexus carcinoma, germinoma and oligodendroglioma. Peritumoural haemosiderin deposits were found only in two cavernous angiomas. Haemorrhage in the astrocytoma series was seen only in glioblastomas.

Table 3 shows a comparision between malignant and benign groups. Only perifocal oedema and mass effect showed a significant difference between malignant and benign groups.

Discussion

MRI is superior to CT in detecting tumours, intratumoural haemorrhage and in assessing precise tumour extent, while CT is useful for detecting calcification, which may be misinterpreted as haemosiderin deposits on MRI. High on unenhanced CT was characteristic of some cases, especially germinoma as compared with nonspecific MR intensity [2]. We believe a combination of CT and MRI is required for differential diagnosis.

The location of tumours is helpful for diagnosis. Germinomas usually occurred in the suprasellar or pineal regions as an extra-axial tumour, but rarely occurred in the basal ganglia and thalamus, as in our cases [2]. In some reports astrocytomas are more likely to be central than peripheral, although glioblastomas are not infrequently peripheral [3].

Cysts and calcification were noted not infrequently in various lesions, although some tumours tend to have a high incidence of these components. Low-grade astrocytomas in children are reported to often have cysts [4]. The enhancement pattern of a cyst wall is helpful to differentiate between benign and malignant groups. Intratumoural haemorrhage was found in various tumours, but peritumoural haemosiderin deposits are typical of cavernous angiomas [5]. Some researchers suggest that haemorrhage should be helpful to separate anaplastic tumours from glioblastoma [3].

Perifocal oedema and mass effect were notable in malignant tumours, which should be subsequent to rapid growth of malignant lesions.

In patients with brain tumours, histological examination is required for final diagnosis. However, some of the points mentioned above were considered to be helpful for prediction of histological types and tumour grade. These are informative for neurosurgeons to plan initial treatment: radical operation with subtotal or total removal, stereotactic biopsy followed by radiochemotherapy, observation, etc.

References

1. Ezura M, Ikeda H, Ogawa A, Yoshimoto T (1992) Intracerebral Schwannoma: case report. Neurosurgery 30:97–100
2. Soejima T, Takeshita I, Yamamoto H, Tsukamoto Y, Fukui M, Matsuoka S (1987) Computed tomography of germinoma in basal ganglia and thalamus. Neuroradiology 29:366–370
3. Fitz C (1993) Magnetic resonance imaging of pediatric brain tumors. Magn Reson Imaging 5:174–189
4. Lee YY, Van Tassel P, Bruner JM, Moser RP, Share JC (1989) Juvenile piocytic astrocytomas: CT and MR characteristics. AJNR 10:363–370
5. Fortuna A, Ferrante L, Mastronardi L, Acqui M, d'Addentta R (1989) Cerebral cavernous angioma in children. Childs Nerv Syst 5:201–207

Intracranial tumors presenting in the first year of life: imaging features

S. Batnitzky[1], D. A. Eckard[1], H. I. Price[1], S. J. Rosenthal[1], P. L. O'Boynick[2]

[1] Department of Radiology, University of Kansas School of Medicine, 3901 Rainbow Boulevard, Kansas City, KS 66160-7234, USA
[2] Department of Neurosurgery, University of Kansas Shool of Medicine, 3901 Rainbow Boulevard, Kansas City, KS 66160-7234, USA

Abstract. Intracranial tumors presenting in the 1st year of life differ from those in later childhood in clinical presentation, anatomical distribution, and histopathological type. Many of these tumors are very large at the time of presentation. Supratentorial tumors are more common in the 1st year of life than posterior fossa tumors. The suprasellar location is more common during the 1st year of life than during the rest of the pediatric age group as a whole.

Key words: Brain tumors – Hypothalamic gliomas – Choroid plexus papillomas – Primitive neural ectodermal tumor

Brain tumors are the most frequent solid tumor of childhood and after leukemia, the most common malignancy of the pediatric population [1]. Intracranial tumors presenting in the 1st year of life differ from those in later childhood in clinical presentation, anatomical distribution, and histopathological type. In most large series of pediatric brain tumors, posterior fossa tumors and supratentorial tumors occur in nearly equal frequency [1]. However, the distribution of primary brain tumors in the 1st year of life is different from the distribution of the entire pediatric period. Supratentorial tumors are more common in the 1st year of life, whereas infratentorial tumors predominate from 4 to 11 years of age [1]. After the age of 11 the incidence in both locations is approximately the same [1].

Correspondence to: S. Batnitzky

Methods and materials

The CT and MRI examinations of 18 patients who presented in the 1st year of life with an intracranial tumor were reviewed and evaluated. There were 12 girls and 6 boys ranging in age from newborn to 12 months.

Results

Of the 18 intracranial tumors, 16 were supratentorial and 2 in the posterior cranial fossa; these were both medulloblastomas. Of the supratentorial tumors, 8 were suprasellar, and comprised 4 hypothalamic gliomas (Fig. 1), 2 teratomas (Fig. 2), and 2 craniopharyngiomas. The other supratentorial tumors included 2 choroid plexus papillomas (Figs. 3, 4), 1 choroid plexus carcinoma, 2 primitive neural ectodermal tumors (PNET) (Fig. 5), 1 hemangiopericytoma, 1 fibrosarcoma, and 1 hemispheric cystic astrocytoma (Fig. 6).

Discussion

In our series the incidence of supratentorial tumors was nearly 90%. Half the supratentorial tumors were suprasellar. There were a number of interesting and unusual features exhibited by these tumors. Many of these tumors were enormous at the time of presentation. This has been attributed to the elasticity of the infant skull and the capacity for functional adaptation of the immature nervous system [2].

Suprasellar tumors are more common during the 1st year of life than in the rest of the pediatric age group as a whole [1]. Of these, the most common are the suprasellar astrocytomas. Most of these are grade II or III [1]. These

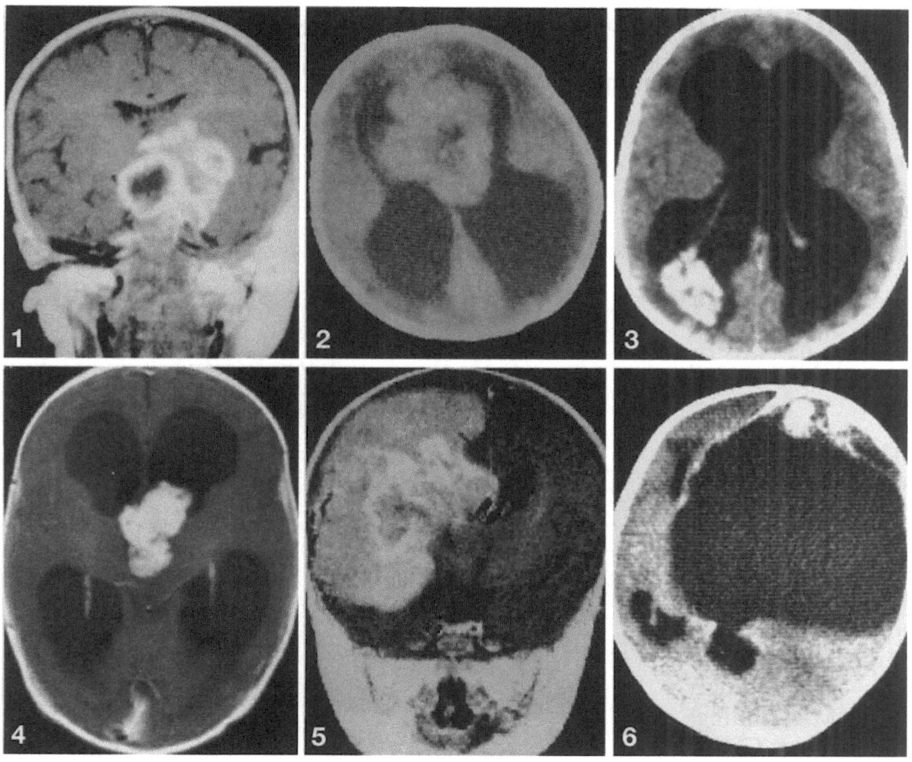

Fig. 1. Hypothalamic glioma in 6-month-old boy. Contrast-enhanced coronal T1-weighted image demonstrates a very large, inhomogeneously enhancing, suprasellar mass with cystic and solid components. The mass extents into the left cerebral hemisphere

Fig. 2. A 1-day-old boy with a suprasellar teratoma. Axial CT demonstrates marked hydrocephalus. There is a dense suprasellar mass containing areas of calcifation, which extends superiorly between the frontal horns of the lateral ventricles

Fig. 3. Choroid plexus papilloma of the trigone of the right lateral ventricle in a 6-week-old boy. Contrast-enhanced CT demonstrates an enhancing mass in the trigone of the right lateral ventricle, with a nodular, cauliflower appearance. Marked hydrocephalus is present

Fig. 4. Choroid plexus papilloma of the third ventricle in 2-month-old boy. Contrast-enhanced T1-weighted axial image demonstrates marked nodular enhancement of a large mass in the third ventricle that extends through the foramen of Monro into the left frontal horn. Marked hydrocephalus is present

Fig. 5. Large supratentorial PNET in 6-week-old girl. Coronal contrast-enhanced T1-weighted image demonstrates inhomogeneous enhancement in an enormous mass occupying almost the entire right cerebral hemisphere

Fig. 6. Enormous cystic astrocytoma in a 7-month-old girl. Contrast-enhanced axial CT demonstrates a large cyst occupying most of the left cerebral hemisphere and extending across the midline. Two small areas of enhancement in the solid portion of the tumor are seen anteriorly

tumors arise in the region of the hypothalamus rather than the benign chiasmal astrocytomas that are seen in later years.

Tumors such as choroid plexus papillomas have a much higher relative incidence in the 1st year of life. In some series they represent approximately 15–20% of brain tumors in this age group [1]. There is a marked male predilection. The trigone of the lateral ventricle, most often the left lateral ventricle, is the most common site of involvement, followed by the third ventricle. Choroid plexus papillomas presenting in adulthood tend to occur in the fourth ventricle.

Teratomas present most frequently within the 1st year of life [1] and most frequently in the first few months after birth. Thereafter, the incidence declines.

The clinical presentation of intracranial tumors presenting within the 1st year of life is also different than in the rest of the pediatric age group. In many cases there is a delay in diagnosis because of the low index of suspicion and nonspecific clinical findings. Because of the relative immaturity of the CNS, they do not present with focal neurological deficits seen in older children and adult. Enlarged head size is the predominant sign of increased intracranial pressure in infants harboring a brain tumor. As these children have unfused cranial sutures and open fontanelles, rapid head growth may be the only sign of increased intracranial pressure.

Both CT and MRI are excellent imaging techniques to evaluate these lesions. However, MRI is the superior imaging technique in the diagnosis and management of these tumors. MRI provides more information about the extent and character of the lesion than does CT and in the posterior cranial fossa MRI does not produce the beam-hardening artifacts seen with CT.

References

1. Barkovich AJ, Edwards MSB (1990) Brain tumors of childhood. In: Barkovich AJ (ed) Pediatric neuroimaging. Raven Press, New York, pp 149–203
2. Koos WT, Miller MH (1971) Intracranial tumors of infants and children. Thieme, Stuttgart

Congenital hypothalamic hamartoma syndrome: a case report

H. Nakagawa[1], S. Iwasaki[1], T. Taoka[1], M. Nakane[1], A. Fukusumi[1], H. Ohishi[2], H. Uchida[1], T. Kakizaki[3], T. Morimoto[3], T. Sakaki[3]

[1] Department of Radiology, Nara Medical University, Nara, Japan
[2] Department of Oncoradiology, Nara Medical University, Nara, Japan
[3] Department of Neurosurgery, Nara Medical University, Nara, Japan

Abstract. The congenital hypothalamic hamartoma or hamartoblastoma syndrome (CHHS) is a rare complex malformation. We report a case of CHHS studied by CT, MRI and angiography.

Key words: Hypothalamic hamartoma – Pallister-Hall syndrome – Magnetic resonance imaging – Computed tomography

The congenital hypothalamic hamartoma of hamartoblastoma syndrome (CHHS), also called the Pallister-Hall syndrome, is a rare malformation comprising hypothalamic hamartoma, craniofacial anomaly, limb anomaly and endocrine anomaly. Few reports on the MRI findings of CHHS are available. We report a case of CHHS focussed on the CT, MRI and angiography of the hamartoma.

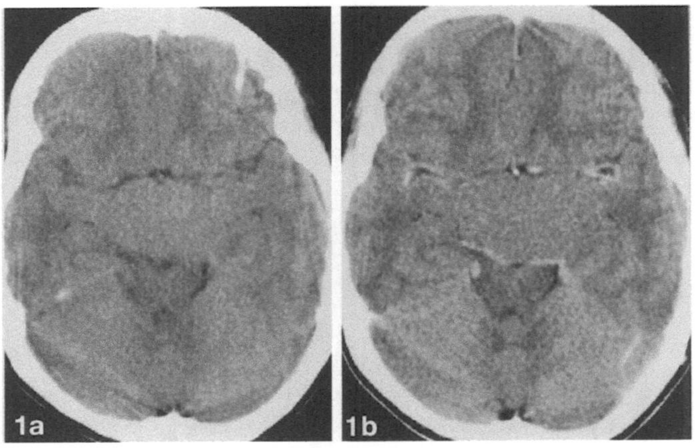

Fig. 1. CT before (**a**) and after (**b**) contrast medium show a suprasellar mass 3 cm in diameter, homogeneous to grey matter, density without abnormal contrast enhancement

Case report

An 11-year-old boy was investigated because of disturbance of visual acuity. He had polydactyly in both hands and feet, concealed penis, phimosis and hypospadias. He has been treated for pituitary dwarfism since the age of 5 years. A neurological examination revealed no abnormality except for visual acuity weakness. He had no precocious puberty. He has no significant familial history of similar disease.

A plain radiograph of both hands showed syndactyly of metacarpal bones of the third and fourth finger. CT showed a suprasellar mass lesion (Fig. 1). High-resolution CT demonstrated a deformity on the left temporal bone (Fig. 2). MRI of the brain was performed at 1.5 T. Both T1- and T2-weighted images revealed that the signal intensity of the mass was iso-intense to the grey matter (Fig. 3 A, B). No contrast enhancement of the mass was demonstrated. The mass lesion was below the anterior commissure, and compressed and displaced the pituitary complex and the optic chiasm anteriorly (Fig. 3C. D). These findings were compatible with a mass lesion arising from the hypothalamic region. Carotid and vertebral angiography showed no abnormal vasculature.

These radiological findings suggested a hamartoma of the base of the hypothalamus. To confirm this, a biopsy by subtemporal craniotomy was done, and the histological findings revealed the mass to be a hamartoma.

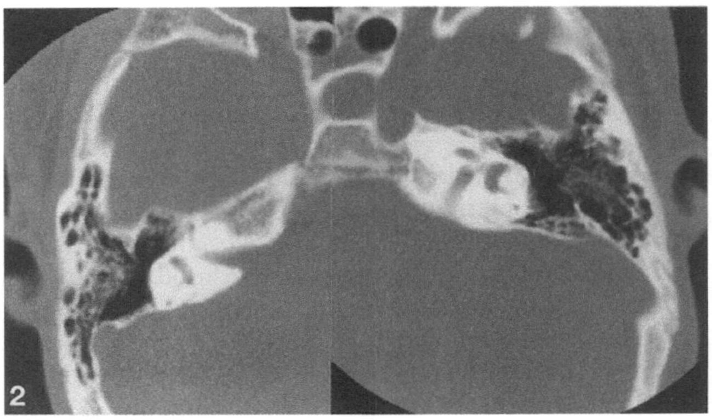

Fig. 2. High-resolution CT demonstrates deformity on the left temporal bone. The internal acoustic meatus shows a posteromedial-to-anterolateral tilt; the cochlear turns were normal

Discussion

The Pallister-Hall syndrome was firstly described by Hall et al. [1, 2] as the lethal malformation syndrome comprising hypothalamic hamartoma, hypopituitarism, and several other malformations in 1980. Although several articles have documented this entity [3, 4], description of CT and MRI of the hypothalamic hamartoma of this syndrome is scarce [5].

The isodense appearance on CT and the iso-intense appearance of grey matter on both T1- and T2-weighted MRI helped to diagnose the suprasellar mass as haematoma. MRI, especially sagittal images, provided the best demonstration of the anatomical relationship of the hamartoma to the surrounding structures, and also demonstrated that the mass originated from the hypothalamus.

Correspondence to: H. Nakagawa

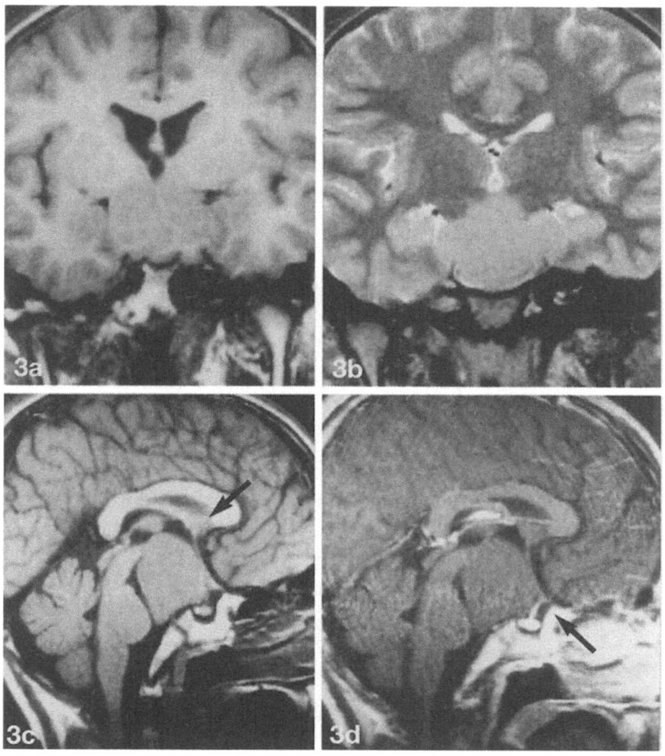

Fig. 3. Coronal T1- (**a**) (TR/TE 550/20) and T2- (**b**) (TR/TE 2000/100) weighted spin-echo images show the signal intensity of the mass to be the same as that of grey matter. A reticular pattern was visible on the T1-weighted images. On sagittal T1-weighted images (**c, d**), the mass was below the anterior commissure (*arrowhead*), and compressed and displaced the pituitary complex (*arrow*) and the optic chiasm anteriorly. No abnormal contrast enhancement was demonstrated (**d**)

CT and MRI are useful to diagnose the hypothalamic hamartoma or CHHS, while high-resolution CT may be useful to show associated craniofacial anomalies.

References

1. Hall JG, Pallister PD, Clarren SK, et al (1980) Congenital hypothalamic hamartoblastoma, hypopituitarism, imperforate anus, and postaxial polydactyly-a new syndrome? I. Clinical, cause, and pathogenic considerations. Am J Med Genet 7:47–74
2. Clarren SK, Alvord EC, Hall JG (1980) Congenital hypothalamic hamartoblastoma, hypopituitarism, imperforate anus, and postaxial polydactyly-a new syndrome? II: Neuropathological considerations. Am J Med Genet 7:75–83
3. Iafolla K, Fraktkin JD, Spiegel PK, et al (1989) Case report and delineation of the congenital hypothalamic, hamartoblastoma syndrome (Pallister-Hall syndrome). Am J Med Genet 33:489–499
4. Encha-Razavi F, Larroche JC, Roume J, et al (1992) Congenital hypothalamic hamartoma syndrome: nosological discussion and minimum diagnostic criteria of a possibly familial form. Am J Med Genet 42:44–50
5. Cheng K, Sawamura Y, Yamauchi T, et al (1993) Asymptomatic large hypothalamic hamartoma associated with polydactyly in an adult. Neurosurgery 32:458–460

Long-term follow-up imaging of subependymal giant cell astrocytoma developing in tuberous sclerosis

H. Shioya[1], K. Mineura[1], J. Sasaki[1], T. Sasajima[1], M. Kowada[1], T. Ogawa[2], J. Hatazawa[2], K. Uemura[2]

[1] Neurosurgical Service, Akita University Hospital, Akita, Japan
[2] Department of Radiology and Nuclear Medicine, Research Institute for Brain and Blood Vessels, 1-1-1 Hondo, Akita-city, Akita, 010, Japan

Abstract. A 13-year-old boy with tuberous sclerosis presented with a syncopal attack. CT and MRI revealed multiple subependymal nodules and cortical tubers. Among the nodules, one on the left anterior horn was more than 2 cm in size. Positron emission tomography revealed the largest nodule and cortical tubers to have low proliferation activity. Thus, the nodules proliferated less and grew gradually over a considerably long period. The largest nodule was resected through a transcallosal approach, and was a subependymal giant cell astrocytoma, with no evidence of malignancy.

Correspondence to: H. Shioya

Key words: Tuberous sclerosis – Subependymal giant cell astrocytoma – Positron emission tomography

Tuberous sclerosis (TS) is well known to be occasionally associated with subependymal giant cell astrocytoma (SGCA). SGCA is considered a benign tumour in its clinical course and morphology. However, it sometimes grows rapidly and causes hydrocephalus. To our knowledge, little is known about circulation and metabolism, particularly in relation to the proliferating activity of TS and SGCA. We report long-term follow-up of subependymal nodules in a patient with TS, together with positron emission tomographic (PET) findings.

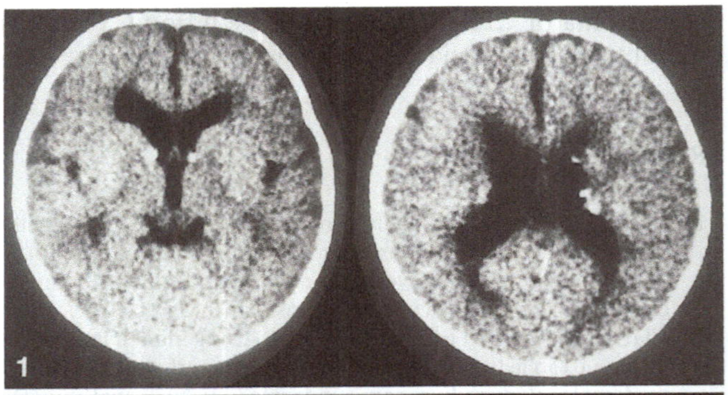

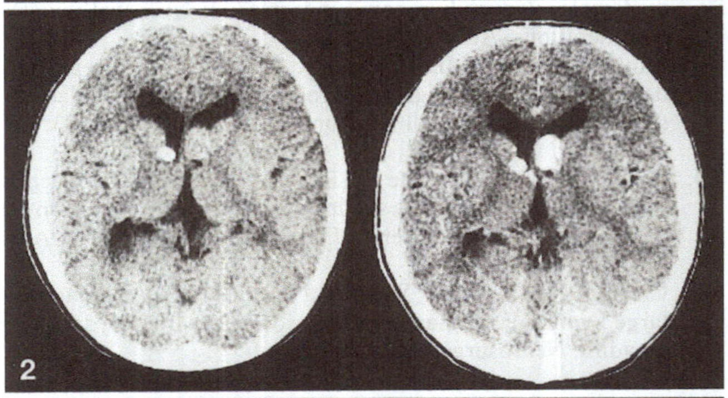

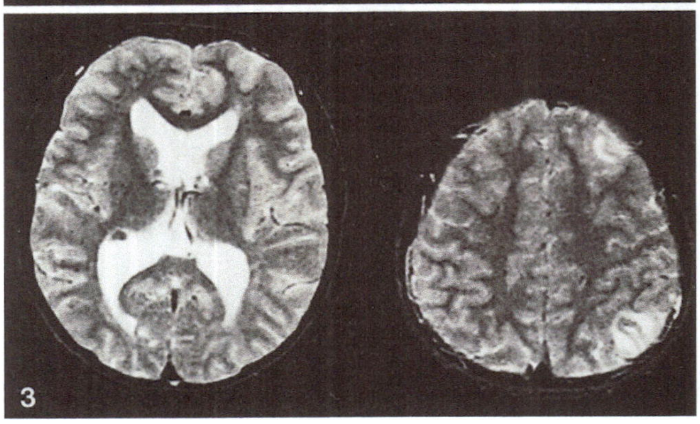

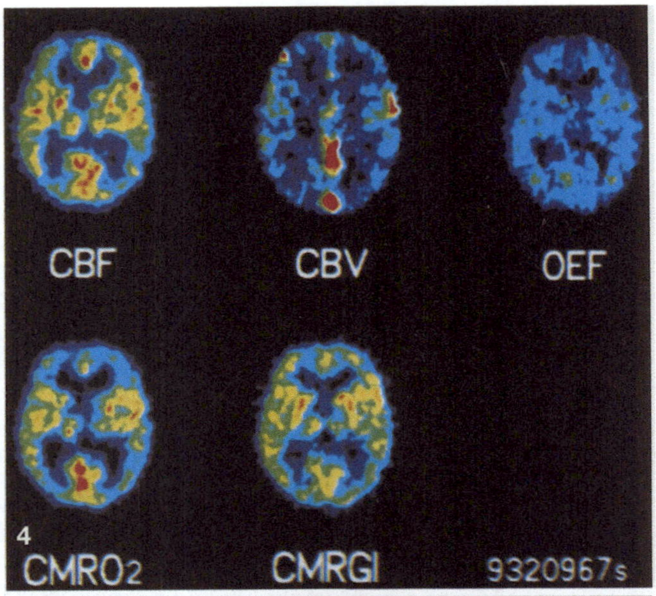

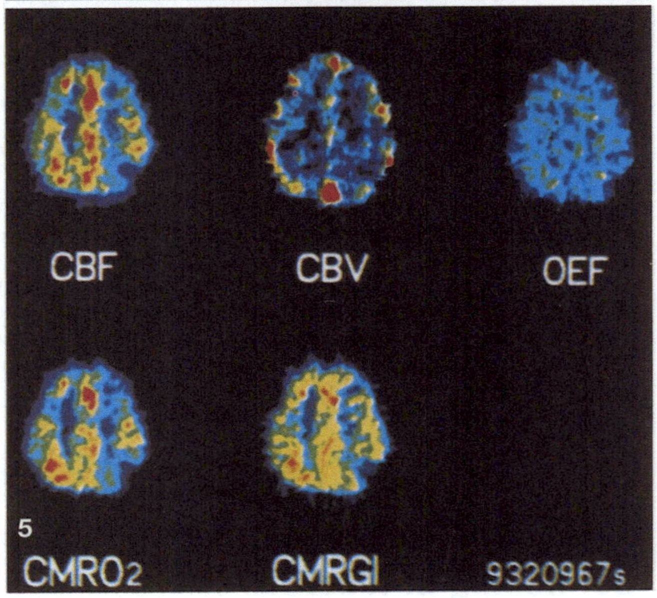

Fig. 1. Multiple areas of subependymal calcification shown by CT, at the age of 5 months

Fig. 2. Large nodule, enhancing homogeneously with contrast medium, adjacent to the foramen of Monro

Fig. 3. T2-weighted images revealed cortical tubers as high-intensity areas in the left frontal and parietal regions

Fig. 4. Blood flow and metabolism of the large nodule were characterised by decrease in all parameters, including rCBF, rCBV, rOEF, $rCMRO_2$ and rCMRGl

Fig. 5. Blood flow and metabolism of cortical tubers were similar to those of the large nodule

Case report

A 13-year-old boy had developed frequent convulsions 4 months after birth. He was diagnosed as having TS and was treated medically with anticonvulsants, since multiple areas of periventricular calcification were detected on CT, at the age of 5 months (Fig. 1). The convulsions had been well controlled. In March 1993, he presented with a syncopal attack and was admitted to hospital. Clinical findings included adenoma sebaceum and depigmented naevi on the trunk. He was alert. There were no focal neurological signs or mental retardation. The EEG showed no focal epileptic discharges.

CT showed multiple subependymal nodules. One on the left anterior horn was more than 2 cm in diameter and obliterated the foramen of Monro, resulting in hydrocephalus. This largest nodule enhanced homogeneously with contrast medium on CT (Fig. 2), and on MRI. T2-weighted images revealed cortical tubers as high intensity areas in the left frontal and parietooccipital regions (Fig. 3).

PET was performed. Regional blood flow (rCBF), blood volume (rCBV), and oxygen extraction fraction (rOEF) metabolic rate of oxygen ($rCMRO_2$) were measured using the ^{15}O-labelled water bolus injection method and the ^{15}O-labelled gas steady-state inhalation method. The regional cerebral metabolic rate of glucose (rCMRG) was measured after an intravenous injection of 256 MBq ^{18}F-fluorodeoxyglucose (FDG) using Phelps's equation with Reivich's constants of normal brain tissue. Blood flow in the largest nodule was lower than that of contralateral grey matter, which suggested poor blood supply. Its oxygen and glucose metabolism were

Table 1. Regional cerebral blood flow and metabolic rates

	rCBF ml/100 ml/min	rCBV ml/100 ml	rOEF	$rCMRO_2$ ml/100 ml/min	rCMRGl mg/100 ml/min
Large nodule	27.2	4.63	0.22	1.35	3.49
Cortical tuber	31.3	4.45	0.32	2.08	3.57
Grey matter	54.9	5.61	0.38	4.44	7.12

decreased compared with the contralateral grey matter, indicative of a low proliferative activity and a clinically benign tumour (Fig. 4, Table 1). In the cortical tubers, blood flow and metabolism were reduced, as in the largest nodule (Fig. 5, Table 1).

The largest nodule was totally resected through a transcallosal approach. Histological diagnosis was SGCA with no evidence of malignancy. The postoperative course was uneventful and the hydrocephalus resolved.

Discussion

SGCA is considered to be a benign tumour, but the possibility of malignancy or bleeding cannot be excluded. Surgical removal of a SGCA increases the chance of relieving intracranial hypertention and achieving prolonged survival.

Analysis of blood flow and metabolism may be useful for interpreting the nature of the tumour and predicting its proliferative activity. Accumulation of FDG is correlated with a proportion of the cells in S + G2M phases of the cell cycle. Enhanced glucose metabolism measured by FDG uptake therefore implies proliferating activity of tumours [1]. Szelies et al. [2] studied four patients with TS using PET. One or two localized cortical foci, with a more than 40% decrease in glucose metabolism compared to the respective contralateral regions, were clearly delineated.

In the present case, tumour rCMFGI remained about 50% lower in the contralateral grey matter. This indicates that both subependymal nodules and cortical tubers seem glucose-hypometabolic as well as hypoperfused. Thus, nodules proliferate less or grow gradually for a considerably long period. 5-Bromodeoxyuridine (BUdR) labelling revealed BUdR-positive cells to be rare, and the DNA histogram demonstrated no aneuploidy and a low percentage of cells in the S and G2M phases [3]. These results also indicate that SGCA has a low proliferative potential.

References

1. Minn H, Joesuu H, Ahonen A, Klemi P (1988) Fluorodeoxyglucose imaging: a method to assess the proliferative activity of human cancer in vivo. Cancer 61:1776–1781
2. Szelies B, Herholz K, Heiss WD, Rackl A, Pawlik G, Wagner R, Ilsen HW, Wienhard K (1983) Hypometabolic cortical lesions in tuberous sclerosis with epilepsy: demonstration by positron emission tomography. J Comput Assist Tomogr 7:946–953
3. Nishizaki T, Orita T, Abiko S, Aoki H, Ito H (1990) Subependymal giant cell astrocytoma associated with tuberous sclerosis: with special reference to cell kinetic studies. Neurol Med Chir 30:695–697

Head and neck causes of newborn respiratory distress

B. Azar-Kia, B. Hotaling, A. J. Horowitz, S. W. Goldberg, M. Fine, R. Neimon

2160 South First Ave., Maywood, IL 60153, USA

Abstract. Early diagnosis and treatment of neonatal respiratory distress is of utmost importance. CT and MRI play a major role in the diagnosis of congenital anomalies in the neck causing respiratory syndrome. We report cases of lesions in the neck causing neonatal airway obstruction.

Key words: Neonatal respiratory distress – Computed tomography – Neck, magnetic resonance imaging – Dermoid

Correspondence to: B. Azar-Kia

Neonatal respiratory distress should be recognized as soon as possible for early treatment to prevent major complications. We present six cases in which neonatal head and neck lesions caused respiratory distress. Most of these lesions have characteristic CT and MRI appearances.

Illustrative cases

Dermoid cyst

Dermoid cysts are usually midline lesions. Only 7% of all dermoid cysts are in the head and neck. Most occur around the orbit and oral

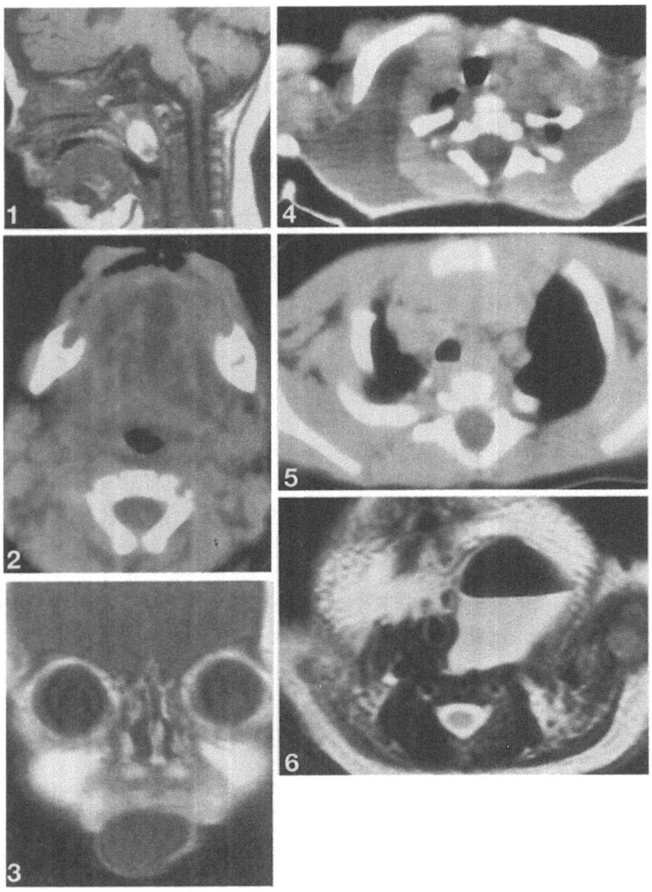

Fig. 1. Nasopharyngeal dermoid cyst. Sagittal T1-weighted image showing a large, mostly high-intensity lesion in the nasopharynx

Fig. 2. Cystic hygroma of the tongue. Axial CT reveals a lobulated cystic lesion infiltrating the tongue muscles

Fig. 3. Lingual cystic hygroma. Coronal T1-weighted image showing a large cyst at the antero inferior aspect of the tongue

Fig. 4. Cystic hygroma. Axial CT demonstrating extension of a large cyst in the neck into the superior part of the chest

Fig. 5. Thyroglossal cyst. Axial CT showing a large, mixed density mass in the anterior mediastinum

Fig. 6. Third branchial arch cyst. Axial T2-weighted image reveals a large cystic lesion extending toward the sternal notch. Note fluid level after aspiration of the cyst

and nasal cavities. Dermoids are commonly cystic, and cannot be easily differentiated from hygromas [1, 2]. Recognition of fatty tissue in the mass is a characteristic finding of dermoid cysts. We present a rare case in which a dermoid cyst in the nasopharynx caused respiratory distress. Physical examination revealed a rounded, well-defined mass in the nasopharynx. MRI showed a mass containing high intensity of fat on T1-weighted images, characteristic of a dermoid (Fig. 1).

Cystic hygroma

Cystic lymphangiomas or cystic hygromas arise from lymphatic tissue; 75% occur in the neck. They comprise 6% of benign tumors of infancy [3, 4]. Only 3–10% extend into the mediastinum. We present three cases. The child was found to have a cystic mass in the floor of the mouth. CT and MRI showed loculated fluid-containing areas in the floor of the mouth with infiltration into the tongue muscle (Fig. 2). The second also had a lingual hygroma. MRI showed a large cyst in the anterior aspect of the neck in the submental region (Fig. 3). The third was born with a large cystic hygroma on the right side of the neck. CT showed a large cyst in the neck extending into the superior fast of the chest (Fig. 4).

Thyroglossal duct cyst

Thyroglossal duct cysts may occur along the course of the migration of the thyroid gland from the foramen cecum at the base of the tongue to the level of the adult thyroid gland. They are usually midline lesions located at the anterior aspect of the neck [5, 6]. We present a case of thyroglossal duct cyst in the superior mediastinum. This patient developed respiratory distress 1 week after birth. CT showed a soft tissue density mass on the anterior aspect of the neck extending into the superior mediastinum (Fig. 5).

Third branchial arch cyst

This cyst occurs along the course of the third branchial arch which extends from the pyriform sinus to the lower third of the sternocleidomastoid muscle. The child we present was born with a large mass on the left side of the neck. MRI showed a large cyst extending down along the left sternocleidomastoid muscle to the sternal notch, characteristic of the third branchial arch cyst [7, 8] (Fig. 6).

Discussion

In all these cases the imaging study, by showing the position, extent and probable nature of the lesion causing respiratory distress, facilitated prompt, appropriate treatment.

References

1. New GB, Erich JB (1937) Dermoid cyst of the head and neck. Surg Gynecol Obstet 65:48
2. Hunter TB, et al (1983) Dermoid cyst of the floor of the mouth. CT appearance. AJR 141:1239
3. Siegel MJ, McAlister WH, Aslam FN (1979) Lymphangiomas in children: report of 121 cases. J Can Assoc Radiol 30:99
4. Silverman PM, Korobkin M, Moore AV (1983) CT diagnosis of cystic hygroma of the neck. J Comput Assist Tomogr 7:519
5. Reede DL, Bergeron RT, Som PM (1985) CT of thyroglossal duct cyst. Radiology 157:121
6. Alland RHB (1982) The thyroglossal cyst. Head Neck Surg 5:134
7. Harnsberger HR, Mancuso AA, Muraki AS, Byrd SE, Dillon WP, Johnson LP, Hanafee WN (1984) Branchial cleft anomalies and their mimics: computed tomographic evaluation. Radiology 152:739
8. Moran AG, Buchanan PR (1978) Branchial cysts, sinuses and fistulae. Clin Otolaryngol 3:77

Spine

Human spinal cord injury: MRI and histopathology

J. L. Becerra, W. R. Pucket, A. E. Marcillo, R. M. Quencer, M. J. D. Post, B. A. Green, R. P. Bunge

The Miami Project to Cure Paralysis and Department of Radiology, University of Miami School of Medicine, 1600 N.W. 10th Avenue, R-48, Miami, FL 33136, USA

Abstract. Detailed changes in the injured spinal cord can be shown by MRI. In many instances, the histopathological basis of the MRI changes is not known. We present observations on the pathology of human spinal cord injury, with post-mortem high-resolution MRI correlation. Specifically, we demonstrate that the central cord syndrome may result from axonal injury primarily in the white matter of the lateral columns; that Wallerian degeneration in the dorsal columns above and the lateral columns below the injury is detectable by MRI as early as 7 weeks after trauma; that intramedullary displacement of crushed cord tissue occurs predominantly in the ventral aspect of the dorsal columns; that post-traumatic intramedullary cavities show variable histological border patterns; and that intramedullary Schwann cells are frequently identified following trauma, probably migrating into the cord from dorsal or ventral roots. These observations explain some of the areas of abnormal signal intensity seen in imaging of spinal cord injury.

Key words: Central cord syndrome – Wallerian degeneration – Spinal cord injury – Post-traumatic spinal cord cysts –Schwannosis

MRI of the injured spinal cord shows areas of abnormal signal intensity that may be difficult to characterize with respect to the underlying pathology. We present observations on the histopathology of human spinal cord injury with high-resolution MRI correlation.

Materials and methods

We obtained 45 spinal cords post-mortem from persons who had suffered spinal cord injury and examined them by means of high-resolution MRI and histopathology. Histological analysis of cord tissue was performed using stains for general histology (hematoxylin-eosin), myelin (solochrome-cyanine), axons (Sevier-Munger) and a stain for connective tissue components (trichrome). The MRI studies were reviewed with a view to areas of abnormal signal intensity. The histological studies were tailored to the areas of abnormal MRI signal intensity.

Correspondence to: R. M. Quencer, The University of Miami School of Medicine, 1115 N.W. 14th Street., Suite 511, Miami, FL 33136, USA

Results and discussion

Central cord syndrome

Published papers [1–3] have ascribed the acute traumatic central cord syndrome (ATCCS) to hemorrhage, necrosis or contusion within the central portion of the spinal cord. However, such findings were lacking in all our specimens. Post-mortem MRI showed areas of increased T2 signal intensity in the lateral columns and no evidence of intramedullary hemorrhage. Histology also showed no evidence of blood or blood products within the cord parenchyma. Axon and myelin loss was seen in the white matter of the lateral columns, particularly in the deeper regions occupied by the corticospinal tracts.

The MRI and pathological observations indicate that ATCCS is predominantly a white matter injury, and that intramedullary hemorrhage is not a necessary feature of the syndrome. We suggest that the most common mechanism of injury in ATCCS is direct compression of the cervical spinal cord caused by buckling of the ligamenta flava into an already narrowed cervical canal; this explains the predominance of axonal injury in the white matter of the lateral columns of the cervical spinal cord [4].

Wallerian degeneration

Wallerian degeneration [5, 6] refers to antegrade degeneration of axons and their accompanying myelin sheaths, which results from injury to the proximal portion of the axon or its cell body.

On MRI, all the spinal cords with post-injury survival of more than 7 weeks showed areas of increased signal intensity in the dorsal columns above and the lateral columns below the injury. Histology showed evidence of Wallerian degeneration in the areas of abnormal signal, manifest in myelin axon breakdown and a predominance of phagocytic cells (Fig. 1).

Recognition of Wallerian degeneration on MRI allows more complete analysis of the injury and explains abnormal signal at sites remote from the site of the injury; it could also be useful in the timing and planning of therapeutic interventions.

Intramedullary displacement of crushed spinal cord tissue

It has been postulated that spinal cord tissue injured by substantial compression can be macerated and forcibly pushed into adjacent cord tissue that is not itself directly damaged [7].

Of the spinal cords studied, six showed histological evidence of intramedullary displacement of crushed spinal

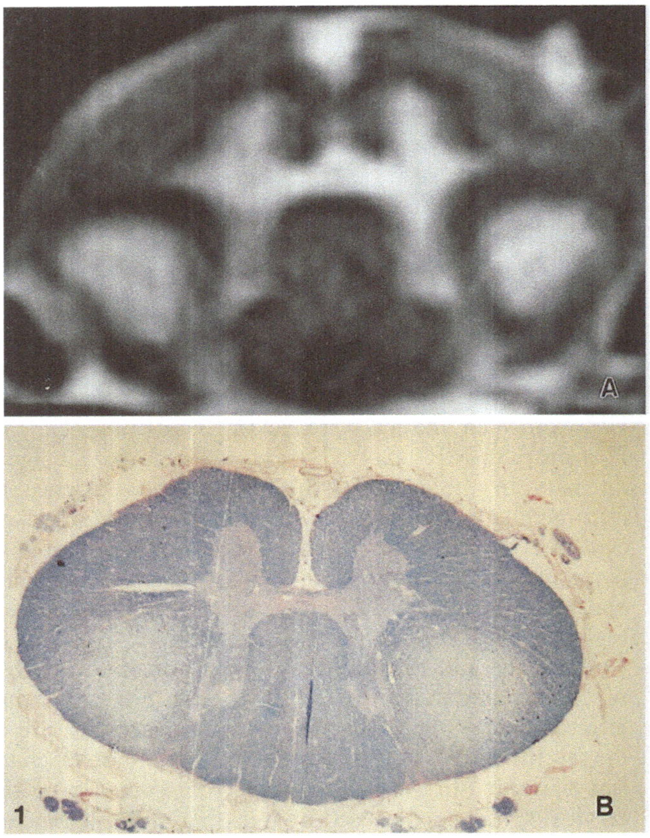

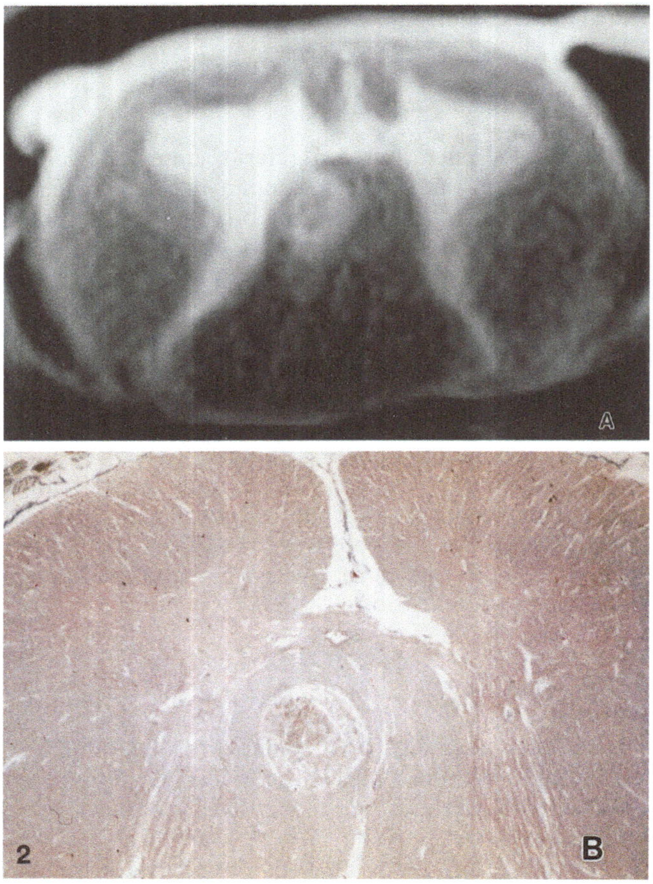

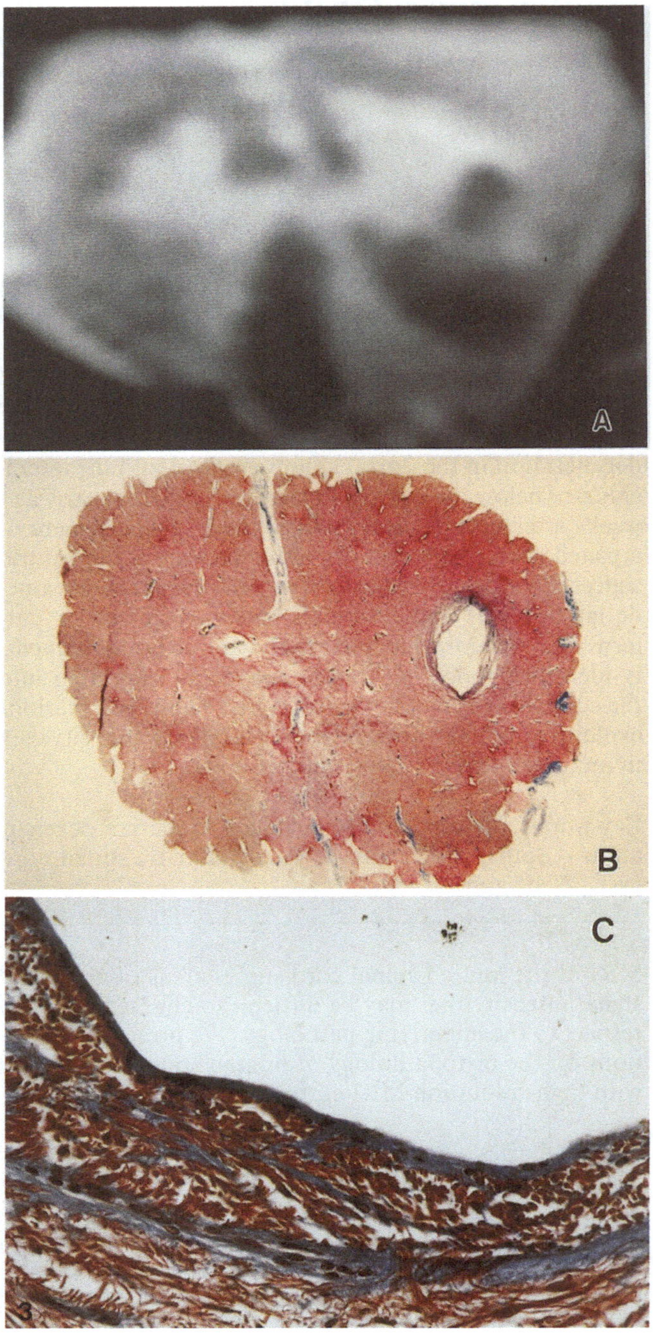

Fig. 1. A Axial T2-weighted (2080/80/2) image at the T2 cord level 4 months after injury shows areas of increased signal intensity in the lateral columns. **B** Myelin staining indicates a loss of axon-myelin units and a large number of phagocytes in both lateral corticospinal tracts, shown by the pallor in those areas

Fig. 2. A Axial T2-weighted (2000/80/2) image of the C8 cord level below a compression injury shows increased signal intensity in the anterior aspect of the right dorsal column, with some mass effect. **B** Histological examination reveals macerated tissue displaced into the dorsal columns

Fig. 3. A Axial T1-weighted (567/26/4) image at the C2 level 10 years after injury and 4 years after shunting shows the proximal extend of an expanding cyst in the left dorsal horn of the gray matter. **B** Trichrome staining shows the cavity at low magnification. **C** Higher magnification shows the fibroblast border (*dark blue*) of the cyst wall

cord tissue, in the anterior aspect of the posterior columns in four. One also showed displaced neural tissue in the anterior horns of the gray matter, and one showed displaced tissue only in the lateral white matter. Most of the lesions were in the cervical cord, and all these spinal cords had suffered severe compression at the center of the lesion. Intramedullary displacement of crushed tissue was seen above and below this in four cases, and only below in two. MRI showed the displaced tissue as focal areas of increased T2 signal intensity (Fig. 2).

We believe that some post-traumatic intramedullary cord cysts may be the end-result, following debris removal, of this intramedullary displacement of crushed cord tissue that occurs at the time of initial injury.

Post-traumatic spinal cord cavities

Following significant trauma to the spinal cord, cavitation is known to occur [8–10], and it was found in 14 of the 45 cords examined: in 4 the lesions were thought to be expanding and in 10, nonexpanding cavities. All the expanding cysts had a defined border, composed primarily of fibroblasts in 3 cases and of astrocytes in 1 (Fig. 3). The borders of 2 nonexpanding cavities also contained fibroblasts. For 8 other nonexpanding cavities no defined borders were apparent.

Schwannosis

Schwannosis is a non-neoplastic proliferation of Schwann cells in the perivascular spaces of the spinal cord, which is seen particularly often in older patients, especially those with diabetes mellitus [11]. Four spinal cords with post-injury survival times between 2 and 23 years showed histological evidence of Schwann cell invasion at the center of the lesion. This manifested on MRI as areas of increased T2 signal intensity.

Theoretically, such accumulations of Schwann cells may be useful for the remyelination of demyelinated axons following spinal cord injury. The clinical significance of these zones of Schwann cell proliferations, in the traumatized spinal cord remains to be elucidated.

Acknowledgements. This investigation was supported in part by a program project grant from the National Institutes of Health/NINDS (NS-28059) and funds from the Miami Project to Cure Paralysis.

References

1. Rand RW, Crandall P (1952) Central spinal cord syndrome in hyperextension injuries of the cervical cord. J Bone Joint Surg [Br] 44:1415–1422
2. Schneider RC, Thompson JM, Bebin J (1958) The syndrome of the acute central cervical spinal cord injury. J Neurol Neurosurg Psychiatry 21:216–227
3. Hopkins A, Rudge P (1973) Hyperpathia in the central cord syndrome. J Neurol Neurosurg Psychiatry 36:637–642
4. Quencer RM, Bunge RP, Egnor M, Green BA, Puckett W, et al (1992) Acute traumatic central cord syndrome: MRI-pathological correlations. Neuroradiology 34:85–94
5. Waller AV (1850) Experiments on the section of the glossopharyngeal and hypoglossal nerves of a frog, and observations of the alterations produced thereby in the structure of their primitive fibre. Philos Trans R Soc Lond (Biol) 140:423–429
6. Kuhn MJ, Mikulis DJ, Ayoub DM, Kosofsky BE, Davis KR, Taveras JM (1989) Wallerian degeneration after cerebral infarction: evaluation with sequential MR imaging. Radiology 172:179–182
7. McVeigh JF (1923) Experimental cord crushes. Arch Surg 7:573–600
8. Green BA, Quencer RM, Post MJD, Eismont F, Pachen S (1990) A review of 100 patients surgically treated for progressive post-traumatic cystic myelopathy. J Neurosurg 72:353A
9. Madsen PW, Green BA, Bowen BC (1991) Syringomyelia. In: Rothman RH, Simeone FA (eds) The spine, 3rd edn. Saunders, Philadelphia, pp 1575–1604
10. Kao CC, Chang LW (1977) The mechanism of spinal cord cavitation following spinal cord transection. J Neurosurg 46:197–209
11. Terzis JK, Smith KL (1990) The peripheral nerve: structure, function and reconstruction. Raven Press, New York, pp 13–15

Delayed onset of neurological deficit caused by post-traumatic incarcerated herniation of the spinal cord

W. Reith [1], M. Forsting [1], V. Tronnier [2], S. Kunze [2], K. Sartor [1]

[1] Department of Neuroradiology, University of Heidelberg Medical School, Im Neuenheimer Feld 400, D-69120 Heidelberg, Germany
[2] Department of Neurosurgery, University of Heidelberg Medical School, Im Neuenheimer Feld 400, D-69120 Heidelberg, Germany

Abstract. We report a patient with progressive paraparesis, where spinal cord had herniated through a dural tear at D4. Over 20 years previously the patient had suffered a back injury, which was the probable cause of the dural tear. Preoperative MRI and postmyelographic CT demonstrated the presence of spinal cord herniation. After successful operation with repositioning of the herniated spinal cord and closure of the dura mater, the patient's clinical status improved markedly.

Correspondence to: W. Reith

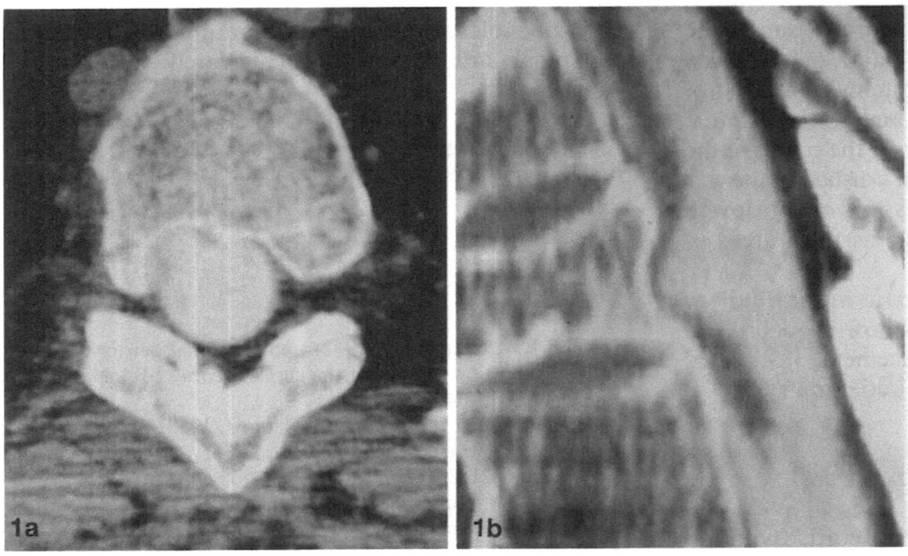

Fig. 1 a, b. Postmyelographic CT **a** with sagittal reformat **b** at the level of T4. The spinal cord is displaced forward and occupies a bony excavation on the deformed body of T4

Key words: Spinal cord herniation – Dural tear – Progressive paraparesis

Spinal cord herniation is a rare pathologic condition with only a few reported cases [1–5]. In our case, the patient had undergone two back operations with lysis of dural adhesions on the dorsal aspect of the dural sac (the ventral aspect was never inspected). Knowledge of spinal cord herniation could have prevented these two operations. The different types of spinal cord herniation – post-traumatic, as in our case, and other, e.g. congenital and postoperative – are discussed.

Case report

A 51-year-old man presented with progressive paraparesis was only able to walk with a crutch. On neurological examination, the patient had a sensory defect with hypalgesia and thermal hypaesthesia below T4, and loss of sensibility below L4; there was hyperreflexia of the legs. In 1967 the patient had a car accident. Plain films of the thoracic spine revealed a compression fracture of the vertebral body of T4, but the patient had no neurological deficit. Ten years later, however, he developed a slowly progressive gait disturbance and weakness of both legs. In 1986 and 1989 he had spinal surgery with lysis of extradural dorsal adhesions at the level of T4. No clinical improvement was noted; rather, the disease worsened. Finally, in 1993, the patient was unable to walk. Myelography and postmyelographic CT with sagittal reformatting were performed and revealed ventral displacement of the spinal cord at the level of T4. The cord appeared to be displaced forward and to occupy a bony excavation of the deformed body of T4. In addition, a slight widening of the dorsal subarachnoid space was seen (Fig. 1). Preoperative MRI showed ventral displacement of the spinal cord at the level of T4, with corresponding widening of the dorsal cerebrospinal fluid (CSF) space. The suspected diagnosis was ventral spinal cord herniation through a dural tear.

At surgery, marked dural thickening with epidural adhesions was evident. Inspection of the ventral aspect of the dura mater revealed an opening about 12 mm in length and 5 mm in width. Portions of the spinal cord that appeared pale and without pulsation projected through this cleft. Careful mobilisation allowed the herniated tissue to be replaced intradurally. Immediately after repositioning, the herniated cord tissue attained its normal red colour and pulsations could be observed. The dural cleft was closed with a suture and fibrin glue. Immediately after operation, transient worsening of the neurological status occurred, which was probably due to postoperative oedema. Three months later, however, the patient was able to walk without an aid.

Discussion

The aetiology of spinal cord herniation varies and can be classified in three groups: traumatic, postoperative and congenital. In our case of delayed onset of paraparesis years after a thoracic compression fracture, a traumatic dural tear was the cause of spinal cord herniation. Twenty years previously our patient had sustained a trauma with a vertebral body fracture exactly at the level of the spinal cord herniation. He had also had two back operations with lysis of dural adhesions at the dorsal aspect of the dural sac (the ventral aspect of the dural sac was never inspected during the two surgical procedures). In our patient, remote trauma thus seemed to be the most likely cause of herniation.

In traumatic spinal cord herniation, the trauma damages the dura mater, causing a tear through which the spinal cord herniates into the epidural space, sometimes resulting in an erosion of the vertebral body [6]. Hoffman et al. [7] reported the case of a 12-year-old boy with paraparesis progressing over a period of 5 years after craniospinal trauma. They noted "loss of a pedicle" at the level of the lesion in plain radiographs. At surgery, a large arachnoid diverticulum extending around the dorsal and lateral aspects of the dural sac and communicating with the subarachnoid space at C5 was discovered. Postoperatively, the patient made an excellent recovery. It appears that the loss of the pedicle was caused by a continuous pulsation effect of the diverticulum, which was communicating with the subarachnoid space. The mechanism of post-traumatic spinal herniation may be as follows: the initial trauma causes a small dural tear but no permanent neurological deficit. Over time, continuous CSF pulsations enlarge this small dural tear and some day spinal cord herniation occurs and neurological symptoms start.

Congenital defects of the dura or other types of spinal malformation may cause spinal cord herniation. Closure defects of the neural tube are generally located dorsally in the cranial or caudal region of the spine, and usually involve the sclerotome or myotome (spina bifida, myelomeningocele, diastomatomyelia). Another group of malformations are arachnoid cysts (intradural and extradural), which tend to be located posterolaterally. Most of these cysts are detected incidentally, while a few cause clinical symptoms [7]. The exact origin of these arachnoid cysts, which may communicate with the subarachnoid space, is still unclear; possible explanations are embryonic cell remnants, local hyperplasia and proliferation, and congenital defects of the dura. The preferred treatment for symptomatic arachnoid cysts is complete resection. The most likely cause of the neurological deficit in these cases is from pressure or traction on the spinal cord exerted by the distended cysts. The increasing neurological deficit is attributed to the fact the cysts enlarge over time. Another cause of delayed spinal cord compression, which is associated with brachial plexus injury, is the tethering effect on the spinal cord of fibrous adhesions.

Postoperative spinal cord herniation most often occurs after laminectomy. The spinal cord herniates through the dural defect caused by surgery or incomplete dural suture. Most often, this kind of lesion appears in the dorsal aspect of the dura mater. The diagnosis of an incarcerated herniation of the spinal cord is decidedly uncommon, but if radiologists are aware of the condition they will be able to recognise its characteristic features on CT or MRI and to suggest an appropriate kind of treatment.

References

1. Burres KP, Conley FK (1978) Progressive neurological dysfunction secondary to postoperative cervical psuedomeningocele in a C-4 quadriplegic. J Neurosurg 48:289–291
2. Cobb C, Ehni G (1973) Herniation of the spinal cord into an iatrogenic meningocele. J Neurosurg 39:533–536
3. Mizuno J, Nagagawa H, Iwata K (1986) Postoperative spinal cord herniation diagnosed by metrizamide CT. Neurol Surg 14:681–685
4. Sachdev VP, Huang YP, Shah CP, Mallis LI (1981) Posttraumatic pseudomeningomyelocele (enlarging fracture?) in a vertebral body. J Neurosurg 54:545-549
5. Tronnier V, Steinmetz A, Albert FK, Scharf J, Kunze S (1991) Hernia of the spinal cord: case report and review of the literature. Neurosurgery 29:916–919
6. Wortzman G, Tasker RR, Rewcastle NB, Richardson JC, Pearson FG (1974) Spontaneous incarcerated herniation of the spinal cord into a vertebral body. J Neurosurg 41:631–635
7. Herskowitz J, Bielwaski MA, Nagagopal V, Sabin TD (1978) Anterior cervical arachnoid cyst simulating syringomyelia. Arch Neurol 35:57–58

MRI in spinal trauma: early and follow-up examinations

T. Kryst-Widzgowska[1], **G. Rejnowski**[1], **J. Ryterski**[1], **J. Bronarski**[2]

[1] Department of Neuroradiology, Institute of Psychiatry and Neurology, Warsaw, Poland
[2] Rehabilitation Centre, Medical Academy in Warsaw, Konstancin, Poland

Abstract. The aim of this study was to study the cervical spine using MRI in acute trauma and in the long-term follow-up. Sixty patients were examined with a 0.38T resistive unit, using spin-echo T1- and T2-weighted sequences in the sagittal and axial planes. The first examination was done within 10 days of injury. The follow-up study was performed within 10–12 weeks. The major findings included dislocation, compression of the thecal sac, vertebral fractures, spinal cord contusion and oedema. In follow-up studies spinal canal stenoses and intramedullary syrines were found. MRI proved to be a very good modality for initial diagnosis and long-term management of cervical spine trauma.

Key words: Cervical spine injury – Magnetic resonance imaging

Correspondence to: T. Kryst, Department of Neuroradiology, Al. Sobieskiego 1/9, 02-957 Warsaw, Poland

A retrospective analysis of magnetic resonance imaging (MRI) studies of 60 patients with acute cord injuries was undertaken to determine which observations were related directly to the follow-up MRI findings. MRI is one of the most valuable imaging modalities for investigation of the spine and is essential to the proper management and therapy [1–3]. The purpose of this study was to assess clinical efficacy of MRI in the diagnosis of spinal injury and in the long-term follow-up. We wanted to examine the relationship between initial MRI findings and the eventual outcome of spinal cord injured subjects.

Patients and methods

Sixty patients (58 males, 2 females) ranging from 13 to 67 years of age (mean age, 33.7 years) were referred to the MRI centre with tetraplegia after cervical spine injury. The causes of the injuries to the spine were falls, jumping into water head-first, traffic accidents and sport injuries. Damage to the spinal cord in the analysed material was observed after trauma involving the flexion, hyperextension and compressive injuries. The first MRI examinations were performed within 10 days of trauma. Patients were treated surgically

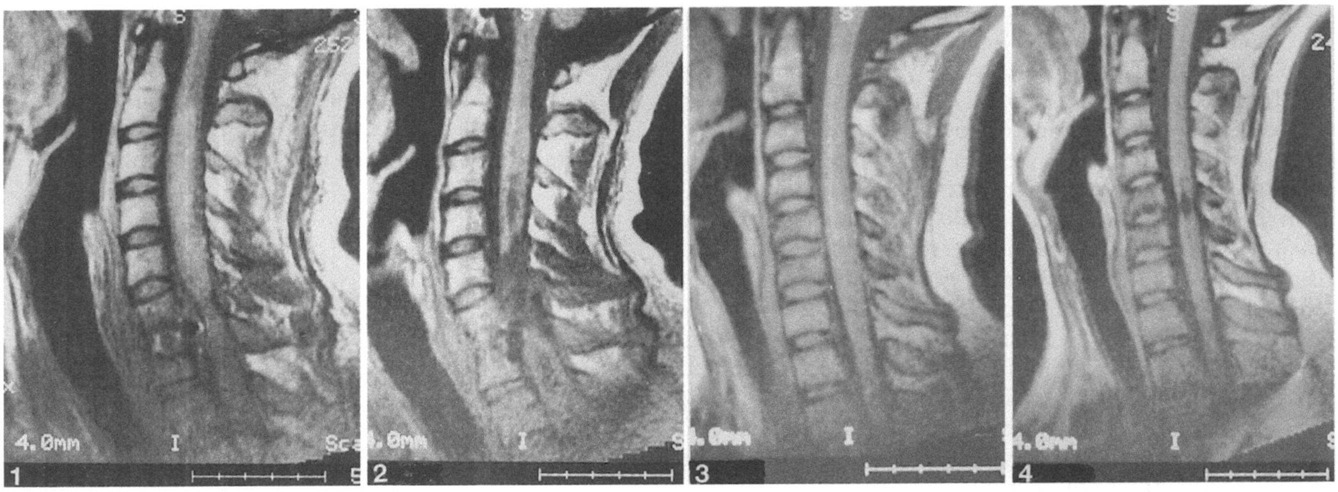

Fig. 1. Young quadriplegic man with hyperflexion injury of C6 and C7. Initial postoperative sagittal T1-weighted image after spinal fusion, showing extensive areas of low signal in the marrow of the bodies of C6 and C7. High signal in the spinal cord, due to ascending oedema, is present

Fig. 2. Initial examination of a patient with cervical spine injury. Early post-traumatic sagittal T1-weighted image revealed widening of the cord at C4–C6 due to contusion and oedema, no spinal canal stenosis and decreased bone marrow signal intensity of the bodies of C5 and C6

Fig. 3. Control examinations after 3 and 6 weeks: sagittal and axial T1-weighted images showing partial cord transsection, with a large cyst

Fig. 4. After 4 weeks of rehabilitation repeat MRI showed intramedullary syrinx at the C5–6 level (same patient as Fig. 3)

or conservatively. On the basis of the results of clinical neurological examinations, plain films and MRI, 30 patients received early exploration and decompression subdivided into: 10 anterior interbody fusions (Cloward's technique), 10 subtotal corpectomies with strut bone graft, laminectomies and laminoplasties. Conservative treatment included collars, skeletal traction with a combination of these methods, and 'halo' fixation. Follow-up studies were carried out within 10–12 weeks after trauma. All MRI studies were performed with a 0.38T resistive magnet. Multisection sagittal and axial T1-weighted (TR 600 ms, TE 30 ms) images were obtained and T2-weighted (TR 2000 ms, TE 25/80 ms) spin-echo images were undertaken in the sagittal plane. Slice thickness was 4 mm, and matrix 192×256.

Results

The injury involved the cervical spine in all patients examined. All were tetraplegic prior to the first MRI examination. Pathological findings on the initial MRI examination included: vertebral dislocation with compression of the thecal sac (24 cases), vertebral dislocation causing spinal cord compression (24), fractures of vertebrae (39), spinal cord oedema (35), intramedullary haemorrhage (9), epidural haematomas (11), damage of the intervertebral discs (26), and cord contusion with focal lesions (35 cases) (Figs. 1, 2). In 11 patients, 2 lesions were found, 48 patients had 3 or 4 lesions, and 1 patient had 5 lesions, as mentioned above.

On the follow-up MRI examinations syrinxes (33 cases), areas of glioses (28), spinal canal stenoses (44), vertebral fractures (39), and damage to intervertebral discs (26 cases) were detected (Figs. 3, 4). Three patients had only one kind of lesion, 48 patients had 2 or 3 pathological findings. In 4 cases, 4 lesions were detected.

Discussion

The main findings on the initial MRI examination of patients with cervical spine injury were vertebral dislocation causing compression with or without affecting the spinal cord, vertebral fractures and spinal cord contusion and oedema. Major lesions on the follow-up MRI studies were stenosis of the spinal canal and intramedullary syrinxes.

Patients who had no lesion in the spinal cord in the follow-up MRI study showed no changes in the spinal cord on retrospective review of the initial MRI examination in spite of post-traumatic narrowing of the spinal canal. MRI findings of an acutely injured cervical spinal cord suggested the prognosis of spinal cord injury and were confirmed by sequential studies [4]. Understanding of the pathophysiology of this injury should enable clinicians to treat spinal cord injuries more effectively and lay the groundwork for continuing investigations aimed at improving neurological recovery after spinal cord injury.

References

1. O'Beirne J, Cassidy N, Raza K, Walsh M, Stack J, Murray P (1993) Role of magnetic resonance imaging in the assessment of spinal injuries. Injury 24:149–154
2. Curati W, Kingsley D, Kendall B, Moseley I (1992) MRI in chronic spinal cord trauma. Neuroradiology 35:30–35
3. Wittenberg R, Boetel U, Beyer H (1990) Magnetic resonance imaging and computer tomography of acute spinal cord trauma. Clin Orthop 260:176–185
4. Silberstein M, Tress BM, Hennessy O (1992) Prediction of neurologic outcome in acute spinal cord injury: the role of CT and MR. AJNR 13:1597–1608

CT of atlanto-occipital dislocation: the "absent atlas" sign

M. Hardjasudarma [1], **R. Prieto** [2], **B. Willis** [2]

[1] Department of Radiology, Louisiana State University Medical Center, Shreveport, Shreveport, LA 71130-3932, USA
[2] Department of Neurosurgery, Louisiana State University Medical Center, Shreveport, Shreveport, LA 71130-3932, USA

Abstract. A case of atlanto-occipital dislocation (AOD) is presented. Lateral cervical spine films, tomography, and computed tomography (CT) with reconstructions were obtained. The Powers ratio produced different values for different imaging procedures. This was probably caused by changes in the position of the craniovertebral junction from one examination to another. Axial CT produced one image that was almost completely devoid of bony craniovertebral structures. The "absent atlas" sign is an important indicator of AOD. Patients with (suspected) AOD should have cervical spine films and CT. Conventional tomography is unnecessary and should be avoided.

Key words: Dislocation, atlanto-occipital – Radiography – Tomography – Computed tomography

We describe a finding on axial computed tomography (CT) that is very specific for atlanto-occipital dislocation (AOD), as well as the advantages and disadvantages of the Powers ratio (PR).

Case report

A 31-year-old woman, was involved in an automobile accident and later admitted with quadriplegia and a Glasgow coma scale of 4. Her lateral cervical spine films did not lend themselves to calculation of the PR, due to obscuration of several reference points. The PR was 1.06 on the lateral cervical spine tomograms, but was 0.77 on sagittal reconstructed CT. On coronal studies, the distraction between the atlanto-occipital joints was asymmetrical. The least affected joint varied between 3.15 mm on the left (as seen on tomography; Fig. 1a) and 4.6 mm on the right (on CT; Fig. 1b).

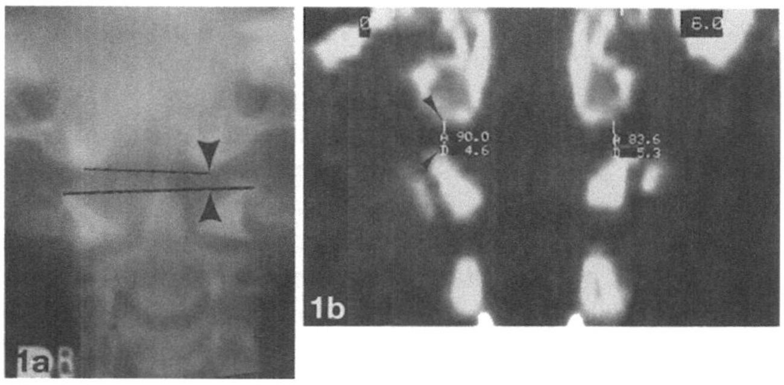

Fig. 1. Minimum cephalocaudad distraction measured 3.15 mm on the left on coronal tomography (**a** *arrowheads*), which changed to 4.6 mm for the right joint on coronal reconstructed CT (**b** *arrowheads*)

Discussion

Frank and unreduced AOD can often be clearly seen on lateral radiographs [1]. However, identification of reference points on the films can be difficult [2]. In our case, the PR could not be established on lateral films of the cervical spine because one or more reference points were obscured. The lateral tomograms and sagittal reconstructed CT were better, but yielded different PR values (1.06 which is slightly abnormal; and 0.77 which rules out anterior, but not posterior AOD [1]). We believe this, as well as the variation between the distracted atlanto-occipital joints on coronal studies (Fig. 1), to be secondary to actual changes in position between the skull base and the atlas. This strongly suggests that AOD can be increased, decreased, and even masked, depending on how the patient is positioned. The distraction of the joint that was

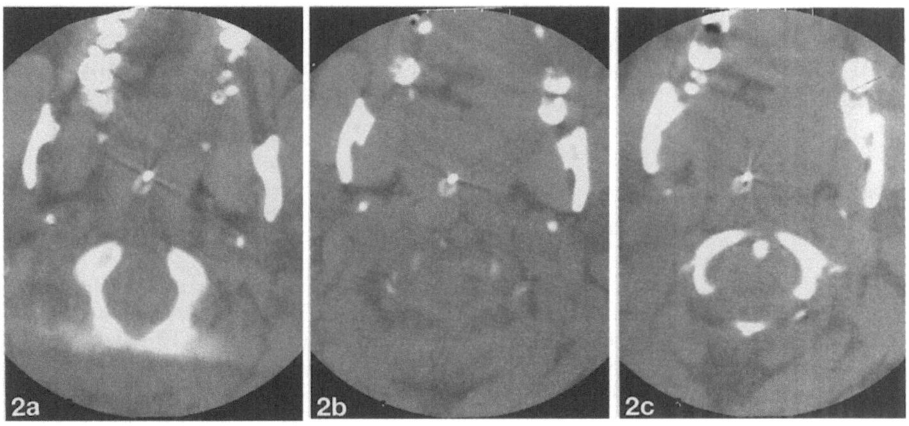

Fig. 2. Axial 3-mm CT images at the level of the occipital condyles (**a**), the atlanto-occipital joints (**b**; 6 mm caudal to **a**) and the atlas (**c**, 12 mm caudal to **a**). **b** Almost totally devoid of bony craniovertebral structures. This "absent atlas" sign is very specific for atlanto-occipital dislocation

Correspondence to: M. Hardjasudarma

least separated on coronal studies (Fig. 1) corresponded to 1–1.5× the thickness of the 3 mm axial CT image. This resulted in one axial CT slice that was almost completely devoid of bony craniovertebral elements (Fig. 2). Since CT scans of the cervical spine are commonly studied in a cephalo-caudad direction, a slice is thus encountered that shows little, if any, of C1. This "absent atlas" sign (Fig. 2b) is a very important finding. Despite the fact that it has undoubtedly been seen on numerous prior occasions [2], we have found no direct reference to it. An "absent atlas" on axial CT by itself is highly suggestive of AOD, and within the context of acute trauma, the patient must be considered as having AOD until proven otherwise. The sign is produced if the separation at the atlanto-occipital joints is at least equal to the thickness of the CT slice and the slice is made within this hiatus without volume averaging. The "absent atlas" sign is highly specific, but not very sensitive. Absence of the sign in a patient with AOD will likely be caused by volume averaging, which may result from too thick a CT slice, too little separation at the atlanto-occipital joints, malpositioning, deformities, or a combination of these factors. Patients with obvious or suspected AOD should undergo a CT scan with thin slices of the craniovertebral junction (occiput – C2), with reconstructions, and measurements done directly on the CT console. Plain film tomography [2], especially in the lateral projection [3], should be avoided.

References

1. Harris JH, Edeiken-Monroe B (1987) The radiology of acute cervical spine trauma. Williams & Wilkins, Baltimore, pp 220–225
2. Gerlock AJ, Mirfakhraee M, Benzel EC (1983) Computed tomography of traumatic atlantooccipital dislocation. Neurosurgery 13:316–319
3. Pang D, Wilberger JE (1980) Traumatic atlanto-occipital dislocation with survival: case report and review. Neurosurgery 7:503–508

Detection of ligamentous and supporting soft tissue injuries using fat-suppressed MRI in acute spinal trauma

L. C. Blake, W. A. Cohen, K. R. Maravilla

University of Washington Department of Radiology – SB.05 1959 NE Pacific, Seattle, WA 98195, USA

Abstract. The MRI examinations of 31 patients with acute cervical spine trauma were retrospectively reviewed. Sagittal T1-weighted, fast spin-echo T2-weighted (FSE-T2) (with and without fat suppression), and short tau inversim recovery (STIR) images were reviewed for the presence of ligamentous and soft tissue injury. MRI findings were correlated with computed tomography and conventional radiography in all patients. Fat-suppressed FSE-T2 and STIR pulse sequences showed the highest sensitivity in detecting disruption of cervical ligaments, facets and intervertebral disks. Increased signal intensity was useful as a marker of ligamentous and soft tissue injury. Preliminary results indicate that MRI utilizing fat-suppression techniques can identify these injuries with a high degree of accuracy.

Key words: Cervical spine – Fat suppression – Ligaments – Magnetic resonance imaging

The clinical and radiological evaluation of patients with suspected cervical spine trauma is focused on detecting the presence of osseous injury, ligamentous instability and spinal cord parenchymal pathology. Conventional radiography and CT are the gold standard for investigating cervical alignment and bony injury. Multiple prior studies have documented the role of MRI in studying intrinsic spinal cord injury [1, 2]. However, the value of MRI in detecting ligamentous disruptions resulting from acute spine trauma has not been as thoroughly assessed.

Recent reports have emphasized the benefit of fat-suppressed pulse sequences in evaluating head, neck and spine pathology [3, 4]. These techniques are useful in removing the high intensity signal that interferes with detection of pathology on T1-weighted and FSE-T2 pulse sequences. The purpose of this study was to assess the use of fat-suppressed pulse sequences in detecting traumatic disruptions of cervical spinal ligaments, facets and intervertebral disks.

Patients and methods

The MRI studies of 31 patients who were referred for evaluation of suspected cervical spine injury were retrospectively reviewed for the presence of ligamentous disruption. Sagittal T2-weighted FSE (3500–4000/68, TR/TE Echo train 8) pulse sequences, with and without fat-suppression, and fast STIR (4000/34/140/, TR/TE/TI, echo train 8) images were compared using a 3-point scale for lesion detection and conspicuity. MRI results in all patients were correlated with findings of bony injury and ligamentous instability found on conventional radiography and CT.

Correspondence to: K. R. Maravilla

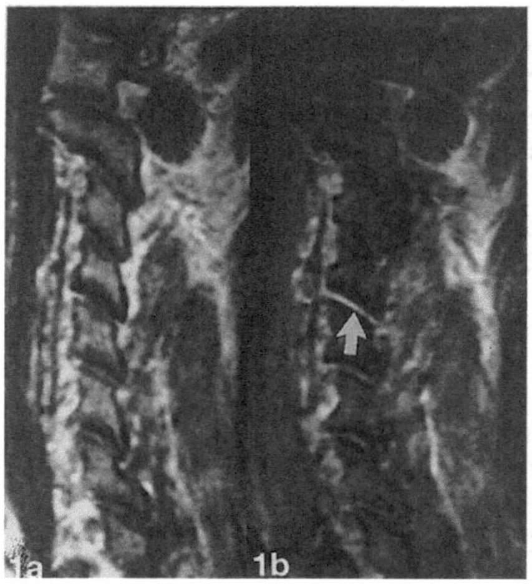

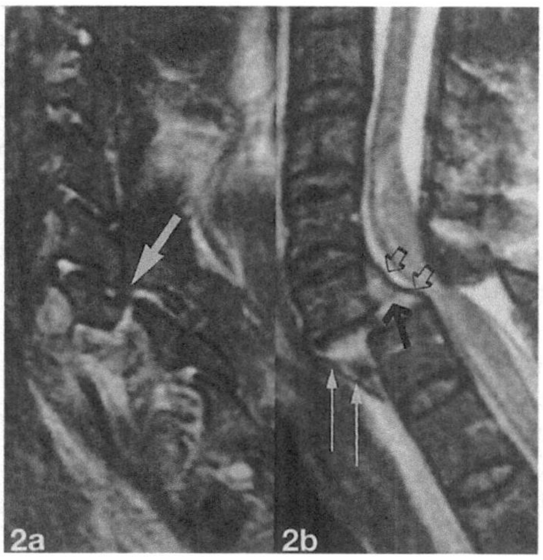

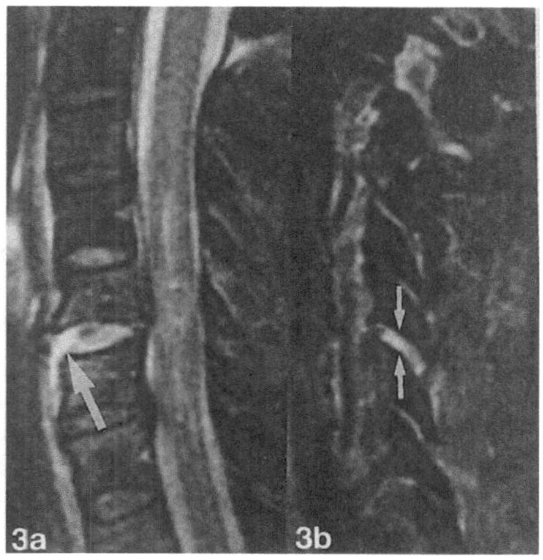

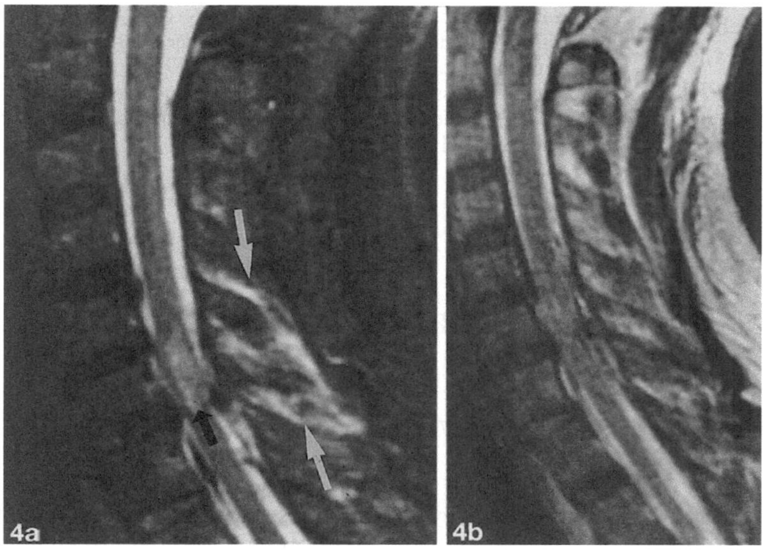

Fig. 1 a, b. Left parasagittal MR images through the facets of a 34-year-old man following reduction of C4–5 subluxation. T2-weighted FSE images without (**a**) and with (**b**) fat-suppression. Alignment is normal. Facet capsular injury is seen in **b** as increased capsular signal at the C4–5 facet (*arrow*) and is detected only on the image with fat suppression

Fig. 2 a, b. Fast-STIR sagittal images of a 36-year-old man with severe spinal cord injury and grade III C6–7 subluxation. **a** C6–7 facet fracture dislocation (*large arrow*). Displacement of the ALL (*long arrows*) and PLL (*open arrows*) is present in **b**. Note acute disc rupture, subligamentous disk derniation (*black arrow*) and extensive spinal cord injury

Fig. 3. **a** Midsagittal fast-STIR image demonstrates disruptions of the ALL (*arrow*). The C5–6 disk space shows signs of acute disk rupture, including abnormal intervertebral disk space widening and increased signal intensity. In **b** the C5–6 facet capsule is wide and gives increased signal intensity (*between arrows*), which correlated with a disrupted facet on CT

Fig. 4 a, b. Midsagittal MRI of the cervical spine after closed reduction of C5–6 subluxation. Interspinous ligament injury was unsuspected in **a**, an FSE-T2-weighted image without fat suppression. Abnormal increased signal in the interspinous spaces from C4–7 (*between arrows*) was clearly demonstrated on the fast-STIR image (**b**) and was thought to represent interspinous ligament injury. Note focal cord contusion (*black arrow*)

Results

Fat-suppressed FSE-T2 and STIR sequences showed the highest sensitivity in detecting liagmentous, facet and intervertebral disk injuries. Facet injury was detected on MRI as increased capsular signal (Fig. 1) and was often accompanied by fracture, joint space widening or dislocation. Using increased facet signal intensity as a marker of injury, MRI correctly identified 43/47 (91%) facet disruptions documented by CT. MRI accurately identified all 7 facet subluxations (Fig. 2), including two cases of bilateral locked facets and one unilateral perched facet, present at the time of MRI. High capsular signal was present in a total of 18 facet levels without CT or plain film evidence of injury. Two patients in this category had subsequently confirmed spine instability.

Anterior (ALL) and posterior (PLL) longitudinal ligaments appeared discontinuous (Fig. 3) or displaced (Fig. 2) when injured. A total of 7 ALL and 8 PLL disruptions were visualized; these lesions were commonly associated with vertebral body subluxation and disk herniation. Three liagmenetum flavum disruptions were detected.

Interspinous ligament (ISL) injuries appeared as focal areas of increased signal intensity within the interspinous space and were more conspicuous on images with fat suppression (Fig. 4). Abnormally high ISL signal was present at 24/26 (92%) cervical spine levels with documented subluxations, wide intervertebral disks or wide interspinous spaces. Diffuse high signal in the ligamentum nuchae/posterior soft tissue complex was common. Ruptured intervertebral disks appeared abnormally wide, demonstrated high signal intensity and were associated with vertebral body subluxations. CT was more effective in demonstrating osseous injuries.

Discussion

Occult cervical spine instability, secondary to traumatic disruption of osseous and ligamentous structures, may result in severe spinal cord injury. The ability of MRI to document potential ligamentous injury is important for appropriate patient care and therapeutic management. Information obtained from MRI concerning soft tissue injury complements plain film and CT imaging studies, which are superior to MRI for the evaluation of osseous injury.

This study demonstrates the value of MRI in detecting disruptions of cervical ligaments, facets and intervertebral disks in acute spine trauma. Fat-suppressed FSE-T2 and STIR pulse sequences are particularly useful in demonstrating subtle areas of increased soft tissue signal intensity, which may be used as a marker of ligamentous injury. Preliminary results indicate that MRI utilizing fat-suppression techniques can detect these injuries with a high degree of accuracy.

Implementation of fat-suppression techniques when imaging cervical spine trauma provides for a more sensitive evaluation of cervical soft tissue structures with only minor modifications in routine pulse sequence protocols and without increased imaging time or cost.

References

1. Silberstein M, Tress BM, Hennessy O (1992) Prediction of neurologic outcome in acute spinal cord injury: the role of CT and MRI. AJNR 13:1597–1608
2. Schaefer DM, Flanders AE, Osterholm IL, Northrup BE (1992) Prognostic significance of magnetic resonance imaging in the acute phase of cervical spine injury. J Neurosurg 76:218–223
3. Tien RD, Hesselink JR, Chu PK, Szumowski J (1991) Improved detection and delineation of head and neck lesions with fat suppression spin-echo imaging. AJNR 12:19–24
4. Georgy BA, Hesselink JR (1994) Evaluation of fat suppression in contrast-enhanced MR of neoplastic and inflammatory spine disease. AJNR 15:409–417

CT changes after conservative treatment for lumbar disc herniation

R. Dullerud, P. H. Nakstad

Section of Neuroradiology, Department of Radiology, Ullevaal University Hospital, N-0407 Oslo, Norway

Abstract. Follow-up CT of 106 pathological disks in 92 patients at a mean interval of 14 months after the initial examination revealed a strong association between the evolution of disc protrusions and clinical results, with a decrease in size of the majority of protrusions in successfully treated patients, whereas the others essentially remained unchanged ($P<0.0001$). A significantly higher proportion of large protrusions diminished as compared to the smaller ones ($P<0.0001$). Diffuse disc bulges were associated with a poor outcome and never regressed. There was a lower incidence of diminution of the central protrusions compared to other locations. Patients with normal disc spaces at the initial examination had better outcome than those with disc space narrowing. Only occasionally was a reduction of the disc space observed at follow-up.

Key words: Computed tomography – Disk protrusion – Physical therapy

Since the first CT demonstration of regression of a disc protrusion after conservative treatment in 1984 [1], several publications have documented that morphological change frequently accompanies the clinical improvement [2–7]. However, little attention has been paid to changes occurring in protrusions associated with a poor clinical outcome [2, 7]. The purpose of the present investigation was to assess changes occurring in the size of protrusions after conservative treatment and to correlate the changes to clinical and radiological parameters.

Correspondence to: R. Dullerud

Patients and methods

There were 92 patients with 106 herniated and bulging discs. Sixty-one of them (66%), 33 women and 28 men aged 20–68 years, mean age 38 years, with 73 pathological discs, had failed to respond to conservative treatment. The other 31 patients (34%), 16 women and 15 men, aged 20–65 years, mean age 42 years, with 33 pathological discs, had responded well to conservative means, such as analgesics, bed rest, physical therapy including traction and exercise. In both groups the patients were included consecutively without exclusions and had a CT follow-up with 6 continuous 5-mm slices through the discs and adjacent vertebra at a mean interval of 14 months after the initial examination.

Results

There was a higher incidence of large and very large protrusions in patients with a good outcome than in failures ($P<0.0001$). All 8 diffuse bulging discs were in patients with a poor outcome. The location of the protrusions was not significantly different in the two populations.

A higher incidence of narrow disc spaces was found in patients who failed to respond to the subsequent treatment, with only 25 of 73 disc spaces assessed to be normal ($P = 0.048$).

After treatment, the incidence of reduced and completely resolved protrusions was significantly higher ($P < 0.0001$) in patients with a good clinical outcome, with 26 of 33 reduced protrusions. In the symptomatic group, on the other hand, only 4 protrusions were reduced and 13 had increased in size, leaving 56 unchanged.

There was a strong association ($P < 0.0001$) between the initial size of the protrusion and alteration after treatment, with a reduction of the majority of the large and very large protrusions. Only 13% of the small protrusions reduced in size. Of the 13 protrusions that increased in size, 8 were originally small and 5 medium sized. There was a tendency towards a higher incidence of reduced size of noncontained protrusions than of the contained ones. The central protrusions were less inclined to diminish in size compared to those in other locations ($P = 0.031$). Four of the 8 diffuse bulging discs remained unchanged; the other 4 increased in size.

Discussion

Consistent with our findings, many authors have observed a reduction in size of the majority of lumbar disc protrusion on CT [3, 4] and MRI [2, 8] after successful conservative treatment. Based on 19 and 5 cases, respectively, two reports [2, 7] indicate, like our results, that a majority of protrusions remain unchanged or increase in size in therapeutic failures.

An association between the initial size of the protrusion and alteration after treatment has also been observed by others, with the largest decreasing most and having the greatest likelihood of total resolution [2–4, 7, 8]. In contrast, our results indicate that an increase in size is more likely to occur in small and medium-sized protrusions.

A less favourable outcome after conservative treatment in patients with disc space narrowing at the initial examination has, to our knowledge, not previously been reported.

References

1. Guinto FC Jr, Hashim H, Stumer M (1984) CT demonstration of disk regression after conservative therapy. AJNR 5:632–633
2. Bozzao A, Gallucci M, Masciocchi C, Aprile I, Barile A, Passariello R (1992) Lumbar disk herniation. MR imaging assessment of natural history in patients treated without surgery. Radiology 185:135–141
3. Bush H, Cowan N, Katz DE, Gishen P (1992) The natural history of sciatica associated with disc pathology. A prospective study with clinical and independent radiologic follow-up. Spine 17:1205–1212
4. Delauche-Cavallier MC, Budet C, Laredo JD, Debie B, Wybier M, Dorfmann H, Ballner I (1992) Lumbar disc herniation. Computed tomography scan changes after conservative treatment of nerve root compression. Spine 17:927–933
5. Fagerlund MKJ, Thelander U, Friberg S (1990) Size of lumbar disc hernias measured using computed tomography and related to sciatic symptoms. Acta Radiol 31:555–558
6. Köhler D, Langer M, Schultz U, Weiss T, Stäbler A (1989) Klinische und computertomographische Verlaufskontrollen konservativ behandelter Diskusvorfälle. Röntgen-Blätter 42:346–351
7. Maigne JY, Rime B, Deligne B (1992) Computed tomographic follow-up study of forty-eight cases of nonoperatively treated lumbar intervertebral disc herniation. Spine 17:1071–1074
8. Saal JA, Saal JS, Herzog RJ (1990) The natural history of lumbar intervertebral disc extrusions treated nonoperatively. Spine 15:683–686

MR myelography using a 2D-fast spin-echo pulse sequence: clinical evaluation including comparison with conventional myelography

S. Matsumoto [1], K. Hasuo [1], A. Mizushima [1], Y. Nakamura [1], A. Uchino [1], M. Oga [2], K. Masuda [1]

[1] Department of Radiology, Kyushu University Hospital, Fukuoka 812, Japan
[2] Department of Orthopedics, Kyushu University Hospital, Fukuoka 812, Japan

Abstract. Seventy-five patients (76 regions) with various spinal diseases underwent MR myelography (MRM) using the 2D-fast spin-echo (FSE) technique. In 52 lumbar examinations, overall image quality was excellent or good in the majority of cases. However, in 24 cervical or thoracic examinations, excellent or good images were obtained in only about one-third of cases. Twenty-eight cases were compared with conventional myelography (MG). In 20 lumbar examinations, MRM was superior to MG in 7, equal in 6 and inferior in 7. However, MRM was inferior to MG in 6, equal in 1 and superior in only 1 of 8 cervical and thoracic examinations. Therefore, MRM may replace MG in the lumbar region. In the cervical and thoracic regions, however, this technique is not satisfactory.

Correspondence to: Dr. S. Matsumoto

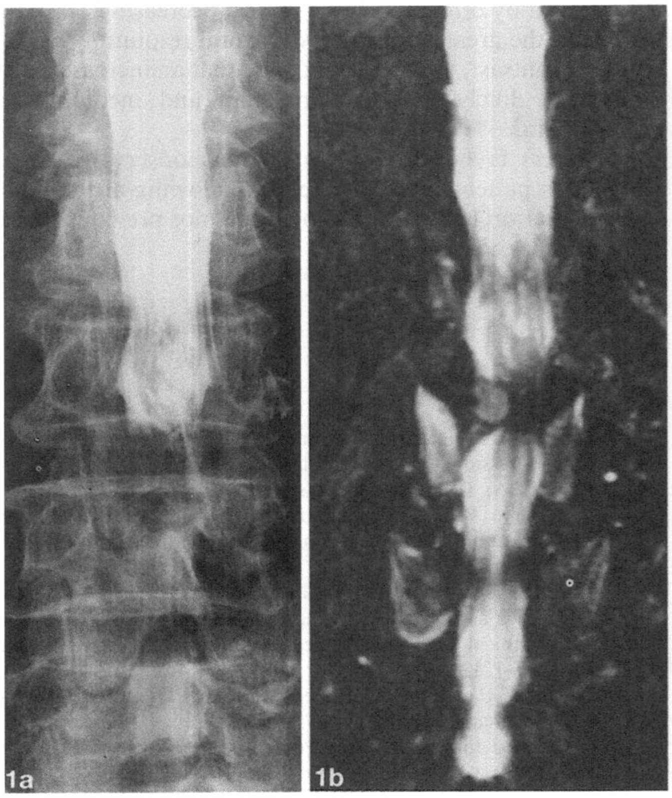

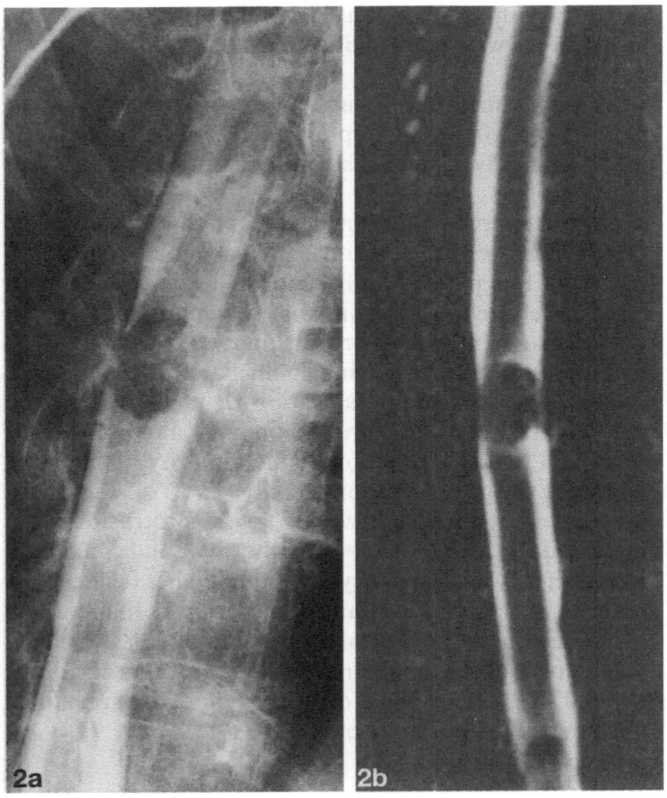

Fig. 1a, b. A 78-year-old woman with a synovial cyst. Anteroposterior myelogram (**a**) shows an extradural mass at L3–4. However, the opacification below L3 is not satisfactory and the margins of the lesion are not clearly defined. Coronal MIP MRM (**b**) shows the relationship between the extradural mass and the thecal sac more clearly. Paravertebral venous structures are also seen in **b**

Fig. 2a, b. A 73-year-old woman with a meningioma. Myelogram (**a**) clearly shows the irregular surface of the intradural-extramedullary mass. Left posterior oblique MRM (**b**) also demonstrates these findings; however, the surface irregularity is slighty less well shown than on the myelogram

Key words: Magnetic resonance imaging – Magnetic resonance myelography – Fast spin-echo pulse sequence – Myelography – Spinal diseases

Myelographic images of the thecal sac can be made by heavily T2-weighted images; however, conventional spin-echo (SE) techniques require a long scanning time. A fast spin-echo (FSE) technique has made it possible to obtain such myelographic images within several minutes [1, 2]. Therefore, we evaluated the clinical usefulness and limitations of MRM in the diagnosis of spinal diseases to clarify the clinical efficacy of MRM.

Materials and methods

Seventy-five patients (76 regions) with various spinal diseases, including 37 spondylosis deformans, 23 disk hernias/disk degenerations, 9 spinal tumours and 7 other diseases, underwent MRM.

Table 1. Image quality on MR and conventional myelography

a Lumbar examination (20 cases)

	Excellent	Good	Fair	Poor
MR myelography				
Thecal sac	15	5	0	0
Nerve root	12	7	1	0
Lesion	13	6	1	0
Conventional myelography				
Thecal sac	16	2	2	0
Nerve root	10	8	2	0
Lesion	12	7	1	0

b Cervical or thoracic examination (8 cases)

	Excellent	Good	Fair	Poor
MR myelography				
Thecal sac	2	5	1	0
Nerve root	1	3	4	0
Lesion	1	4	2	1
Conventional myelography				
Thecal sac	5	3	0	0
Nerve root	4	3	1	0
Lesion	3	5	0	0

c Overall evaluation of MRM and MG

	MRM > MG	MRM = MG	MRM < MG
Lumbar (20)	7	6	7
Cervical or thoracic (8)	1	1	6

There were 38 men and 37 women, aged 20–90 years (mean: 55.5 years). Twenty-seven patients (28 regions) also underwent myelography (MG). A 1.5-T imager was used for image acquisition. A two-dimensional (2D) FSE sequence with a 16-echo train was used with 5500/240–255 (TR/TE), 3-mm slice thickness, no interslice gap, 256×256 or 256×192 matrix, 2 excitations, and a 16-cm or a 24-cm field of view. Fat presaturation and the no phase-wrap technique were also used. Coronal individual images and maximum-intensity projection (MIP) images were routinely obtained in all cases. Oblique sagittal images were also obtained in the majority of cases. The image quality was evaluated according to the following parameters: delineation of thecal sac; delineation of nerve roots; lesion delineation. Comparison with MG was also made.

Results

Image quality of MRM

In 52 lumbar examinations, excellent or good images were obtained in the majority of cases (50 for thecal sac and nerve roots, and 43 for lesion delineation). In 24 cervical and thoracic examinations, however, excellent images were obtained in only 10 cases (6 for thecal sac, 1 for nerve roots and 3 for lesion delineation). The delineation of nerve roots was especially poor when compared with lumbar MRMs.

Comparison of MRM and MG (Table 1)

In 20 lumbar examinations, MRM was superior to MG in 7 (Fig. 1), equal in 6 and inferior in 7. Delineation of the thecal sac, nerve roots and lesion was excellent or good on both MRM and MG in the majority of cases. The thecal sac and the nerve root sheath, distal to the spinal block, were better delineated on MRM than on MG. In contrast, MRM was inferior to MG in 6 (Fig. 2), equal in 1 and superior in only 1 of 8 cervical and thoracic examinations. MRM was definetely inferior to MG in the delineation of the thecal sac, the nerve roots and the lesion.

Discussion

MRM can provide high-quality images in the lumbar region. The major advantage of MRM over MG is excellent delineation of the thecal sac and nerve roots, irrespective of the presence or absence of spinal block [2]. The signals from paravertebral vessels may be troublesome in evaluating the nerve root sheath, but it can be diagnosed without difficulty by adding oblique MRM. In the 2D-FSE technique, evaluation of the nerve root is not satisfactory using coronal MRM alone, so oblique sagittal images are needed in the majority of cases. In cervical and thoracic regions, however, MRM is less useful. Although the margins of the thecal sac are visible, compression of the thecal sac or nerve root is poorly delineated. Signal loss in the cervical and thoracic regions is probably due to higher flow and relatively lower quantities of CSF, compared to the lumbar region [2]. In summary, MRM using the 2D-FSE technique may replace MG in the lumbar region. In the cervical and thoracic regions, this technique is not satisfactory. 3D techniques and flow-compensation techniques may be required in order to obtain better images and minimize the flow artefacts.

References

1. Friedburg H, Henning J, Schumacher M (1987) Clinical application of RARE-MR myelography as a routine MR examination: experience with 175 cases. Fortschr Roentgenstr 146:584–590
2. Adrian GK (1992) MR myelography using heavily T2-weighted fast spin-echo pulse sequences with fat presaturation. AJR 159:1315–1320

Magnetization transfer 3D MR radiculography

I. Berry [1,2], J. M. Franconi [3], C. Manelfe [1,4], Ph. Arrué [4], P. Hollenbach [5], F. Châ [1], M. Thorn-Kany [4], A. Bonafé [1]

[1] Neuroradiology, University Hospital Purpan, Toulouse, France
[2] Biophysics, University Hospital Rangueil, Toulouse, France
[3] Siemens, Saint-Denis, France
[4] Neuroradiology, University Hospital Rangueil, Toulouse, France
[5] Siemens, UB Med, Erlangen, Germany

Abstract. Three-dimensional MR radiculography is achievable in less than 11 min with magnetization transfer radiofrequency pulses for further suppression of unwanted paravertebral signals. Visualization of the thecal sac and dural sheaths is adequate and this technique may be competitive to X-ray radiculography, although so far the later is the only technique permitting dynamic studies. This technique was used in ten patients suffering from lumbar degenerative disease.

Correspondence to: I. Berry, Service de Neuroradiologie, Hôpital Purpan, F 31059 Toulouse, France

Key words: Magnetic resonance imaging – Myelography – Magnetization transfer – Lumbar spine – Degenerative disc disease

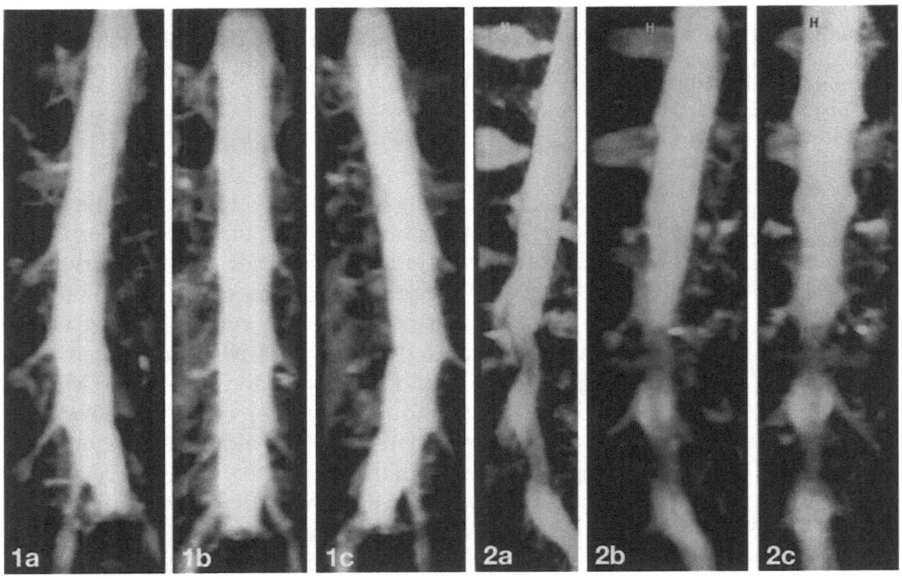

Fig. 1 a–c. Normal MR radiculography. **a** Left nerve roots; **b** coronal reconstruction; **c** right nerve roots. Excellent separation of dural sheaths emerging from the dural sac

Fig. 2 a–c. Narrow lumbar canal a 64-year-old man with claudication of the lower limbs. Saggital (**a**) oblique, (**b**) and coronal (c) reconstructions. Constitutionally narrow lumbar canal is further accentuated by L3–4 and L4–5 stenosis impinging on the thecal sac and lateral recesses. At these levels turbulence decreases the signal of CSF on both T2-weighted images and on MR radiculography. The nerve root sheaths were not seen to be compressed in the foramina on T1- and T2-weighted sequences and MR radiculography confirmed adequate visualization of the dural sheaths

Three-dimensional magnetic resonance imaging (3D MRI) is now routinely used with the widespread availability of fast sequences. The multiplanar reformation capabilities are extremely interesting and allow for visualization of various projections in the postprocessing phase. Radiculography can be obtained from magnetic resonance without any contrast enhancement if sequences selectively enhancing the signal of the cerebrospinal fluid (CSF) are designed. This was achieved in our system by P. Hollenbach. To produce a bright signal intensity of cerebrospinal fluid in the thecal sac we combined a steady-state gradient echo fast 3D sequence (FISP) and magnetization transfer radio-frequency pulses [1, 2] used to decrease the signal of all components except fluid. The parameters of the FISP sequence are optimized for maximum reduction of T1 contrast and enhancement of T2 contrast (small flip angle and relatively long TR for a 3D acquisition). The dataset is subsequently treated with maximum intensity projection algorithm to further select the brighter signals.

Materials and methods

Ten patients were examined with MR radiculography, 8 men and 2 women aged 36–76 years old (mean age: 58.8 years). Clinical presentation was lumbar pain (1 case), neurological claudication (6 cases), and sciatica (3 cases).

Examinations were performed at 1.5 Tesla. Conventional T1- and T2-weighted sagittal and axial imaging was obtained prior to MR radiculography with a turbo-spin-echo technique. T1-weighted images were 4-mm-thick, high resolution (matrix 168 × 512, FOV 188 × 300) slices with TR 788 and TE 12 ms, 4 excitations (acquisition time 3 min). T2-weighted images were also 4 mm thick and high-resolution (matrix 224 × 512, FOV 263 × 300) slices with TR 4000 and TE 96 ms, 1 excitation (acquisition time 4 min 25 s).

Optimization of MR radiculography was achieved with the following parameters: FISP gradient echo (remaining transverse magnetization not destroyed prior to the repeated radiofrequency pulse) TR 79 ms, TE 21 ms, flip angle 7°, 5-cm-thick slab, 32 sagittal partitions (1.56 mm reconstructed slices), bandwidth of data sampling: 33 Hz/pixel, field of view 300 in a rectangular data matrix (192 phase encoding steps × 256 frequency encoding steps in the readout direction), 1 excitation, acquisition time 10 min 47 s. Magnetization transfer was produced by an off-resonance radiofrequency pulse (duration 7.,68 ms, gaussian shaped, offset 1.5 KHz downfield from free water resonance frequency, bandwidth 500 Hz). Cerebrospinal fluid flow compensation and a prevertebral coronal radiofrequency saturation slab were also used to further eliminate artefacts. Twelve projections were reconstructed from one sagittal view through coronal to the other sagittal.

The ten examinations were classified to their image quality: excellent, good, average and poor.

Results

Magnetization transfer markedly decreases the signal of the perivertebral tissues and allows for an excellent radiculographic effect on 3D MRI (Fig. 1). Image quality was excellent in 5 cases, good in 2 cases and average in 3 cases.

The calibre of the dural canal is well appreciated (Fig. 2). Nevertheless, the degree of stenosis seems to be somewhat overestimated by flow artefacts. In 7 cases the delineation of the nerve roots and radicular dural sheaths is superior on MR radiculography as compared to conventional T1- and T2-weighted sequences. In 3 cases, nerve roots and dural sheaths are not adequately seen in relation to average quality of the data.

Optimization of the MR radiculography produced absence of signal in the vertebral bodies that do not superimpose on the thecal sac. On the other hand, signal coming from the annulus and outer nucleus is better seen and allows interesting delineation of disk compromise of the radicular dural sheaths. Finally, the paravertebral venous structures are visualized and superimpose onto the signal of the radiculography.

Discussion

MR radiculography obtains images similar to X-ray after intrathecal injection of water-soluble contrast medium. The advantages are its noninvasiveness and acquisition time limited to less than 11 min. The 3D reconstruction algorithm permits an interesting display of the dataset with several projections. Dynamic display on the MR-console may be achieved in the cine mode and allows for careful study of the thecal sac and dural sheaths under various incidences. Dural sac compressions and impingements on dural sheaths are adequately visualized. In 7/10 cases, the quality of their delineation is better than conventional T1- and T2-weighted sequences.

When CSF turbulences occur, particularly in the case of stenosis, they produce dephasing and lower signal intensity. This may overestimate the degree of stenosis on MR radiculography (Fig. 2). Nevertheless, this problem is limited by comparison with morphological images.

The diagnostic capabilities are increased by the absence of signal of the vertebral bodies, which do not superimpose on the thecal sac, and the persistence of signal coming from the annulus and outer nucleus showing disk conflicts with the radicular dural sheaths.

On the other hand, dynamic studies are not achievable contrary to conventional-radiculography where standing and flexion/extension studies can be performed.

Several groups have already described radiculographic images obtained with MRI. For example, the PSIF sequence (CE Fast) allows for highly T2-weighted images in which cerebrospinal fluid is very intense [3]. These techniques use stimulated echos (spin-echos), which are not influenced by magnetic susceptibility differences between tissues, but achieve only a limited signal-to-noise ratio inherent to this type of sequence which samples stimulated echos. The sequence we used here is based on gradient echos (FISP) with steady-state of both longitudinal and transverse magnetizations. Zero-order refocusing in the slice selection, readout and phase encoding directions are added, as well as first-order flow compensation in the readout direction. The narrow bandwidth (33 Hz/pixel) improves signal-to-noise ratio. Although the gradient-echo technique (FISP) is more sensitive to magnetic susceptibility artefacts than a spin-echo technique, like PSIF, it is not an issue here because of the small voxel size obtained with the 3D acquisition. Indeed, it did not interfere with our application, although the lumbar spine presents many interfaces.

The optimized parameters (small flip angle i.e. 7°, long TR) decrease the T1 weighting of the contrast and enhance T2-weighted effect with bright cerebrospinal fluid signal.

The magnetization transfer radiofrequency pulse decreases the signal of tissues that contain macromolecules accessible to free water (i.e. muscles). On the other hand, the signal of fluids (i.e. cerebrospinal fluid) and fat is minimally decreased. The bright signal of fat will subsequently be further reduced with the use of a selective radiofrequency pulse, centered on the resonance frequency of fat. Preliminary assessment of such saturation pulse shows improvement of the quality of the radiculography. It reduces the signal of the fatty marrow of the vertebral bodies without increased radiofrequency power deposition in the patient over the tolerance limits.

One of the remaining problems is the persistent visualization of the veins that superimpose on the lumbar structures in the 3D data set. They appear very bright because they benefit from the flow compensation pulse applied for enhancement of the signal of cerebrospinal fluid. Additionally, the signal of slowly flowing blood is not affected, and therefore cannot be decreased, either by magnetization transfer or by fat saturation. Non-selective radiofrequency saturation pulse, used as an example to decrease motion artefact generated by moving structures, cannot suppress their signal because the blood does not originate from a limited number of feeders. On the other hand, visualization of the epidural venous plexuses and their displacements are diagnostic information that may be of importance in the discussion of subtle epidural compression.

References

1. Wolff SD, Balaban RS (1989) Magnetisation transfer contrast (MTC) and tissue water proton relaxation in vivo. Magn Reson Med 10:135–144
2. Balaban RS, Ceckler TL (1992) Magnetization transfer contrast in magnetic resonance imaging. Magn Reson Q 8:116–117
3. Schnarkowski P, Wallner B, Goldmann A, Friedrich JM (1993) MR-myelographie der Lendenwirbelsäule mit einer PSIF-Sequenz: erste Erfahrungen. Aktuelle Radiol 3:53–56

Gd-DTPA enhancement of herniated discs: its pathological meaning and influence on prognosis

M. Gallucci[1], **A. Bozzao**[1], **R. J. Galzio**[2], **A. Ricci**[2], **T. Ventura**[3], **G. Calvisi**[3], **E. Ferone**[1], **C. Micheli**[1]

[1] Department of Radiology, University of L'Aquila, I-67100 L'Aquila, Italy
[2] Department of Neurosurgery, Teramo, Italy
[3] Department of Pathology, ULSS, L'Aquila, Italy

Abstract. An MRI-pathological correlation was obtained in 15 disc herniations from 15 patients undergoing surgery. The study showed that when peridiscal enhancement was evident on MRI, granulation tissue with macrophagic cells was present histopathologically. Disc fragment infiltration by this tissue appeared as diffuse enhancement of the disc itself on MRI. High signal on T2-weighted images was related to hyperhydration of the fragment. These data indicate that high signal on T2-weighting and peridiscal enhancement are features typical of the first phases of disc herniation.

Key words: Disc herniation – Magnetic resonance imaging

Spontaneous reduction of lumbar disc herniation and back pain or sciatica in conservatively treated patients has been widely described [1, 2]. However, there is still little known about the mechanisms of reduction of disc herniation. Dehydration and phagocytosis have been suggested as possible causes of disc material reduction [1]. The observation of epidural enhancement associated with disc herniation and the presence of newly formed vessels in the periphery of herniated disc material corroborate the hypothesis that epidural inflammation may be potentially relevant in the evolution of disc herniation [3]. We performed a perspective follow-up MRI study in 15 patients with diagnosed disc herniation. All MRI examinations were performed using Gd-DTPA. All the patients were operated upon and histopathology was performed on disc material.

Patients and methods

Fifteen patients with lumbar disc herniation were studied by MRI before and after Gd-DTPA administration. The patients underwent surgery within 36 h of the study. The surgically removed disc material was immediately fixed in formalin solution and examined by a pathologist to explain the T2-weighted signal charges and the type of enhancement.

Results

In all cases nice correlations were found between the T2-signal intensity obtained on SE, sequences and the hydration (mucopolysaccharide content) of the discs

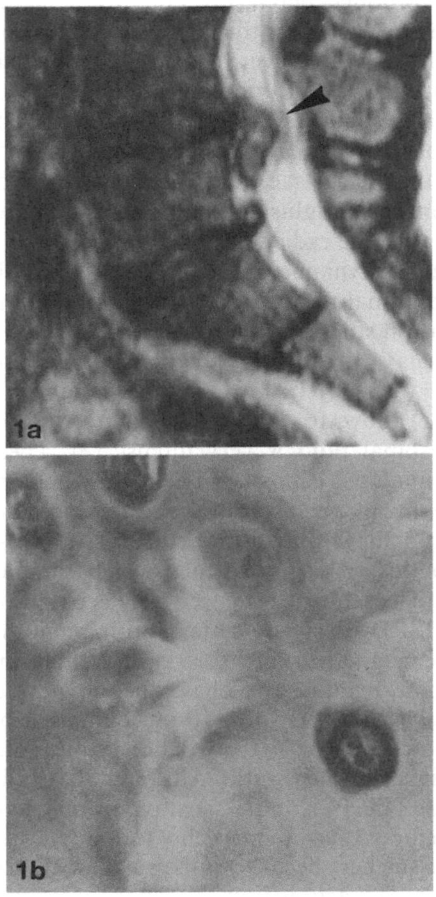

Fig. 1. Disc protrusion giving high signal (**a** *arrow*) on T1-weighted image. Histological examination (**b**) demonstrates highly hydrated mucopolysaccharide material

(Fig. 1). Low signal material appears less hydrated and prevalently constituted by fibrous structure (3 cases), while high signal correlated on histopathology with highly hydrated mucopolysaccharide material. Three different behaviours after contrast administration were found and attributed to corresponding anatomical patterns.

1. No disc enhancement (3 cases): little or no inflammatory response; macrophages few or absent
2. Peridiscal enhancement (8 cases): inflammatory response, peripheral to the disc, mostly evident in acute phases (Fig. 2)
3. Diffuse discal enhancement (4 cases): inflammatory infiltration of the herniated material, with abundant macrophages

Correspondence to: M. Gallucci

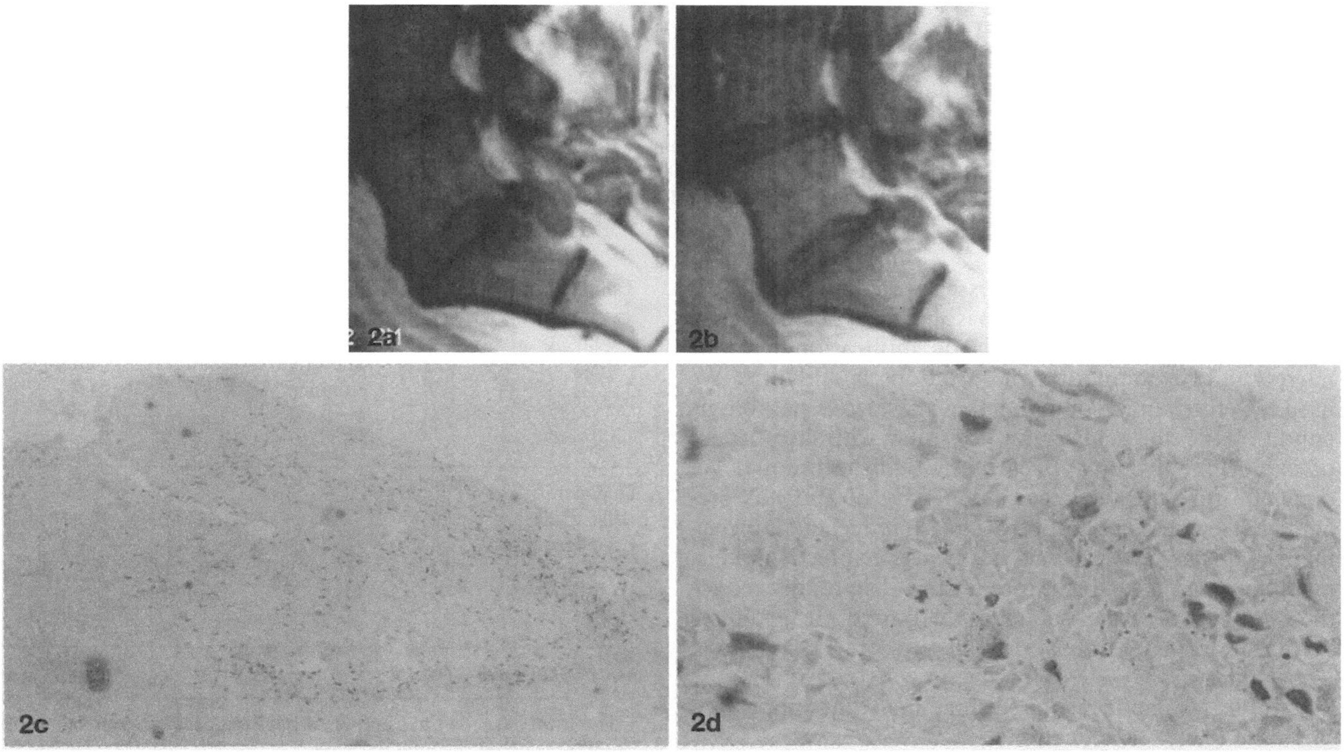

Fig. 2. MRI of an extruded fragment before and after Gd-DTPA, showing evident enhancement surrounding the disk fragment (**a, b**). Histology (**c, d**) (low and high magnification) shows newly formed vessels with pigmented macrophages infiltrating the disc fragment itself

Discussion

Recent studies emphasize the possibility of spontaneous reduction of disc herniations [1–3]. The mechanisms of this reduction are still unknown [4]. Dehydration and shrinkage of the disk material, refraction of the disc into the annulus and fragmentation have been advocated as possibly being responsible. Since MRI has been considered able to identify possible prognostic patterns in the evolution of disc herniation (high signal on T2-weighting and peridiscal enhancement), we performed a perspective MRI study in 15 patients suffering from disc herniation who underwent surgery. All MRI studies were performed after i.v. injection of Gd-DTPA. This allowed us to assess epidural inflammatory tissue, known from other studies to cause peridiscal enhancement

Our data confirmed the assumption that the high signal intensity on T2-weighted images in disk fragments is related to hyperhydration, thus suggesting the acute onset of the disease. Although impossible to demonstrate in our patient population (since all underwent surgery), this could represent only the acute and transient phase of the disease. Peridiscal enhancement, known to be present from other studies [5] and observed in 8 of our cases, was mostly related to the presence of granulation tissue and newly formed vessels around the disc fragment. These data have also been reported by other pathological studies [6], indicating that the vessels in the periphery of herniated disc material are newly formed around the extruded tissue. The role of this tissue in the evolution of the disc fragment is debatable, although it could indicate the first phase of an active reaction towards the disc fragment.

The diffuse enhancement observed in 4 cases could be an expression of the process of disc fragment infiltration since it was found in cases in which histopathology demonstrated the presence of macrophages and granulation tissue inside the disc fragment itself. In 3 cases no enhancement was observed around disc material. In these cases no inflammatory tissue was evident around the disc material; the disc fragment also showed a more fibrous structure than in the other specimens. A possible explanation of this might be related to the presence of an "old" disc herniation with exacerbation of symptoms (anatomically old and clinically new disc herniation).

References

1. Bozzao A, Gallucci M, Masciocchi C, Aprile I, Barile A, Passariello R (1992) Lumbar disk herniation: MR imaging assessment of natural history in patients treated without surgery. Radiology 185:135–141
2. Bush K, Cowan N, Katz DE, Gishen P (1992) Spine 17:1205–1212
3. Gallucci M, Bozzao A, Orlandi O, et al (in press) Enhanced MR in lumbar disk herniation. Is there a prognostic role? Comput Assist Tomogr
4. Lindblom K, Hultqvist G (1950) Absorption of protruded disc tissue. J Bone Joint Surg [Am] 32:557–560
5. Ross JS, Modic MT, Masaryk TJ, Cater J, Marcus RE, Bohlman H (1990) Assessment of extradural degenerative disease with Gd-DTPA-enhanced MR imaging: correlation with surgical and pathologic findings. AJNR 10:1243–1249
6. Yasuma T, Arai K, Yamauchi Y (1993) The histology of lumbar intervertebral disc herniation. The significance of small vessels in the extruded tissue. Spine 18:1761–1765

Fat-suppressed MRI in spinal disease

A. E. Rosenbaum[1], S. F. Yu[1], C. S. Collins[2], M. C. Formikell[2], S. E. Joy[1], R. S. Caruso[1], J. K. Chang[1]

[1] MR Research Laboratory and Neuroradiology Division, Department of Radiology, SUNY Health Science Center as Syracuse, 750 E. Adams Street, Syracuse, NY 12310, USA
[2] MR/CT of Syracuse, 550 Harrison Stree, Suite 125, Syracuse, NY 13202, USA

Abstract. The use of fat-suppressed spinal imaging (FSI) has so far been limited largely to isolation of postoperative scarring, assessment of neoplastic infiltration of bone narrow, and examination of infections spondylitis. We used FSI to examine 40 patients with various pathologic conditions of different sections of spine, with the purpose of exploring further applications of the technique. We conclude that the technical complexity of FSI has precluded its wider use hitherto and that recent improvements to the software and hardware involved make it much more manageable. Since it can substantially reduce the number of MRI sequences required, it promises savings in terms of time and of direct cost.

Key words: Magnetic resonance imaging - Fat-suppressed spinal imaging - Applications

Despite the capacity of MRI to separate aliphatic from water protons readily by use of a presaturation offset pulse to suppress fat, fat-suppressed spinal imaging (FSI) has largely been applied to isolating postoperative scarring from residual or recurrent disc material [1–3], assessing neoplastic infiltration of bone marrow [4–6], and investigating infectious spondylitis [4]. Our purpose was to explore additional applications for FSI in the spine.

Materials and methods

We examined 40 patients using 1.5-T imagers: Intravenous contrast enhancement was used in 38 patients employing fat-suppressed (FS) T1-weighted sequences while in 2 a T2-weighted FS sequence was used without contrast medium. The patients' age range was 9–78 years, the majority (31) being 30–49 years of age. There were 24 men and 16 women. The spinal regions examined were lumbar (36), thoracic (2), and cervical (2).

Intravenous contrast enhancement at 0.1 mmol/kg was with a gadolinium-chelate (gadopentetate dimeglumine) with imaging performed immediately thereafter with a conventional T1-weighted sequence followed by a T1-weighted sequence with a fat-saturation pulse. The majority of our patients, 28/40, were examined following discectomy; this was the usual indication for intravenous enhancement. The specific fat-saturation pulse used was determined empirically/visually following prescanning interrogation of the spinal region. In the Siemens FSI menu, offset frequencies vary from −600 Hz to +50 Hz at 50-Hz intervals (14 steps); −250 or −300 Hz was the RF pulse usually selected. With the 63 SP system, the additional time required for shimming, tuning, and selection of the "appropriately saturated" preliminary imaging from the prescan profile prolonged the image process by at least 5 min before the actual fat-saturated sequence could be initiated. To reduce the overall FS examination time, the matrix size was reduced to 192×256 for the majority of cases.

Correspondence to: A. E. Rosenbaum

Table 1. Findings in spinal fat-suppressed MRI

Diagnosis	Patients	Postoperative enhancement (%)	End-plate changes (%)	End-zone changes (%)
Degenerative disc disease	20	17 (85)	11 (55)	9 (45)
Disc herniation	4	2 (50)	1 (25)	3 (75)
Scarring	12	12 (100)	5 (42)	4 (33)
Neoplasm	3	0	3 (100)	2 (67)
Other	7	2 (28)	0	2 (40)
Total[a]	46	33	17	20

[a] The total exceeds the number of patients because more than one finding occurred in some patients

Results

Diagnostic quality imaging was obtained in 38 of the 40 patients, both with T1-weighted parameters and with gadolinium enhancement. Two examinations were judged unsatisfactory because of shimming/tuning difficulties resulting in images (Figs. 4, 5) that contained much less morphologic detail than the unsuppressed images, especially where larger quantities of adjacent air were present: lung with respect to the thoracic spine and trachea on cervical imaging. The disease processes examined were reduced to five categories (Table 1).

Discussion

New and additional information

Presuming a merit of advancement in methodology is based on its supplying new information, FSI complies readily in degenerative disc disease. An instance of this was the unanticipated frequency of peridiscal enhancement, i.e., contrast enhancement in the region of the cartilaginous end-plates, immediately superficial to the vertebral body end-plate. This subtle imaging information advances pathogenetic microscopic and biochemical evidence of altered vascularization and metaplasia of the end-plates and the resultant cartilaginous end-plate reception of nutrients. This increased "permeability" to the contrast medium is demonstrable in degenerative disc disease (Fig. 1), which the peridiscal vertebral body metaplastic changes [7] that occur (fibrovascular, fatty, and bony) [8, 9], are also better demonstrated by FSI (Fig. 1);

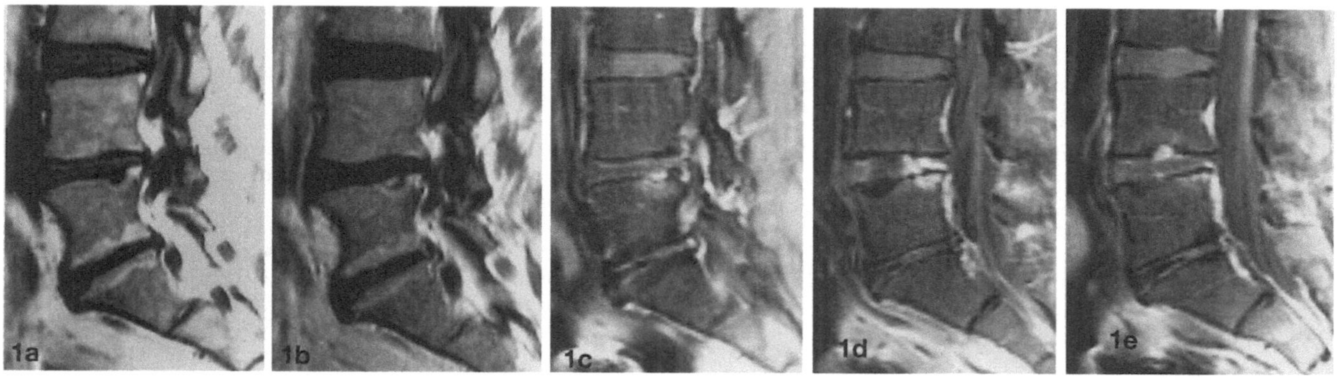

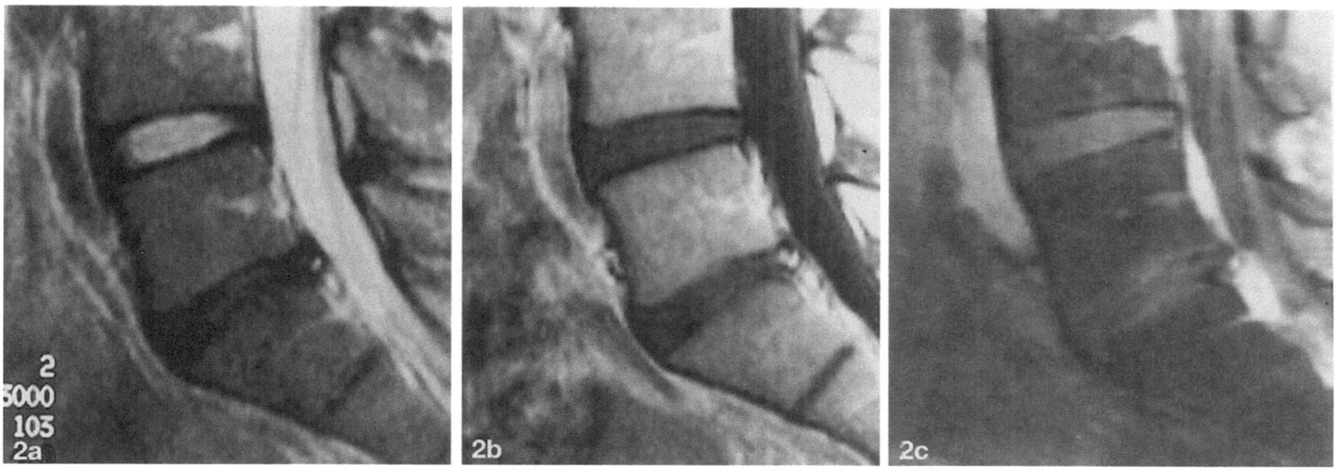

Fig. 1a–e. Multiple findings in lumbar disc degeneration. A 40-year-old man with chronic low back pain and prior L4–5 and L5–S1 disc surgery. **a** Sagittal T1-weighted image. Extensive fatty replacement of the marrow of the end-zones of L5–S1 is present (MSR type II); the operated discs are reduced in height. The superior end-plate of L5 shows a Schmorl's node. **b** There is contrast enhancement of portions of the Schmorl's node and perhaps also along its "fat-replaced" perimeter. **c** Fat-suppressed contrast-enhanced T1-weighted image. The Schmorl's node enhances intensely and beyond its perimeter there is also considerable enhancement. At L5–S1 there is extensive "bivalve" enhancement of the degenerate disc with a vacuum phenomenon anteriorly between the enhancing "valves"; the residual disc tissue, and the end-plate betweeen the gas and the vertebral body are well shown. Note the fat suppression of the L5 and S1 end-zones. A posterior annular tear also enhances. **d** Extensive contrast enhancement of the L4–5 posterior annulus relates to previous surgical exploration. A thin band of anterior disc enhancement is seen. Again, the low signal of the suppressed fat of the L5 end-zone is clearly seen. **e** A second Schmorl's node involving L4 inferiorly also enhances intensely. The end-zone adjacent to the node enhances subtly while thin enhancement of the L5 end-zone superiorly and posteriorly, and of the region of the opposite end-plates of L4–5 is evident

Fig. 2a–c. New information regarding a surgical scar. **a** Sagittal T2-weighted image. The L5–S1 posterior annular tear is discrete within the protruding disc. **b** The tear enhances and has two discrete portions. **c** With fat-suppression the L5–S1 disc is seen to enhance mildly, but diffusely. The annular tear is shown to enhance, but the low signal of hemosiderin along the superior and inferior portion of the curetted disc becomes very evident

the complexity shown by mixed fibrovascular (modic type I) and fatty metaplasia (type II) patterns is well seen using FSI. St. Amour et al. [10] indicate that marginal enhancement occurs in Schmorl's nodes (Fig. 1a–c), but FSI shows that the metaplastic changes as demonstrated by contrast enhancement are broader (Fig. 1c).

Another unanticipated finding was extensive vascularization of the fibrous septum adjacent to the bony spike in diastematomyelia. Scar detail (Fig. 2), nerve root enhancement both normal (subtle) and pathologic, and improved capsular definition of a mass of tuberculous spondylitis were shown.

Technical considerations

We believe the reason FSI has not been more widely used is its technical complexity to date: the need in some MRI systems to integrate multiple programming menus, non-automated or nonsubstantial shimming, problems in obtaining body part isocentricity of the region to be saturated, and intrinsic magnetic susceptibility variations among subjects. Recently released hard- and software advances in MRI accomplish multiaxis shimming and respond to the other difficulties enabling rapid high-quality FSI at the touch of a button, key, or plasma screen.

Economic considerations

In spinal imaging, contrast-enhanced T1-weighted FSI can obviate the need for conventional contrast-enhanced imaging. Moreover, in the clinical dilemma of postoperative scarring versus recurrent disc herniation, the sole MRI sequences it may be necessary to obtain is contrast-enhanced FSI. This could markedly reduce the time required for and cost engendered by MRI.

References

1. Bobman SA, Atlas SW, Listerud J, Grossman RI (1991) Postoperative lumbar spine: contrast-enhanced chemical shift MR imaging. Radiology 179:577–562
2. Mirowitz SA, Shady KL (1992) Gadopentetate dimeglumine-enhanced MR imaging of the postoperative lumbar spine: comparison of fat-suppressed and conventional T1-weighted images. AJR 159:385–389
3. Simon JH, Rubinstein D (1994) Contrast-enhanced fat suppression neuroimaging. Neuroimaging Clin North Am X:153–173
4. Georgy BA, Hesselink JR (1994) Evaluation of fat suppression in contrast-enhanced MR of neoplastic and inflammatory spine disease. AJNR 15:409–417
5. Rahmouni A, Divine M, Mathieu D, Golli M, et al (1993) Detection of multiple myeloma involving the spine: efficacy of fat-suppression and contrast-enhanced MR imaging. AJR 160:1049–1052
6. Jones KM, Schwartz RB, Mantello MT, Ahn SS, et al (1994) Fast spin-echo MR in the detection of vertebral metastases: comparison of three sequences. AJNR 15:401–407
7. Schmorl G, Junghanns H (1959) The human spine in health and disease. Grune & Stratton, New York, p 188
8. Modic MT, Steinberg PM, Ross JS, et al (1988) Degenerative disk disease: assessment of changes in vertebral body marrow with MR imaging. Radiology 166:193–199
9. Modic MT (1994) Degenerative disorders of the spine. In: Modic MT, Masaryk TJ, Ross JS (eds) Magnetic resonance imaging of the spine. Mosby, St. Louis, pp 88–150
10. St Amour TE, Hodges SC, Laakman RW, Tamas DE (1994) MRI of the spine. Raven Press, New York, pp 35; 569

Recurrent disc herniation versus scar: triple- versus single-dose gadoteridol

S. W. Horowitz, B. Azar-Kia, M. Fine, K. Goldberg

Department of Radiology, Section of Neuroradiology, Loyola University Medical Center, 2160 S 1st Ave., Maywood, IL 60153, USA

Abstract. We carried out MRI to evaluate possible recurrent herniated nucleus pulposus (HNP) before and after i.v. infusion of 0.1 mmol/kg gadoteridol, immediately followed by an additional 0.2 mmol/kg and repeat imaging in 21 patients. In comparison with standard 0.1 mmol/kg gadoteridol, images at a cumulative 0.3 mmol/kg demonstrated increased epidural enhancement, increased enhancement of intradural and affected S1 nerve roots. The level of certainty in MRI diagnosis of recurrent HNP at 0.3 mmol/kg was decreased in 5, increased in 1, and unchanged in 4 patients compared with standard dose. The triple dose was not advantageous for identification of recurrent HNP, owing to the increased peridiscal and S1 nerve root enhancement, which masked the displaced S1 nerve root and decreased the conspicuity of HNP.

Key words: Magnetic resonance imaging – Contrast enhancement – Spine

---

MRI before and after i.v. contrast medium is best to evaluate recurrent HNP in post-laminectomy patients [1–3]. Epidural scar tissue enhances, contrasting with HNP that does not enhance or enhances to a lesser extent than scar. In an experimental dog model, a triple dose of i.v. MRI contrast medium, viz. 0.3 mmol/kg, showed greater intensity of scar than disc enhancement, providing greater conspicuity of the disc fragment than at standard dose [4].

As far as we know, the use of triple-dose MRI contrast medium to diagnose postoperative recurrent HNP in humans has not been studied, to our knowledge. The purpose of this study was to see whether differentiation of recurrent HNP from scar would be better with 0.3 mmol/kg of gadoteridol i.v. than with the 0.1 mmol/kg dose.

Patients and methods

We studied 21 consecutive patients with a history of lumbar laminectomy or microdiscectomy using a 1.5 T imager. Of the 21 patients, 11 were male and 10 were female; the average age was 49 years. The time since prior surgery ranged from 9 days to 25 years, with a mean of 6 years. Protocol included preinfusion sagittal T1-weighted, sagittal fast spin echo T2-weighted, and axial T1-weighted sequences. Postinfusion T1-weighted sagittal and axial sequences were obtained immediately after 0.1 mmol/kg gadoteridol i.v. Immediately after image acquisition, an additional 0.2 mmol/kg gadoteridol i.v. was followed by T1-weighted axial and sagittal sequences. The time needed for each T1-weighted sequence was approximately 5 min. Analysis by visual qualitative inspection included grading of the extent of enhancing epidural fibrosis (none mild, moderate, or severe) and intensity (mild, moderate, or very bright). Diagnostic certainty of HNP on MR was graded as possible, probable, or definite by the neuroradiologist. Criteria for recurrent HNP included posterior protrusion of nonenhancing disc material (frequently with a rim of enhancing peridiscal fibrosis), mass effect on the thecal sac, and nerve root displacement.

Correspondence to: S. W. Horowitz

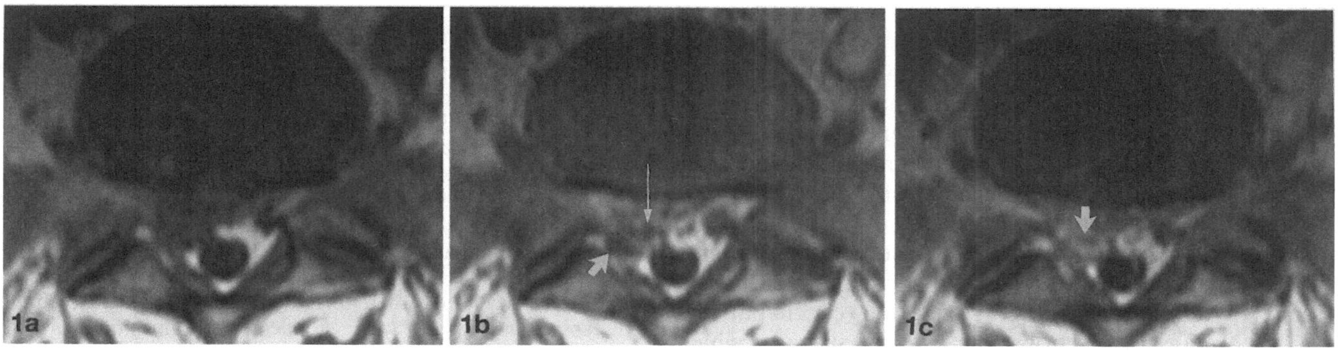

Fig. 1a–c. Patient with L5-S1, right laminectomy 3 years before. **a** Unenhanced T1-weighted image (TR 450, TE 11). **b** Following injection of 0.1 mmol/kg gadoteridol, the axial image shows posterior displacement of right S1 nerve root (*short arrow*) by surgically confirmed low-signal HNP (*long arrow*) surrounded by enhancing fibrotic scar. **c** Triple-dose-enhanced axial T1-weighted image fails to show the right S1 nerve root, due to its enhancement blending with that of peridiscal scar. Decreased conspicuity of the low-signal disc (*arrow*) within the enhancing scar, the latter appearing larger

Results

Of the 21 patients examined, 2 were eliminated from the final analysis for HNP, as they were imaged in the early postoperative period (9 and 17 days postoperatively) when MRI is indeterminate for HNP. Of the remaining 19 patients, recurrent herniated nucleus pulposus was diagnosed on MRI in 10 patients, 1 of whom had two-level HNP. Surgical confirmation of the HNP was obtained in 3 patients for a total of four levels, including 1 patient with HNP at both L4–5 and L3–4.

In the 10 patients with a MRI diagnosis of HNP, the level of certainty of HNP diagnosis at 0.3 mmol/kg was lower in 5 patients and higher in 1 patient than with the standard 0.1 mmol/kg study; in 4 patients the level of certainty was the same. The reasons for decreased certainty in HNP diagnosis at 0.3 mmol/kg included: S1 nerve root enhancement blending with peridiscal enhancement (3 patients); increased extent and intensity of peridiscal enhancement, simulating greater amount of scar tissue (3 patients); and central fill-in of the disc fragment (2 patients). More than one of these factors were seen in some cases (Fig. 1). Mass effect on the thecal sac was important in HNP diagnosis in cases with increased peridiscal enhancement at the triple dose.

In the total patient group, at the 0.3 mmol/kg dose epidural enhancement was increased in intensity in 11 patients and in area (extent) in 4 patients. The group of 11 patients with increased intensity of enhancement at 0.3 mmol/kg included 5 of 11 patients without disc protrusion and 6 of 10 with disc protrusion. The group of 4 patients with increased area of enhancement at 0.3 mmol/kg included only 1 of the 12 patients without disc protrusion and 3 of the 10 with disc protrusion.

S1 nerve root enhancement was seen in 4 patients at 0.1 mmol/kg, and in 7 patients at 0.3 mmol/kg. These 7 showed greater S1 nerve root enhancement at the higher than at the lower dose. Intrathecal nerve root enhancement was diffuse in 5 patients at 0.1 mmol/kg and in 11 patients at 0.3 mmol/kg. Focal intrathecal nerve root enhancement was seen in 3 patients at 0.1 mmol/kg (2 of the 3 patients showed greater enhancement at the higher dose) and 5 patients at 0.3 mmol/kg (4 of 5 showed greater enhancement at the higher dose), and was seen only at the higher dose in 2 patients. In a case of spinal stenosis with small HNP, both the intensity and the extent of clumped nerve root enhancement were greater at the higher dose.

Discussion

The distinction of recurrent HNP from enhancing epidural scar on MRI has been well described [1–3]. Herniated discs show little or no enhancement, but are generally surrounded peripherally by enhancing peridiscal fibrosis, frequently with a large amount of scar relative to the small central non-enhancing disc, even in the spine that has not been surgically treated.

Experimental dog models have been used to compare the conspicuity of enhancing scar and the conspicuity of disc fragment vs scar at the triple dose vs standard dose of MRI contrast media [4, 5]. In the model, epidural scar at the laminectomy site showed greater enhancement at the triple dose, with the degree of scar enhancement dependent on the scar age and on the time after infusion. The conspicuity of inerted disc fragment vs epidural scar was increased at the triple dose in the dog model at the L3–L4 level 15–90 days postoperatively, the greatest difference between scar and disc being at 15 days after surgery at 2 min after infusion.

Studies of nerve root enhancement have shown selective, unilateral intradural enhancement of nerve roots affected by a large HNP [6]. Radicular neural enhancement was seen in the postoperative MR of symptomatic patients, but was absent in asymptomatic patients in the chronic postoperative period, beyond 6 months [7]. Triple dose in unoperated patients with HNP showed increased incidence, intensity, and extent of nerve root enhancement compared with single dose [8]. Furthermore, the triple dose MR study in asymptomatic, unoperated, normal volunteers showed enhancement of normal nerve roots both on early scans and with a delay of 30–60 min, and intervertebral disc enhancement parallel to the end-plates.

Our study of postoperative symptomatic patients confirmed the increased incidence and intensity of affected nerve root enhancement at S1 and intradurally, and greater intensity and extent of epidural enhancing tissue at the triple dose compared with the standard dose. However, the combination of increased enhancement of the S1 nerve root and increased peridiscal enhancement was a disadvantage in conspicuity of recurrent HNP, sometimes masking the posterior displacement of the S1 nerve root and decreasing the conspicuity of the nonenhancing disc fragment. The situation in these postoperative patients differed significantly from that in the experimental dog model in: time since surgery (average of 6 years in patients vs 15–90 days in the dogs; the level of surgery, which included L5–S1, as opposed to L3–4 in the experimental dog model; and nature of the disc fragments, which were degenerate in the patients while normal disc fragments were inserted in the dog [4].

The limitations of our study are conditioned by the small number of patients and the unavoidable time-lag between the single-dose injection and the triple-dose scans. Despite immediate scanning after the injection, the addition of a second dose immediately after the initial dose resulted in imaging compatible with the higher dose at 13–30 min after injection of the 1st dose. This delay may have contributed to the increased extent of peridiscal enhancement and to the few cases of central fill-in of HNP with triple dose. Additional factors in disc enhancement may have included granulation tissue or vascularity in the degenerate disc fragment.

Acknowledgement. This study was supported in part by a grant from Bracco Diagnostics.

References

1. Ross JS, Delamarter R, Hueftle MG, Masaryk TJ, Aikawa M, Carter J, Vandyke C, Modic MT (1989) Gadolinium-DTPA-enhanced MR imaging of the postoperative lumbar spine: time course and mechanism of enhancement. AJNR 10:37–46
2. Bundschuh CV, Stein L, Slusser JH, Schinco FP, Ladaga LE, Dillon JD (1990) Distinguishing between scar and recurrent herniated disk in postoperative patients: value of contrast-enhanced CT and MR imaging. AJNR 11:949–958
3. Ross JR, Masaryk TJ, Schrader M, Gentili A, Bohlman H, Modic MT (1990) MR imaging of the postoperative lumbar spine: assessment with gadopentetate dimeglumine. AJNR 11:771–776
4. Nguyen C, An H, Ho KC, Haughton VM, Hasegawa T (1994) Utility of high-dose contrast enhancement for detecting recurrent herniated intervertebral disks. AJNR 15:1291–1297
5. Nguyen CM, Haughton VM, Ho KC, An HW (1993) MR contrast enhancement: an experimental study in postlaminectomy epidural fibrosis. AJNR 14:997–1002
6. Crisi G, Carpeggiani P, Trevisan C (1993) Gadolinium-enhanced nerve roots in lumbar disk herniation. AJNR 14:1379–1392
7. Jinkins JR, Osborn AG, Garrett D Jr, Hunt S, Story J (1993) Spinal nerve enhancement with Gd-DTPA: MR correlation with the postoperative lumbosacral spine. AJNR 14:383–394
8. Jinkins JR, Gee GT, Rauch RA, Bazan C (1993) MR evaluation of gadolinium in the evaluation of the unoperated patient with clinical lumbosacral radiculopathy: comparison of 0.1 mmol/kg intravenous gadopentetate dimeglumine with 0.3 mmol/kg intravenous gadoteridol. JMRI 3(P):114

3D-FT true FISP (fast imaging with steady-state precession) MRI of intraspinal abnormalities in complex spinal dysraphism

J. Straiton[1], **J. Ridgway**[2], **J. Ward**[2]

[1] Neuroradiology Section, Department of Radiology, General Infirmary, Leeds, UK
[2] MR Unit, St. James's University Hospital, Leeds, UK

Abstract. The 3D-FT (3-dimensional fourier transformation) true FISP (fast imaging with steady-state precession) sequence has been assessed in 20 patients with spinal dysraphism investigated by MRI. The true FISP sequence generates high signal intensity from cerebrospinal fluid and the 3D-FT acquisition allows multiplanar displays of reformatted images. A combination of true FISP acquisition and conventional T1-weighted spin-echo sagittal images provided full demonstration of the intrathecal structures and limits of the thecal sac in all cases. Site and level of cord termination, cord splitting, cord cavitation and intraspinal masses were readily detected. The T1-weighted images allowed identification of lipomatous masses. Extra conventional sequences were required in 4 patients for more complete assessment of associated extrathecal disease. 3D-FT true FISP imaging is advocated in the MRI assessment of spinal dysraphism, replacing sequences traditionally used, to improve demonstration of spinal contents and reduce imaging time.

Key words: Spinal dysraphism – Magnetic resonance imaging

Correspondence to: J. Straiton

The utility of MRI in the assessment of spinal dysraphism is established [1], and MRI is the definitive imaging investigation for this indication. Conventionally, intraspinal abnormalities are demonstrated by obtaining a series of 2D-FT T1- and T2-weighted sections. A series of 20

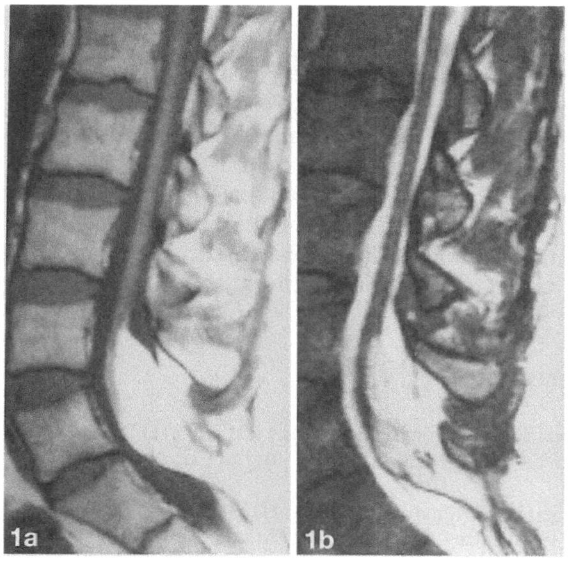

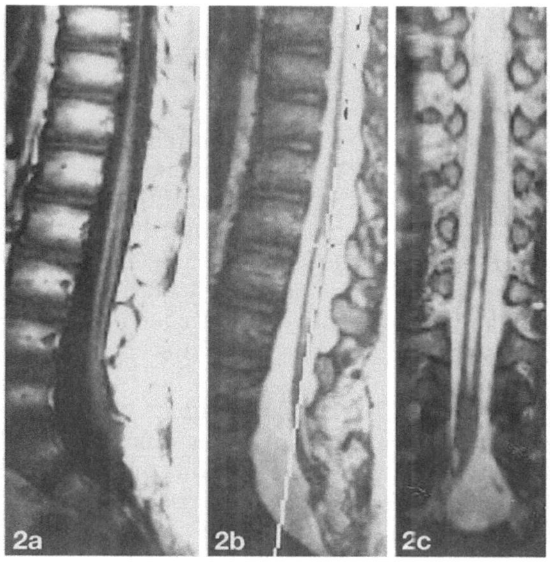

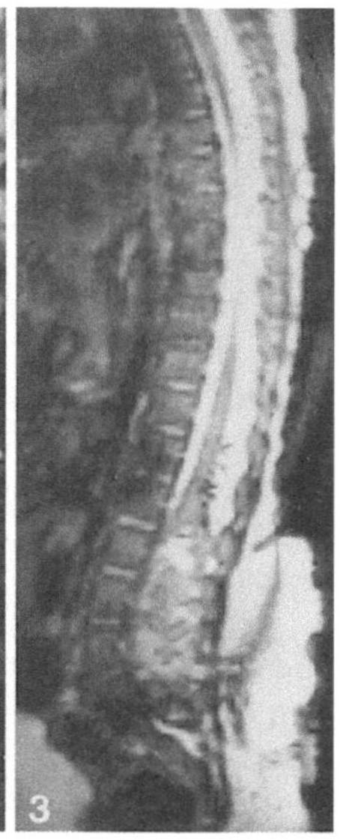

Fig. 1 a, b. Spinal cord tethering, lipomeningocoele. **a** T1-weighted, **b** true FISP sagittal images

Fig. 2 a–c. Spinal cord tethering and cavitation. **a** T1-weighted sagittal image. **b** Sagittal FISP and **c** reformatted coronal image

Fig. 3. Spinal cord tethering, lipomeningocoele, vascular malformation. True FISP sagittal image. Multiple small areas of signal void posterior to the lower cord are highlighted

Table 1. 3D-FT true FISP sequence: technical parameters

Repetition time	14 ms
Echo time	7 ms
Flip angle	40°
Matrix	160 × 256
Field of view	300 mm rectangular
Acquisition time	2 m in 24 s × 2 = 4 m in 48 s

patients is described in which a three-dimensional Fourier transformation true FISP (fast imaging with steady-state precession) sequence was included in the examination, to determine if this sequence could beneficially replace any of those normally used.

Patients and methods

We examined 20 patients (14 children, 6 adults) referred for MRI to assess spinal dysraphic syndromes. A 3D-FT true FISP sequence (Table 1) was added to the examination protocol determined by the supervising neuroradiologist. Images from the true FISP sequence were acquired in the sagittal plane, with further images derived by the reformatting of images on an on-line independent console.

Images were retrospectively reviewed to assess if the true FISP images could provide sufficient demonstration of abnormalities present to replace any sequence normally used. The true FISP and T1-weighted sagittal spin echo images were presented for the purposes of this analysis. The neuroradiologist was asked to determine the adequacy of the examination as presented, and to indicate what, if any, further sequences might be needed.

Results

MRI including true FISP was carried out successfully in all 20 patients (Table 2). In 16, a combination of true FISP and sagittal T1-weighted images was considered a complete examination, and no further sequences would have

Table 2. Diagnosis – complete assessment by T1-weighted/ true FISP combination

Cord tethering/lipoma	6
Cord tethering/syrinx	3
Split cord	2
Lipoma of filum terminate	1
Syrinx	1
Scoliosis/split cord	1
Fibrolipoma/abnormal intraspinal vessels	1
Normal intraspinal appearances	1
Diagnosis – supplementary sequences required	
Cord tethering/myelomeningocoele	3
Cord tethering/intervertebral disc protrusion	1

been necessary. In 4 patients, additional T2-weighted sagittal and T1-weighted axial images were required. The true FISP images identified cord tethering, cavitation or splitting, intraspinal masses and level of cord termination (Figs. 1, 2). The T1-weighted images allowed distinction of lipomatous masses. In 1 patient, focal signal void within the thecal sac was highlighted and correctly attributed to the presence of a vascular anomaly (Fig. 3).

In 4 patients, the combination of true FISP and T1-weighted sequences was judged inadequate; 3 patients had meningocoeles, the extraspinal component being poorly defined by true FISP, and a fourth had focal lumbar disc protrusion with only focal constriction of the theca of the undetermined cause apparent on true FISP.

Discussion

The underlying physical principles of the true FISP sequence are complex [2, 3], but the result is images with "myelogram effect" contrast, due to preservation of the steady state and compensated for the effects of cerebrospinal fluid (CSF) motion. A 3D-FT acquisition allows multiplanar reformatting of images with 2 mm effective slice thickness. True FISP is distinguished from other "steady state" sequences by the greater number of signal elements that contribute to the final image; two acquisitions (with alternating and nonalternating radiofrequency) and maximum intensity projection postprocessing are necessary to avoid artefact.

The high signal intensity of CSF defines the limits of the subarachnoid space and intrathecal structures which can be displayed with relatively high resolution, and signal/noise ratio. The capacity for tissue characterisation is otherwise limited, and in the absence of CSF, insufficient contrast is present in the extrathecal soft tissues to produce images of any value. This limited capacity for tissue characterisation can be offset by incorporating a T1-weighted sequence with true FISP, to distinguish lipomatous masses.

The display of many of the abnormalities seen in the spectrum of spinal dysraphism is facilitated by the true FISP sequence, and reduced examination time can result by eliminating combinations of 2D-FT sequences. While the intrathecal structures may be clearly outlined, the lack of soft tissue contrast limits the value of true FISP in extrathecal disease. High-intensity CSF techniques have been used for other indications [4, 5], but the fundamental weakness of true FISP and similar 3D-FT sequences is the lack of extraspinal soft tissue contrast.

True FISP can be used advantageously in spite of these limitations in selected cases of spinal dysraphism where the principal aim is to define the anatomical relationships of the spinal cord within the thecal sac.

References

1. Byrd SE, Darling CF, McLone DG (1991) Developmental disorders of the pediatric spine. Radiol Clin North Am 29:711–752
2. Oppelt A, Graumann R, Barfuss H, Fischer H, Hartl W, Schajor W (1986) FISP – a new fast MRI sequence. Electromedica 54:15–18
3. Haacke EM, Wielopolski PA, Tkach JA, Modic MT (1990) Steady state free precession in the presence of motion: application for improved visualization of the cerebrosinal fluid. Radiology 175:545–552
4. Ross JS (1992) MR imaging of the cervical spine – techniques for two- and three-dimensional imaging. AJR 159:779–786
5. Van Dyke CW, Modic MT, Beale SM, Amartur S, Ross JS (1992) J Comput Assist Tomogr 16:497–500

Cervical occult spinal dysraphism with vascular marker: MRI

M. Boukobza[1], **O. Enjolras**[1], **A. Pierre-Kahn**[2], **JJ. Merland**[1]

[1] Department of Neuroradiology and Therapeutic Angiography, Hôpital Lariboisière, Paris, France
[2] Department of Neurosurgery, Hôpital Necker-Enfants Malades, Paris, France

Abstract. We emphasize the value of MRI in the detection of occult spinal dysraphism (OSD) in infants with a cervical midline vascular marker. Two infants aged 8 and 14 months with vascular birthmarks of the cervical midline, normal limb growth and neurological examinations were examined by CT and MRI using axial and sagittal T1- and T2-weighted images. In both MRI revealed a fibrous band tethering the spinal cord to a cutaneous pit. One had cervical syringomyelia and the other had a possible dermoid cyst. MRI provided sufficient information to diagnose OSD confidently and to define the extent of the lesions. In one child a thick fibrous band was found running from the skin to the dura mater and a syrinx, and in the second, a dermoid cyst from the skin pit through the spine, ending intradurally. Postoperative MRI and neurological examinations were normal. Cervical OSD is rare. Beause of the risk of neurological impairment due to a traction effect on the developing spinal cord, early prophylactic surgery is useful and MRI is required as early as possible.

Key words: Occult spinal dysraphism – Spinal cord – Magnetic resonance imaging – Vascular marker

Spinal dysraphism is an embryophathy consisting of incomplete fusion or malformation of midline structures. There are two major forms: the open type (spinal bifida aperta) with meningocele, myelomeningocele or myeloschisis, exhibits abnormal embryogenesis throughout the central nervous system is easily diagnosed at birth, the closed type (spina bifida occulta, or occult spinal dysraphism (OSD)) involves predominantly the spine, spinal cord and cauda equina and does not expose neural tissue. It is associated with various combinations of cutaneous, muscular, bony, vascular and nervous abnormalities. Most cases occur at the lumbosacral level [1].

A midline posterior cutaneous anomaly is often the clue to underlying OSD and may take the form of a lipoma [2], hairy patch, skin dimple, pit, dermal sinus, faun tail [3]

Correspondence to: M. Boukobza

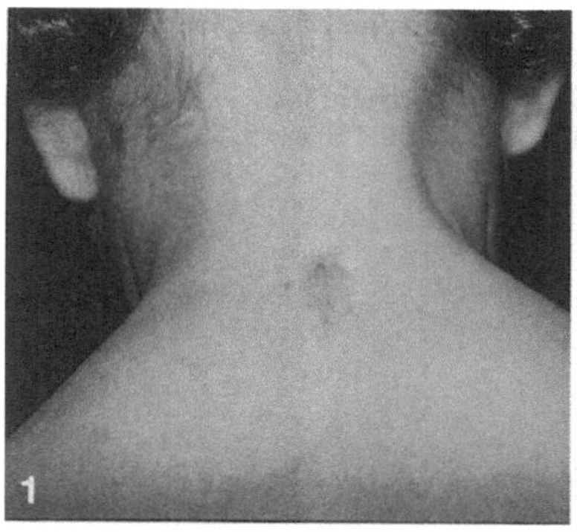

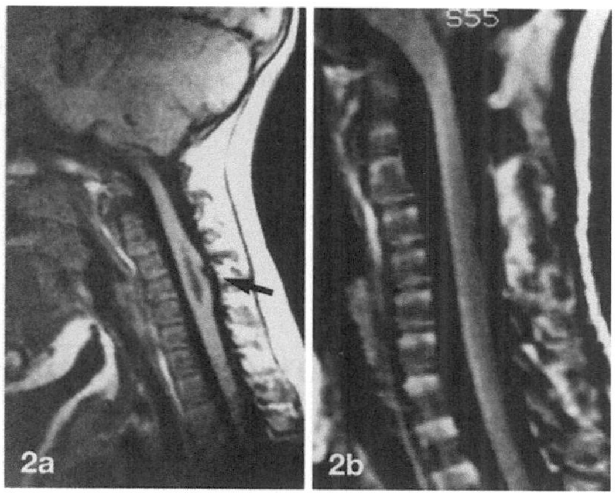

Fig. 1. Vascular birthmark. Low on the neck there is a capillary malformation with a small cutaneous pit inside it, a white halo and a small hairy tuft

Fig. 2a, b. T1-weighted sagittal images. **a** A fibrous band extends from the cutaneous pit, to tether the spinal cord to the vertebral column. A C3–C5 syrinx is present. **b** Postoperatively the appearances are normal

or vascular birthmark, most commonly a port-wine capillary malformation, or rarely a haemangioma. Skin changes are present in about half of cases of OSD [4]. However, OSD may go unnoticed until neurological complications, e.g. bladder disturbance or progressive difficulty in walking occur. We describe two rare cases of cervical OSD and discuss the usefulness of MRI and a cutaneous naevus in their recognition.

Case reports

We examined children with cervical occult spinal dysraphism: a girl 18 months and a boy 14 months of age. Each had an almost identical vascular birthmark: capillary malformation low on the neck with a small cutaneous pit inside. The girl (Fig. 1) also had a white halo and a small hairy tuft while in the boy a small mass could be palpated deep to the skin pit. The two children had normal neurological examinations, and their limb growth was normal.

MRI was performed to assess the clinically suspected OSD, and in preparation for surgical treatment; sagittal and axial sections were obtained with T1- and T2-weighted sequences. These confirmed the diagnosis of OSD and defined the extent of the lesions. Both children had a fibrous band extending from the cutaneous pit and tethering the spine to the spinal cord. The girl also had a C3–C5 syrinx (Fig. 2). The boy had a mass indicating a possible dermoid cyst in contact with the spine.

Prophylactic surgery was performed. In the girl a dermal sinus, a thick fibrous band running transversely from the skin pit to the dura mater and a cervical syrinx were found. In the boy there was an intradural, extramedullary dermoid cyst at C1–C2 with a fibrous attachment extending ventrally from the skin pit through the dysraphic spinal elements and ending intradurally. The fibrous tracts and dermoid cyst were removed; the syrinx was left. Histopathologically, the specimen from the girl contained thick fibrous tissue made up of schwann cells, collagen and elastic bundles and numerous nerve fibres, without a cyst. In the boy, a Malpighian dermoid cyst was filled with cutaneous annexa and there was a dense fibrovascular tract. Postoperative MRI studies were normal; the cervical syrinx in the girl was no longer visible. The two children have had normal neurological examinations over a 2-year follow-up period.

Discussion

Ultrasonography may be used for screening infants less than 6 months old if OSD is suspected. However, MRI is the definitive study. MRI provides an excellent preoperative investigation of these patients. In a patient with a previously diagnosed, or clinically suspected dysraphic spinal anomaly, MRI clearly defines the type and extent of the anomalies, before surgical treatment [5]. Most reports stress the need for early recognition and early surgical treatment of OSD in order to prevent neurological deterioration.

OSD can cause varying degrees of neurological impairment. Neurological symptoms usually occur by adolescence or young adulthood. The developing spinal cord and spine can be affected either by traction, or by pressure, or by both, depending on the type of OSD.

In our two cases, an early preventive operation was decided upon because of the neurological risks, particularly at these high cervical spinal levels, and of the risk of infection proceeding from the skin pit and dermal sinus to the meninges.

A single vascular birthmark for OSD, whatever the spinal level involved is very rare – only one pure vascular stain was seen in 200 cases [4]. In most patients, as in our cases, there are two or more median cutaneous warning signs of a developmental defect in the neural axis. For these patients MRI is required as early as possible.

OSD occurs rarely in the cervical region [3]. Of 462 cases only 5.5% were in the cervical and dorsal regions [6]; surgical treatment was undertaken for 287, only 4 of which were cervical. Thus, in the neck, it is important not to confuse a vascular marker for OSD, which is almost always associated with other cutaneous midline skin changes, and the very frequent vascular birthmark, occuring in more than 50% neonates, and known variously as naevus of Unna, salmon patch, naevus flammeus neonatorum, stork bite, fading macule, etc. The latter is not a clue to OSD and does not need investigation.

References

1. Serna MJ, Vasquez-Doval J, Vanaclocha V, Zubieta J: Quintanilla E (1993) Occult spinal dysraphism: a neurosurgical problem with a dermatologic hallmark. Pediatr Dermatol 10:149–152
2. Pierre-Kahn A (1991) Les spina lipomes. Arch Fr Pediatr 48:45–51

3. Miyamoto T, Hagari S, Mihara M, Hagari Y, Shimao S (1993) Tail-like protrusion on the nape with cervical spina bifida. Arch Dermatol 129:918–919
4. Tavafoghi V, Ghandchi A, Hambrick GX, Udverhelyi GB (1978) Cutaneous signs of spinal dysraphism. Report of a patient with a tail-like lipoma and review of 200 cases in the literature. Arch Dermatol 114:573–577
5. Brunberg JA, Latchaw RE, Kanal E, Burk L, Albright L (1988) Magnetic resonance imaging of spinal dysraphism. Radiol Clin North Am 26:181–204
6. Schiffer J, Till K (1982) Spinal dysraphism in the cervical and dorsal regions in childhood. Child's Brain 9:73–84

A case of syringomyelia investigated by cine-MRI and intraoperative ultrasonography

M. Takamura [1], K. Moritake [1], A. Fukuma [1], H. Shiraisi [2], M. Ito [2]

[1] Department of Neurosurgery, Shimane Medical University, Izumo, Japan
[2] Department of Pediatrics, Shimane Medical University, Izumo, Japan

Abstract. A 14-year-old girl had been suffering from a progressive decrease in the grasping force of the hands and sensory disturbance in the left C8 dermatome.

MRI revealed a syrinx from C2 to T11 and a downward protrusion of the cerebellar tonsils and the lower part of the medulla oblongata through the foramen magnum.

Posterior decompression was performed and a syringo-subarachnoid (SS) shunt constructed. After a C3 and C4 laminectomy, ultrasonography showed that the syrinx was still moving in the same cycle with pulsation. After the SS shunt, placement of the shunt tube in the syrinx and a decrease of its size were also confirmed by ultrasonography. Furthermore, a dynamic flow study of the cerebrospinal fluid (CSF) using cine-MRI disclosed that the CSF velocity had improved. It was thus suggested that both posterior decompression and SS shunt were effective in this case.

Key words: Syringomyelia – Ultrasonography – Cine-MRI – CSF dynamics

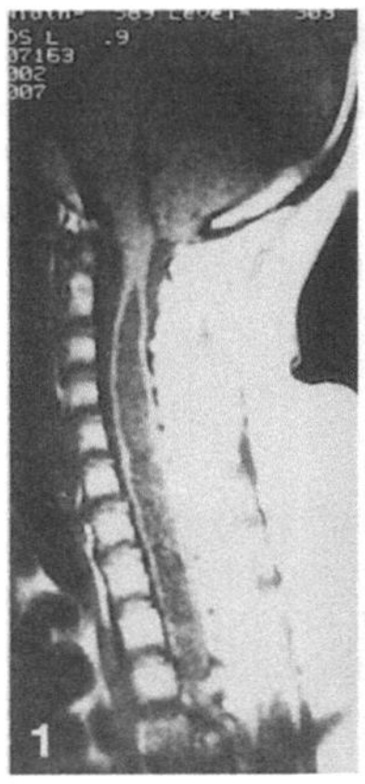

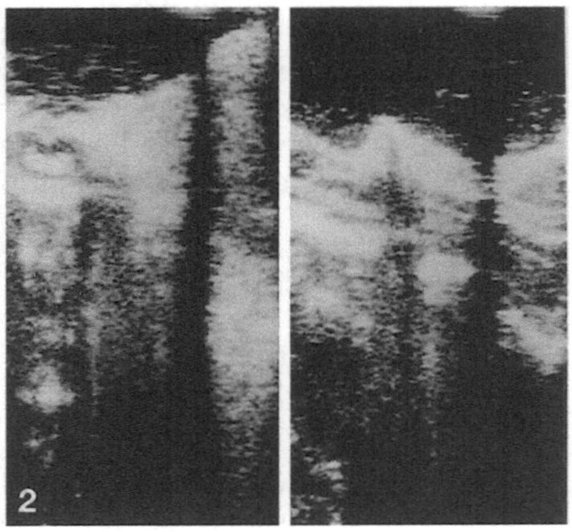

Fig. 1. Midsagittal T1-weighted MRI demonstrates the ectopic cerebellar tonsils and the distended syrinx from C2 downwards

Fig. 2. Intraoperative ultrasonography: before syringosubarachnoid shunting, a distended syrinx with pulsation was found

Since the introduction of MRI, syringomyelia is now more easily diagnosed. However, opinions on operative indications and methods differ greatly [1–4]. A patient with syringomyelia, Chiari I malformation and basilar impression underwent posterior decompression and syringo-subarachnoid (SS) shunting. Cine-MRI and intraoperative ultrasonography were used to estimate the operative method and its effect.

Case report

A 14-year-old girl noted disturbance of flexion and hypoaesthesia of her left fingers in February 1991. In June 1991, an orthopedic surgeon performed ulnar nerve stripping and diagnosed entrapment. However, the clinical signs were progressive, and the same signs appeared in the right fingers in February 1993. She was then admitted to hospital.

MRI demonstrated ectopic cerebellar tonsils and an expanded syrinx from C2 to T11 (Fig. 1).

As we thought the formation of the syrinx was caused by Chiari malformation, posterior decompression was performed, and as the syrinx had been large and the clinical signs progressive an SS shunt was also constructed.

When the inferior edge of the occipital bone was removed and C1 laminectomy was performed, we found a firm epidural band compressing the dura mater at the level of foramen magnum. It was then removed. After the C3 and C4 laminectomy, ultrasonography was performed through the dura mater [5]. It showed pulsation of the spinal cord and the syrinx (Fig. 2). The dura mater and arachnoid membrane were incised and adhesion was recognized between the inner surface of the skull and the dura mater, the dura mater and the arachnoid membrane were incised and adhesion was recognized between the inner surface of the skull and dura mater, the dura mater and the arachnoid membrane, and the arachnoid membrane and the spinal cord. After myelotomy, an SS shunt was performed with a shunt tube developed in Hokkaido University. The shunt tube was sutured with a soft membrane. Ultrasonography was performed

Correspondence to: M. Takamura, Department of Neurosurgery, Shimane Medical University, F693 89-1, Enya-cho, Izumo City, Shimane pref., Japan

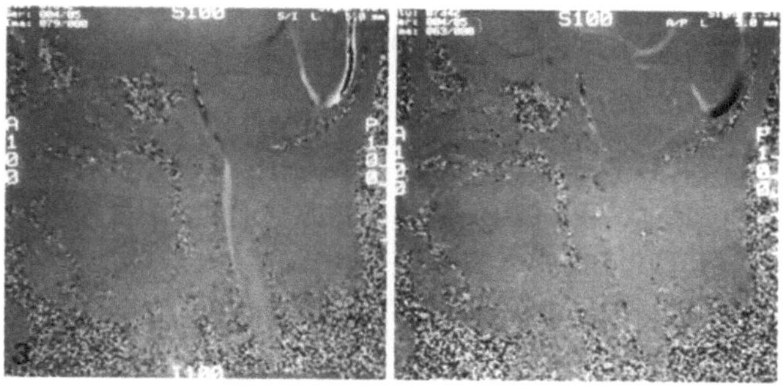

Fig. 3. Cine-MRI: cerebrospinal fluid movement was shown dynamically

again. It showed that the syrinx had decreased markedly in size and that the tip of the shunt tube was in the syrinx.

The postoperative course was uneventful, with improvement of symptoms and signs. MRI 1 month after the operation revealed a decrease in size of the syrinx.

Discussion

The therapeutic effects were estimated by cine-MRI showing CSF flow [6–8] (Fig. 3). CSF flow velocities are dependent on factors that vary between individuals, such as the volume produced, the volume emerging from the intracranial space and the form and area of the subarachnoid space. Therefore, comparison by velocity alone is generally impossible. However, we think it is useful to estimate the therapeutic effect. In this case, the CSF flow within the anterior subarachnoid space became slower, and it was thought that this result indicated an increase in subarachnoid space.

The number of patients found to have syringomyelia without clinical signs has been increasing recently. They include some in whom the syrinx has disappeared. Therefore patients to be operated on must be selected precisely [9]. Our protocol for the treatment of syringomyelia is shown in Fig. 4.

References

1. Abe T (1992) Operative procedure for syringomyelia associated with chiari malformation. Spinal Cord 5:659–663
2. Iwasaki Y, Hida K, Cho KH, Imamura H, Abe H (1992) Surgical treatment of syringomyelia associated with chiari malformation. Spinal Cord 5:645–649
3. Takahashi T, Hattori K, Kobayashi Y, Imagawa K, Asai A, Kuwayama A (1992) Operative methods for chiari malformation associated with syringomyelia. Spinal cord 5:651–657
4. Yamaura A (1992) Surgical technique for Chiari malformation I associated with syringomyelia: foramen magnum decompression with lateral extention. Spinal Cord 5:665–670
5. Moritake K, Takaya M, Minamikawa J, Ishikawa M, Kikuchi H, Minami S (1989) Hydrodynamic study of syringomyelia by MRI and intraoperative ultrasonography. Child's Nerv Syst 14:259–265
6. Matsuzawa H, Hida K, Houkin K, Yoshinobu I, Abe H, Akino M (1992) Quantitative analysis of cerebrospinal fluid dynamics in syringomyelia using cine-MRI with pre-saturation. Brain Nerve 44:24–29
7. Quencer RM, Post MJD, Hinks RS (1990) Cine-MR in evaluation of normal and abnormal CSF flow: cranial and intraspinal studies. Neuroradiology 32:371–391
8. Nitz WR, Bradley WG, Watanabe AS, Lee RR, Burgoyne B, O'Sullivian RM, Herbst MD (1992) Flow dynamics of cerebrospinal fluid: assessment with phase-contrast velocity MR imaging performed with retrospective cardiac gating. Radiology 183:395–405
9. Mii K (1988) Surgical treatment of syringomyelia. Spinal Cord 1:219–226

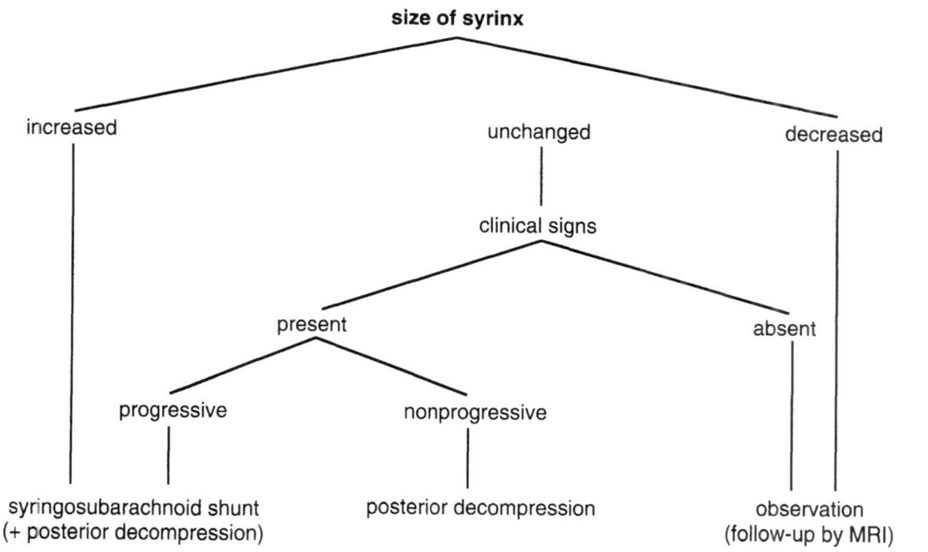

Fig. 4. Protocol for the treatment of syringomyelia

Percutaneous shunt insertion for assessment and treatment of syringomyelia in the radiology department

A. G. Clifton[1], **D. Uttley**[2]

[1] Department of Neuroradiology, Atkinson Morley's Hospital, Wimbledon, London SW20 ONE, UK
[2] Department of Neurosurgery, Atkinson Morley's Hospital, London, UK

Abstract. The management of syringomyelia is often difficult because of its uncertain pathogenesis and the many therapeutic options available. Many procedures, including foramen magnum decompression, plugging the obex, and various shunting procedures are used with varying success rates. In order to assess both the symptomatic and anatomic responses to the placement of a shunt prior to more invasive placement of syringoperitoneal or syringopleural shunts, we have placed a shunt catheter via a Touhy needle into the syrinx cavity. This was done under local anaesthetic via percutaneous puncture with the patient in the prone position under screening in the X-ray suite. We have performed this procedure in four patients, in one twice. In all patients the symptoms improved. In one of these patients, after two temporary shunt placements, a permanent shunt was placed in situ percutaneously and tunnelled to the pleura. In a second of these patients a standard surgical syringopleural shunt was placed. In a third patient there was some improvement in symptoms but the patient did not wish a permanent shunt. In the fourth patient there was only a transient improvement in symptoms and his permanent shunt was found to be patent.

Key words: Syringomyelia – Percutaneous shunt insertion

There are many surgical options for the treatment of syringomyelia [1]. The condition may be congenital (usually with an associated Chiari malformation), secondary to tumour, post-traumatic or idiopathic. The hydrodynamics of cerebrospinal fluid in syringomyelia are still poorly understood [2–7]. Treatment methods may include: plugging of the obex, decompression of the posterior fossa with duraplasty, lysis of arachnoid adhesions, drainage of the fourth ventricle [1]. Alternative procedures include shunting, including syringo-subarachnoid shunts, syringo-peritoneal shunting, syringo-pleural shunting and lumbo-peritoneal shunting. Symptoms and signs are variable. They include: dissociated sensory loss, long tract signs and muscular atrophy. Patients complain of pain and stiffness in the legs, and weakness in the legs and hands along with pain (in less than 50%). Lower cranial nerve signs may be present if the syrinx extends into the brain stem [8]. In patients with Chiari I malformation, posterior fossa decompression is regarded as the procedure of choice. Improvement of pre-operative symptoms may occur in up to 50% of patients [9]. The second treatment protocol is of syrinx shunting; this procedure is associated with a failure rate of 25–50% [10, 11].

In view of this high failure rate and the unpredictable response to shunting, we aimed to assess the symptomatic and anatomic result from inserting a temporary percutaneous shunt prior to possible insertion of a permanent syringo-pleural or peritoneal shunt.

Methods

The patient is placed in the prone position on a standard X-ray screening table with a facility for biplane screening. The patient is sedated with the appropriate neuroleptic analgesia. The syrinx is punctuated at the site of maximum distension but ideally below the level of T1 in order to avoid damaging innervation to the upper limbs. Under screening, a 22 G lumbar puncture needle is inserted into the syrinx cavity, fluid aspirated, and a few millilitres of contrast injected gently to outline the syrinx. This needle is then removed and a 14 G Touhy needle is inserted into the syrinx cavity. Through this needle, over a guide wire, a standard lumbar drainage system or pleural shunt system is inserted into the syrinx. For temporary shunting, the drain is sutured to the skin and the end connected to a drainage bag.

In our last case, we performed an elective combined percutaneous insertion of the syrinx with tunnelling of the distal end of the drain to the pleura. This was performed under a general anaesthetic with screening facilities in the theatre. The procedure was rapid and obviated the need for laminectomy and formal myelotomy.

Case reports

Case 1

A 49-year-old man sustained a fracture at L1 leading to a large ascending cervico-thoracic post-traumatic syrinx. He had symptoms of increasing weakness of the right arm and leg with marked sweating and a burning sensation on the right side of the face. He had two temporary percutaneous drainages with arrest of symptoms and improvement of pain and sweating. These were performed at 6-monthly intervals. He was reluctant to have a permanent shunt.

On return of the symptoms for the third time, a permanent shunt was inserted in theatre using a percutaneous shunt approach with tunnelling of the shunt tubing to the pleura. MRI, after shunt insertion, has shown reduction in the distension of the syrinx.

Case 2

A 52-year-old man presented with increasing weakness of the left hand and a tendency to drag his left hand and leg. MRI showed a cervical and upper thoracic syrinx with a narrow spinal canal but with marked distension at the lower end. The syrinx was punctuated at the level of distension and drained for 3 days, this resulting in good improvement in his symptoms. No permanent shunt was inserted and he remains stable at 6 months. MRI shows continued collapse of the distended segment.

Correspondence to: A. G. Clifton

Case 3

A 34-year-old man with a large, distended cervico-thoracic syrinx presented with increasing weakness in both arms and legs. Percutaneous drainage was performed for 5 days, with marked subjective improvement in his symptoms. The shunt had to be removed due to low pressure headaches after 5 days. This was then converted to a permanent syringo-pleural shunt. Follow-up MRI showed continued collapse of the syrinx with stable neurological state.

Case 4

A 63-year-old man with a Chiari I malformation with a large distended cervico-thoracic syrinx had marked meningeal fibrosis. He had a foramen magnum decompression, leading to worsening symptoms. A syringo-pleural shunt was inserted with no improvement. There was rapid deterioration. The shunt was revised with continued deterioration. Two locules of syrinx were aspirated percutaneously and a drain was inserted into the upper loculus. This showed patency of the shunt and there was also transient improvement of his symptoms.

Discussion

In view of the high failure rate and unpredictable response to formal shunting procedures for the treatment of syringomyelia we have performed a total of seven percutaneous shunt procedures in four patients with one permanent procedure. The procedure allows rapid and effective symptomatic and anatomic assessment of the response to shunt placement in a syrinx allowing for later placement of a permanent shunt which can be performed as a combined radiological and surgical procedure at a later date.

References

1. Milhorat TH, Johnson WD, Miller JI, Bergland RM, Hollinberg-Sher J (1992) Surgical treatment of syringomyelia based on magnetic resonance imaging criteria. Neurosurgery 31:231–244
2. Clifton AG, Stevens JM, Kendall BE (1991) Idiopathic and Chiari-associated syringomyelia in adults: observations on cerebrospinal fluid pathways at the foramen magnum using static MRI. Neuroradiology 33:167–169
3. Williams B (1980) On the pathogenesis of syringomyelia: a review. Proc R Soc Med 73:789–806
4. Gardner WJ, Angel J (1975) The mechanism of syringomyelia and its surgical correction. Clin Neurosurg 6:131–140
5. Aboulker J (1979) La syringomyélie et les liquides intrarachidiens. Neurochirurgie 25 [Suppl 1]:9–144
6. Ball MJ, Dayan AD (1972) Pathogenesis of syringomyelia. Lancet II:799–801
7. Barnet HSM, Foster JB, Hudgson D (1973) Syringomyelia. Saunders, London
8. Cahan LD, Bentson JR (1982) Consideration in the diagnosis and treatment of syringomyelia and the Chiari malformation. J Neurosurg 57:24–31
9. Pillay PK, Awdin A, Little JR, Hahn JF (1991) Symptomatic Chiari malformation in adults: a new classification based on magnetic resonance imaging with clinical and prognostic significance. Neurosurgery 28:639–645
10. Barbaro NM, Wilson CB, Gutin PH, Edwards MS (1984) Surgical treatment of syringomyelia: favourable results with syringo-peritoneal shunting. J Neurosurg 61:531–538
11. Matscino T, Symon L (1989) Surgical management of syringomyelia: current results. Surg Neurol 32:258–265

Functional MRI of the cervical spine

K. E. W. Eberhardt[1], H. P. Hollenbach[2], B. Kiefer[2], W. J. Huk[1]

[1] Division of Neuroradiology, Department of Neurosurgery, University of Erlangen, Erlangen, Germany
[2] Siemens Medical Engineering Group, Erlangen, Germany

Abstract. We prospectively studied 35 patients with degenerative spinal canal stenosis and functional disorders using a new MRI procedure that allows demonstration of movement in the cervical spine, a 1.0 T whole-body MR system. The patients were positioned in a Helmholtz neck coil, with special device for measuring different positions of the neck. T2-weighted single-shot HASTE sagittal images were acquired. For display the images were loaded into a cine loop. Our experience shows that functional aspects play an important role in bony canal stenosis as well as in movement disorders.

Correspondence to: K. E. W. Eberhardt, Division of Neuroradiology, Department of Neurosurgery, University of Erlangen, Schwabachanlage 6, D-91054 Erlangen, Germany

Key words: Magnetic resonance imaging – Cervical spine – Single-shot technique – Spinal stenosis

Functional aspects play an important part in diseases of the cervical spine. We present a new MRI procedure, which allows demonstration of movements of the cervical spine.

Materials and methods

In a prospective clinical case study we examined 35 patients with degenerative spinal canal stenosis and spondylolisthesis, medial disc herniation, post-traumatic changes, occipitocervical changes and functional disorders, using functional MRI; the results were com-

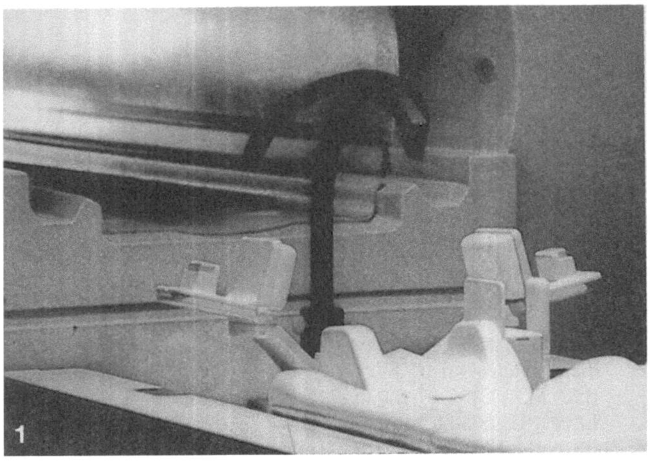

Fig. 1. The measuring device attached to the Helmholtz neck coil

pared with the findings in 15 volunteers. The average age of the patients (volunteers) was 51.6 (22.8) years; there were 19 men and 16 women in the clinical group and 7 men and 8 women volunteers. Fifteen patients with spinal canal stenoses underwent an operation, the interval between MRI and surgery varying from 2 to 14 days (mean 7.8 days). The investigation was performed using 1.0 T or 1.5 T whole-body systems. The subjects were positioned in a Helmholtz receive-only neck coil, where the body resonator served as a transmitter. A special device (Fig. 1) was added to the coil to measure the position of the neck. A strongly T2-weighted single shot HASTE [1] sequence (TE 87 ms) was used for sagittal images. Spatial resolution was 1.04 × 1.17 × 5.00 mm. All patients were examined supine. Between 12 and 18 different positions of the neck were measured in 5° steps (range: 50–170°). The acquisition time for each position was 1.2 s. We measured the diameter of the spinal cord and the bony canal in relationship to the cerebrosinal fluid (CSF) space at different levels between C1 and T1. To analyse pathological changes the images were also loaded into a cine loop.

Table 1. Findings in 35 patients with degenerative disease and disorders of movement in the cervical spine. Comparison between functional and conventional MRI

Disease	Functional	Conventional
Spinal stenosis/Spondylolisthesis	14/15	10/15
Medial disc herniations	4/5	2/5
Post-traumatic postoperative changes	4/6	1/6
Chiari I malformation	3/4	1/4
Disorders of movement	3/10	0/10

Results

Initial studies indicate that functional aspects play an important part in diseases of the cervical spine (Table 1). In medial disc herniations the extent of protrusion is dependent on the position in which patients are examined (Fig. 2). Of 5 patients 3 showed significant displacement of the spinal cord and nerve roots only on functional MRI. In spinal stenosis and spondylolisthesis we were able to classify the patients into 3 groups. Group 1 contained 5 patients with functional stenosis in extreme flexion or extension. In groups 2 and 3 there were 10 patients with an incomplete or complete CSF block in positions. Figures 3 and 4 show clinical examples. In 3 of 4 patients with post-traumatic or postoperative changes we could pinpoint dislocation of implants only on functional MRI. In 4 of 6 patients with a Chiari I malformation herniation of

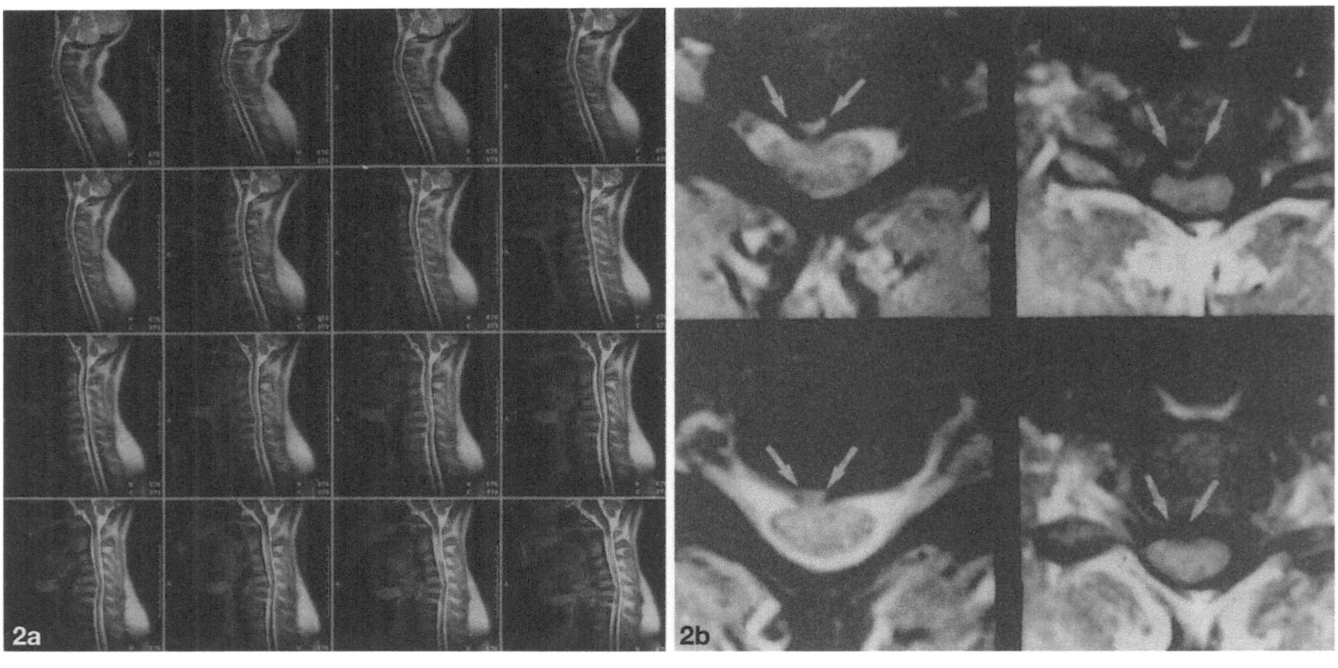

Fig. 2. Sagittal dynamic study with 16 single-shot images, the range of movement being 80°. Axial T1- and T2-weighted images show in flexion *top* a clear protrusion of disc material (*arrows*) and dorsal displacement of the spinal cord due to this. In extension *bottom* only circumscribed constriction of the CSF space can be seen

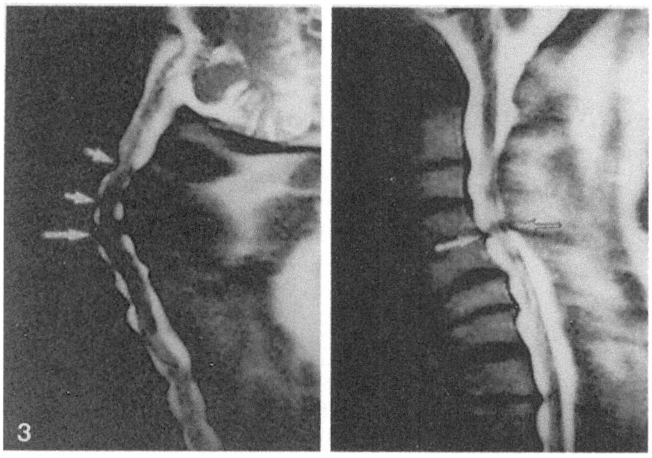

Fig. 3. Functional stenosis at two levels in flexion and an organic stenosis at one level with an incomplete CSF block *arrows*, classified as group 2

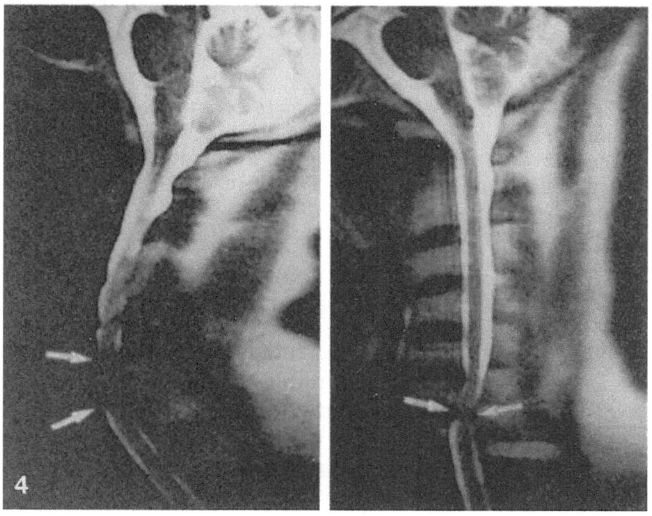

Fig. 4. Extreme canal stenosis with a complete loss of signal on MRI *arrows*, associated with a clinical spinal cord lesion; severe organic stenosis, classified as group 3

cerebellar tonsil was seen on functional MRI only. In 2 of 10 patients with functional disorders were found pathological changes in the craniocervical region.

Discussion

Functional aspects seem to play an important part in diseases of the cervical spine and the craniocervical resion. Currently, a precondition for analysing movement in this region is fast or ultrafast sequences combined with standardised measurement devices. Coordinated movements can then be demonstrated and pathological changes observed. We used a half-Fourier single-shot technique (HASTE) to produce multiple midline sagittal single slices. We showed that functional MRI allows classification of functional and organic spinal stenosis. Medial disc herniations, post-traumatic and postoperative changes depend on functional aspects as well as changes in the cranio-cervical region Disorders of movement can be analysed in dynamic studies and pathological changes can be found. Standard X-ray myelography, with functional imaging only in flexion and extension, is inadequate for analysing complex disorders [2]. Functional MRI can be combined with 3D-MR myelography. In the future this new technique might be helpful for surgeons deciding whether an operation is necessary or not.

References

1. Kiefer B, Hausmann R (1993) Fast imaging with single shot MRI imaging techniques based on Turbo SE and Turbo GSE. Radiology 189 [Suppl]:289
2. Langlotz M (1981) Myelographie mit wasserlöslichen Kontrastmitteln. Thieme, Stuttgart

Correlation of clinical features and high-dose steroid therapy in spinal multiple sclerosis with MRI

M. Nomura[1], **H. Anno**[2], **K. Katada**[2], **A. Suzumura**[3], **H. Osawa**[3], **Y. Ogura**[1], **G. Takeshita**[1], **H. Yamamoto**[3], **S. Koga**[1]

[1] Division of Radiology, Fujita Health University School of Medicine, Toyoake, Japan
[2] Fujita Health University School of Hygiene, Toyoake, Japan
[3] Department of Neurology, Fujita Health University School of Medicine, Toyoake, Japan

Abstract. MRI is useful for detecting spinal lesions in multiple sclerosis (MS). We have performed MRI in 14 patients (26 attacks) with clinically definite MS and investigated correlations between neurological and MRI findings and their changes before and after high-dose steroid "pulse therapy". The spinal level at which the lesion was suspected on the basis of neurological examinations was located as high-intensity areas on T2-weighted images. The lesions on Gd-DTPA enhanced T1-weighted images correlated better with clinically suspected lesions. Since the Gd-DTPA enhancing area disappeared after treatment in most cases, the enhancing lesions were useful for our understanding of the activity and the reaction to therapy in MS.

Key words: Multiple sclerosis, spinal cord – Magnetic resonance imaging – Relapse phase, high-dose steroid therapy

To investigate whether MRI can show clinically suspected spinal lesions in MS and be a useful tool in seeing the effects of steroid therapy, we examined serial MRI in the spinal form of MS before and after pulse therapy.

Methods

We studied 14 patients (26 attacks) with a clinically definite spinal form of MS. MRI was performed in the acute phase of clinical relapse (within 5 days) and after pulse therapy (during tapering steroid administration). The patients were all women aged between 15 and 65 (mean 37.8) years. MRI was performed on a 1.5 T MRI system using a T2-weighted (TR/TE = 2000–2600/90 ms). 5 mm sagittal slice without Gd-DTPA. For 17 attacks T1-weighted (TR/TE = 500–710/20 ms), 5 mm sagittal and axial slices, with 5 min later administration of Gd-DTPA (0.1 mmol/kg) were also obtained. The highest level of spinal cord lesions was estimated by neurological examination for weakness or subjective and objective sensory disorder.

Results

High-intensity areas were detected in T2-weighted images in 22 of 26 attacks. The spinal levels at which the lesions were suspected were located in these high-intensity areas. Contrast-enhancing areas in T1-weighted images were found in 12 of 17 attacks, and in 9 of 12 with symptoms (Figs. 1, 2).

In all cases, as the symptoms improved after pulse therapy, the high-intensity and contrast-enhancing areas

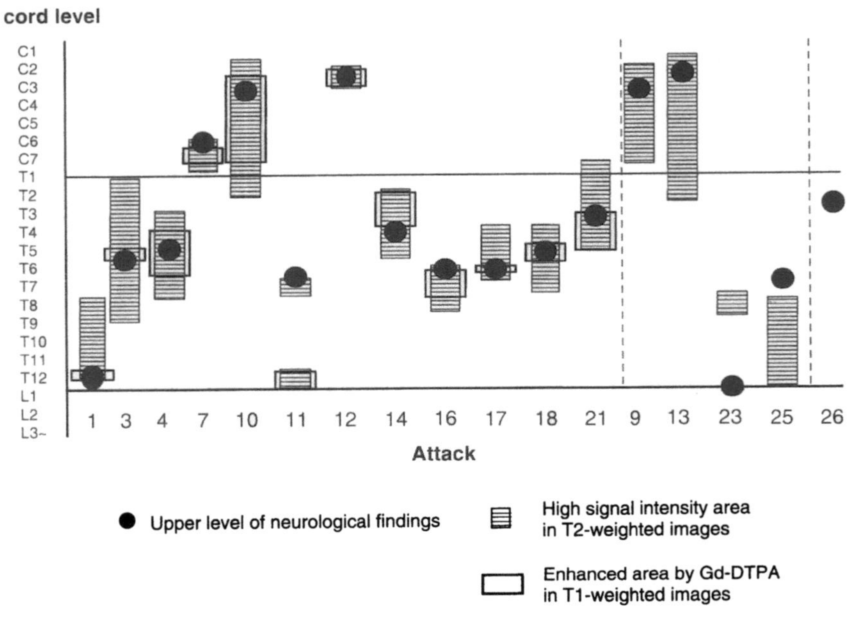

Fig. 1. The upper level of neurological deficit, contrast-enhancing area on T1-weighted images and high-intensity area on T2-weighted images

Correspondence to: M. Nomura, Department of Radiology, Fujita Health University School of Medicine, 98-1 Dengakugakubo Kutsukake-cho, Toyoake City, Aichi pref., Japan 470-11

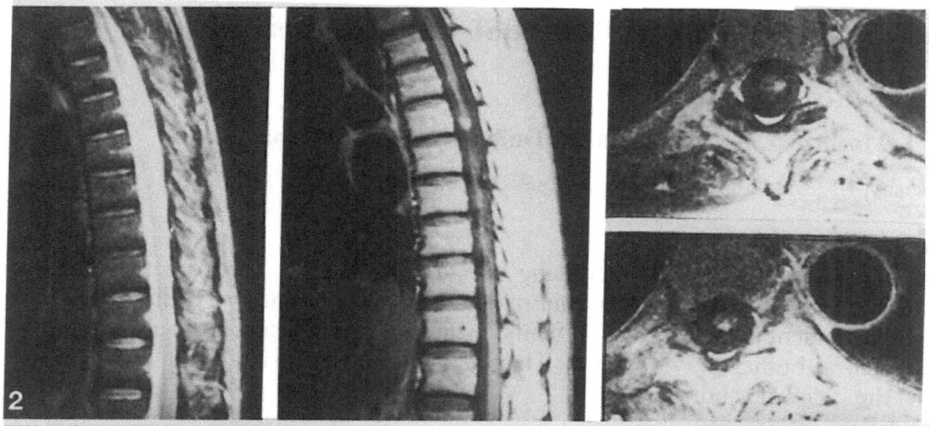

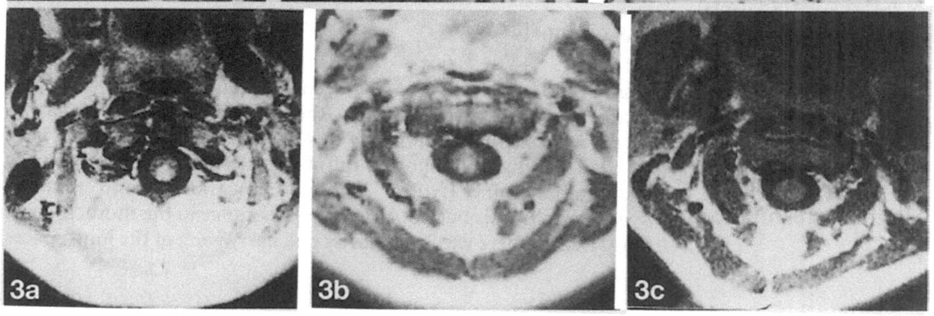

Fig. 2a–d. Patient was a 54-year-old woman. On T2-weighted images, **a** increased signal intensity was seen from T5 to T9 and
b there was contrast enhancement at T7 and T8 in the acute phase. On axial images, an enhancing lesion can be seen **c** on the right of the spinal cord at T7 and **d** posteriorly at T8 neurological examination indicated a spinal cord lesion at the same level

Fig. 3. A 24-year-old woman in her second attack and first episode of cervical disease. There is contrast enhancement at C2 (**a**) in the acute phase. After first pulse therapy, the enhanced lesion had changed little **b**. After a second course, no enhancing lesion could be seen (**c**)

became less distinct. The contrast enhancement disappeared after pulse therapy in 6 of 9 attacks, and in the other 3 the enhancing lesions became smaller. In 1 of these 3 attacks, the enhancing lesions disappeared after a 2nd or 3rd burst of pulse therapy. Two attacks relapsed clinically when the dose of prednisolone was reduced, but the patients received additional pulse therapy and showed good responses both clinically and radiologically (Fig. 3).

Discussion

We recognised the plaques of MS as high-intensity areas on T2-weighted images and contrast enhancement with Gd-DTPA T1-weighted images in acute phase L1–7. Because of its anatomical characteristics, parenchymal oedema in the spinal cord is often more extensive than in the brain [1, 2, 4, 8, 9]. Therefore, high-intensity areas on T2-weighted images were larger than had been suspected clinically. The changes in MRI findings and the course of symptoms suggest that the pathologic changes in spinal MS are caused not only by demyelination, but also by parenchymal oedema.

Since gadolinium-enhanced had a closer relationship to clinically suspected lesions than high-intensity areas on T2-weighted images, contrast enhancement seems to be useful for identifying actual inflammatory lesions in spinal cord MS. T1-weighted images are also very useful for our understanding of the reaction to the therapy and the activity in MS.

References

1. Capra R, Marcino N, Cotti Comrtti V, Vignolo LA, Bettinzioli M, Airo P, Cattaneo R, Gasparotti R (1992) Immunological and gadolinium-DTPA MRI evaluation of relapsing remitting multiple sclerosis. Acta Neurol Scand 86:342–345
2. Hawkins CP, Munro PMG, Mackenzie F, Kesselring J, Tofts PS, du Boulay EPGH, Landon D, McDonald WI (1990) Duration and selectivity of blood-brain barrier breakdown in chronic relapsing experimental allergic encephalomyelitis studied by gadolinium-DTPA and protein markers. Brain 113:365–378
3. Paradopoulpos A, Gatzonis S, Gouliamos S, Takadas S, Kalodouris A, Sgouropoulos P, Vlachos L, Papavasiliou C (1993) Correlation between spinal cord MRI and clinical features in patients with demyelinating disease. Neuroradiology 36:130–133
4. Smith ME, Stone LA, Albert PS, Frank JA, Martin R, Armstrong M, Maloni H, McFarlin DE, McFarland HF (1993) Clinical worsening in multiple sclerosis is associated with increased frequency and area of gadopentetate dimeglumine-enhanced magnetic resonance imaging lesions. Ann Neurol 33:480–489
5. Wiebe S, Lee DH, Kaarlik SJ, Hopkins M, Vandervoort MK, Wong CJ, Hewitt L, Rice GPA, Ebers GC, Noseworthy JH (1992) Serial cranial and spinal cord magnetic resonance imaging in multiple sclerosis. Ann Neurol 32:643–650
6. Kojima S, Hirayama K (1984) Spinal cord edema and its treatment: In multiple sclerosis and the other spinal cord disease. Shikei Kenkyu no Shinpo 28:644–653
7. Okasawa H, Inoue K, Yoshikawa K, Mannen T (1986) Magnetic resonance imaging of spinal lesions in multiple sclerosis. Clin Neurol 26:1157–1164
8. Ingrid VA, John K (1992) Demyelinating disease. In: Adams JH, Duchen LW (eds) Greenfield's neuropathology, 5th edn. Arnold, London, pp 447–520
9. Kojima S, Yagisawa T, Hirayama K, Mii K (1984) Neuroradiological studies on the brain and spinal cord in multiple sclerosis: edema and mass effect due to demyelinated plaques. Clin Neurol 24:165–171

MRI in ankylosing spondylitis: abnormal contrast enhancement in the thoracic spine

K. Mochizuki, Y. Inoque, Y. Nemoto, T. Mochizuki, K. Nakayama, H. Daikokuya, Y. Onoyama

Department of Radiology, Osaka City University, 1-5-7 Asaki-machi Aendo-ku, Osaka 545 Japan

Abstract. We performed Gd-DTPA enhanced MRI in two patients with ankylosing spondylitis (AS), and noticed interesting long T1 and T2 lesions and enhancement in the cephalad and caudal portions of the vertebral bodies in one case, particularly prominent in the ventral and dorsolateral aspects. These seemed to reflect inflammatory changes in active AS (enthesitis and osteitis). Knowledge of these characteristic long T1 and T2 lesions and enhancement may help not only in early diagnosis of AS, but also in differentiation of this from other diseases involving the spine.

Key words: Ankylosing spondylitis – Magnetic resonance imaging – Gadfolinium – Spine

Ankylosing spondylitis (AS) is a chronic, progressive inflammatory diesease. We present obervations on MRI in two patients, which are evidence of the inflammatory process. They may aid in diagnosis.

Case reports

Case 1: A 34-year-old man had been suffering from back pain for 7 years. HLA B-27 was positive. Rheumatoid factor was negative. Erythrocyte sedimentation rate was about 20 mm/h (40 mm/2 h).

Plain radiographs showed diffuse syndesmophyte formation in the lumbar spine (typical bamboo appearance), and minimal syndesmophytosis but not bamboo appearance in the thoracic spine (Fig. 1a, b). There was irregularity and narrowing of the joint spaces

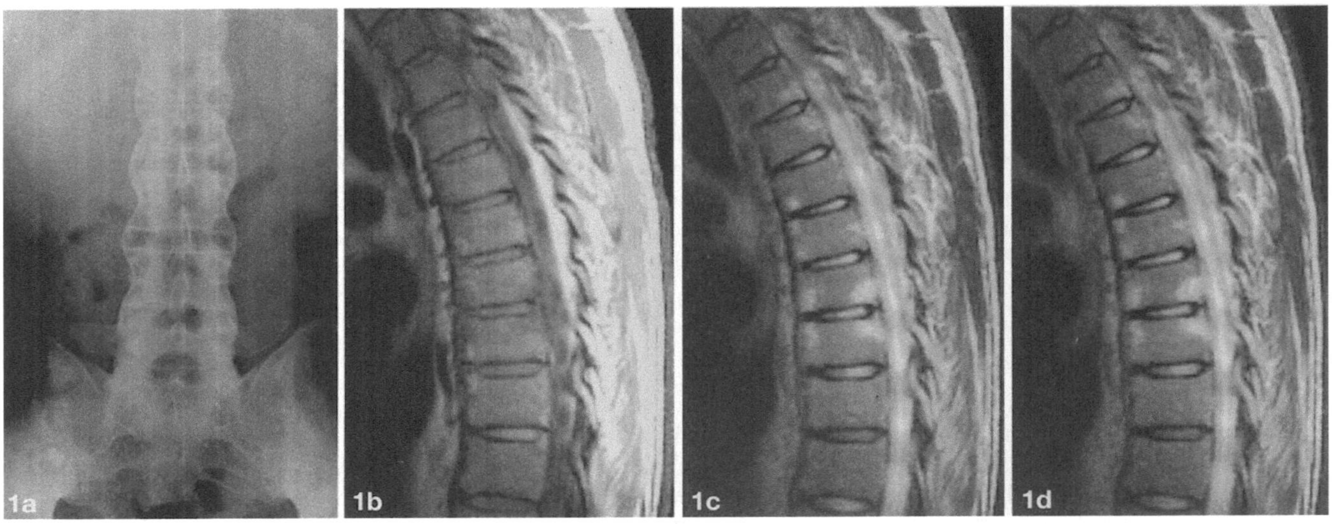

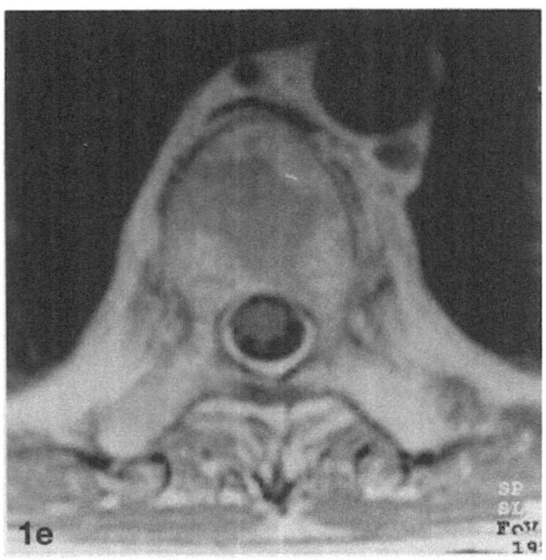

Fig. 1 a–e. Case 1. 34-year-old man. Plain radiography **a** showed a typical bamboo lumbar spine and irregularities of the joint spaces and subchondral sclerotic changes in both sacroiliac joints particularly on the left). Sagittal **b** T1- and **c** T2-weighted spin-echo images showed localised long-T1 and T2 lesions in the cephalad and caudal portions of several thoracic vertebral bodies. Abnormal gadolinium enhancement was seen on sagittal **d** and axiale T1-weighted images, in exactly the areas where long T1 and T2 changes were demonstrated on unenhanced images. The changes were especially prominent in the ventral and dorsolateral aspects near the costovertebral aspects joints **e**

Correspondence to: K. Mochizuki

and subchondral sclerotic changes (predominantly on the left) in both sacroiliac joints (Fig. 1a). These findings are typical of AS. We later noticed some erosions and sclerotic changes in costovertebral joints.

MRI showed localised long T1 and T2 changes in the cephalad and caudal portions (near the junction of the outer layer of the annulus fibrosis) of the vertebral bodies from T to T11 (Fig. 1c, d).

After intravenous Gd-DTPA, abnormal enhancement was noted in the same areas (Fig. 1e). These changes were especially prominent in the ventral and dorsolateral aspects near the costovertebral joints (Fig. 1f). There was no abnormal intensity or enhancement in the lumbar spine, which showed a complete ankylosis on plain radiographs. CT of the thoracic spine showed sclerosis consistent with the abnormal intensity on MRI.

Case 2. A 55-year-old man had been suffering from AS for more than 15 years. He had had no back pain for several years. Plain radiographs of his thoracolumbar spine showed a complete bamboo appearance. MRI of his thoracolumbar spine demonstrated neither abnormal signal intensity nor abnormal enhancement.

Discussion

AS is a disease characterised by enthesitis (inflammation around the enthesis, the ligamentous attachment) and reactive bone formation in its reparative process. It involves primarily the axial joints, such as the sacroiliac joints and the spine, but may affect peripheral joints and ligamentous attachments [1].

Pathologically, in the spine, there is inflammatory change, with infiltration of lymphocytes and plasma cells, at the junction of the outer layer of the annulus fibrosis and the vertebral body in its early stages (enthesitis). The inflammation also spreads to the bone marrow (osteitis) and the soft tissue around it, and may cause some bone erosion. The erosion in the bone surface is repaired by deposition of reactive bone. The reactive bone not only fills the defect but also spreads to the ligamentous structures (the outer layer of the annulus fibrosis and the connective tissue around it, which connects the vertebral bodies) and leads to syndesmophyte formation [2]. This process usually starts in the lumbar spine and then ascends to the thoracic spine. The cervical spine tends to be the last to be affected [3]. The inflammation also affects the apophyseal joints and the costovertebral joints [1].

In case 1, there were long T1 and T2 changes and abnormal enhancement in the vertebral bodies of the thoracic spine near the junction of the outer layer of the annulus fibrosis. Although not proved pathologically, we believe these reflect the inflammatory changes in active AS; enthesitis and osteitis. On the other hand, there was no abnormal intensity or enhancement in the lumbar spine, which was thought to be inactive.

In case 2, the thoracolumbar spine was completely ankylosed and thought to be inactive. We found no abnormal intensity or enhancement.

Although further studies should be made, MRI was useful in assessing the activity and distribution of inflammatory change in AS. The pattern of abnormal intensity and enhancement in vertebral bodies is so characteristic as to be potentially valuable in differentiating this from other kinds of spondylitis (pyogenic, tuberculous etc.). MRI can possibly detect early inflammatory change that may not be demonstrated by plain radiographs or CT [4], and may therefore also be useful for early diagnosis of AS.

References

1. Resnick D (1989) Bone and joint imaging. Saunders, Philadelphia, pp 299–319
2. Ball J (1979) Articular pathology of ankylosing spondylitis. Clin Orthop Rel Res 143:30–37
3. Wilkinson M, Bywaters EGL (1958) Clinical features and course of ankylosing spondylitis as seen in a follow-up of 222 hospital referred cases. Ann Rheum Dis 17:209–228
4. Murphey MD, Wetzel LH, Bramble JM, Levine E, Simpson KM, Lindsley HB (1991) Sacroiliitis: MR imaging findings. Radiology 180:239–244

Intradural ventral nerve root enhancement in disease of the conus medullaris

C. Takahashi, K. Miyasaka

Department of Radiology, School of Medicine, Hokkaido University, N-15 W-7, Kita-ku, Sapporo, Japan

Abstract. We report ventral nerve root enhancement with Gd-DTPA in patients with non-neoplastic lesions of the conus medullaris. The enhancement probably resulted from a breakdown of the blood-nerve barrier, which might represent a manifestation of Wallerian degeneration.

Key words: Magnetic resonance imaging – Gd-DTPA – Spinal nerve root – Blood-nerve barrier

MRI is one of the best methods for demonstration not only of spinal cord disease but also of nerve root involvement. We report on three patients with non-neoplastic and noninfectious lesions of the conus medullaris with ventral nerve root enhancement after Gd-DTPA

Correspondence to: C. Takahashi

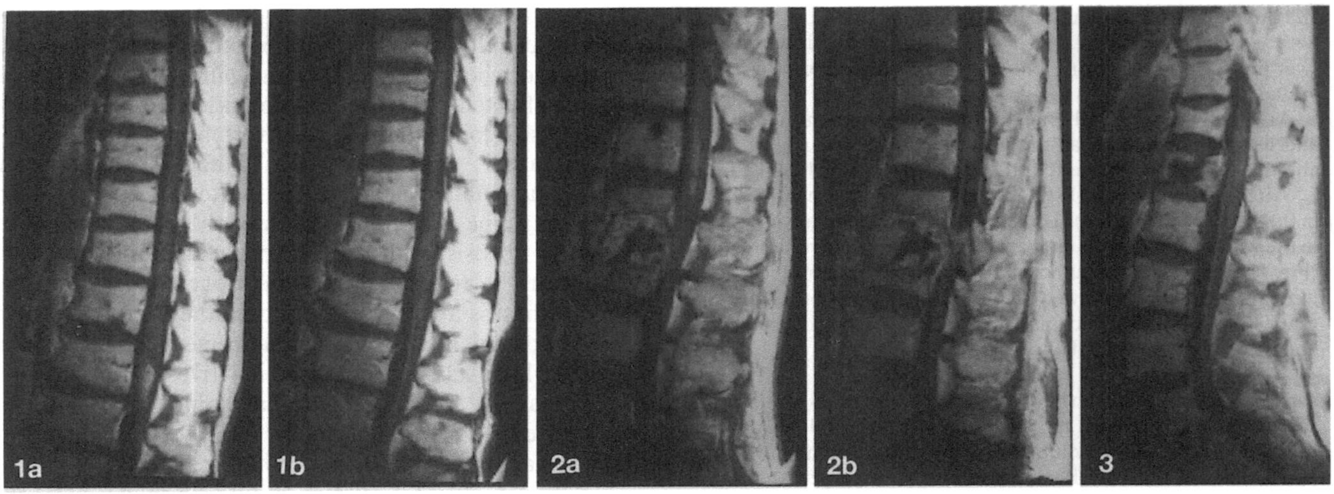

Fig. 1. Case 1. Gd-enhanced T1-weighted (SE600/15) sagittal images show **a** spinal cord swelling with intramedullary enhancement at L1 on the 9th day; **b** almost complete disappearance of cord swelling and intramedullary enhancement by day 20, when ventral nerve root enhancement is seen

Fig. 2. Case 2. Gd-enhanced T1-weighted sagittal images show **a** intramedullary enhancement at T12–L1 level on the 9th day; **b** abnormal enhancement of the ventral nerve roots but not of spinal cord on the 24th day

Fig. 3. Case 3. Gd-enhanced T1-weighted sagittal image shows spinal cord deformity at L1 and abnormal enhancement of ventral nerve roots on the 50th day

administration. As far as we know, enhancement has not been described previously. We also discuss the mechanism behind this finding.

Case reports

Case 1: A 69-year-old woman presented with a sudden onset of urinary and gait disturbance and was clinically diagnosed as having had a conus medullaris infarction. Nine days after clinical onset, sagittal images revealed swelling of the conus medullaris with intramedullary abnormal signal on T2-weighted images and enhancement after Gd-DTPA administration (Fig. 1a). After 20 days, the cord swelling and abnormal signal had almost disappeared. There was abnormal contrast enhancement of ventral nerve roots (Fig. 1b); this was also seen at 36 and 62 days.

Case 2: A 57-year-old man who had presented with urinary disturbance and paraparesis immediately after an L1/2 anterior fusion was clinically diagnosed as having spinal cord infarction. Nine days after the clinical onset abnormal findings like those in case 1 at 9 days were present in the lower spinal cord, above the level of the operation (Fig. 2a). After 24 days, cord size was normal, and intramedullary contrast enhancement had disappeared, but ventral nerve root enhancement appeared (Fig. 2b), which was still present at 45 days.

Case 3: A 74-year-old woman had an L1 burst fracture; the spinal cord was compressed by a bone fragment. Fifty days after the fracture there was abnormal enhancement of the nerve roots (Fig. 3).

The cerebrospinal fluid (CSF) of all three patients was normal. Examinations were performed on a 1.5 T MR unit. T1-weighted (SE600/15 ms), before and after Gd-DTPA 0.1 mmol/kg administration and T2-weighted (SE3000/90 ms or GE23/18 ms, FL12°) images were obtained.

Discussion

The blood-nerve barrier (BNB) regulates the microenvironment of the nerves [1]. Since each nerve of the cauda equina has this barrier, it does not normally enhance with Gd-DTPA. Enhancement ofnerve roots suggestsa change in the permeability of the BNB. CSF dissemination of malignant tumours, infection, trauma, compression, toxins or other regions may be the direct cause for this change. In our cases of infarction, the history, CSF, and MRI findings indicate that nerve root enhancement is the result of these causes. Considering that enhancement was seen only in ventral nerve roots when that in the conus medullaris had already disappeared, the defect of the BNB might represent a manifestation of Wallerian degeneration secondary neuronal to abnormality in the anterior horn of the spinal cord [2]. It is probable that the enhancement in the patient with the fracture was due to the same reason, as in the other two cases, since her conus medullaris was compressed by a bone fragment. However, this cause is still questionable, as nerve root enhancement remained after neurological deficits had disappeared. For a solution to this question, it is necessary to investigate more cases.

References

1. Rechthand E, Rapoport SI (1987) Regulation of the microenvironment of peripheral nerve: role of the blood-nerve barrrier. Prog Neurobiol 28:303–343
2. Mizisin AP, Kalichman W, Myers RR, Powell CP (1990) Role of the blood-nerve barrier in experimental nerve edema. Toxicol Pathol 18:170–185

MRI of subarachnoid seeding from cerebral glial tumors

C. C. Leite[1], J. R. Jinkins[1], C. Bazan[1], S. Reddy[1], L. Xiong[1], K. S. Kagan-Halle[1], W. T. C. Yuh[3], T. Simonson[3], M. Castillo[4], M. I. Rothman[5]

[1] Neuroradiology Section, The University of Texas Health Science Center, San Antonio, Tex., USA
[2] Department of Pathology, The University of Texas Health Science Center, San Antonio, Tex., USA
[3] The University of Iowa, Iowa City, Iowa, USA
[4] Department of Radiology, University of North Carolina Hospital, Chapel Hill, N.C., USA
[5] Department of Radiology, University of Maryland, Baltimore, USA

Abstract. We illustrate the spectrum of findings in subarachnoid spread of glial neoplasms originating in the brain, as revealed by gadolinium-enhanced MRI. The 12 patients in our series show that subarachnoid spread of cranial glial tumors occurs more commonly than may be supposed. Longer patient survival may portend an increasing incidence of this phenomenon. Gadolinium-enhanced MRI is the method of choice for both primary and sequential post-therapeutic investigation of patients with glial tumors of the central nervous system.

Key words: Cranium spine – Magnetic resonance imaging – Contrast medium, paramagnetic – Glioma, cerebral

Subarachnoid dissemination of primary intracranial glial tumors is well documented [I–II]. It was our impression that it occurs more frequently than is widely appreciated. We report a series of 12 patients.

Patients and methods

We reviewed the records of 12 patients with histologically proven primary cerebral glial tumors and remote areas of abnormal enhancement on gadolinium-enhanced MRI: 4 with grade 1–II astrocytomas, 2 with pilocytic astrocytomas, 1 with malignant transformation of an oligodendroglioma, 1 with anaplastic astrocytoma, and 4 with glioblastoma multiforme. T1- and T2-weighted spin echo acquisitions and contrast-enhanced T1-weighted spin echo images of the cranium or craniospinal region were performed in multiple planes (Fig. 1).

Results

Contrast-enhanced MRI-revealed various patterns of subarachnoid space seeding: intraventricular (3 patients), cranial extraventricular subarachnoid space only (4), spinal subarachnoid space alone (4) and cranial and spinal subarachnoid space seeding (1). Deposits not observed on unenhanced images were seen after intravenous gadolinium administration in 7 patients following a dose of 0.1 mmol/kg, and in 1 patient studied with an augmented dose of 0.3 mmol/kg. The diagnosis of cerebrospinal fluid (CSF) seeding was confirmed in 11 of 12 patients by CSF

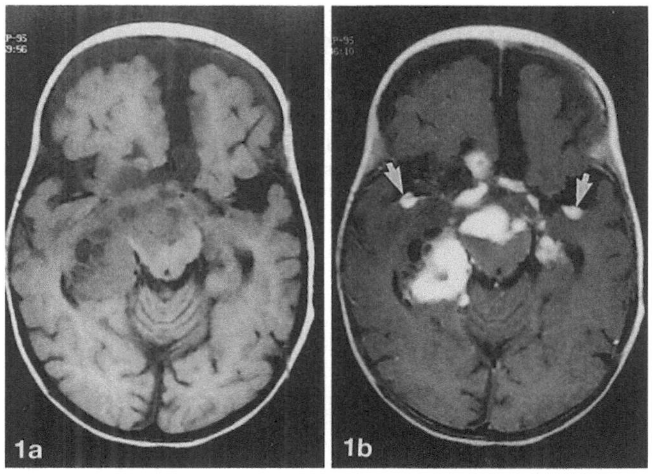

Fig. 1. CSF seeding of juvenile pilocytic astrocytoma without previous treatment in an 11-month-old boy. **a** Axial T1-weighted (660/15) spin-echo image shows a complex lesion in the suprasellar region extending posterolaterally to the right. **b** An image following 0.1 mmol/kg intravenous gadolinium shows intense enhancement of the hypothalamic tumor as well as multiple superficial enhancing cerebrospinal fluid seed nodules (*arrows*)

analysis (5), by direct open biopsy or resection of an area of seeding (5) or by autopsy (1).

Because there are false-negative CSF cytology studies for malignancy [5, 12], a positive gadolinium-enhanced MRI study in patients with persistently negative CSF cytologic findings may suggest that further diagnostic studies (e.g., dural biopsy) should be performed [8, 13, 14]. On the other hand, in the absence of other predisposing factors (e.g., immunocompromise, immunosuppression) or concomitant disease (e.g., fever, infection, other known peripheral primary neoplasm) gadolinium-enhanced MRI may be sufficient to suggest conclusively CSF spread of the primary neoplasm. Contrast-enhanced MRI showed evidence of subarachnoid space seeding in 7 patients in this series, in the face of negative CSF cytologic examinations. For this reason a gadolinium-enhanced MRI examination may ultimately become the study of choice for noninvasive survey of the central nervous system for tumor seeding in the subarachnoid space in patients with or without relevant clinical signs and symptoms. The detection of early tumor seeding, even in the unoperated patient, will obviously alter the course of therapy in this subset of patients with glial tumors of the central nervous system [10].

Correspondence to: J. Randy Jinkins, Director of Neuroradiology, Department of Radiology, The University of Texas Health Science Center, 7703 F Curl Drive, San Antonio, TX 78284-7800, USA

References

1. Awad I, Bay JW, Rogers L (1986) Leptomeningeal metastasis from supratentorial malignant gliomas. Neurosurgery 19:247–251
2. Obana WG, Cogen PH, Davis RL, Edwards MSB (1991) Metastatic juvenile pilocytic astrocytoma. Case report. J Neurosurg 75:972–975
3. Saleh J, Afshar F (1987) Spinal cord astrocytoma with intracranial spread: detection by magnetic resonance imaging. Br J Neurosurg 1:503–508
4. Natelson SE, Dyer ML, Harp DL (1992) Delayed CSF seeding of benign oligodendroglioma. South Med J 85:1011–1012
5. Mishima K, Nakamura M, Nakamura H, Nakamura O, Funata N, Shitara N (1992) Leptomeningeal dissemination of cerebellar pilocytic astrocytoma. J Neurosurg 77:788–791
6. McLaughlin JE (1976) Juvenile astrocytomas with subarachnoid spread. J Pathol (Lond) 118:101–107
7. Bell WO, Packer RJ, Seigel KR, et al (1988) Leptomeningeal spread of intramedullary spinal cord tumors. J Neurosurg 69:295–300
8. Bryan P (1974) CSF seeding of intracranial tumours: a study of 96 cases. Clin Radiol 25:355–360
9. Onda K, Tanaka R, Takahashi H, Takeda N, Ikuta F (1989) Cerebral gliobastoma with cerebrospinal fluid dissemination: a clinico-pathological study of 14 cases examined by complete autopsy. Neurosurgery 25:533–540
10. Kandt RS, Shinnar S, D'Souza BJ, Singer HS, Wharam MD (1984) Cerebrospinal metastases in malignant childhood astrocytomas. J Neuro-Oncol 2:123–128
11. Lam CH, Cosgrove GR, Drislane FW, Sotrel A (1991) Spinal leptomeningeal metastasis from cerebral glioblastoma. Appearance on magnetic resonance imaging. Surg Neurol 35:377–380
12. Glass JP, Melamed M, Chernik NL, Posner JB (1979) Malignant cells in cerebrospinal fluid (CSF): the meaning of a positive CSF cytology. Neurology 35:1369–1375
13. Twijnstra A, Visser BWO de, Zanten AP van (1987) Diagnosis of leptomeningeal metastasis. Clin Neurol Neurosurg 89:79–84
14. Phillips ME, Ryals TJ, Kambhu SA, Yuh WTC (1990) Neoplastic vs inflammatory meningeal enhancement with Gd-DTPA. J Comput Assist Tomogr 14:536–541

Spinal vessels: normal and abnormal findings on CT

O. Sakai, M. Furuse, N. Nakashima, C. Ogawa, T. Shinozaki, M. Kikuno

Department of Radiology, Jichi Medical School, 3311-1 Yakushiji, Minamikawachi, Kawachi, Tochigi, 329-04 Japan

Abstract. We describe the normal and abnormal CT appearances of the spinal vessels. Our control group consisted of 180 patients without known spinal diseases, who underwent CT study for a visceral survey. Contiguous 10-mm-thick incremental scans were obtained 30–60 s after intravenous injection of contrast material (100 ml, 300 mgI/ml, 2–3 ml/s). Abnormal cases were three arteriovenous malformations (AVMs). Scans showing a normal CT appearance of the spinal vessels were divided into seven groups. Anterior spinal arteries were identified in 88.3%. The arteria radicularis magna was seen in 26.7% and its location was identified. It is important to avoid misinterpretation to recognise that spinal vessels are normally demonstrated on contrast-enhanced CT. The nidus of a glomus-type vascular malformation and its intraparenchymal location were clearly demonstrated. A single-coil-type malformation was seen, but diagnosis by CT only would be difficult.

Key words: Anatomy – Computed tomography – Spinal artery – Arteriovenous malformation

The normal spinal arteries are not routinely bought on CT studies. There is a misconception that they are not visible. We studied patients undergoing contrast-enhanced abdominal CT, to assess the frequency with which these vessels can be identified. We also compared the normal findings with those in patients with vascular malformations.

Correspondence to: O. Sakai

Methods

The control group consisted of 180 patients undergoing abdominal CT for various visceral diseases. Contiguous 1-cm collimation incremental scans were obtained 30–60 s after intravenous administration of 100 ml of nonionic contrast medium (300 mgI/ml, rate; 2–3 ml/s). All scans were obtained with a 2 s scanning cycle (scanning time, 1 s; incremental time, 1 s).

Results

Normal findings

Scans showing normal CT appearance of the spinal vessels were divided into seven groups (Fig. 1). An 'enhanced dot' located in the midline on the anterior surface of the cord was considered to be the anterior spinal artery, and an 'accompanying dot', to be a radicular artery (Fig. 2). The vessels on the posterior surface of the spinal cord were thought to be posterior spinal arteries or veins. Anterior spinal arteries were seen in 159 of the 180 patients (88.3%). The arteria radicularis magna was identified in 48 patients (26.7%), emerging at the T10 to L2 level; 29 (60.4%) were on the left and 19 (39.6%) on the right.

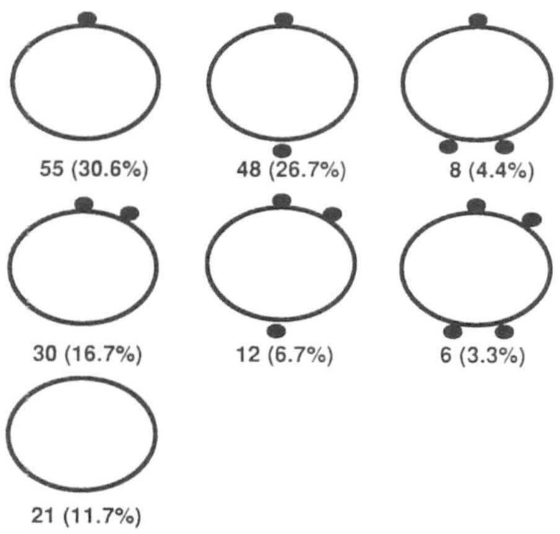

Fig. 1. Patterns of the spinal vessels in 180 patients and their frequency. *Dots* indicate contrast-enhanced vessels

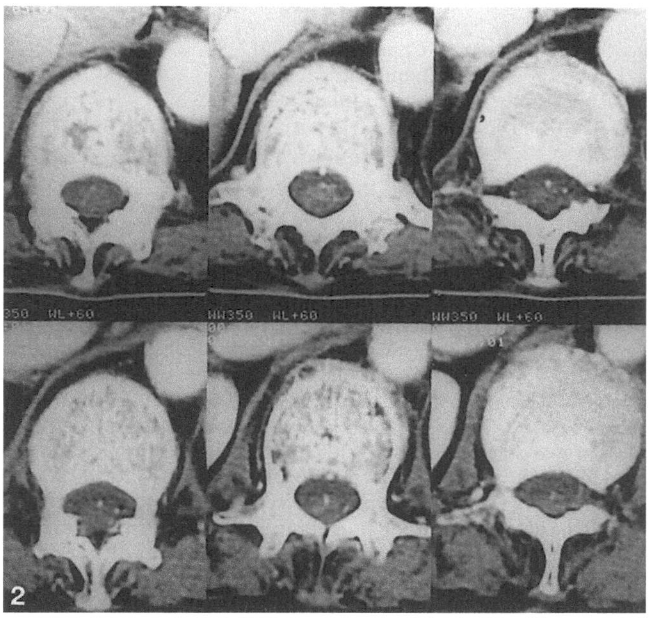

Fig. 2. Sequential contrast-enhanced CT. The anterior spinal artery and the arteria radicularis magna are demonstrated on contiguous slices

Spinal AVMs

Glomus-type. Contrast-enhanced CT demonstrated a significantly dilated anterior spinal artery and the nidus (glomus) of the AVM; the intraparenchymal location of the nidus was clearly demonstrated (Fig. 3a). Selective spinal angiography confirmed the diagnosis (Fig. 3b).

Single-coil type. The anterior spinal artery was seen on enhanced CT, but no anomalous vessels could be identified. Selective spinal angiography revealed a single-coil-type spinal AVM.

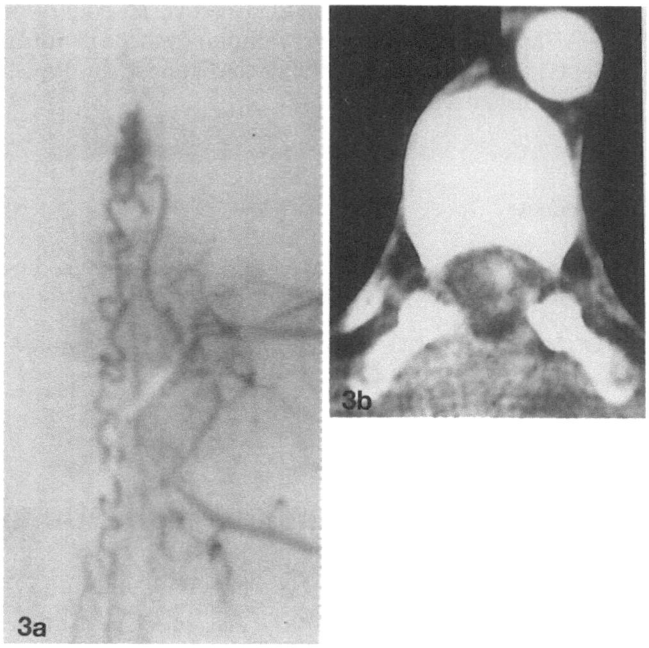

Fig. 3a, b. Glomus type of spinal AVM. **a** Contrast-enhanced CT. Significantly dilated anterior spinal artery and anomalous vessels are seen. The intramedullary location of the anomalous vessels is clearly demonstrated. **b** Selective spinal angiography. The AVM is clealy demonstrated. Its intraparenchymal location is not unequivocal on the frontal projection alone

Discussion

Recent improvements in CT scanners and the use of a power injector have facilitated demonstration of the spinal vessels, though this has been considered difficult in normal patients [1–4]. Recognition that spinal vessels are normally demonstrated on contrast-enhanced CT is important, so that they will not be misinterpreted as vascular abnormalities. The patterns of these vessels, and the frequency with which they are identified, depend on various factors, including the rate and amount of contrast medium injection and the interval between administration and scanning. The enhanced dots on the anterior surface of the spinal cord near the midline in our study were considered to be anterior spinal arteries and the accompanying dots, to be radicular arteries. Those on the posterior surface could not be identified as either arteries or veins. They may be interpreted as arteries or veins based on their shape and on the degree and timing of enhancement compared with that of the anterior spinal artery or aorta.

Although conventional selective spinal angiography is still used in investigation of vascular abnormalities of the spinal cord, it is associated with some risk of spinal cord damage [1, 2, 5]. In practical terms, prior knowledge of the gross location of the arteria radicularis magna, which can be gained by CT before conventional spinal angiography, is very useful in simplifying the procedure.

Large spinal vessels may suggest AVMs or other vascular lesions [1, 2, 4]. The typical glomus type of AVM was clearly seen on enhanced CT, and its intraparechymal location was well demonstrated. However, a single-coil-type AVM showed findings very similar to those in normal patients, and it would be difficult to diagnose this type by contrast-enhanced CT alone.

References

1. Di Chiro G, Doppman JL, Wener L (1977) Computed tomography of spinal cord arteriovenous malformation. Radiology 123:351
2. Di Chiro G, Rieth KG, Oldfield EH, Tievsky AL, Doppman JL, Davis DO (1982) Digital subtraction angiography and dynamic computed tomography in the evaluation of arteriovenous malformation and hemangioblastomas of the spinal cord. J Comput Assist Tomogr 6:655
3. Haughton VM, Syvertsen A, Williams AL (1980) Soft-tissue anatomy within the spinal canal as seen on computed tomography. Radiology 134:649
4. Miyamoto S, Kikuchi H, Karasawa J, Nagata I, Shishido H, Naitoh H, Imakita T, Sakashita Y (1987) Application of spinal dynamic computed tomography in the diagnosis of spinal cord arteriovenous malformation. Neurol Surg (Jpn) 15:523
5. Di Chiro G, Wener L (1973) Angiography of the spinal cord. A review of contemporary techniques and applications. J Neurosurg 39:1

CT-guided percutaneous aspiration biopsy of solitary vertebral lesions

N. Khandelwal[1], P. B. Roy[1], V. K. Kak[2], R. Nijhawan[3], S. Suri[3]

[1] Department of Radiodiagnosis, Postgraduate Institute of Medical Education and Research, Chandigarh 160012, India
[2] Department of Neurosurgery, Postgraduate Institute of Medical Education and Research, Chandigarh, India
[3] Department of Cytology, Postgraduate Institute of Medical Education and Research, Chandigarh, India

Abstract. CT-guided percutaneous aspiration biopsy (PAB) of solitary vertebral lesions was performed in 50 patients. The lesions were in the cervical (7), dorsal (21), lumbar (16) and sacrococcygeal (6) regions. Tuberculosis (30%) and metastases (30%) were the commonest pathological findings. A positive cytological diagnosis was obtained in 46 patients (92%). PAB is a simple outpatient procedure with very low morbidity and an effective alternative to open biopsy.

Key words: Computed tomography – Biopsy, percutaneous – Spine

Percutaneous aspiration biopsy (PAB) has emerged as a valuable technique for the diagnosis and evaluation of vertebral lesions prior to therapy [1]. This is of particular importance in suspected infection where a chemotherapeutic agent may be indicated and in suspected metastatic disease where it may be helpful in identifying the nature and probable site of the primary tumour [2]. Moreover, a solitary vertebral lesion in a patient with known malignant disease does not always indicate metastasis [3]. Accurate delineation of the site, size and extent of vertebral lesions has become possible with advances in medical imaging (CT/MRI) but the nature of the lesion still cannot be ascertained in all the cases [3]. The present study was undertaken using as a guiding modality for PAB in solitary vertebral lesions.

Correspondence to: N. Khandelwal

Patients and methods

We carried out 52 PAB in 50 patients (32 men, 18 women), 18–70 years of age, with evidence of a solitary vertebral lesion on routine spinal radiographs and/or CT. A detailed clinical examination was carried out in all patients. Laboratory examination included complete haemogram and coagulation profile. Prebiopsy radiological investigations included spine and chest radiography, CT of the spine or CT-myelography. Informed consent was obtained in all cases. Preliminary CT was obtained and an appropriate approach to the lesion was selected. A posterior, posterolateral, transpedicular or anterolateral approach was used depending on the location of the lesion, using the shortest needle trajectory as the guiding principle. With the help of a radio-opaque skin marker in the form of a grid, an 18–19 G lombar puncture needle was advanced into the vertebral lesion under local anaesthesia and aseptic precautions. Aspiration of material was done with the help of an aspiration handle. Gross (quantity, nature) and cytological examinations (with May Grunwald Giemsa stain) were performed. The aspirated material was also examined bacteriologically including acid-fast staining and culture.

The patients were observed for at least 6 h after the procedure and analgesics were used whenever indicated. A chest radiograph was obtained in all cases of PAB of the thoracic spine, to exclude a pneumothorax. All complaints following the procedure were recorded and managed appropriately.

Results

The anatomical distribution of the lesions and the cytological findings are shown in Tables 1 and 2. Osteolytic lesions were seen in 40 patients (80%), osteoblastic in 4 (8%) and mixed lesions in 6 (12%). PAB was repeated in 2 cases where scanty material was obtained at the initial attempt. Tuberculous infection and metastases, 15 (30%) cases each, were the commonest pathological findings encountered (Figs. 1, 2). Staphylococcal osteomyelitis was seen in 5 (10%), followed by giant cell tumour (6%) and plasmacytoma (6%). All osteolytic lesions showed posi-

Table 1. Anatomical site of lesions for aspiration biopsy and needle approaches in 50 patients

Site	Cases	Needle approach	
Cervical	7	Anterolateral	5
		Posterior	1
		Posterolateral	1
Thoracic	21	Posterolateral	15
		Transpedicular	4
		Transcostovertebral	2
Lumbar	16	Posterior	6
		Posterolateral	10
Sacrococcygeal	6	Posterior	2
		Posterolateral	4

Table 2. Cytological findings in 50 cases

Cytological findings	Cases
Tuberculosis	15
Metastasis	15
Staphylococcal	5
Giant cell tumour	3
Plasmacytoma	3
Degenerative bone	1
Fibrous band	2
Trauma (normal osteoid)	2
Necrotic or scanty materal	4

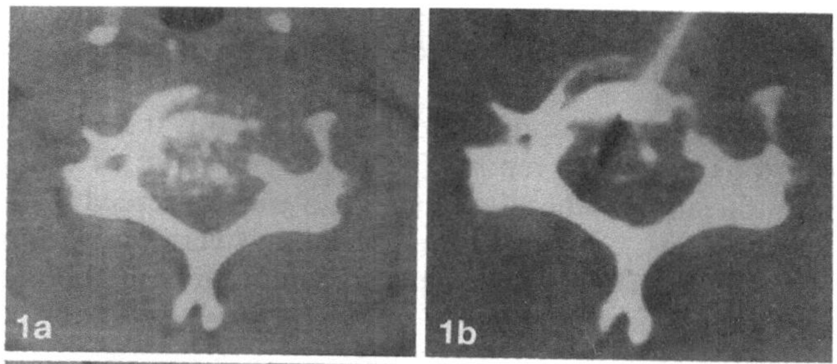

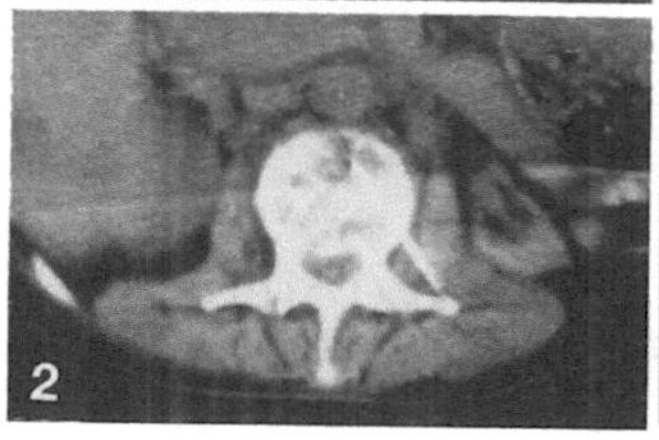

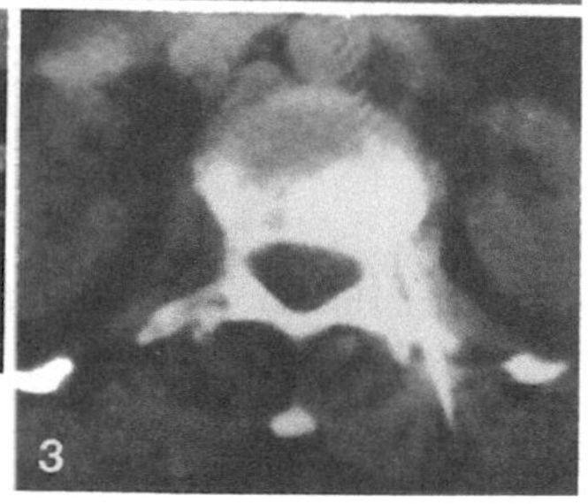

Fig. 1. a CT showing gross destruction of C6 vertebral body. b Anterolateral approach showing the needle tip with distal artefact. Diagnosis: tuberculosis

Fig. 2. Posterolateral approach showing the needle tip in L2 vertebral body (metastasis)

Fig. 3. Posterolateral approach showing the needle tip in a sclerotic tumour

tive cytological findings. One of 6 mixed lesions had necrotic material and thus could not be categorised. Of 4 osteoblastic lesions, only one had positive cytological findings, viz. metastasis (Fig. 3). Cytological studies were thus inconclusive in 4 cases. Six patients had known malignant disease elsewhere in addition to the solitary vertebral lesion; cytological examination demonstrated tuberculous infection in 2 of them. Surgery was performed in 22 patients and subsequent histopathological examination confirmed the cytological findings in all of them. No major complications occurred.

Discussion

Vertebral lesions vary from the innocuous benign lesions to life-threatening malignancies [4]. The ultimate optimal therapy in such situations depends on the histopathological nature of the lesion [2]. PAB is a simple non-surgical technique resulting in early diagnosis and institution of therapy. Moreover in patients with medically treatable benign conditions or with inoperable advanced malignancies, the discomfort, mortality and morbidity inherent in surgical "open" biopsy can be avoided [2–4].

The maximum diagnostic yield from PAB can be achieved via accurate localisation of the lesion prior to and during the procedure [2]. CT can be used accurately not only to detect the lesions but also to guide needle placement at the time of PAB and provides a safe access route to the lesion [5, 6].

The overall accuracy of PAB varies from 72.3% to 96% [3, 7]. In our study the accuracy was 92%. Metastases and tuberculous infection (30% each) were the most commonly encountered pathological findings in this study. This is consistent with other reported studies in our country [10]. Staphylococcal osteomyelitis (10%), giant cell tumour (6%) and plasmacytoma (6%) were the other lesions encountered in this series. One patient had a small lytic lesion in the posterior edge of the vertebral body along with degenerative changes. Cytological examination showed evidence of degenerative disease. Two patients presented with lytic lesions following laminectomy with a clinical and radiological diagnosis of postoperative osteomyelitis. Cytological examination demonstrated a fibrous band in one case and normal osteoid tissue in the other. Re-exploration was done and histopathological examination confirmed the cytological findings. Two cases of collapsed vertebrae with some lytic areas were biopsied for possible infection or malignancy. Cytological examination showed fibrous tissue in one and normal osteoid tissue in the other, and retrospectively a distant history of trivial trauma could be elicited. In 4 patients, cytological examination was negative and no specific diagnosis could be reached. The lesion was sclerotic in 3 of these and adequate tissue could not be obtained. In 1 patient with a mixed density lesion, the material was very necrotic and thus a proper cytological diagnosis could not be established. Six patients of known malignancy had lytic lesions, of which 2 turned out to be tuberculous infection. This suggests that lytic destruction of vertebrae in a patient with known malignant disease does not always indicate metastasis [2].

The average complication rate of PAB is 0.2–0.7% in various published reports [1, 9, 10]. No major or minor complications other than local pain were observed in our study. Thus, CT-guided PAB of solitary vertebral lesions is a safe, reliable, inexpensive and quick method of reaching a tissue diagnosis.

References

1. Murphy WA, Destonet JM, Girula LA (1981) Percutaneous skeletal biopsy. A procedure for radiologists – results, review and recommendations. Radiology 139:545–549
2. Stoker DJ, Kissin CM (1985) Percutaneous vertebral biopsy: a review of 135 cases. Clin Radiol 36:569–577
3. deSantos LA, Lukeman JM, Wallace S, Murray JA, Ayala AG (1978) Percutaneous needle biopsy of bone in cancer patients. AJR 13:641–649
4. Findlay GFG, Sundeman DR, Buxton DR, Buxton P (1988) The role of needle biopsy in the management of spinal compression. Br J Neurosurg 2:479–484
5. Brugieres P, Gaston A, Heran F, Voisin MC, Marsault C (1990) Percutaneous biopsies of the thoracic spine under CT guidance: transcostovertebral approach. J Comput Assist Tomogr 14:446–448
6. Renfrew DL, Whitten CG, Wiese JA, El-Khoury GY, Harris KG (1991) CT guided percutaneous transpedicular biopsy of the spine. Radiology 180:574–576
7. Georges Y, Khoury EL, Terepka RH, Michael MR, Rainville KL, Zaleski MS (1983) Fine needle aspiration biopsy of bone. J Bone Joint Surg [Am] 65:522–525
8. Schweitzer ME, Deely DM (1993) Percutaneous biopsy of osteolytic lesions: use of a biopsy gun. Radiology 189:615–616
9. Kattapuram SV, Rosenthal DI (1987) Percutaneous biopsy of cervical spine using CT guidance. AJR 149:539–541
10. Jayakumar PN, Arya BYT, Vasudev MK, Rao TV, Srikanth SG, Dinakar S (1994) Fine needle aspiration of spinal lesion. Neurol India 42:97–99

Bevel- versus pencil-point needles for myelography

J. M. Prager[1], S. Roychowdhury[1], M. T. Gorey[1], G. Lowe[2], W. Ankenbrandt[1], A. Ragin[1]

[1] Department of Radiology, Evanston Hospital/Northwestern University Medical School, 2650 Ridge Ave, Evanston, IL 60201, USA
[2] Stanford University Medical Center, Palo Alto, California, USA

Abstract. The frequency of spinal headache following myelography was assessed comparing the pencil-point side-hole spinal needle (Sprotte) with the bevel-tip end-hole spinal needle (Quincke). All needles were 22 gauge. The quality of the myelogram was also studied. We reviewed 100 patients referred for myelography: 4 of 47 (8.5%) patients in the pencil-point needle group and 13 of 53 (24%) in the bevel needle group experienced spinal headaches. There was no difference in myelographic quality between the two groups.

Key words: Myelography – Sprotte needle – Spinal headache

Headache is a common complication of myelography; when patients are questioned more than 2 days after their examination, the reported frequency is between 17% and 60% [1]. The hallmark of spinal headache is postural dependence [2]. Current research done to examine the complications of myelography involve comparisons of different needle sizes. These studies tend to show a decrease in frequency of headache when the smaller needles are used [3, 4]. A spinal needle with a tapering pencil-point tip and side-hole has been studied in the anesthesiology [5, 6] and neurology [2, 7] literature with generally favorable results. This study examines the use of pencil-point needles (Sprotte) compared to bevel-tip needles (Quincke) for myelography.

Correspondence to: J. M. Prager

Patients and methods

We studied 100 patients referred for myelography, randomized to either 22 gauge bevel- or pencil-point spinal needles. The only exclusion parameters were inability to sit or stand pre-existing headache. Patient data included age, sex, and area of spine. All myelograms were performed by a neuroradiologist. Spinal puncture was done with the patient prone on a fluoroscopy table with a pillow under abdomen. Puncture was slightly off-midline with the patient slightly rotated except for an occasional patient with wide open inter spinous spaces. In this case, puncture was in the midline. Puncture was at the L2–3 level regardless of the part of the spine being studied. Spinal fluid was not collected, and routine recommended dose of contrast material, iohexol, was injected into the subarachnoid space. Standing and prone images were obtained. CT always following myelography. Routine orders included bedrest with the head elevated 45° for 6 h following the myelogram. Patients were contacted by phone by an independent observer between 5 days and 2 weeks after myelography. Headache severity was graded on a 1–10 scale by the patient. A headache of grade 3 was effectively treated with over-the-counter medication, 5 was somewhat controlled but too severe for the patient to go to work, 8 was "miserable", and 10 was hospitalized.

The myelograms were examined by an independent neuroradiologist for extra-arachnoid injection of contrast medium. Mixed injection was graded as: 1, questionable; 2, slight; 3, examination quality limited but still diagnostic; and 4, nondiagnostic.

Table 1. Spinal headache and needle type

Needle type	Pa-tients	Number with spinal headache (%)	Average grade of headache severity	Average duration (days) of headache
Pencil-point	47	4 (8.5)*	5.3	4.4
Bevel-tip	53	13 (24)	6.2	5.0

* Chi square $P=0.03$

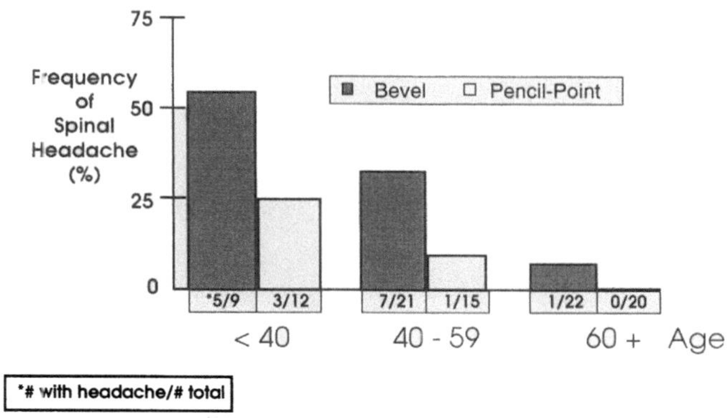

Fig. 1. The frequency of postmyelogram spinal headache with respect to patient age. The number of patients in each age group (with headache and total) is shown

Results

Follow-up was obtained in all 100 patients. We examined 53 with the end-hole needle and 47 with the side-hole needle. There were 52 women and 48 men, whose ages ranged from 25 to 88 years with an average of 56 years.

Spinal headaches (Table 1) occurred in 4 of the 47 patients in the side-hole group (8.5%) and 13 of the 53 patients in the end-hole group (24%). This is a statistically significant difference with $P=0.03$ using chi squared analysis. The frequency of spinal headache was inversely proportional to the ages of the patient examined (Fig. 1).

There were 82 lumbar, 1 thoracic, and 16 cervical studies and 1 combined cervical and lumbar study.

We reviewed only 65 myelograms for extra-arachnolid injection: 32 with side-hole and 33 with end-hole needles. There were only 2 definite mixed injections, one grade 2 with an end-hole needle and one grade 3 with a side-hole needle. Four injections were questionable, 3 with end-hole and 1 with the side-hole needle.

Discussion

Spinal headache, as a complication of dural puncture, was first described by August Bier, the pioneer of spinal anesthesia, in 1898 [1]. The frequency of spinal headaches in myelography is decreased when smaller gauge needles are used [3, 4]. Keeping the bevel parallel to the fibers of the dura mater may also be helpful [6]. Although the etiology of spinal headache is not fully understood, the most commonly accepted hypothesis is that leakage of cerebrospinal fluid (CSF) from the tear in the dura mater made by the spinal needle results in reduction in the CSF volume and thereby a fall in CSF pressure [1–4].

In a study of patients having a lumbar puncture for CSF examination, 4% of 50 patients with the pencil-point Sprotte needle had spinal headaches, compared to 36% of 25 patients with a bevel-tip needle [2]. The anesthesiology literature also suggests a decreased frequency of spinal headaches with the use of a side-hole needle [5, 6, 8].

Our study adds weight to the argument that pencil-point side-hole needles are less likely to be associated with spinal headache and provides data to support their routine use in myelography with younger patients.

References

1. McGann GM, Gleeson FV, Kelly I, Valentine AR, Platts A, Butler P, Crump BJ (1992) The influence of needle size on post-myelography headache: a controlled trial. Br J Radiol 65:1102–1104
2. Raskin NH (1990) Lumbar puncture headache. A review. Headache 30:197–200
3. Sand T (1989) Which factors affect reported headache incidences after lumbar myelography) Neuroradiology 31:55–59
4. Vezina JL, Fontaine S, Laperriere J (1989) Outpatient myelography with fine-needle technique: an appraisal. AJR 153:383–385
5. Sprotte G, Schedel R, Pajunk H (1987) An atraumatic needle for single shot regional anesthesia. Reg Anesth 10:104–108
6. Cesarini M, Torrielli R, Lahaye F, Mene JM, Cabiro C (1990) Anaesthesia 45:656–658
7. Engelhardt A, Oheim S, Neundorfer B (1990) Lumbar puncture with a new atraumatic needle. J Neurol 237:54
8. Ross BK, Chadwick HS, Mancuso JJ, Benedetti C (1992) Sprotte needle for obstetric anesthesia: decreased incidence of post dural puncture headache. Reg Anesth 17:29–33

Sella

Dynamic MRI versus dynamic CT in the diagnosis of pituitary microadenoma

J. F. Bonneville, F. Cattin, M. Piotin, M. L. Franck, S. Miralbes, K. Ghedas

Department of Neuroradiology, Jean Minjoz Hospital, F-25000 Besançon, France

Abstract. Dynamic MRI is today the most precise technique for detecting the smallest pituitary microadenomas. If MRI is not available or if patients are uneligible for MRI, dynamic CT remains a very acceptable competitive imaging modality.

Key words: Computed tomography – Magnetic resonance imaging – Pituitary, neoplasms

MRI is now considered the first-choice technique for detection of pituitary tumours. In some situations, for instance for pituitary adenomas less than 4 mm in diameter (picoadenomas), T1-weighted spin-echo (SE) sequences alone are clearly positive in as few as 40% of cases and T2-weighted fast SE is diagnostic in 70% of the T1-weighted negative cases. Gadolinium-enhanced coronal T1-weighted images are then often mandatory, but the hypersignal created by the ferromagnetic agent can also completely blur a small lesion. For all these reasons, dynamic MRI is frequently considered today as the most promising technique for imaging the smallest pituitary adenomas [1–4].

The purpose of this study is to compare dynamic MRI with dynamic CT which, up until now, was considered the most precise imaging technique [5, 6].

Patients and methods

Twenty patients all harbouring a prolactinoma less than 7 mm in diameter were selected. The pituitary adenoma has been proven anteriorly through the demonstration of some tumour shrinkage with bromocriptine treatment. This homogeneous series of patients was studied during the same week with dynamic CT and dynamic MRI.

In all patients, MRI study included a coronal T1-weighted sequence (500/14/3, 3 mm slice thickness, 300 × 512 acquisition matrix and a 23 cm field of view) and a coronal T2-weighted sequence (turbo SE 5000/90/2, 3 mm slice thickness 288 × 512 matrix and 26 cm field of view).

Coronal dynamic MRI was acquired with parameters of 230/15/1, 3 mm slice thickness, 145 × 256 acquisition matrix and a 23 cm field of view. There was no delay time between images and the temporal resolution was 36.95 s. Three different planes were obtained in each stage of the dynamic study. Immediately after a bolus injection of 0.05 mmol/kg gadopentetate dimeglumine, dynamic MRI was initiated and continued for a total of 5 min. Coronal dynamic CT was obtained in the midsellar plane with a 1.5 mm section thickness and 2 s scan time. The interval between the initial sections was 2.3 s and between the last few sections, 8, 15 and 30 s. A dose of 80 ml of 32% iodinated contrast medium (26 g iodine) and 30 ml saline solution were mechanically injected at 15 ml/s in an arm vein 8 s before the first slice of the dynamic acquisition.

Table 1. Positivity of various imaging techniques in the diagnosis of 20 residual pituitary adenomas less than 7 mm in diameter

Technique	Cases	Positive	(%)
Coronal T1-weighted SE	20	9	(45)
Coronal T2-weighted fast SE	9	4	(44)
Contrast-enhanced T1-weighted	20	6	(30)
Dynamic MRI	20	17	(85)
Contrast-enhanced CT	20	5	(25)
Dynamic CT	20	16	(80)

Results

Dynamic MRI was considered positive when an abnormal or asymmetrical focal enhancement was demonstrated and dynamic CT was considered positive in the presence of a displayed or compressed tuft, a delayed focal enhancement or in contrast, an early transient focal enhancement indicating a direct arterial supply (Fig. 1).

Coronal T1-weighted images alone were definitely diagnostic in only 9 of 20 cases (45%). An additional fast SE T2-weighted sequence was positive in 4 of 9 cases. Gadolinium-enhanced T1-weighted sequence had a very low rate of positivity (4 of 9 patients or 30%). On the other hand, dynamic MRI appeared to be an excellent technique, giving a positive result in 17 of 20 cases (85%).

Dynamic CT remains a very acceptable, competitive method with a positive rate of 80%. Post-contrast CT alone was positive in only 5 of 20 patients (25%) (Table 1).

Discussion

Dynamic MRI and dynamic CT scan are much more reliable than plain enhanced techniques for the diagnosis of pituitary tumours that are less than 7 mm in diameter. Moreover, both techniques have a complementary diagnostic value because, in 15–20% of the cases, either dynamic MRI or dynamic CT is clearly diagnostic.

Correspondence to: J. F. Bonneville

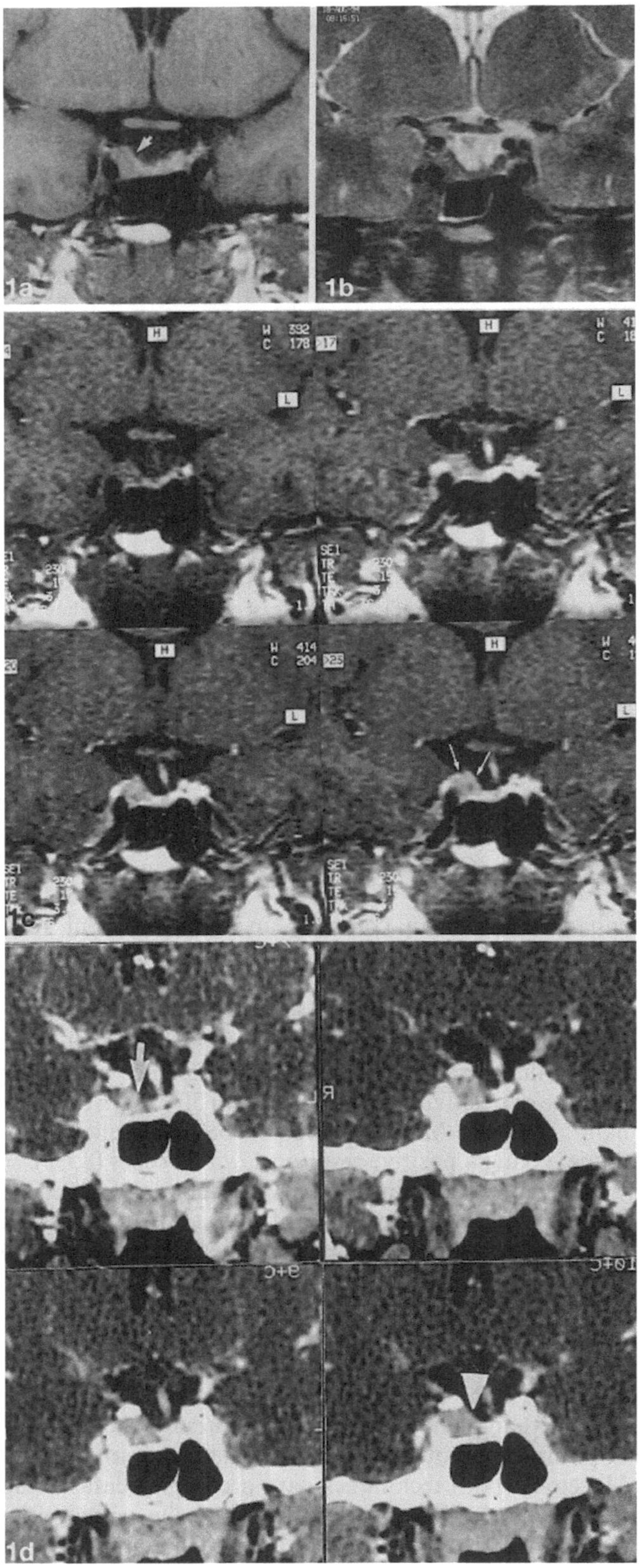

Fig. 1a–d. Bromocriptine-treated microprolactinoma in a 32-year-old woman. **a** Coronal T1-weighted SE image demonstrates more abundant pituitary tissue in the right half of the sella turcica (*arrow*) but no obvious signal abnormality. **b** Coronal T2-weighted SE image does not show any signal abnormality. **c** Dynamic MRI. Delayed enhancement of the right half of the pituitary (*arrows*) in favour of residual tumour. **d** Dynamic CT. Displacement of the pituitary tuft and early enhancement of the adenoma (*arrow*). At the end of dynamic CT, the lesion appears hypodense (*arrowhead*)

References

1. Miki Y, Matsuo M, Nishizawa S, Kuroda Y, Keyaki A, Makita Y, Kawamura J (1990) Pituitary adenomas and normal pituitary tissue: enhancement patterns on gadopenteate-enhanced MR imaging. Radiology 177:35–38
2. Sakamoto Y, Takahashi M, Korogi Y, Bussaka H, Ushi Y (1991) Normal and abnormal pituitary glands: gadopenetate dimeglumine-enhanced MR imaging. Radiology 178:441–445
3. Tien RD (1992) Sequence of enhancement of various portions of the pituitary gland on gadolinium-enhanced MR images: correlation with regional blood supply. AJR 158:651–654
4. Finelli DA, Kaufman B (1993) Varied microcirculation of pituitary adenomas at rapid, dynamic, contrast-enhanced MR imaging. Radiology 189:205–210
5. Bonneville JF, Cattin F, Moussa-Bacha K, Portha C (1983) Dynamic computed tomography of the pituitary gland: the "tuft sign". Radiology 149:145–148
6. Bonneville JF, Cattin F, Gorczyca W, Hardy J (1993) Pituitary adenomas: early enhancement with dynamic CT – implications in arterial blood supply and potential importance. Radiology 187:857–861

Perfusion enhancement of anterior pituitary gland with MRI: a functional study

H. M. Liu, Y. W. Li, Ch. T. Su

Department of Medical Imaging, National Taiwan University Hospital, 1 Chan-Te Street, Taipei, Taiwan

Abstract. In assessing the dynamic enhancement curves of the anterior pituitary gland with T1-weighted MRI in normal and pathological conditions such as idiopathic pituitary dwarfism, anterior lobe adjacent to microadenomas, haemosiderosis, post-irradiation, and empty sella, we found that different types of lesion had different dynamic enhancement curves, and this possibly represented their different blood perfusion condition and also their functional state.

Key words: Pituitary – Dynamic enhancement – Magnetic resonance imaging

Hypopituitarism is one of the most important endocrinological problems. Prior reports about MRI of hypopituitarism only mention findings of the idiopathic type [1–4]. The possibility of other aetiologies such as haemosiderosis, post-irradiation, empty sella, glands compressed by microadenomas, was not fully studied before. The purpose of this paper is to study those conditions with dynamic enhancement and to correlate them with pituitary function.

Materials and methods

From October 1991 to December 1993, we encountered 27 cases of idiopathic hypopituitarism (male:female = 21:6), 7 cases of haemosiderosis (male:female = 3:4), 68 cases of pituitary microadenomas (male:female = 3:65), 15 cases post-irradiation (male:female = 12:3), 8 patients with an empty sella (male:female = 2:6), and 3 cases of metastasis (male:female = 2:1). Their ages ranged from 3 to 74 years with a mean age of 38.1. Laboratory examinations were performed in cases with suspected hypopituitarism. Another 250 cases were studied as a normal control group (male:female = 1:1; mean age = 41.3).

All MRI examinations were performed with a 1.5 T unit as described before [5]. In brief, the dynamic study was performed with TR = 50–67 ms, TE = 20 ms with a matrix of 128 × 256 and one excitation. It took about 8 s per image. There was no delay time between images and a total 8–9 images were obtained. The dynamic studies began with the manual bolus intravenous injection of the contrast medium, gadopentetate dimeglumine (0.1 mmol/kg body weight), with a 21-gauge plastic cannula or needle. The injection duration time was less than 10 s.

The enhancement of various portions of the pituitary gland was assessed quantitatively. The signal intensity (SI) of the anterior lobe was measured by the region-of-interest method (minimum, 0.2 cm × cm) on sequential dynamic images. The data were obtained by averaging repeated measurements to decrease variability. Enhancement difference was defined as the difference of SI in the same region of interest before and after injection of contrast medium.

Correspondence to: H. M. Liu

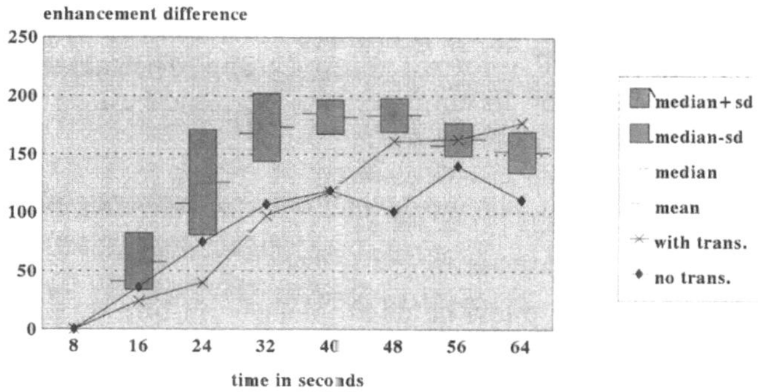

Fig. 1. Comparison of dynamic enhancement between normal and pituitary dwarfism (sd, standard deviation; trans, transection of stalk)

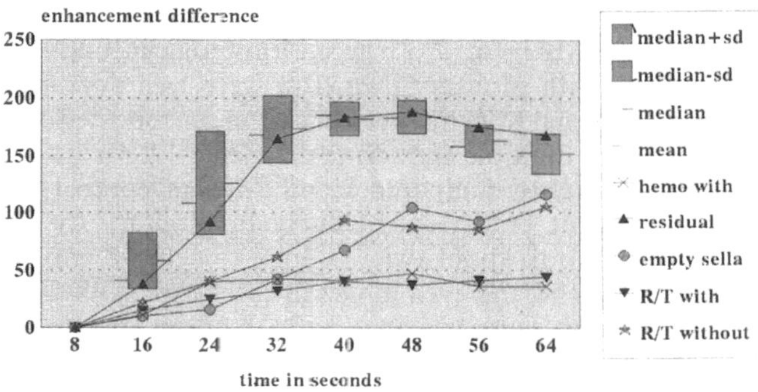

Fig. 2. Comparison of dynamic enhancement between normal and various acquired lesions (sd, standard deviation; hemo with, haemosiderosis with hypogonadism; R/T with, post-irradiation with hypofunction; without, without hypofunction)

Results

Normal control group (Figs. 1, 2)

The maximum enhancement occurred after about 32–40 s, and the time for half-maximum enhancement ($t_{\frac{1}{2}}$) after about 10–24 s.

Pituitary dwarfism (Fig. 1)

In cases with transection or without transection of pituitary stalk, the maximum enhancement occured after about 48–56 s (cases without transection), or later than 64 s (cases with transection), and the $t_{\frac{1}{2}}$ was after about 24–32 s. The height of maximum enhancement was approximately normal in cases with stalk transection.

Microadenomas (Fig. 2)

There was no difference between the dynamic enhancement curve of this group and that of the normal group.

Empty sellae and post-irradiation with hypopituitarism (Fig. 2)

The curves had maximum enhancement as low as half to two-thirds of the normal control group. The maximum enhancement of the empty sella bases could be after 64 s.

Haemosiderosis and post-irradiation with hypopituitarism (Fig. 2)

The curves were low in height, delayed in time and they never reached half of the maximum enhancement shown on the normal control group.

Discussion

Due to the lack of an intact blood-brain barrier and its unique blood supply, the pituitary gland enhances on dynamic MRI [6, 7]. The morphological findings in patients with pituitary dwarfism were well documented [1–4]. Normal MRI has been occasionally reported even in cases with multiple endocrine deficiency [2, 4].

In our study, compared with the normal control group, the dynamic enhancement curve in pituitary dwarfism generally took about twice as long to achieve maximum enhancement, and even longer in cases with stalk transection. This was also true in cases with normal height of the anterior lobes. However, their difference in maximum enhancement was slight. So far, we still cannot determine whether such findings are the result of etiology or of pituitary dwarfism. However, at least with the cases of normal height, we suggest that relatively less perfusion may play a part in cases of pituitary dwarfism.

In cases of microadenoma, the function of the anterior lobes was usually preserved. The normal appearance of their dynamic enhancement curves can therefore be expected.

Hypopituitarism can occur after irradiation of the head and neck due to damage to vascular stroma [8, 9]. Our study demonstrated the perfusion damage in them in different degrees.

Considerable defect of the diaphragm sellae was present in 20% autopsy [10]. Its relationship to hypopituitarism was previously described [11, 12]. In patients with hypopituitarism, either their functioning tissue is presumbly less than the necessary minimum 10%, or the hypothalamic and vascular connections have been lost [10]. We have not encountered cases of hypopituitarism caused by empty sella syndrome, so we cannot comment on this.

In cases of haemosiderosis due to thalassaemia, Bergeron and Kovacs [13] found that there was more iron deposition in the gonadotrophin-secreting areas. Our data possibly represented the low metabolism and low perfusion demand in them.

In addition to morphological findings, dynamic MRI study, which is easy to perform and not time-consuming, may be one of the most important parts of integral functional MRI examinations of pituitary anterior lobes.

References

1. Kelly WM, Kucharczyk W, Kucharczyk J, Kjois B, Peck WW, Normal D, Newton TH (1988) Posterior pituitary ectopia: an MR feature of pituitary dwarfism. AJNR 9:453–460
2. Abrahams JJ, Trefelner E, Boulware SD (1991) Idiopathic growth hormone deficiency: MR findings in 35 patients. AJNR 12:155–160
3. Kuroiwa T, Okabe Y, Hasuo K, Yasumori K, Mizushima A, Masuda K (1991) MR imaging of pituitary dwarfism. AJNR 12:161–164
4. Cacciari W, Zucchini S, Carla G, Pirrazzoli P, Cicognani A, Mandini M, Busacca M, Trevisan C (1990) Endocrine function and morphological findings in patients with disorders of the hypothalamo-pituitary area: a study with magnetic resonance. Arch Dis Child 65:1199–1202
5. Liu HM, Li YW, Tsai WY, Su CT (in press) Dynamic enhancement MRI of anterior lobe in pituitary dwarfism. Neuroradiology
6. Miki Y, Matsuo M, Nishizawa S, Kuroda Y, Keyaki A, Makita Y, Kawamura J (1990) Pituitary adenomas and normal pituitary tissue: enhancement patterns on gadopentetate-enhanced MR imaging. Radiology 177:35–38
7. Sakamoto Y, Takahashi M, Korogi Y, Bussaka H, Ushio Y (1990) Normal and abnormal pituitary glands: gadopentetate dimeglumine-enhanced MR imagings. Radiology 178:441–445
8. Travis EL (1975) Primer of medical radiobiology. Yearbook Medical, Chicago
9. Duncan W, Nias AHW (1977) Clinical radiobiology. Churchill Livingstone, London
10. Adams JH, Corsellis JAN, Duchen LW (1984) Greenfield's neuropathology, 4th edn. Arnold, London
11. Farber M, Turksoy RN, Rogers J (1977) The primary empty sella syndrome. Obstet Gynecol 49:2s–5s
12. Shapiro S, Herzog P, Sarto G (1977) Pseudo-pseudohypoparathyroidism, empty sella syndrome, and hypopituitarism in a young woman. Obstet Gynecol 49:6s–8s
13. Bergeron C, Kovacs K (1978) Pituitary siderosis. Am J Pathol 93:295–310

Use of fast spin-echo sequence in T2-weighted and dynamic contrast-enhanced MRI of sellar lesions

K. Migita, T. Uozumi, K. Arita, M. Sumida, H. Satoh, F. Ikawa

Department of Neurosurgery, Hiroshima University School of Medicine, Hiroshima, Japan

Abstract. We evaluated fast spin echo (FSE) sequences in dynamic and T2-weighted MRI of sellar lesions. We examined 25 patients with sellar lesions by dynamic FSE imaging (400/17, ETL 8, 256 × 128, 2 signal averages every 20 s on a 1.5 T MR unit. In 10 patients, dynamic FSE images were compared with dynamic standard spin echo (SSE) images. Thirty-eight patients were imaged with a T2-weighted FSE sequence (6000/76, ETL 16, 512 × 256, 2 signal averages). In 10 patients, T2-weighted FSE images were compared with SSE images. FSE dynamic imaging enables a two-slice acquisition and thin slice imaging without sacrificing the image quality and the acquisition time. High-resolution imaging of a T2-weighted FSE sequence enables the detection of the diaphragm in 80% of patients and the chiasm in 95%. Therefore, an FSE sequence is valuable in detecting sellar lesions and adjacent structures.

Key words: Magnetic resonance imaging – Fast spin echo – Pituitary – Contrast enhancement

Magnetic resonance imaging (MRI) is accepted as the most sensitive imaging method in the diagnosis of sellar lesions. Most importantly, dynamic contrast-enhanced MRI is indispensable to find the small adenoma. However, dynamic standard spin echo (SSE) images do not have enough spatial resolution or signal-to-noise ratio (SNR) because of the limitations of their acquisition time. In a patient with a large sellar tumour, it is desirable to know the margins of the tumour and its relationship to adjacent structures such as optic apparatus, diaphragma sellae and the cavernous sinus, before surgery. We evaluated the value of a fast spin echo (FSE) sequence in dynamic contrast-enhanced imaging to detect a small lesion and in T2-weighted imaging to identify the surrounding structure of the tumour.

Patients and methods

We studied 38 patients with sellar lesions on a 1.5 T MR imaging system (Table 1).

In 25 patients, T1-weighted FSE images with a repetition time (TR) of 400 ms, an effective TE of 16 ms (400/16), an echo-train length of 8 echoes, 2 excitations, a 256 × 128 matrix, 3-mm slice thickness and 16-cm field of view (FOV) (imaging time, 14 s), were obtained during the bolus injection of 0.1 mmol/kg gadopentetate dimeglumine for the dynamic contrast-enhanced study. In 10 of these patients, T1-weighted SSE images with 100/, 16 1 excitation, a 256 × 128 matrix, 5-mm slice thickness and 16-cm FOV (imaging time, 16 s), were obtained to compare with the FSE images.

Coronal T2-weighted FSE images of the sellar region were obtained with a 6000/76, an echo-train length of 16 echoes, a 512 × 256 matrix, 2 excitations, 3-mm slice thickness with a 1-mm intersection gap and 16-cm FOV (imaging time, 3 min 12 s). T2-weighted SSE images with 2000/80, a 256 × 192 matrix, 2 excitations, 3-mm slice thickness with 1-mm intersection gap (imaging time, 57 s) were acquired in addition to FSE images in 10 patients to compare the detectability of optic apparatus, diaphragma sellae and the medial wall of the cavernous sinus which surrounds the tumour and pituitary gland (Fig. 1).

Correspondence to: K. Migita, Department of Neurosurgery, Hiroshima University, 1-2-3 kasumi, Minami-ku, Hiroshima, 734, Japan

Table 1. Types of lesions

Diagnosis	Number
Microadenoma	8
Macroadenoma	23
Meningioma	2
Rathke's cleft cyst	2
Germ cell tumour	2
Craniopharyngioma	1
Total	38

Table 2. Detectability of structures surrounding the sella in ten patients

Structure visualised	Spin-echo technique	
	Fast (%)	Standard (%)
Optic chiasm	10/10 (100)	7/10 (70)
Diaphragma sellae	8/10 (80)	3/10 (30)
Medial wall of cavernous sinus	2/20 (10)	0/20 (0)

Results

Dynamic contrast-enhanced images

FSE dynamic imaging with prolonged TR and an increased number of excitations, could raise signal intensity without sacrificing the acquisition time. A thin slice section was possible while still maintaining good image quality, and prolonged TR made two slice acquisition possible. In 1 case, the tumour was detected only by FSE dynamic images; it was not visible on SSE dynamic images (Fig. 2).

T2-weighted images

The optic chiasm was visible in 95% of 38 cases, the diaphragm in 80% and the medical wall of the cavernous

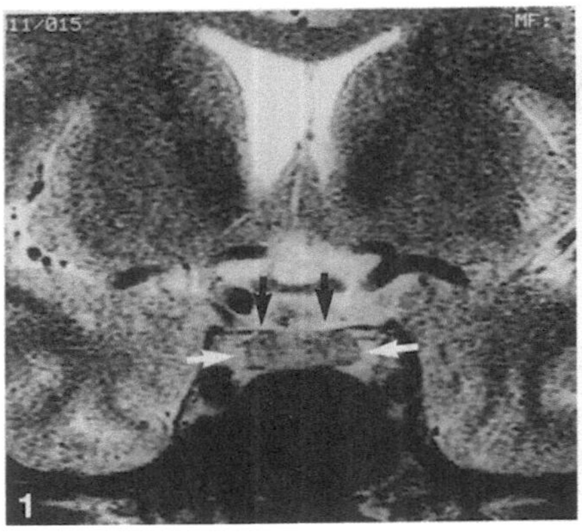

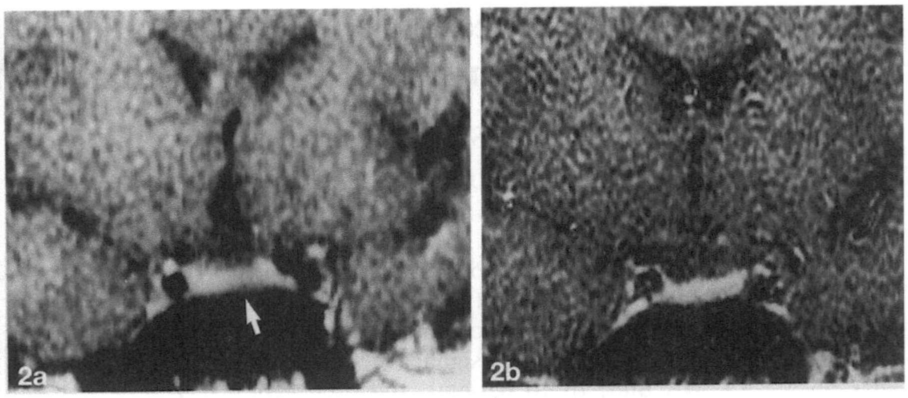

Fig. 1. T2-weighted FSE image of a normal volunteer. The optic chiasm is seen clearly as an isointense bar. The low-intensity line between pituitary gland and cavernous sinus (*arrow*) is the medial wall of the cavernous sinus, and the horizontal low-intensity line (*arrowhead*) contiguous with the medial wall the diaphragma sellae

Fig. 2. **a** FSE and **b** SSE images of a microadenoma imaged after bolus injection of contrast medium. The tumour is seen on the FSE image whereas it is not visible on the SSE image

stinus was detected in only 8%. In comparison with SSE imaging, the optic chiasm was detected in all cases on FSE images but in only 70% on SSE images. The diaphragm was detected in 80% by FSE images but in only 30% by SSE images. The medial wall of the cavernous sinus was visible in only 10% by using the FSE sequence and it was not visible in any cases using the SSE sequence (Table 2).

Discussion

Dynamic contrast-enhanced MRI is indispensable in finding the small adenoma. As the best contrast, the enhancement difference between the normal pituitary gland and pituitary adenoma had occurred by the 1st or 2nd min [1, 2], we think temporary resolution must be less than 30 s. Because of this limitation in acquisition time, dynamic SSE images do not have enough spatial resolution and SNR. Increased signal intensity and the thin slice section of FSE imaging contributed to the detection of a small lesion. In addition, FSE might be useful to visualise a lesion located on the sellar floor because it reduces susceptibility to artefacts caused by sphenoid sinus interface. Gradient-recalled echo imaging has a high temporal resolution but has limitations at the sella because of its sensitivity to magnetic susceptibility effects. Therefore, we think that the FSE sequence is most suitable for the dynamic study of sellar lesions at present.

A higher resolution study using larger matrices is desirable for sellar lesions but was impractical with the SSE technique because of time constraints. The faster acquisition time of FSE can be traded off for increased spatial resolution while still maintaining short imaging times [3]. T2-weighted FSE imaging made it possible to identify the optic chiasm and diaphragma sellae faster than with SSE imaging but visualisation of the medial wall of the cavernous sinus was difficult even when using the FSE sequence. Thus, T2-weighted FSE imaging is helpful in recognising the relationship between the sellar lesion and its surrounding structures but might have limitations in estimating the cavernous sinus invasion.

References

1. Miki Y, Matsuo M, Nishizawa S, Kuroka Y, Keyaki A, Makita Y, Kawamura J (1990) Pituitary adenomas and normal pituitary tissue: enhancement patterns in gadopenterare-enhanced MR imaging. Radiology 177:35–38
2. Sakamoto Y, Takahoshi M, Korogi Y, Bussaka H, Ushio Y (1991) Normal and abnormal pituitary glands: gadopentate dimegulumine-enhanced MR imaging. Radiology 178:441–445
3. Ahnn SS, Mantello MR, Jones KM, Mulkern RV, Melki PS, Higuchi N, Barnes PD (1992) Rapid MR imaging of pediatric brain using fast spin-echo technique. AJNR 13:1169–1177

Dynamic contrast-enhanced MRI of the pituitary gland

M. Thorn-Kany[1], I. Berry[2,3], C. Manelfe[1,2], P. Arrué[1], J. M. Franconi[4], A. Bonafé[2]

[1] Department of Neuroradiology, University Hospital Rangueil, Toulouse, France
[2] Department of Neuroradiology, University Hospital Purpan, Toulouse, France
[3] Department of Biophysics, University Hospital Rangueil, Toulouse, France
[4] Siemens, Saint-Denis, France

Abstract. Dynamic contrast-enhanced MRI of the pituitary gland was used in ten patients. It is interesting in our preliminary series because it could appreciate the contrast kinetics of the sellar, laterosellar and parasellar components as well as adenomas. In one case, it discovered a lesion. In another, it suspected cavernous sinus invasion. The dynamic contrast-enhanced sequence was equivalent to conventional sequences in the other four lesions in terms of diagnosis and extent. Subtraction of precontrast images and the use of lower-dose boluses could improve these techniques further.

Key words: Magnetic resonance imaging- Gadolinium - Pituitary gland - Pituitary adenomas

Fast MRI greatly improves the exploration of the pituitary gland, which benefits from high spatial resolution. Nevertheless, it has not been possible, so far, to combine a sufficiently high resolution imaging time for tracking interstitial contrast medium arrival in the parenchyma. In this study, paramagnetic bolus of contrast medium could be followed by 24 sequential MRI fast acquisition of 3D-T1-weighted data sets every 18 s.

Methods

Ten patients (7 females, 3 males) aged between 16 and 83 years (mean age 43.5 years) were examined with dynamic contrast-enhanced MRI of the pituitary gland. They were suspected of having pituitary adenomas on clinical and biological data: hyperprolactinaemia in 7 cases, hypotestosteronism in 1 case, hypersecretion of FSH-LH in 1 case and a visual deficit (non-secreting adenoma) in 1 case.

MRI was performed at 1.5 T with the acquisition of three sequences:

1. Dynamic study: 3D-T1-weighted gradient-echo with suppression of the residual transverse magnetisation between pulses (FLASH) was used with the following parameters: TR 20 ms, TE 6 ms, flip angle 15°, 30.4-mm-thick slab, 8 coronal partitions (3.8 mm reconstructed slices), field of view 113 mm × 150 mm, data matric size 92 phase-encoding steps in the left-right direction × 128 frequency-encoding steps.
2. T2-weighted sequence: turbo spin echo TR 3500 ms, TE 96 ms, 11 coronal slices 2 mm thick, matrix 392 × 512, 2 excitations, acquisition time 6.4 min.
3. T1-weighted sequence: turbo spin echo TR 600 ms, TE 12 ms, 11 coronal and sagittal slices 3 mm thick, matrix 256 × 512, 2 excitations, acquisition time 5.1 min, before and after contrast bolus injection (0.1 mmol/kg body weight).

Correspondence to: C. Manelfe, Servide de Neuroradiologie, Hôpital Purpan, F-31059 Toulouse, France

Results

Dynamic contrast-enhanced MRI was normal in 4 cases and abnormal in 6 cases: 3 microadenomas (one postoperative recurrence), 2 macroadenomas and 1 inhomogenous pituitary hyperplasia.

Morphological and kinetic aspects

Arteries. In all cases, intracavernous internal carotid arteries are the first enhancing structures, seen 18 s after bolus injection.

Cavernous sinus. In 8 of 10 cases, the venous plexuses of the cavernous sinuses are delineated. They enhance 18–36 s after contrast injection.

Second pituitary capillary bed ("tuft") [1]. In 3 of the 3 normal cases, it appears twice at 36 s and one at 18 s after contrast injection. Among the microadenomas, the "tuft" is still seen but impinged on the side of the adenoma.

Normal anterior hypophysis. This begins in all cases 36 s after contrast injection and is maximum at 1.12 min twice and at 2.20 min twice; it decreases after 2.7–5 min. Among the 4 normal hypophyses, enhancement is homogeneous twice and inhomogenous twice. In the 2 laterosellar microadenomas, enhancement is delayed and less intense than on the normal side; this asymmetry is striking during the initial 3 min.

Comparison with conventional sequences

In the 6 abnormal cases, conventional sequences always describe the topography and the extension of the lesions well. Nevertheless, in 1 case, dynamic sequence showed a lesion (associated microadenoma in pituitary by perplasia) (Fig. 1). Dynamic sequence did not miss any lesions although the extent was less clear in 1 case.

Cavernous sinus invasion was confirmed in 1 case and was equivocal in another on the dynamic sequences.

Dynamic sequences show contrast medium kinetics in adenomas. The 3 microadenomas enhance with delay, well after the maximum enhancement of the normal anterior hypophysis (i.e. 3.6, 2.4 and 1.2 min for microadenomas, compared with 1.12–2.20 min for normal anterior hypophysis). The 2 macroadenomas enhance earlier than microadenomas, like the normal parenchyma (beginning of enhancement at 36 s and maximum enhancement at 1.12 min). However, no normal pituitary tissue can be delineated.

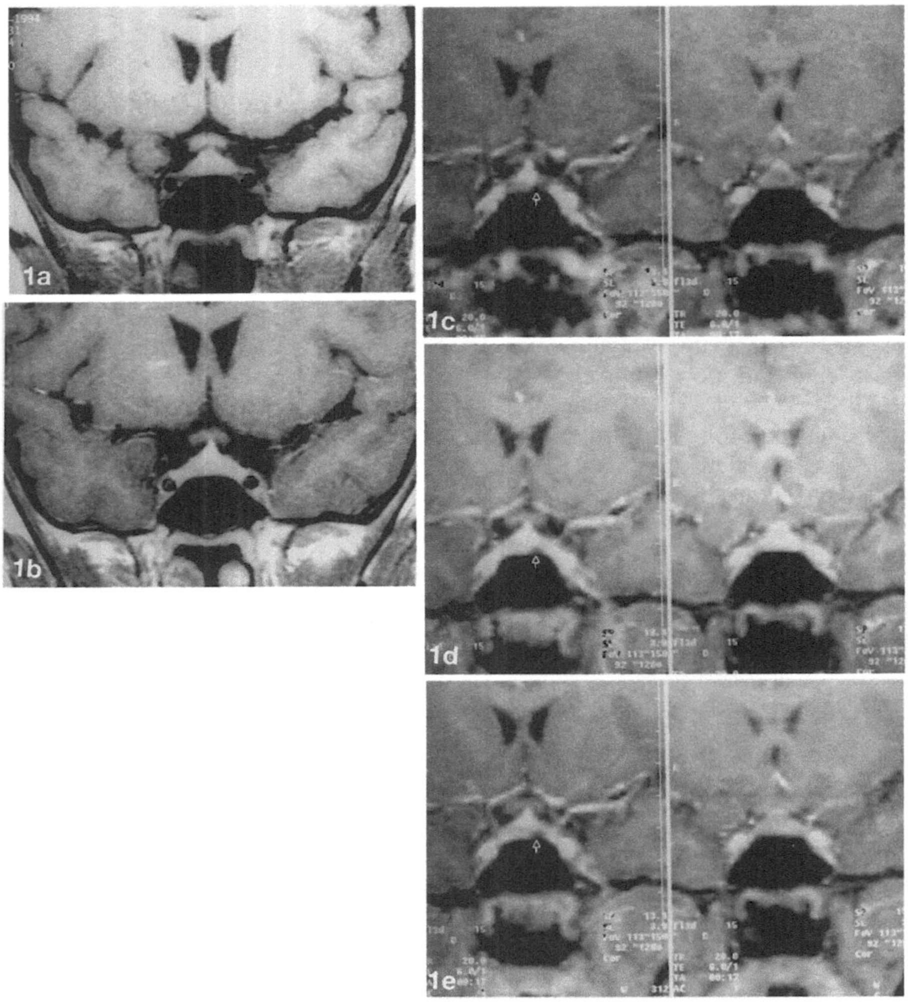

Fig. 1 a–e. a Inhomogeneous pituitary hyperplasia. **a** Conventional T1-weighted spin-echo image. Increased volume of the pituitary gland without abnormality of signal intensity. **b** Conventional T1-weighted spin-echo image after contrast medium injection. Inhomogeneous enhancement of the hyperplastic parenchyma. **c** 3D T1-weighted gradient-echo dynamic study 36 s after contrast medium bolus injection. The "tuft" is seen medially and on the right. Lack of diffusion of contrast medium on the left suggests the presence of a lesion (*arrow*). **d** At 1 min 12 s, maximum enhancement of anterior pituitary is seen. The left sided lesion is still suspected (*arrow*). **e** At 6 min wash-out of the normal anterior pituitary occurs. No significant change is seen in the suspected microadenoma

Discussion

Dynamics of enhancement derive from the special vascularisation of the hypophysis. The anterior hypophysis is vascularised by a portal system originating from superior hypophyseal arteries. This portal system generates a capillary bed located at the superior and medial aspect of the gland, anterior to the emergence of the pituitary stalk. The posterior hypophysis is directly vascularised by the hypophyseal inferior arteries. Dynamic MRI findings are similar to dynamic computed tomography as described by Bonneville et al. [1, 2]. It allows visualisation of: (1) intracavernous internal carotid arteries and their intracranial branches 10 s after the end of injection; (2) second pituitary capillary bed (so-called "tuft") after maximum enhancement of internal carotid arteries; (3) anterior pituitary from the capillary 20 and 40 s after injection, regular and symmetrical centrifugal enhancement; (4) laterosellar vein enhancement 5 s after injection of the internal carotid arteries. The cavernous sinus is homogeneously enhanced 10 s later.

Early dynamic images can demonstrate the contrast difference between adenomas and normal structures better than conventional sequences. Indeed, the normal pituitary tissue and cavernous sinus show early and progressive enhancement, whereas enhancement of pituitary adenomas and postoperative packing materials are slightly delayed. In our experience of 3 confirmed microadenomas, the dynamic sequence was beneficial only for the contrast kinetics of pituitary components. Only in a single case (Fig. 1) did the dynamic sequence discover a lesion that was not seen on the conventional sequences.

Enhancement of macroadenomas is in relation to their direct arterial supply. However, they enhance less intensely than the normal anterior pituitary gland. It has been shown that dynamic sequences appreciate the size and location of the normal pituitary tissue within macroadenomas. Yuh et al. [8] confirms that in 10 patients with macroadenomas tumour enhancement was noted to occur slightly, although not significantly, before the posterior pituitary and significantly before the anterior pituitary.

Early tumoural invasion of the cavernous sinus is indirectly suspected from visualisation of the venous compartment, especially the internal venous plexuses. Lack of enhancement is not specific of early tumoural invasion or compression because of their high variability and is missing in more than 70–80% of cases [2]. In our series, we could confirm sinus invasion in only one case out of two. A half-dose dynamic study yielded superior contrast between cavernous sinus and pituitary and was particularly useful in evaluating sinus invasion by adenomas.

References

1. Bonneville J, Cattin F, Dietemann JL (1986) Computed tomography of the pituitary gland. Springer, Berlin Heidelberg New York
2. Bonneville JF, Cattin F, Tang YS (1991) Radioanatomy of the laterosellar veins. Value of dynamic computerized tomography. J Neuroradiol 18:240–249
3. Yuh W, Fisher DJ, Nguyen HD, et al (1994) Sequential MR enhancement pattern in normal pituitary gland and in pituitary adenoma. AJNR 15:101–108

Sequential inferior petrosal sinus sampling: a simplified technique for the diagnosis of Cushing's disease

M. Nelson[1], J. T. Lamb[1], J. P. Sebastian[2], S. M. Orme[2], P. E. Belchetz[2]

[1] Section of Neuroradiology, General Infirmary, Leeds, LS1 3EX, UK
[2] Department of Neuroradiology, General Infirmary, Leeds, UK

Abstract. Sequential inferior petrosal sinus sampling after corticotropin-releasing hormone stimulation was applied to 16 patients with surgically confirmed adrenocorticotropin (ACTH) hypersecretion of pituitary origin using a catheter designed to permit rapid venous sampling. The findings had diagnostic and lateralising value comparable with the "gold-standard" technique, bilateral simultaneous sampling. Sequential sampling is the simplest and most cost-effective technique for diagnosing a pituitary source of ACTH hypersecretion.

Key words: Catheters and catheterisation, technology – Sinuses, dural – Cushing's disease

Whatever its cause, hypercortisolism carries high morbidity and significant mortality, which should be improved by earlier diagnosis and appropriate treatment. Non-invasive biochemical tests of the pituitary-adrenal axis are not reliable for planning treatment [1]. Demonstration of a pituitary microadenoma by CT or MRI cannot establish a diagnosis of Cushing's disease, since there is a high incidence (12–27%) of incidental pituitary adenomas in the general population [2]. Simulteaneous inferior petrosal sinus (IPS) sampling for adrenocorticotropin (ACTH) after corticotropin-releasing hormone (CRH) stimulation is the "gold-standard" technique for distinguishing pituitary and non-pituitary causes of hypercortisolism. In the largest published series an IPS: peripheral vein ratio (IPS: P ratio) for ACTH of $\geqslant 3.0$ had 100% accuracy, sensitivity and specificity for differentiating pituitary (Cushing's disease) and non-pituitary (adrenal and ectopic Cushing's syndrome) causes of hypercortisolism. Comparing the right and left sides, an intersinus ratio for ACTH of $\geqslant 1.4$ correctly predicted the side of the microadenoma in about 70% of patients [2].

Since a high IPS:P ratio of ACTH after CRH stimulation is maintained much longer than the early (2–5 min) peak of ACTH release, we have used sequential IPS sampling after CRH stimulation to investigate patients with suspected Cushing's disease.

We present the results of sequential IPS sampling after CRH stimulation, using a catheter designed to facilitate rapid sampling, in 16 patients with Cushing's syndrome, caused by pituitary hypersecretion of ACTH, subsequently confirmed by surgical resection.

Correspondence to: M. Nelson

Patients and methods

Sixteen consecutive patients with Cushing's syndrome, as shown by elevated 24-h urinary cortisol and lack of suppression following low-dose dexamethasone, were studied prospectively. There were 4 males and 12 females with a mean age of 37 years (range 22–60). Imaging of the pituitary gland excluded macroadenoma in all patients. An abnormality compatible with the presence of microadenoma was found in 7 of 13 CT scans and in 9 of 10 MRI scans; all patients who had both CT and MRI showed a focal abnormality compatible with the presence of microadenoma in at least one of the two studies. In all patients, the diagnosis of pituitar-dependent hypercortisolism (Cushing's disease) was established by sequential IPS sampling and was confirmed by biochemical remission following pituitary surgery.

The Leeds IPS sampling catheter is designed to permit rapid sampling of the IPS and other suprathoracic veins. A 5F high-flow nylon-braided shaft construction imparts a combination of suppleness and pushability that are desirable for catheterisation in the venous system with a high degree of torque control for accurate placement of the catheter tip. Angulation of the tip facilitates catheterisation of the IPS and a two-hole design permits aspiration of blood from large veins or small tribularies, such as the IPS, without delay or any need for further manipulation of the catheter (Fig. 1).

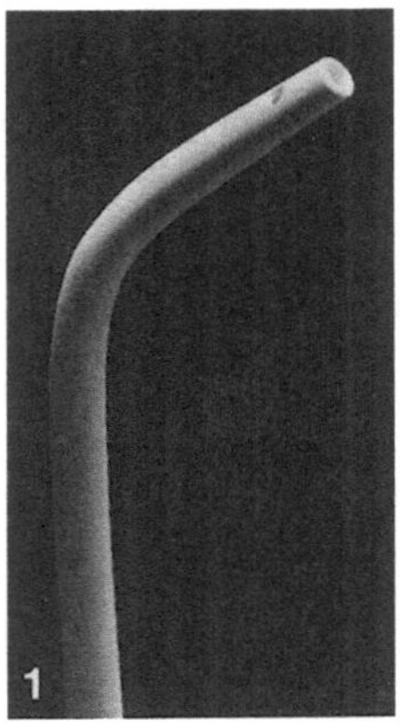

Fig. 1. The Leeds inferior petrosal sinus sampling catheter; view of catheter tip shows taper and angulation to facilitate catheterisation of the inferior petrosal sinus and two-hole design which permits prompt aspiration from veins of any size

Table 1. ACTH ratio between inferior petrosal sinus (IPS) and peripheral vein for right and left sides (larger value underlined for each pair) and the intersinus ratio

Patient	IPS:P ratio of ACTH		Intersinus ratio
	Right	Left	
1	1.09	*12.57*	11.53
2	*12.10*	7.36	1.64
3	0.91	*2.84*	3.12
4	*3.58*	1.05	3.41
5	0.96	*5.99*	6.24
6	*9.40*	0.97	9.69
7	1.57	*5.03*	3.20
8	*4.48*	3.26	1.38
9	*10.31*	0.88	11.72
10	*14.65*	1.21	12.08
11	0	0	0
12	2.60	*3.02*	1.16
13	*13.75*	5.09	2.70
14	1.92	*3.56*	1.85
15	*14.39*	1.01	14.25
16	*2.76*	1.19	2.32

Sampling can be undertaken without sedation as a day-case procedure. After inserting an indwelling cannula in an antecubital vein and in IPS sampling catheter through a femoral vein, 100 µg human CRH is given through the peripheral vein. In turn, the right and left inferior petrosal sinuses are sampled. During catheterisation check venograms are done with gentle injection to limit the reflux of contrast medium to the IPS only. After sampling a further venogram confirms the sample site and defines the venous anatomy, avoiding reflux to the opposite cavernous sinus if it has yet to be sampled. Samples for ACTH measurement are collected in EDTA tubes on ice; plasma is separated by centrifugation within 30 min and stored at −20 °C until radioimmunoassay.

Results

Both inferior petrosal sinuses were sampled in all 16 patients. Using a variety of catheters after the injection of CRH, the right IPS was sampled in a mean time of 23 min (range 8–32 min), the left IPS in a mean time of 50 min (range 30–94 min). Using the Leeds IPS sampling catheter, the interval between the right and left IPS samples has been as litte as 5 min and no interval has been greater than 40 min.

A biochemical diagnosis of pituitary-dependent disease was established in all cases (Table 1). Fifteen of the 16 patients had IPS:P ratios for ACTH of >2.5. All had biochemical remission following transphenoidal hypophysectomy. Thirteen patients had IPS:P ratios >3.0. One patient had a rare disorder characterised by undectable ACTH levels in each IPS and peripherally caused by adrenal hypersensity to ACTH associated with macronodular adrenal hyperplasia; the hypercortisolism remitted after hypophysectomy, confirming the pituitary cause of the disorder [3].

The intersinus ratio (the ratio of the IPS:P for the right and left sides) showed a ratio ⩾1.4 in 13 patients (Table 1).

Discussion

Sequential IPS sampling after CRH stimulation is diagnostic in patients with Cushing's disease and identifies intersinus ratios that assist surgical planning for partial hypophysectomy. The magnitudes of the IPS:P and intersinus ratios are similar to those found using the "gold-standard" bilateral simultaneous sampling technique [2].

Sequential sampling employs a single femoral venepuncture and uses a single sampling catheter to obtain only four ACTH assays and does not require systemic heparinisation. The sequential sampling technique is simpler and more cost-effective than other IPS sampling techniques. It avoids the complexity and cost of techniques that use multiple catheters with heparinisation [2], catheters shaped individually for each IPS [4], or coaxial catheter systems for bilateral cavernous sinus sampling.

References

1. Orth DN (1991) Differential diagnosis of Cushing's syndrome. N Engl J Med 325:957–959
2. Oldfield EH, Doppman JL, Nieman LK, et al (1991) Petrosal sinus sampling with and without corticotropin-releasing hormone for the differential diagnosis of Cushing's syndrome. N Engl J Med 325:897–905
3. Hermus AR, Pieters GF, Smals AG, et al (1988) Transition from pituitary-dependent to adrenal-dependent Cushing's syndrome. N Engl J Med 318:966–970
4. Miller DL (1991) Selective catheterization of the inferior petrosal sinuses; new catheter design. Radiology 178:281–282

Imaging of Rathke's cleft cysts

M. Fukuchi[1], K. Mineura[1], N. Kuwahara[1], M. Kowada[1], S. Fushimi[2], M. Yoneya[2]

[1] Neurosurgical Service, Akita University Hospital, Akita, Japan
[2] Department of Neurosurgery, Hiraka General Hospital, Akita, Japan

Abstract. Clinical and radiographic findings were studied in seven patients with Rathke's cleft cysts. The age of patients varied from 14 to 73 years with a mean age of 53. They had presented with polyuria, headache, and visual disturbance. CT revealed a cystic mass with varying densities located in the intra- and suprasellar region. One tumour had homogeneous enhancement, and two tumours had ring enhancement. MRI was performed in five patients. The signal intensities of the cysts on T1-weighted images varied considerably from case to case. The cysts were high intensity on T2-weighted images in four of five patients. An injection of gadolinium-DTPA enhanced signal intensity at the margin of the cyst in one patient. MRI had a high sensitivity supplementing CT in detection of lesions and in determining the relationship between tumour and surrounding brain structures.

Key words: Rathke's cleft cysts – Computed tomography – Magnetic resonance imaging

Accurate diagnosis is an import issue in the management of cystic sellar and parasellar diseases such as craniopharyngioma, Rathke's cleft cysts, or pituitary adenoma.

In the current study, we retrospectively reviewed radiological findings including CT and MRI in patients with histologically proven Rathke's cleft cysts.

Patients and methods

The present study included seven patients with histologically verified Rathke's cleft cysts. There were three men and four women with a mean age of 53 years (range, 14–73 years). Initial symptoms were polyuria in three patients, headache in three, and visual disturbance in one. One patient showed optic atrophy, and the remaining patients were free of neurological deficits.

CT was performed before and after contrast medium in all patients. Five patients underwent MRI.

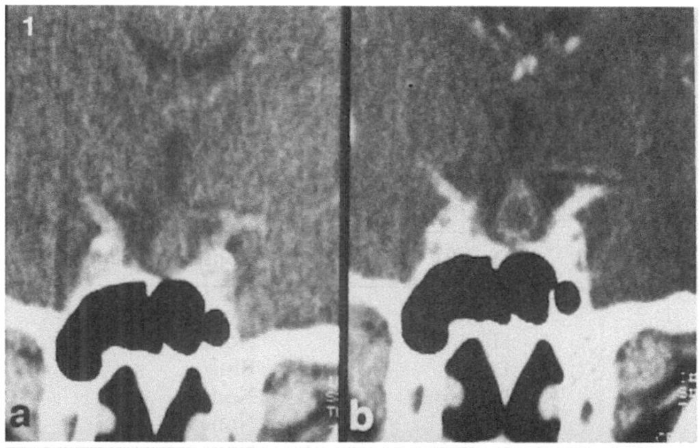

Fig. 1 a, b. Case 7. **a** Coronal CT showing an isodense intra- and suprasellar mass. **b** Contrast-enhanced image reveals ring enhancement

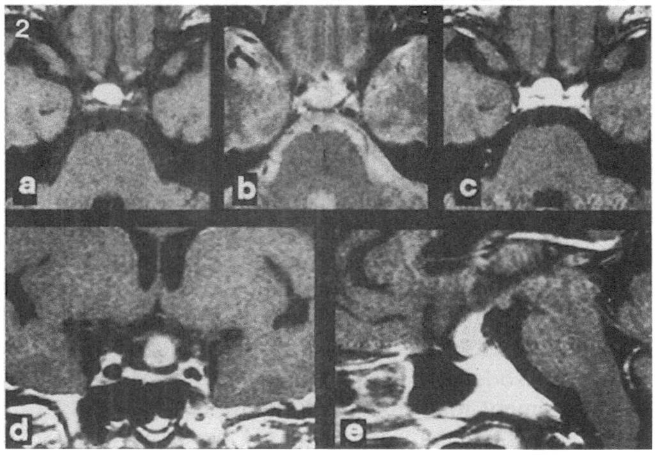

Fig. 2 a–e. Case 7. **a, b** T1- and T2-weighted axial MRI demonstrating a high intensity intra- and suprasellar mass. **c–e** T1-weighted axial, coronal and sagittal images after gadolinium administration showing ring enhancement

Results

Table 1 gives the clinical presentations. The cysts varied in diameter between 8 and 20 mm. All cysts were located in the intra- and suprasellar region.

The CT and MRI findings are summarised in Table 2. Representative cases are shown in Figs. 1 and 2. CT showed a low-density lesion in two patients, a high-density lesion in two, and an isodensity lesion in three. One region enhanced homogeneously with intravenous contrast medium and two regions had ring enhancement. There was no evidence of calcification or hydrocephalus on CT in any case. Two (cases 3 and 4) of five cysts had a low intensity on T1-weighted images and a high intensity on T2-weighted images. Another two cysts (cases 5 and 7) had a high intensity on both T1- and T2-weighted images. The cysts of case 2 had isointensity on T1- and low intensity on T2-weighted images. In only one case (case 7) did the cyst have ring-like enhancement with gadolinium-DTPA.

Compared with CT, MRI provided better spatial resolution of cysts, and clarified more accurately a relationship of cysts, optic tracts, and hypothalamus.

Correspondence to: M. Fukuchi

Table 1. Clinical findings in seven patients with Rathke's cleft cysts

Case	Age (years)	Sex	Symptoms	Size (mm)	Endocrinology
1	46	F	Headache	16 × 16 × 14	Normal
2	14	M	Polyuria	12 × 17 × 14	Diabetes insipidus
3	64	M	Polyuria	10 × 10 × 10	Diabetes insipidus
4	52	F	Headache	20 × 16 × 14	Normal
5	59	F	Headache	14 × 14 × 20	Normal
6	73	M	Visual disturbance	15 × 20 × 20	Normal
7	60	F	Polyuria	12 × 10 × 10	Diabetes insipidus

Table 2. Radiographic findings

Case	CT		MRI		
	Density	Contrast enhancement	T1-weighted	T2-weighted	Contrast enhancement
1	Isodense	Homogenous	Not done	Not done	Not done
2	High	None	Isointense	Low	None
3	Low	Ring	Low	High	Not done
4	Isodense	None	Low	High	None
5	High	None	High	High	None
6	Low	None	Not done	Not done	Not done
7	Isodense	Ring	High	High	Ring

Discussion

The CT and MRI appearances of Rathke's cleft cysts have recently been reported with the advance in neurimaging methods [1–8]. They are derived from remnants of the embryologic Rathke's pouch, and are biologically benign tumours located in the sellar and/or parasellar region [9].

On CT, Rathke's cleft cysts most frequently appear as a low or isodensity mass with or without a contrast-enhancement margin [6]. Okamoto et al. [10] suggested that ring-like enhancement on CT occurred when stratified squamous epithelium or inflammation was present in the cyst wall. In two cases (nos. 3 and 7) in our series, CT showed ring enhancement. In case 7, the cyst wall was histopathologically composed of ciliated cuboidal or columnar cells, and was lined by granulation tissue which consisted of inflammatory cells.

In the present study, MRI findings were not specific, because they had variable signal intensities. It is difficult to differentiate Rathke's cleft cysts from other sellar or suprasellar cystic tumours by signal intensity only. However, MRI had a high sensitivity, supplementing CT in the detection of lesions and in determining the relationship of cysts and surrounding brain structures.

Thus, neuroimaging knowledge provides useful information on the management of Rathke's cleft cysts and other sellar lesions.

References

1. Steinberg GK, Koenig GH, Golden JB (1982) Symptomatic Rathke's cleft cysts. Report of two cases. J Neurosurg 56:290–295
2. Ito H, Shoin K, Hwang W, Oonishi H, Hasegawa T, Yamamoto S (1987) Preoperative diagnosis of Rathke's cleft cyst. Child's Nerv Syst 3:225–227
3. Maggio WW, Cail WS, Brookeman JR, Persing JA, Jane JA (1987) Rathke's cleft cyst: computed tomographic and magnetic resonance imaging appearances. Neurosurgery 21:60–62
4. Kucharczyc W, Peck WW, Kelly WM, Norman D, Newton TH (1987) Rathke's cleft cysts: CT, MR imaging, and pathologic features. Radiology 165:491–495
5. Nemoto Y, Fukuda T, Shakudo M, Katsuyama J, Hakuba A, Nishimura S, Onoyama Y (1988) MR appearance of Rathke's cleft cyst. Neuroradiology 30:155–159
6. Nahasu Y, Isozumi T, Nakasu S, Handa J (1990) Rathke's cleft cyst: computed tomographic scan and magnetic resonance imaging. Acta Neurochir (Wien) 103:99–104
7. Voelker JL, Campbell RL, Muller J (1991) Clinical, radiographic, and pathological features of symptomatic Rathke's cleft cysts. J Neurosurg 74:535–544
8. Sumida M, Uozumi T, Mukada K, Arita K, Kurisu K, Eguchi K (1994) Rathke's cleft cysts: correlation of enhanced MR and surgical findings. AJNR 15:525–532
9. Fager CA, Carter H (1966) Intrasellar epithelial cysts. J Neurosurg 24:77–81
10. Okamoto S, Handa H, Yamashita J, Ishikawa M, Nagasawa S (1985) Computed tomography in intra- and suprasellar epithelial cysts (symptomatic Rathke's cleft cysts). AJNR 6:515–519

Cranial nerve enhancement on three-dimensional MRI in patients with ophthalmoplegia

T. Hosoya, N. Watanabe, K. Yamaguchi

Department of Radiology, Yamagata University School, 990-23 Iidanishi 2-2-2 Yamagata, Japan

Abstract. We investigated abnormal enhancement of the oculomotor, trochlear and abducens nerves in patients with ophthalmoplegia using contrast-enhanced three-dimensional (3-D) MRI, which offered high-quality images delineating the cisternal portion of the cranial nerves. In 23 patients with ophthalmoplegia, 12 nerves of 7 patients definitely enhanced. The causes of the cranial nerve enhancement were tumour, vertebral artery dissection, trauma, multiple sclerosis and Fisher's syndrome. Contrast-enhanced 3-D MRI is an extremely useful examination in patients with ophthalmoplegia and the abnormality of the oculomotor and abducens nerve can be detected in living humans.

Key words: Cranial nerve - Ophthalmoplegia - Contrast enhancement - Three-dimensional magnetic resonance imaging

Our aim was to demonstrate and point out the clinical significance of abnormal enhancement of the cisternal portion of the cranial nerves in patients with ophthalmoplegia due to various causes using three-dimensional (3-D) MRI.

Materials and methods

Our study included 23 consecutive patients (17 men, 6 women) aged between 14 and 77 years (mean age, 47.3) who underwent contrast-enhanced-3D MRI because of opthalmoplegia (12 with unilateral oculomotor, 1 with unilateral trochlear, 6 with unilateral abducens, 2 with bilateral oculomotor and 2 with bilateral oculomotor, trochlear and abducens nerve palsy), except those without any abnormality in the orbit or the cavernous sinus.

Contrast-enhanced 3-D MRI was obtained by spoiled gradient-recalled acquisition in a steady state using a 1.5 T system after injection of 0.1–0.15 mmol/kg (up to 20 ml) Gd-DTPA.

The incidence and causes of cranial nerve enhancement were investigated.

Results

In 23 patients with ophthalmoplegia, cranial nerve enhancement was seen in 12 nerves of 7 patients. Of the 12 enhanced cranial nerves, 8 (5 oculomotor and 3 abducens nerves) were symptomatic and 4 (2 oculomotor and 2 abducens nerves) were asymptomatic.

The causes were tumours (2 patients; leukaemic infiltration and neuroma), vertebral artery dissection (Fig. 1) (2), trauma (Fig. 2) (1), multiple sclerosis (1) and Fisher's syndrome (1). There was no cranial nerve enhancement in patients with myasthenia gravis (4), diabetic neuropathy (1), pituitary apoplexy (1), and in those with unknown causes (10).

In 2 patients with cranial nerve enhancement due to vertebral artery dissection and multiple sclerosis, brainstem lesions in the mid-brain and medulla oblongata were associated as focal enhancement on contrast-enhancement 3-D MRI and high-intensity lesions on T2-weighted images.

In 5 patients, all with cranial nerve enhancement, except those with tumours, MRI was performed 7 days to 3 months after the onset of ophthalmoplegia. All 5 patients made full recoveries during 1–3 months, except for 1 with vertebral artery dissection. In 2 patients with multiple sclerosis and Fisher's syndrome, follow-up MRI was performed and resolution of the enhancement, correlated with recovery of the cranial nerve palsy, was observed.

Discussion

Contrast enhancement of the cranial nerves, such as optic, oculomotor [1], trigeminal and facial nerve, has been reported recently. In this paper, we have described Gd-DTPA enhancement of the abducens nerve in addition to the above cranial nerves using contrast-enhanced 3-D MRI, which has been shown to offer high-quality images for delineating the cisternal portion of the cranial nerves [2].

As the causes of cranial nerve enhancement, neoplastic or inflammatory processes are well known. We encountered various causes such as tumour, vertebral artery dissection, trauma, multiple sclerosis and Fisher's syndrome. Cranial nerve enhancement on MRI caused by ischaemia has not been well described, although ischaemia is a common cause of cranial nerve palsy. Vertebral artery dissection is considered to be an important cause of brainstem ischaemic disease as well as Wallenberg's syndrome [3]. Head trauma may also cause ischaemic processes due to disturbance of the microvascular circulation. Demyelinating or inflammatory processes of the cranial nerves may occur in cases of multiple sclerosis and Fisher's syndrome, MRI findings which have not been well described. It seems important that definite abnormality of the cisternal portion of the cranial nerves should be confirmed in patients with ophthalmoplegia, because the affected lesion becomes clear and a correct diagnosis is made. Furthermore, contrast-enhanced 3-D MRI is appropriate for detecting aneurysms compressing the cranial nerve as it shows them as small vessels [2]. Thus, con-

Correspondence to: T. Hosoya

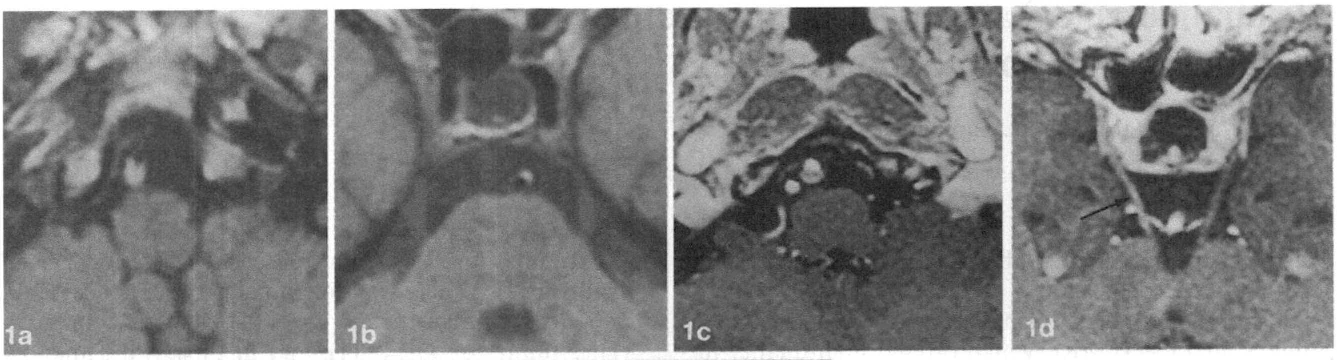

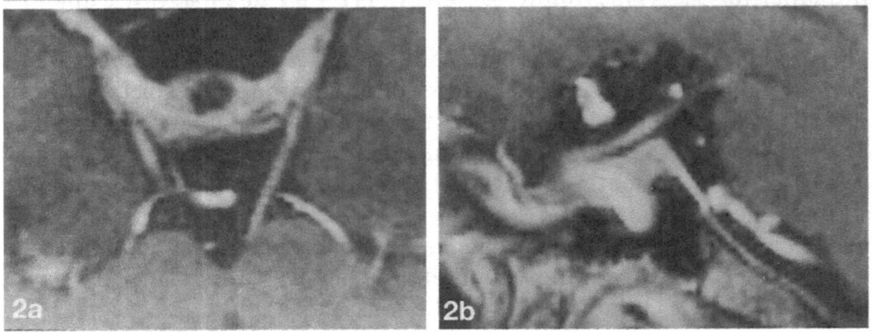

Fig. 1a–d. Vertebral artery dissection. A 45-year-old man complained of severe frontal headache preceding left, occipital head dullness and incomplete right oculomotor palsy. Subarachnoid haemorrhage was confirmed by lumbar puncture despite negative CT. No aneurysm was detected by angiography but left vertebral artery dissection was shown. MRI was performed 30 days after the onset. T1-weighted images (**a, b**) show semicircular high-intensity lesions with eccentric flow void of the left vertebral and basilar artery, which disappeared on follow-up. Contrast-enhanced 3-D MRI shows double lumen of the left vertebral artery (**c**) and contrast enhancement (*arrow*) of the right oculomotor nerve (**d**)

Fig. 2a, b. Trauma. A 43-year-old man fell down the stairs and hit his head. The next morning, he had a right oculomotor palsy. Contrast-enhanced 3-D MRI (**a, b**) shows abnormal enhancement of the oculomotor nerves

trast-enhanced 3-D MRI examination is extremely useful in patients with ophthalmoplegia.

References

1. Mark AS, Blake P, Atlas SW, Ross M, Brown D, Kolsky M (1992) Gd-DTPA enhancement of the cisternal portion of the oculomotor nerve on MR imaging. AJNR 13:1463–1470
2. Hosoya T, Sato N, Yamaguchi K, Sugai Y, Ogushi M, Kubota H (1992) MR imaging of the cranial nerves and the intracranial vessels using 3D-SPGR. J Magn Reson 12:245–252
3. Hosoya T, Watanabe N, Yamaguchi K, Kubota H, Onodera Y (1994) Intracranial vertebral artery dissection in Wallenberg syndrome. AJNR 15:1161–1165

MRI morphometric study of the quadrigeminal plate

R. Poniatowska, J. Ryterski, R. Krawczyk, E. Grochowska, T. Kryst

Institute of Psychiatry and Neurology, Warsaw, Poland

Abstract. The aim of this study was to assess the anatomy of the quadrigeminal plate in normal brain and abnormal conditions. Examinations were carried out on 0.38 T resistive magnet, using spin-echo sequences in T1- and T2-weighted images in sagittal and axial planes. The width and length of the tectum were measured, as were the angles of inclination of tectum to clivus and to Chamberlain's line. The patients were divided into four groups: one group with normal brains and three with pathological findings – hydrocephalus, supratentorial tumours and posterior fossa tumours. The exact localisation of the lesions, involvement of the tectum and its displacement were assessed. Marked displacement and involvement of the tectum were observed in pineal and peduncular tumours. The most significant finding in hydrocephalus was elevation of the tectum.

Correspondence to: R. Poniatowska, Department of Neuroradiology, Institute of Psychiatry and Neurology, Al. Sobieskiego 1/9, 02-957 Warsaw, Poland

Key words: Midbrain – Quadrigeminal plate – Morphometry – Brain neoplasms – Hydrocephalus

The purpose of this study was to develop a method of measuring the size of the quadrigeminal plate by routine MRI and to assess its dimensions and position in a normal brain compared with pathological conditions. The quadrigeminal plate, the tectum of the midbrain, consists of the paired superior and inferior colliculi and brachia.

The large group of lesions can involve the tectal region of the brain [1]. Our goal was to determine the impact of local and distant pathological brain lesions on the quadrigeminal plate. We compared our measurements with those of previous studies [2, 3].

Subjects and methods

A retrospective study of 200 MRI head examinations was performed. Patients (aged 6 months to 70 years) were divided into four groups: 75 without pathological findings (group 1), 20 with normotensive hydrocephalus (group 2), 75 with supratentorial tumours (group 3) and 30 with infratentorial tumours (group 4). T1-weighted SE sagittal images (TR 0.5 s, TE 20 ms) and T2-weighted SE axial images (TR 2.0 s, TE 25/80 ms) were obtained with a 0.38 T resistive unit. Slice thickness was 5–6 mm, matrix size 192 × 256, and field of view 24 cm.

The width of the quadrigeminal plate was measured in the axial, the length in the midsagittal plane, in which other measurements were also taken: the angle of inclination of the longitudinal axis of the tectum to the clivus (angle A) and the angle of its inclination to Chamerlain's line (angle B). To determine interobserver variation, all midsagittal and axial dimensions and angles were measured by two authors. The mean value (M) and standard deviations (SD) were calculated for tectum dimensions in each group. A mean from range (M – SD, M + SD) was considered to be normal.

Results

Interobserver variation was small. The difference between the dimensions was less than 1 mm in 84% of the measurements, and the difference between angles was less than 5° in 93% of the cases. In group I (Fig. 1) the length of the tectum varied between 10 and 18 mm (M 14.76, SD 0.97), the width between 13 and 20 mm (M 15.76, SD 1.57) (Table 1). The values of angle A were 0–28° (M 13.98, SD 6.25). The values of angle B were 30–70% (M 51.02, SD 3.33). In group 2 (Fig. 2) the length of the tectum varied from 10 to 14 mm (M 11.4, SD 1.39), the width from 9 to 19 mm (M 14.35, SD 2.46). The values of angle A were 0–47° (M 21.85, SD 10.33), and of angle B were 24–80° (M 47.35, SD 14.36). The group of brain tumours consisted of haematomas, benign and malignant neoplasms. In group 3 (Fig. 3) the length of the tectum was 9–16 mm (M 14.48, SD 1.35) and the width was 10–17 mm (M 15.21, SD 1.78). The values of angle A were 5–35° (M 15.64, SD 6.97); the values of angle B were 30–70°C, M 51.02, SD 10.79). Tumours of the pineal gland caused the most significant impact on the tectum. In the group of 7 patients, horizontal dislocation of its longitudinal axis was observed. Tumours compressed the whole tectum and decreased its distance from the clivus. Group 4 was divided in two subgroups: 15 patients with brain-stem tumours (Fig. 4) and 15 with cerebellar tumours (Fig. 5). The length of the tectum was 11–16 mm (M 14.08, SD 1.75), width 12–16 mm (M 13.88, SD 1.39), angle A 15–30° (M 22.13, SD 7.29), angle B 40–85° (M 49.58, SD 10.68). Tumours located in the pons compressed the tectum and caused horizontal inclination of its longitudinal axis. The distance between the inferior colliculi and the clivus was increased. In the second subgroup, compression of the tectum was caused by neoplasms of vernis and superior parts of cerebellar hemispheres, which dislocated them upwards and changed the shape of the tectum from linear to crescentic, decreasing the sagittal dimension. Moreover, the fourth ventricle and the lower part of the aqueduct were compressed, which caused supratentorial hydrocephalus, and changed the location of the tectum to a more vertical position.

Table 1. Mean length (mm) and width (mm) of quadrigeminal plate and mean values of angles A and B

	Length (mm)	Width (mm)	Angle A°	Angle B°
Group 1	14.76	15.76	13.98	51.02
Group 2	11.40	14.35	21.85	47.35
Group 3	14.48	15.21	15.64	51.02
Group 4	14.08	13.88	22.13	49.58

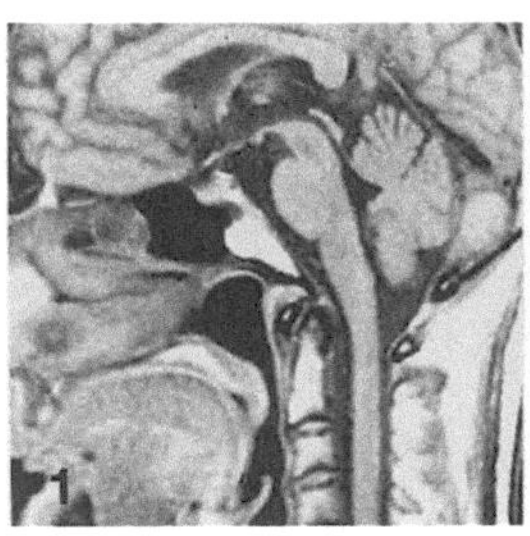
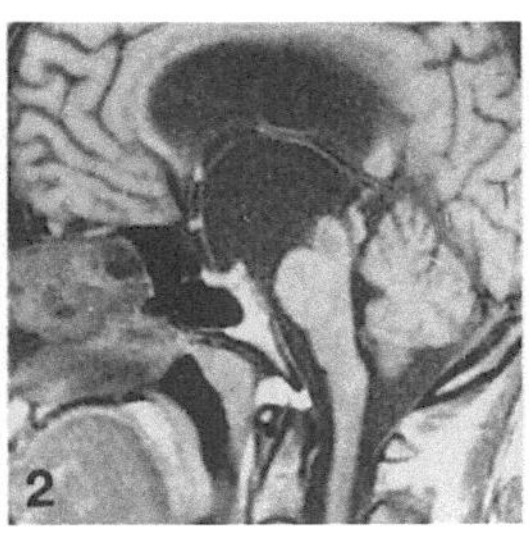
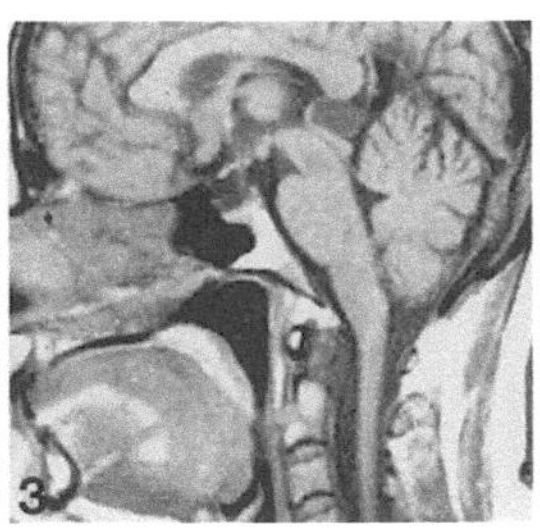
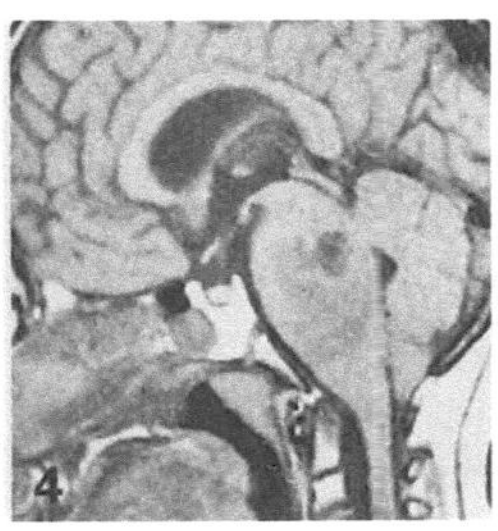
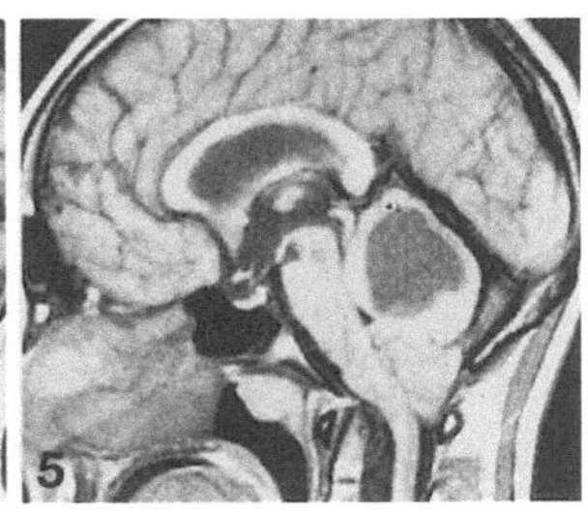

Fig. 1. Quadrigeminal plate of normal brain

Fig. 2. Triventricular hydrocephalus: vertical dislocation of the superior colliculi

Fig. 3. Pineal cyst: compression of superior colliculi, horizontal quadrigeminal plate

Fig. 4. Pontive neoplasm: elevation of inferior colliculi and upward dislocation of whole quadrigeminal plate

Fig. 5. Cystic tumour of vernis: compression of the inferior colliculi and vertical dislocation of the tectum

Discussion

The shape of the tectum was affected by neoplastic disease of the pineal gland and by cerebellar tumours. The dimensions were unaltered in both groups. Pineal and pontal tumours have a significant effect on the localisation of the tectum. Tumorus of pons and cerebral peduncles changed the position of the tectum to a more horizontal position. In four ventricles, hydrocephalus distance from the clivus to the tectum increased. In supratentorial hydrocephalus, the position of the tectum became vertical.

The analysis of our investigations leads to the conclusion that the superb sensitivity of MRI and its multiplanar imaging capability allowed unparalleled diagnostic accuracy in this region.

References

1. Fiedman DP (1992) Extrapineal abnormalities of the tectal region: MRI findings, AJR 159:859–866
2. Raininko R, Autti T, Vanhanen SL, Ylikoski A, Erkinjutti T, Santavouri P (1994) The normal brain stem from infancy to old age. A morphometric MRI study. Neuroradiology 36:364–368
3. Doraiswamy PM, Na C, Husain MM, Figiel GS, McDonald VM, Ellinwood EH Jr, Boyko OB, Krishnana KR (1992) Morphometric changes of the human midbrain with normal aging – MR and stereologic findings. AJNR 13:383–386

Orbit

New MRI methods in the diagnosis of orbital lesions

K. E. W. Eberhardt[1], H. P. Hollenbach[2], B. Beck[3], W. J. Huk[1]

[1] Division of Neuroradiology, Department of Neurosurgery, University of Erlangen, Erlangen, Germany
[2] Siemens Medical Engineering Group, Erlangen, Germany
[3] Departement of Ophthalmology, University of Erlangen, Erlangen, Germany

Abstract. We studied 30 patients with retrobulbar lesions preoperatively with a 1.0 T whole-body MR system. The examinations were evaluated according to histological grading, grade of malignancy and delineation from neighbouring anatomical structures. Axial T1-weighted spin-echo sequences before and after contrast medium and a T2-weighted double-echo spin-echo sequence were obtained using a circular polarised head coil. MRI, especially with fat-suppressing techniques, is superior to ultrasound and CT as regards delineation, and comparable to CT as regards the grade of malignancy.

Key words: Orbital lesions – Fat suppression – Computer tomography – Ultrasound

Ultrasound and CT have become powerful modalities in the diagnosis of diseases of the orbit. MRI on the other hand, has as yet not established itself as a routine diagnostic study. We present MRI techniques: fat-suppression [1] and constructive interference in steady state (CISS) and compare the results with those of ultrasound and CT.

Materials and methods

We prospectively examined 30 patients with orbital masses and 10 volunteers and compared the results concerning histological grading, and delineation from neighbouring anatomical structures, with respect to intraoperative findings or biopsy. The average age of the patients (volunteers) was 52.1 (23.1) years. In the clinical group there were 16 men and 14 women, and we had 6 women and 4 men volunteers. The interval between the diagnostic examinations and the MRI was performed using a 1.0 T whole body system. The patients and volunteers were positioned in a circular polarised head coil used for transmitting and receiving. The patients were given pinhole blinders to suppress eye movement. Axial T1-weighted (TR/TE/α 370/15/90 ms/ms/deg), T2-weighted (TR/TE/α 5000/22–90/90 ms/ms/deg) and CISS (TR/TE/α 14/6/80 ms/ms/deg) sequences were used with and without fat suppression. The T1-weighted spin-echo sequence was repeated after medium. The highest spatial resolution was $1.10 \times 0.57 \times 3.00$ mm. The examination time was about 30 min.

Correspondence to: K. E. W. Eberhardt, Division of Neuroradiology, Department of Neurosurgery, University of Erlangen, Schwabachanlage 6, D-91054 Erlangen, Germany

Table 1. Diagnostic sensitivity in 30 patients with orbital lesions; comparison of ultrasound, CT, MRI and fat-suppressed (FS) MRI

Disease	Patients	Lesions adequately assessed			
		Ultrasound	CT	MRI	FS MRI
Haemangiomas	8	6	7	6	8
Lymphangiomas	4	2	3	3	4
Schwannomas	2	0	2	2	2
Meningiomas	4	0	3	3	4
Dermoid cysts	3	2	3	2	3
Carcinomas	2	0	1	1	1
Lymphomas	3	1	2	1	2
Metastases	4	2	2	2	2

Results

Delineation

CT and MRI using fat suppression are confirmed to be superior to ultrasound. Small lesions in the retrobulbar space and infiltration via the superior orbital fissure and optic cana are shown best on MRI using fat suppression (Figs. 1–4) or CISS sequences.

Degree of malignancy

Vascular lesions such as haemangiomas and lymphangiomas, which are in general well defined show strong contrast enhancement on CT or MRI, clear delineation and on T2-weighted MRI a strong signal, which makes a diagnosis possible. The sensitivity of CT and MRI is comparable. Benign tumours such as menigiomas and schwannomas show extension into the retrobulbar space or along the optic nerve and strong enhancement on CT in most cases. On MRI these lesions give intense signal on T2-weighting. The diagnostic sensitivity of CT and MRI with fat suppression is comparable. Lipomas and dermoid cysts can be identified by CT or MRI. In malignant tumours contrast enhancement and signal behaviour are nonspecific. The results are summarised in Table 1.

Discussion

MRI of the orbit has not yet reached the high level generally achieved in the diagnosis of intracranial diseases. Reasons for this are the relatively long examination times and the motion artefacts caused by eye movement [2]. In addition, changes of signal intensity in the retrobul-

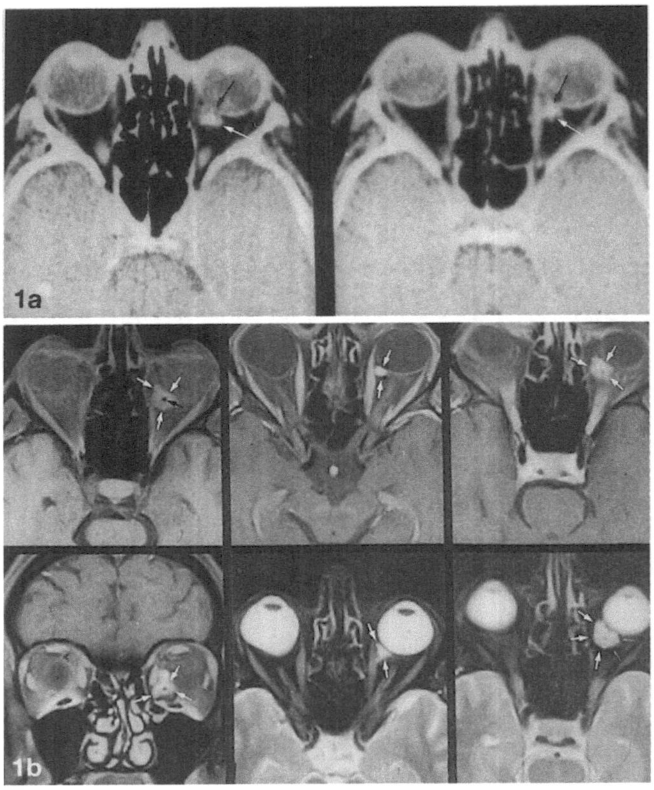

Fig. 1 a, b. CT and MR both show a small mass clearly separate from the optic nerve. This shows mild contrast-enhancement in T1-weighted and high signal intensity on T2-weighted images. Minor internal calcification can be suspected (*arrows*). This was histologically confirmed as a haemangioma

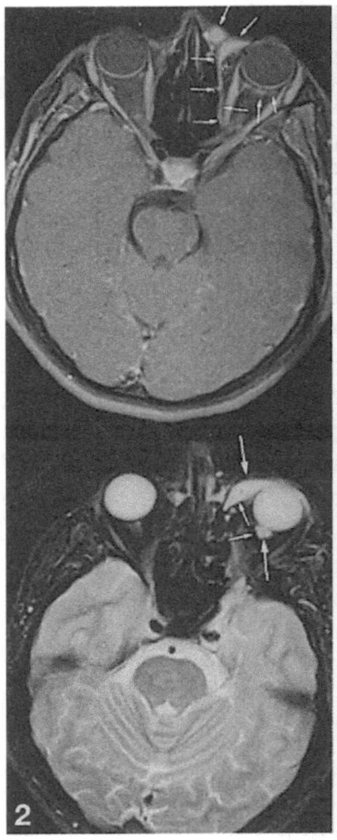

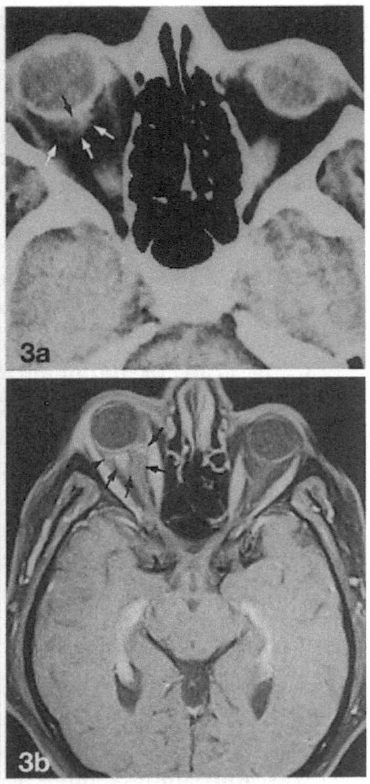

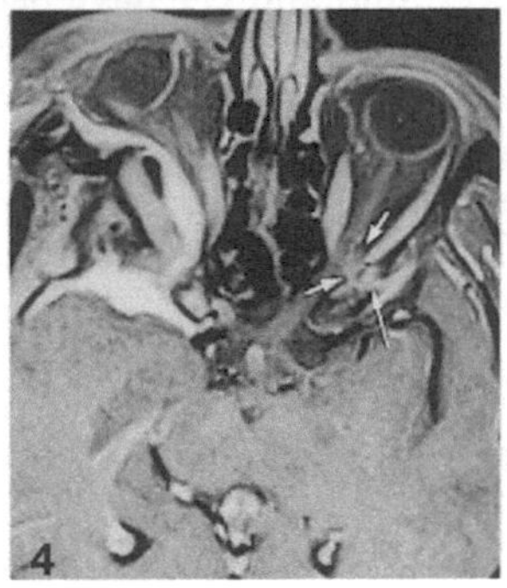

bar space, particularly small changes, are often difficult to detect in the isointense signal of fat [3]. With the development of fat-suppression sequences there has been a noticeable improvement in the use of MRI. T2-weighted images using fat suppression have advantages over T2-weighted inversion recovery sequences based on the shorter measurement time. CISS sequences allow excellent delineation of the sheath of the intracanalicular part of the optic nerve due to its reduced motion sensitivity. CT, new MRI techniques with fat suppression, and CISS sequences have a higher diagnostic sensitivity than ultrasound. However, demonstration of the relationship of pathological changes to anatomical structures is better on MRI than on CT, if fat suppression and CISS are used. In malignant tumours, the differential diagnostic sensitivity is low with all modalities.

Fig. 2. Patient with a infratemporal lymphangioma. T1-weighted images with fat suppression indicate orbital infiltration via the inferior orbital fissure there was contrast enhancement medially and in the retrobulbar space (*arrows*)

Fig. 3 a, b. Histiocytoma. CT and MRI with fat suppression both demonstrate a small lesion laterally and in the retrobulbar space. The retrobulbar fat enhances on T1-weighted images (*arrows*)

Fig. 4. Patient with a meningioma of the right lesser wing of the sphenoid. The patient developed scotoma of the left eye. T1-weighted images show a small enhancing tumour (*arrows*) adjacent to the intracanalicular segment of the left optic nerve

References

1. Hore PJ (1983) Solvent suppression in Fourier transform nuclear magnetic resonance. J Magn Reson 55:166
2. Atlas SW, Zimmermann RA, Bilaniuk LT (1987) In: Lee SH, Rao KCVG (eds) Cranial computed tomography and MRI. 2nd edn. McGraw-Hill, New York
3. Simon JH, Szumowski J, Tottermann SEA (1988) Fat-suppression MR imaging of the orbit. AJNR 6:259

Gd-DTPA enhancement of the optic nerve/sheath complex in fat-suppression MRI

H. K. Lee, K. H. Yoon, G. Choi, D. C. Suh

Department of Radiology, Asam Medical Centre, University of Ulsan College of Medicine, 388-1 Poognap-dong, Songpa-gu, Seoul 138-040, Korea

Abstract. To assess the clinical significance of enhancement of the optic nerve/sheath complex (ONC) in fat-suppression MRI, orbit MRI was performed in 58 patients. Fast suppression was accomplished with a frequency-selective presaturation pulse (ChemSat) with and without Gd-DTPA enhancement. All MRI findings were reviewed in a blind fashion on the basis of orbital compartments. ONC enhancement was seen in cavernous sinus lesions (86%), intraconal lesions excluding the ONC (80%), ONC lesions (57%), ocular lesions (38%), normal orbits (2%) and conal and extraconal lesions (0%). Among the ONC lesions, ONC enhancement was common in optic nerve/sheath tumours (100%), optic nerve contusion (67%) and optic neuritis (21%). ONC enhancement in fat-suppression MRI may be seen not only in optic neuritis and perioptic meningioma, but also in various other cases including cavernous sinus lesions, intraconal and ocular lesions.

Key words: Optic nerve – Orbit – Magnetic resonance imaging – Fat suppression

Fat-suppression MRI with a paramagnetic agent is required for assessment of the optic nerve/sheath complex (ONC). Gd-DTPA enhancement of the ONC is well known in optic neuritis and optic nerve sheath meningioma [1–3]. We report various types of orbital pathology producing contrast enhancement of the ONC.

Methods

From April 1992 to May 1994, orbital MRI was performed in 58 consecutive patients (116 orbits). All MRI studies were performed on a 1.5 T imager with a quadrature head coil. Fat suppression was accomplished with a frequency-selective presaturation pulse (ChemSat). All images were obtained with both the pre- and post-enhanced T1-weighted images with ChemSat using Gd-DTPA. Twenty-one patients were surgically proven and 37 were diganosed clinically. All MR images were interpreted retrospectively on the basis of orbital compartments.

Results

ONC enhancement was noted in 35 sites of a total 116 (30%): 16 of 28 ONC lesions (57%), 8 of 10 intraconal lesions excluding the ONC (80%), none of 8 conal and extraconal lesions (0%), 3 of 8 ocular lesions (38%), 6 of 7 cavernous sinus lesions (86%) and 1 of 55 normal orbits (2%). Of the ONC lesions (Fig. 1), enhancement was common in optic nerve/sheath tumours (9/9) and optic contusion (2/3), and less common in optic neuritis (3/14). Of the cavernous sinus lesions (Fig. 2), ONC enhancement was seen in 2 of 2 dural arteriovenous malformations, 2 of 2 cases of cavernous sinus thrombosis, and 2 of 3 cases of Tolosa-Hunt syndrome. Of the intraconal lesions excluding ONC (Fig. 3), ONC enhancement was seen 6 of 6 pseudotumours, 1 retrobulbar lymphoma, and 1 case of orbital cellulitis.

Discussion

In the study of orbital lesions, fat-suppression MRI techniques have been widely used because they can show improved anatomical detail, decreased chemical shift artefact, and increased grey scale width [4]. The use of a paramagnetic contrast agent in combination with the fat-suppression technique has advanced the contrast between pathological lesions and normal structure. To detect ONC enhancement precisely, we obtained both the pre- and post-enhancement fat-suppression T1-weighted imaged comparing them with other reports [1, 2] using post-enhanced fat suppression only.

Hendrix et al. [2] initially reported the usefulness of the fat-suppression technique using Gd-DTPA in the evaluation of the optic nerve meningioma and Tien et al. [1] applied it to optic neuritis. In addition, we noted enhancement of ONC in other pathologies such as optic nerve contusion, retinoblastoma, dural arteriovenous malformations, cavernous sinus thrombosis, etc.

Various MRI techniques have been used in patients with acute optic neuritis. Larsson et al. [5] reported a 19% rate of detection using chemical shift selective sequences. Guy et al. [6] showed a higher rate (54%) of optic nerve enhancement in patients with optic neuritis (54%) and radiation induced optic neuritis (100%) on T1-weighted images. Our results showed a lower rate (21%) of ONC enhancement. Several factors may have contributed to our results. Firstly, these patients took oral corticosteroids before MRI. Corticosteroids are well known to reduce the permeability of endothelial cells forming the blood-brain barrier. Secondly the lesions of these patients were too small to be detected by our current MRI techniques.

There were various orbital pathologies inducing ONC enhancement on the base of orbital compartments, including optic neuritis and perioptic meningioma. Higher rates of ONC enhancement were in cavernous sinus lesions and intraconal lesions excluding ONC. It is interesting that

Correspondence to: H. K. Lee

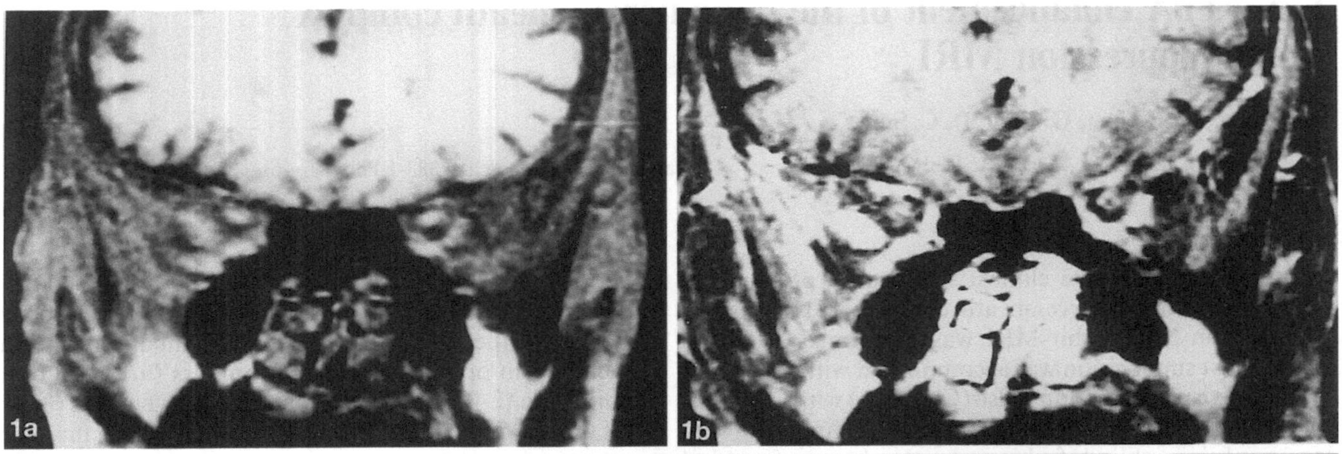

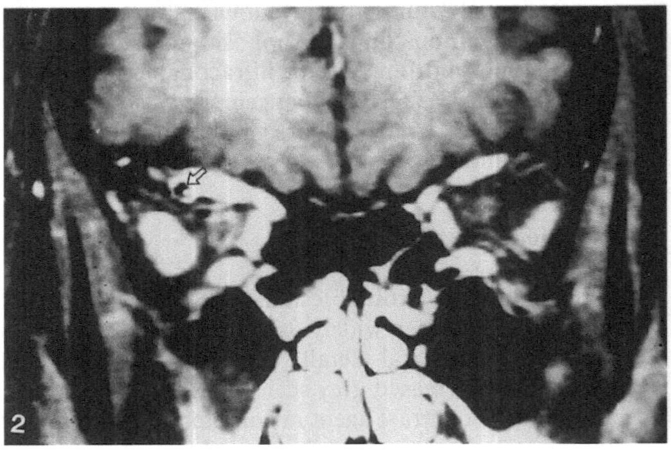

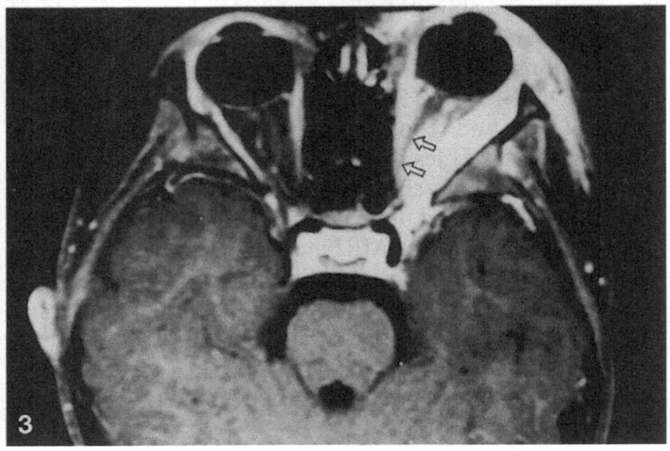

Fig. 1 a, b. Bilateral optic neuritis. **a** Relatively high signal intensity of the optic nerve/sheath complex on a T1-weighted image. **b** Bilateral perioptic contrast enhancement

Fig. 2. Dural arteriovenous malformation on the right cavernous sinus. Perioptic enhancement and swelling of whole extraocular muscles. Note dilated superior ophthalmic vein (*arrow*)

Fig. 3. Left orbital cellulitis. Involvement of preseptal space and retrobulbar fat. Nasal displacement of optic nerve (*arrows*)

cavernous sinus lesions showed the highest rate. We thought it might be caused not by disruption of the blood optic nerve barrier [7], but by the hyperemic state of the optic nerve sheath.

Gd-DTPA-enhanced MRI with fat suppression is a powerful adjunct in MRI of optic nerve pathology. ONC enhancement in fat-suppression MRI may be seen not only in ONC lesions including optic neuritis and perioptic meningioma, but also in various other cases including cavernous sinus lesions and intraconal and ocular lesions.

References

1. Tien RD, Hesselink JR, Szumowski J (1991) MR fat suppression combined with Gd-DTPA enhancement in optic neuritis and perineuritis. J Comput Assist Tomogr 15:223–227
2. Hendrix LE, Kneeland JB, Haughton VM, Daniels DL, Szumowski J, Williams AL, Mark LP, Czervionke LF (1990) MR imaging of optic nerve lesions: value of gadopentetate dimeglumine and fat-suppression technique. AJNR 11:749–754
3. Lindblom B, Truwit CL, Hoyt WF (1992) Optic nerve sheath meningioma: definition of intraorbital, intracanalicular, and intracranial components with magnetic resonance imaging. Ophthalmology 99:560–566
4. Tien RD (1992) Fat-suppression MR imaging in neuroradiology: techniques and clinical application. AJR 158:369–379
5. Larsson HBW, Thomsen C, Frederiksen O, Olesen J (1988) Chemical shift selective magnetic resonance imaging of the optic nerve in patients with acute optic neuritis. Acta Radiol 29:629–632
6. Guy J, Mancuso A, Quisling RG, Beck R, Moster M (1990) Gadilinium-DTPA-enhanced magnetic resonance imaging in optic neuropathies. Ophthalmology 97:592–600
7. Guy J, Fitzsimmons, Ellis EA, Mancuso A (1990) Gadolinium-DTPA-enhanced magnetic resonance imaging in experimental optic neuritis. Ophthalmology 97:601–607

Gd-DTPA in blood-ocular barrier damage: a new diagnostic tool for future application in MRI?

L. Manfré[1], A. Mangiameli[1], G. Cardella[1], G. Giuffre[2], F. Ponte[2], R. Lagalla[2], A. E. Cardinale[1]

[1] Institute of Radiology, University of Palermo, Palermo, Italy
[2] Institute of Ophthalmology, University of Palermo, Palermo, Italy

Abstract. The blood-brain barrier is not the only neuro-epithelial blood filter in the body: the eye too is supported by a highly specialised microvascular filter, the so-called blood-ocular barrier (BOB). The BOB is actually divided into a blood-aqueous (BAB) and a blood-retinal (BRB) barrier, filtering the aqueous fluid and biological supplies, respectively, to the retina. The authors' purpose was to study the possibility of imaging BAB or BRB damage by contrast-enhanced MRI: they examined 21 patients with a 0.5 T system and surface coil. Despite the normal findings in the damaged eyes immediately after a Gd-DTPA bolus, delayed contrast-enhanced MRI was able to show focal or diffuse barrier damage.

Key words: Magnetic resonance imaging – Gadolinium – DTPA – Blood-ocular barrier – Eye

Human or animal eyes are known to be supported by a microvascular complex filter, the blood-ocular barrier (BOB). Damage to the BOB can cause severe ocular sequelae, resulting in the patient's loss of vision. For this reason, the accurate diagnosis of BOB damage is always important.

The purpose of this study was to prove the possibility of imaging BOB breakdown in different human diseases, using a simple middle-field MRI unit and contrast-enhanced imaging.

Materials and methods

Using a 0.5 T MRI unit and a surface coil, 21 patients with proven blood-retinal barrier (BRB) damage (from fluorangiography) or supposed blood-aqueous barrier (BAB) breakdown were examined. The technique consisted of T1-weighted axial, coronal or sagittal image (530/20), centred on the bulb of the patients. Contrast-enhanced examination consisted of T1-weighted images immediately after Gd-DTPA injection and delayed images performed 40 min after the paramagnetic contrast medium bolus.

The control group consisted of 10 patients who underwent contrast-enhanced MRI for different diseases not involving the eye.

Results

On normal contrast-enhanced images marked, homogeneous enhancement of the choroidal layer and the ciliary bodies is usually seen, related to the rich vascular structure of the uveal membrane.

In patients suffering from BRB damage as a result of diabetic retinopathy, MRI was always able to demonstrate diffuse (Figs. 1, 2) or irregular and focal (Figs. 3, 4) enhancement spreading inside the vitreous body on delayed images, although no abnormal findings were seen in MRI performed immediately after Gd-DTPA administration. Similarly, patients with neovascular glaucoma showed evident anterior and posterior chamber hyperintensity when delayed post-contrast scans were performed, related to the leakage of Gd-DTPA from the ciliary bodies and iris neovessels inside the enhancing aqueous fluid (Fig. 5).

Discussion

The central nervous system is not the only human system supporting a blood-tissue barrier, the blood-brain barrier in this case. In fact, the eye also contains a highly specialized microvascular filter, the BOB, selectively straining nutritional elements to the bulb. The BOB is acutally divided into a BAB, made of small endothelial capillary cells, that filters the aqueous fluid from the ciliary bodies to the posterior chamber, communicating with the anterior on through the "foramen" of the pupil; and a BRB, resulting from the combination of retinal endothelial capillary cells and epithelium pigmentatum layer, filtering biological factors to the retina.

Many different pathological conditions can cause BOB damage. With regard to the BAB, neovascular glaucoma (usually in diabetic ophthalmopathy) [1] is one of the most common diseases responsible for the opening of the BAB, but post-surgical intra-ocular lens implantation for cataract eye surgery has recently been supposed to do the same. BAB alterations have been documented during intravenous chemotherapy too [2]. BRB breakdown can be demonstrated in severe diabetic [3] or hypertensive retinopathy, retinopathy of prematurity, retinal detachment, systemic chemotherapy [2], and iathrogenic diode or argon laser endophotocoagulation [4]. All of these conditions can cause an increase of BRB permeability to exogenous proliferative substances and inflammatory cells, responsible for subsequent proliferative vitreoretinopathy. Therefore, an early diagnosis of BOB breakdown is essential to preserve the visual acuity of the patient [3].

Fluorescein angiography (FA) is undoubtedly the "gold standard" in the assessment of BRB, while vitreous photometry has been proposed for quantifying the BRB opening and monitoring intravitreous leakage of fluorescein dye. However, these methods are problematic when the optic media – cornea, lens, vitreous body – are unclear (cataract, haemovitreous, intraocular silicone oil).

Correspondence to: L. Manfré, via Duca degli Abruzzi 40, I-95127 Catania, Italy

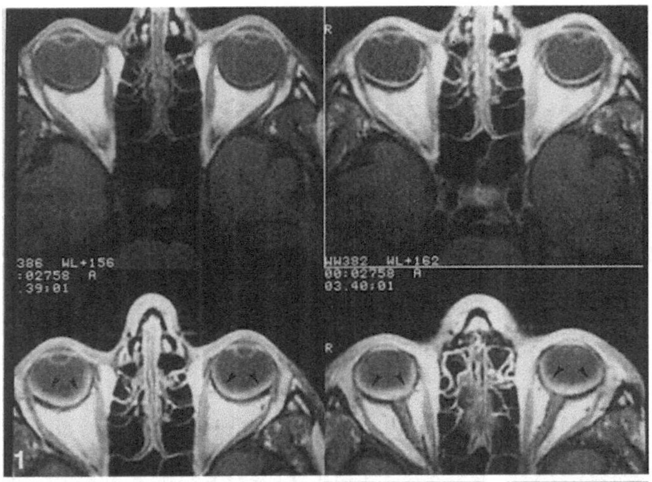

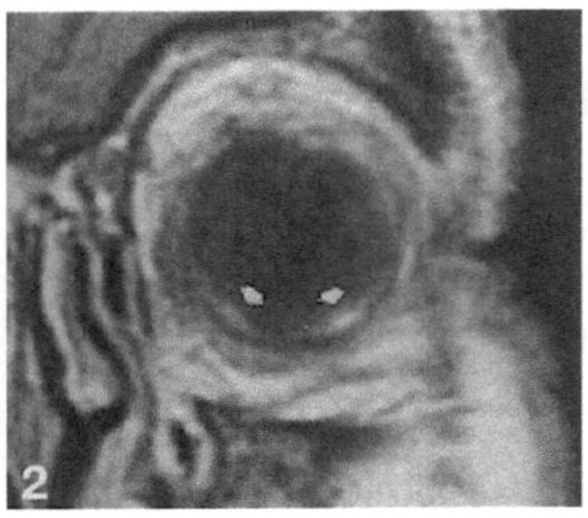

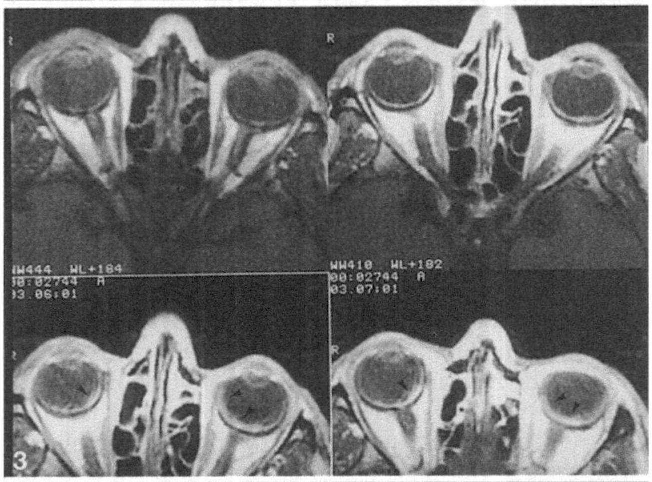

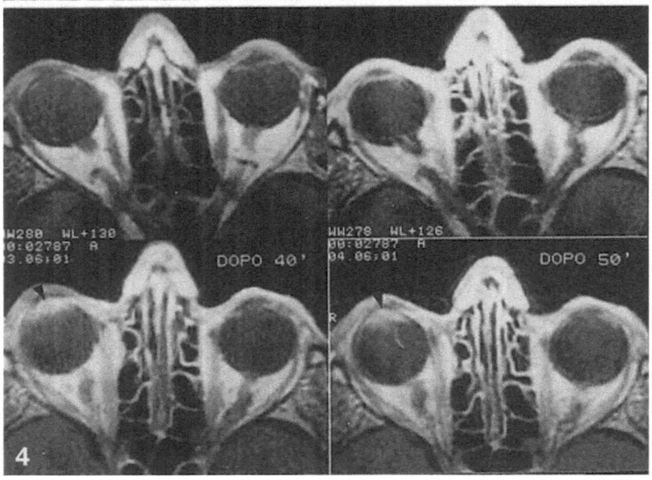

Fig. 1. *Diffuse blood-retinal (BRB) damage in severe diabetic retinopathy.* T1-weighted images before (*top left*), immediately after (*top right*) and 40 min after GD-DTPA injection (*bottom*). Uniform diffusion of paramagnetic contrast medium inside the vitreous is seen (*arrows*) on the delayed images

Fig. 2. *Focal BRB opening in diabetic disease.* Delayed T1-weighted coronal image: note small inferior temporal and nasal retina foci of enhancement (*arrows*), due to gadolinium leakage into the vitreous

Fig. 3. *Multifocal BRB damage in diabetic disease.* T1-weighted axial before (*top left*), immediately after (*top right*) and 40 min after (*bottom*) GD-DTPA injection. Despite the normal appearance of choroidal enhancement after GD-DTPA injection, delayed images show bilateral irregular diffusion of gadolinium into the vitreous, more evident in the nasal retina (*arrows*)

Fig. 4. *Right eye blood-aqueous barrier (BAB) opening in central retinal vein thrombosis.* T1-weighted axial images before (*top left*), immediately after (*top right*) and 40 min after (*bottom*) GD-DTPA injection. The delayed images clearly show enhancement of the anterior and posterior chambers related to the diffusion of Gd-DTPA into the aqueous (*arrows*)

Furthermore, all of these diagnostic tools allow only a one-plane sight of the retina, with difficult visualization of the peripheral retina, the preferential site of diabetic retinal alteration. Moreover, slow reabsorption of macromolecular complex made of fluorescein dye prevents the continuous use of FA in monitoring the evolution of BRB opening.

Iridography can show BAB damage, but it is rarely performed in patients with a neovascular glaucoma.

Recently, using high filed MRI units, different authors have tried to prove the capability of contrast-enhanced scans in demonstrating ocular barrier damage in rabbits [5] or monkeys [6], but only three cases of human BRB openings have been described [7].

In our preliminary study, delayed contrast-enhanced MRI seems to be sufficiently reliable in demonstrating focal or diffuse BRB opening.

Similarly, the diffusion of Gd-DTPA inside the aqueous fluid at the level of the anterior and posterior

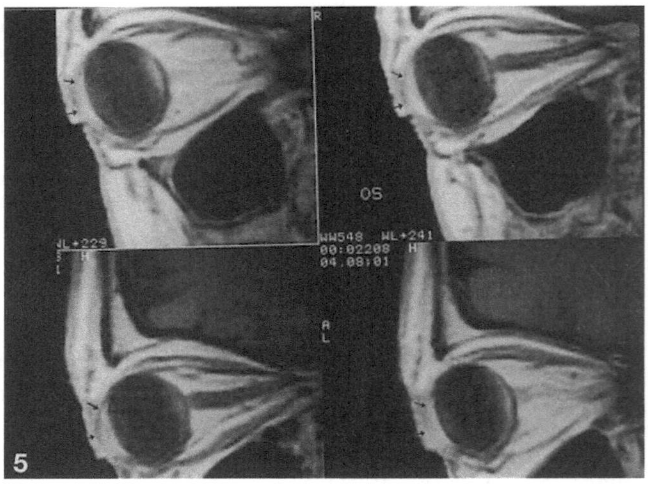

Fig. 5. *Bilateral BAB damage in severe diabetic neovascular glaucoma. Top left* and *bottom right* delayed sagittal T1-weighted images. Note high-signal aqueous just behind the cornea (*arrow*) and over the lens

chambers was evident in patients with BAB breakdown for neovascular glaucoma.

In conclusion, although FA remains the modality of choice in the detection of focal or diffuse BRB damage, delayed contrast-enhanced MRI seems to be an interesting, easy-to-perform and repeatable alternative imaging technique for demonstrating BAB or BRB opening, especially useful in conditions where FA is of no use.

References

1. Cunha-Vaz JG (1980) Blood-retinal barriers in health and disease. Trans Ophthalmol Soc UK 100:337–340
2. Kapp JP, Ross RL, Tucker EM (1983) Supraophthalmic carotid infusion for brain-tumor therapy. J Neurosurg 58:616–618
3. Davis MD (1989) Proliferative diabetic retinopathy. In: Ryan SJ (ed) Retina. Mosby, ST. Loius, pp 367–402
4. Sato Y, Berkowitz BA, Wilson CA, Juan E de (1992) Blood-retinal barrier breakdown caused by diode vs argon laser endophotocoagulation. Arch Ophthalmol 110:227–281
5. Sen HA, Berkowitz BA, Ando N, Juan E de (1992) In vivo imaging of breakdown of the inner and outer blood-retinal barriers. Invest Ophthalmol 33:3507–3512
6. Frank JA et al (1986) Opening of blood-ocular barrier demonstrated by contrast-enhanced MR imaging. J Comput Assist Tomogr 10:912–916
7. Wilson CA, Fleckenstein JL, Berkowitz BA, Green ME (1992) Preretinal neovascularization in diabetic retinopathy: a preliminary investigation using contrast-enhanced magnetic resonance imaging. J Diabetes Complications 6:223–229

CT in retinoblastoma

J. L. Chen, S. Q. Chen

Department of Radiology, Sun Yat-sen University of Medical Sciences, Guangzhou, People's Republic of China, 510080

Abstract. Fifty-four patients with retinoblastoma were reviewed. The main CT findings were: (1) tumour calcification (89%) – one rare case appeared as arcuate calcification at the posterior pole of the globe; (2) the intraocular tumour always appeared as a mass, sometimes cloud-like; (3) all the masses showed various degrees of contrast enhancement; a few demonstrated necrotic areas without enhancement; (4) intracranial invasion of the tumour in three ways: spread along the optic nerve to the suprasellar area, blood metastasis and intracranial ectopic development; (5) spontaneous regression of the tumour seen in one involved eye.

Key words: Retinoblastoma – Tomography, X-ray computed

Retinoblastoma (Rb) is the most common malignant tumour of the eye. CT is an important assistant examination. In this paper, we summarise the CT findings of 54 cases.

Materials and methods

Of 54 cases, there were 26 boys and 28 girls. Their age ranged from 2 months to 9 years: 43 patients were younger than 3 years (80%), and the mean age was 2 years 4 months. Forty-five underwent enucleation and the diagnosis was proved histologically. Nine were not operated on, but their clinical appearances and CT findings were typical.

The patients were scanned continuously from the orbit to the top of the orbit with 2–5 mm thickness and interval, and up to the peneal area with 5–10 mm. Forty-six cases were examined both before and after contrast enhancement. Eight cases were examined either before or after contrast enhancement. Sedatives were routinely used.

CT measurement of the transverse diameter of the optic nerve of 40 eyes of healthy children was made for reference of the diagnosis. The normal diameter ranged from 4 mm to 5 mm, averaging 4.7 mm.

Results

Forty-three of 54 cases were unilateral, 20 on the left and 23 on the right. Eleven cases were bilateral. One was trilateral Rb, i.e. bilateral Rb with an ectopic intracranial focus.

According to Danziger and Price [1], Rb can be divided into three stages. Stage I (36 cases) – the tumour is limited to the globe; stage II (13 cases) – the tumour has invaded the optic nerve or retrobulbar tissue, stage III (5 cases) – the tumour has invaded intracranially or at a distant. Among 45 cases proved histologically, 5 cases were diagnosed as stage I with CT, but the histological diagnosis was stage II. Diagnosis of histology and CT was concordant in the other 40 cases.

The mass was usually large, occupying half or more of the vitreous (50/60). Most of the masses had clear margins. A few showed cloud-like, poorly defined masses in the vitreous (Fig. 1). Thirty-six eyes had tumour at the posterior pole. Only 5 eye tumours were near the equator. The other 24 eye tumours filled the whole vitreous. If the tumour was huge, the eyeball was enlarged. Fifteen eyes had exophthalmos. One eye had ophthalmatrophia due to spontaneous regression of the tumour.

Of 24 foci, 48 (89%) were seen to be calcified (135–328HU). About half of the calcification showed irregular patches; the rest showed masses or spots. One case showed arcuate calcification at the posterior pole of the sclera (Fig. 2).

In 46 cases, the tumours showed various degrees of enhancement after injecting contrast medium. There were

Correspondence to: J. L. Chen

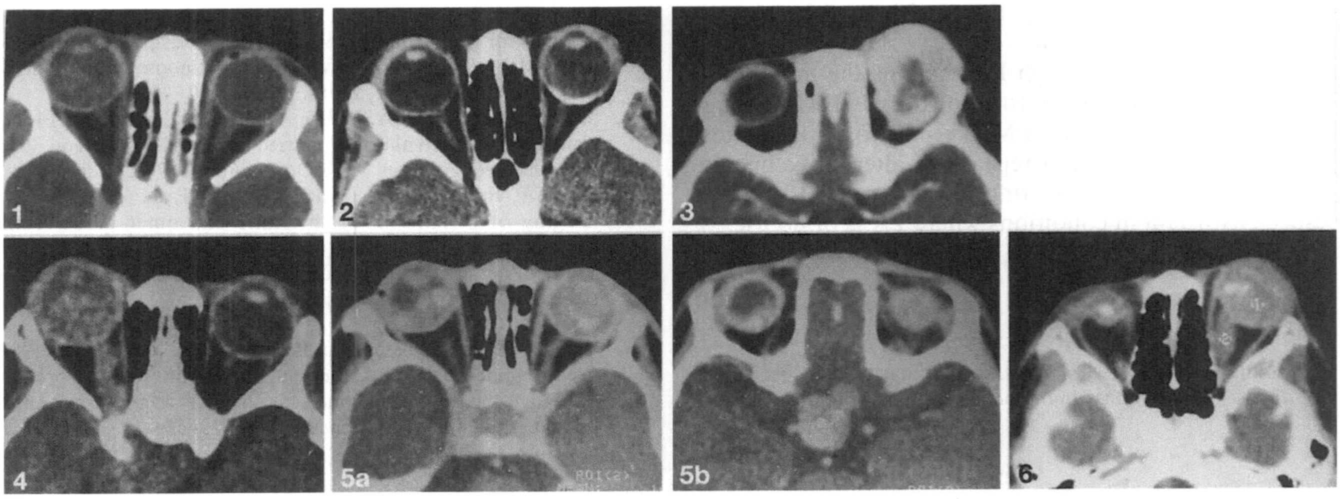

Fig. 1. Stage I. A cloud-like, poorly defined mass with mild contrast enhancement. No calcification

Fig. 2. Stage II. Arcuate calcification at the posterior pole. The optic nerve is enlarged

Fig. 3. Stage II. Mass with marked contrast enhancement with a nonenhancing necrotic area

Fig. 4. Stage III. A dumbbell mass. The optic canal is enlarged

Fig. 5. Trilateral retinoblastoma. **a** Tumours in both eyes are solely intraocular. **b** Lobulated, ectopic suprasellar tumour

Fig. 6. Bilateral retinoblastoma. Tumour in the right eye has spontaneously regressed. Tumour in the left stage II; the optic nerve is enlarged

37 cases of mild (10–20HU), 7 of moderate and 2 of marked enhancement. Two cases had a large area of nonenhancing necrosis within the enhancing mass (Fig. 3).

Of 18 cases of stage II and III diagnosed with CT, 17 had extraocular invasion. Among them, 7 cases only had enlargement of the optic nerve and 10 cases had enlargement of the optic nerve with scleral destruction and an intraorbital mass.

Among 36 stage I cases diagnosed with CT, tumour cells in the proximal-end of the optic nerve were found in 5 cases. The histological diagnosis was stage II.

Among the 5 stage III cases, 3 tumours extended to the intracranium through the enlarged optic nerve and appeared as a dumbbell-like orbital-cranial combined mass. The optic canal was enlarged to a mild-to-moderate degree in all cases (Fig. 4). One case showed the posterolateral bone of the orbit destroyed by an oval mass stradding the orbit, middle cranial fossa and infratemporal fossa. Blood borne metastasis occurred, and two masses arose on the other side of the face a week after the orbital tissue was cut out. Another case of bilateral Rb demonstrated an isolated mass in the chiasmatic cistern which was considered as an ectopic intracranial focus of Rb. The optic nerve was of normal size and the sclera was in tact in this patient (Figs. 5, 6).

Discussion

Rb is common in children: 80 percent of the patients were younger than 3 years. The typical finding in Rb is an intraocular mass and calcification of the focus. Most of the masses have clear margins. A few have cloud-like poorly-defined margins caused by the exudation of tumour cells that seed into the vitreous. With contrast medium, most of the masses enhance mildly (37/46, 80.5%); a few have moderate to marked enhancement. Contrast-enhanced CT is helpful in detecting small foci and making cloudlike masses look clearer.

The reported incidence of calcification of Rb found by CT is 86 ~ 96% [2, 3]. In our material, it was 89%. The shape and the number of foci of calcification vary. In this series, one patient had an arc of calcification at the posterior pole of the sclera, which has never been reported. Histological examination showed that tumour tissue had almost filled up the whole vitreous; calcific substance piled up in an arc-like fashion around the optic disc, similar to the finding 3 on CT. We believe that as the tumour grew, the previous calcification was pushed to the posterior pole.

In general, if a child with leukocoria is younger than 3 years and CT shows calcification in the tumour, Rb can be diagnosed. Rb without calcification is difficult to differentiate from many other diseases like Coats' disease, persistent hyperplastic primary vitreous and retinal detachment etc., because those diseases also show masses in the vitreous on CT [3]. According to our material, the following signs can help us to differentiate Rb from other non-neoplastic diseases: (1) the cloud-like mass floats in the vitreous cavity and is not definitely connected to the sclera: (2) the mass can be enhanced, which means it is a solid mass; in particular, the mass has a necrotic area in the enhanced focus: (3) an intraocular mass accompanies the enlarged optic nerve or the tumour has destroyed the sclera and extends to the extraocular tissues, having these signs. Rb can be diagnosed even without calcification.

The ways that Rb invades the intracranial space include immediate extension to the suprasellar area along the optic nerve, blood metastasis and intracranial ectopic tumour. The first mentioned is most common. Intracranial ectopic tumour commonly happens in bilateral Rb cases, when it is called trilateral Rb [4]. The intracranial ectopic tumour is located in the pineal or suprasellar area [5], so CT must be routinely performed not only at the orbit, but also in the pineal area.

A few Rb spontaneously regress [6, 7]. There was one case in our series where a 4-year-old girl was found to have leukocoria of the right eye 2 months after birth. Without any treatment, the ill-eye ophthalmatrophia itself. Her left eye was found to be leukocoric for 1 year and was exophthalmic for 3 months. CT showed the right eye was phthisical with a spot of calcification (Fig. 6). The left eye showed typical CT appearance of Rb; the tumour had destroyed the sclera and had extended to one suprasellar cistern through the optic nerve. The reason for Rb spontaneous regression may be tumoural necrosis, organisation and atrophy caused by insufficient of blood supply.

In our material, 5 cases were diagnosed to be stage I Rb with CT, but histologic examination found that the tumour cells had passed the amina cribrosa of the sclera and had invaded the proximal end of the optic nerve. Among them, three optic nerves of excised specimens were not enlarged and hardened under gross examination. This means that CT cannot show early invasion of the optic nerve.

References

1. Danziger A, Price HI (1979) CT findings in retinoblastoma. AJ R 133:695
2. Char DH, et al (1984) Retinoblastoma: CT diagnosis. Ophthalmology 91:1347
3. Lindahl S (1986) Computed tomography of retinoblastoma. Acta Radiol Diagn 27:513
4. Bader JL, et al (1982) Bilateral retinoblastoma with ectopic intracranial retinoblastoma: trilateral retinoblastoma. Cancer Gene Cytogenet 5:203
5. Kingston JE, et al (1985) Ectopic intracranial retinoblastoma in childhood. Br J Ophthalmol 69:742
6. Brodwall J (1981) Spontaneous regression of a retinoblastoma. Acta Ophthalmol 59:430
7. Sanborn GE, et al (1982) Spontaneous regression of bilateral retinoblastoma. Br J Ophthalmol 66:685

Head and neck

New Horizons Special Lecture II

Recent advances in head and neck imaging

William P. Dillon

University of California, San Francisco, California, USA

MRI is currently the technique of choice for the investigation of many disorders of the head and neck. Most authors feel that MRI is superior to CT for studies of the nasopharynx, upper oropharynx, and internal auditory canal. MRI and MRA have also proven useful in assessing lesions of the skull base and temporal bone. I shall highlight some of the recent advances in head and neck imaging, emphasizing oncologic imaging, and those areas which are under development.

Malignant adenopathy

Advances in imaging must address the important clinical issues. Several situations remain difficult for head and neck clinicians. These include the detection of nonpalpable disease in the clinical stage NO neck, contralateral adenopathy, mediastinal adenopathy and microscopic disease in otherwise normal size nodes and earlier identification of treatment responders or nonresponders so that other treatment options can be instituted prior to clinical signs of relapse or failure.

Contrast-enhanced CT is still the gold standard against which other modalities must be compared. In the detection of adenopathy of the neck, MRI, while capable of differentiating lymph nodes from vascular structures, is often not as specific as CT in elucidating the internal architecture of nodes. Several newer MRI techniques may prove useful in this regard. Higher resolution imaging using phased-array surface coils with fast spin-echo techniques may improve our ability to detect smaller "micrometastases". While size criteria for malignant adenopathy are still in use, it is worth emphasizing that direct evidence of tumor invading a node is better than indirect evidence based on size or morphologic changes.

Positron emission tomography

Several groups have had positive results using 2-Defluroxyglucose positron emission tomography (PET) for the detection of recurrent disease as well as microscopic malignant adenopathy. The basis of this technique depends on the difference in metabolic activity of tumor and surrounding tissues tumor generally having a higher activity than other tissues. The drawback with this technique has been inadequate spatial resolution, but newer generation PET scanners have <2 mm in-plane resolution and may finally make an impact on clinical oncology. A potential advantage is the ability to image of a variety of tracers, which may indicate the biologic activity as well as the sensitivity to treatment of a particular tumor. For example, work performed at University of Washington using PET imaging with fluoromidonizadol, a hypoxic cell marker, may indicate which tumors are hypoxic and therefore will not respond to radiation therapy.

MR lymphangiography

Another technique being investigated for the detection of adenopathy is MR lymphangiography using intravenous administration of ferrous particles, which selectively accumulate within normal nodes over a 24-h period following injection. Early results from the Department of Radiology at the University of California, Los Angeles suggest that this technique may be useful in detection of occult metastases within normal-sized lymph nodes. It has, however, been found that the specificity appears lost, despite the high sensitivity of the examination. Normal nodes take up this agent, which gives low signal on T2-weighted images. Nodes involved with metastases demonstrate filling defects within them at the site of the metastases.

MR spectroscopy

The role of spectroscopy in oncologic imaging is as yet undefined. The hopes are that this technique will permit earlier recognition of neoplasms which will fail to respond to therapy, allowing alternative therapies to be instituted at an earlier juncture. Improvements in spectroscopic imaging include better resolution through the use of specialized surface coils, 3D proton spectroscopy, and computerized analysis of data with better registration models so that data can be more easily interpreted. At the University of California, San Francisco, we are embarking on a prospective analysis of proton and phosphorous spectroscopy in tumors of the brain and of the head and neck. Early results have indicated that elevated choline/creative ratios signify more highly malignant areas of brain tumors. We are just beginning a study of patients with squamous cell carcinoma of the head and neck with ^{31}P and ^{1}H spectroscopy.

Fast spin-echo

The main advantage of this new technique is that higher resolution images can be obtained in a time-efficient fashion. For example, 512×512 matrix images, field of view 17 cm, TR/TE 4000/102, 2 excitatims, 16 echo-train can be obtained in under 5 min. This is particularly useful for studies of smaller structures in the head and neck, such as the temporal bone, the 7th and 8th cranial nerves, and the temporomandibular joint. Our protocol includes the use of fast spin-echo in most routine head and neck cases; using a single echo and fat saturation, 256×256 matrix images are routinely obtained through the suprahyoid neck in under 4 min.

Dynamic MRI

The use of fast imaging in combination with rapid administration of gadolinium has proven advantageous in certain situations in the head and neck. Although it is not a routine sequence at our facility, others have demonstrated its utility in differentiating tumors from scar tissue and normal mucosa (e.g.), in paranasal sinus tumors. It may also be possible to infer the adequacy of blood supply and oxygenation of a neoplasm – factors that may influence the response to therapy with radiation.

Normal CT appearances of the subarcuate fossa and petromastoid canal

H. Nakagawa[1], S. Iwasaki[1], T. Taoka[1], M. Nakane[1], K. Kichikawa[1], A. Fukusumi[1], H. Ohishi[2], H. Uchida[1]

[1] Department of Radiology, Nara Medical University, Nara, Japan
[2] Department of Oncoradiology, Nara Medical University, Nara, Japan

Abstract. To determine the normal CT appearances of the subarcuate fossa and petromastoid canal, the 136 temporal bones of 68 patients, without injuries or anomalies, were scanned with high-resolution CT. The subarcuate fossa was visualised in 48.6%. The average width of the fossa was 8.3 mm (SD 3.1) and the depth 1.9 mm (SD 0.6). The petromastoid canal was visualised in 48.6%. The diameter of the canal was 0.6 mm, (SD 0.1) and the total length was 9.3 mm (SD 1.7). The canal connected the subarcuate fossa and the mastoid antrum with the appearance of an anteriorly convex curve, 15.6° (SD = 12.2) anteriorly then bent 44° (SD = 16.0) posteriorly. In the coronal plane, the canal inclined 2.9° (SD = 6.3) from the horizontal plane. It is important to understand these structures to diagnose fracture and to estimate the pathological nature of the intracranial spread of mastoiditis.

Key words: Subarcuate fossa – Petromastoid canal – Temporal bone – Computed tomography

The purpose of this study was to define the normal CT appearances of the subarcuate fossa and petromastoid canal (Fig. 1). The subarcuate fossa is large in the fetal era and located on the superior and posterior aspect of the internal auditory canal. With growth, the fossa regresses into the petromastoid canal, which connects with the mastoid antrum and includes the subarcuate artery and vein.

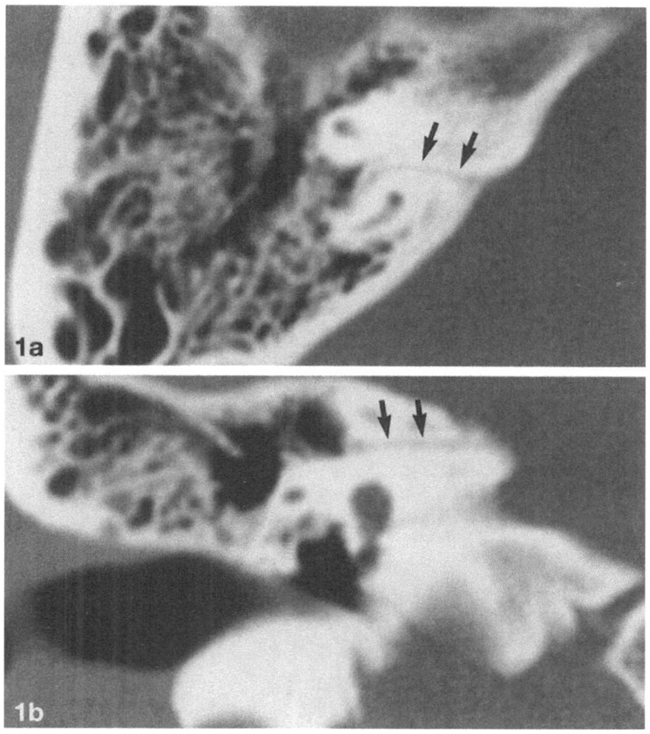

Fig. 1. Axial (**a**) and coronal (**b**) CT of the right temporal bone. The subarcuate fossa (*arrow*) and petromastoid canal (*arrowhead*) are shown

Materials and methods

The 136 temporal bones of 68 patients, aged 6–81 years (15 males and 43 females) without injuries or anomalies, we scanned with high-resolution bone target CT. The slice thickness and interval were 1.5 mm, and the planes were parallel and 110° to Reid's base line. A total of 136 transaxial and 123 coronal images were reviewed (Table 1).

Detectability and size of the subarcuate fossa and the petromastoid canal were measured. The size of the subarcuate fossa and the size and angle of the petromastoid canal were measured by using Vernier calipers and a semicircular protractor on the CT images which were printed life-size.

On axial CT, the petromastoid canal shows posteromedial concave bend. We defined the segment from orifice to bending point (B) as the "first segment" and the segment from bending point to the mastoid antrum as the "second segment". The diameter of the petromastoid canal was measured at the centre of the first segment. Figures 2–4 show the measurement points and methods.

Table 1. Diagnoses of patients examined

	Temporal bones	
	Axial	Coronal
Normal	78	67
Chronic otitis media	46	44
Acute otitis media	1	1
Cholesteatoma	11	11
Total	136	123

Results

Table 2 shows the detectability of the subarcuate fossa and the petromastoid canal and their size.

Discussion

Although there are several pathological reports about the development and maturation of the subarcuate fossa and the petromastoid canal [1–3] there is no radiological

Correspondence to: H. Nakagawa

Table 2. Measurements obtained

Subarcuate fossa	
Detectability	48.6%
Width	8.3 ± 3.1 mm
Depth	1.9 ± 0.6 mm
Petromastoid canal - axial	
Detectability	48.6%
Diameter	0.6 ± 0.1 mm
Angulation	
1st segment	15.6 ± 12.2°
2nd segment	−44.0 ± 16.0°
Lenght	
1st segment	6.0 ± 1.5 mm
2nd segment	4.0 ± 1,2 mm
Total	9.3 ± 1.7 mm
Petromastoid canal - coronal	
Detectability	48.6%
Diameter	0.6 ± 0.1 mm
Angulation	2.9 ± 6.3°
Length	8.7 ± 1.7 mm

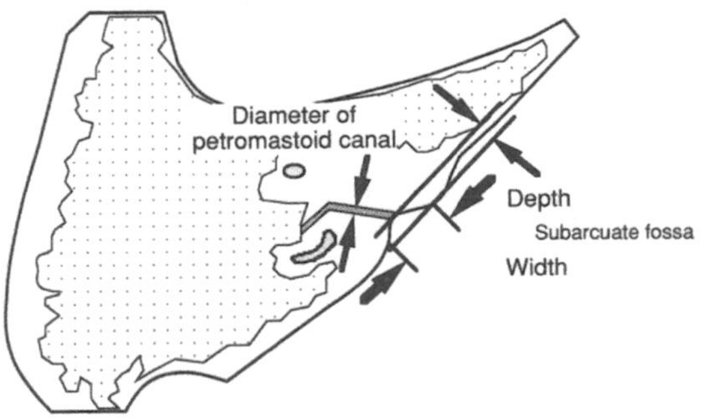

Fig. 2. Diagram of the temporal bone shows measurement of the size of the subarcuate fossa and the petromastoid canal

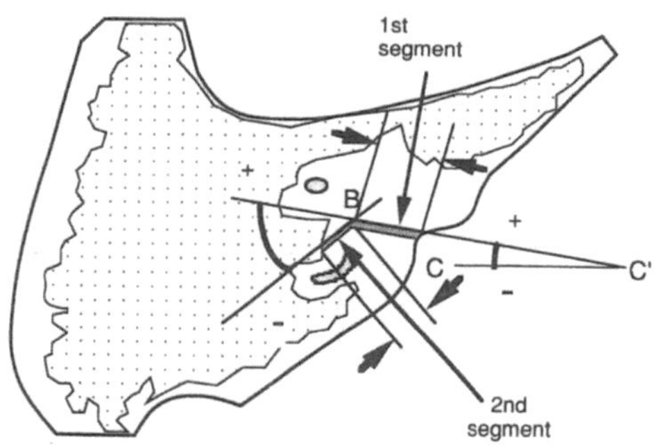

Fig. 3. Measurement of angulation and length of each segment of the petromastoid canal on axial CT. Angulation of the first segment was taken as that subtended by coronal plane (*C–C'*) and a line tangential to this segment (*B–C'*). Angulation of the second segment was taken as subtended by a line (*B–C'*) and a line tangential to this segment. Nasal direction and occipital direction of angulation were defined as plus and minus respectively

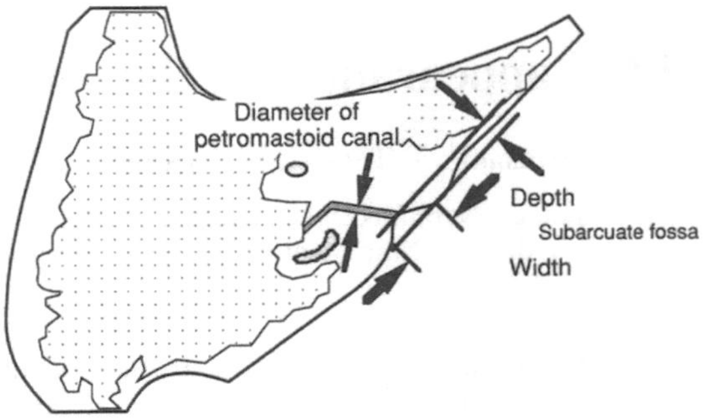

Fig. 4. Measurement of diameter, angulation and length of the petromastoid canal on coronal CT. Angulation of the canal was taken as that subtended by horizontal plane (*H–H'*) and a line tangential to this segment. Cranial direction of angulation was defined as plus

report about the measurement of these normal structures, to the best of our knowledge. Proctor [2] reported that the length of the petromastoid canal varied from 6 to 10 mm. The results of our investigation are compatible with this measurement.

The petromastoid canal may be the route for infections to pass from the tympanum to the meninges [4]. If the subarcuate vessels are large, they may be of some surgical significance when removing acoustic nerve tumours [1].

In a case of temporal bone fracture, the petromastoid canal may be misinterpreted as a fracture line. For this reason, basic knowledge of the normal subarcuate fossa and petromastoid canal is necessary.

This study revealed normal appearances of the subarcuate fossa and petromastoid canal. It is important to understand these structures to diagnose the fracture and to estimate the pathological nature of the intracranial spread of mastoiditis.

References

1. Hilding D (1987) Petrous apex and subarcuate fossa maturation. Laryngoscope 97:1129–1135
2. Proctor B (1983) The petromastoid canal. Ann Otol Rhinol Laryngol 92:640–644
3. Gacek R, Leipzig B (1979) Congenital cerebrospinal otorrhea. Ann Otol 88:358–365
4. Dolan K (1989) Temporal bone fractures. Semin Ultrasound CT MR 10:262–279

Fat-suppression MRI: clinical applications in orbital and skull base neoplasms

A. M. Wang, A. N. Shetty, D. P. Wesolowski, S. Noujaim

Department of Diagnostic Radiology, William Beaumont Hospital, 3601 West 13 Mile Road, Royal Cak, MI 48073, USA

Abstract. In the high fat-content regions of orbits and skull base, as well as in the regions of fat implanation from surgery, the anatomic details and the detection of contrast enhancement are not optimally appreciated on a conventional T1-weighted contrast-enhanced image. We performed T1-weighted MRI with selective presaturation of fat signal following intravenous administration of paramagnetic contrast medium for investigation of neoplasms in these regions. The results are encouraging in that it is particularly useful in the investigation of orbital neoplasms and of the postoperative status of acoustic schwannoma.

Key words: Orbit – Skull base – Neoplasm – Magnetic resonance imaging – Fat suppression

Paramagnetic contrast enhancement has proved invaluable for improving the ability to differentiate between a neoplasm and the surrounding structures. However, in regions with high fat content, the distinction between paramagnetic contrast enhancement and fatty tissue can be difficult. This is due to the short T1 of the fat, causing high intensity signal that is isointense with contrast-enhanced neoplasms. Fat-suppression MRI techniques have proved useful in several areas of the body to improve significantly the depiction of anatomic details and highlight the visualization of the paramagnetic contrast enhanced neoplasms [1, 2]. We performed selective presaturation fat technique coupled with a conventional T1-weighted pulse sequence following paramagnetic contrast medium in the examination of orbital and skull base neoplasms as well as the postoperative status of patients with schwannoma and assessed its value by comparing it with conventional T1-weighted MRI.

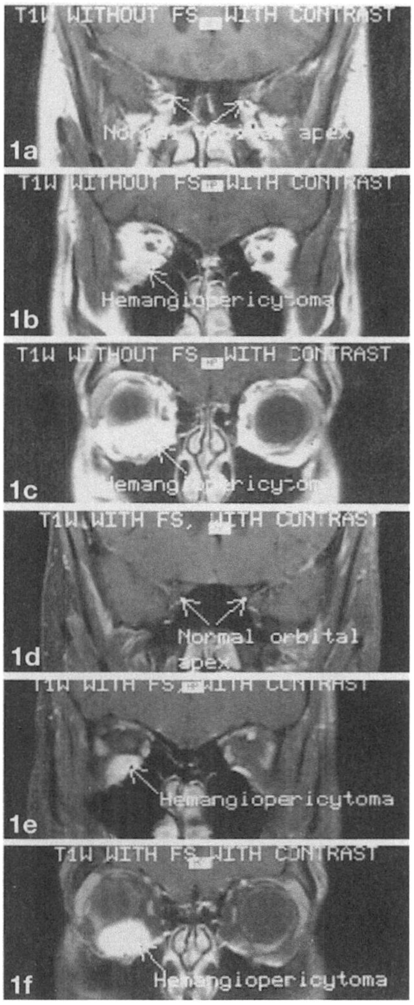

Fig. 1 a–f. Hemangiopericytoma. Coronal contrast-enhanced T1-weighted images **a–c**. Fat-suppressed (FS) images (**d–f**). The hemangiopericytoma was better defined on FS images. It lay extraconally and inferiorly without evidence of extension to the orbital apex: surgical intervention was successful

Materials and methods

MRI of the orbit and skull base for assessment of tumor extension or postoperative status was performed on 23 patients on a 1.5 T unit. All patients were imaged with conventional (NFS) as well as fat suppression (FS) spin-echo T1-weighted (short TR, short TE) images before (WOC) and after (WC) gadopentetate dimeglumine. The TS technique used a spatially nonselective and frequency-selective Gaussian radio frequency pulse with a narrow bandwidth. A circularly polarized head coil was used.

Results

Based on four lesion conspicuity grades (0: not visible; 1: poorly visualized; 2: moderately apparent; 3: very apparent) the visibility of six orbital neoplasms was graded as 1 for T1-weighted, NFS, WOC; 2 for T1-weighted, NFS, WC; 2 for T1-weighted, FS, WOC; and 3 for T1-weighted, FS, WC. The FS technique is clearly superior to the NFS technique in defining the extent of the orbital tumor (Fig. 1). In 6 patients with acoustic schwannoma, the contrast-enhanced FS technique was at least equal to and may better than the contrast-enhanced NFS technique in detecting the presence of acoustic schwannoma (Table 1). In 10 patients with acoustic neuroma who underwent surgical intervention with tumor resection and fat impaction, the FS technique was much better than NFS in detecting residual tumor (Table 1, Fig. 2). For the patient

Correspondence to: A. M. Wang

Table 1. Conspicuity of 17 skull base tumors

Tumor	Cases	Score	Fat-suppression			
			No		Yes	
			T1WI	T1WI+Gd	T1WI	T1WI+Gd
Acoustic schwannoma						
preoperative	6	0	2	–	–	–
		1	4	–	6	–
		2	–	2	–	–
		3	–	4	–	6
postoperative residual tumor	6	0	2	–	–	–
		1	4	2	6	–
		2	–	4	–	–
		3	–	–	–	6
no residual tumor	4	0	4	4	4	–
		1	–	–	–	–
		2	–	–	–	–
		3	–	–	–	4
Glomus jugulare tumor	1	0	–	–	–	–
		1	1	1	1	–
		2	–	–	–	1

T1WI, T1-weighted images; + *Gd*, contrast-enhanced

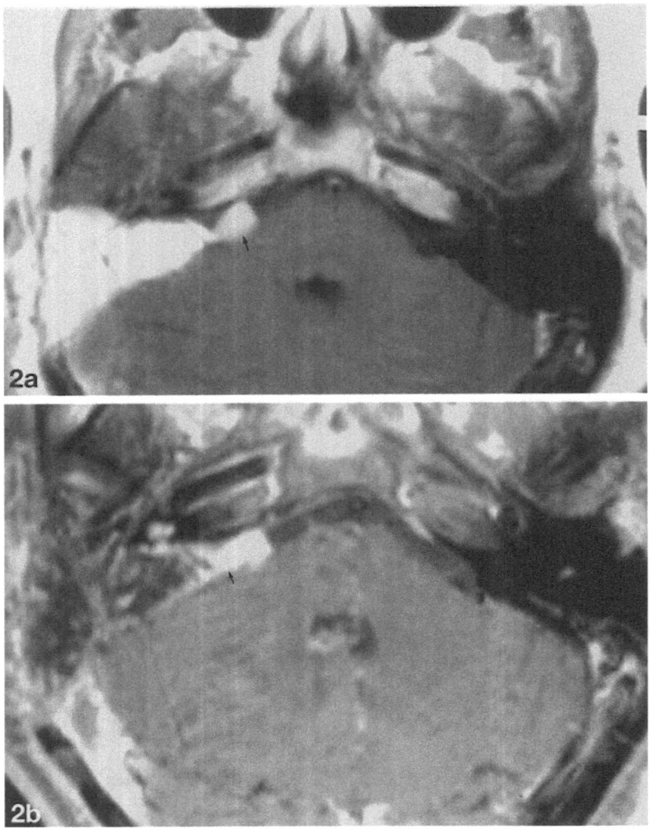

Fig. 2a, b. Residual acoustic schwannoma. **a** Axial contrast-enhanced T1-weighted image. **b** A fat-suppressed image shows the entire mass which was partially obscured in **a** by the high signal intensity from the surgically implanted fat

with paraganglioma in the skull base, it was easier to define the tumor and to separate it from the surrounding structures using the contrast-enhanced FS technique (Table 1).

Discussion

Contrast enhanced T1-weighted MRI investigation of the neoplasms in the orbits and skull base can be difficult sometimes due to the presence of surrounding high-fat structures. Contrast-enhancing neoplasms may appear isointense with fat. Several techniques for fat suppression have been used in MRI studies in the body. The fat suppression technique we used in this study is a simple spatially nonselective, frequency-selective radiofrequency pulse to presaturate the fat signal followed by conventional T1-weighted sequence. The technique being sensitive to magnetic field inhomogeneity, additional time was spent in shimming the magnet with the patient inside the magnet to ensure homogeneous suppresson of fat. We found that contrast-enhanced fat suppression T1-weighted MRI appears to be a valuable technique for imaging orbits and skull base neoplasms.

References

1. Tien RD, Chu PK, Hesselink JR, Szumowski J (1991) Intra- and periorbital lesions: value of fat suppression MR imaging with paramagnetic contrast enhancement. AJNR 12:245–253
2. Barakos JA, Dillon PW, Chew WM (1991) Orbit, skull base, and pharynx: contrast enhanced fat suppression MR imaging. Radiology 179:191–198

Chondrosarcoma of the head and neck

B. Azar-Kia, S. W. Horowitz, M. Fine, K. Goldberg, R. Neimon

2160 S. First Ave, Maywood, IL 60151, USA

Abstract. Head and neck chondrosarcoma involving the skull base is rare. We present our experience of five cases. CT and MRI findings varied with the degree of malignancy. Low-grade chondrosarcomas are less invasive, showing a well-defined mass with heavy calcificaton. High-grade chondrosarcomas are more destructive with a lower degree of calcification. Low-grade skull base chondrosarcoma should be differentiated from chordoma and meningioma. High-grade chondrosarcoma may mimic metastasis, carcinoma arising from facial sinuses and eosinophilic granuloma.

Key words: Chondrosarcoma – Skull – primary neoplasm – Magnetic resonance imaging – Computed tomography

Skull base cartilaginous tumors arise from embryonal rest which forms cartilaginous matrix. Chondrosarcomas usually occur along the petro-occipital fissure in the parasellar of cerebello pontin cisterns [1]. They are slow-growing tumors and locally invasive. Low-grade chondrosarcomas are well-defined lesions with numerous foci of calcification. Higher grade of malignancy is demonstrated by lower degree of calcification and more destructive changes in adjacent bone. Low-grade chondrosarcoma at the base of the skull may grow to a large mass with no or few clinical symptoms.

Methods

We reviewed the clinical, radiologic and pathologie details in five cases.

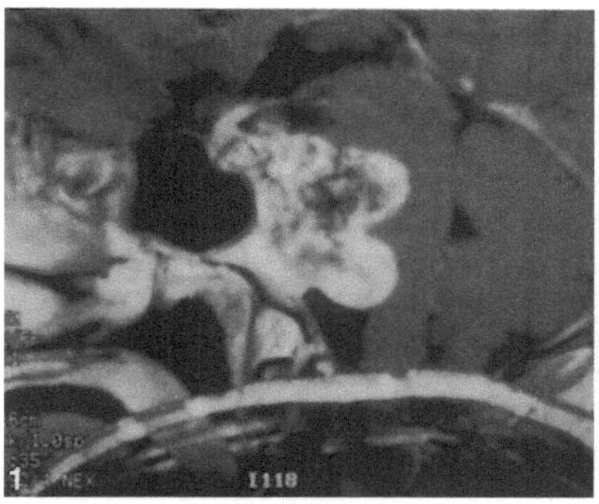

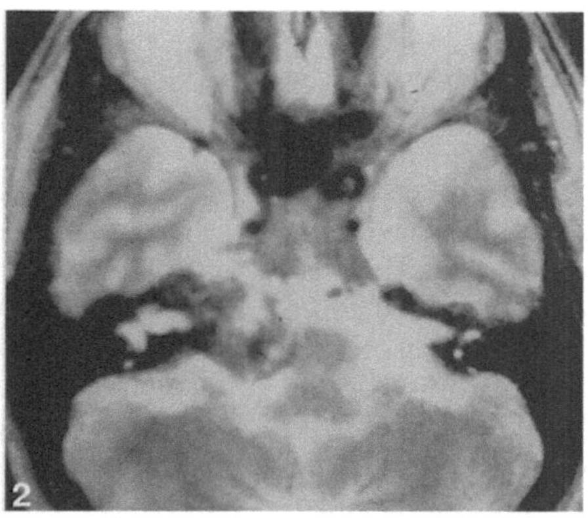

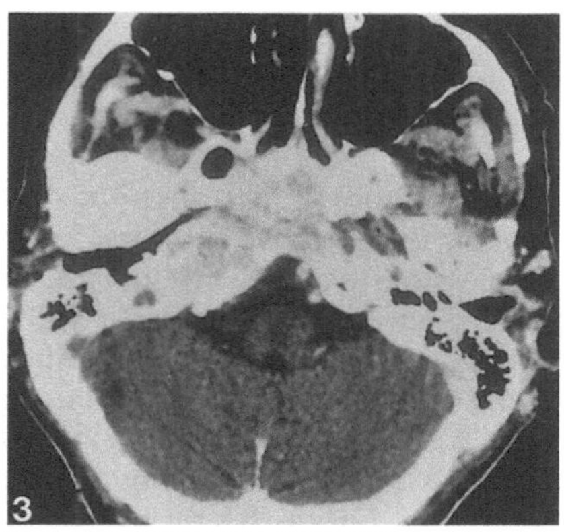

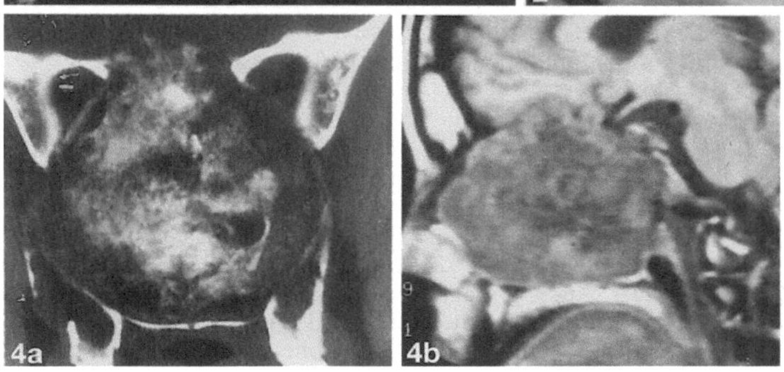

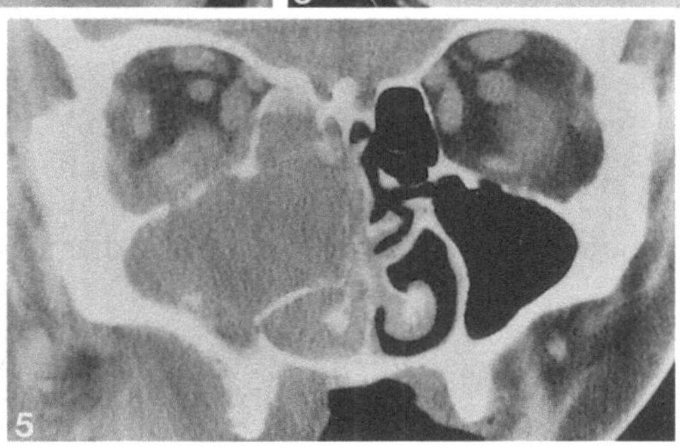

Fig. 1. Grade I chondrosarcoma. Sagittal contrast-enhanced T1-weighted image showing a well-defined, inhomogenously enhancing mass. Note involvement of clivus and dorsum sellae

Fig. 2. Grade I chondrosarcoma. Axial T2-weighted image showing a large inhomogeneous mass involving the tip of the petrous bone with extension into the cerebelloepontine cistern

Fig. 3. Grade II chondrosarcoma. Axial contrast-enhanced CT showing a large, enhancing, destructive midline mass in the base of the skull. Note invasion of clivus, sphenoid sinus and the tip of the petrous bone

Fig. 4 a, b. Grade II chondrosarcoma. **a** Coronal CT showing a large, partially calcified, midline facial mass. **b** Sagittal T1-weighted MRI revealed an inhomogeneous midline mass. Note involvement of skull base, orbits and facial sinuses

Fig. 5. Grade III chondrosarcoma. Coronal CT showing a large destructive mass with minimal calcification involving right ethmoid and maxillary sinuses. Note extension into right nasal cavity and orbit

Correspondence to: B. Azar-Kia

Results

Of our five patients, a 22-year-old woman with a large midfacial mass had a history of right-sided nasal obstruction until she developed double vision; a 55-year-old man with a large clival mass was referred for MRI for recent diplopia; a 35-year-old woman with a history of an exostosis of the hand complained of photophobia; a 53-year-old had a recent history of nasal obstruction and proptosis, and a 59-year-old man presented with right facial numbness. CT and MRI findings varied in our cases. A well-defined, highly calcified mass with slight adjacent bone involvement showed a pathologic diagnosis of grade I chondrosarcoma (Figs. 1, 2). Mild calcification with moderate expansion is demonstrated in a case of grade II chondrosarcoma (Figs. 3, 4). T1- and T2-weighted images revealed mainly intermediate to mixed intensity. Highly destructive lesions with minimal calcification were grade III chondrosarcoma (Fig. 5). All of these cases showed marked contrast enhancement on CT and MRI [2–4].

Discussion

Differential diagnosis of low-grade chondrosarcoma is from chordoma and meningioma. Chordomas are mainly midline lesions arising from the clivus, in contrast to chondrosarcomas, which are usually off the midline. Meningiomas may show thickening or sclerosis of adjacent bone. Enhancement of the adjacent dural mater (tail sign) [5] on MRI is in favor of meningioma. High-grade chondrosarcomas should be differentiated from metastasis, squamous cell carcinoma or adenocarcinomas [6] arising from facial sinuses.

References

1. Berkman YN, Blatt ES (1918) Cranial and intracranial (path) cartilaginous tumors. Clin Radiol 19:327–333
2. Grossman RI, Davis KR (1981) Cranial computes tomographic appearance of chondrosarcoma of the base of the skull. Radiology 141:403–408
3. Bourgouin PM, Tampieri D, Robitaille Y, Robert F, et al (1992) Low-grade myxoid chondrosarcoma of the base of the skull: CT, MR, and histopathology. J Comput Assist Tomogr 16:268–273
4. Meyers S, Hirsch WL, Curtin HD, Barnes L, et al (1992) Chondrosarcoma of the skull base: MR imaging features. Radiology 184:103–108
5. Meyer JE, Oat RF, Lindfors KK (1986) CT appearance of clival chondromas. J Comput Assist Tomogr 10:34–38
6. Sze G, Uichanlo LS, Brant-Zawadzki M, et al (1988) Chordomas: MR imaging. Radiology 166:187–191

Petrous bone: low-dose high-resolution CT

H. Becker, B. Dietrich

Department of Neuroradiology, Medical School, Hannover, Germany

Abstract. Since the petrous bone shows large differences in density, the objective of the study was to establish whether it is possible to reduce the dose used in high-resolution CT. A hard plastic phantom, with drill holes 1.3 mm–0.2 mm in diameter, was used to determine the spatial resolution in different radiaton doses and image algorithms. On the GE CT 9800, it was possible to reduce the dose from 510 mAs to 120 mAS using the bone algorithm and a voltage of 120 kV. These parameters were applied prospectively in patients. The reduced dose value proved to be adequate for a definitive diagnosis of pathological changes. A further reduction of dose to 80 mAs was possible with the recently installed GE CT HiSpeed Advantage RP. The dose could thus be reduced to about one-sixth without loss of anatomical details or diagnostic information.

Key words: Computer tomography – Petrous bone – Dose reduction

Correspondence to: H. Becker, Abteilung Neuroradiologie, Medizinische Hochschule Hannover, D-30625 Hannover, Germany

CT is the method of choice for differentiated imaging of the osseous structures of the petrous bone. High-resolution (HR) petrous bone CT is usually done with the same dose, of about 400–600 mAs, necessary for imaging the cerebral parenchyma. However, in the petrous bone there are large differences in contrast between the bony structures, air-containing spaces and soft tissue. We were prompted by the publications on low-dose CT of the paranasal sinuses [1, 2] to investigate whether it is possible to reduce the radiation dose in a similar way, without loss of anatomical and diagnostic information.

Materials and methods

A hard plastic phantom of grey PVC with a mean density of +1200 HU was made, containing drill holes 1.3 mm–0.2 mm in diameter with a graduation of 0.1 mm each, in 12 rows. With this phantom, measurements were carried out with the doses 60, 120, 210 and 510 mAS using the standard, bone and edge algorithm on the GE CT 9800 (slice thickness 1.5 mm) and CT HiSpeed Advantage RP (slice thickness 1.0 mm). The parameters determined for investigations of the petrous bone in patients were applied in prospective studies.

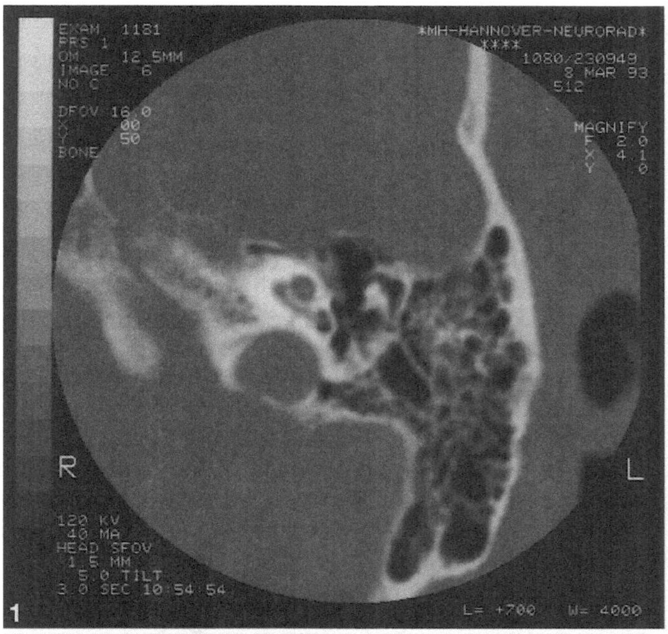

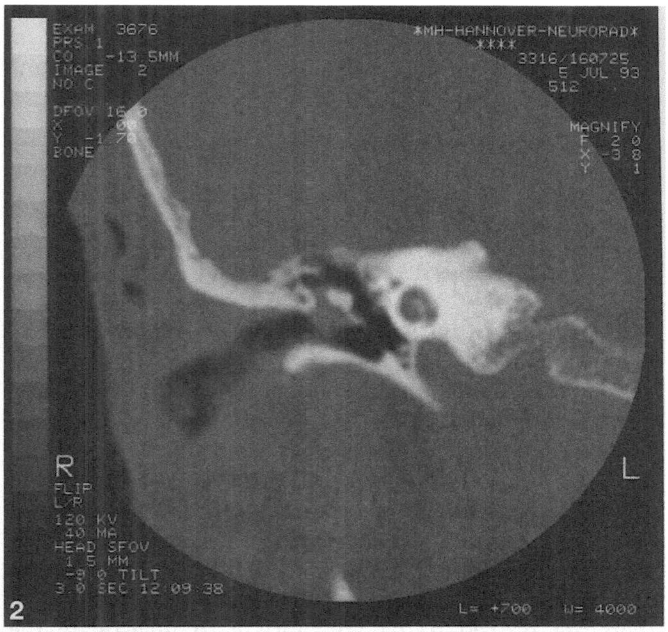

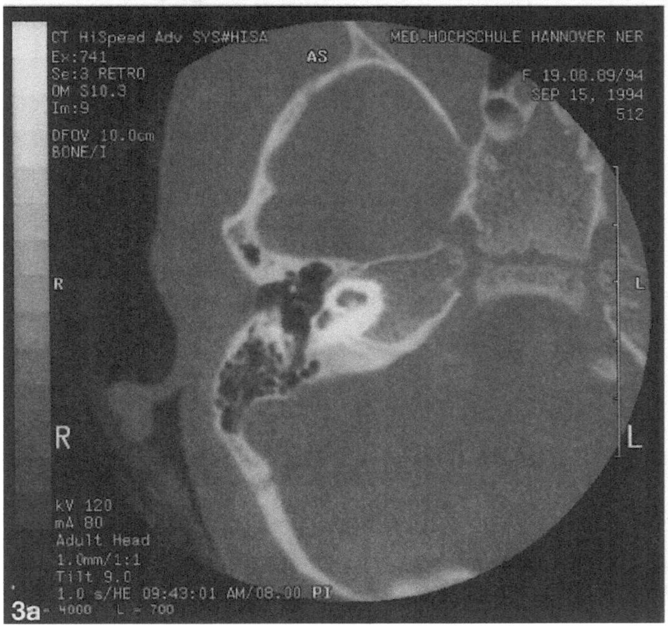

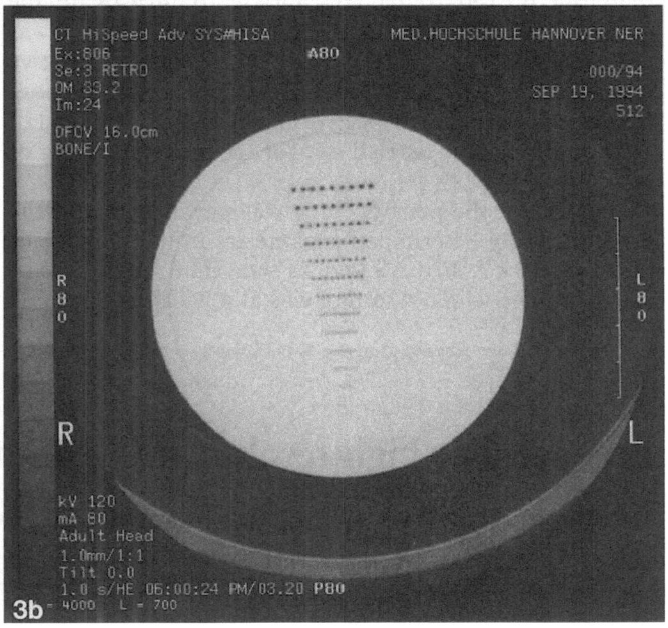

Fig. 1. Secondary cholesteatoma

Fig. 2. Transverse pyramidal fracture

Fig. 3. Helical CT of the phantom and the petrous bone of a patient at 80 mAs. Note the precise demonstration of the stapes

Results

The best resolution was obtained at the maximum dose with the edge algorithm (Table 1). The same resolution was obtained with a minimum dose of 60 mAs in the edge algorithm as was measured with 120 mAS in the bone algorithm. No difference was found in comparing 120 and 510 mAS in the bone algorithm. On the other hand, the

Table 1. Phantom measurements with different doses and algorithms

Drill-holes TD/per cm	Algorithm dose standard	Algorithm dose bone	Algorithm dose edge
1.3/ 4	60/120/210/510	60/120/210/510	60/120/210/510
1.2/ 5	60/120/210/510	60/120/210/510	60/120/210/510
1.1/ 5	60/120/210/510	60/120/210/510	60/120/210/510
1.0/ 6	60/120/210/510	60/120/210/510	60/120/210/510
0.9/ 6	60/120/210/510	60/120/210/510	60/120/210/510
0.8/ 7	510	60/120/210/510	60/120/210/510
0.7/ 8	*	60/120/210/510	60/120/210/510
0.6/ 9	*	120/210/510	60/120/210/510
0.5/11	*	*	510
0.4/13	*	*	*
0.3/18	*	*	*
0.2/22	*	*	*

Table 2. Standard deviation of the cerebellar parenchyma adjacent to the petrous bone for different doses and algorithms

Algorithm \ Dose	510 mAS	210 mAS	120 mAS
Standard	9	12	16
Bone	33	50	62
Edge	67	91	121

standard algorithm was very much poorer in terms of resolution.

The edge algorithm could not be applied in clinical use, due to increased noise in the form of interfering marginal blurring. The degree of noise was determined on the basis of the standard deviation for the dose values 510, 210 and 120 mAS and the three kernels used in the adjacent cerebellar parenchyma. As expected, the standard deviation increases most substantially in the pronounced edge emphasis of the kernel in the edge algorithm (Table 2). It therefore proved to be appropriate to investigate the patient with 120 mAS in the one algorithm. This was performed with a field of view of 16 cm, for comparative imaging of both petrous bones. Enlargement with a zoom factor of 2, or the retrospective calculation with a field of view of 10 cm, was carried out for secondary imaging of the petrous bone.

The CT of the petrous bone was performed with the experimentally determined parameters in the bone algorithm at 120 kV, 40 mAS and 3 s scan time, i.e. a dose of 120 mAs. The window setting was at a width of 4000 HU and a level of +700 HU. The reduced dose values proved to be sufficient for definitive diagnosis of pathological alterations in the petrous bone.

Conclusions

Two examples demonstrate the effectiveness of low-dose HR CT: a secondary cholesteatoma after chronic otitis media with destruction of the attic spur (Fig. 1), and transverse pyramidal fracture with a fracture line passing into the cochlea in labyrinthine deafness which occurred after trauma (Fig. 2).

Using the newly installed CT HiSpeed Advantage RP scanner, it was possible to reduce the dose even further. It was established with the phantom used before that the same resolution can be obtained in the bone algorithm with a dose product of 80 mAs as with 120 mAs on the GE scanner CT 9800. This was possible both with conventional CT and helical CT (Fig. 3).

To summarise: with roughly a sixfold reduction of the radiation dose, a highquality CT imaging of the petrous bone can be obtained without loss of anatomical details or diagnostic information.

References

1. Duvoisin B, Landry M, Chapuis L, Krayenbuhl M, Schnyder P (1991) Low-dose CT in inflammatory disease of the paranasal sinuses. Neuroradiology 33:403–406
2. Marmolya G, Wiesen EJ, Yagan R, Haria CH, Shab AC (1991) Paranasal sinuses: low-dose CT. Radiology 181:689–691

Preoperative high-resolution CT of the temporal bone in microtia

T. E. Mayer [1], H. Brückmann [1], R. Siegert [2], A. Witt [2], H. Weerda [2]

[1] Institut für Radiologie-Neuroradiologie, Medizinische Universität, D-23538 Lübeck, Germany
[2] HNO-Klinik, Medizinische Universität, D-23538 Lübeck, Germany

Abstract. One hundred and forty temporal bones of microtic patients were examined by high-resolution CT. In minor microtia auditory canal stenosis and in major microtia atresia was predominant. The middle ear malformation depended on the severity of the auricular dysplasia. There were middle ear cavity anomalies in 90%, ossicle dysplasias in 97% (stapes 70%), oval window absence in 32%, labyrinth malformations in 16%, closed round window in 7%, facial canal displacement in up to 75% and vascular canal aberrations in 22% of microtia grade III. Multiplaner scanning or reformation of 1-mm slices (spinal CT) is necessary for preoperative planning. A neuroradiological score can be obtained.

Correspondence to: T. E. Mayer

Key words: Ear, congenital malformations – Computed tomography

Congenital aural atresia occurs in 1 in 10,000 births [1] except in the era of thalidomide embryopathy (1959–1962) in Germany when it was diagnosed in 1 in 900 neonates [2].

Surgery of congenital aural atresia is one of the most difficult ear operations. It consists of reconstructive surgery of the auricle, often by skin and rib cartilage grafts [3] and if necessary restoration of hearing by drilling a new auditory canal and reconstruction of the ossicle chain. Other reasons for operation are: congenital cholesteatoma, labyrinth fistula and infection or facial nerve palsy from previous surgery [4]. Even if there is some labyrinth involvement by the malformation, inner ear function is normally preserved (and patients are not candidates for cochlea implants). Endoscopy is not possible in stenotic or atretic auditory canals. CT staging is necessary to avoid the risk of facial nerve lesions, hearing worsening and bleeding and to obtain a valid prognosis of success.

We reviewed, 70 CT studies of patients with microtia and external auditory canal dysplasia.

Methods

All patients had high-resolution CT, 67 of 70 with 1-mm slices (3 with 2-mm slices) in the axial plane, reconstruction of coronal, oblique or sagittal planes was sometimes done. Twelve patients were also scanned in the coronal plane and 5 of them in the sagittal plane by low-dose (85 mAs) spiral CT. In these case 3-D surface reconstructions were also made.

Results

Of 140 ears examined, 86 were microtic: 16 of 70 patients had bilateral microtia. We classified 75% of the microtic ears as grade III and added 1 case of anotia to the group of major microtia; 13% had microtia grade I and 11% grade II, grouped as minor microtia [3].

External auditory canal (EAC)

In major microtia 78% of the ears had atresia, 22% stenosis and none were normal. In minor microtia EAC stenosis predominated (75%); in 10% there was an atretic and in 15% a normal EAC. Of the patients with normal outer ears (contralateral to a microtic ear), 6% had EAC stenosis and none bad atresia. Stenotic auditory canals often had a distinct more angulated course than normal from caudal lateral to cranial medial. Atretic canals varied from a fibrous closure to thick atresia plates.

EAC stenosis and atresia were often combined with tympanic masses of solid tissue of fat density and sometimes a destructive aspect, suggesting an epidermoid cyst or congenital or secondary cholesteatoma.

Other skull dyplasias

Atresia is associated with aplasia or hypoplasia of the tympanic part or mastoid process of temporal bone (serve changes in 25% of minor and 63% of major microtia). The mandibular condyle is dysplastic in 21% of minor and 62% of major microtia, the zygomatic arch is interrupted in 18% versus 44%. In genetic disorders such as Franceschetti (Treacher-Collins) or Crouzon's disease the whole skull, or in Klippel-Feil syndrome the cervical spine, are dysplastic.

Temporal bone vessels

The carotid canal is often asymmetrical in unilateral aural atresia, and slightly rotated or elevated in relation to the hypoplastic base of the skull. In 1 case there was an additional cranial directed loop, and in 2 cases it was missing; but there was no dehiscence into the middle ear, and no remnant stapedial artery. The sigmoid sinus and jugular vein showed in addition to normal asymmetry and emissaries often a high-riding jugular bulb. In cases of severe hypoplasia of the tympanic part of the temporal bone, the sigmoid was slightly displaced ventral. Only 3 patients had a bony erosion of the squamous part of the temporal bone by venous structures, but no dehiscence into the tympanum.

Pneumatisation of the temporal bone

It is strongly correlated to the degree of anomalies of the outer ear; 6% of normal contralateral ears had reduced mastoid pneumatisation. In cases of minor microtia 30% had reduced, including 20% with no pneumatisation of the mastoid and middle ear cavity. In severe microtic ears pneumatisation was reduced in 63%, including 46% where it was missing.

The Eustachian tube had a dyplastic appearance in 24% of the minor and 47% of the major microtic ears. It could be enlarged excessively to a sagittally-orientated space.

Tympanic space

Normal outer ears were combined with a normal middle ear space in 98%. Minor microtia showed a (severely) reduced epitympanic space in 30 (25)%, mesotympanic space in 45 (5)% and hypotympanic space in 35 (15)%. Major microtia was accompanied by (obliteration or severe) reduction of the epitympanum in 62 (41)%, of the mesotympanum in 89 (43)% and of the hypotympanum in 88 (71)%. In obliterated middle ears there was usually a small residual cleft of the mesotympanum. The epitympanum could be totally obliterated; the hypotympanum could be reduced to a knob-like ending Eustachian tube.

Malleus-incus complex

In 8% of normal contralateral ears there were dysplastic changes. In minor microtia 45% were dysplastic, 5% absent. In severe microtia only 3% were normal. Nearly two-thirds were dysplastic and one-third absent.

Incus-stapes joint

This was dysplastic in 65% of minor and 87% of major microtia. In case of stapes absence the remnant incus was always malformed.

Stapes

This was not involved as frequently as the rest of the ossicular chain. Even in severe microtia, 29% remained normal, 16% were dysplastic (thickened) and 54% absent.

In minor microtia 10% were dysplastic and 40% absent, so there was no significant dependence on the degree of the auricular anomalies.

Oval window

This was always open in normal ears. Minor microtic ears showed closure of the oval window in 45%, major microtic ears in 33% and there was no correlation to the degree of the outer ear changes.

Facial nerve canal

Aberration of the labyrinthine segment occured in 5% of minor and 23% of major microtia. In 4 cases it was hypoplastic. The tympanic segment was caudally displaced in 25% of minor and 29% of major microtia; it could be dehiscent, reaching down till the round window. Two patients showed moderate thickening of the facial nerve along its tympanic course. The mastoid segment was ventrally displaced in 50% of minor and 75% of major microtia. Not only the facial nerve but also the dorsal attic wall often stood far ventral. Consecutively the tympanic sinus reached very deep. In some of these cases the facial nerve left the mastoid cranial to the stylomastoid foramen in ventral direction to the mandibular joint or there was an exit in lateral direction. In 2 patients the facial nerve canal showed an extremely anterior course straight down from the geniculate ganglion. In 1 patient the mastoid segment went medially to the tympanic sinus just dorsal to the round window. The mastoid facial nerve canal was often split in two or three parts on the normal as well as on the pathological side.

Internal auditory canal

This was dysplastic in 13% of all cases of microtia. The entrance could be distended. A highly inclined course from cranial lateral to caudal medial was typical.

Round window

This was absent in only 6% of the microtic ears. Bony closure of the round window was not correlated to other anomalies. It could also happen in well-pneumatised middle ear cavities.

Labyrinth

Except in one case it was mildly dysplastic in 16% of the microtic ears, as it was in all patients with Franceschetti syndrome. In 12 cases the lateral semicircular canal was hypoplastic, in 5 cases the vestibulum. In 1 case of thalidomide embryopathy only rudiments of the whole labyrinth, including the cochlea, were present. The cochlear and vestibular aqueducts were sometimes slightly thickened with fluent limits to normal. On the pathological side the cochlear canaliculus frequently went more horizontal than on the normal side.

Discussion

There is a strong correlation between anomalies of the auricle, the EAC, the pneumatisation and eustacian tube, the middle ear cavity, malleus and incus, and the facial nerve canal in its mastoid segment. This might be due to its common origin of the first and second branchial arch, first branchial groove and first branchial pouch. Less well correlated are malformations of stapes and the oval window. Although not rare, dysplasia of the labyrinth and the round window have no connection with the severity of the microtia. The cause might be their origin of the otic capsule.

The ventral dislocation of the mastoid segment of the facial nerve might be caused directly by the hypoplasia of Reichert's cartilage and the consecutively ventrally moved mastoid bone, joining the atresia plate. The ventral placement of the dorsal tympanic wall leads to a deep tympanic sinus. The chorda tympani then courses lateral to the atresia plate [5]. Facial nerve canal doubling, ventral dehiscence of the mastoid segment, caudal displacement and dehiscence of the tympanic segment are also frequent [6]. A detailed classification of the facial nerve anomalies based on anatomical specimens and collected clinical literature is given by Fowler [7]. His types of facial nerve courses can all be demonstrated by CT.

Only in one case of thalidomide embryopathy was the cochlea involved (bilateral). Other derivates of the otic capsule such as the lateral semicircular canal, were involved in up to 16%. A detailed description of the inner ear malformations was published by Mündnich and Terrahe [1].

Major vessel anomalies were rare but a ventrally dislocated sigmoid sinus in an a-p reduced mastoid could be dangerous for surgery.

The majority of our patients were admitted for reconstructive surgery because of severe auricular anomalies [8]. This selection leads to a high number of patients with microtia grade III and corresponding severe changes of the middle ear.

The current most important preoperative scoring for hearing repair surgery [9], invented by Jahrsdoerfer [10], includes the clinical appearance of the outer ear and facial nerve function but only partially the CT results.

We propose a thorough neuroradiological score containing:

1. Pneumatisation of the middle ear. Otherwise occlusion of the artifacial EAC is probable. Complete opacification of the tympanum almost excludes hearing repair surgery.
2. Pneumatisation of the mastoid. It may be not so important, but reduced air content in the mastoid is associated with frequent infections.
3. Extent of the tympanic space. It should be sufficient for the ossicular chain.
4. Preserved malleus, incus and above all stapes.

5. Open oval and round window.
6. Cochlea and labyrinth. Even changes of the vestibular organ seem to be a sign for inner ear dysfunction [11].
7. Facial nerve. Dehiscence of the tympanic part may obscure the stapes. Ventrally displaced mastoid segment could be dangerous, if there is little space for drilling the EAC.
8. Aberrant vessels. They could involve a bleeding risk for surgery.
9. Cholesteatoma. It can destroy the middle ear and facial nerve and requires surgery [12]. It may itself be an indication for surgery.

The ear surgeon is interested in multiplanar, especially sagittal views, before drilling an artificial EAC. Therefore direct scanning in these planes or reconstruction of a 3-D data set, acquired by spinal CT, is necessary.

References

1. Mündnich K, Terrahe K (1979) Mißbildungen des Ohres. In: Berendes, Link, Zöllner (eds) Hals-Nasen-Ohrenheilkunde, 2nd edn. Thieme, Stuttgart, pp 1–49
2. Lenz W (1963) Das Thalidomid-Syndrom. Fortschr Med 81:148
3. Weerda H (1988) Classification of congenital deformities of the auricle. Facial Plast Surg 5:385–388
4. Jahrsdoerfer RA (1992) Clinical aspects of temporal bone anomalies. AJNR 13:821–825
5. Mattox DE, Nager GT, Levin LS (1991) Congenital aural atresia: embryology, pathology, classification, genetics and surgical management. In: Paparella MM, Shumrick DA (eds) Otolaryngology, 3rd edn. Saunders, Philadelphia, pp 1191–1225
6. Swartz JD (1984) The facial nerve canal: CT analysis of the protruding Tympanic segment. Radiology 153:443–447
7. Fowler EP (1961) Variations in the temporal bone course of the facial nerve. Laryngoscope 71:937
8. Weerda H (1988) Reconstructive surgery of the auricle. Facial Plast Surg 5:399–410
9. Aguilar EA, Jahrsdoerfer RA (1988) The surgical repair of congenital microtia and atresia. Otolaryngol Head Neck Surg 98:600–606
10. Jahrsdoerfer RA, Yeakley JW, Aguilar EA, Cole RR, Gray LC (1992) Grading system for the selection of patients with congenital aural atresia. Am J Otol 13:6–12
11. Murata K, Isono M, Ohta F, Yoshida A, Ishida O (1987) Quantitative analysis of inner ear anomalies by high resolution CT scanning of the temporal bone. J Otolaryngol 16:133–136
12. Mehra YN, Dubey SP, Mann SBS, Suri S (1988) Correlation between high-resolution computes tomography and surgical findings in congenital aural atresia. Arch Otolaryngol Head Neck Surg 114:137–141

Heavily calcified petrous lesions

B. Azar-Kia, S. W. Horowitz, K. Goldberg, M. Fine, R. Neimon

2160 S. First Av., Maywood, IL 60153, USA

Abstract. We present four cases of heavily calcified masses in the area of the petrous bone. These cases have similar radiological findings on plain film, CT, MRI and angiography, with different histopathologic diagnoses: a rare papillary cystadenocarcinoma arising from the endolymphatic sac; two meningiomas, one with extracranial extension into the neck; one low-grade chondrosarcoma.

Key words: Meningioma – intracranial neoplasm – Skull – Computed tomography – Magnetic resonance imaging

Radiological apperances are rarely pathognomonic. We present four cases with similar imaging features, but significantly different histology.

Case reports

Case 1: meningioma

A 41-year-old man was surgically explored for a left parotid region mass. A biopsy proved it to be a meningioma. Examination revealed slight weakness of the left shoulder and partial paralysis of the left vocal cord, with a large, firm mass at the left angle of the mandible. CT showed a large calcified mass in the left petrous bone extending into the posterior cranial fossa, jugular foramen and the left side of neck (Fig. 1). MRI revealed intermediate intensity on T1- and T2-weighted images. CT and MRI both demonstrated marked contrast enhancement. Angiography showed a moderately vascular lesion.

Case 2: meningioma

An 81-year-old woman with a history of diabetes was referred for treatment of coronary artery disease. She complained of occasional headaches and CT of the head showed a large, lobulated, calcified mass in the left temporal bone extending into the posterior and middle cranial fossae and suprasellar region. Mild contrast enhancement was noted (Fig. 2).

Case 3: papillary cystadenocarcinoma of endolymphatic duct

A 16-year-old girl had conductive hearing loss on the left, left facial weakness and occasional headaches. Examination also showed a diminished left corneal reflex. The remainder of the cranial nerves were entirely normal. CT showed a large calcified mass in the petrous bone extending into the posterior and middle cranial fossae. T1-weighted MRI (Fig. 3a, b) revealed signal void of calcification along with intermediate intensity. T2-weighted images showed mixed low and high intensity (Fig. 3c). CT and MRI demonstrated

Correspondence to: B. Azar-Kia

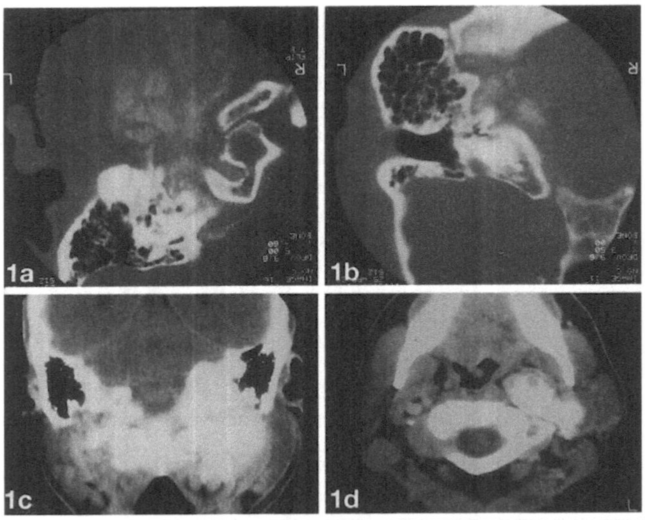

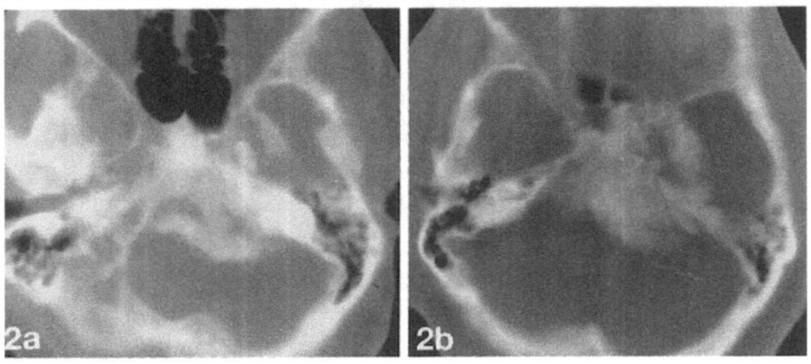

Fig. 1 a–d. Meningioma. Axial (**a**) and coronal (**b**) CT showing a large calcified mass in the petrous bone extending into the posterior cranial (**a**) and neck (**b**). Note marked contrast enhancement in petrous bone and neck (**c, d**)

Fig. 2 a, b. Meningioma. Axial CT showing heavily calcified mass involving petrous bone, parasellar region, cerebellopontine angle cistern (**b**) with extension into foramen magnum (**a**)

marked contrast enhancement (Fig. 3b). Angiography demonstrated a highly vascular lesion.

The surgical specimen proved to be papillary cystadenocarcinoma arising from endolymphatic duct, a very rare tumor of the temporal bone.

Case 4: low-grade chondrosarcoma

A 35-year-old woman gave a history of photophobia. CT showed a large calcified mass arising from the petro-occipital fissure and extending into the tip of the petrous bone and posterior cranial fossa (Fig. 4). MRI revealed mixed intensity on T1- and T2-weighted images, with marked contrast enhancement.

Discussion

A heavily calcified lesion with a broad base on the posterior aspect of the petrous bone is usually a meningioma, but chondrosarcoma, hemangioma, laterally located chordoma and choroid plexus papilloma with extension into the cerebellopontine angle cistern may also show heavy calcification [1, 2]. Chordoma and chondrosarcoma are usually associated with destructive changes in the adjacent bone [3]. Hemangiomas are mainly along the course of the seventh nerve with the same characteristic bone spicules as in meningioma and papillary cystadenomas. We report a rare case of papillary cystadenocinoma arising from endolymphatic duct showing all radiologic features similar to meningioma. Papillary cystadenomas are slow-growing invasive tumors. Distant metastases have not been reported although local recurrence is common [4–6].

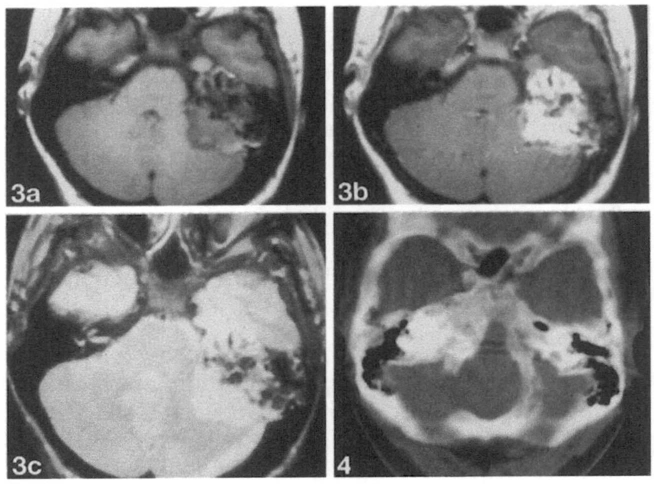

Fig. 3 a–c. Papillary adenocarcinoma of endolymphatic duct. **a, b** Axial T1-weighted images showed mixed low and intermediate intensity with marked contrast enhancement (**b**) A T2-weighted image revealed central signal void with peripheral high intensity (**c**)

Fig. 4. Low-grade chondrosarcoma. Axial CT revealed a calcified mass at the top of the petrous bone, extending into the posterior cranial fossa

References

1. Valvanis A, Schubiger O, Hayek J, Pauliadis G (1982) CT of meningiomas on the posterior surface on the petrous bone. Neuroradiology 22:111
2. Møller A, Hatam A, Olivercrona H (1978) The differential diagnosis of petrous angle meningioma and acoustic neuroma with computed tomography. Neuroradiology 17:21
3. Zimmermann RD, Fleming CA, Saint Louis LA, Lee BCP, Manning JJ, Deck MDF (1985) Magnetic resonance imaging of meningioma. AJNR 6:149
4. Lo WM, Applegate CJ, Carberry JN, Solti-Bohman LG, et al (1993) Endolymphatic sac tumors: radiologic appearance. Radiology 189:199
5. Meyer J, Geharski SS, Blaivas M (1993) Cerebellopontine angle invasive papillary cystadenoma of endolymphatic sac origin with temporal bone involvement. AJNR 14:1319
6. Heffner DK (1989) Low-grade adenocarcinoma of probable endolymphatic sac origin; a clinicopathologic study of 20 cases. Cancer 64:2292

MRI of inner ear fluids using modified GRASS sequences: a useful tool in the assessment of the normal and pathological labyrinth

L. Manfré, R. Lagalla, A. E. Cardinale

Institute of Radiology, University of Palermo, Palermo, Italy

Abstract. MRI is acquiring a progressively more important role in the investigation of petrous bone disease. Nevertheless, despite the extensive use of MRI in the detection of inflammatory or neoplastic involvement of the seventh and eighth cranial nerves, conventional spin-echo images cannot be considered the modality of choice in inner ear imaging "Steady-state sequences" are known to be motion sensitive. By setting a very short repetition time, a large flip angle and a long echo time, one can obtain a sequence sufficiently sensitive to the slow movement of endo- and perilymph. We report our experience in MRI of normal and pathological inner ear with modified GRASS sequences.

Key words: Inner ear – Magnetic resonance imaging – GRASS – Pathology

Materials and methods

MR images centered on the membranous labyrinth were performed using a 0.5 T unit and a 14 cm diameter surface coil. For the anatomical study, ten healthy volunteers (6 male and 4 female) were examined. We also examined four patients with cholesteatoma, whose CT findings suggested a labyrinthine fistula and inner ear symptoms – sensorineural hearing loss (SNHL) and vertigo; three with tympanic cholesteatoma, with identical CT findings but no symptoms; four with malformations (Mondini, cholea/aplasia, large vestibular aqueduct and Noonan's syndrome, with bilateral semicircular canal aplasia and Mondini deformity) and one with labyrinthine sclerosis.

GRASS sequences were obtained using a 3D 22.5-mm-thick slab (0.8 mm single partition tickness), TR 35/TE 17 and flip angle 90°. The matrix was 128×256, with a 20 cm field of view and 4 excitations, in 8 min 35 s. Finally, a comparison between GRASS findings and CT in the patients was performed

Results

Thanks to the high signal intensity of the slowly moving labyrinth fluids and the thin (0.8 mm) no-gap imaging technique, GRASS images appear to be able to show all the main labyrinthine components seen on a CT study.

Patients with acquired tympanic cholesteatoma destroying the otic capsule (Fig. 1) suffering from SNHL and vertigo showed abnormal decrease in signal intensity in the damaged membranous labyrinth. In particular, patients with high-tone, SNHL showed loss of physiological high signal intensity only in the basal turn of the cochlea, where acute tones are usually codified (Fig. 2). In patients with CT findings compatible with lybyrinthine fistula, but no inner ear symptoms, normal high signal intensity from the slow movement of the endo- and perilymph fluids was seen. A thin low signal line separating the normal inner ear from the cholesteatomatous mass was also visible (Fig. 2).

The patient with Noonan's syndrome [1] complained of bilateral SNHL [2]. MRI and CT both demonstrated bilateral semicircular canal aplasia, anomalous vestibules and a Mondini malformation, with a dysplastic modiolus (Fig. 3). Another patient had an incidental CT finding of unilateral cochlear aplasia, a rare malformation probably due to premature arrest of development of the otic bud in the 5th week. GRASS images showed total absence of the cochlea (Fig. 4), proving the presence of a normal cochlear nerve.

The patient suffering with labyrinthine sclerosis showed severe otic capsule ossification with only a residual basal turn on CT. GRASS imaging was similar, showing the loss of the normal labyrinthine fluid signal intensity in all but the basal turn.

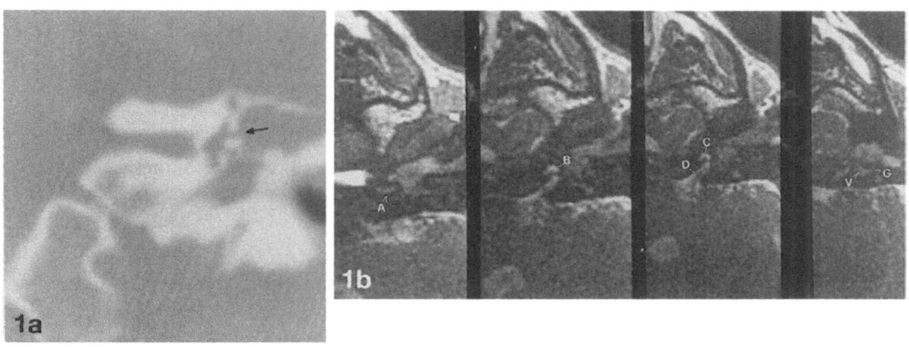

Fig. 1. a Cholesteatoma and lateral canal fistula with vertigo and high-tones sensorineural hearing lass. *Coronal CT of left temporal bone.* The mass has eroded the lateral wall of the lateral semicircular canal (*arrows*). Nothing can be said about the membranous labyrinth. **b** Axial *GRASS* image (*left to right, caudo-cranial*). Note decreased signal intensity of the basal turn of the cochlea (*A*), the vestibule (*V*) and semicircular canal (*G*). Normal high signal intensity in middle (*B*) and apical turn (*C*) of the cochlea and internal auditory meatus (*D*)

Correspondence to: L. Manfré, via Duca degli Abruzzi 40, I-95127 Catania, Italy

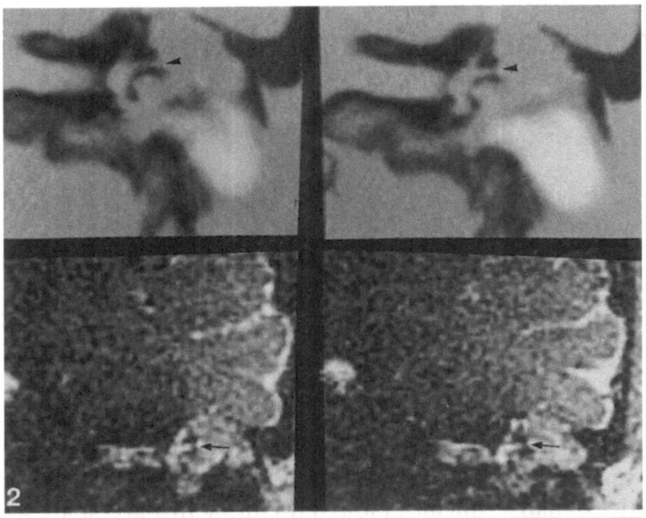

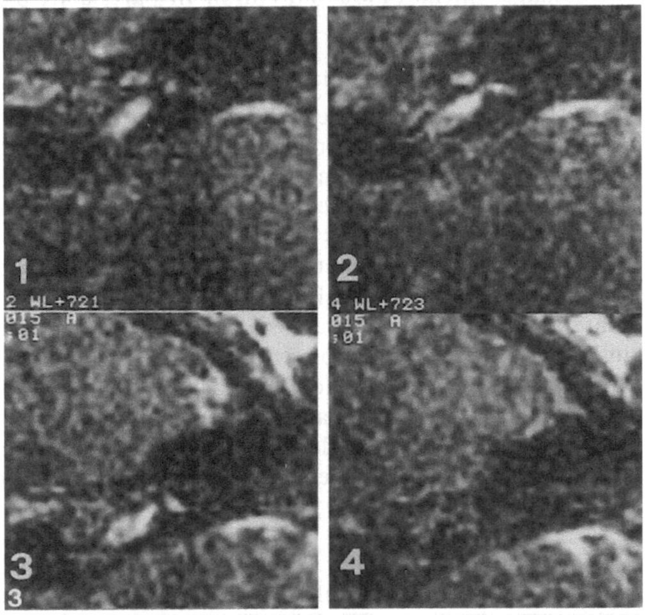

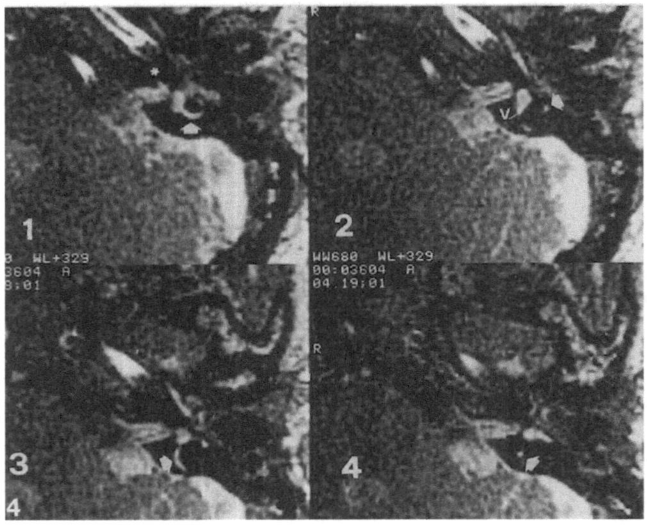

Discussion

MRI has become increasingly useful in the investigation of many temporal bone diseases: Conventional spin-echo (SE) T1-weighted images can readily show intralabyrinthine high signal, a result of old cochlear of vestibular haemorrhage [3], while contrast-enhanced MRI is important in detecting inflammatory or neoplastic seventh and eighth cranial nerve changes [4–9] as well as discease of the cochlea of vestibule [10]. Recently, otic capsule enhancement in otospongiosis has been described. However, the poor contrast between the inner ear fluids and the background on T1-weighted images, or the relatively thick slice and long acquisition for T2-weighted images make conventional SE not a competitive imaging technique in comparison to high-resolution CT in the analysis of small membranous labyrinth components.

"Steady-state" sequences are known to be motion sensitive [11]. By using a GRASS pulse sequence with a very short repetition time to saturate the stationary tissue, a large flip angle to avoid the saturation of residual transversal magnetisation, and a large echo time (always useful when long T2-decay tissue must be examined), one can obtain a sequence sufficiently sensitive to the slow flow of the endo- and peri-lymphatic fluids of the inner ear.

By using this method, three major advantages are found. Firstly, the possibility of obtaining a very thin sectioning (0.8 mm) of the inner ear enables demonstration of the main components of the membranous labyrinth. Secondly, considering that a volume acquisition is acquired, multiplanar reconstruction can be performed. Thirdly, the application of the maximum intensity projection (MIP) software allows the building up of three-dimensional imaging of the membranous labyrinth freely rotating in the space, exactly as for vascular imaging.

The GRASS sequence seems to be very reliable in the investigation of membranous labyrinth damage. The absence of the normal high signal intensity inside pathological membranous labyrinth in symptomatic patients with a labyrinthine fistula could be related to the leakage of inner ear fluids and/or focal soft tissue degeneration. Taking this into consideration the selective SNHL for the acute tones in one of our patients in the series could be referred to as a focal basal cochlear turn involvement, demonstrated by the loss of physiological slow flow signal inside it. In contrast, the normal GRASS findings at the

Fig. 2. Cholesteatoma and apparent lateral semicircular canal fistual, without relevant symptoms. *Top CT, bottom GRASS images.* Although CT proves destruction of lateral semicircular canal bony canal (*arrowheads*), MRI reveals a normal high signal intensity labyrinth and a thin low signal line (*arrows*) separating the inner ear from the cholesteatoma

Fig. 3. Noonan syndrome *Axial GRASS images* (1–4, caudocranial) show a one-turn cochlea, a displastic modiolus and a small vestibule. No semicircular canal can be detected

Fig. 4. Cochlear aplasia. *Axial GRASS images* (1–4, caudocranial). Despite normal vestibule (*v*) and semicircular canals (*arrows*) high signal, no inner ear fluid can be appreciated in the region of the cochlear (*)

level of inner ear in asymptomatic patients should suggest the integrity of the membranous labyrinth.

GRASS sequences were also quite reliable in the detection of morphological changes of malformative membranous labyrinths, and sclerotic changes of the otic capsule resembling traditional CT studies.

References

1. Levine B, Skope L, Parker R (1991) Cherubism in a patient with Noonan syndrome. J Oral Maxillofac Surg 49:1014–1018
2. Cohen MM, Gorlin RJ (1991) Noonan like/multiple giant cell lesion syndrome. Am J Med Genet 40:159–166
3. Mark AS, Seltzer S, Harnsberg KR (1993) MRI of sensorineural hearing loss: more than meets the eye? AJNR 14:37–45
4. Brogan M, Chakeres DW (1990) Gd-DTPA-enhanced MR imaging of cochlear schwannoma. AJNR 11:407–408
5. Mafee MF et al (1990) CT and MR imaging of intralabyrinthine schwannoma: report of two cases and review of the literature. Radiology 174:395–400
6. Tash R, DeMerrit J, Sze G, Leslie D (1991) Hemifacial spasm: MR imaging features. AJNR 12:839–842
7. Tali ET, et al (1993) Cystic acoustic schwannomas: MR characteristics. AJNR 14:1241–1247
8. Stack JP, et al (1988) Magneitc resonance imaging of acoustic neuromas: the role of gadolinium-DTPA. Br J Radiol 61:800–805
9. Weissmann JL, et al (1992) High signal form otic labyrinth on unenhanced magnetic resonance imaging. AJNR 13:1183–1187
10. Seltzer S, Mark AS (1991) Contrast enhancement of the labyrinth on MR scans in patients with sudden hearing loss and vertigo: evidence of labyrinth disease. AJNR 12:13–16
11. Casselman JW, Kuhweide R, Ampe W, Meeus L, Steyaert L (1993) Pathology of the membranous labyrinth: comparison of T1- and T2-weighted and gadolinium enhanced spin-echo and 3DFT-CISS imaging. AJNR 14:59–69

Clinical role of fast-spin echo MRI of the temporal bone in inner ear dysfunction

J. I. Chung, D. I. Kim

Department of Diagnostic Radiology, Yonsei University, College of Medicine, 134 Shinchondong, Seodaemun-ku, Seoul, 120 752 Korea, Fax. 82c2c393 3035

Abstract. To assess the clinical effectiveness of high-resolution fast spin-echo (FSE) MRI in the study of the normal and pathological cochleovestibular and neural structures, we examined 19 patients with clinically diagnosed inner ear dysfunction. Contiguous interleave 3-mm-thickness axial and coronal T2-weighted images were obtained by using 16 echo train length (ETL) and FSE with surface dual temporomandibular at joint 1.5 T. Imaging parameters were as follows: TR 4500 ms, effective TE 100 ms, 2 excitations field of view 16 cm, and 512 matrix. Fine inner ear structures including the osseous spiral lamina and labyrinthine segment of the facial nerve were exceptionally shown in all cases. Bundles of the cochlear and vestibular branches of the acoustic nerve were resolved in 79–92%: cochlear branch 92% (35/38), 79% (30/38) on axial and coronal images; superior vestibular branch 89% (34/38) on coronal images; inferior vestibular branch 82% (31/38) on axial images respectively. The vestibular aqueduct was also visualised in 16% (6/38) on axial images only. Five patients were shown to have inner ear pathology, including 2 intracanalicular acoustic schwannomas, 2 congenital anomalies and 1 labyrinthitis.

Key words: Tempral bone – Magnetic resonance imaging

Correspondence to: J. Chung

Fast spin-echo (FSE) T2-weighted MRI allows us to obtain high-resolution images in a clinically acceptable time for the assessment of small anatomical structures such as the inner ear. We investigated the clinical usefulness of FSE MRI in the diagnosis of inner ear dysfunction.

Patients and methods

Nineteen patients (10 male, 9 female), aged from 4 to 66 years with a clinical diagnosis of inner ear dysfunction were included for FSE MRI using a 1.5 T magnet. Imaging parameters were as follwos: TR 4000 ms, effective TE 100 ms, echo train length (ETL 16, field of view 16 cm, 3 mm slice thickness with contiguous interleave acquisition and 2 excitations, 512×512 matrix size, and bandwidth 32 kHz. Surface dual temporomandibular joint coils were applied to the temporal bone area for the acquisition of better signal to noise ratio (SNR). Axial and coronal images were obtained, each parallel to the plane of internal acoustic meatus. Gadolinium-enhanced axial T1-weighted images (TR 500 ms, TE 25 ms, FOV 16 cm, 256 matrix) were also obtained with head coil.

Results

Fine inner ear structures including osseous spiral lamina and labyrinthine segment of facial nerve were visualised in all cases. Bundles of cochlear and vestibular branches of the eights nerve were seen in 79–92%. The cochlear branch of the eighth nerve was seen in 92% (35/38) and 79% (30/38) on axial and coronal FSE T2-weighted images respectively. The superior vestibular branch of the eighth nerve

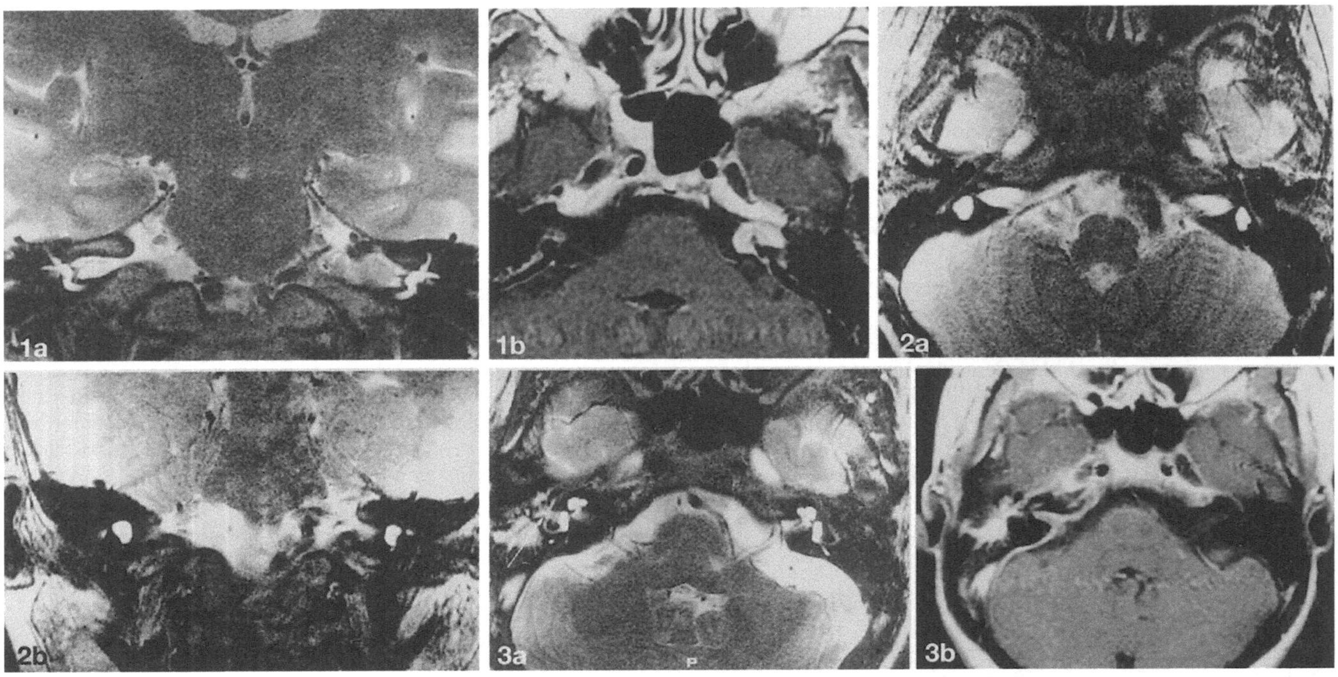

Fig. 1 a, b. Vestibular schwannoma in a 56-year-old woman with a 2-year history of hearing loss of left sided and dizziness. **a** Coronal FSE T2-weighted image demonstrates oval low signal intensity mass occupying left internal auditory canal, replacing normal high-signal membranous labyrinth structures. **b** Gadolinium-enhanced T1-weighted image shows comma-shaped mass with strong contrast enhancement, suggesting intracanalicular acoustic schwannoma

Fig. 2 a, b. Congenital malformation of inner ear in a 4-year-old boy with bilateral deafness and blue sclerae. Axial and coronal T2-weighted images show absence of semicircular canals and common vestibular channels with underdevelopment of cochlear canals

Fig. 3 a, b. Labyrinthitis with perilymph fistula in a 50-year-old woman with a 3-months history of headache and right sensorineural hearing loss. **a** Axial FSE T2-weighted image shows high signal fistula on the right lateral semicircular canal (*long arrow*), with irregular high signal change in the mastoid antrum, associated with mastoiditis. **b** Axial Gd-enhanced T1-weighted image shows enhancement of mastoid lesion and perilymph fistula, connected to the membranous labyrinth and tentorium. Biopsy of right mastoid lesion revealed a chronic inflammatory reaction

was seen in 89% (34/38) on coronal images. The inferior vestibular branch of the eighth nerve was seen in 82% (31/38) on axial images. Vestibular aqueduct was also depicted in 16% (6/38) on axial FSE T2-weighted images only. Of 19 patients, 5 were shown to have inner ear diseases, including 2 acoustic schwannomas (Fig. 1), 2 congenital inner ear malformations (Fig. 2) and 1 chronic labyrinthitis (Fig. 3).

Discussion

The usefulness of FSE imaging is reduction of scan time due to successive 180° pulses representing a factor of ETL [1, 2]. Moreover, a surface coil can improve the SNR; thus, high resolution for inner ear imaging is possible [3]. Heavily T2-weighted, longer TR/TE images are possible within a clinically acceptable time using a 512 matrix for adequate tissue contrast between the cochleovestibular structures and the membranous labyrinth. Our imaging parameters make it possible for a voxel size of about 0.3 mm in plane resolution and continuous interleave scan with thin (3 mm) slice imaging which can prevent omitting the interslice gap. Small anatomical structures of inner ear are clearly visualised, including osseous spiral lamina and vestibulum and labyrinthine segments of the facial nerve. In some patients, the cisternal segment of the seventh cranial nerve was demonstrated parallel to the superior vestibular branch of the eighth cranial nerve above the level of the superior part of the internal auditory canal [4, 5]. The superior and inferior vestibular branch were better depicted on coronal and axial images due to the parallel course of the nerve bundles to the imaging plane. Subsequently, acoustic schwannomas which mainly arise from the inferior vestibular branch, would be detected easily in this high-resolution MRI without additional gadolinium-enhanced study (Fig. 1).

It is known that the endolymphatic sac plays a role in the aetiology of Ménière's disease [6, 7]. Tanioka et al. [6] reported that the visualisation of the ipsilateral side of the membranous endolymphatic duct and sac, running through the vestibular aqueduct using three-dimensional Fourier-transform FLASH imaging, failed in 83% of affected patients. These findings may suggest the pathogenesis of endolymphatic duct and sac, which consists of early endolymphatic duct hydrops and late progressive obliteration of endolymphatics in Ménière's disease. Since our study protocol involves two-dimensional images with a 3 mm slice thickness, endolymphatic sacs like small structures are not identified in all cases and only 16% (6/38) of patients demonstrated the high signal structure of endolymphatic duct. A three-dimensional volume imaging study, such as 3D FSE including echo planar image, is recommended for further definitive evaluation of this endolymphatic sac abnormality. Clinical suspicion of labyrinthine abnormality such as perilymph fistula which is not well demarcated on temporal CT can be definitely delineated in these high resolution MRI (Fig. 3). The congenital inner ear malformations are well recognised in FSE MRI due to superior visualisation of the vestibulum and membranous labyrinth.

References

1. Tien R, Felsberg GJ, Macfall J (1992) Fast spin echo high-resolution MR imaging of the inner ear. AJR 159:395–398
2. Henning J, Nauerth A, Friedburg H (1986) RARE imaging: a fast imaging method for clinical MR. Magn Reson Med 3:823–833
3. Kumakawa K, Takemori S (1989) High resolution MR imaging of the inner ear. Acta Otolaryngol (Stockh) [Suppl] 468:391–397
4. Tanioka H, Shirakawa T, Machida T, Sasaki Y (1991) Three dimensional reconstructed MR imaging of the inner ear. Radiology 178:141–144
5. Casselman JW, Kuhweide R, Deimling M, Ampe W, Dehaene I, Meeus L (1993) Constructive interference in steady state (CISS)-3DFT MR imaging of the inner ear and cerebellopontine angle. AJNR 14:47–57
6. Tanioka H, Zusho H, Machida T, Sasaki Y, Shirakawa T (1992) High resolution MR imaging of the inner ear: findings in Meniere's disease. Eur J Radiol 15:83–88
7. Brogan M, Chakeres DW, Schmalbrock P (1991) High resolution 3DFT MR imaging of the endolymphatic duct and soft tissues of the otic capsule. AJNR 12:1–11

Three-dimensional MRI in acoustic neuroma

H. Miki, Y. Ishimaru, K. Kikuchi, K. Hamamoto

Department of Radiology, Ehime University School of Medicine, Shigenobu-cho, Onsengun, 791-02 Ehime, Japan

Abstract. Twenty-four patients with acoustic neuroma were studied with 1.5 T MRI. Tumour extirpation was performed in all cases. We evaluated the detectability of tumour, cyst formation, deposits of haemosiderin, and residual tumour on MRI. MRI diagnoses were compared with histological findings and operative records. The detectability of acoustic neuroma by three-dimensional (3D) MRI and spin echo was the same; however, the characteristics of a tumour such as a cyst formation and deposits of haemoside in were depicted in greater detail by 3D MRI. 3D MRI was considered to be able to detect a residual tumour in the postoperative state. 3D MRI was very useful for the preoperative diagnosis of acoustic neuroma, but should also be used in the postoperative management of such patients.

Key words: Acoustic neuroma – Three-dimensional magnetic resonance imaging – Cyst formation

The usefulness of T1-weighted spin-echo using gadolinium (Gd) DTPA in the detection of acoustic neuroma has been reported [1]. The recently developed three-dimensional (3D) rephased spoiled GRASS (SPGR) sequence gives good T1-weighted images. The purpose of our study is to evaluate the clinical utility of 3D MRI for the pre- and postoperative examination of acoustic neuroma by comparing it with the SE method, histological findings, and operative results.

Correspondence to: H. Miki

Patients and methods

The study group includes 24 patients (10 men and 14 women) with acoustic neuroma. Tumour extirpation was performed in all cases. 3D MRI, enhanced 3D MRI, and enhanced T1-weighted SE (Gd-DTPA 0.1 mmol/kg) were performed in all cases. T1-weighted SE was performed in 22 cases. T2-weighted SE was performed in 10 cases. T2-weighted fast SE was performed in 14 cases. Seventeen cases were examined after operation (1 week–1 month). All studies were performed with a 1.5 T MRI unit. 3D MRI was performed with a SPGR sequence at TR 40 ms, TE 4.7 ms, flip angle 30°, field of view (FOV) 18 cm, 1 excitation (NEX) and matrix 256 × 192. Slice thickness was 1.5 mm. T1-weighted SE was performed with TR 400–500 ms, TE 12–14 ms, slice thickness 3–5 mm and 1 NEX. T2-weighted SE was performed with TR 2000 ms, TE 90 ms, slice thickness 5–10 mm and 1 NEX. T2-weighted fast SE was performed with TR 3000 ms, TE 100 ms, slice thickness 3–5 mm and 1 NEX.

We assessed the detectability of tumour, cyst formation and deposits of haemosiderin on MRI. Deposits of haemosiderin were recognised by the detection of black dots as in small cavernous haemangiomas [2]. Furthermore, we compared MRI and histological findings. We assessed the detectability of the residual tumour on contrast-enhanced 3D MRI. Four patterns of abnormal enhancement [A: enhancing mass or the enhancement of tumour capsule in the cerebello pontine (CP) angle; B: solid enhancement of the internal auditory canal (IAC); C: the peripheral enhancement of the IAC; D: dural enhancement of the CP angle] were observed on postoperative 3D MRI. Patterns A and B were diagnosed as the patterns of residual tumour. Pattern C and D were diagnosed as the patterns of no residual tumour. These MRI diagnoses were compared with operative records.

Results

All tumours were detected by 3D MRI, enhanced 3D MRI and enhanced T1-weighted SE. On T1- and T2-weighted SE, 2 of 4 tumours small than 10 mm were not detected.

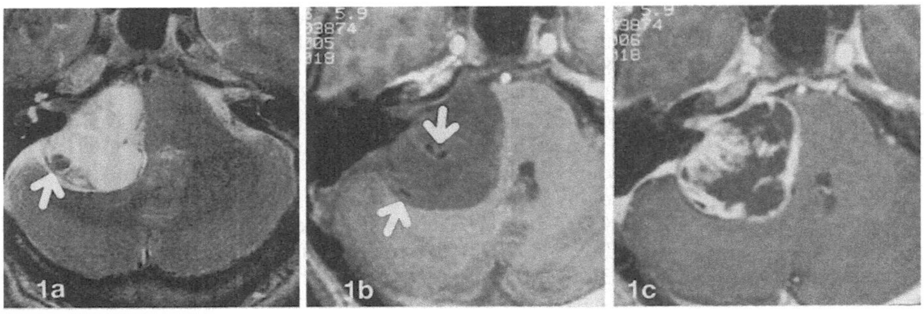

Fig. 1a–c. A 52-year-old man with right acoustic neurinoma. A cystic component could be detected on T2-weighted fast spin echo (**a**), 3D MRI (**b**), and contrast-enhanced 3D MRI (**c**). Contrast-enhanced T2-weighted fast spin echo and 3D MRI demonstrated cystic components more clearly than 3D MRI. Black dots were detected in **a** (*arrow*) and **b** (*arrow*)

Table 1. Cyst formation on MRI

	Apparent	Proven histologically	Histology (12 cases)
T2-weighted spin-echo	7	4	
T2-weighted fast spin-echo	10	8	Antoni A 2
3D MRI	13	12	Antoni B 3
3D MRI + Gd	17	12	Antoni A + B7

Table 2. Black dots suggesting haemosiderin on MRI

Technique	MRI	Proven histologically	Histology (14 cases)
T2-weighted spin-echo	4	4	
T2-weighted fast spin-echo	6	10	Antoni A 1
3D MRI	15	14	Antoni B 2
3D MRI + Gd	15	14	Antoni A + B11

For detection of tumours, enhanced 3D MRI had the same ability as enhanced T1-weighted SE. However, 3D MRI detected tumours more clearly than T1-weighted SE. We considered that 3D MRI should be useful for screening of acoustic neuroma. Cyst formation of tumour was detected in 13 cases by 3D MRI and in 17 cases by enhanced 3D MRI (Fig. 1). Enhanced 3D MRI was equal to T2-weighted or T2-weighted fast SE in the detection of cyst formation (Table 1). Small cysts were only detected by enhanced 3D MRI and thin slice T2-weighted fast SE. Twelve cases were proved to be cyst formations by histological examination, using small specimens of tumour. However, 7 cases without cyst formation (on MRI) were not proved to be cyst formation. Black dots that reveal deposits of haemosiderin were detected in 15 cases by 3D MRI and enhanced 3D MRI (Fig. 1). 3D MRI was superior to T2-weighted fast SE in detecting haemosiderin because of the lower susceptibility of the latter technique (Table 2). Fourteen cases were proved to be deposits of haemosiderin by histological examination. Antoni A + B type of acoustic neuroma tended to deposit haemosiderin.

Five cases were diagnosed as having no residual tumour on enhanced 3D MRI. Total resection was performed in all 5 cases. Twelve cases were diagnosed as residual tumour on enhanced 3D MRI. Subtotal resection was performed in 8 of 12 cases, but total resection was performed in another 4 cases. On follow-up MRI, however, the size of the enhancing mass was increased in 1 of another 4 cases. 3D MRI should be useful for following up patients with patterns A and B.

Discussion

The ability of 3D MRI and SE to detect acoustic neuroma was the same. However, the characteristics of a tumour such as cyst formation and deposits of haemosiderin were depicted in greater detail by 3D MRI. Furthermore, 3D MRI was considered to be able to detect residual tumour in the postoperative state. 3D MRI was very useful both in the preoperative diagnosis of acoustic neuroma, but should also be used in the postoperative management of such patients.

References

1. Press GA, Hesselink JR (1988) MR imaging of cerebellopontine angle and internal auditory canal lesions at 1.5 T. 150:1371–1381
2. Gomori JM, Grossman RI, Goldberg HI, Hackney DG, Zimmerman RA, Bilaniuk LT (1986) Occult cerebral vascular malformations: high-field MR imaging. Radiology 158:707–713

Malignant astrocytoma causing trigeminal neuralgia: positron emission tomography

T. Sasajima[1], K. Mineura[1], M. Kowada[1], J. Hatazawa[2], T. Ogawa[2], K. Uemura[2]

[1] Neurosurgical Service, Akita University Hospital, Akita, Japan
[2] Department of Radiology and Nuclear Medicine, Research Institute for Brain and Blood Vessels-Akita, Akita, Japan

Abstract. We report a right temporal malignant astrocytoma associated with trigeminal neuralgia, with positron emission tomography (PET) findings. CT and MRI revealed a heterogeneous enhancing mass in the right temporal lobe and mild hydrocephalus. PET disclosed right temporal hyperperfusion and glucose hypermetabolism, characteristic of malignant tumour. In the contralateral grey matter, haemocirculation and metabolism were depressed, whereas oxygen extraction fraction was markedly increased, suggesting intracranial hypertension. A sagittal PET image clearly demonstrated high ^{18}F-fluorodeoxyglucose uptake in the uncus as much as in the posterior part of parahippocampal gyrus, which was equivocal on CT. Histological examination confirmed subarachnoid and leptomeningeal seeding. PET is useful for delineating tumour localisation and understanding haemocirculatory and metabolic aspects of communicating hydrocephalus caused by leptomeningeal seeding.

Key words: Malignant astrocytoma – Trigeminal neuralgia – Positron emission tomography

Recently, many patients with trigeminal neuralgia have been successfully treated with microvascular decompression of the trigeminal root. Symptomatic trigeminal neuralgia of different aetiollogies has also been reported [1, 2]. Posterior fossa tumours and meningiomas are most likely to cause trigeminal neuralgia [3]. In the current study, we report a case of right temporal malignant astrocytoma associated with trigeminal neuralgia, together with positron emission tomography (PET) findings.

Case report

A 14-year-old girl presented with a 3-month history of nausea and vomiting. One month before admission, she developed a right trigeminal neuralgia. On admission, neurological examination disclosed a facial sensory deficit. CT demonstrated a heterogeneously enhancing mass in the right medial temporal lobe and mild hydrocephalus without sheath-like enhancement along ventricular and cerebral surfaces (Fig. 1). T1- and T2-weighted MRI demonstrated a heterogeneous mixed intensity mass in the right temporal lobe (Fig. 2). We used ^{15}O-labelled gas and ^{18}F-fluorodeoxyglucose (FDG) tracers for quantitative measurement of haemocirculation and metabolism. Cerebral blood flow (CBF), blood volume (CBV) and metabolic rate of glucose (CMRGl) values in the lesion were 20.9 ml/100 ml/min, 6.7 ml/100 ml, and 5.8 mg/100 ml/min, respectively. These values were higher than those for the contralateral grey matter (CBF: 18.6 ml/100 ml/min; CBV: 2.4 ml/100 ml; CMRGl: 3.7 mg/100 ml/min). Metabolic rate of oxygen ($CMRO_2$) of the lesions was 1.7 ml/100 ml/min, lower than that for the contralateral grey matter (2.9 ml/100 ml/min). In the contralateral grey matter, haemocirculation and metabolism were suppressed, whereas oxygen extraction fraction (OEF: 0.78) was markedly increased (Fig. 3). Coronal and sagittal PET images were reconstructed by reslicing of original axial images employing an imaging analysis system. A sagittal FDG-PET image clearly revealed increased accumulation of tracers not only in the uncus but also in the posterior part of the parahippocampal gyrus, which was equivocal on CT (Fig. 4). The temporal mass, where FDG tracers had accumulated, was extirpated. Unter the microscope, the surgical specimens were seen to contain pleomorphic cells with hyperchromatic nuclei and endothelial proliferation. The histologic findings corresponded to malignant astrocytoma. Tumour cells infiltrated into the subarachnoid space and spread throughout the intracranial leptomeninges. In spite of postoperative radiotherapy and medical treatment, neurological symptoms and performance status deteriorated progressively. One month after the surgery, the patient died.

Discussion

Tumours causing trigeminal neuralgia are located throughout the course of the trigeminal nerve between the gasserian ganglion and the root entry zone in the pons [1]. Bullitt et al. [2] reported that posterior fossa tumours were most likely to cause trigeminal neuralgia and usually gave rise to other symptoms and neurological deficits in addition to trigeminal neuralgia. Middle fossa tumours were often manifestated by atypical facial pain associated with progressive neurological deficits [2, 4, 5]. Nijensohn et al. [5] reported on 12 cases of Meckel's cave meningioma and found that the tumour compression caused trigeminal neuralgia without destruction of the ganglion. When the causative factors were benign tumours such as meningiomas and neurinomas, not only gross total removal but also debulking and exploration were useful for relief of pain [2, 3, 5]. Moreover, a variety of the tumours producing trigeminal neuralgia are found in the middle fossa [1–5], so neuroradiological and histological diagnoses are significant landmarks in determining the therapeutic strategy.

In the present case, PET demonstrated hyperperfusion and glucose hypermetabolism, characteristic of malignant tumours [6]. FDG is a promising tracer for qualitative diagnosis of histological malignancy [6, 7] and the prediction of survival [8] in patients with gliomas. The coronal and sagittal FDG-PET images clearly revealed viable portions within the tumour infiltrating the posterior part of parahippocampal gyrus, which was equivocal on CT. The temporal malignant astrocytoma affected the gasserian ganglion, which was confirmed by the operative findings.

Correspondence to: T. Sasajima

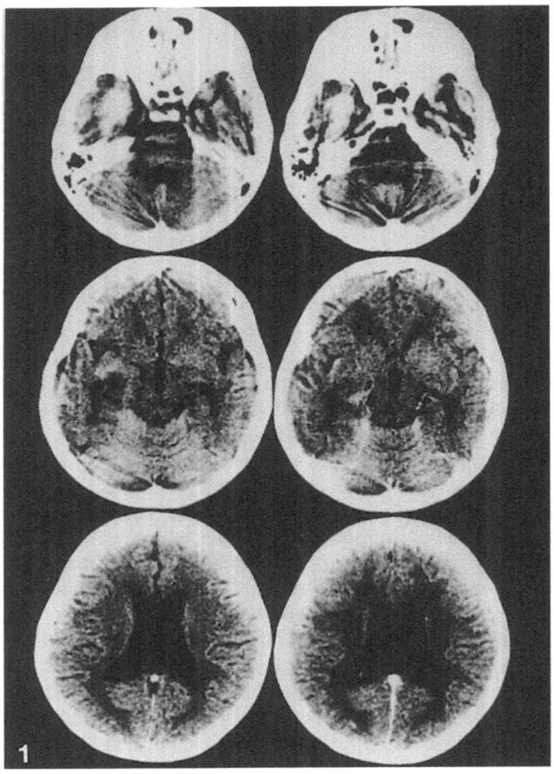

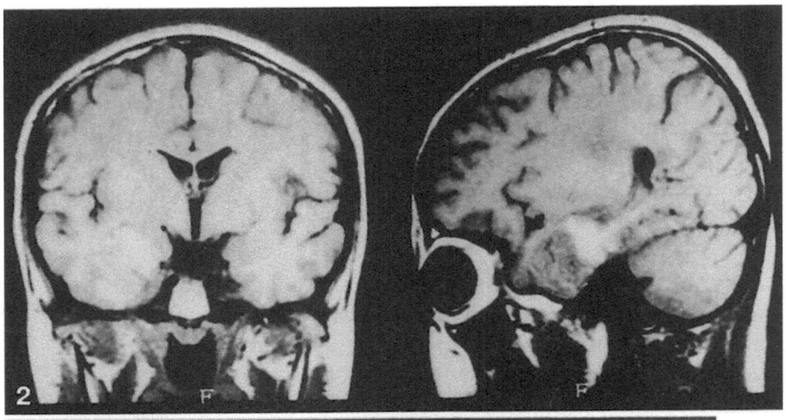

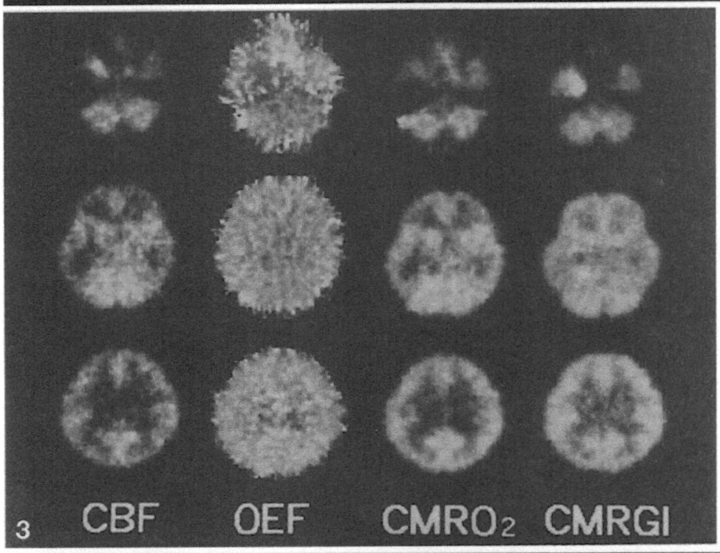

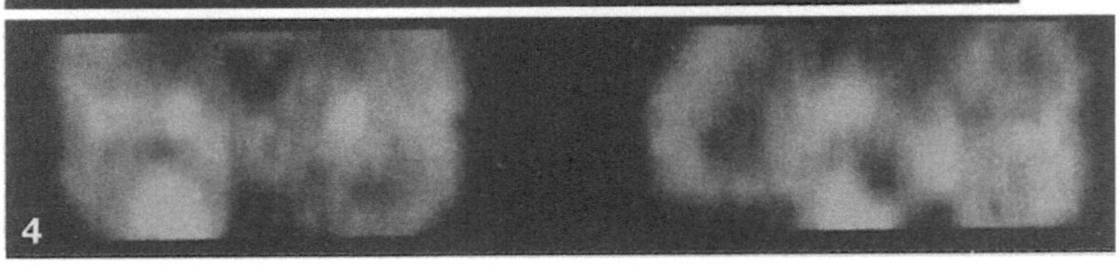

Fig. 1. CT before (*left*) and after (*right*) contrast medium shows heterogeneous enhancing lesion in the right temporal lobe and mild hydrocephalus

Fig. 2. T1-weighted (TR 600, TE 25 ms) MRI; *left*, sagittal; *right*, coronal) shows a mixed intensity mass extending to the parahippocampal gyrus

Fig. 3. PET hyperperfusion and FDG-hypermetabolism in the medial part of the right temporal lobe (*top*). Haemocirculation and metabolism of the contralateral grey matter shows marked depression due to intracranial hypertension caused by communicating hydrocephalus

Fig. 4. A coronal FDG-PET image clearly delineates increased activity in the medial part of the right temporal lobe (*left*). A sagittal image reveals another hypermetabolic lesion posteriorly in the parahippocampal gyrus (*right*)

In the contralateral grey matter, the reduction of haemocirculation and metabolism and the increased OEF indicated intracranial hypertension. Communicating hydrocephalus caused by leptomeningeal and ependymal seeding may be responsible for intracranial hypertension, because mass signs such as midline shift did not appear on either CT or MRI. Contralateral grey matter haemocirculation and oxygen metabolism are also well correlated with survival time and performance status [8]. Our patient showed poor performance status and short survival time. PET, using various tracers, multifariously elucidates the biochemical characteristics and pathogenesis of brain tumours.

References

1. Wilkins RH (1985) Trigeminal neuralgia: introduction. In: Wilkins RH, Rengachary SS (eds) Neurosurgery. McGraw-Hill, New York, pp 2337–2344
2. Bullitt E, Tew JM, Boyd J (1986) Intracranial tumors in patients with facial pain. J Neurosurg 64:865–871
3. Cheng TMW, Cascino TL, Onofrio BM (1993) Comprehensive study of diagnosis and treatment of trigeminal neuralgia secondary to tumors. Neurology 43:2298–2302
4. Vassilakis D, Phylaktakis M, Selviaridis P, Karavelis A, Sirmos C, Vlaikidis N (1988) Symptomatic trigeminal neuralgia. J Neurosurg Sci 32:117–120
5. Nijensohn DE, Araujo JC, MacCarty CS (1975) Meningiomas of Meckel's cave. J Neurosurg 43:197–202
6. Mineura K, Yasuda T, Kowada M, Shishido F, Ogawa T, Uemura K (1986) Positron emission tomographic evaluation of histological malignancy in gliomas using oxygen-15 and fluorine-18-fluorodeoxyglucose. Neurol Res 8:164–168
7. Di Chiro G (1987) Positron emission tomography using [^{18}F] fluorodeoxyglucose in brain tumors: a powerful diagnostic and prognostic tool. Invest Radiol 22:360–371
8. Mineura K, Sasajima T, Kowada M, Ogawa T, Hatazawa J, Shishido F, Uemura K (1994) Perfusion and metabolism in prediction the survival of patients with cerebral gliomas. Cancer 73:2386–2394

Three-dimensional computed tomography of skull base lesions

H. Tomita, K. Ehara, H. Eguchi, M. Sugimoto, A. Takahashi, A. Kawamura, A. Tanimoto, T. Nagashima, N. Tamaki

Department of Neurosurgery, Kobe University School of Medicine, 5-1 Kusunoki-cho 7-chome, Chuo-ku, Kobe 650, Japan

Abstract. Three-dimensional (3D) images reconstructed from the data obtained by helical volume computed tomography (CT) clearly demonstrated the spatial relationship among complex structures, such as bones, vessels and tumours in the skull base. It was helpful for surgical planning and postoperative studies of skull base lesions. We present our early experience using 3D CT images in 11 patients with skull base lesions. The structures of major arteries, veins and skull base bone were clearly and accurately visualised on 3D images. Among the skull base tumours, well-enhanced tumours, such as meningiomas were easily reconstructed by routine procedures. However, less enhanced tumours or cystic tumours such as epidermoids or cystic neuromas were difficult to visualise on 3D images. Some techniques can improve the 3D image, but it is important to keep in the mind that the 3D image has pitfalls and should be checked by original slice image.

Key words: Three-dimensional reconstruction – Computed tomography – Skull base surgery – Meningioma – Neuroma

It is well known that computed tomography (CT) is useful in the diagnosis of intracranial lesions. However, it is usually inadequate for surgical planning and postoperative studies of skull base lesions. Three-dimensional (3D) images, reconstructed from the data obtained by helical volume CT, clearly display the spatial relationship of complex structures, such as the skull base bone, vessels and tumours, and are helpful for surgical planning and postoperative evaluation of skull base lesions [1]. We present our early experiences using 3D CT images in 11 patients with skull base lesions.

Materials and methods

Spiral CT was used in 11 patients with skull base lesions. There were 9 tumours (1 foramen magnum meningioma, 2 clival meningiomas, 1 tentorial meningioma, 3 acoustic neuromas, 1 trigeminal neurinoma, 1 prepontine epidermoid), 1 aneurysm and 1 cavernous angioma.

The scan parameters were as follows: table speed of 1–2 mm/s, slice thickness of 1–2 mm. A total of 60–100 ml contrast material (300 mg/ml) was injected at a rate of 2–3 ml/s. 3D images were reconstructed from CT data of every 0.3–0.5 mm slice using a workstation.

The degree and accuracy of the visualisation of the major vessels, skull base bone and tumours were evaluated and the utility for skull base surgery was discussed.

Correspondence to: H. Tomita

Results

The structures of major arteries, veins and skull base bone were clearly and accurately visualised on 3D images (Fig. 1). However, some techniques were required to improve the 3D images. The well-enhanced tumours, such as meningiomas were easily reconstructed by routine procedures, but the less enhanced tumours or cystic tumours such as epidermoids or cystic neuromas were difficult to visualise on 3D images. When a larger volume or a higher concentration of contrast material was injected at a higher speed, the tumours were more clearly visualised on 3D images. In such cases, 3D images were sometimes reconstructed separately and were mixed together to abolish the relatively large noise from the brain. The skull base bone was easily reconstructed by the routine procedure. However, the bone must be reconstructed separately from other structures, because it was sometimes necessary to the bone cut for the simulation of skull base surgery. In regard to the vessels, smaller arteries were more difficult to visualise. They were more clearly visualised when a larger volume or a higher concentration of contrast material was injected at a higher speed. When it is necessary to visualise the vessels separately from surrounding bony structures, a smaller volume of contrast material should be injected. The CT number of the arteries decreased more than the skull base bone and they were separated from each other. For the arteries, the scan was performed from the base to the top, and for veins from the top to the base. This allowed scanning of arteries or veins at their peak CT number

Discussion

It is important for the simulation of skull base surgery that the structures of major arteries, veins and skull base bone and tumours be clearly and accurately visualised on 3D images preoperatively. However, slightly enhanced tumours, cystic tumours, and smaller vessels are difficult to visualise on 3D images [2, 3]. In these cases, the above-mentioned techniques are helpful in making a 3D image. Postoperatively, the utility of 3D CT for skull base surgery is limited. The size and character of an object are observed more precisely on the original image before reconstruction, because many procedures are needed to make 3D images. The area of the skull base bone, which was drilled out at surgery, could easily be assessed on 3D images, because few procedures were needed to make this 3D image. However, the size of residual tumour could be evaluated on the original image before reconstruction rather than on 3D images.

Whether preoperatively or postoperatively, it is important to bear in mind that the 3D image is not the real image and must be checked against the original slice image.

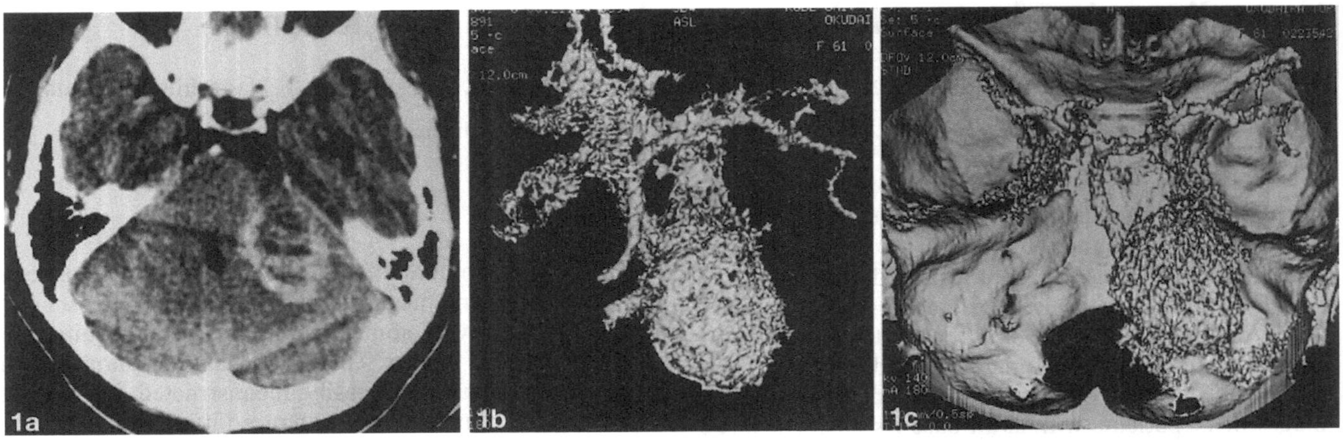

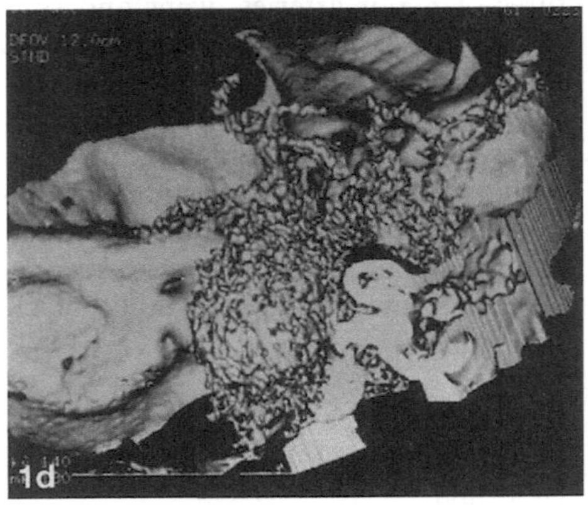

Fig. 1a–d. Acoustic neuroma. **a** Enhanced CT showing cystic tumour in the right cerebellopontine angle. **b** 3D image of tumour and vessels is helpful in reducing the noise from the brain. **c** 3D image of the tumour, vessels and skull base bone. **d** 3D image: operative view

References

1. Katada K, Anno H, Koga S (1990) Three-dimensional angio-imaging with helical scanning CT. Radiology 177:364
2. Harbaugh RE, Schlusselberg DS, Jeffery R, Hayden S, Cromwell LD, Pluta D (1992) Three-dimensional computerized tomography angiography in the diagnosis of cerebrovascular disease. J Neurol Sci 76:408–414
3. Polacin A, Kalender WA, Marchal G (1992) Evaluation section sensitivity profiles and image noise in spiral CT. Radiology 185:29–35

Diagnosis of cerebrospinal fluid fistulae using a 3D-PSIF sequence

K. E. W. Eberhardt[1], **H. P. Hollenbach**[2], **W. J. Huk**[1]

[1] Division of Neuroradiology, Department of Neurosurgery, University of Erlangen, Erlangen, Germany
[2] Siemens Medical Engineering Group, Erlangen, Germany

Abstract. CT cisternography was compared with a new MRI method, so-called MR cisternography, to detect cerebrospinal fluid (CSF) fistulae in patients with post-traumatic and postoperative dural lesions. The MRI examinations were performed using a 1.0 T whole-body system. A strongly T2*-weighted 3D-PSIF sequence and a 3D-CISS sequence were in the coronal plane. We examined 30 patients with CSF fistulae, and the results of the CT and MRI methods were compared and assessed with respect to intraoperative findings. The sensitivity of the MRI technique was higher than that of CT cisternography. MR cisternography was also possible in patients without rhinorrhoea.

Key words: Cerebrospinal fluid fistulae – MR cisternography – CT cisternography

Fractures of the skull base and the paranasal sinuses complicated by lacerations of the dura mater have a high risk of subsequent intracranial infection; about 20–30% of post-traumatic meningitis follows this type of injury. It is therefore important to find out whether the dura mater has been damaged when assessing a patient preoperatively. We present a new MRI method that makes it possible to demonstrate cerebrospinal fluid (CSF) fistulae.

Correspondence to: K. E. W. Eberhardt

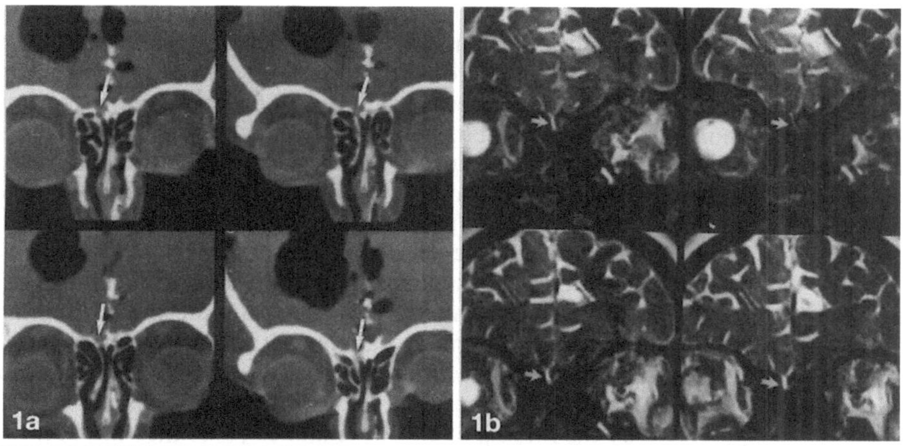

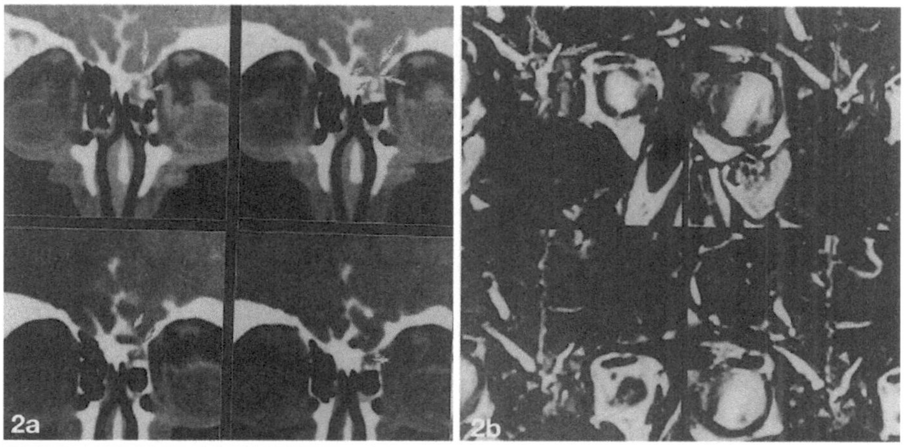

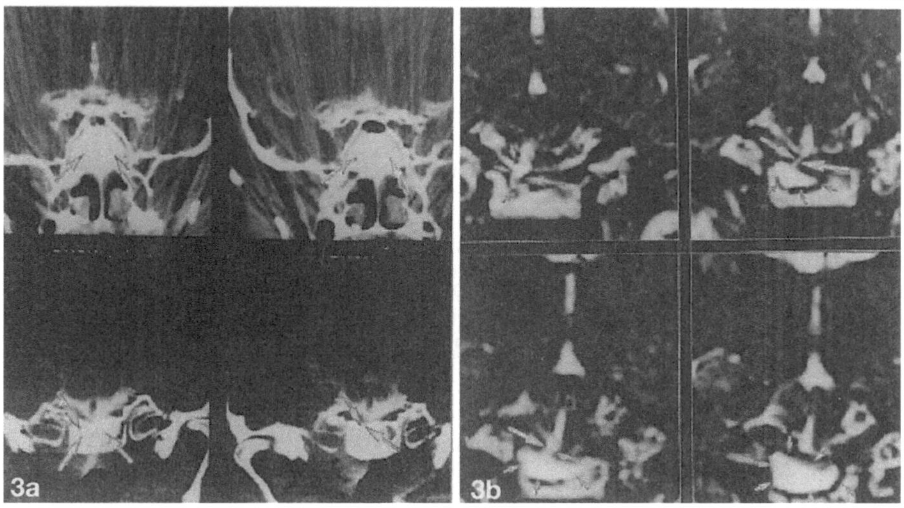

Fig. 1 a, b. Patient with a 2-mm-wide Escher type 2 fracture in the vicinity of the cribiform plate. While CT cisternography showed only a bony defect, MR cisternography revealed a dural lesion. *Arrows* "CSF channel"

Fig. 2 a, b. Patient with persistent CSF rhinorrhoea after trauma. On high-resolution CT 3- to 4-mm-wide Escher type 2 fracture of the ethmoid bone was found. Both CT and MR cisternography showed a dural tear and demonstrated its exact location (*arrows*), confirmed at operation

Fig. 3 a, b. Patient with a CSF fistula from a fracture of the petrous temporal bone, with extension into the dorsum sellae and pituitary fossa. The fracture of the dorsum sellae was about 2 mm wide. CSF rhinorrheoa was present. CT cisternography confirmed a dural lesion. MRI showed CSF tracking from the basal cisterns through the roof of the sphenoid and into the sphenoid sinus (*arrows*); this was confirmed at operation

Material and methods

In 25 patients with post-traumatic and 5 with postoperative CSF fistulae, we compared the diagnostic sensitivity of a new MRI method, so-called MR cisternography, with CT cisternography in a prospective clinical study. The average age of the patients was 35.7 years (6–68 years). The sex distribution was homogeneous (19 men, 11 women). The interval between the initial CT cisternography and subsequent MR cisternography ranged from 1 to 3 days (mean 1.7 days). Subsequently, the patients had surgery within the next 1 to 5 days (mean 2.5 days).

The surgical results were compared with both methods. The MRI examinations were performed on a 1.0 T whole-body MR system. The patients were positioned both prone and supine. A strongly T2*-weighted 3D-PSIF sequence (TR/TE/α 17/7/80 ms/ms per degree) and 3D-CISS sequence (TR/TE/α 14/6/80 ms/ms per degree were used to obtain transverse and coronal images. A circular polarized head coil was used, and the resolution in both sequences was 0.9 × 0.9 × 1.00 mm. The aquisition time for the PSIF sequence was 4 min/41 s and for the CISS 8 min.

Results

We found MR cisternography to be more sensitive (100%) than CT cisternography (72.0%) in detecting dural lesions. Both MRI techniques were able to do this, but PSIF sequence has the disadvantage that it is inherently more sensitive to flow, which can cause signal voids. The CISS sequence overcomes this disadvantage. The diagnostic sensitivity of CT cisternography depends strongly on the location of the CSF fistula (roof of the ethmoid; 80%, roof of the sphenoid; 85.6%; cribriform plate: 50%, and the CT technique can only be used in patients with persistent CSF leakage (Figs. 1–3).

Discussion

Popa described in 1936 the dura mater of the skull base as containing three groups of fibres. In our early anatomical studies, we determined the thickness of the dura mater and the orientation and width of fractures in the skull base, finding a relationship between fracture width and dural lesions. In order to demonstrate dural lesions directly, numerous techniques have been proposed. Recently, intrathecal instillation of water-soluble contrast medium combined with CT (CT cisternography) has been used and considered the best diagnostic procedure for tracing CSF leakage. We found CT cisternography to be less sensitive in patients with slight CSF leakage and with fractures in the region of the cribiform plate, because intrathecal contrast medium rarely shows the dural lesion directly; it often only shows a paranasal sinus containing contrast medium. In patients with sinusitis, CT cisternography can give false-positive results. 3D-MR cisternography, however, is able to show the CSF fistula directly by the finding of a "CSF-channel", a connection between the subarachnoid space and the paranasal sinus or nasal cavity. The MRI method is noninvasive, anodyne requires little measurement time, and has advantages in patients who have no rhinorrhoea.

MRI of rhabdomyosarcoma in the head and neck

T. Mochizuki, H. Isoda, T. Masui, M. Takahashi, M. Kaneko

Department of Radiology, Hamamatsu University School of Medicine, 3600 Handa, Hamamatsu 431-31, Japan

Abstract. The purpose of this study was to determine the typical MR signal intensity characteristics of rhabdomyosarcomas in the head and neck and to establish their signal changes after therapy. MRI studies of six patients with rhabdomyosarcomas of the head and neck, three embryonal and three alveolar type, were retrospectively reviewed. Four patients received contrast medium before chemotherapy or surgery. The most common MRI appearance was that of a homogeneous mass, hyperintense to both muscle and fat on T2-weighted images and isointense to muscle on T1-weighted images. All lesions of the patients who received contrast media showed remarkable enhancement. Only one lesion had intratumoral haemorrhage. Similar MR signal intensity patterns have been reported for other malignant tumours. MRI provides information on the extent of the rhabdomyosarcoma.

Key words: Rhabdomyosarcoma – Head and neck – Magnetic resonance imaging

Correspondence to: T. Mochizuki

The purpose of this investigation was to determine the characteristics of the MR signal intensity of rhabdomyosarcomas in the head and neck and to establish their signal changes during treatment.

Patients and methods

Six patients with histopathologically proven rhabdomyosarcomas were included in this study. There were two female and four male patients ranging in age from 1 to 71 years. Three of the rhabdomyosarcomas were of the embryonal type and the other three were alveolar (Table 1).

MRI was obtained with a 1.5 T unit. T1-weighted, proton density-weighted and T2-weighted images were obtained with axial spin-echo sequences. Coronal images were also obtained to assess intracranial and intraorbital extension with T1-weighted images with/without frequency-selected fat suppression. Five patients received an injection of gadopentetate dimeglumine (0.1 mmol/kg) and were imaged with conventional T1-weighted or frequency-selected fat suppression T1-weighted images. The lesions were assessed for size, signal intensity, homogeneity, the presence of haemorrhage, degree of contrast enhancement and the existence of intracranial extension.

Table 1. Findings in six patients with rhabdomyosarcoma

Case	Sex	Age (years)	Months from 1st study	Type	Site	SI (vs muscle)			SI (vs fat)		Enhancement		
						T1-WI	PDI	T2-WI	PDI	T2-WI	Y/N	Staining	Homo/ Hetero
1	M	14	3	Alveolar	Tonsil-soft palate	+	+	+	−	+	Y	+	Homo
			3			+	+	+	−	+	N		
			5			+	+	+	−	+	Y	+	Homo
			19			+	+	+	−	+	Y	+	Homo
			21			+	+	+	−	+	Y	+	Hetero
			26			+	+	+	−	+	Y	+	Hetero
			34			+	+	+	−	+	Y	+	Hetero
2	F	71		Alveolar	Pterygopalatine fossa	=	=	+	−	+	Y		Hetero
3	M	24		Alveolar	Cheek	=	+	+	−	+	Y	+	Homo
			2		(resected)						Y		
			5		(resected)						Y		
			11		(resected)						Y		
4	M	11		Embryonal	Massete	=	+	+	−	+	N		
5	M	19		Embryonal	Ethmoid sinuses	=	+	+	−	+	Y	+	Hetero
			1			=	+	+	−	+	Y	+	Hetero
			3			=	+	+	−	+	Y	+	Hetero
			4			=	+	+	−	+	Y	+	Hetero
			5		(Vanished on MRI)						Y		
6	F	6		Embryonal	Petrous vone, clivus	=	+	+	−	+	N		
			1			=	+	+	−	+	Y	+	Hetero
			3			=	+	+	−	+	Y	+	Homo
			4			=	+	+	−	+	Y	+	Homo
			6			=	+	+	−	+	Y	+	Homo

Case	Sex	Age (years)	Months from 1st study	Dural enhancement	Homo/ hetero on T2WI	Intratumoral haemorrhage	Size			Therapy	Status
							Width	Height	Length		
1	M	14		−	Homo	−	55	45	70	Chemo + RT + Surg.	
			3	−	Homo	−	25	35	25		
			5	−	Homo	−	25	10	25		
			19	−	Homo	−	30	20	20		
			21	−	Hetero	−	45	30	50		
			26	+	Hetero	−	95	90	150		Local recurrence and lung metastases
			34	+	Hetero	−	95	90	150		
2	F	71		+	Hetero	−	30	50	25	Chemo	Died from leukaemoid reaction
3	M	24		−	Homo	+	40	25	60	Chemo + surgery	
			2								
			5								
			11								CR
4	M	11		−	Hetero	−	40	70	60	Surgery + Chemo	CR
5	M	19		+	Hetero	−	75	75	70	Chemo + RT	
			1	+	Hetero	−	60	40	15		
			3	−	Hetero	−	25	15	5		
			4	−	Hetero	−	15	15	5		
			5				0	0	0		CR
6	F	6		+	Homo	−	40	40	40	Chemo + RT	
			1	+	Homo	−	50	40	40		
			3	−	Homo	−	50	40	40		
			4	−	Homo	−	50	40	40		
			6	−	Homo	−	50	40	40		

SI, signal intensity; T1WI, PDI, TsWI: T1-, proton density and T2-weighted images; Y, yes; N, no; Homo, homogeneous; Hetero, heterogeneous; Chemo, chemotherapy; RT, radiotherapy; CR, complete remission

Results

The rhabdomyosarcomas were isointense (five cases) or very minimally hyperintense (in 1) in relation to muscle on T1-weighted images. One case demonstrated partial hyperintensity in the tumour, which represented haemorrhage due to its heterogeneous intensity and fluid-fluid level. The non-haemorrhagic part of the tumour was isointense in relation to the muscle. Proton density images revealed five tumours with increased signal intensity compared to that of muscle and one with isointensity. In three of six cases, the signal intensity was significantly heterogeneous on T2-weighted images before treatment. T2-weighted images revealed that all lesions were hyperintense to both muscle and fat. In all of five cases in which contrast medium was used (four of them were examined before therapy), contrast-enhanced images demonstrated enhancement of the tumour. Three of four tumours revealed homogeneous enhancement and the other showed a heterogeneous appearance. In one case, homogeneity was changed to heterogeneity because the recurrent tumour grew extremely rapidly and invaded intracranially after chemotherapy and operation (case 1).

The tumour showed dural enhancement along the tumour, which suggested intracranial extension, in three cases (through the ethmoid sinus in one and through the infratemporal fossa in two before therapy (cases 2, 5, 6).

No differences in signal intensity characteristics or invasiveness were noted when the embryonal and alveolar subtypes of head and neck rhabdomyosarcomas were compared.

Discussion

Rhabdomyosarcoma is not only the most common soft tissue sarcoma in children under 15 years of age but also in adolescents and young adults. However, it is rare in persons over 45 years of age. Rhabdomyosarcoma is the most common soft tissue sarcoma in children, occurring most frequently in children under 12 twelve years of age; 40% of rhabdomyosarcomas occur in the head and neck. The orbits, nasopharynx and middle ear are the most commonly affected sites. Histologically, the most common forms found in the head and neck are the embryonal and botryoid type, which rarely arise in skeletal muscle.

Embryonal rhabdomyosarcoma, the first and most common of the four categories, accounts for 70–80% of all rhabdomyosarcomas. It affects mainly children between birth and 15 years of age and occurs predominantly in the head and neck, the genitourinary tract, and the retroperitoneum. It may also be encountered in the limbs. It bears a close resemblance to various stages in the development of normal muscle tissue and ranges in its morphological spectrum from poorly differentiated tumours with hardly any rhabdomyoblasts to extremely well-differentiated neoplasms, consisting almost entirely of rhabdomyoblasts with cross-striations.

Alveolar rhabdomyosarcoma is less frequent. It accounts for 10–20% of all rhabdomyosarcomas, is found predominantly in subjects between 10 and 25 years of age, and has an anatomical distribution similar to that of embryonal rhabdomyosarcoma, except for a much greater incidence in the upper and lower extremities.

The prognosis of rhabdomyosarcoma has improved dramatically over the past few decades. As a rule, treatment is carried out after biopsy and resection and after careful assessment of the tumour stage or tumour group with plain films, CT and MRI. Recommendations for therapy chiefly depend on the stage or clinical group of the disease and the site of the tumour following resection or biopsy.

It is known that rhabdomyosarcomas in parameningeal regions may invade the meninges in 35–55% of patients and may cause death in 90% with meningeal invasion. Coronal MRI is the best method for demonstrating intracranial extension. Furthermore, a frequency-selected fat-saturated T1-weighted image with enhancement is superior to any other image in delineating the tumour extension because it shows the clear margin of the tumour and attains better contrast between fat and enhanced mass lesions. We detected intracranial spread of the tumours in three of six patients. The information provided by images is valuable in deciding on therapeutic methods and estimating the prognosis of the patient. It is necessary to inform radiation therapists about the boundary of the tumour. As in a previous report [1], no differences in signal intensity were noted between embryonal or alveolar rhabdomyosarcomas in this study. The findings that tumours are isointense or nearly isointense to muscle on T1-weighted images, variable in signal intensity on proton density images, and high in intensity on T2-weighted images may be of use in the differential diagnosis of head and neck malignancies. It has been reported that high-grade malignancies of the paranasal sinuses and salivary glands may have lower signal intensity on T2-weighted images. Relatively common tumours of the head and neck lymphoma and nasopharyngeal carcinoma usually have the same signal intensity characteristics as rhabdomyosarcomas. MRI provides information as to the extent of the rhabdomyosarcoma.

Reference

1. Yousem DM, Lexa FJ, Bilaniuk LT, Zimmerman RI (1990) Rhabdomyosarcomas in the head and neck: MR imaging evaluation. Radiology 177:683–686

Dynamic MRI of head and neck carcinomas

S. Abe, K. Minowa, T. Sawamura, C. Takahashi, S. Terae, Y. Kikuchi, K. Miyasaka

Department of Radiology, Hokkaido University School of Medicine, N 15, W 7, Kita-ku, Sapporo 060, Japan

Abstract. To evaluate the utility of dynamic MRI, we reviewed 28 patients with head and neck carcinomas. Dynamic images demarcated the extension of tongue carcinomas more clearly than spin-echo images. Time-intensity curves were useful to distinguish tumours from other tissues and to predict the vascularity and recurrence of the tumours.

Key words: Carcinoma, head and neck - Magnetic resonance imaging - Dynamic study

Dynamic MRI of head and neck carcinomas following injection of gadolinium (Gd)-DTPA was evaluated for its clinical value.

Materials and methods

We examined 28 patients with carcinoma proven by biopsy or surgery in the head and neck region; half had tongue carcinoma. Just after injection of Gd-DTPA (0.1 mmol/kg), serial MR images were obtained every 7–30 s up to 4–6 min. Dynamic MRI was compared with conventional spin-echo (SE) images. Dynamic time-intensity curves of the tumours and adjacent tissues were examined.

Results

Table 1 shows the results of comparing dynamic images and conventional SE images. In 14 cases of tongue carcinoma (all squamous cell type), dynamic images were better than T2-weighted SE images in 9, and they were equally good in 5. Dynamic enhanced images also revealed dilated vessels in affected sides of tongue cancers (Fig. 1). In 14 cases of other head and neck carcinomas, dynamic images were superior to T2-weighted SE images in only 3. They were equally good in 2 cases. In 9 cases, T2-weighted SE images were better than dynamic images. All dynamic images were better than plain and contrast-enhanced T1-weighted SE images. In 9 operated cases of tongue carcinoma, pathological specimens were compared with MRI; all tumours were within early-enhancement areas on dynamic MRI. Thus, dynamic MRI slightly overestimated tumour extent.

Time-intensity curves of tongue carcinomas are quite similar. They enhanced rapidly and reached maximum intensities within 60–120 s, then maintained their plateaux. Mucous membrane also enhances rapidly, like tumours, but muscle and granuloma enhance gradually and to not show their peaks within 6 min. Necrosis and

Table 1. Comparison of dynamic and conventional T2-weighted spin-echo (SE) images

Tongue carcinomas	14 cases
Dynamic > SE	9
Dynamic = SE	5
Dynamic < SE	None
Other carcinomas	14 cases
Dynamic > SE	3
Dynamic = SE	2
Dynamic < SE	9

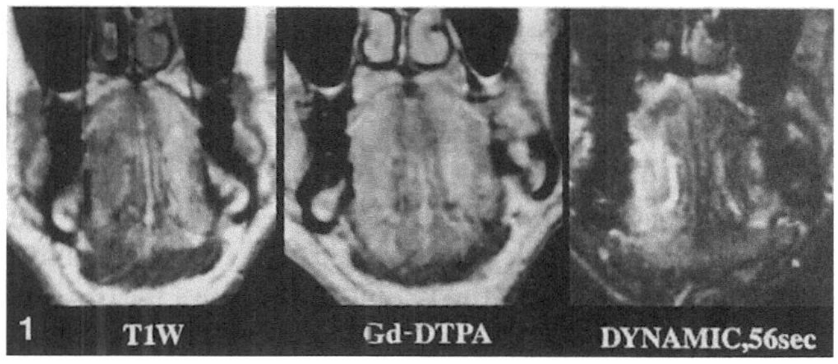

Fig. 1. T2NO tongue cancer after 40 Gy radiation. T1-weighted image shows the tumour as low signal. On conventional contrast-enhanced T1-weighted images, it is difficult to localise the tumour. Dynamic MRI showed the extent of the tumour clearly. There is a dilated vessel at the medial margin of the tumour

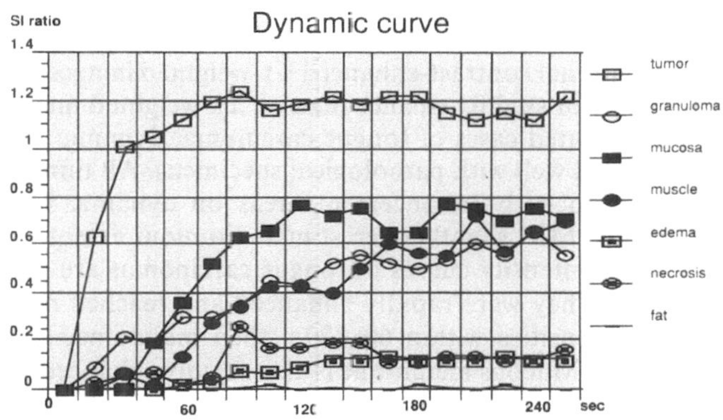

Fig. 2. Comparison of time-intensity curves of a tongue cancer and other tissues. SI (signal intensity) ratio = {SI (post) - SI (pre)}/SI (pre)

Correspondence to: S. Abe

oedema enhance slightly. Fat does not enhance (Fig. 2). Malignant tumours other than squamous cell carcinoma and benign tumours show various patterns in time-intensity curves.

Discussion

MRI is an indispensable examination in the management of extracranial malignant tumours of the head and neck [1]. Although unenhanced images allow us to delineate malignant tumours in most cases, the use of Gd-DTPA improves the diagnostic information significantly. We often overestimated tumour size on T2-weighted images as compared with the surgical findings, probably due to surrounding oedema and inflammation [2, 3]. Vogl et al. [2] reported that administration of Gd-DTPA gives significant additional information and aids in the determination of tumour extent in the head and neck, especially in patients with tongue base carcinomas. In our experience, however, tongue carcinomas show low to isointense signal on T1-weighted images and iso- to high-signal intensity on T2-weighted images [4]. Conventional contrast-enhanced T1-weighted images show only slight enhancement; therefore, the tumours become isointense with the residual tongue tissue.

Administration of Gd-DTPA sometimes obscures the extension of tongue tumours [4, 5] (Fig. 1). T2-weighted images usually depict the extent of tumours more clearly than plain and contrast-enhanced T1-enhanced images, they take much more time to examine and are vulnerable to motion artefact. Zoarski et al. [6] reported their experience with fast spin-echo (FSE) MRI; FSE pulse sequences are rapid alternative to conventional T2-weighted SE sequences when imaging pathological conditions of the head and neck [6]. In cases in which we could not obtain good T2-weighted images, dynamic enhanced images played a very important role in depicting tumour extent. They are less influenced by motion artefact. Areas of early enhancement are smaller than on plain and conventional contrast-enhanced T1-weighted images, and the same or slightly smaller than on T2-weighted images. In 9 operated cases of tongue carcinoma, dynamic MRI correlated well with pathological specimens. All tumours are within early-enhancement areas on dynamic MRI. Dynamic MRI slightly overestimated tumour extent.

Time-intensity curves of tongue carcinomas are quite similar. They were rapidly enhanced and reached maximum intensities within 60–120 s, then maintained their plateaux. Mucous membrane is also rapidly enhanced like tumours, so tumours adjacent to mucosa are difficult to distinguish on dynamic images. This seems to be a reason why T2-weighted SE images are better than dynamic images in patients with malignant tumours other than tongue cancers.

Malignant tumours other than squamous cell carcinoma and benign tumours show various patterns in time-intensity curves. Therefore, it seems difficult to differentiate between benign and malignant tumours. Takashima et al. [7] classified time versus signal intensity curves into five types depending on peak time. They concluded that although use of dynamic MRI contributes little in predicting malignancy in head and lesions, it can limit the differential diagnosis and has potential in predicting vascularity and recurrence. They reported that the same dynamic pattern in a tumour was present in recurrences and metastasis. In our series, residual or recurrent tumours (four tongue cancers after radiotherapy and one malignant transformation of inverted papilloma) all had signal peaks within 120 s. Surgical scar did not show signal peaks for at least 180 s. Therefore, recurrent or residual tumours seem to have the same dynamic curve as original tumours, but we could not compare the dynamic curve with the initial one, because we did not perform a dynamic study before treatment in these cases. At present we cannot obviate the need for biopsy of suspect tissue with dynamic MRI. If tumours have an early and high peak, we can predict hypervascularity.

References

1. Hudgins PA, Gussack GS (1992) MR imaging in the management of extracranial malignant tumors of the head and neck. AJR 159:161–169
2. Vogl T, Bruning R, Grevers G, Mees K, Bauer M, Lissner J (1988) MR imaging of the oropharynx and tongue: comparison of plain and Gd-DTPA studies. J Comput Assist Tomogr 12:427–433
3. Takashima S, Ikezoe J, Harada K, Akai Y, Hamada S, Arisawa J, Morimoto S, Masaki N, Kozuka T, Maeda H (1989) Tongue cancer: correlation of MR imaging and sonography with pathology. AJNR 10:419–424
4. Minowa K, Abe S, Ohmori K, Hosokawa Y, Yamasaki M, Hirano M (1992) MR imaging diagnosis of tongue tumors – including dynamic enhanced MR imaging (in Japanese) Jpn J Oral Maxillofac Surg 38:974–981
5. Minowa K, Abe S, Sawamura T, Ohmori K, Hosokawa Y, Yamasaki M, Chu B, Terae S, Takahashi C, Miyasaka K (1994) A study of magnetic resonance imagings of tongue tumors, focusing on signal intensity changes after Gd-DTPA injection (in Japanese) Jpn J Cancer Clin 40:161–167
6. Zoarski GH, Mackey JK, Anzai Y, Hanafee WN, Melki PS, Mulkern RV, Jolesz FA, Lufkin RB (1993) Head and neck: initial clinical experience with fast spin-echo MR imaging. Radiology 188:323–327
7. Takashima S, Noguchi Y, Okumura T, Aruga H, Kobayashi T (1994) Dynamic MR imaging in the head and neck. Radiology 189:813–821

Tumefactive fibroinflammatory disease of the head and neck

B. Azar-Kia, O. Al-Mefty, S. W. Horowitz, K. Goldberg, M. Fine, R. Neimon

2160 S. First Ave, Maywood, IL 60153, USA

Abstract. Tumefactive fibroinflammatory lesions of the head and neck are benign invasive masses simulating malignancy. We present three cases of fibroinflammatory lesions in the parapharyngeal space, posterior aspect of the neck and at the base of the skull.

Key words: Fibromatosis - Desmoid - Neck - Computed tomography - Magnetic resonance imaging

Tumefactive fibroinflammatory lesions, desmoid, fibromatosis and fibrosclerosing disorders are terms applied to histologically benign lesions consisting of infiltrative fibrous tissue. In the same histologic group are retroperitoneal fibrosis, sclerosing cholangitis, mediastinal fibrosis, Riedel's thyroiditis and pseudotumor of the orbit. These lesions are locally aggressive with extension into adjacent soft tissue. They may show erosion of the bone and invasion of adjacent vessels. They are treated by high doses of steroids, surgical excision and radiation therapy. The local recurrence rate after any type of treatment is high.

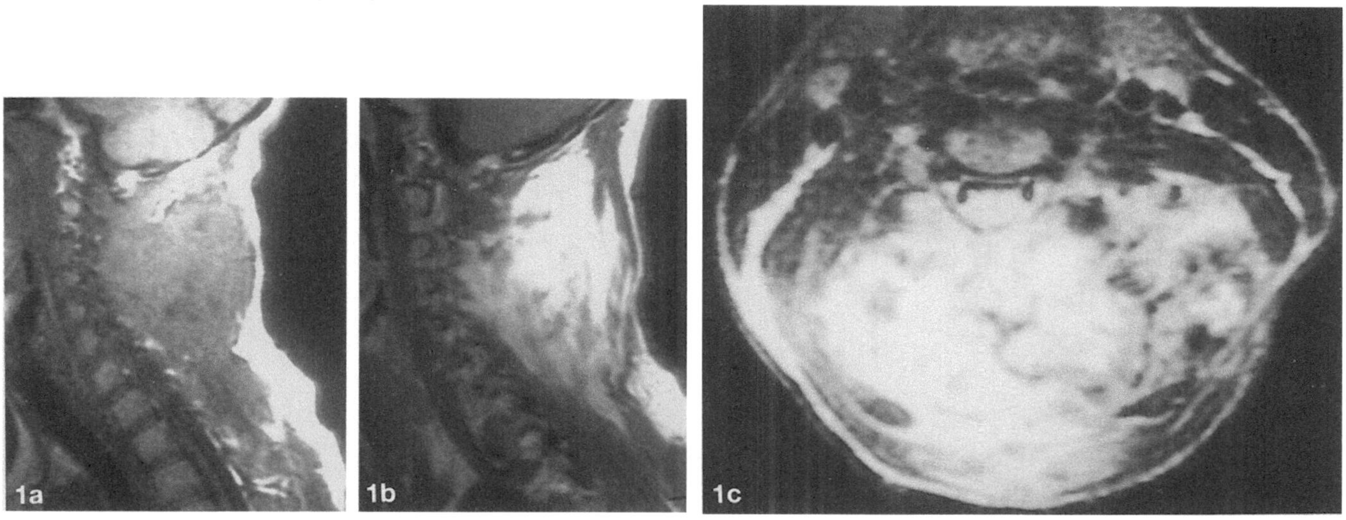

Fig. 1. Case 1. Sagittal T1-weighted images (**a**) show an intermediate and low intensity mass at the posterior aspect of the neck with erosion of spinous processes. Contrast-enhanced T1-weighted images revealed marked enhancement (**b**). Axial T2-weighted images show high intensity (**c**)

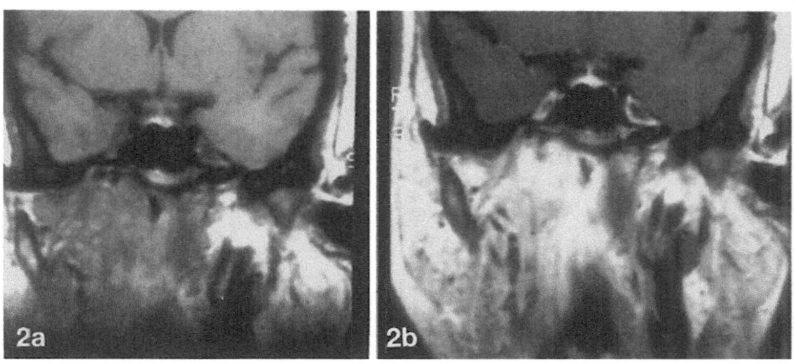

Fig. 2. Case 2. Coronal T1- (**a**) and T2-weighted images demonstrate a large intermediate intensity mass in the right parapharyngeal space. Marked contrast-enhancement was seen (**b**)

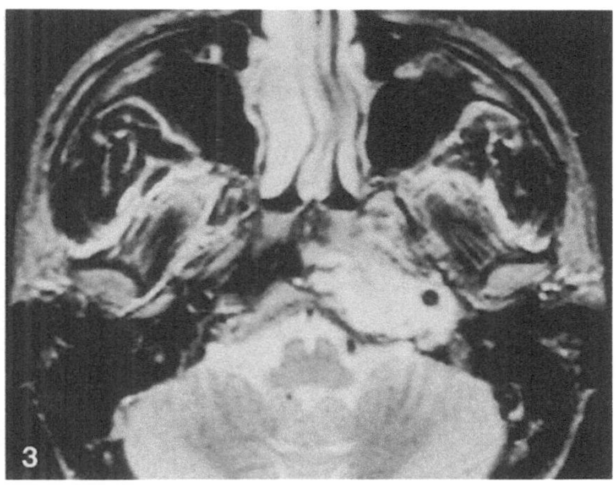

Fig. 3. Case 3. Axial T2-weighted image revealed high intensity mass in the base of the skull, involving the petrous bone

Correspondence to: B. Azar-Kia

Case reports

Case 1

A 20-year-old man presented with a progressively enlarging posterior neck mass. Plain films showed a large soft tissue mass in the posterior aspect of the neck with erosion of spinous processes in the midcervical spine. MRI revealed a large ill-defined mass with low to intermediate intensity on T1-weighted images (Fig. 1a) and high intensity on T2-weighted images (Fig. 1b). There was marked contrast-enhancement (Fig. 1c). This tumor was surgically removed and proved to be desmoid [1].

Case 2

A 52-year-old woman gave a history of 5 months of right tonsillar discomfort, of trismus and slight right hearing loss. CT demonstrated an ill-defined soft tissue lesion in the right parapharyngeal space, involving the right tonsil. There was moderate contrast-enhancement. MRI revealed an intermediate intensity lesion in the right parapharyngeal space on T1- and T2-weighted images (Fig. 2a, b). Marked contrast-enhancement was noted (Fig. 2c). This patient underwent radiation and steroid therapy, and repeat CT and MRI showed marked improvement.

Case 3

A 28-year-old man's chief complaint was spasm, pain and numbness on the left side of the face and jaw for about 1 year. CT showed a soft tissue mass in the left parapharyngeal space with erosion of the adjacent skull base. MRI revealed an intermediate intensity extending into the base of the skull (Fig. 3). There was slight contrast enhancement.

Discussion

We present CT and MRI findings in three cases of fibromatosis of the head and neck. These locally invasive lesions should be differentiated from malignant tumors. The CT and MRI findings in case 2 are similar to an infiltrative squamous cell carcinoma or adenocarcinoma [2–4]. CT-guided biopsy showed no evidence of malignancy. Angiography in cases 2 and 3 showed no abnormal vessels or tumor stain. Encasement of the left internal carotid was noted in case 3. All showed contrast enhancement on both cT and MRI. The findings on MRI depend mainly on the histologic nature of the lesion. Predominance of inflammatory changes is demonstrated by higher intensity on T2-weighting (case 1). Extensive fibrotic changes are manifest as intermediate or low intensity on T2-weighted images (case 2).

References

1. Masson JK, Soule EH (1966) Desmoid tumor of the head and neck. Am J Surg 112:615
2. Olsen KD, Desanto LW, Wold LE, Weiland LH (1986) Tumefactive fibroinflammatory lesions of the head and neck. Laryngoscope 96:940
3. Esdaile J, Murray D, Hawkins D, et al (1980) Idiopathic fibrosis of the lateral compartment of the neck. Arch Intern Med 140:1386
4. Rice DH, Batsakis JG, Coulthard SW (1975) Sclerosing cervicitis. Homologue of sclerosing retroperitonitis and mediastinitis. Arch Surg 110:120

New Horizons Special Lecture III

What will be the future of interventional neuroradiology?

L. Picard

University Hospital, Nancy, France

If we try to give some ideas about the future of interventional neuroradiology (INR), we must first define interventional neuroradiology. For many people, INR is mainly a technique but it could also be a way of life, a specific behaviour of a neuroradiologist, a possibility of grasping the opportunity to create a subspeciality etc; it seems like a kaleidoscope, in which everybody can see what he wishes to see.

Over the past three decades, many advances have occurred in the treatment of several neurological and neurosurgical diseases due to the very rapid development of interventional neuroradiological techniques. INR has entered multidisciplinary therapeutic discussion and daily practice. A series of improvements in angiographic equipment, microcatheters, embolic agents and knowledge of microvascular anatomy have all played an important role in this advance.

Expansion of INR varies across the world. In Europe and North America, INR is performed mainly by neuroradiologists but in most of the countries of Asia, the procedures are done by neurosurgeons. In other continents like Africa, INR has not developed because of financial difficulties. We have no precise data on the number of neurointerventional teams in the world. According to the manufacturers, about 100 centres were using Guglielmi detachable coils in 1994. In fact, there are probably about 200 centres working to a greater or lesser extent in INR. If we include all interventional techniques on the spinal canal, the number of centres becomes greater. One aspect of this extreme diversity is the competence of interventional neuroradiologists appears very variable and often insufficient.

We are facing a crisis of development due to an overly rapid evolution of techniques. Consequently, there is no real validation, since a new technique appears before we are able to perform long-term follow-up. The interventional neuroradiologist is daily confronted with many problems: he must improve his clinical and anatomical knowledge, he must work more and more in emergencies, he must find money to buy more and more complex machines and the number of indications is increasing.

This dramatic evolution is due to improvement in techniques mainly digital subtraction angiography (DSA) and MRI, but also to progress in equipment: microcatheters, embolic agents, and so on. For many reasons, these things must immediately be highly efficient: they must be reliable, and are obviously more and more expensive.

Correspondence to: L. Picard

To embolise safely, we need modern DSA equipment with a biplane C-arm, high resolution fluoroscopy, real-time subtraction and road-mapping facilities. Without these, the risks obviously become higher. We must be able to see on fluoroscopy very small vessels inside the brain and spine. With the most sophisticated new equipment we can catheterise and embolise vessels about 300–400 μm across.

Indications for stereoangiography will certainly become increasingly frequent in the future; the best way to treat intracranial aneurysms would be to see the neck from the inside. New experimental machines like the "morphometer" will give us such information and this technique must be adapted to biplane C-arms. Interventional MRI is appearing on the market. It cannot yet be used for endovascular procedures, but it can be used for all kinds of stereotactic procedures and also for open cranial surgery: to use MRI for the endovascular approach, we need an improvement in spatial resolution and real-time MR fluoroscopy.

With regard to embolic agents, we know that almost one century ago, Dawborn was the first to perform an embolisation by injection of paraffin for a facial tumour supplied by external carotid branches. Many embolic agents have since been used: pieces of muscle, Fogarty catheters, detachable balloons, miscospheres, and now "glue", detachable coils, etc.

The scope of interventional neuroradiology

With all the technical progress, the field of INR is very large. It can be divided into three main chapters: vascular disease; diseases of the spinal canal, oncology.

Vascular diseases

Endovascular INR has two main techniques: occlusion (embolisation) and reopening (angioplasty and fibrinolysis).

Embolisations formed the beginning of INR. During the 1970s embolisation was used to treat inoperable cases; it was the "last chance" treatment for some arteriovenous malformations (AVMs) which were large or in eloquent areas.

From an ethical point of view, it is interesting to know that our goals have changed. Thirty years ago, a patient presenting with an AVM of the brain was considered "cured" when the AVM was totally removed even if the patient was hemiplegic. Now, more and more teams give priority to function, even if the radiographic result is not perfect.

Today the challenge is more difficult: even when using a new technique, we must immediately treat with the same efficiency and reliability as neurosurgery; obviously, the risks of complications must not be higher. Consequently, the value of the endovascular approach is not only to treat lesions which are difficult or impossible to reach by neurosurgery, such as a caroticocavernous fistula, but to offer less discomfort and, if possible, less functional sequelae. INR does not consist in treating a picture or a disease but a patient with specific symptoms and specific risks that we know about according to the natural history of his condition.

What is the goal of the endovascular approach? Is it only an associated treatment, a palliative treatment or is it a true therapeutic alternative? We need more maturity for out indications: INR cannot remain a repeated technical exploit. To illustrate our opinion, we can discuss some examples.

What are the persisting problems in treating intracranial aneurysms? Over the last few decades, we have successively used occlusion of the parent artery, then endosaccular occlusion with balloons, and more recently endosaccular occlusion with detachable microcoils. When we are faced with a giant aneurysm of the carotid siphon, we can occlude the siphon or introduce multiple microcoils into the aneurysm sac; some neuroradiologists will try first to preserve the patency of the carotid siphon because they think it is more "elegant"! However, experience proves that the chance of obtaining a regression of ocular motor palsies and visual acuity deficit is higher after total occlusion of the carotid siphon. In such cases, the decision must be based on clinical, not technical concepts.

In the same field, it is interesting to recall that the international study initiated for Guglielmi detachable coils concerned "nonsurgical" aneurysms. Is this only for ethical reasons? Some years after the beginning of this international trial, it appears obvious that most "surgical" aneurysms are excellent indications for endovascular coiling. The risk of secondary recurrence is certainly less after packing of a small aneurysm than after packing of a medium-sized or a large one.

Working with neurosurgeons, we must determine the best time to treat a recently ruptured aneurysm. It seems that an emergency endovascular treatment offers several advantages and avoids the feared early rebleeding. This point represents an important argument in consideration of the endovascular approach; indeed, everybody knows that surgery is very dangerous in the acute phase when there is already vasospasm. Although spasm can complicate the endovascular approach, it is not an absolute contraindication; we can use chemical angioplasty with papaverine or mechanical angioplasty with specific balloons.

To answer all these questions, we need randomised studies in comparison with surgery. But one of the most important questions is not solved: what exactly is long-term follow-up? Long-term follow-up is not 6 months or 1 year, but 5 or 10 years. Today, we can only hope that this real long-term follow-up will be favourable!

A new problem arises with the new devices now on the market: who is able to use them safely for the patient? When there is no complication, it seems very easy to treat an intracranial aneurysm with microcoils. I confess I am scared to see young neuroradiologists beginning to use microcoils even though they are completely unable to use a detachable balloon: they are slaves to one technique and consequently unable to choose the best one for the patient. We cannot leave the manufacturers to choose the operators; we must organise appropriate training.

The treatment of intracranial aneurysms epitomises most of the problems of INR. We know that the indications depend on size (small, so-called "surgical" aneurysms are excellent indications) and topography (the best indications are the carotid siphon, vertebrobasilar system, anterior and posterior communicating arteries; aneurysms of the middle cerebral are more difficult). We know that we must treat ruptured aneurysms as emergencies and consequently have to create interventional teams able to attend to these needs. However, many questions must be studied and among them: is reopening or regrowth predictable? Are there contraindications to the use of detachable coils?

For brain AVMs, the discussion is almost the same. Some problems are solved by the endovascular approach: small AVMs and direct arteriovenous fistulae. For direct arteriovenous fistulae, the difficulty is to choose the best site to inject glue and to avoid reflux in normal branches proximal to the shunt. We know that intranidal glue embolisation is certainly the best way to obtain a permanent occlusion of the nidus: we must inject the glue inside the nidus and can then hope for a complete radiological cure. This technique is useful mainly for eloquent areas: if we inject inside the nidus, we can obtain an occlusion without deficit, if we are able to avoid embolisation of normal branches around the nidus. One of the persisting debates concerns the criteria of complete cure. What is a good criterion? Is it disappearance of the arteriovenous shunt or of all abnormal vessels? Probably the disappearance of any arteriovenous shunt is sufficient, but this hypothesis must be proved. To obtain a complete anatomical cure, we know that, in many cases, we can combine embolisation, radiotherapy and surgery, but what about partial embolisation? In my own experience, after 15 years, when I have embolised more than two thirds of the initial nidus, the risk of bleeding seems reduced, but if we have embolised less than two thirds, the risk of bleeding does not really seem diminished.

The techniques suggested for reopening vessels can be divided into two main areas: thrombolysis and angioplasty.

Fibrinolytic agents can be injected through the veins or directly inside the clot via an arterial approach. When faced with an embolic complication during an interventional procedure, in most cases we can reopen the vessel without side effects if hyperselective fibrinolysis is performed urgently. But, when we discuss the treatment of strokes, we need large randomised studies to demonstrate the real efficiency of these techniques. Is the arterial approach better than the intravenous? What is the reasonable delay before beginning treatment? If we are able to probe real efficiency of fibrinolysis in the treatment of ischaemic strokes, it will be necessary to find the money and the teams to apply these techniques in the emergency setting for a lot of patients. The field of INR will be yet larger if we confirm the efficiency of hyperselective fibrinolysis in the opthalmic artery in acute amaurosis of the venous sinuses in thrombophlebitis.

What will be the future of intracerebral angioplasty for atheromatous disease? This is a new problem to evaluate. We know that sometimes it can be very efficient but the equipment must be improved. These procedures are technically difficult and dangerous, needing a wide experience of catheterisation. We have to prove the efficiency of hyperselective angioplasty in comparison with anticoagulation. For that, we need randomised studies with long-term follow-up.

Spinal disease

The diseases of the spinal canal are of interest not only to neuroradiologists, but also to rheumatologists, neurosurgeons and orthopaedic surgeons. These specialists mainly use their own techniques, explaining the difficulty of organising a good evaluation. It is more difficult and complex because the goal of this treatment is often to reduce pain, but everybody knows that pain includes multiple psychological parameters very difficult to evaluate. To take the everyday example of disc herniation, the choice between surgery, nucleolysis and nucleotomy remains open. To take the best decision, we need good clinical training and a multidisciplinary approach.

Oncology

This will perhaps be an important part of INR in the future, but is now mainly a research field. It seems that survival time is slightly increased by some hyperselective chemotherapy but many new techniques are tested: some teams try to heat the tumour, others to increase the photosensitivity of cells by chemical agents to use the laser. It is probably in this field that stereotactic interventional MRI will be useful.

How can we develop and improve INR throughout the world?

During the next few years, we have to create a standard of training, organise the practice of INR, formalise accrediation, organise continuing education and to develop research.

The world federation of therapeutic and interventional neuroradiology has proposed a standard of training including 1 year in general radiology, 2 years in neuroradiological sciences, 2 years in diagnostic neuroradiology and finally 2 years in INR. This is a long training period, but includes anatomy, physiology, neuropathology, clinical, radiological, technical and neurosurgical training.

What about stereotaxy? Stereotaxy has been the domain of neurosurgeons, but can and will be used more and more without a frame. For many reasons, stereotaxy must be included in neuroradiological training, not only for intervention but also for diagnosis: if we wish to be able to appreciate the progression of cerebral tumours, we should perform the different neuroradiological examinations in stereotactic conditions. Stereotaxy will certainly be more and more important in some difficult endovascular procedures. It may be impossible to know if the tip of the microcatheter is inside or outside the brain stem: superimposition of stereotactic MRI and hyperselective angiographic data should be very useful. When we discuss the indications for nucleolysis for lumbar disc herniation, it is not simply a technical discussion, it is treatment of pain which needs multiple expertise. This is the reason interventional neuroradiologists must be clinicians, responsible for indications, procedures and follow-up, working in close co-operation with a multidisciplinary team.

Patients undergoing interventional procedures should be followed daily by interventional neuroradiology staff members. A clinician must be able to listen to the patient, to do a clinical examination, to know the diseases of the nervous system and also to be considered as a consultant. For the latter the clinician must be competent from a technical and clinical points of view. This is a heavy load, which is why we can discuss if interventional neuroradiologists should be part-time or full-time.

This concept includes an ethical responsibility. This concerns the indications, informing the patient and family about the goals, the protocol and the risks of complications. The responsibility of the interventional neuroradiologist includes performing the procedure, the subsequent management, and long-term follow-up. This responsibility is a medical rule but also an ethical one. From an ethical point of view, we must be able to know when to abstain, when to proceed would be futile (like occlusion of a vein of Galen aneurysm when the brain is destroyed). We must also be able to avoid choosing a particular technique because it is the only one we know how to use.

We cannot forget the importance of patient management. We need general anaesthesia or neuroleptanalgesia and it is absolutely necessary to work with a team of neuroanaesthetists.

For all these reasons, a department of neuroradiology must be organised appropriately to interventional necessities. We need offices for consultation, angiographic rooms, organised like surgical rooms, recovery rooms, access to beds for hospitalisation and to intensive care units. The department must be close by those of neurosurgery and neurology.

Finally we have to organise research, both technical and clinical. Technical research includes stereoangiography to see inside the vessels; we must develop all the possibilities of superimposition of hyperselective angiography with MRI and CT. For that we must work stereotactically. We need interventional MRI and also frameless stereotaxy. We must improve our equipment and maintain discussions with the manufacturers to obtain smaller microcatheters, new embolic agents, more supple stents; perhaps we will use hyperselective endovascular fibroscopy.

We must develop clinical research to define the indications for treatment after international multidisciplinary randomised studies, including long-term follow-up. We must compare the results of INR with those of neurosurgery and radiotherapy. This clinical concept of INR implies a clinical training to work as a consultant, a specific architecture, access to beds for hospitalisation and intensive care units. Finally, the department of neuroradiology is a part of the neurological hospital.

To overcome the challenge of INR, we must maintain the continuity between diagnostic and interventional neuroradiology and open the door to other specialities.

Intervention: aneurysms

Interventional neurovascular treatment of giant intracranial aneurysms

R. T. Higashida, Van V. Halbach, C. F. Dowd, C. McDougall, D. Larsen, J. M. Higashida, G. B. Hieshima

Department of Radiology and Neurological Surgery, Interventional Neurovascular Radiology Division, University of California, San Francisco Medical Center, San Francisco, CA 94143-0628, USA

Abstract. Interventional neurovascular treatment of giant intracranial aneurysms is now being performed in selected cases utilizing detachable balloons, microcoils, and electrolytic detachable coils. Of the 321 cases treated by interventional techniques by our group, 95 (29.6%) were giant aneurysms, >2.5 cm in diameter. In 74 cases, the aneurysm was on the anterior circulation, and in 21 involved the posterior circulation. The patients presented with mass effect in 81 cases (85.3%), subarachnoid hemorrhage in 11 (11.6%), and thromboemboli in 3 (3.1%). In 64 cases (67.4%), the aneurysm was treated by parent vessel occlusion, and in 31 (32.6%), direct treatment of the aneurysm with preservation of the parent artery was attained. Complications related to treatment included 11 cases (11.6%) of stroke, transient cerebral ischemia in 6 (6.3%), and 9 deaths (9.5%). Treating giant intracranial aneurysm is technically feasible by interventional techniques. Continued advances in endovascular therapy should expand the indications and decrease associated morbidity.

Key words: Giant intracranial aneurysms – Endovascular therapy – Balloon occlusion of aneurysms

Methods

All procedures were performed in the interventional neurovascular radiology suite from a transfemoral arterial approach. In the majority of cases, light neuroleptic anesthesia was given so that patients were awake and neurological testing could be performed throughout the procedure. A complete four-vessel cerebral angiogram was performed to assess the size, anatomical site, the diameter of the aneurysm neck, and collateral circulation. Systemic anticoagulation with heparin, 70 units/kg, was administered to prevent thromboembolic occurrence during the procedure.

For patients with aneurysms without a well-defined neck, test occlusion of the parent artery was performed with a double-lumen latex balloon, inflated to occlude the parent artery. The test occlusion was performed for 30 min while full neurological testing was performed to insure patient tolerance, and arterial back-pressures were measured. For patients who did not tolerate test occlusion, an extracranial-to-intracranial bypass procedure was performed to increase cerebral perfusion to the distal cortical vessels. Following successful test occlusion, permanent occlusion of the parent vessel was performed using the silicone detachable balloon occluder system. Detachable balloons were placed across, or just proximal to, the neck of the aneurysm [1] (Fig. 1).

Patients with a well-defined aneurysm neck were treated by direct placement of either detachable silicone balloons filled with 2 hydroxy-ethyl-methacrylate, platinum microcoils, or electrolytic detachable platinum microcoils, directly into the aneurysm lumen, with preservation of the parent artery [2] (Fig. 2). All patients were then monitored in the neurological observation unit for 24–72 h, and follow-up angiography, MRI, and/or CT were performed at 1–3 months and 6–12 months, to document continued occlusion of the aneurysm.

Results

A total of 321 patients have been treated for an intracranial aneurysm by our group. In 95 (29.6%), the aneurysm was considered to be giant, measuging greater than 25 mm diameter. In 74 (77.9%) of these, the aneurysm was on the anterior cerebral circulation and in 21 (22.1%) cases it was on the posterior cerebral circulation. The presentation of these patients was mass effect in 81 (85.3%) cases, subarachnoid hemorrhage in 11 (11.6%), and symptoms of thromboemboli in 3 (3.1%). Treatment consisted of parent artery vessel occlusion in 64 cases (67.4%) and direct occlusion of the aneurysm in 31 (32.6%).

Complications related to treatment included stroke in 11 (11.6%) patients, transient cerebral ischemia in 6 (6.3%), and 9 (9.5%) deaths. Five deaths were due to subtotal occlusion of the aneurysm with subsequent rebleeding, 2 to large strokes with resultant cerebral edema and herniation; 1 was due to perioperative myocardial infarction, and 1 to rupture of a second untreated aneurysm 2 months after endovascular therapy of the primary aneurysm.

Discussion

Treatment of intracranial aneurysms by endovascular therapy was initially reported in the early 1970s by Serbinenko [3]. Later series were reported utilizing detachable latex and silicone balloons, fibered microcoils, and in the late 1980s electrolytic detachable coils [4–6]. In the mid 1980s, Higashida and Fox reported in separate series, the safety and efficacy of treating giant aneurysms by parent vessel occlusion [7, 8]. The ability to perform test occlusion in the awake patient, followed by parent artery occlusion with detachable balloons for aneurysms involving the petrous, cavernous, and supraclinoid internal carotid artery, or vertebral artery, compared favorably with previous surgical reports.

Direct aneurysm occlusion, surgically or from an endovascular approach, has been more difficult. This is due to the wide neck of the aneurysm making it more difficult technically to completely exclude all the aneurysm, while not encroaching upon the parent vessel. In addition, placement of coils or balloons directly into the lumen of giant aneurysm is not always stable; once detached, the devices may shift, migrate, or compact, thus causing subtotal occlusion. Giant aneurysms also may

Correspondence to: R. T. Higashida

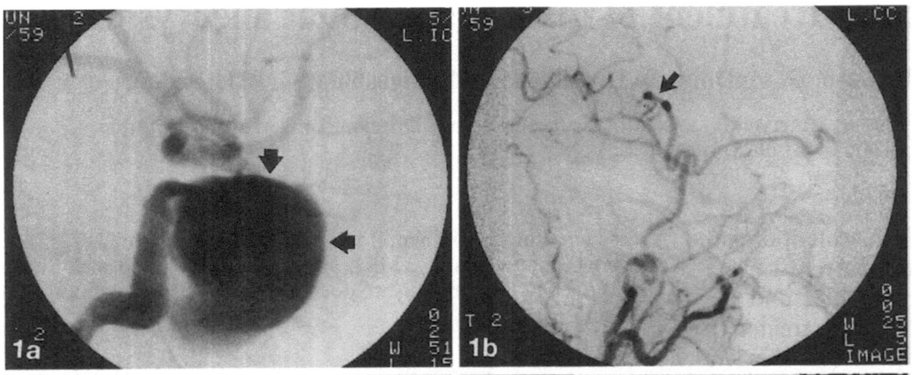

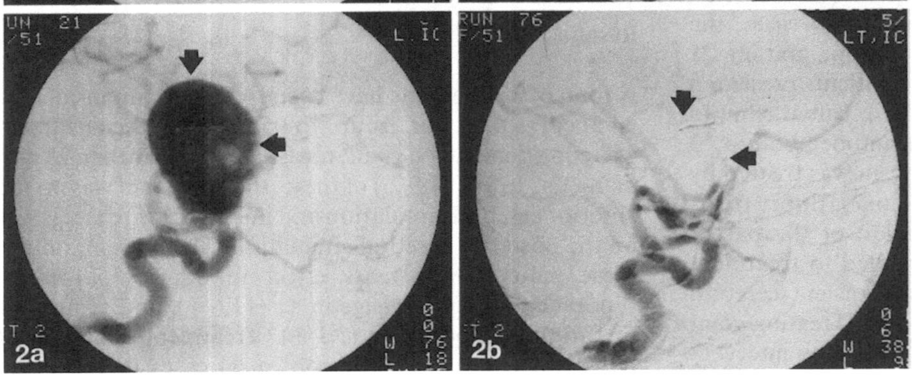

Fig. 1. **a** Giant, fusiform, ectatic aneurysm (*arrows*) arising from the cavernous internal carotid artery. This patient failed initial test occlusion, an extra- to intracranial bypass graft was therefore performed prior to treatment. **b** Following balloon occlusion of the internal carotid artery, the aneurysm is now completely occluded, and the bypass graft fills normal cortical of the middle cerebral artery (*arrow*)

Fig. 2. **a** Giant 3-cm-diameter aneurysms (*arrows*) arising from the supraclinoid internal carotid artery, at the level of the ophthalmic artery. **b** Following direct balloon occlusion *arrows*, there is complete obliteration of the aneurysm with preservation of the normal distal intracranial circulation

have intraluminal thrombus and during deposition of devices, distal embolization may infrequently occur. Other potential complications include rupture of the aneurysm during treatment due to perforation, spasm of vessels due to intimal damage, and, if the aneurysm is not completely excluded from the circulation, then delayed aneurysm rupture or continued aneurysm expansion may occur.

References

1. Higashida RT, Halbach VV, Dormandy B, et al (1990) Endovascular treatment of intracranial aneurysms with a new silicone microballoon device: technical considerations and indications for therapy. Radiology 174:687–691
2. Guglielmi G, Vinuela F, Dion J, et al (1991) Electrothrombosis of saccular aneurysms via endovascular approach. 2. Preliminary clinical experience. J Neurosurg 75:8–14
3. Serbinenko FA (1974) Balloon catheterization and occlusion of major cerebral vessels. J Neurosurg 41:125–145
4. Moret J, Benlin A, Mawad M, et al (1991) Endovascular treatment of berry aneurysms by endosaccular balloon occlusion. Neuroradiology 33:135–136
5. Romodanov AP, Shchegelov VI (1982) Intravascular occlusion of saccular aneurysms of the cerebral arteries by means of a detachable balloon catheter. In: Krayenbuhl H (ed) Advances and technical standards in neurosurgery. Vol 9. Springer, Wien New York, pp 25–49
6. Higashida RT, Halbach VV, Barnwell SL, et al (1990) Treatment of intracranial aneurysms with preservation of the parent vessel: results of percutaneous balloon embolization in 84 patients. AJNR 11:633–640, 1990
7. Fox AJ, Vinuela F, Pelz DM, et al (1987) Use of detachable balloons for proximal artery occlusion in the treatment of unclippable cerebral aneurysms. J Neurosurg 66:40–46
8. Higashida RT, Halbach VV, Dowd CF, et al (1990) Endovascular detachable balloon embolization therapy of cavernous carotid artery aneurysms: results in 87 cases. J Neurosurg 72:857–863

Treatment of intracranial aneurysms with Guglielmi detachable coils

D. Kühne, H. C. Nahser, H. Henkes

Department of Neuroradiology, Alfried Krupp Krankenhaus, Alfried-Krupp-Strasse 21, D-45117 Essen, Germany

Abstract. We treated 160 intracranial aneurysms in 148 patients (109 female, 39 male, mean age 48) by endovascular means using the Guglielmi detachable coils (GDC) system. The aneurysms were in the anterior and posterior circulation with almost equal frequency. In 26 patients a failed neurosurgical attempt or partial clipping had been undertaken. Based on early angiographic findings, coil occlusion resulted in total obliteration of 93 aneurysms. A small remnant of the neck persisted in 58 aneurysms, and only partial obliteration could be obtained in 6 cases. In 3 cases coil migration forced us to occlude the aneurysm-bearing vessel with a detachable balloon. In 11 cases with large or giant aneurysms, reduced mass effect led to an improved neurological status. We encountered the following complications: transient neurological deterioration (21 patients); permanent neurological deficit (5); perforation of the aneurysm during chatheterisation or coil insertion without serious clinical sequelae (8); secondary occlusion of the parent vessel (10); fatal thrombosis of the basilar artery subsequent to the coil occlusion of a basilar tip aneurysm (1); recurrent subarachnoid haemorrhage from a partially embolised giant aneurysm (1). In small aneurysms (13 patients) angiography 1 year after the initial treatment confirmed permanent occlusion of the aneurysm in 11 cases; a small recurrent neck was detected in 2. In large and giant aneurysms (29 patients), 12 were obliterated, 2 showed a slight filling. Fifteen partially thrombosed aneurysms required retreatment. Endovascular treatment of small and middle-sized aneuryms is most promising. In partially thrombosed large and giant aneurysms in haemodynamically critical locations, coil occlusion bears a significant risk of recurrence.

Key words: Aneurysm – Intracranial artery – Coil occlusion – Endovascular therapy – Interventional neuroradiology

Endovascular treatment of inoperable or technically difficult intracranial aneurysms by platinum microcoils was introduced by Hilal et al. in 1988 [1]. The advent of electrolytically detachable coils [2–4] improved both the efficacy and the safety of this technique. The treatment results presented here are intended to contribute to the evaluation of this endovascular method. This paper will focus on the following aspects: can this technique be used with an acceptable risk? and are long-term results satisfactory?

Correspondence to: D. Kühne

Table 1. Locations of 160 intracranial aneurysms treated with coil, Guglielmi detachable coils

Cavernous internal carotid artery (ICA)	16	Middle cerebral artery	11
Supraclinoid ICA	14	Posterior cerebral artery	7
Ophthalmic artery	15	Basilar tip	47
Posterior communicating artery	9	Midbasilar artery	2
ICA bifurcation	2	Basilar artery origin	9
Anterior cerebral artery	3	Vertebral artery	3
Anterior communicating artery	14	Posterior interior cerebral artery	5
		Superior cerebellar artery	3
Additional aneurysms	32 (11 neurosurgical)		
Additional arteriovenous malformations	4		

Patients and methods

Between November 1992 and August 1994, we treated 160 aneurysms in 148 patients (109 female, 39 male, mean age 48 years). Ninety-two patients presented with a subarachnoid and 8 with intracerebral haemorrhage. Thirty-five patients had symptoms due to aneurysms-related mass effect. In 5 patients, large, partially thrombosed aneurysms had caused transient ischaemic deficits and in 17 the aneurysm had been found incidentally. The angiographically detected aneurysms were on the posterior and the anterior circulation with almost equal frequency (Table 1). Additional aneurysms were found in 32 patients. In 4 cases, the aneurysm was associated with a cerebral arteriovenous malformation.

According to the GDC study protocol, indications for, and timing of, endovascular treatment were decided upon with the referring neurosurgeon. Failed neurosurgical attempts and incomplete clipping prior to the endovascular treatment had been performed in 26 cases.

The treatment was performed under general anaesthetic with standard heparinisation. Calcium antagonists were given intravenously, if required (e.g., in cases of angiographic evidence of vasospasm). All procedures were performed using a biplane, high-resolution digital subtraction unit. If technically feasible, small and middle-sized aneurysms were catheterised with a microcatheter, introduced via a soft 6F guiding catheter. Once the aneurysm sac was catheterised, it was packed as far and densely as possible. Follow-up angiograms were obtained 1 week and 1 year after treatment.

Results

The immediate postprocedural angiography and follow-up examination 1 week later showed complete occlusion of the aneurysm sac in 13 of 18 aneurysms (58%). A small remnant of the aneurysm neck remained in 58 (36%). Only a partial occlusion was the result in 6 aneurysms (3.7%). Balloon occlusion of the parent vessel was necessary in 3 cases.

The treatment of large and giant aneurysms resulted in improvement of the neurological deficit in 11 cases. One patient with a giant aneurysm of the basilar tip, treated several times with balloons and coils, experienced a nondisabling recurrent subarachnoid haemorrhage. Another with a basilar tip aneurysm died due to retrograde thrombosis of the basilar artery. Three patients in poor condition (Hunt and Hess stage IV or V), who underwent endovascular coil occlusion of their middle cerebral artery aneurysms, died from the sequelae of the heaemorrhage. A total of 21 patients (14%) experienced transient neurological deficits during or immediately after the aneurysm treatment. These may be ascribed to emboli dislodged from the coil-containing aneurysm sac. Catheterisation of the aneurysm or insertion of a coil caused rupture of the aneurysm sac in 8 cases. The bleeding could be stopped in all patients and caused mild and transient clinical deterioration in only a few. During the first week after endovasular treatment, secondary occlusion of the aneurysm-bearing vessel was observed in 10 patients. The position of the coil appeared unchanged. Thus, excessive thrombosis might have been the cause of secondary parent vessel occlusion.

Angiograms 1 year after the initial endovascular treatment have been performed, to date, in 42 patients. In 11 of 13 with smaller aneurysms, the occlusion of the aneurysm sac was permanent. A recurrence or remnant of a small aneurysm neck was oberseved in 2 patients. Twelve of 29 large or giant aneurysms remained entirely occluded 1 year after the treatment. Insignificant filling deemed not to necessitate treatment was observed in 2 patients. Pre-embolisation MRI revealed a partially thrombosed large or giant aneurysm sac in 15 patients. In these cases, recurrence of perfused aneurysm lumen required treatment.

Discussion

Using the GDC system, endovascular occlusion of small and middle-sized aneurysms, even in surgically difficult locations, yields favourable short- and long-term results. Wide-necked and partially thrombosed large and giant aneurysms in haemodynamically critical locations have a strong tendency to recur. Definitive obliteration of an aneurysm requires dense packing of the coils.

Planitum coils are not very thrombogenic and the thrombotic effect of electrolysis is partially suspended by the required heparinisation.

One might speculate whether this drawback can be compensated by adding fibres to the detachable coils or coating [5] their surface, in order to increase their thrombogenicity.

References

1. Hilal SK, Khandji AG, Chi TL, Stein BM, Bello JA, Silver AJ, Schumacher KJ (1988) Synthetic fiber-coated platinum coils successfully used for endovascular treatment of arteriovenous malformations, aneurysms and direct arteriovenous fistulas of the CNS. AJNR 9:1030
2. Guglielmi G, Viñuela F, Sepetka I, Macellari V (1991) Electrothrombosis of saccular aneurysms via endovascular approach. I. Electrochemical basis, technique, and experimental results. J Neurosurg 75:1–7
3. Guglielmi G, Viñuela F, Dion J, Duckwiler G (1991) Electrothrombosis of saccular aneurysms via endovascular approach. II. Preliminary clinical experience. J Neurosurg 75:8–14
4. Guglielmi G, Viñuela F, Dion J, Duckwiler G, Dion J, Lylyk P, Berenstein A, Strother C, Graves V, Halbach V, Nichols D, Hopkins N, Ferguson R, Sepetka I (1992) Endovascular treatment of posterior circulation aneurysms by electrothrombosis using electrically detachable coils. J Neurosug 77:515–524
5. Ahuja AA, Hergenrother RW, Strother CM, Rappe AA, Cooper SL, Graves VB (1993) Platinum coil coatings to increase thrombogenicity: a preliminary study in rabbits. AJNR 14:794–798

Early endovascular treatment with coils for ruptured cerebral aneurysms

S. Miyachi, S. Bracard, R. Anxionnat, J. C. Marchal, A. Per, L. Picard

Department of Diagnostic and Therapeutic Neuroradiology, University of Nancy, Saint-Julien Hospital, Nancy, France

Abstract. We treated 47 patients presenting with a subarachnoid haemorrhage due to rupture of an intracranial saccular aneurysm, within 1 week of the onset of symptoms, using microcoils via an endovascular approach. Total occlusion was obtained in 19 cases following the initial embolisation. In forty-one of (87%) all cases significant occlusion was eventually achieved. No postoperative bleeding occured. Overall morbidity and mortality rates were 21% and 30%, respectively. Complications related to treatment were observed in 5 cases: 3 distal embolisations, 1 intraoperative rupture and 1 premature detachment of the coil. Early coil embolisation is a valuable alternative for the treatment of ruptured aneurysms.

Key words: Aneurysms – Coils

Correspondence to: S. Miyachi, Nagoya Eksaikai Hospital, 4–66. Shoren-cho, Nakagawa-Icu, Nagoya 454, Japan

Recent advances in endovascular treatment have made it possible to occlude aneurysms safely and less invasively using mirocoils [1, 2]. We have aggressively treated

Table 1. Clinical data

Patient characteristics		
Male/female	25/22	
Age (years)	21–75 (mean 48.6)	
Neurological condition		
Hunt and Hess grade I, II	18	
III	4	
IV, V	25	
Location of aneurysms		
Anterior circulation	33	
ICA (C1)		9
ACA		2
AcomA		14
MCA		8
Posterior circulation	14	
VA-Pica		1
BA bifurcation		11
BA-SCA		1
PCA (P2)		1
Size of aneurysms		
small (< 10 mm)	31	
(particularly small (< 5 mm)	(6)	
large (11–25 mm)	14	
giant (> 25 mm)	2	
Angiographic vasospasm		
yes	25	
no	22	

ICA, Internal carotid artery; ACA, anterior cerebral artery; AcomA, anterior communicating artery; MCA, middle cerebral artery; VA, vertebral artery; PICA, posterior inferior cerebellar artery; BA, basilar artery; SCA, superior cerebellar artery; PCA, posterior cerebral artery

Table 2. Initial angiographic results

Coil	Initial angiographic occlusion		
	Partial	Subtotal	Total
Platinum microcoil	5 (36%)	9 (64%)	0 (0%)
GDC	4 (12%)	10 (30%)	19 (58%)
Total	9 (19%)	19 (40%)	19 (40%)

GDC, Guglielmi detachable coil

Table 3. Degree of occlusion on angiography according to the size of the aneurysm

Size of aneurysm	Final angiographic occlusion		
	Partial	Subtotal	Total
Small	2 (6%)	7 (23%)	22 (71%)
Large or giant	4 (25%)	3 (19%)	9 (56%)
Total	6 (13%)	10 (21%)	31 (66%)

ruptured aneurysms inaccessible to surgery using coils, in the early stage, based on the conviction that early intervention must prevent rebleeding and be followed by maximum treatment for delayed vasospasm [3, 4]. We present our experiences in 47 patients and discuss the benefits of early treatment of ruptured aneurysms.

Materials and methods

We treated 47 ruptured intracranial saccular aneurysms via an endovascular approach with coils, within a week of the onset of bleeding: 37 were treated within 3 days and 10 were treated on days 4–7. The patients ranged in age from 21 to 75 years (mean 48.6 years); 22 were women. Eighteen were classified as having Hunt and Hess neurological grade I or II, four grade III, and 25 grade IV or V. The origin and size of the aneurysms are shown in Table 1. Embolisation of the aneurysms was by placement of microcoils through a microcatheter using the road-map technique. Fourteen patients were initially treated with platinum microcoils and the remaining 33 cases were treated with Guglielmi detachable coils (GDC). Both types of coil were used in two cases. All embolisations were performed by one of three neuroradiologists.

When follow-up angiography revealed inadequate embolisation, further therapy (supplementary coils or surgical clipping) was performed to achieve complete exclusion of the aneurysm.

Results

Radioanatomical results

Angiographic follow-up studies were carried out 1–15 months postoperatively. Total aneurysmal occlusion after initial embolisation was achieved in 19 cases, and subtotal (70–95%) and partial (< 70%) occlusions were obtained in 19 and 9, respectively. In patients treated only using the GDC, the rates of total, subtotal and partial occlusion were 58%, 30%, and 12%, respectively (Table 2). Three subtotally embolised aneurysms appeared totally occluded on follow-up angiography as a result of intra-aneurysmal thrombosis. Eleven patients required additional treatment: supplementary coils in 6 and surgical clipping in 5, which resulted in complete cure. However, 4 aneurysms showed a reopacification of the aneurysmal sac due to coils compacting or migrating to the top of the dome. The final overall results were 31 total (66%), 10 subtotal (21%) and 6 partial occlusions (13%). Smaller aneurysms were more likely to be totally occluded than large and giant aneurysms (Table 3).

Clinical results

Clinical follow-up ranged from 1 to 16 months. The overall results are presented in Table 4. Twenty-three patients (49%) had a good outcome without neurological deficit. There was no significant difference between the two stages (acute and subacute) of treatment; overall morbidity and mortality rates were 21% (10 cases) and 30% (14 cases), respectively (Table 4).

Complications

There were no cases of postoperative rupture or deaths from complications. A distal embolism occured in two patients treated using the GDC. Coil migration occured in one patient with a basilar bifurcation aneurysm but who had no symptoms. Protrusion of the GDC into the parent artery due to premature detachment was observed in one

Table 4. Clinical outcome vs. Hunt and Hess grade

Outcome	Hunt and Hess grade			Total
	I, II	III	IV, V	
Good	15	1	7	23 (49%)
Moderately disabled	1	2	4	7 (15%)
Severely disabled	0	0	3	3 (6%)
Dead	2	1	11	14 (30%)
Total	18	4	25	47

patient. Intraoperative rupture of a pericallosal artery aneurysm appeared as extravasation during aneurysmography. Fortunately, it resulted in only a small haematoma in the interhemispheric fissure due to uninterrupted coil packing, and had little effect on the patient.

Discussion

The timing of surgery for ruptured intracranial aneurysms remains controversial, in spite of many recent studies [4]. However, it is desirable to prevent rebleeding and should be followed by maximum treatment for delayed vasospasm [1, 3, 5].

Almost all patients with ruptured aneurysms undergo surgery in the acute stage if they can tolerate it. During the acute stage, however, it is technically difficult to provide access to and expose aneurysms associated with high-grade subarachnoid haemorrhage (SAH), and deep-seated ones, especially those on the basilar artery, because of the tight, angry, red brain [5]. However, patients with high-grade SAH often have hydrocephalus needing acute ventricular drainage [6]. In cases of untreated ruptured aneurysm, however, external drainage can induce rebleeding [6].

Endovasular "haemostasis" may be more valuable in these situations, being less invasive than open surgery and offering the chance of another treatment [1]. The rupture site of saccular aneurysms is at the dome and sac in 98% of cases [2]. Therefore, making the most fragile part of the dome thrombose by inserting coils may be a reasonable way to obtain "haemostasis". Our results may suggest the advantage of GDC [2]. Although our series included many more patients (25 cases) with high-grade SAH than in other series [3, 6], the percentage of patients in Glasgow outcome scale I and II using the coils (44%) may be similar to the 42%–45% obtained with surgery [7, 3]. Patients with a high-grade SAH, and in poor general condition, may be good candidates for endovascular treatment.

Intra-arterial papaverine infusion is a very effective way of reducing intense vasospasms and making catheterisation easier. Vasospasm does not therefore appear to be contraindication to the endovascular approach [1].

References

1. Casasco AE, Aymard A, Gobin P, Houdart E, Rogopoulus A, George B, Hodes JE, Cophignon J, Merland JJ (1993) Selective endovascular treatment of 71 intracranial aneurysms with platinum coils. J Neurosurg 79:3–10
2. Guglielmi G, Viñuela F, Dion J, Duckwiler G (1991) Electrothrombosis of saccular aneurysms via endovasular approach. 2. Preliminary clinical experience. J. Neurosurg 75:8–14
3. Gilsbach JM, Reulen HJ, Ljunggren B, Brandt L, Holst H von, Mokry M, Essen C von, Conzen MA (1990) Early aneurysms surgery and preventive therapy with intravenously administrated nimodipine: a multiventer, double-blind, dose-comparison study. Neurosurgery 26:458–464
4. Kassel NF, Torner JC, Jane JA, Haley EC, Adams HP et al (1990) The International Cooperative Study on the timing of aneurysm surgery. II. Surgical results. J Neurosurg 73:37–47
5. Peerless SJ, Nemoto S, Drake CG (1987) Acute surgery for ruptured posterior circulation aneurysms. In Symon L (ed) Advances and technical standards in neurosurgery. Springer, Berlin Heidelberg New York, pp 115–129
6. Gijn J van, Hijdra A, Wijdicks FM, Vermeulen M, Crevel H van (1985) Acute hydrocephalus after aneurysmal subarachnoid hemorrhage. J Neurosurg 63:355–362
7. Auer LM (1991) Unfavorable outcome following early surgical repair of ruptured aneurysms – a critical review of 238 patients. Surg Neurol 35:152–158

Intravascular neurosurgery for intracranial aneurysms using detachable coils

A. Takahashi[1], T. Yoshimoto[2]

[1]Division of Intravasular Neurosurgery, Department of Neurosurgery, Hohnan Hospital, Sendai, Japan
[2]Department of Neurosurgery, Tohoku University, Sendai, Japan

Abstract. Thirty-nine patients who underwent detachable coil embolization for cerebral aneurysms were investigated. Twenty-two small-necked cases were performed by intra-aneurysmal embolization and 17 broadnecked or dissection cases were performed by parent artery occlusion. Anticoagulation was used during and after the therapy (48 h). Complete obliteration, neck remnant and body filling were obtained in 24, 6 and 5 cases at follow-up. Most complications were related to post-therapeutic anticoagulation; unintended parent artery obstruction with persistent neurological deficits (under-dosage) in 2, and haemorrhagic tendency (over-dosage) in 2. In conclusion, embolization using detachable coils is a safer and more definitive way to treat aneurysms by the intravascular route than by more usual ways such as balloon occlusion. Thromboembolic complications will be overcome by intensive post-therapeutic anticoagulation therapy.

Key words: Anticoagulation - Detachable coils - Embolization - intravascular neurosurgery - parent artery occlusion

Recent technological advances allow clinical application of detachable coils for neurosurgical intervention. We report our clinical experiences of detachable coil embolization in cases of cerebral aneurysm.

Patients and methods

Thirty-nine patients who had surgically difficult aneurysms (site, shape, etc.) and/or who were in a poor clinical condition (age, cancer, etc.) underwent detachable coil embolization for cerebral aneurysms. Guglielmi's detachable coils (GDC; Targe Therapeutics, San Jose, Calif.) [1] or interlocking detachable coils (IDC; Target Therapeutics) were used. Clinical presentation, site, type and size of aneurysms are shown in Tables 1–3. In 22 small-necked (<4 mm) cases intra-aneurysmal embolization was carried out and in 17 broad-necked or dissection cases, parent artery occlusion following a balloon occlusion test. Anticoagulation (heparin or argatroban) was used during and up to 48 h after the therapy.

Results

Angiographic results and clinical outcome are summarized in Figs. 1 and 2. In 7 patients a second embolization procedure was performed. In 11 cases presenting with subarachnoid haemorrhage (SAH), there was no rebleeding after the embolization. Of 11 cases with mass effect, 8 improved markedly (Table 4). The only patient whose condition deteriorated after embolization was treated by intra-aneurysmal embolization. Unintended obstruction

Correspondence to: M. Ezura, Department of Neurosurgery, Kohnen Hospital 4-20-1, Nagamachi-mininami, Taihaku-KJ, Sendai 982, Japan

Table 1. Clinical presentation

Subarachnoid haemorrhage	
Acute stage:	4
Chronic stage:	7
Mass effect:	11
No symptoms:	15
Infarction:	2
Total	39

Table 2. Site of aneurysms

Internal carotid artery:	14
Anterior communicating artery:	4
Middle cerebral artery:	2
Vertebral artery:	12
Basilar artery:	6
Posterior cerebral artery:	1
Total	39

Table 3. Type and size of aneurysms

Saccular:	31	
Small (< 10 mm):		6
Large (10–25 mm):		15
Giant (> 25 mm):		10
Dissection	8	
Total	39	

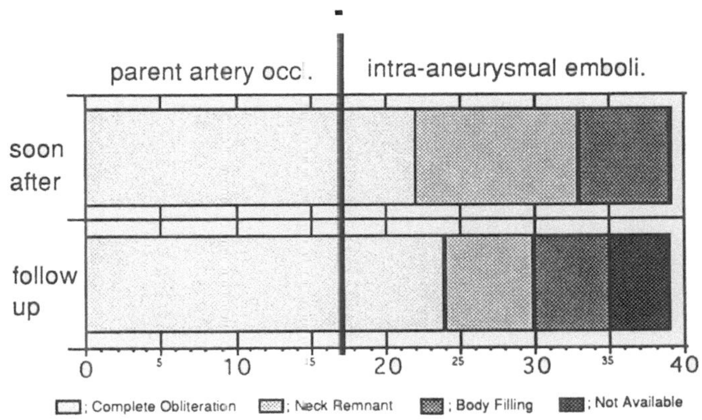

Fig. 1. Angiographic results

Table 4. Symptom change

Mass effect	11
Improved	8
Unchanged	2
Worsened	1
SAH	11
Rebleeding	0

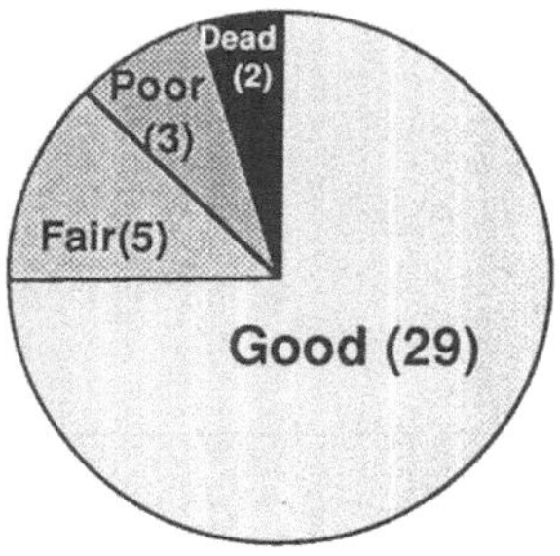

Fig. 2. Clinical outcome

of the parent artery occurred in 4 cases with persistent hemiparesis (2) or homonymous hemianopsia (2), presumably due to inadequate anticoagulation in 2 cases. Two cases showed a haemorrhagic tendency due to an overdosage of anticoagulant.

Discussion

Detachable balloons have been used for intravascular neurosurgery of cerebral aneurysms [2–4]. However, a detachable balloon has several drawbacks: (1) every kind of detachable balloon leads to minor difficulties during the detaching process, (2) a detachable balloon is shaped in such a way that it may asymmetrically press against the aneurysm wall. A newly developed detachable coil would overcome these drawbacks. A detachable coil has a simpler detaching process and a more precise configuration than a balloon. In our experience, GDCs are superior to IDCs. GDCs are accompanied by a flexible shaft and can be applied through a Tracker 10 catheter (Target Therapeutics). Above all, IDS are not repeatable precisely because they do not allow trial fixation in the last 3 or 4 mm.

Guglielmi et al. [5] treated 42 aneurysms by GDCs [5], 24 of which presented as SAH; in no case did rerupture occur after embolization. Complete aneurysm occlusion was achieved in 13 of 16 small-necked aneurysms and 4 of 26 wide-necked aneurysms, and 70–98% thrombosis occured in 3 and 22 respectively. This suggests that GDC embolization would protect against rerupture of aneurysms even if embolization was not complete. Application in cases of wide-necked and/or giant aneurysms should be limited. For parent artery occlusion, there is little difference between detachabe coils and detachable balloons.

GDCs also have several drawbacks, especially thromboembolic complications. In general, thromboembolic complications would be overcome by systemic heparinization. However, too much heparinization could cause haemorrhagic complications. Thus, it is essential that post-therapeutic anticoagulation therapy be monitored closely. Further long-term follow-up should clarify the problems concerning coil compaction, regrowth of aneurysms and rebleeding.

References

1. Guglielmi G, Viñuela F, Sepetka I, et al (1991) Electrothrombosis of saccular aneurysms via endovascular approach, part 2. Preliminary clinical experience. J Neurosurg 75:8–14
2. Romodanov AP, Shcheglov VI (1982) Intravascular occlusion on saccular aneurysms of the cerebral arteries by means of a detachable balloon catheter. In: Krayenbuhl (ed) Advances and technical standards in neurosurgery. Springer, Vienna, pp 25–49
3. Fox AJ, Viñuela F, Pelz DM, et al (1987) Use of detachable balloons for proximal artery occlusion in the traetment of unclippable cerebral aneurysms. J Neurosurg 66:40–46
4. Higashida RT, Halvach VV, Cowd C, et al (1990) Endovascular detachable balloon embolization therapy of cavernous carotid artery aneurysm: result in 87 cases. J Neurosurg 72:857–863
5. Guglielmi G, Viñuela F, Duckwiler G, et al (1992) Endovascular treatment of posterior circulation aneurysms by electrothrombosis using electrically detachable coils. J Neurosurg 77:515–524

Unclippable aneurysms of the internal carotid artery treated by balloon occlusion of the parent vessel: late clinical outcome

E. Berg-Dammer[1], H. Henkes[2], H. C. Nahser[2], W. Heienbrok[3], D. Kühne[1]

[1] Department of Neurology, Alfried-Krupp-Krankenhaus, Essen, Germany
[2] Department of Neurosurgery, Alfried-Krupp-Krankenhaus, Essen, Germany
[3] Department of Neurosurgery, Alfried-Krupp-Krankenhaus, Essen, Germany

Abstract. The late clinical outcome after balloon occlusion of the internal carotid artery (ICA) as treatment for unclippable aneurysms arising from this vessel was studied. Between 1984 and 1994, 60 patients underwent this treatment. In 19 patients, an extra-intracranial bypass was established before the endovascular procedure. After ICA occlusion, 18 patients experienced a deterioration in their neurological status, which was fatal in 1 patient, permanently disabling in 3 and of a transient nature in 14 patients. Compared to their state at admission, 25 patients were discharged in an unchanged condition, and 24 had improved. Improvements were primarily related to early regressions of pain and cranial nerve palsies. A clinical follow-up examination including MRI was performed 1–122 months (mean ± SD: 53 ± 34) after ICA occlusion. No recurrence of the presenting symptoms was encountered and 25 patients were asymptomatic. Compared with their pre-therapeutic status, 24 out of 57 patients had improved but were still symptomatic, 8 were basically unchanged and no patient was worse in terms of aneurysm-related symptoms. In 2 patients, new neurological symptoms had emerged, related to the aneurysm or its treatment in 1 patient and unrelated in the other. MRI follow-up studies revealed a remnant of the aneurysm sac with shrinkage and thrombosis in 9 patients. In 27 patients the mass effect of the aneurysm was entirely resolved. Ischaemic parenchymal lesions that were not present before the balloon occlusion were detected in 1 patient. The immediate mortality and morbidity risks of therapeutic ICA occlusion are 1–2% and 5 respectively.

Key words: Aneurysm – Internal carotid artery – Balloon occlusion

---

Direct surgical approach to clinoidal region aneurysms of the internal carotid artery (ICA) confined to the cavernous sinus [1], with transitional projection into the intradural space [2], or with intradural origin [3] is a major procedure with serious potential complications. Thus the treatment of these patients has become a multidisciplinary task considering, and possibly combining, microsurgical and endovascular methods [4]. With the refinement of interventional techniques, some dedicated centres were able to treat over 40 patients with ICA aneurysms during the 15 years [5, 6]. The indications for the treatment are well defined and include progressive ophthalmoplegia, visual impairment, severe facial or orbital pain, confirmed aneurysm enlargement during follow-up, carotid-cavernous sinus fistula due to aneurysm rupture, epistaxis, or subarachnoid haemorrhage [4]. There is limited knowledge, however, about the long-term tolerance to ICA occlusion and the efficacy of the procedure to ameliorate the symptoms. This prompted us to re-examine our 60 patients who underwent endovascular balloon occlusion of one ICA for aneurysm treatment between April 1984 and August 1994.

Patients and methods

Between April 1984 and August 1994, a total of 60 patients (43 female, 17 male; age range, mean ± SD 46 ± 17 years, 16–81 years) underwent endovascular balloon occlusion of one ICA as treatment of a cavernous or intradural aneurysm of this vessel.

Pre-therapeutic work-up included MRI, four-vessel angiography with cross compression studies, and temporary balloon test occlusion (BTO) of the ICA with clinical surveillance for 20 min under systemic heparinisation. With the BTO tolerated, or after EC-IC bypass operation and repeated BTO, the parent vessel was occluded with a detachable balloon via a transfemoral route or via direct puncture of the ICA. Balloon inflation and detachment was proximal to the aneurysm [5, 6]. The balloon trapping technique [7] was not performed; balloon packing of the aneurysm in order to preserve the parent vessel is beyond the scope of this article. We followed 57 patients for 1–122 months (mean ± SD; 53 ± 34 months) after the procedure, including neurological examination and MRI.

Results

Aneurysm size and site, as well as presenting symptoms, are summarised in Table 1. BTO was not tolerated by 7 patients. In these patients, and for other reasons such as advanced age, large aneurysm sac, etc., in 12 additional patients who passed the BTO, an extra-intracranial (EC-IC) bypass operation was performed. At the time of discharge from the hospital, 3–23 days after the ICA occlusion, 25 patients were unchanged and 24 were improved compared to their pre-therapeutic status. Ten patients were completely asymptomatic whereas 8 patients were in a worse clinical condition. When reexamined for a second time 1–122 months after ICA occlusion, 8 patients were diagnosed unchanged, 24 were improved, 25 were asymptomatic and no patient had deteriorated. In 2 patients, the presenting symptoms had regressed, but new signs or symptoms had occurred.

MRI was performed in 37 patients. The size of the aneurysm was reduced in 9 patients. In 27 patients, the

Correspondence to: E. Berg-Dammer, Department of Neurology, Alfried-Krupp-Krankenhaus, Alfried-Krupp-Strasse 21, D 45117 Essen, Germany

Table 1. Size and site of the aneurysm and presenting symptoms in 60 patients who underwent balloon occlusion of one internal carotid artery

Aneurysm size (diameter, cm)	patients	Site of aneurysm origin (ICA segment)	patients	Presenting symptoms	patients
≤1	1	C1	2	Headache	20
>1–2	7	C2	5	Visual field loss	9
2–3	17	C3	5	Impaired vision	13
3–4	24	C4	13	Diplopia	32
4–5	8	C5	2	Neuralgia	8
>6	3	C1, 2	5	Sensory deficit V1	3
		C2, 3	7	Horner's syndrome	3
		C3, 4	11	Epistaxis	3
		C3, 4, 5	2	Transient ischaemic attack/stroke	8
		C4, 5	5	Subarachnoid haemorrhage	5
		extracranial	3	Trauma	6

aneurysm sac had undergone significant involution and was visible as a discrete focus of different signal intensity in the area of the cavernous sinus without any mass effect. In 1 patient, MRI revealed parenchymal lesions not present of less pronounced at the time of ICA occlusion.

Discussion

The frequently benign nature of cavernous ICA aneurysms is well known and was recently re-emphasised [8]. Intradural ICA aneurysms and traumatic ICA pseudoaneurysms, however, may cause life-threatening haemorrhagic complications. Therefore exact anatomical localisation of the aneurysm, a patient's history and present symptoms, and findings must be considered. The acute, short-term and late tolerance, as well as the therapeutic efficacy of balloon occlusion of the ICA, are addressed by several authors. Treatment of ICA aneurysms in patients who do not tolerate the BTO can be accomplished by endovascular parent vessel occlusion after EC-IC bypass [4]. Early relief of trigeminal neuralgia and regression of retrobulbar pain followed by an improved function of extraocular muscles has been reported [7] and is confirmed by our data. Since alleviation of the mass effect of the aneurysm sac may require several months [9] or remains incomplete with calcification of the vessel wall [5], even delayed improvement of cranial nerve function may be expected. Our series includes 35 out of 57 patients with significant amelioration of cranial nerve function between ICA occlusion and late follow-up. As experienced by others [10], however, the prognoses of patients with complete ophthalkmoplegia is less favourable.

Embolic complications may occur during BTO [6] or in the early and intermediate post procedural phase due to premature deflation of the balloon, dural collateral supply to the C4 and C5 ICA segments [7], or external carotid branches to the distal ICA bearing the aneurysm. Another mechanism leading to cerebral ischeamia is haemodynamic compromise. Transient deterioration of cranial nerve palsy in the first days after the balloon occlusion is ascribed to an increase of mass effect of the thrombosing aneurysm [11] and was oberved in 2 of our patients. The concern that occlusion of an ICA will cause long-term cerebral ischaemia is not supported by our data.

Traumatic aneurysms of the cavernous ICA have no arterial wall. They are pseudoaneurysms. Potentially life-threatening epistaxis and cavernous sinus syndrome are the most frequent presenting symptoms [12]. When epistaxis has stopped at the time of elective treatment, ICA occlusion appears to be easier and as safe as the trapping procedure by others [4].

Neither the formation of de novo aneurysms nor the growth of contralateral pre-existing aneurysms, as it has been reported subsequent to ICA ligation [13, 14], was observed by us. One might speculate whether the follow-up period was too short for aneurysm development, since the relevant publications generally report intervals of several (3–22) years between ICA ligation and the above-mentioned complications.

References

1. Diaz FG, Ohaegbulam S, Dujovny, Ausman JI (1988) Surgical management of aneurysms in the cavernous sinus. Acta Neurochir (Wien) 91:25–28
2. Al-Rodhan NRF, Piepgras DG, Sundt TM (1993) Transitional cavernous aneurysms of the internal carotid artery. Neurosurgery 33:993–998
3. Diraz A, Kyoshima K, Kobayashi S (1993) Dorsal internal carotid artery aneurysm: classification, pathogenesis, and surgical considerations. Neurosurg Rev 16:197–204
4. Linskey ME, Sekhar LN, Horton JA, Hirsch WL, Yonas H (1991) Aneurysms of the intracavernous carotid artery: a multidisciplinary approach to treatment. J Neurosurg 75:525–534
5. Higashida RT, Halbach VV, Dowd C, Barnwell SL, Dormandy B, Bell J, Hieshima GB (1990) Endovascular detachable balloon embolization therapy of cavernous carotid artery aneurysms: results in 87 cases, J Neurosurg 72:857–863
6. Vazquez Añon V, Aymard A, Gobin YP, Casasco A, Rüffenacht D, Khayata MH, Abizanda E, Redondo A, Merland JJ (1992) Balloon occlusion of the internal carotid artery in 40 cases of giant intracavernous aneurysm: technical aspects cerebral monitoring, and results. Neuroradiology 34:245–251
7. Berenstein A, Ransohoff J, Kupersmith M, Flamm E, Graeb D (1984) Transvascular treatment of giant aneurysms of the cavernous carotid and vertebral arteries. Functional investigation and embolization. Surg Neurol 21:3–12
8. Kupersmith MJ, Hurst R, Berenstein A, Choi IS, Jafar J, Ransohoff J (1992) The benign course of cavernous carotid artery aneurysms. J Neurosurg 77:690–693

9. Triebel HJ, Grzyska U, Frehrking M, Zeumer H (1989) Klinische und MRT-Verlaufskontrollen von Karotisaneurysmen nach Ballonembolisation. Radiologe 29:427–431
10. Raymond J, Théron J (1986) Intracavernous aneurysms: treatment by proximal balloon occlusion of the internal carotid artery. AJNR 7:1087–1092
11. Fox AJ, Viñuela F, Pelz D, Peerless SJ, Ferguson GG, Drake CG, Debrun G (1987) use of detachable balloons for proximal artery occlusion in the treatment of unclippable cerebral aneurysms. J Neurosurg 66:40–46
12. Liu MY, Shih CJ, Wang YC, Tasi SH (1985) Traumatic intracavernous carotid aneurysm with massive epistaxis. Neurosurgery 17:569–573
13. Drapkin AJ, Rose WS (1992) Serial development of 'de novo' aneurysms after carotid ligation: case report. Surg Neurol 38:302–308
14. Fujiwara S, Fujii K, Fukui M (1993) De novo aneurysm formation and aneurysm growth following therapeutic carotid occlusion for intracranial internal carotid artery (ICA) aneurysms. Acta Neurochir (Wien) 120:20–25

Endovascular treatment of giant intracranial carotid artery aneurysms

P. Karapurkar, R. Ramakantan

Departments of Neurosurgery and Radiology, Seth G. S. Medical College and K. E. M. Hospital, Bombay, India 400012

Abstract. We treated 22 patients presenting with ocular palsies and periorbital pain due to giant aneurysms of the cavernous internal carotid artery (ICA) by the endovascular route. In 7, the ICA was occluded with balloons and in 11 with Gianturco coils. In 3 patients the balloon could not be negotiated past the arch due to kinks in the catheter. They refused treatment by the cervical route.

Key words: Aneurysms, giant – Endovascular treatment

Proximal occlusion of the internal carotid artery (ICA) is a well-accepted form of treatment of giant aneurysms of the cavernous segment of the (ICA) [1–4]. The commonly practised method of endovascular treatment is placement of a balloon in the cavernous ICA, opposite the aneurysm, to occlude the mouth of the aneurysm. If the balloon cannot be placed opposite the mouth of the aneurysm, then it is placed as close to the aneurysm as possible. One or two safety balloons are detached proximally in the ICA. The protocol includes performing an angiogram of the opposite carotid artery with compression of the carotid to be occluded, and of any one vertebral artery with the carotid compressed to check cross-flow through the anterior and middle cerebral arteries respectively. Particular attention is paid to the venous phase. If the cross-flow is satisfactory, the ICA is occluded temporarily with a balloon catheter for 30 min under full heparinization. Clinical and EEG monitoring is carried out. If the patient is able to tolerate the occlusion, the balloons are detached.

Due to bureaucratic delay and problems of importing balloons, we were forced to occlude the ICA with Gianturco coils instead of balloons in a patient who was in severe pain. Subsequently this has become the procedure of choice. A balloon catheter with a 0.38-inch guide-wire lumen is used to occlude the ICA. If the patient tolerated the occlusion, two 38-5-5 of 38-5-8 Gianturco coils are detached in such a manner that they intertwine, confirming that the patient can tolerate balloon occlusion.

Correspondence to: P. Karapurkar

Materials and methods

There were 28 patients who had presented with giant aneurysms of the cavernous ICA between 1986 and 1993. Twenty-two of these were taken up for endovascular treatments. All patients had presented with ocular palsy of varying degrees and had periorbital pain suggesting affection of the trigeminal nerve. The youngest patient was 14 years of age and the oldest 75. After following the standard angiographic protocol the patient was monitored clinically for 30 min with the ICA occluded by a balloon under full heparinization. In 2 patients EEG monitoring was also done.

Results

In 3 earlier patients a balloon was then detached opposite the mouth of the aneurysm. In 4 patients the balloon could not be placed opposite the mouth because of narrowing of the ICA, just proximal to the aneurysm, due to compression by the aneurysmal mass. In all these patients one balloon was detached proximal to the first balloon. In the remaining 11 patients, two coils were detached easily and uneventfully at the skull base. In 3 patients, balloons could not be negotiated beyond the arch of the aorta as the thin-walled guiding catheter had become kinked at the arch. The 3 patients refused treatment by percutaneous puncture in the neck.

There were no neurological complications. Technical complications included premature detachment of balloon in 1 patient with no neurological sequelae. All successfully treated patients showed recovery in their neurological deficit. The relief of the periorbital pain was most dramatic. Ocular palsies recovered completely in all patients except in 1 where the recovery was partial. Radiological follow-up was either by static CT scan, dynamic CT scan, angiogram or MRI. Every treated aneurysms has disappeared on follow-up.

Discussion

Proximal balloon occlusion of the cervical ICA is a safe procedure if the circle of Willis is open. If it is not, then some form of extra-intracranial vascular bypass is necessary. This was not necessary in any of our patients. Coil occlusion is technically very easy. Occasionally, though the diagnostic catheter can be manipulated past tortuous arteries, the thin-walled catheters become kinked and do not allow a balloon to pass. There is a theoretical risk of distal embolization by the thrombus around the coil becoming dislodged. However, control angiogram done after 20 min with gentle manual injection is safe. No evidence of any vascular insult was seen in any of our patients on long-term follow-up. Atraumatic investigation is preferable for follow-up. Dynamic CT and MRI are useful, but MRA may provide the best information.

References

1. Berenstein A, Ransohoff J, Kupersmith M, et al (1984) Transvascular treatment of giant aneurysms of the cavernous carotid and vertebral arteries. Functional investigations and embolization. Surg Neurol 21:3–12
2. Debrun G, Fox A, Drake C, et al. (1989) Giant unclippable aneurysms: treatment with detachable balloons. AJNR 2:167–173
3. Fox AJ, Viñuela F, Pelz DM, et al (1987) Use of detachable balloons for proximal artery occlusion in the treatment of unclippable cerebral aneurysms. J Neurosurg 66:40–46
4. Serbinenko FA (1974) Balloon catheterization and occlusion of major cerebral vessels. J Neurosurg 41:125–145

Percutaneous transluminal angioplasty for prevention of symptomatic vasospasm following aneurysmal subarachnoid haemorrhage

H. Katoh[1], K. Wada[1], A. Shimizu[1], H. Takiguchi[1], K. Shima[1], H. Chigasaki[1], T. Kaji[2], K. Makita[3], K. Tsuchiya[4]

[1] Department of Neurosurgery, National Defense Medical College, 3-2 Namiki Tokorozawa, Saitama 359, Japan
[2] Department of Radiology, National Defense Medical College, Toleorozawa, Japan
[3] Department of Radiology, Shakai-Hoken Chuo General Hospital, Tokyo, Japan
[4] Department of Radiology, Kyorin University, Tokyo, Japan

Abstract. We investigated the efficacy of percutaneous transluminal angioplasty (PTA) for prevention of symptomatic vasospasm after subarachnoid haemorrhage. Thirty patients were treated with angioplasty (PTA group). In 12 of them angioplasty was done as early as possible after neurological decline by vasospasm (treatable PTA group). In 18 of them, angioplasty was performed for asymptomatic angiograhic vasospasm (preventive PTA group). Another 40 patients were treated without angioplasty (non-PTA group). The outcome of the preventive PTA group was excellent. The mortality was significantly lower in the PTA group than in the non-PTA group. The combination of preventive PTA and treatable PTA seemed to be useful for the treatment of symptomatic vasospasm.

Key words: Percutaneous transluminal angioplasty – Vasospasm – Subarachnoid haemorrhage – Cerebral aneurysm

Vasospasm still remains a major cause of neurological deficit after subarachnoid haemorrhage, even though many new treatments have been attempted. In this report, the clinical usefulness of percutanous transluminal angioplasty (PTA) was investigated for the prevention of symptomatic vasospasm following aneurysmal subarachnoid haemorrhage.

Correspondence to: H. Katoh

Patients and methods

Between 1990 and 1993, 77 patients underwent early operation (within 72 h of aneurysm rupture) and were treated with hypertensive hypervolaemic therapy postoperatively in our hospital. Seven patients whose condition became poor mainly because of massive haematomas and/or operative complications were excluded. Angioplasty was performed in 30 patients (PTA group). Twelve of them underwent angioplasty as early as possible after neurological decline caused by vasospasm (treatable PTA group). In 18 patients, angioplasty was performed to prevent their asymptomatic angiographic vasospasm from becoming symptomatic vasopasm (preventive PTA group). In principle, angioplasty was performed even for patients in whom CT had already revealed low-density areas. The other 40 patients were treated without angioplasty (non-PTA group). Among these three groups, there was no significant difference in age, gender, Junz and Hess grade and location of aneurysms.

Results

There were 6 good recoveries, 2 moderate deficits, and 4 severe disabilities in the treatable PTA group; 15 good recoveries and 3 moderate deficits in the preventive PTA group; 21 good recoveries, 9 moderate dificits, 4 severe

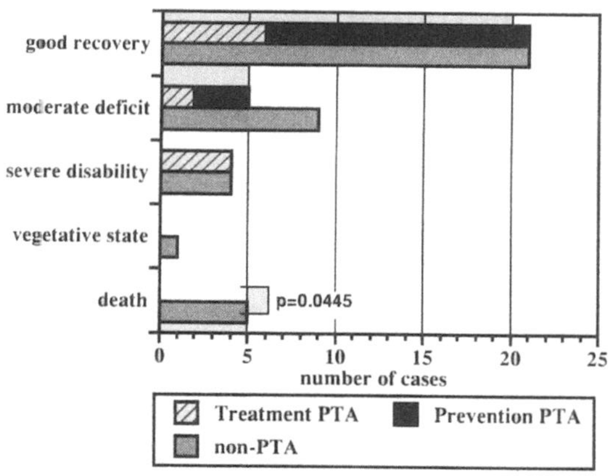

Fig. 1. Although there was no significant difference in outcome between the PTA group and the non-PTA group as a whole, the mortality was significantly lower in the PTA group than in non-PTA group (<0.05)

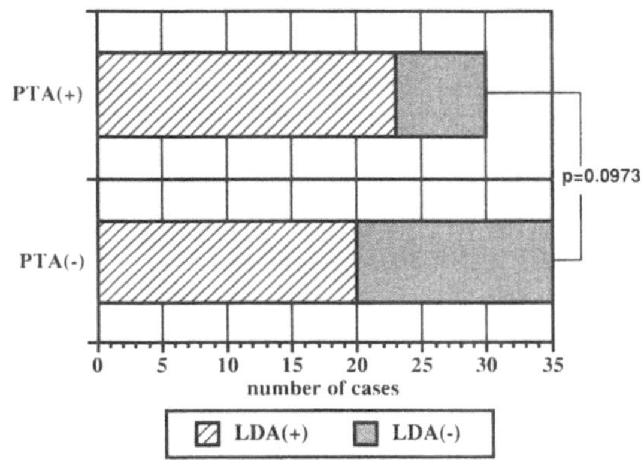

Fig. 2. Residual low-density areas caused by vasospasm on follow-up CT. Low-density areas tend to be less in the PTA group than in the non-PTA group on follow-up CT of 65 living patients. Low-density areas caused by haematomas were excluded

disabilities, 1 vegetative state and 5 deaths in the non-PTA group. In the preventive PTA group, no patient had a residual deficit caused by vasospasm. Although there was no significant difference in outcome between the PTA group and the non-PTA group, the mortality was significantly lower in the PTA group than in the non-PTA group ($P<0.05$) (Fig. 1). Residual low-density areas tended to be less in the PTA group than in the non-PTA group on follow-up CT scans (Fig. 2). We have not experienced any complication associated with the procedure of angioplasty.

Discussion

The usefulness of PTA for the treatment of vasospasm after subarachnoid haemorrhage has recently been discussed [1–3]. It is considered to be better to perform angioplasty as early as possible after neurological decline. However, if angioplasty can be performed in the early period of vasopasm, it might prevent an occurrence of symptomatic vasospasm. Vasopasm most frequently breaks out in the period between day 6 and day 9 [4], so we carried out preventive angioplasty in the period between day 5 and day 8, just before the vasospasm reached maximum levels and became symptomatic, even if the patients had no neurological decline by vasospasm. Our attempt in this matter had an excellent outcome. The results are not yet sufficient to conclude whether the preventive angioplasty symptomatic vasospasm, since little is known about the time span of the vasospasm. However, combining preventive and treatable angioplasty did seem to decrease the mortality form vasospasm and diminish residual low-density areas on follow-up CT scans. The combination of preventive angioplasty and treatable angioplasty may reduce the mortality from vasospasm following subarachnoid haemorrhage. Angioplasty may diminish low-density areas on follow-up CT after subarachnoid haemorrhage. The right timing for preventive angioplasty seemed to be between day 6 and day 8.

References

1. Randoll TH, Van VH, Leslie DC, Mickael BZ, Stanley B, Christopher D, Grant BH (1989) Transluminal angioplasty for treatment of intracranial vasospasm. J Neurosurg 71:648–653
2. Michael FB, Richard CH (1990) Intrancranial angioplasty for treatment of vasospasm after subarachnoid hemorrhage: technique and modifications to improve branch access. AJNR 11:239–247
3. Bracard S, Picard L, Marchal JC, Ducrocq X, Per A, Czorny A, Islak C, Roy D, Roland J, Lepoire J (1990) Role of angioplasty in the treatment of symptomatic vascular spasm occuring in the postoperative course of intracranial ruptured aneurysms. J Neuroradiol 17:6–19
4. Saito I, Sano K (1980) Vasospasm after aneurysm rupture: incidence, onset, and course. In: Wilkins RH (ed) Cerebral arterial spasm. Williams and Wilkins, Baltimore, pp 77–81

Intra-arterial infusion of high-dose papaverine for cerebral vasospasm

S. Yoshimura, N. Hashimoto, T. Tsukahara, K. Kazekawa, K. Sampei, S. Nishi, T. Iwama, Y. Gotoh

Department of Neurosurgery, National Cardiovascular Center, 5-7-1 Fujishirotai, Suita, Osaka 565, Japan

Abstract. We treated 14 patients with cerebral vasospasm with intra-arterial infusion of high-dose papaverine without balloon angioplasty. When cerebral vasospasm was diagnosed on angiography after confirmation of absence of major infarct on CT, superselective infusion of papaverine was performed. High-dose (80–120 mg) of papaverine was infused in the M1 or A1 segment, or a higher dose (160–320 mg) of papaverine was infused at the top of the internal carotid artery. Of the 14 patients treated by this method, 12 improved angiographically and clincally; 2, treated more than 6 h after the onset of neurological deficits, did not improve. Temporary neurological deficits during infusion appeared in 2 of 14 cases but disappeared within 30 min after infusion. A small haemorrhage without clinical manifestation was recognised in 1 case on the follow-up CT. Infusion of high-dose papaverine is considered to be safe and effective and it should be performed without delay.

Key words: Cerebral vasospasm – Papaverine – Subarachnoid haemorrhage

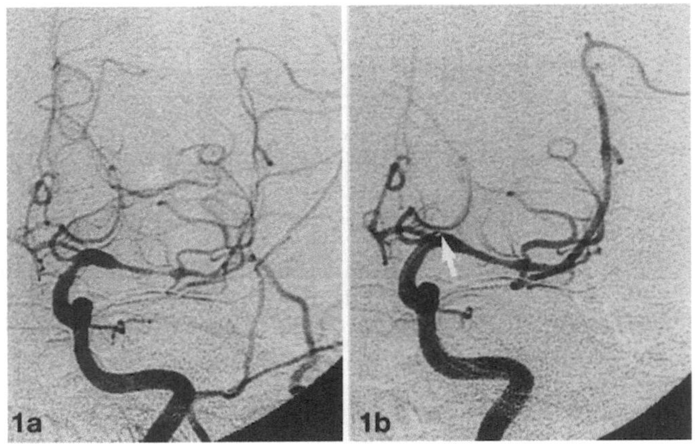

Fig. 1. a Left internal carotid arterery angiogram demonstrating diffuse severe of the left middle and anterior cerebral arteries. **b** Angiogram after infusion of high-dose (160 mg/10 min) papaverine at the top of the ICA demonstrating dilated vessels with evidence of improved perfusion. The tip of the microcatheter can be seen (*arrow*) at the top of the ICA

Intra-arterial infusion of papaverine has been shown to dilate spastic cerebral arteries after subarachnoid haemorrhage (SAH) [1–3]. Superselective infusion of papaverine just proximal to the affected site is considered to be necessary to obtain an effective concentration (10^{-4} M) at the lesion. When superselective infusion is difficult, a higher dose of papaverine will be required. Recently 14 patients with cerebral vasospasm were treated with infusion of high-dose papaverine. We discuss the timing, site of infusion, and the optimum dose of papaverine with these clinical experiences.

Materials and methods

When symptomatic vasospasm was suspected clinically, angiography was performed as soon as possible after confirmation of absence of a major infarct on CT. A microcatheter was introduced into the M1 or A1 segment and 80–120 mg of papaverine was infused within 10 min. When it was difficult, 160–320 mg papaverine was infused at the top of the internal carotid artery (ICA) within 10 min. Follow-up angiography was performed 48–72 h after treatment.

Results

Papaverine was infused at the M1 or A1 segment in 8 of 14 patients and at the top of the ICA in 6 of 14 patients. Twelve of 14 patients (86%) improved angiographically and clinically after infusion of papaverine (Fig. 1). Two patients (14%) treated over 6 h after the onset of neurological deficit improved angiographically but not clinically. The follow-up angiography showed recurrences of vasospasm in 4 of 14 cases, who were then treated with the same method again (Table 1). Cerebral infarction due to vasospasm occurred in 2 of these 4 recurrent cases. We experienced slight side effects in 3 patients. Two were temporary neurological deficits during infusion that disappeared within 30 min, after infusion. A small haemorrhage without clinical manifestation was recognized in 1 case on the follow-up CT.

Discussion

Papaverine (10^{-4} M) induced a maximal vasodilatation on control and spastic arteries following SAH, and it was used for the treatment of the already constricted artery after SAH [1–3]. To obtain a sufficient concentration of papaverine in the affected artery, it may be necessary to infuse it just proximal to the spastic arteries. In such a condition, 40 mg or less of papaverine may be enough to dilate the artery. However, when it is difficult to insert the microcatheter into the relevant artery, papaverine should be infused at the more proximal portion, such as the top of the ICA, and the same amount of papaverine may be insufficient because it may pass more into the normal artery than into the spastic artery in proportion to the blood flow. In this study, infusion of high-dose (160–

Correspondence to: S. Yoshimura

Table 1. Clinical summary of 14 patients

Case no.	Age sex	Location of aneurysm	H&H grade	Fisher group	Days after SAH	Location of vasospasm	Grade of vasospasm	Site of infusion	Dose of papaverine	Result	Complication
1	55, F	lt. ICA	III	4	8	lt. MCA & ACA	Severe	lt. MCA & ACA	40	Improved	–
2	45, M	Rt. MCA	IV	2	8	Rt. MCA	Severe	Rt. MCA	200	Improved	Small ICH
3	49, M	ACoA	IV	3	3	Bil. MCA & ACA	Moderate	Bil. IC top	80, 80	Improved	Temporary deficit
4	49, M	ACoA	IV	3	6	lt. MCA & ACA	Moderate	lt. IC top	80	Improved	–
					9	lt. MCA & ACA	Moderate	lt. IC top	80	Improved	–
5	46, M	lt. ACA	IV	4	7	Bil. MCA	Moderate	Bil. MCA	120, 120	Improved	–
6	78, F	ACoA	IV	4	5	Bil. ACA	Moderate	Bil. IC top	120, 120	Unchanged	–
					8	Bil. MCA & ACA	Severe	Bil. IC top	120, 120	Unchanged	Infarction
7	69, M	ACoA	IV	4	6	lt. MCA	Severe	lt. MCA	160	Improved	–
					9	Rt. MCA	Severe	Rt. MCA	320	Improved	–
					12	Bil. MCA & ACA	Severe	Bil. MCA & ACA	240, 240	Improved	–
8	48, F	ACoA	III	3	5	Rt. PCA	Moderate	BA	80	improved	–
						lt. MCA	Mild	lt. IC top	160	Improved	–
9	63, F	lt. ICA	II	2	7	Bil. MCA & ACA	Moderate	Bil. IC top	160, 80	Improved	–
10	69, M	ACoA	II	3	7	lt. MCA & ACA	Severe	lt. IC top	160	Improved	–
11	65, F	lt. ACA	III	3	12	Rt. MCA & ACA	Mild	Rt. IC top	320	Improved	–
12	46, M	lt. ICA	II	3	7	lt. MCA	Severe	lt. IC top	240	Improved	Temporary deficit
13	77, M	Rt. MCA	IV	3	7	Rt. MCA	Mild	Rt. MCA	160	Improved	–
14	54, M	ACoA	IV	4	5	Bil. MCA & ACA	moderate	bil. IC top	200, 200	Improved	–
					10	lt. MCA	Severe	lt. MCA	320	Unchanged	Infarction

ICA, Internal carotid artery; MCA, middle cerebral artery; ACA, anterior cerebral artery; ACoA, anterior communicating artery; BA, basilar artery; PCA, posterior cerebral artery; SAH, subarachnoid haemorrhage

320 mg) papaverine was effective and safe in 12 of 14 patients. Although infusion just proximal to the narrowing segment may be ideal, infusion of high-dose papaverine at the top of the ICA may also be effective when superselective catheterization is difficult.

These experiences suggested that intra-arterial infusion of high-dose (up to 320 mg/10 min) papaverine seemed to be effective and safe even when it was infused at the top of the ICA, and it should be performed before neurological deficits are irreversible.

References

1. Kaku Y, Yonekawa Y, Tsukahara T (1992) Superselective intraarterial infusion of papaverine for the treatment of cerebral vasospasm after subarachnoid hemorrhage. J Neurosurg 77:842–847
2. Kassell NF, Sasaki T, Colohan ART (1985) Cerebral vasospasm following aneurysmal subarachnoid hemorrhage. Stroke 14:562–572
3. Yoshimura S, Hashimoto N, Tsukahara T (1993) Treatment of cerebral vasospasm after subarachnoid hemorrhage with high-dose nicardipine and intra-arterial papaverine. In Findlay JM (ed) Cerebral vasospasm, vol 3. Elevier, Amsterdam, pp 365–368

MRI and phase-contrast MRA after selective Guglielmi detachable coil embolisation for intracranial aneurysms: preliminary results

M. Boukobza, C. Hoeffel, J. Guigui, E. Houdart, A. Casasco, J. P. Guichard, F. Lafitte, D. Reizine, J. J. Merland

Department of Neuroradiology and Therapeutic Angiography, Hôpital Lariboisière, 2 rue Ambroise Paré, F-75010 Paris, France

Abstract. We prospectively examined the utility of MRI (0.5 T) and of MRA in patients who underwent Guglielmi detachable coil (GDC) embolisation for intracranial aneurysms, postembolisation digital subtraction angiography serving as the standard. Fourteen patients with 16 aneurysms were treated. Thirteen aneurysms were small (< 12 mm), 2 were large (12–25 mm) and 1 was giant (> 25 mm). MRI and MRA, using the phasecontrast technique, were performed in all cases at a mean post-embolisation interval of 3.7 days. On T1- and T2-weighted images, the artefacts produced in most cases had a characteristic appearance. MRI is better than CT, particularly for demonstrating small zones of ischaemia. MRI and (phase contrast) MRA are not accurate in assessing residual lumen, but the parent vessel may be asseessed by MRA.

Key words: Intracranial aneurysm – Detachable coil – MRA – postoperative MRI

CT alone does not ideally assess the complications of endovascular treatment of aneurysms. Coil artefact is extensive and small infarcts, which may be clinically significant, are not well shown. This report describes our experience with MRI and MRA after endovascular treatment by electrothrombosis of intracranial aneurysms. This treatment used first-generation electrically detachable coils.

Patients and methods

We prospectively assessed the CT, MRI, MRA and arteriograms of 14 patients whose intracranial aneurysms were treated using the Guglielmi detachable coil (GDC) [1]. The patients included 6 men and 8 women with a mean age of 49 years (range 33–73 years). Preoperative CT was available in all patients. Postoperative CT was performed at a mean postoperative interval of 1 day. Preoperative angiography revealed a total of 18 aneurysms in 14 patients, and 16 were treated.

The origin of the aneurysms was as follows: the basilar artery bifurcation in 4, the anterior communicating artery in 4 (1 at the A1–A2 junction), the posterior communicating artery in 3, the certebrobasilar junction in 1, the P1 segment of the posterior cerebral artery (PCA) in 1, the origin of the anterior inferior cerebellar artery in 1, the superior cerebellar artery in 1, the middle cerebral artery in 1, the carotid-ophthalmic junction in 1 and the internal carotid artery at the bifurcation in 1. Thirteen aneurysms were small (< 12 mm), 2 were large (12–25 mm) and 1 was giant (> 25 mm).

The number of GDCs used ranged from 1 to 13 (average 4). Postoperative angiography was performed in all patients. Postoperative MRI and MRA were obtained at a mean interval of 3.7 days (range 1–14). MRI and MRA were performed solely to provide a non-invasive assessment of the status of the aneurysm, and to assess the cerebral parenchyma. Following treatment, MRI and MRA were obtained with a 0.5 T unit. In all cases, routine spin-echo sagittal 5-mm T1-weighted sections at 600/25 (TR/TE) and axial 5-mm T2-weighted sections at 3000/30,90. Preoperative MRI and MRA were available for comparison in 2 patients.

Results

On postoperative angiography, complete non-filling of the aneurysm was demonstrated in 10 aneurysms. A residual lumen was found in 6. The parent vessel was preserved. The MR examination was well tolerated by all patients. In 2 cases there were movement artefacts because MRI was performed early after the treatment.

The artefact produced by the coils had a characteristic appearance (Fig. 1).

On T1-weighted images there was complete absence of signal centrally, of variable shape, but usually round or oval, and depending on the scan plane. Usually there was a rim of high signal in the frequence-encoding axis, at one or both margins. On T2-weighted images the artefact was greater than on T1 weighting, and more important at the second echo. In a few cases, the artefact was patchy with areas of bright signal, and areas of signal void on T1-weighted images (Fig. 2). On T2 weighting small areas of highsignal appear in the core of the artefact, more marked on the first echo, with a halo of highsignal which is brighter on the second echo (Fig. 2). Coil artefact averaged 15 mm in size (range 10–60 mm). Because of these artefacts, in all cases but one MRI did not provide a good study of the lumen of the aneurysm (residual lumen, thrombosis). In 2 other cases, asymptomatic ischaemic lesions where seen on T2-weighted images but were missed by CT.

Except in 2 cases, (because of movement artefarcts) MRA showed a signal void in the area of the coils, but parent vessels were well visualised (Fig. 1).

Discussion

The artefact produced by coils appears very similar to that produced by non-magnetic clips [2]. The artefact significantly obscures regional anatomy, particularly the treated aneurysm, but in case of giant aneurysm, luminal thrombosis may be visible. Despite this, postoperative MRI is more informative than CT for several reasons. Ischaemic lesions are more readily detectable and the reconstruction mode used in MRI produces much more limited metallic

Correspondence to: M. Boukobza

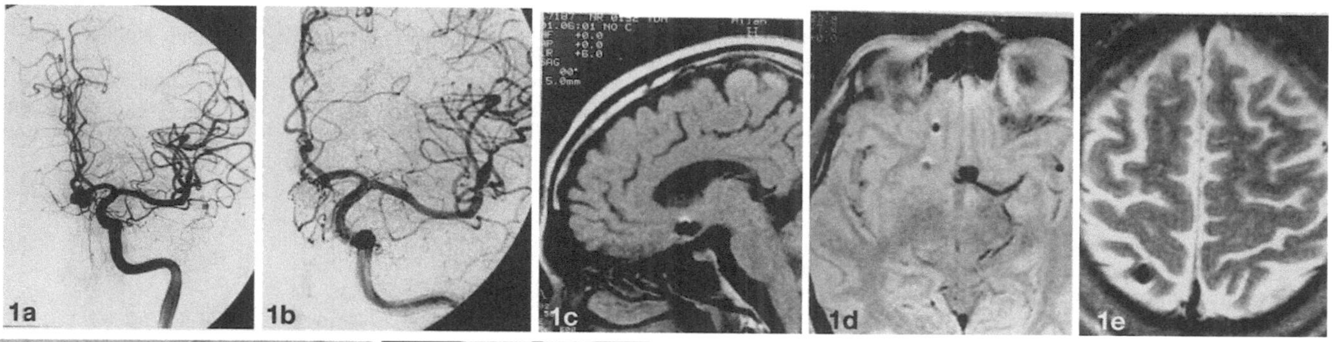

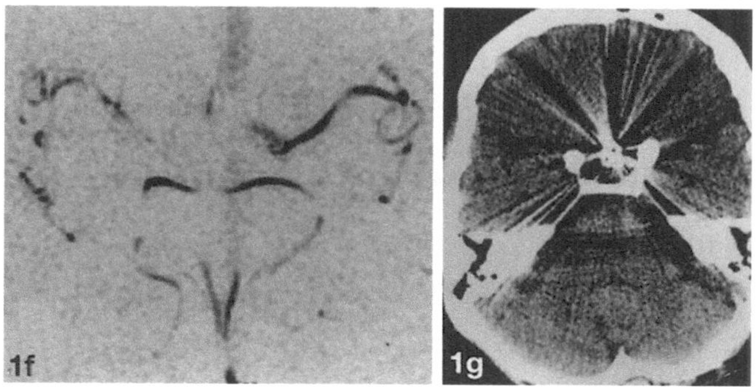

Fig. 1 a–g. Anterior communicating artery aneurysm left A1–A2 junction. **a** Large anterior communicating artery aneurysm (9 mm in the maximum diameter). **b** Left carotid arteriogram after endovascular treatment, showing complete obliteration of the aneurysm. Not disappearance of the right anterior cerebral artery, filled from the right internal carotid artery. **c** T1-weighted sagittal MRI 2 days after embolisation with five GDCs shows moderate artefact (11 mm diameter) with complete absence of signal, and a superior rim of high signal. **d** T2-weighted image, first echo, shows a multibular signal void corresponding to the occluded aneurysm. There is no rim of highsignal. On the right, two punctiform artefacts, the posterior centrally of lowintensity with a highintensity anterior rim, the anterior round with contral signal void and a peripheral high-intensity rim. **e** Second echo showing a round artefact of signal void with anterior and posterior high signal rim. The two artefacts are in the anterior cerebral artery territory, corresponding to distal migration of metallic components of coil juntion released during electrothombosis. **f** Axial MRA shows absence of signal in the area of the treated aneurysm. The anterior cerebral arteries are visible below. g CT scan 3 days after treatment. Both aneurysm and frontal lobes are obscured by artefact

Fig. 2 a–d. Large aneurysm, (20 mm) of the right posterior communicating artery. **a** post-embolization (13 coils, total length 325 mm) right carotid arteriogram. **b–d** Three days after treatment. T1-weighted image (**b**) shows a patchy artefact. On T2-weighting (**c** 1st, **d** 2nd echo) a few areas of highsignal are seen inside the signal void, which is also surrounded by a halo of highsignal

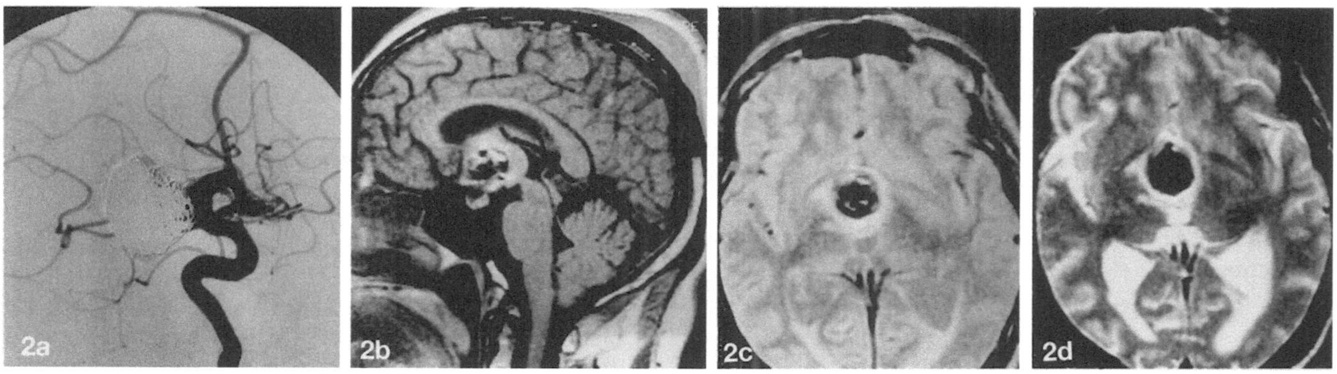

artefact from the coils than that used with CT [3]. The artefact from basal skull bone which degrades CT images is not present on MRI, so that postoperative MRI may demonstrate ischaemic lesions close to the coils and near the skull base.

In our experience, local artefacts produced by GDCs are small (ranging from 10 to 60 mm, average 15 mm). The most helpful sequence is spinecho T1 weighting. Measurements were made in the sagittal plane, but the size might be smaller depending on the relative orientation of the imaging plane.

In the patients studied by Brother et al. [2], clip artefacts averaged 29 mm in size, dependent on the number and size of aneurysm clips used. In our study the size of artefact produced by GDCs is independent of their total length.

These preliminary results must be confirmed by an additional study which compares the artefact volume to the volume of the GDC.

In 2 patients, artefacts were found distally in the territory of the parent vessel with the same characteristic appearance of local artefacts. These artefacts correspond to distal migration of metallic components at the coil junction during electrothrombosis.

In all cases MRA showed a signal void in the area of the GDCs; however, the parent vessel was well visualised. It nevertheless remains difficult to show vasospasm with the phase-contrast technique.

MRI is not accurate for assessing residual lumen and neck occlusion and conventional angiographs remains the gold standard. In cases of giant aneurysms, luminal thromboses may be visible.

References

1. Guglielmi G, Viñuela F, Duckwiler G, Dion J, et al (1992) Endovascular treatment of posterior circulation aneurysms by electrothrombosis using electrically detachable coils. J Neurosurg 77:515–524
2. Brother MF, Fox AJ, Lee DH, Pelz DM, Deveikis JP (1990) MR imaging after surgery for vertebrobasilar aneurysm. AJNR 11:149–161
3. Kelly W (1987) Image artifact and technical limitations. In: Brant-Zawadzki M, Normal D (eds) Magnetic resonance imaging of the central vervous system. Raven Press, New York, pp 43–82

Long-term follow-up of embolised aneurysms using MRI

M. Tsuura, T. Terada, Y. Nakamura, S. Tanaka, K. Nakai, T. Itakura

Department of Neuroradiology Surgery, Wakayama Medical College, 7-bancho-27, Wakayama City, Wakayama, Japan 640

Abstract. To determine when and how the size and characteristics of intracranial aneurysms change following endovascular treatment, MRI was employed to follow up five patients for 2 or 3 years after interventional procedures. In parent artery occlusion group, the size of the aneurysm reduced to approximately 30% of the intial volume between 4 months and 1 year following the treatment, when hyperintense area in the aneurysm on T1-weighted images changed to the isointense area. There were only slight decreases in volume after 1 year. In the intra-aneurysmal occlusion group, the volume reduction and signal intensity changes were less than those of parent artery occlusion on postembolisation MRI. Parent artery occlusion tends to decrease the aneurysmal volume faster than intra-aneurysmal occlusion and may be better treatment for the patients with mass effect due to the aneurysm.

Key words: Aneurysm – Embolisation – Magnetic resonance imaging

Recently, intracranial aneurysms, which compress surrounding tissue and cause symptoms or signs, have been treated by the endovascular approach. However, there have been few reports on the changes in size and characteristics after the treatment. To determine when and how the size and characteristics change, following embolisation, MRI was employed to follow up the embolised aneurysms for 2 or 3 years after the interventional procedures.

Patients and methods

Five patients who had aneurysms compressing the surrounding structures three internal carotid (IC) cavernous giant aneurysms, one IC cavernous large aneurysm and one vertebral artery (VA) giant aneurysm underwent endovascular treatment: proximal balloon occlusion of the parent artery in three cases (group 1) and intra-aneurysmal occlusion with microcoils or balloons followed by parent artery occlusion in two cases (group 2). Three aneurysms were partially thrombosed and two were not thrombosed. MRI (T1-weighted and T2-weighted imaging) were performed employing 0.5 T or 1.5 T clinical machines every 2–4 months in order to evaluate the volume of the aneurysm and the signal intensity changes in the aneurysm. The volume was calculated using the following formula: $V = 4\,pi/3\,(a/2)\,(b/2)\,(c/2)$, where V is the volume of the aneurysm, pi the circular constant, and a, b, c the maximum diameter of the aneurysm on the axial, sagittal and coronal view, respectively.

Results

Volume changes of the aneurysms

In group 1 the mean volume of the aneurysms reduced to 30% of the initial values between 4 months and 1 year following treatment. The final volumes in the follow-up period were about 30% of the initial values. In group 2, the mean volume decreased to 78% after 1 year and tended to reduce more slowly that in group 1. The final mean volume was 50% of the initial values in this group.

Signal intensity changes

After embolisation, signal intensity in the aneurysm tended to be hyperitense on both T1-weighted and T2-weighted images. When the volume of the aneurysm reduced rapidly (from 4 months to 1 year in group 1), the hyperintense area in the aneurysm turned isointense of hypointense on T1-weighted images. On T2 weighting, the isointense of hypointense area appeared in the hyperintense area of the aneurysm and it tended to be shown as a mixed intensity area.

Correspondence to: M. Tsuura

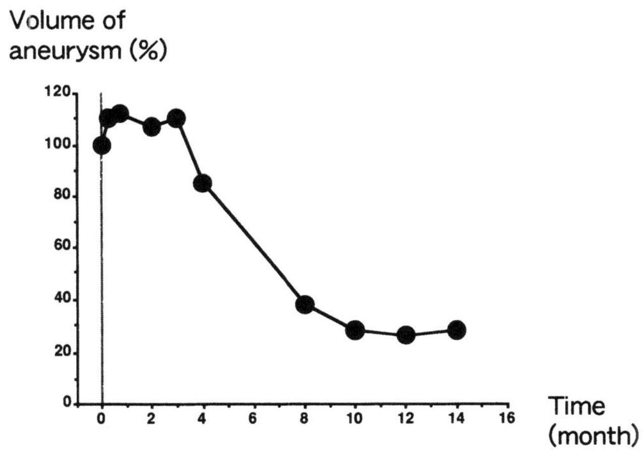

Fig. 1. Time-volume curve of the aneurysms in case 1. The aneurysm reduced rapidly to 30% of its volume between 4 months and 1 year after embolisation

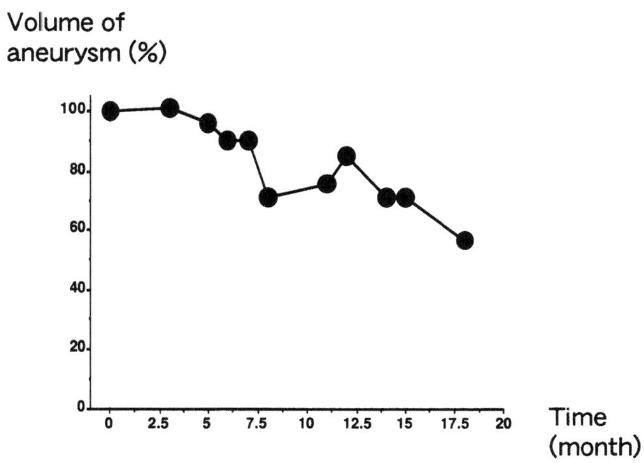

Fig. 2. Time-volume curve of the aneurysm in case 5. The volume of the aneurysm reduced gradually and was approximately 57% of its initial volume 18 months later

Case reports

Case 1 (group 1)

A 58-year-old woman who had complained of facial pain came to our hospital. She showed right oculomotor nerve palsy and right abducens nerve palsy in addition to pain and dysaesthesia in the ophthalmic nerve territory of the trigeminal nerve. A partially thrombosed IC cavernous giant aneurysm was detected by MRI and angiography. Proximal IC occlusion was performed using two detachable balloons. Figure 1 demonstrates the time course of the volume of the aneurysm following treatment. The volume reduced rapidly to about 30% of the pre-embolisation volume from 4 months to 1 year after the embolisation and there has been almost no change since a year after treatment. On MRI, both T1- and T2-weighted images showed a hyperintense area in the aneurysm 3 weeks after the treatment. Four to 8 months later, when the volume reduced rapidly, the hyperintense area on T1-weighted images turned isointense of hypointense, while isointense or hypointense areas apperared in the aneurysm on T2 weighting. The final volume was 28% of the pre-embolisation value 14 months later.

Case 5 (group 2)

A 19-year-old woman with a 3 year history of occipital pain complained of dizziness. A partially thrombosed giant VA aneurysm was detected by MRI and angiography. After intra-aneurysmal occlusion using microcoils, proximal VA occlusion using detachable balloons was performed following test occlusion of the VA, because small lumen remained after coil embolisation. Figure 2 shows the time course of the volume of the aneurysm. The volume began to decrease 4 months later and was approximately 85% a year following embolisation. The volume reduced slowly to 57% 18 months later. Signal intensity in the aneurysm turned hyperintense 3 months after the embolisation and isointense areas appeared gradually on T1-weighted images. On T2 weighting, hyperintense areas appeared in the hypointense area of the aneurysm 3 months later.

Discussion

Recently, surgically unclippable aneurysms have been treated via the endovascular route using detachable balloons or microcoils [1]. In this report, we studied changes in volume and signal intensity of the aneurysm on MRI following the intravascular procedures.

Shrinkage (volume reduction) and absorption of intra-aneurysmal thrombi after embolisation depends on several factors: (1) the surrounding tissue, (2) the aneurysmal wall, i.e. intramural thrombi, calcification, fibrosis and vascularity (vasa vasorum) [4], (3) intraluminal condition, i.e. whether the intraluminal contents are embolic materials such as coils or new thrombus caused by trapped blood, whether the pulsation (driving force) from the parent artery is transmitted to the aneurysmal lumen or not [5], and so on.

Considering these factors, we can summarise some advantages on parent artery occlusion: (1) the pulsation from the parent artery is transmitted less than that in cases of intra-aneurysmal occlusion and (2) the aneurysm with only thrombus in the lumen may decrease in size more rapidly than that including platinum coils or balloons, because thrombus seems to be easily absorbed. Morever, growth of thrombosed aneurysm has been reported [4, 5] and the mechanisms seem to be (1) transmission of the pulsation from the parent artery and (2) intramural haemorrhage from the vasa vasorum. Therefore, parent artery occlusion may have more advantages in preventing the growth and recanalisation of embolised aneurysms, in spite of the possibility of ischaemia in the distal territory. Based on our results, the aneurysm after parent artery occlusion tends to reduce in volume more rapidly than that after intra-aneurysmal occlusion (with resultant parent artery occlusion). Although intra-aneurysmal occlusion will come to the goal of embolisation according to the development of embolic materials like the Guglielmi detachable coil [1], parent artery occlusion or parent artery occlusion with bypass surgery may be the first choice in some patients with aneurysms compressing surrounding tissue who need rapid volume reduction of the aneurysm.

On MRI, signal intensity of the aneurysm tended to be hyperintense on both T1- and T2-weighted images after embolisation. Then isointense or hypointense areas on both T1- and T2-weighted images appeared in the aneurysm when the volume decreased rapidly. These signal intensity changes seem to be similar to those of intracerebral haematoma. Accordingly, hyperintense areas on both T1- and T2-weighted images probably result from free methaemoglobin [6]. The volume of the aneurysm may reduce rapidly when intra-aneurysmal free methaemoglobin is absorbed or degraded.

References

1. Guglielmi G, Viñuela F, Duckwiler G, et al (1992) Endovascular treatment of posterior circulation aneurysms by electrothrombosis using electrically detachable coils. J Neurosurg 77:515–524
2. Schubinger O, Valvanis A, Wichmann W (1981) Growth mechanism of giant intracranial aneurysms; demonstrated by CT and MR imaging. Neuroradiology 29:266–271
3. Kwan ESK, Heilman CB, Shucart WA, et al (1991) Enlargement of basilar artery aneurysm following balloon occlusion – "water hammer effect". J Neurosurg 75:963–968
4. Hecht S, Horton JA, Yonas H (1991) Growth of a thrombosed giant vertebral artery aneurysm after parent artery occlusion. AJNR 2:449–451
5. Katayama Y, Tsubokawa T, Miyazaki S, et al (1991) Growth of totally thrombosed giant aneurysm within the posterior cranial fossa. Neuroradiology 33:168–170
6. Atlas SW, Grossman RI, Goldberg HI, et al (1987) Partially thrombosed giant intracranial aneurysms: correlation of MR and pathologic findings. Radiology 162:111–114

Intervention: angioplasty

Percutaneous transluminal angioplasty for atherosclerotic stenosis of intracranial or skull base arteries

A. Hyodo[1], Y. Matsumaru[1], I. Anno[2], H. Onitsuka[1], A. Matsumura[1], Y. Yoshii[1], T. Nose[1], A. Tsukada[3], E. Kobayashi[4]

[1] Department of Neurosurgery, University of Tsukuba, Tsukuba, Japan
[2] Department of Radiology, University of Tsukuba, Tsukuba, Japan
[3] Department of Neurosurgery, Kennan Hospital, Tsukuba, Japan
[4] Department of Neurosurgery, Tsukuba Memorial Hospital, Tsukuba, Japan

Abstract. Percutaneous transluminal angioplasty (PTA) was performed in 14 patients for atherosclerotic stenotic lesions involving the intracranial or skull base cerebral arteries. The stenotic lesions involved the middle cerebral artery in 6 cases, the internal carotid artery in 4 cases, the basilar artery in 3 cases, and the intracranial vertebral artery in 1 case. PTA was performed using Stealth or Angel balloon angioplasty catheters. After PTA, the stenotic lesion dilated successfully in all cases (0–50% residual stenosis; mean 20%). No symptomatic complications occurred after PTA. After PTA, patients were followed up clinically for 5–28 months (mean: 15 months), and no clinical deterioration such as transient ischaemic attacks or stroke occurred. A follow-up angiogram was performed in 12 cases. Four out of 12 cases showed restenosis to an extent roughly equal to the original stenosis, but remained asymptomatic.

Key words: Percutaneous transluminal angioplasty – Atherosclerosis – Intracranial arteries

---

With recent advances in the devices and techniques of intravascular neurosurgery, percutaneous transluminal angioplasty (PTA) can be performed for treatment of symptomatic stenoses of the cerebral arteries [1–5]. But in most reported cases, stenotic lesions involve the extracranial cerebral arteries [3–5]. We present our results in PTA of the intracranial or skull base cerebral arteries.

Materials and methods

From May 1992 to February 1994, PTA was performed in 14 cases of atherosclerotic stenosis of the intracranial or skull base cerebral arteries, and all the cases were followed up for at least 6 months after the PTA procedure (Table 1). The age of the patients varied from 42 to 75 years, with a mean of 60 years, and included 10 men and 4 women. The site of the stenotic lesion was in the middle cerebral artery (MCA; M1 portion) in 6 cases, the basilar artery in 3 cases, the internal carotid artery (petrous-cavernous portion) in 4 cases, and the intracranial vertebral artery in 1 case. Almost all cases were symptomatic, such as transient ischaemic attacks (TIA) or minor stroke, and the degree of stenosis ranged from 70 to 90%, with a mean of 80%.

PTA was performed under local anaesthesia, and with digital subtraction angiography (DSA) control using the road map function. The patient was fully heparinised and ACT monitoring was used. For PTA, a Stealth or an Angel balloon was inflated to a pressure of 2–6 atm for 20–120 s. After the PTA, systemic heparinisation continued for 24 h, and antiplatelet therapy continued before and after PTA.

Correspondence to: A. Hyodo

Results

As shown in Table 1, initial stenosis ranged from 70 to 90% with a mean of 80%. After PTA, stenosis ranged from 0 to 50%, mean 20%. In one case, dissection occlusion of the anterior cerebral artery occurred during PTA for MCA stenosis, but remained asymptomatic. This was the only complication we encountered in this group. Regarding the clinical results, no symptomatic complications arose, but one severe occlusion intolerance occurred during PTA of the basilar artery.

Follow-up angiography was performed in 12 of 14 cases, 3 months or more after PTA was carried out. Restenosis to an extent roughly equal to the original stenosis occurred in 4 cases, but these remained asymptomatic. Clinical follow-up was performed for 5–28 months after PTA. One patient died 5 months after PTA due to myocardial infarction, but no other clinical deterioration, such as TIA or stroke, occurred.

Representative case

A 63-year-old man (case 1) suffered from a residual ischaemic neurological deficit because of right MCA stenosis (Fig. 1). PTA was performed using the 2.5-mm-diameter (Angel catheter, at a pressure of 3–4 atm for 80 s. The 90% stenosis initially observed improved to 20% after PTA (Fig. 1, right). Figure 2 shows the follow-up angiogram. No obvious restenosis occurred within a year after PTA.

Discussion

There are several advantages to PTA, especially compared to surgical procedures, such as a bypass operation or endarterectomy. Firstly PTA is much less invasive. Secondly, we are able to monitor the patient's neurological state and consciousness. Thirdly, we are able to continue anticoagulant and antiplatelet therapy. And lastly, we can recover adequate orthograde blood flow. On the other hand, there are several shortcomings of PTA. Preoperative problems that may be encountered include distal emboli, dissection, acute occlusion and a problem of the perforating artery. Post-PTA difficulties include resteno-

Table 1. Summary of patients treated

Case	Age (years)	Sex	Site of stenosis	Initial stenosis (%)	Stenosis after PTA (%)	Angiographic follow-up (months)	Re-stenosis	Clinical follow-up (months)
1	44	M	MCA	70	20	6, 15	No	28
2	75	M	(Cavernous) ICA	80	50	MRA only	?	22
3	68	M	Basilar	90	40	6, 13	No	19
4	73	F	Basilar	80	20	6, 16	No	18
4	73	F	Basilar	80	20	6, 16	No	18
5	52	M	MCA	70	10	6, 13	Yes	17
6	42	M	Cavernous ICA	70	0	3, 15	No	17
7	52	M	Basilar	70	40	3, 14	No	17
8	69	F	MCA	90	20	13	Yes	15
9	48	F	MCA	70	10	4, 13	No	15
10	64	F	MCA	80	0	3	Yes	12
11	63	M	90	20	3, 6, 12	No	12	
12	63	M	VA (V4)	70	10	-	?	5 (died of myocardial infarction)
13	58	M	Petrous ICA	90	0	3, 7	Yes	8
14	63	M	(Cavernous) ICA	80	30	3	No	7

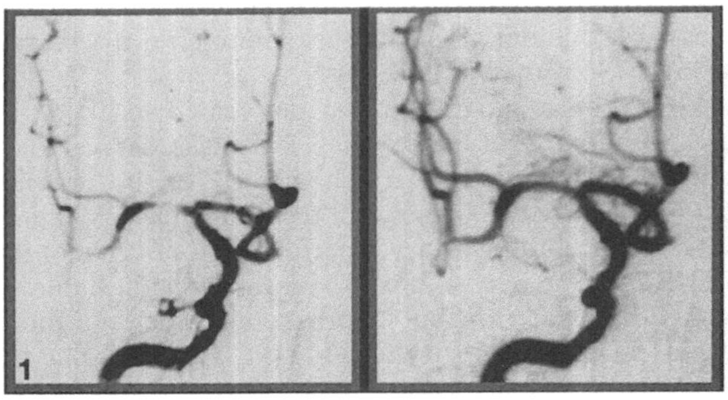

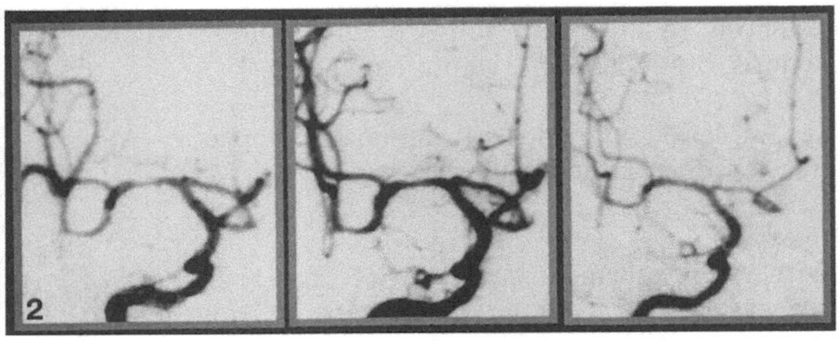

Fig. 1. Case 1. Right internal carotid angiogram before (*left*) and after (*right*) percutaneous transluminal angioplasty (PTA). The 90% stenosis initially observed improved to 20% after PTA

Fig. 2. Right internal carotid angiogram 3 (*left*), 6 (*centre*) and 12 (*right*) months after PTA. No obvious restonis

sis and distal emboli, but perhaps the biggest problem is that there are no data on effectiveness, frequency of complications and long-term follow-up.

From the results described here, we conclude that PTA of the intracranial or skull base cerebral artery is technically feasible, and it can be performed with relatively low morbidity. From our experience it may be a useful procedure, but the results from a larger number of patients and more long-term follow-up data are necessary in order to evaluate the safety and usefulness of this method.

References

1. Higashida RT, Tsai FY, Halbach VV, et al (1993) Transluminal angioplasty for atherosclerotic disease of the vertebral and basilar arteries. J Neurosurg 78:192–198
2. Purdy PD, Devous MD, Unwin DH, et al (1990) Angioplasty of an atherosclerotic middle cerebral artery associated with improvement in regional cerebral blood flow. AJNR 11:878–880
3. Kachel R, Basche S, Heerklotz I, et al (1991) Percutaneous transluminal angioplasty (PTA) of supra-aortic arteries especially the internal carotid artery. Neuroradiology 33:191–194
4. Theron J, Courtheoux P, Alachkar F, et al (1990) New triple coaxial catheter system for carotid angioplasty with cerebral protection. AJNR 11:869–874
5. Tsai FY, Matovich V, Hieshima GB, et al (1986) Percutaneous transluminal angioplasty of the carotid artery. AJNR 7:349–358

Carotid angioplasty: the Atkinson Morley's/St. George's Hospital experience and the results of transcranial Doppler monitoring for emboli and assessment of middle cerebral artery flow and CO_2 reactivity before and after angioplasty

A. G. Clifton[1], **M. M. Brown**[2], **H. Markus**[2], **T. Buckenham**[3]

[1] Department of Neuroradiology, Atkinson Morley's Hospital, London
[2] Department of Clinical Neuroscience, St. George's Hospital, London, UK
[3] Department of Radiology, St. George's Hospital, London, UK

Abstract. The European Carotid Surgery Trial and the North American Carotid Endarterectomy Trial have recently shown the value of carotid endarterectomy in patients with 70–90% stenosis who have had recent cerebrovascular symptoms in that carotid artery territory. Percutaneous transluminal angioplasty (PTA) may offer an alternative. We have, to date, performed 25 PTA, 21 being randomised to PTA from our participation in the Carotid and Vertebral Artery Transluminal Angioplasty Study, the others being elective procedures. We have performed successful dilatations in 21, being unable to cross the stenosis in 4; 1 patient suffered a stroke. Transcranial Doppler ultrasound (TCD) was used to monitor for embolic signals and to assess middle cerebral artery flow velocity and ipsilateral CO_2 reactivity. Asymptomatic emboli were detected and cerebral haemodynamics were shown to be improved following angioplasty. The risk of stroke or death from carotid PTA is thus thought to be similar to that of carotid endarterectomy; it may offer a practical alternative. TCD has shown embolisation usually occurs but is asymptomatic. This is consistent with a low risk of stroke and successful PTA results in improved cerebral haemodynamics.

Key words: Carotid artery stenosis – Angioplasty – Transcranial Doppler – Cerebral haemodynamics – Cerebral embolisation

---

Internal carotid artery stenosis is associated with an increased risk of stroke; in symptomatic patients with 70% or greater diameter stenosis carotid endarterectomy has been shown to result in a significant reduction in subsequent stroke risk [1, 2]; however, surgery also carries a significant morbidity in addition to risks of anaesthesia, which include myocardial ischaemia in patients with coexistent coronary heart disease. Risks of stroke or death of 7.5% have been shown in the European Carotid Surgery Trial (ECST) [2] and 5% in the North American Carotid Endarterectomy Trial (NASCET) [1]. Preliminary results suggest that percutaneous transluminal angioplasty (PTA) of carotid and vertebral stenosis also has an acceptable complication rate and may provide an alternative to surgery [3, 4]. PTA also requires a short hospital stay and avoids the risk of anaesthesia. The Carotid And Vertebral Artery Transluminal Angioplasty Study (CAVATAS) is an internal, multi-centre, randomised trial which has been established to evaluate angioplasty in patients with cerebral vascular disease. Its aims are to determine the risks and benefits of carotid and vertebral angioplasty and compare the risks and benefits of carotid and vertebral angioplasty, with surgical treatment in patients who are eligible for surgery or best medical treatment alone in patients ineligible for surgery.

An understandable concern about distal embolisation has led to the reluctance to use carotid angioplasty; it has been demonstrated that circulating atheroma, platelet and thrombus emboli can be detected using Doppler ultrasound where they appear as short-duration, high-intensity signals in the Doppler spectrum [5]. In order to investigate the effectiveness of carotid PTA on both immediate and short-term cerebral embolisation, we performed a prospective study in patients undergoing carotid PTA. We used transcranial Doppler ultrasonography of the middle cerebral artery to monitor for high-intensity embolic signals.

Methods

All patients were pretreated with aspirin. A 6 French sheath was inserted into the right femoral artery; a 5 French guiding catheter was inserted into the appropriate common carotid or vertebral artery. After systemic heparinisation intravenously (heparin 5000 IU), the stenosis was crossed with a standard or hydrophylic wire. The guide catheer was passed across the stenosis. After ascertaining that the guide catheter was intraluminal, an exchange wire was placed through the guide catheter distal to the stenosis and an angioplasty catheter exchanged across the stenosis. A 100 cm length shaft – 2 cm long × 5, 6 or 7 mm diameter balloon, depending on the diameter of the normal internal carotid artery – was used to dilate the stenosis. Hand inflation was performed up to 3 times for a duration of up to 30 s depending on the results seen on fluoroscopy. The balloon catheter was then removed and a check angiogram performed. Anticoagulation, heparin 20,000 U/24 h, was continued for 48 h after PTA. During the procedure simple neurological examination was performed, ECG and blood pressure monitored. Patients were also studied using transcranial Doppler sonography. The middle cerebral artery was insonated via the transtemporal route at a depth of 46–54 mm using a sample volume of 10 mm.

Correspondence to: A. G. Clifton, Department of Neuroradiology, Atkinson Morley's Hospital, London, SW20 ONE, UK

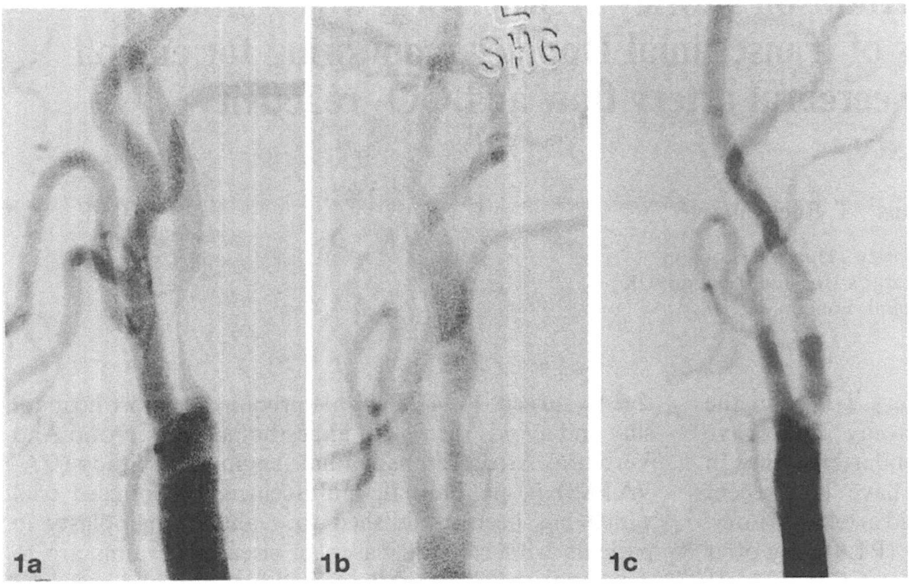

Fig. 1. a Long, 99% stenosis of the internal carotid artery.
b Angiogram immediately after dilatation showing an excellent result with a degree of subintimal dissection and a residual 40% stenosis.
c One year later there is excellent remodelling with no discernible residual stenosis

Results and discussion

To date we have performed 25 angioplasties, 19 being part of the CAVATAS trial and 6 elective. These comprise 18 carotid artery bifurcations, 2 vertebral artery origins, 2 brachiocephalic, 1 carotid syphon, 1 distal cervical internal carotid and 1 external carotid artery. We have performed successful dilatations in 21, being unable to cross the stenosis in 4; 1 of these latter 4 suffered a stroke. Embolic signals were detected by sonography immediately following balloon deflation in 9 of 10 patients; neurological symptoms (transient ischaemic attack which resolved within 24 h) occurred in only 1. Further embolic signals were detected in the first postoperative week but were asymptomatic: immediately following arterial line removal in 8 of 10 subjects; at 2 h, in 5 of 6; at 4 h, in 1 of 5; at 2 days, in 2 of 10; and at 4 weeks, in 1 of 10. Ipsilateral middle cerebral artery flow velocity (VMCA) fell transiently during balloon inflation (greater than 50% in 5 of 10) but was otherwise unchanged. Before the procedure (pre), it was 45.9; at 2 days, 44.1; and at 4 weeks, 40.3 cm/s (P = not significant). In contrast, ipsilateral CO_2 reactivity, expressed as the percentage change in velocity between 8% CO_2 and hyperventilation compared to resting velocity, increased (pre, 87.9%; 2 days 105.5%; 4 weeks 112.3%: pre V 4 week, $P < 0.05$). Ipsilateral MCA pulsatility index increased (pre 0.85; 2 day, 1.02; 4 weeks, 0.97; pre V 2 day, and V 4 week, $P < 0.05$).

Several of the immediate postangioplasty angiograms showed a degree of subintimal dissection with the angiographic lumen being less than the degree of dilatation achieved by the angioplasty balloon. We have performed follow-up angiograms in 2 of these patients, which have shown excellent remodelling and restoration to near-normal lumen on angiograms 1 year after angioplasty. We intend to perform repeat angiograms on all our patietns (Fig. 1).

References

1. North American Symptomatic Carotid Endarterectomy Trial Collaborators (1991) Beneficial effects of carotid endarterectomy in symptomatic patients with high grade carotid stenosis. N Engl J Med 325:445–453
2. European Carotid Surgery Trial Collaboration Group (1991) MRC European Carotid Surgery Trial: interim results for symptomatic patients with severe (70–99%) or with mild stenosis (0–29%) carotid stenosis. Lancet 337:1235–1243
3. Kachel R, Basche S, Heerlotz I, Grossmane K, Endler S (1991) Percutaneous transluminal angioplasty (PTA) of supra-aortic arteries especially the internal carotid artery. Neuroradiology 33:191–194
4. Eckert B, Zanella FE, Steinmetz J, Thie A, Zeumer H (1994) 53 Carotid angioplasties: results, complications, follow-up. Cerebrovasc Dis 4:259
5. Markus HS, Clifton A, Buckenham T, Brown M (1994) Carotid Angioplasty: immediate and short term embolic consequences. Stroke (in press)

A simple technique for minimising complications of percutaneous transluminal angioplasty for internal carotid stenosis

T. Hirayama[1], Y. Katayama[1], T. Tsubokawa[1], K. Himi[2]

[1] Department of Neurological Surgery, Nihon University School of Medicine, Tokyo, Japan
[2] Department of Radiology, Nihon University School of Medicine, Tokyo Japan

Abstract. The application of percuteneous transluminal angioplasty (PTA) to the treatment of cerebrovascular diseases risks complications caused by emboli flowing into the intracerebral arteries. We report here a simple technique to prevent such complications of PTA for internal carotid artery stenosis. The principle of the technique is to occlude the common carotid artery with a latex balloon mounted on a guiding catheter during the PTA procedures. This usually gives rise to retrograde flow from the internal carotid artery, which carries debris away to the external carotid artery. We treated 18 cases of internal carotid artery stenosis by this technique. It was confirmed before the PTA procedure that slow injection of contrast medium through the guiding catheter demonstrated retrograde flow from the internal carotid artery. Excellent results were obtained in all cases, without any complications. We found that the proximal occlusion technique was much easier to perform than the distal occluion technique. The present technique appears to offer a practical and useful procedure for treating internal carotid artery stenosis.

Key words: Angioplasty – Carotid artery, stenosis

Percutaneous transluminal angioplasty (PTA) has become a common procedure for the treatment of extremity and coronary arteries, and clinical evaluations have been attempted [1, 2]. This technique, however, has rarely been applied to stenosis of the internal carotid artery because of the resultant embolisation with debris following balloon manipulation. We report here a simple proximal occlusion technique employing a newly devised guiding catheter with a balloon, in order to prevent such complications of PTA when treating internal carotid artery stenosis.

Materials and methods

The principle of this technique is to occlude the common carotid artery with a latex balloon mounted on a 9 F guiding catheter during the PTA procedure. This usually gives rise to retrograde flow from the internal carotid artery, which carries debris away to the external carotid artery. Furthermore, this technique minimises any blood pressure-induced movement of the PTA balloon along the ulcerated vessel wall and the formation of debris.

The new 9 F polyethylene catheter used is illustrated in Fig. 1. A latex balloon (11 mm in external diameter) was attached. This was made on an experimental basis. To keep the interior of the whole catheter large, CO_2 gas was employed to inflate the balloon. In addition, a PTA balloon 6 mm in diameter and 2 cm in length with a 3.5 F shaft was manufactured.

The operation was carried out according to Seldinger's method in every case, We gave 3000 U heparin systemically, and the guiding catheter with the balloon was inserted near to the stenosis, into the common carotid artery. Blood flow was shut off for 10 min under

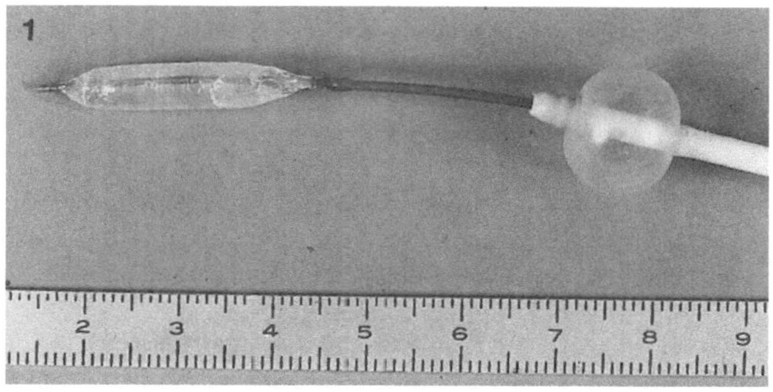

Fig. 1. The new 9 F polyethylene catheter used in this study. A latex balloon (11 mm external diameter) is attached. To keep the inside of the catheter large, CO_2 gas was employed to inflate the balloon. In addition, a PTA balloon 6 mm in diameter and 2 cm in length with a 3.5 F shaft was manufactured

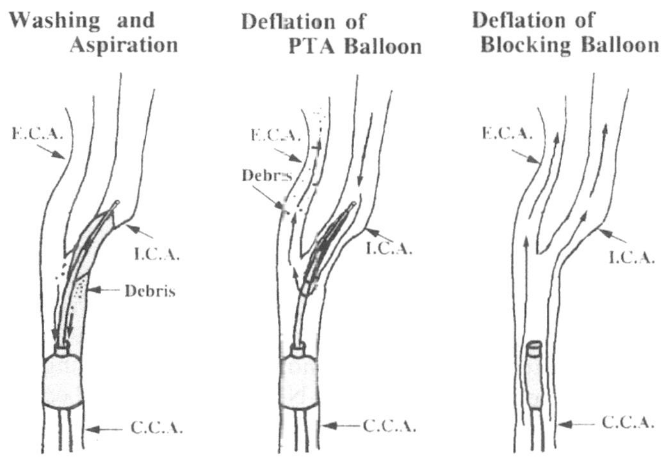

Fig. 2. First, the proximal portion of the artery was shut off with the guiding catheter and balloon. The PTA catheter was inserted into the stenosis site, and PTA was performed. Before deflation of the PTA balloon, debris was washed and aspirated with physiological saline solution through the balloon guiding catheter. After this debris had been washed out, the PTA ballcon was deflated. By utilising the back-flow of blood, all remaining debris was flushed into the external arterial system, and occlusion by the balloon was then terminated. *ICA,* Internal carotid artery; *ECA,* external carotid artery; *CCA,* common carotid artery

Correspondence to: T. Hirayama

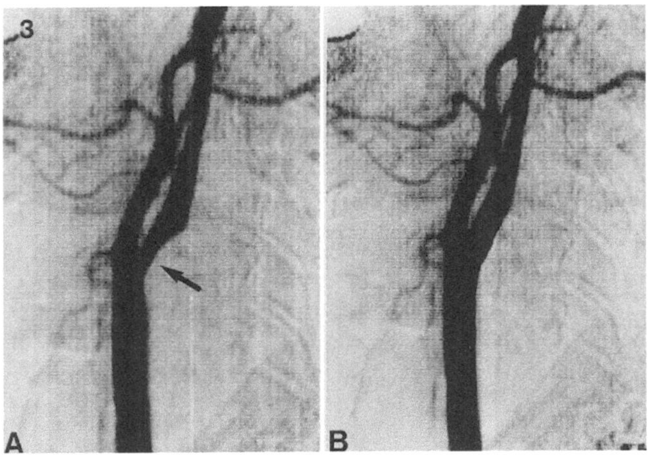

Fig. 3. Subtotal occlusion of the right internal carotid artery before (**A**) and after (**B**) PTA

electroencephalographic monitoring. After confirmation of no abnormal neurological findings and no changes in the electroencephalogram, PTA was performed. In addition, it was confirmed before the PTA procedure that slow injection of contrast medium through the guiding catheter demonstrated retrograde flow from the internal carotid artery.

First, the proximal portion of the artery was shut off with the guiding catheter and balloon (Fig. 2). The PTA catheter was then inserted into the stenosis, and PTA was performed. Before deflation of the PTA balloon, the guiding catheter with the balloon was washed with physiological saline solution introduced from its open end. After debris had been washed out, the PTA balloon was deflated. By utilising the back-flow of blood, all remaining debris was flushed into the external arterial system, and the occlusion by the balloon was then terminated (Fig. 2).

Results

We treated 18 cases of carotid stenosis ranging between 50 and 85%. The normal vessel calibre was restored in 11 cases. In the other 7 subjects, post-PTA angiography demonstrated a residual stenosis, but not exceeding 10% of the prestenotic lumen. No complications occurred during or after the PTA procedures. We found that the proximal occlusion technique was much easier than the distal occlusion technique.

A typical case is described. A 57-year-old man, who suffered from transient left hemiparesis from about May 1991 onwards, was given a platelet antiaggregant (100 mg aspirin daily). Since 70% stenosis was observed in the right carotid on preoperative angiography, PTA was performed employing the guiding catheter with occlusion balloon described above. Following the PTA, the stenosis mostly disappeared, and no complications were encountered (Fig. 3).

Discussion

In a previous PTA technique, prevention of debris scattering was accomplished by occlusion of the distal part of the stenosis [3]. With such a technique, however, an occlusion balloon catheter should be inserted distal to the stenotic lesion, in addition to a PTA balloon catheter. This procedure may release plaque whilst ascending the catheter distal to the lesion, and may not be effective for preventing cerebral embolisation. We believe that our simple proximal occlusion technique, with a newly devised guiding catheter and occlusion balloon, may offer several advantages, as follows.

There is no need to site the blocking balloon in the distal part of the stenosis site. Debris is therefore not flushed into the peripheral region at the time of insertion of the blocking balloon. Since blood flow is shut off with the blocking balloon in advance, flow of debris into the peripheral region can be avoided by utilising the back-flow at the time of insertion of the PTA balloon into the stenosis site. At the time of inflation or deflation of the PTA balloon, flow of debris into the peripheral region can be avoided by utilising the blood back-flow. Since blood flow is shut off by the blocking balloon, migration of the PTA balloon with blood flow can be prevented.

References

1. Gruentig AR, King SB, Schlumpf M, Siegenthaler W (1987) Long-term follow-up after percutaneous transluminal coronary angioplasty: the early Zurich experience. N Engl J Med 316:1127–1132
2. Whitaker SC, Gregson RH (1991) Case report: occlusion of subclavian artery treated by percutaneous angioplasty. Clin Radiol 44:199–200
3. Theron J, Raymond J, Casasco A, Courtheoux F (1987) Percutaneous angioplasty of atherosurgical stenosis of carotid arteries. AJNR 8:495–500

Percutaneous transluminal angioplasty of extra- and intracranial cerebral vascular disease

R. T. Higashida[1], F. Y. Tsai[2], Van V. Halbach[1], C. F. Dowd[1], D. Larsen[1], C. McDougall[1], J. M. Higashida[1], G. B. Hieshima[1]

[1] Departments of Radiology and Neurological Surgery, Interventional Neurovascular Radiology Division, University of California, San Francisco Medical Center, San Francisco, CA 94143-0628, USA
[2] Department of Radiology, Truman Medical Center, Kansas City, MO 64108, USA

Abstract. Cerebral percutaneous transluminal angioplasty (PTA) is being performed with increasing frequency in patients with angiographically documented stenosis of greater than 70%, who are symptomatic and are not good candidates for surgical endarterectomy. The initial reports of cerebral PTA were described in the early 1980s. Over the past decade, with the development of microballoons and guidewires which have allowed the interventional neuroradiologists safer access to the head and neck vessels, more centers have been performing angioplasty for both extra- and intracranial lesions including atherosclerosis, fibromuscular dysplasia, ateritis, vessel dissection, and postsurgical intimal hyperplasia. We report our experience in treating 274 patients with stenosis of the brachiocephalic vessels treated by balloon angioplasty techniques.

Key words: Cerebral angioplasty – Stroke treatment – Balloon angioplasty – Interventional neuroradiology

Methods

All patients were examined by a neurologist or internist, and initially managed by medical treatment including antiplatelet or anticoagulation medication, control of blood pressure, and screened by computed tomography or magnetic resonance imaging to document previous infarcts and areas of cortical ischemia [1, 2]. Only patients who continued to remain symptomatic in spite of medical therapy and who were not considered candidates for surgical revascularization procedures were treated by percutaneous transluminal angioplasty (PTA) techniques. Cerebral angiography was performed initially to document the lesion site, and to assess distal perfusion, cortical branch occlusions, and collateral circulation. Close radiographic assessment of the lesion was performed using rapid-sequence, high-resolution, magnification angiography, with reference markers to measure the diameter of the adjacent normal lumen as well as the stenotic segment. For extracranial lesions the balloon diameters utilized ranged from 3.0 to 10.0 mm and an over wire balloon catheter system was used, and for intracranial lesions, balloon diameters ranging from 2.0–4.5 mm, in 0.5 mm increments were used (Fig. 1). The balloon size chosen approximated the normal lumen diameter proximal to the lesion site [3].

Systemic anticoagulation by intravenous heparin, 70 U/kg, was given in all cases prior to crossing the lesion with the guidewire. The balloon was then gently navigated across the lesion under road mapping guidance, and the balloon was usually inflated to the maximum recommended pressure, ranging from 6 to 18 atmospheres, for 10–30 s. Close monitoring of the patient was performed

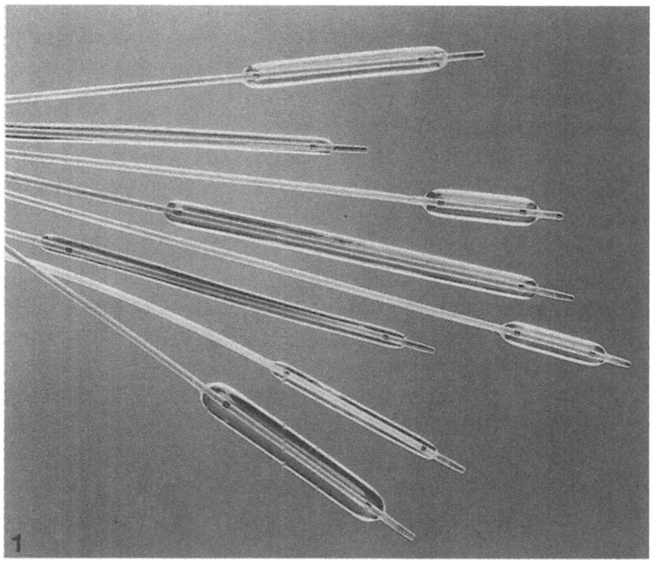

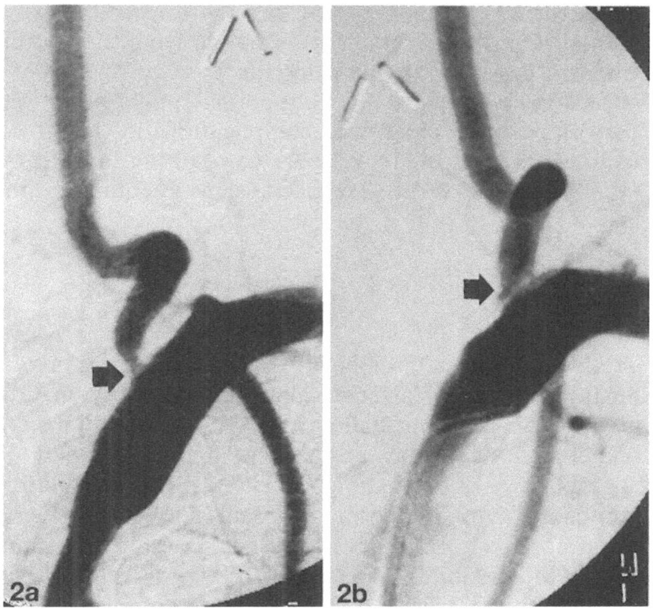

Fig. 1. Percutaneous transluminal angioplasty balloons, available in sizes from 2.0 to 10.0 mm in diameter, which can be inflated to 8–16 atmospheres of pressure

Fig. 2. a Left subclavian arteriogram, showing a high-grade stenosis of the proximal vertebral artery (*arrow*), in a patient with posterior cranial fossa ischaemia. **b** Following successful angioplasty with a 6.0 mm balloon, there is return to normal luminal diameter (*arrow*) with improved blood flow

Correspondence to: R. T. Higashida

throughout the procedure by a trained neurological specialist. Angiography was performed immediately after balloon dilatation and at 3–12 months to document continued patency at the angioplasty site. Patients were discharged on anti-platelet medications consisting of either aspirin, 5 grains/day, or dipyridamole, 50 mg/day, for a minimum of 6 months.

Results

A total of 274 patients, ranging in age from 9 to 78 years, were treated by PTA techniques. The majority were treated for atherosclerotic lesions, although some patients were treated for symptomatic fibromuscular dysplasia, arteritis, postsurgical intimal hyperplasia, and vessel dissection. In the anterior circulation, 125 patients were treated including the innominate artery in 7 cases, common carotid artery in 58 cases, external carotid artery in 11 cases, internal carotid artery in 42 cases, and the middle cerebral artery in 7 cases. In the posterior circulation a total of 149 procedures were performed including the subclavian artery in 102 cases, proximal vertebral artery in 36 cases, the distal intracranial vertebral artery in 8 cases, and the basilar artery in 3 cases (Fig. 2a, b). Complications associated with the procedure included 7 patients with stroke, 3 of whom died. There were 9 patients with transient cerebral ischemia occurring within 24 h of the procedure and which resolved with volume expansion, anticoagulation, and/or antispasmodic agents. Clinical and radiological follow-up ranged from 3 months to 7 years.

Of the 274 procedures, 256 were performed for extracranial stenosis with transient ischemic symptoms occurring in 5 cases (2.0%), restenosis in 15 cases (5.9%), and stroke in 1 case (0.4%). Intracranial angioplasty was performed in 18 cases, and complications in this group included 6 cases of stroke (33.3%) resulting in 3 deaths (16.7%) and 4 cases (22.2%) of transient cerebral ischemia [4].

Discussion

Treatment of hemodynamically significant lesions involving the cervical and intracranial vascular territory can now be approached using balloon angioplasty techniques to dilate stenotic lesions. Since the mid-1970s, balloon angioplasty has been shown to be effective for dilating lesions involving the coronary, renal, iliac, femoral, and distal popliteal areas. Several recent series have demonstrated the feasibility, safety, and long-term results utilizing balloon angioplasty techniques in the extracranial and intracranial territories [4–9]. Overall, these results have demonstrated a technical success rate of greater than 90%, with a less than 5% permanent morbidity and mortality rate. The best results for PTA have been those involving the proximal subclavian, cervical carotid, and proximal vertebral artery lesions. These vessels tend to have short, focal areas of stenosis, and can be accessed relatively easily with the newer PTA balloon devices now available for treating other vascular territories by these techniques.

The development of smaller PTA devices which are now available on 2 and 3 French microcatheters has allowed access to the intracranial circulation. However, angioplasty in this territory is more difficult due to the inherent tortuousity of these vessels, their smaller diameter, and the critical perforating branches that arise from the distal vertebral, basilar, and middle cerebral arteries. Occlusion of one of these critical perforating branches may lead to a devastating stroke involving the spinal cord, brain-stem, or basal ganglia. Other potential complications include vessel rupture, stroke, dissection, thromboemboli, and restenosis.

Thus far, the results of PTA for stenosis of the brachiocephalic territory appear encouraging and technically feasible. As more experience is gained in these techniques, the safety, efficacy, and long-term results of cerebral angioplasty will be further elucidated.

References

1. Marshall J (1989) Clinical aspects of stroke. In: Fisher M (ed) Medical therapy of acute stroke. Decker, New York, pp 1–11
2. Inoue Y, Takemoto K, Miyamoto T, et al (1980) Sequential computed tomography scans in acute cerebral infarction. Radiology 135:655–662
3. Tsai FY, Hieshima GB, Higashida RT (1989) Percutaneous transluminal angioplasty for the treatment of stroke. In: Fisher M (ed) Medical therapy of acute stroke. Dekker, New York, pp 203–239
4. Higashida RT, Tsai FY, Halbach VV, Dowd CF, Hieshima GB (1993) Cerebral percutaneous transluminal angioplasty. J Heart Dis Stroke 2:497–502
5. Théron J (1992) Angioplasty of brachiocephalic vessels. In Viñuela F, Halbach VV, Dion JE (eds) Interventional neuroradiology: endovascular therapy of the central nervous system. Raven Press, New York, pp 167–180
6. Higashida RT, Tsai FY, Halbach VV, Dowd CF, Smith T, Fraser K, Hieshima GB (1993) Transluminal angioplasty for atherosclerotic disease of the vertebral and basilar arteries. J Neurosurg 78:192–198
7. Tsai FY, Higashida RT, Matovich V, et al (1991) Seven years experience with percutaneous transluminal angioplasty for carotid stenosis. Neuroradiology 33:397–398
8. Tsai FY, Matovich V, Hieshima G, et al (1986) Percutaneous transluminal angioplasty of the carotid artery. AJNR 7:349–358
9. Higashida RT, Halbach VV, Dowd CF, et al (1993) Endovascular management of acute carotid artery dissection. Surg Cereb Stroke 21:407–412

Percutaneous transluminal angioplasty for arteriosclerotic lesions of extra- and intracranial arteries

T. Mori, K. Mori, M. Arisawa, M. Fukuoka, S. Honda

Department of Neurosurgery, Kochi Medical School, Kohasa, Okoh-chyo, Nankoku-city, Kochi, 783 Japan

Abstract. A total of 60 lesions, involving the extracranial artery in 32 cases and the intracranial artery in 28 cases, were treated by percutaneous transluminal angioplasty (PTA). Angiographic follow-up was performed 3 months after successful PTA. Forty-nine of 60 lesions were adequately dilated. The technical success rate was 81.7% (49/60). Complications occurred in 3 patients undergoing intracranial angioplasty. The procedural morbidity rate was 5.0% (3/60). The angiographic restenosis rate at 3 months was 20.4% (10/49). Although PTA is an effective alternative to reconstructive vascular surgery for the supra-aortic artery, intracranial PTA may be more often followed by complications. It is a new problem to determine whether a patient with asymptomatic angiographic restenosis 3 months after PTA should undergo repeat PTA or other revascularization therapy.

Key words: Angioplasty - Extracranial arteries - Intracranial arteries

Percutaneous transluminal angioplasty (PTA) may currently be a treatment of choice for supra-aortic arteriosclerotic lesions [1–3]. Although the development of microballoon catheter technology could make PTA possibly applicable to intracranial [4–6] as well as to extracranial arteriosclerotic lesions, some problems associated with PTA of the supra-aortic arteries remain unsolved. Although the long-term efficacy after PTA is limited by restenosis, the incidence of restenosis after successful PTA is uncertain.

Patients and methods

In patients with transient ischaemic attacks (TIAs) or a history of minor stroke more than 2 weeks old, we treated a total of 60 lesions by PTA between January 1991 and December 1993. The lesions involved the subclavian artery in 5 cases, the proximal vertebral artery (VA) in 7 cases, the intermediate VA in 1, the distal (intracranial) VA in 3, the posterior cerebral artery in 2, the ostium of the left common carotid artery in 2 s, the external carotid artery in 1, the proximal internal carotid artery in 14, the diatal internal carotid artery in 8, the middle cerebral artery (MCA) in 16 and the basilar artery in 1. Angiographic follow-up was performed 3 months after successful PTA. This study did not include patients suffering from acute ischaemic stroke. Therefore, the purpose of performing PTA in this study was a prophylactic treatment to prevent a major stroke.

Correspondence to: T. Mori

Angioplasty procedure. Low-molecular weight dextran was given by intravenous infusion starting 1 h before the procedure. PTA was performed by the percutaneous transfemoral approach. Heparin (10,000 U) was administered to prevent thrombus formation during the procedure. After administration of isosorbide dinitrate (2.5 mg) to prevent catheter-induced vasospasm, a guidewire was inserted to the target vessel. Following confirmation of correct and distal wire positioning by contrast injections, a balloon catheter was advanced over the wire and across the lesion. Inflations of 60 s duration, at pressures ranging from 6 to 8 atm for the extracranial artery and from 4 to 6 atm for the intracranial artery, were routinely performed over the lesion.

Definition of successful angioplasty. Modifying the recommendations of the ISFC/WHO Task Force [7] for coronary angioplasty, a successful PTA was defined as: an absence of major complications, including death or permanent neurological deficits; a 50% or greater pre-PTA stenosis diameter reduced to less than 50% immediately after PTA; and a change of at least 20% from initial to post-PTA stenosis diameter.

Definition of restenosis. According to the recommendations of the ISFC/WHO Task Force for coronary angioplasty, restenosis was defined as a 50% or greater stenosis at follow-up, despite an immediate post-PTA stenosis diameter of less than 50%.

Angiographic follow-up. Patients were observed every month at outpatient clinics for general and neurological symptoms. Because invasive examination involves procedural risks and high costs, the authors used the experience of percutaneous transluminal coronary angioplasty (PTCA). They suggested that the most important time may be approximately 3 months after PTCA [8], and performed initial angiographic follow-up 3 months after successful PTA [9] in order to investigate angiographic morphological changes. If restenosis, ranging from a $\geq 50\%$ to $\leq 70\%$ stenosis diameter, a second angiographic follow-up was performed a further 3 months later, namely 6 months after PTA. If restenosis did not occur at 3 months, a second angiographic follow-up was performed 12 months after PTA.

Results

Successful and unsuccessful PTA

Forty-nine of 60 lesions were successfully and adequately dilated (Fig. 1). Eleven unsuccessful cases included 2 lesions of total occlusion > 3 months old, 1 ostial lesion, 2 lesions with excessive tortuosity of the proximal segment, 3 lesions with heavy calcification, and 3 complications. The technical success rate was 81.7%. Because complications occurred in 1 patient undergoing PTA of the distal carotid artery (dissection) and 2 patients undergoing PTA of the MCA (1 aprupt closure and 1 vessel rupture), the procedural morbidity rate was 5.0% (3/60).

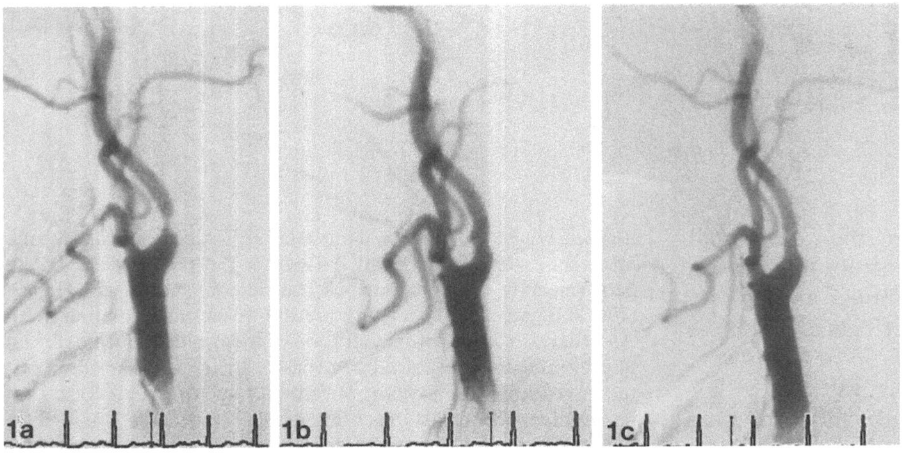

Fig. 1. Right carotid angiogram, demonstrating a lesion of the internal carotid artery before (**a**), immediately after (**b**) and 3 months after (**c**) percutaneous transluminal angioplasty

Angiographic restenosis

Restenosis occurred in 10 out of 49 lesions at 3 months. The restenosis rate at 3 months was 20.4%. Restenosis occurred in 1 left common carotid artery lesion, 2 of 7 proximal VA lesions, 1 of 11 proximal internal carotid artery lesions, 2 of 5 distal internal carotid artery lesions, and 4 of 14 MCA lesions.

Repeat PTA

Nine patients underwent repeat PTA at 3 months, 1 patient at 6 months.

Discussion

We found that complications might occur more often in patients undergoing intracranial PTA, and that restenosis occurred in 20.4% of patients at 3 months.

Although a restenosis rate ranging from 20% to 50% after successful coronary angioplasty (PTCA) has been reported, PTCA is now widely accepted as a revascularization procedure for the coronary artery. Therefore, the incidence of restenosis after successful PTA cannot interfere with application of an angioplasty procedure to the extracranial and intracranial artery.

Complications occurred in patients undergoing intracranial PTA utilizing a Stealth balloon catheter. Dissection was associated with replacement of a valve wire. Balloon inflation at a pressure of 6 atm led to an intracranial vessel rupture. Because the Stealth balloon catheter requires a different technique from orthodox types, more information about the Stealth should be given (e.g. about balloon compliance).

Of 10 patients in whom restenosis occurred at 3 months, only 1 patient suffered a recurrence of TIA. This patient underwent repeat PTA. However, the other 9 patients did not experience a recurrence of neurological disorders, despite angiographic restenosis at 3 months. Consequently, all 9 patients without a recurrence of neurological disorders underwent repeat PTA. It is a new problem to determine whether a patient with asymptomatic restenosis should undergo invasive retreatments (i.e., repeat PTA or other revascularization surgery) or when these re-treatments should take place.

References

1. Tsai FY, Matovich V, Hieshima G, Shah DC, Mehringer CM, Tiu G, Higashida R, Pribram HF (1986) Percutaneous transluminal angioplasty of the carotid artery. AJNR 7:349–358
2. Kachel R, Basche ST, Heerklotz T, Grossman K, Endler S (1991) Percutaneous transluminal angioplasty (PTA) of supra-aortic arteries especially the internal carotid artery. Neuroradiology 33:191–194
3. Mori T, Arisawa M, Honda S, Fukuoka M, Mori K (1993) Percutaneous transluminal angioplasty of supra-aortic arterial stenoses in patients with comcomitant cerebrovascular and coronary artery disease. Neurol Med Chir (Tokyo) 33:368–372
4. Higashida RT, Tsai FY, Halbach VV, Dowd CF, Smith T, Fraser K, Hieshima GB (1993) Transluminal angioplasty for atherosclerotic disease of the vertebral and basilar arteries. J Neurosurg 78:192–198
5. Honda S, Mori T, Fukuoka M, Kajita K, Arisawa M, Nishimura T, Mori K (1994) Successful percutaneous transluminal angioplasty of the intracranial vertebral artery 1 month after total occlusion. Neurol Med Chir (Tokyo) 34:551–554
6. Ahja A, Guterman LR, Hopkins LN (1992) Angioplasty for basilar artery atherosclerosis. Case report. J Neurosurg 77:941–944
7. Bourassa M, Alderman EL, Bertrand M, Fuente LDL, Gratsianski A, Kaltenbach M, King SB, Nobuyoshi M, Romaniuk P, Ryan TJ, Serryus PW, Smith HC, Sousa JE, Boethig S, Rapaport E (1988) Report of the joint ISFC/WHO task force on coronary angioplasty. Circulation 78:780–789
8. Nobuyoshi M, Kimura T, Nosaka H, Mioka S, Ueno K, Yokoi H, Hamasaki N, Horiuchi H, Ohishi H (1988) Restenosis after successful percutaneous transluminal coronary angioplasty: serial angiographic follow-up of 229 patients. J Am Coll Cardiol 12:616–623
9. Mori T, Arisawa M, Honda S, Fukuoka M, Kurisaka M, Mori K (1933) Three-month angiographic follow-up after successful percutaneous transluminal angioplasty (in Japanese). No Shinkei Geka 21:141–146

Stealth balloon angioplasty for intracranial atheromatous stenosis: Factors affecting clinical and angiographic outcome

M. Nelson, G. Bonsor, J. Straiton

Section of Neuroradiology, General Infirmary, Leeds LS1 3EX, UK

Abstract. We have treated three patients with a severe atheromatous stenosis in a proximal segment of an intracranial artery, using the Stealth balloon angioplasty system. Each presented with a haemodynami ischaemic syndrome which did not resolve with anticoagulation. All improved clinically and there was no new neurological deficit. The anatomy of the atheromatous stenosis appeared to determine the quality of the angiographic outcome. Oedema, haemorrhage or spasm in the artery wall caused by angioplasty and the proximity of perforating arteries are likely to be limiting factors in the application of angioplasty to atheromatous stenoses in smaller and more distal intracranial arteries.

Key words: Atheroma – Stenosis, intracranial artery – Balloon angioplasty

Balloon angioplasty is an effective technique for the treatment of extracranial atheromatous stenosis [1, 2]. Applied to patients who are considered high-risk for surgical endarterectomy, balloon angioplasty carries a low risk of neurological deficit [3]. Improved technologies, such as the Stealth balloon angioplasty system, permit treatment of more distal stenoses in smaller arteries, including intracranial lesions. However, there has been a relatively high incidence of neurological complications in the small number of patients who have had intracranial angioplasty for atheromatous stenosis in the basilar and middle cerebral arteries [4–6].

We believe the high risk of neurological deficit with intracranial angioplasty occurs when oedema, haemorrhage or spasm in the artery wall further impairs blood flow either by producing temporary lengthening of the stenosis or by obstructing adjacent perforator branches. For this reason, we have restricted the use of angioplasty to intracranial atheromatous stenoses in larger proximal arteries remote from perforator branches. We present three patients whose angiographic and clinical outcomes support our hypothesis.

Methods

We use neuroleptanalgesia to ensure patient comfort and immobility and to allow neurological examination during angioplasty. Hypovolaemia is avoided by an IV saline infusion of 1–2 before the procedure. Antithrombotic measures in all patients compromise aspirin (600 mg given 12 h and 1 h before the procedure) and heparin in a bolus dose of 5,000 U given immediately after placement of the coaxial catheter. Postangioplasty treatment where the stenosis was relieved comprised subcutaneous heparin (5,000 U 8-hourly for 3 weeks). Where there was haemodynamically significant residual stenosis, full anticoagulation was used for 3 months first with heparin, then warfarin, combined with a short course of high-dose dexamethasone and of nimodipine.

In each case, a coaxial catheter was placed as close as possible to the stenotic lesion without reducing flow. Stealth balloon size was the estimated diameter of the normal artery near the stenotic lesion. In one patient, predilatation with a smaller balloon was necessary before a balloon of the chosen size could be passed. On each occasion, the Stealth balloon catheter was introduced as far as the stenosis on either a Taper-14 or Dasher-10 guidewire, using a pressurised flush of heparinised saline to avoid blood contamination of the balloon valve seat. The guidewire was passed across the stenosis, followed by the full length of the balloon segment of the Stealth catheter. Then the guidewire was replaced with the Stealth valve wire, and the combination was drawn back to lie across the stenosis for the angioplasty. Two or three dilatations were made by hand injection for 15 s, each using sufficient force to produce complete balloon dilatation.

Case reports

Case 1 (Fig. 1)

A 73-year-old male arteriopath had a 20-year history of angina and an 8-year history of treated hypertension. Six years previously he had angioplasty for intermittent claudication in the left leg. In the 5 weeks before admission, he had five episodes of transient weakness affecting the right hand, each lasting approximately 5 min. In the 6 days before admission, he developed a progressive numbness of the right hand that spread to the neck and face, associated with weakness of the right arm and hand. Despite treatment with aspirin and full heparinisation, fluctuating weakness of the right arm and hand persisted. Angiograms showed a severe stenosis of the inferior limb of the left carotid siphon with an isolated left internal carotid supply to the left middle cerebral territory, caused by a grossly eccentric plaque.

Angioplasty with a 2.5-mm Stealth catheter failed to relieve the stenosis, though the lumen was slightly increased. The weakness of the right arm and hand were reduced immediately after the procedure and continued to improve for 2 months, by which time stable minimal residual weakness was present. The improvement was maintained to the latest clinical follow-up at 6 months.

Case 2 (Fig. 2)

A 48-year-old woman presented with a 4-month history of episodes of hemianaesthesia and weakness affecting the right face, arm leg and associated with dysphasia. Episodes lasting about 5 min had occurred on an approximately daily basis, with seven episodes of profound weakness lasting about 30 min. Some episodes had occurred while she was taking aspirin. Between attacks, neurological findings were normal.

Angiography showed a severe stenosis of the inferior limb of the left internal carotid siphon, with an isolated supply to the left anterior and middle cerebral artery territories.

Correspondence to: M. Nelson

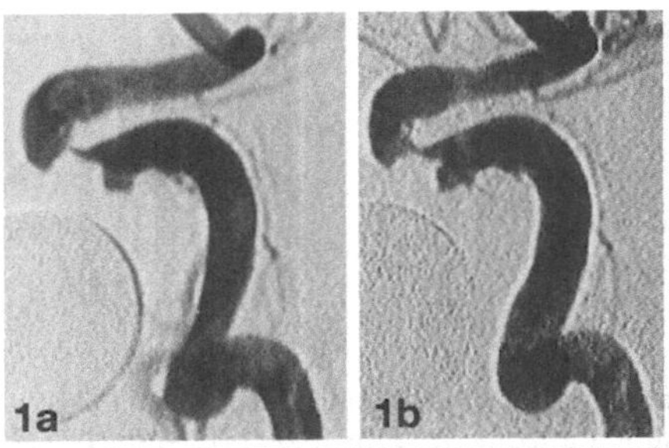

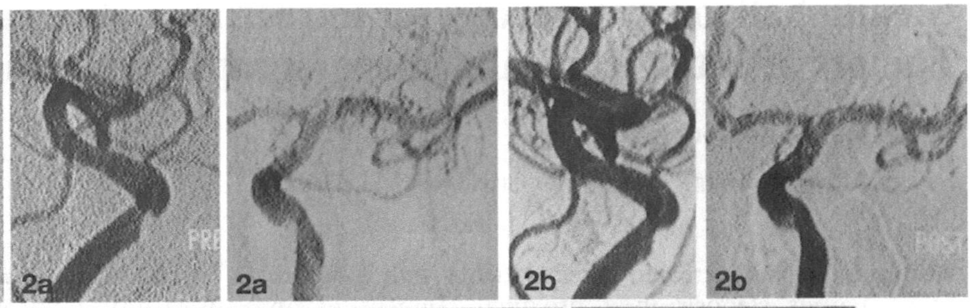

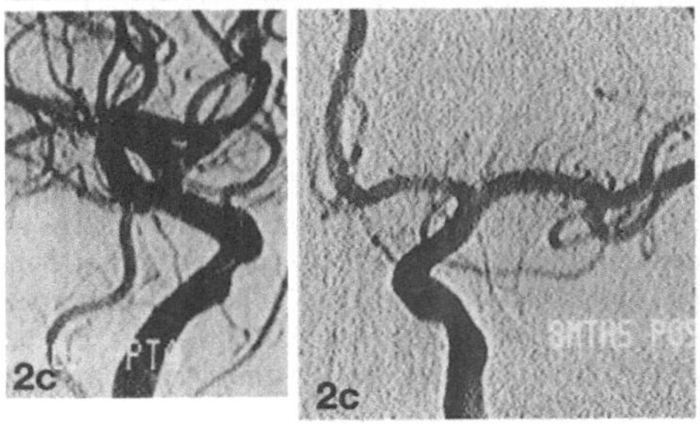

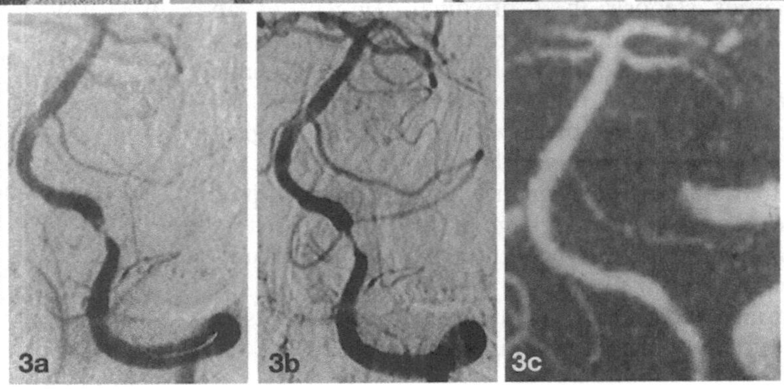

Fig. 1a, b. Case 1. **a** Left internal carotid angiogram shows grossly eccentric stenosis of inferior limb of the carotid siphon. **b** Angiogram immediately after third 2.5-mm Stealth balloon dilatation shows minimally improved lumen diameter with persisting severe stenosis. MRA at 2 months showed patency but did not resolve the lumen at the site of stenosis

Fig. 2a–c. Case 2. **a** Left carotid angiogram (lateral and posteroanterior shows severe stenosis of inferior limb of siphon. **b** Angiogram immediately after 3-mm Stealth angioplasty shows stenosis reduced to approximately 50%. **c** Angiogram at 8 months shows further remodelling, with a wider lumen and a haemodynamically insignificant residual stenosis. The improvement was maintained on MRA at 15 months

Fig. 3a–c. Case 3. **a** Left vertebral angiogram shows extreme stenosis of the intracranial segment. **b** Angiogram immediately after 3-mm Stealth angioplasty shows slightly increased lumen at the stenosis, with persisting severe stenosis, which is longer than previously. **c** MRA 29 months after angioplasty shows extensive remodelling, with no residual stenosis

Angioplasty to 3.0 mm reduced the stenosis to less than 50%. The episodes of hemianaesthesia, hemiparesis and dysphasia resolved. The patient continued to experience episodes of numbness in the right arm and hand, lasting a few seconds only at invervals of about 1 week. There was further remodelling at 8 months, with a haemodynamically insignificant residual stenosis. The improvement was maintained on magnetic resonance angiography (MRA) at 15 months. At the latest clinical follow-up at 21 months, the patient's symptoms were unchanged.

Case 3 (Fig. 3)

A 64-year-old man gave a history of completed stroke causing a left homonymous inferior quadrantanopia, treated with daily aspirin. Subsequently, he experienced transient episodes of visual blurring affecting the entire visual field and, separately, several episodes of transient global amnesia. He was admitted after a 10-day period in which he experienced severe headache and fluctuating constriction of the visual field. He had become inattentive, forgetful and vague. On examination he was dyshasic and disorientated in time and space. He performed poorly on tests of short- and long-term memory. Angiography showed a severe stenosis of the intracranial segment of the left vertebral artery, with an isolated left vertebral supply to the basilar artery and both posterior cerebral arteries.

Angioplasty to 3 mm caused an extensive local reaction in the artery wall. The stenosis was slightly reduced, though a severe degree of stenosis remained. The length of stenosis remained. The length of stenosis increased. Induced hypertension was required to maintain flow across the residual stenosis. On this regime there was resolution of the severe headache and of the fluctuating visual field constriction. Within 24 h the patient became alert and oriented in time and space, with improved memory. Hypertensive-hypervolaemic support was withdrawn gradually within 3 days. There was no new neurological deficit at the time of angioplasty or thereafter. At 4 months, there was some restoration of vision peripherally in the previously fixed quadrantanopia. MRA at 29 months showed no residual stenosis. At the latest clinical follow-up at 33 months there has been no new neurological problem, although the patient is now receiving treatment for angina.

Discussion

In all three patients, the atheromatous stenoses situated in proximal intracranial arteries were readily accessed, crossed and dilated using the Stealth system.

The outcome, judged angiographically, was determined by the anatomy of the atheromatous stenosis. Where there was a grossly eccentric stenosis (case 1), the morphological result of the angioplasty was poor and haemodynamically insignificant. With a less eccentric stenosis (case 2), a better morphological and haemodynamically significant dilatation were achieved. With a tight symmetrical, concentric stenosis (case 3), the acute angioplasty response in the artery wall caused temporary lengthening of the stenosis, after which there was late remodelling to a good morphological result, with no haemodynamically significant residual stenosis.

Symptoms of haemodynamic origin were relieved where the degree of stenosis was reduced. Despite suboptimal early angiographic outcomes in two of the three patients, no new neurological deficit occurred.

We think two factors account for the absence of new neurological deficits despite the angiographically suboptimal immediate results of angioplasty in our patients. First, it was possible to maintain perfusion despite persisting stenosis, using induced hypertension and hypervolaemia until intramural oedema, heamorrhage and spasm had resolved. Second, there were no perforating arteries near the treated stenoses. We believe these two factors account for the higher instance of new neurological deficits complicating angioplasty in smaller and more distal intracranial arteries.

References

1. Higashida RT, Tsai FY, Halbach VV, Heishima GB, Dowd CF, Barnwell SL (1991) Percutaneous transluminal angioplasty of the subclavian, vertebral and basilar arteries: technical considerations. Neuroradiology 33 [Suppl]: 394–396
2. Tsai FY, Higashida R, Matovich V, Alfieri K, Kobayashi (1991) Seven years' experience with percutaneous transluminal angioplasty for carotid stenosis. Neuroradiology 33 [Suppl]: 397–398
3. Kachel R, Basche St, Heerklotz I, Grossmann K, Endler S (1991) Percutaneous transluminal angioplasty (PTA) of supra-aortic arteries especially the internal carotid artery. Neuroradiology 33:191–194
4. Sundt TM, Smith HC, Campbell JK, Vlietstra RE, Cucchiara RF, Stanson AW (1980) Transluminal angioplasty for basilar artery stenosis. Mayo Clin Proc 55:673–680
5. Higashida RT, Hieshima GB, Tsai FY, Halbach VV, Norman D, Newton TH (1987) Transluminal angioplasty of the vertebral and basilar artery. AJNR 8:745–749
6. Purdy PD, Devous MD, Unwin DH, Giller CA, Batjer HH (1990) Angioplasty of an atherosclerotic middle cerebral artery associated with improvement in regional cerebral blood flow. AJNR 11:878–880

Percutaneous transluminal angioplasty of the carotid artery: clinical outcome and follow-up

H. Yokote[1], T. Terada[2], Y. Nakamura[2], H. Tsuura[2], Y. Kinoshita[2], R. Takehara[2], R. Nakai[2], K. Nakai[2], T. Nishiguchi[1], S. Hayashi[2], T. Itakura[2], N. Komai[2]

[1] Department of Neurosurgery, Hashimoto Municipal Hospital, Wakayama, Japan
[2] Department of Neurological Surgery, Wakayama Medical College, Wakayama, Japan

Abstract. We present our experience with 20 patients in whom percutaneous transluminal angioplasty (PTA) was performed in 23 stenotic carotid arteries. We used an angioplasty technique involving temporary distal balloon occlusion of the internal carotid artery to prevent cerebral embolism during carotid angioplasty. This distal occlusive technique was applied to 10 irregular and ulcerated stenotic lesions. To detect distal embolism related to PTA, magnetic resonance imaging (MRI) was performed in 16 cases (19 lesions) before and after angioplasty. Twenty-one stenotic lesions were successfully dilated. Two lesions were insufficiently dilated. No distal embolism was detected by MRI in 6 cases (9 lesions) with the distally occlusive balloon system. However, new cerebral infarctions possibly related to PTA were detected by MRI in 4 of ten cases (10 lesions) without the distal occlusive balloon system. The infarctions were not associated with any new neurological deficits. During follow-up observation of 1–38 months (average 14 months), 2 patients died of acute myocardial infarction and 4 patients developed restenoses. Three months after PTA, carotid artery stenosis can be treated safely and effectively by PTA. In addition, the distal internal carotid occlusive balloon technique may help prevent PTA-related cerebral embolisation.

Key words: Percutaneous transluminal angioplasty – Carotid artery – Embolism – Protective balloon

Percutaneous transluminal angioplasty (PTA) has been increasingly applied to supra-aortic arteries. However, cerebral embolisation during the procedure is still a serious potential risk. We performed carotid angioplasty utilising temporary balloon occlusion of the distal internal carotid artery (ICA) to prevent this complication. We report our experiences with PTA of the carotid artery.

Patients and methods

We have carried out PTA on 20 patients with 23 stenotic lesions of the ICA and common carotid artery. There were 17 men and 3 women, and the age range was from 52 to 77 years (average 67 years). Six patients presented with transient ischaemic attacks, and 14 presented with minor or major strokes. All stenoses were atherosclerotic. A distal ICA balloon occlusion technique was used during PTA of 10 stenotic lesions showing irregular luminal narrowing and ulceration. Haemodynamic ischaemia was the most common indi-

Correspondence to: H. Yokote, 1-3-8, Touge, Hashimoto City, Wakayama, Japan, 648

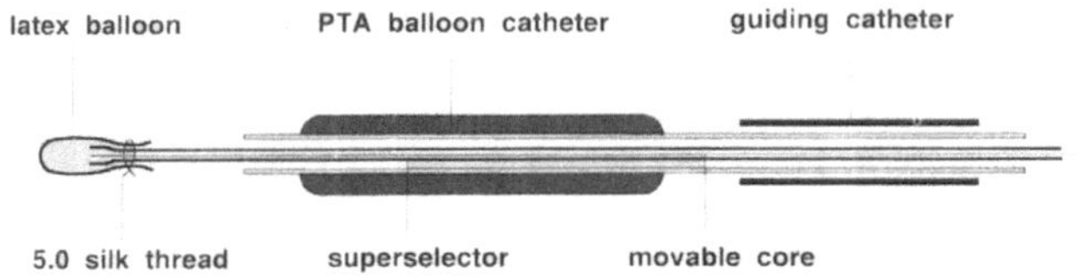

Fig. 1. Diagram of our PTA catheter with distal occlusive balloon. A latex balloon, used as an occlusive balloon, is attached to the top of an infusion-type superselector with a silk thread. A moveable core inserted into the lumen of the superselector gives torque control. An Accent or ultra-thin balloon is used as a PTA balloon catheter

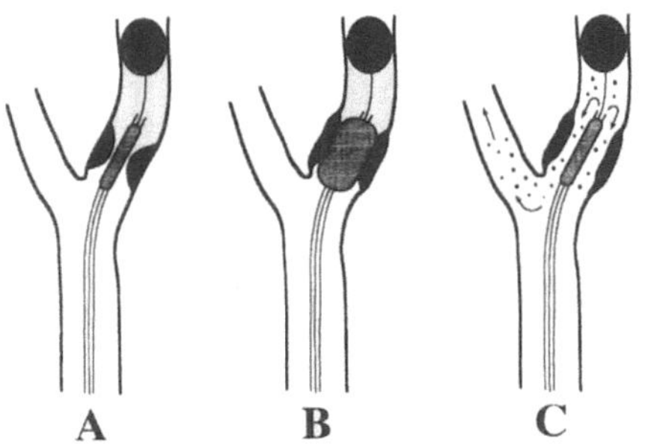

Fig. 2A–C. Diagram of PTA procedure with distal occlusive balloon system. **A** An occlusive balloon is inflated in the internal carotid artery, distal to the stenotic segment, after a PTA balloon has been positioned at the stenosis. **B** A PTA balloon is inflated. **C** The PTA balloon is deflated, while the distal occlusive balloon remains inflated. Potential emboli from the atheromatous plaque are flushed into the external carotid artery by injecting saline through the lumen around the infusion guidewire

cation. Plaque ulceration was not considered to be a contraindication to PTA. PTA was performed for surgically inaccessible stenoses and, in high-risk patients, for surgical endarterectomy (e.g. bilateral ICA stenoses, ischaemic heart disease or severe hypertension).

The balloon system is illustrated in Fig. 1. A latex balloon, which was used for distal ICA occlusion, was attached with a 3-0 silk suture to the distal tip of a 0.035″ superselector, infusion-type guidewire. A movable core inserted into the infusion guidewire afforded the system torque control. Accent or Ultra-thin PTA balloon catheter were used.

The procedure with our balloon system is shown in Fig. 2. A balloon was inflated in the ICA, distal to the stenotic vascular segment, after a PTA balloon was positioned and inflated at the stenotic site. Following a PTA balloon deflation, the distal occlusive balloon remained inflated. Any thrombus and atheromatous material from the plaque, trapped by the distal occlusive balloon, were flushed into the external carotid artery by injecting saline through the lumen around the infusion guidewire. After the distal occlusive balloon was deflated, the PTA balloon catheter together with the distal balloon were withdrawn. PTA required inflation pressures of 6–8 atm. Inflation times for PTA were 30 to 120 s. Two to three dilatations were usually required to treat the stenosis adequately. Angioplasty was carried out under systemic heparinization.

Before and after angioplasty, cerebral blood flow was examined by xenon-enhanced CT and/or SPECT and MRI was performed. All patients were given anti-platelet aggregants (200 mg ticlopidine/day) for 2 weeks prior to angioplasty. Each patient was heparinized (10,000–15,000 U i.v./day) for 1 week after the procedure. Follow-up angiography was performed at 1 week, 3 months, 6 months, and 1 year after angioplasty.

MRI was performed in 16 of 20 cases (19 lesions) before and after angioplasty, to assess for new cerebral infarcts, denoted by high signal intensity on T2-weighted images, possibly signifying PTA-related embolisation. In 6 of these 16 cases (9 lesions), the distal occlusive balloon system was used. In the remaining cases (10 lesions), no temporary distal occlusive balloon was used.

Results

Twenty-one of 23 stenotic lesions were successfully dilated. In 2 lesions residual stenoses > 50% were present, and these were considered to be insufficient dilatation. The distal occlusive balloon system was applied to 10 irregular and ulcerated stenotic lesions. MRI revealed no distal embolisation in 6 cases (9 lesions) in which a distal occlusive balloon system was used. However, new cerebral infarcts presenting as spotty high signal intensity foci, which might be related to PTA, were detected by MRI in 4 of 10 cases (10 lesions) not using the distal occlusive balloon system. These new cerebral infarctions did not cause any new neurological deficit. During a follow-up period of 1–38 months (average 14 months), 2 patients died of acute myocardial infarction and 4 patients had developed restenosis 3 months after PTA. Three of these were treated by surgical endarterectomy and 1 was successfully treated by repeat PTA. No major procedural complication occurred.

Representative Cases

Case 1. A 67-year-old man with a history of mild right hemiparesis was admitted to our hospital. An infarct in the left frontal watershed area was found on MRI. A left carotid angiogram showed ICA stenosis. PTA with distal occlusive balloon was performed. The stenosis was successfully dilated. A new infarct detected by T2-weighted MRI was not revealed. Follow-up angiography at 3 months demonstrated restenosis of the left ICA. Successful repeat PTA was then performed.

Case 2. A 69-year-old woman with a history of cerebral embolism was admitted to our hospital. High signal intensity in the area of the left frontal lobe was seen on T2-weighted imaging. A left carotid angiogram revealed moderate left ICA stenosis, with obvious ulceration suggesting the origin of cerebral embolism. Right carotid angiography showed severe right ICA stenosis. A cerebral blood flow study revealed impaired cerebrovascular reserve in both the right and the left hemispheres. Angioplasty without our distal occlusive balloon was performed on the right ICA stenosis, which was successfully dilated. MRI post-angioplasty showed no new right cerebral infarct. Restenosis had not been demonstrated within the 5 months following the procedure.

Discussion

Distal embolisation is a serious potential complication of PTA for supra-aortic arteries. We experienced 4 cases in which new infarcts occurred following angioplasty performed without the distal occlusive balloon system. However, no infarct was demonstrated in 6 cases in which the system was used. This suggests that our distal occlusive balloon system could prevent distal embolisation which might have occurred without our system. It is thought that PTA with no protection has a higher risk of distal embolisation than with protection. Carotid artery stenosis can be treated safely with PTA using the distal occlusive balloon technique.

Successful balloon angioplasty of postendarterectomy restenosis of the internal carotid artery

H. F. Kong[1], J. M. Bartoli[2], G. Moulin[2], M. Kasbarian[2]

[1] Department of Radiology, Shandong Province Hospital N° 1, 250021 Jinan, People's Republic of China
[2] Department of Radiology, Timone Hospital, C.H.U. Marseille, F-13385 Marseille, France

Recurrent stenosis >50% of the internal carotid artery after endarterectomy occurs in 13% [1] of cases. Its treatment usually involves surgical intervention, which is difficult for the surgeon. We report successful balloon dilatation of an internal carotid restenosis after endarterectomy.

Case report

A 71-year-old man, who had undergone endarterectomy of the left internal carotid for severe stenosis 10 years previously presented with a recent transient cerebral ischaemic attack. Echography showed a restenosis at the site of endarterectomy because of intima hyperplasia (thickened intima). No calcification or thrombus was observed in the left common and internal carotid arteries. Arteriography revealed a severe focal stenosis (>90%) of the left internal carotid artery about 1.5 cm from the bifurcation. The right carotid arteriogram, while compressing the left carotid, demonstrated that both cerebral arteries had opacified well. Dilatation was performed from a common femoral artery approach. The left common carotid artery was selected, a 6-F diagnostic catheter was advanced over the wire, and contrast medium was injected to confirm the intraluminal location. Then, a 0.035-in. floppy-tipped guidewire was used to cross the lesion. No antispasmodic agents were given prophylactically. The selective catheter was then exchanged for a 5-F catheter equipped with a 5-mm balloon to dilate the lesion. The balloon was inflated for approximately 5 s to a pressure sufficient to eliminate the "waist" in the balloon. The balloon catheter was then withdrawn to the common carotid and a further arteriogram was obtained, which showed successful dilatation. Satisfactory postdilatation flow in the left internal carotid artery was detected. A standard check of neurological status was carried out after the procedure. No neurological symptoms or signs were evident. After the procedure, the patient was given an oral antispasmodic (Fonzylane 300 mg/day) and an anti-aggregation agent (Tichid 500 mg/day). Follow-up was peformed with carotid Doppler sonography. Fifteen months after the dilatation, the patient is in good condition, and no recurrent stenosis has been seen on carotid arterography.

Discussion

The major technical surgical difficulty in the management of restenosis encountered during operative repair occurs when the common carotid bifurcation is dissected out from surrounding scar tissue. In addition to the difficulty of mobilising the artery from scar tissue and the jugular vein, the vague and hypoglossal nerves may be incorporated in the scar tissue, resulting in potential injury to these structures during reoperation.

Percutaneous transluminal angioplasty is, technically, a well-established treatment for a variety of arterial occlusions and stenoses. The best results and long-term clinical success are found in the vessels of high flow. However, the exact role of angioplasty in the carotid artery remains to be defined. Following the dilatation of innominate arteries, investigators extrapolated their results and concluded that proximal lesions in the carotid artery might be amenable to angioplasty [2, 3], but the thrombus from the atherosclerotic lesion always puts the cerebral arteries at risk.

The most frequent causes of recurrent stenosis or occlusion of the reconstructed carotid artery after operation are intimal and subintimal fibrosis and intimal hyperplasia at the distal end of the endarterectomy, which in pathology are different from atherosclerotic lesions. Thus, a low prevalence of stroke following angioplasty may certainly be expected. But the patient should be carefully examined before the procedure. Vascular echography and arterography are useful for verifying the absence of thrombus in the carotid. The contralateral carotid arterography, which involves compressing the carotid (stopping the flow), is necessary to observe the perfusion of the cerebral arteries to both hemispheres and the patient's clinical tolerance. Otherwise, the size of the balloon should be slightly smaller than the lumen of the dilated artery, to avoid irritating the carotid sinus. From our results, we think that angioplasty is feasible for postendarterectomy restenosis of the carotid artery.

References

1. Mattos MA, Hodgson KJ, Londrey GL, et al (1992) Carotid endarterectomy: operative risks, recurrent stenosis and long-term stroke rate in a modern series. J Cardiovasc Surg 33:387–400
2. Selby JB Jr, Matsumoto AH, Tegtmeyer CJ, et al (1993) Balloon angioplasty above the aortic arch: immediate and long-term results. AJR 160:631–635
3. Kachel R, Basche S, Heerklotz I, Grossmann K, Endler S (1991) Percutaneous transluminal angioplasty (PTA) of supra-aortic arteries, especially the internal carotid artery. Neuroradiology 33:191–194

Correspondence to: H. F. Kong

Local fibrinolysis in central retinal artery occlusion: follow-up in 36 cases

M. Schumacher[1], D. Schmidt[2]

[1] Department of Neuroradiology, University Clinic, Freiburg, Germany
[2] Eye Hospital, University Clinic, Freiburg, Germany

Abstract. Since central retinal artery occlusion treated conservatively has a poor prognosis, intra-arterial thrombolysis has been introduced. Fibrinolysis with urokinase or recombinant tissue plasminogen activator was carried out through a microcatheter placed supraselectively within the ophthalmic artery. Initially 29% of the patients showed a marked improvement or total recovery, and 37% partial recovery, with improvement of the visual acuity or a field defect. The worst results were obtained in those patients in whom there was a longer latency between the appearance of symptoms and initiation of treatment (34%). Long-term results, with a follow-up of 22–50 months, show a stable visual acuity except in those patients suffering from a deterioration caused by cataract. Local intra-arterial thrombolysis has a better outcome than conservative treatment. The best results can be achieved if at the beginning of the treatment there is slight, nonprogressive oedema of the central retina, good perfusion of the perimacular arterioles, few retinal emboli with some residual vision and if the patient is younger than 65 years of age and the interval between onset of symptoms and treatment is short.

Key words: Central retinal artery occlusion – Local intra-arterial fibrinolysis – Urokinase – Interventional neuroradiology

The prognosis of central retinal artery occlusion (CRAO) caused by an embolus or local thrombus is unfavourable. For several years it has been generally accepted, that patients with occlusion of the basilar artery benefit from intra-arterial fibrinolytic treatment [1, 2]. Since 1977 [3] several attempts have been made to treat CRAO with systemic fibrin-selective thrombolytic agents. Early studies [4–6] did not show a significant improvement in recanalisation and clinical outcome after systemical fibrinolysis. Additionally, systemic fibrinolysis can lead to cerebral haemorrhage, as has been observed following the administration of tissue plasminogen activator (TPA) [7]. To avoid those complications local intra-arterial fibrinolysis was carried out through a microcatheter placed in the proximal opthalmic artery.

Patients and methods

Since 1990, we have treated 35 patients with acute CRAO, mean age 65 years (range 45-87 years). Two additional patients were excluded because after treatment vasculitis was diagnosed. One patient has been treated twice. The diagnosis was made if the patient had acute visual loss of one eye and if ophthalmoscopically cherry-red-macular and/or cattle trucking could be observed. The diagnosis was additionally confirmed by a mancula oedema and in some patients also by hypoperfusion in fluorescein angiography. Exclusion criteria for fibrinolytic treatment were coagulopathies, stroke, myocardial infarction, vascular malformation, vasculitis, fixed arterial hypertension, surgery, trauma, bleeding or pregnancy within the first 12 weeks.

The technical procedure has been described before [8–10]. According to our initial concept of treatment the total amount of urokinase was not more than 1.2 Mio units in a maximum of 2 h followed by heparinisation for 2–3 days with 20000–25000 U/day. We treated 7 patients with TPA. In most patients, fluorescein angiography was performed before and after treatment to enable changes in retinal perfusion to be judged (Fig. 1).

Results

Significant return of visual auity may be expected if treatment is started during the first 10 h following CRAO. In all cases except one (Fig. 2), the opthalmic artery was not included in the thromboembolic CRAO. Regarding the clinical outcome after fibrinolysis, three groups can be distinguished: in group 1 (10/35) a distinct improvement of vision or complete recovery could be observed. In group 2 (13/35) a definite but less marked improvement could be seen. In some patients the visual field defect recovered more clearly than visual acuity (Fig. 3). In the third group (12/35) the worst results were obtained showing no or only slight improvement or even deterioration of vision in 2 patients. The results are summarised in Fig. 4.

In a small number of patients long-term results from 22 to 50 months (mean 38 months) after initial fibrinolysis, revealed a stable therapeutical effect in most patients. A slight deterioration in 5 patients was due to increasing cataract, except in one who had no cataract.

Complications after lysis occurred in 3 patients, 2 with thromboembolic occlusion of branches of the anterior cerebral artery and middle cerebral artery, which were also treaed by local intra-arterial fibrinolysis. There was no neurological deficit after complete recanalisation. One patient developed a local haematoma at the puncture site, which had to be removed.

Discussion

Compared with other treatment modalities, intra-arterial local fibrinolysis is more effective in CRAO, leading to distinct improvement in visual acuity and/or visual field defects in two-thirds of patients. As expected, different conditions can be discerned that point to a good or poor

Correspondence to: M. Schumacher, Sektion Neuroradiologie, Universitätsklinik Freiburg, Breisacher Strasse 64, D-79106 Freiburg, Germany

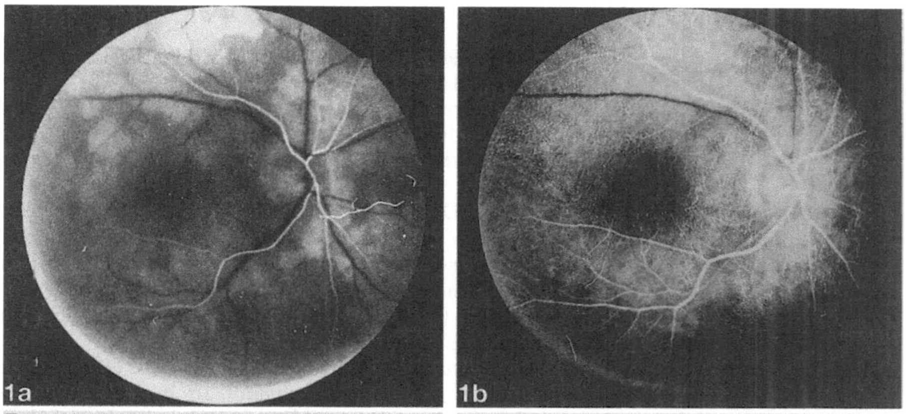

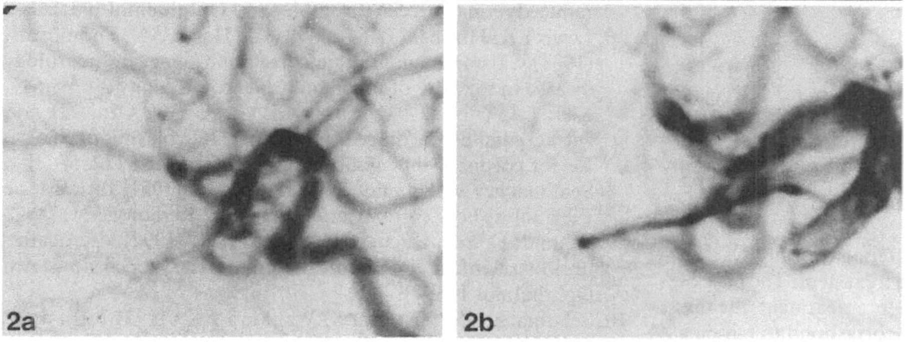

Fig. 1 a, b. Fluorescein angiogram of right eye: **a** 27.9 s after injection of contrast medium and after treatment with urokinase; **b** 27.6 s after injection. Reperfusion of the small retinal vessels

Fig. 2. a Right internal carotid angiogram showing reduced perfusion of the ophthalmic artery. **b** Reperfusion of the artery after treatment with urokinase

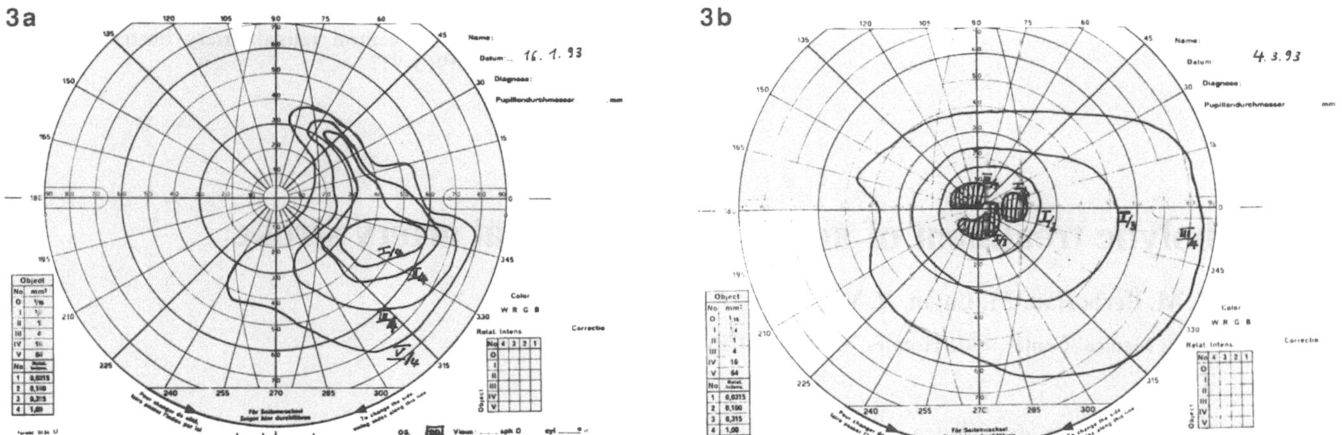

Fig. 3 a, b. Goldmann perimetry of the right eye: only temporal island for the biggest targets prior to treatment (**a**). Restitution of the nasal and central field with two small paracentral scotomas. Improvement visual acuity from hand movements to 20/50

clinical outcome. The prognosis is good if severe retinal oedema is not present and if initial visual acuity is at least better than perception of hand movements. Factors suggesting good changes for fibrinolysis are nonprogressive oedema, perfusion of the perimacular arterioles, no or few retinal emboli and patient's age less than 65 years. The interval between onset of symptoms and fibrinolysis plays a major role as known from treatment in the vertebrobasilar and carotid system. It is known that in monkeys the retina can tolerate up to 100 min of ischaemia [11]. In contrast to experimental results, experience in man has shown that CRAO is seldom complete [12]. Therefore therapy should be begun even after several hours, in order to achieve at least the essential blood supply of the peripheral retina. Although the best results were obtained in patients treated within the first 10 h, a definite time-window for fibrinolysis cannot be defined as yet. Since we have not observed any retinal haemorrhage within 4–60 h delay between of CRAO and treatment, the risk of bleeding can be regarded as low. Compared with other methods, including systemic thrombolysis, intra-arterial treatment seems to be more effective with an acceptable complication rate (5.5% transient neurological deficits).

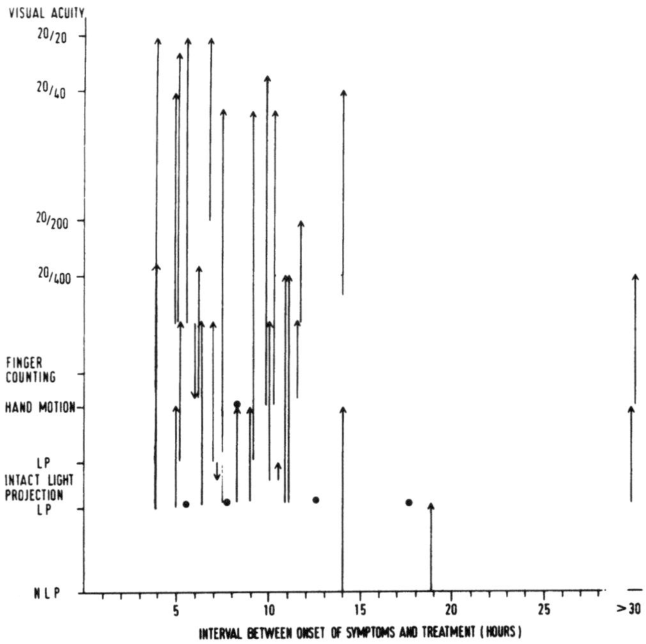

Fig. 4. Results in 35 patients after intra-arterial thrombolysis in relation to delay between onset of CRAO and treatment. The base of the *arrows* corresponds to the visual acuity before treatment, the tips to the outcome after fibrinolysis. The *circles* correspond to patients with no improvement

References

1. Sloan MA (1987) Thrombolysis and stroke. Past and future. Arch Neurol 44:748–768
2. Zeumer H, Freitag HJ, Grzyska U, Neunzig HP (1989) Local intra-arterial fibrinolysis in acute vertebrobasilar occlusion. Technical developments and recent results. Neuroradiology 31:336–340
3. Kwaan HC, Dobbie JG, Fethenhour CL (1977) The use of anticoagulants and thrombolytic agents in occlusive retinal vascular disease. In: Paoletti R, Sherry S (eds) Thrombosis and urokinase. Academic Press, London, pp 191–198
4. Rossmann H (1980) Treatment of retinal arterial occlusion. Ophthalmologica 180:68–74
5. Vine AK, Maguire PT, Martongi C, Kincaid MC (1988) Recombinant tissue plasminogen activator to lyse experimentally induced retinal arterial thrombi. Am J Ophthalmol 105:266–270
6. Lewis LK, Hinshaw DB Jr, Will AD, Hasso AN, Thompson JR (1988) CT and angiographic correlation of severe neurological disease in toxemia of pregnancy. Neuroradiology 30:59–64
7. Kase CS, O'Neal AM, Fisher M, Girgis GN, Ordia JI (1990) Intracranial hemorrhage after use of tissue plasminogen activator for coronary thrombolysis. Ann Intern Med 112:17–21
8. Schumacher M, Schmidt D, Wakhloo AK (1991) Intraarterielle Fibrinolyse bei Zentralarterienverschluß. Radiologe 31:240–243
9. Schmidt D, Schumacher M, Wakhloo AK (1992) Microcatheter urokinase infusion in central retinal artery occlusion. Am J Ophthalmol 113:429–434
10. Schumacher M, Schmidt S, Wakhloo AK (1993) Intra-arterial fibrinolytic therapy in central retinal artery occlusion. Neuroradiology 35:600–605
11. Hayreh SS, Colder HE, Weingeist TA (1980) Central retinal artery occlusion and retinal tolerance time. Ophthalmology 87:75–78
12. Augsburger JJ, Magargal LE (1980) Visual prognosis following treatment of acute central retinal artery obstruction. Br J Ophthalmol 64:913–917

Thrombolytic treatment of acute middle cerebral artery stroke

F. Y. Tsai, B. M. Berberian, M. Lavin, V. Matovich

UMKC – Truman Medical Center, 2301 Holmes, St. Kansas City, MO 64108, USA

Abstract. We report our experience with intra-arterial thrombolysis in 33 patients, combined with transluminal angioplasty.

Key words: Stroke – Thrombolysis – Urokinase – Middle cerebral artery thrombosis

The sequelae of untreated acute thrombosis of the middle cerebral artery (MCA) can be devastating. Although anticoagulation and systemic thrombolysis have been used to treat acute MCA stroke, the results have not been favorable [1–5]. Recently, intra-arterial thrombolysis has been used to treat patients with acute thrombosis of the MCA [6–11]. We report our experience using urokinase in 33 patients.

Methods

Thrombolysis was performed through a Tracker 18 catheter advanced to the occluded segment of the MCA utilizing a coaxial technique through a 5F catheter. The procedure for urokinase treatment was an intermittent injection of 80,000 IU over 2–3 min every 15 min following an initial dose of 250000 IU. All patients were given 3000 U heparin intravenously and an additional 1000 U hourly. Heparinization was not reversed after thrombolysis. Oral anticoagulation was continued for 3 months. Angioplasty was performed with a Stealth angioplastic catheter with balloon size 2 × 1,5 cm or 3 mm × 1.5 cm. Nitroglycerin 100 mg was given intra-arterially before a Stealth catheter was advanced to the stenosis [12].

Correspondence to: F. Y. Tsai

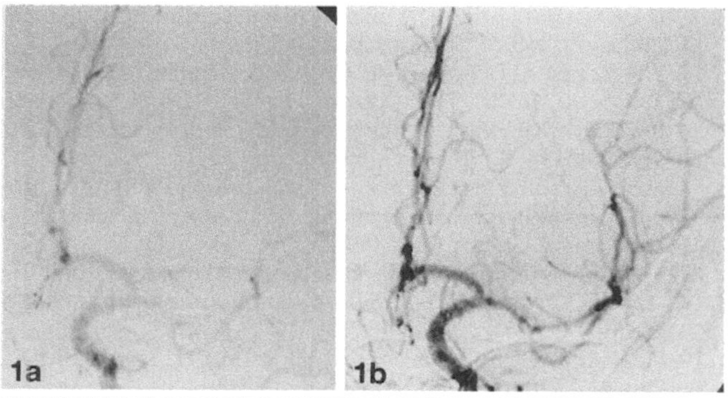

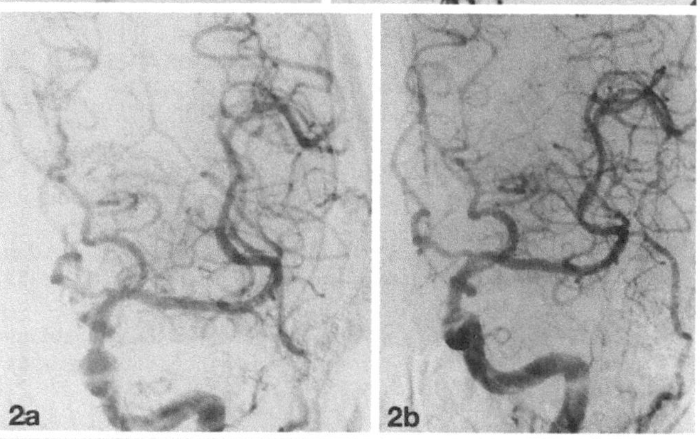

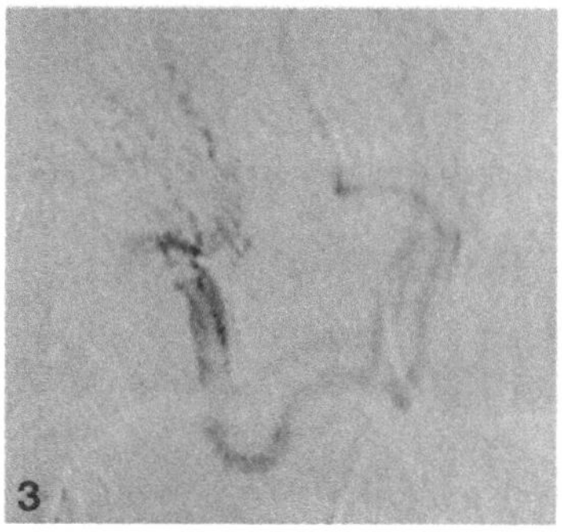

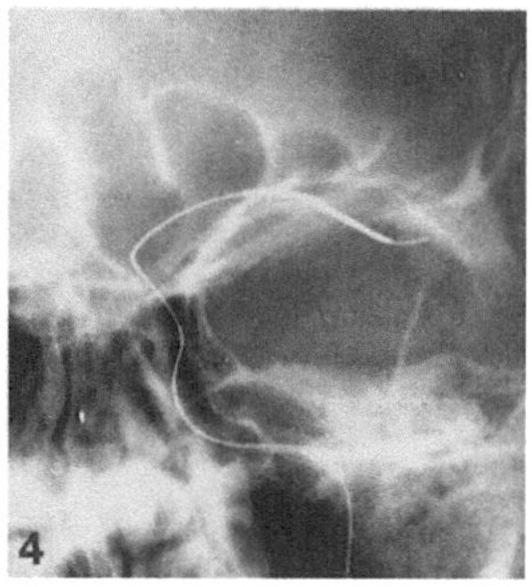

Fig. 1. a Left carotid angiogram showed occlusion of the proximal middle cerebral artery (MCA). **b** After thrombolysis, the MCA was open, but with stenosis of the distal trunk and proximal branches

Fig. 2. a Left carotid angiogram showed multiple thrombi in the anterior, middle and posterior cerebral arteries. The patient suddenly became unresponsive with right hemiparesis. **b** After thrombolysis with 250000 IU urokinase, the thrombi were completely dissolved

Fig. 3. Digital subtraction angiography of the MCA showed the tip of the catheter at the origin of a lenticulostriate artery

Fig. 4. Anteroposterior radiograph showed Stealth catheter in the left MCA during angioplasty

Results

Over the past 8 years, we have treated 33 patients with acute MCA occlusion. Of these, 16 were women and 17 were men. Their ages ranged from 42 to 67 years, with an average age of 54. Seven patients had hemorrhagic complications, of which 4 were small hemorrhages without clinical deterioration, but 3 were severe. Of these 3 patients, 2 died from massive hemorrhage and 1 had a poor recovery with complete left hemipareisis. In 2 patients, recanalization of the occluded vessels failed. Of the remaining 28 patients, 21 made a good to excellent recovery, but 7 showed only mild improvement.

Ten of the 33 patients had mild to severe stenosis (Fig. 1), and 5 patients had severe stenosis. Four rethrombosed immediately after the first thrombolytic treatment. Percutaneous transluminal angioplasty (PTA) was performed adjunct to the thrombolysis to preserve the success of thrombolysis. One patient did not receive a second thrombolytic treatment and PTA failed in another patient due to technical difficulty. The result was a massive left cerebral infarct in both patients. Although 2 of the patients who rethrombosed had a second successful thrombolysis and PTA, their recoveries were less complete than those who did not rethrombose. The fifth patient received PTA after initial thrombolysis.

The site of occlusion or thromboemboli may be divided into three groups: (a) proximal M_1 segment - 11 patients; (b) main trunk but distal to lenticulostriate artery - 14 patients; (c) proximal branch - 7 patients; (d) multiple sites due to angiographic complications - 1 patient (Fig. 2).

Discussion

Acute stroke from MCA occlusion may be the result of dislodging of thromboembolus from the heart or atherosclerotic carotid bifurcation stenosis [1–5]. Local intra-arterial thrombolysis has been more effective and safer for those patients with an acute onset of MCA occlusion than systemic treatment of thrombolysis. Thrombolysis with continuous infusion may be easier for physicians. However, it may not allow for the continuous monitoring of the progression of the thrombolytic treatment or monitoring of the tip of the catheter [6–11]. The tip of the catheter may migrate from the initial site of infusion. It may become lodged in an opening of the lenticulostriate arteries (Fig. 3). Overinfusion of urokinase may result, unless the tip of the catheter is checked periodically [9, 12]. This complication may be more prevalent with continuous infusion. Our three patients with massive hemorrhagic complications were treated with this technique. With intermittent injection, we are able to finish the treatment more quickly than with continuous infusion [6–11]. We believe the time lapse from the onset of symptoms is important for thrombolysis but the duration of thrombolysis should be a concern too. Both can delay reperfusion and lead to potential complications [9].

We found that the site of the occlusion has no bearing on the outcome of treatment. Occlusion of the MCA may be the result of dislodged thromboemboli from a carotid bifurcation or the heart, or the result of the propagation of thrombus locally from stenosis [12–14]. Rethrombosis may occur after initial thrombolysis and PTA may be performed as an adjunct to the thrombolysis to avoid rethrombosis [12, 13]. Since those patients who rethrombosed after thrombolysis did not recover as well as those who did not rethrombose, we believe PTA may be required to prevent rethrombosis in severe stenotic MCA

[8, 9, 12, 13]. We need more experience in evaluating the need for MRI before thrombolysis. The potential risk of thrombolytic treatment is hemorrhage, but it is not overwhelming. Thrombolytic treatment may be performed with reasonable safety to treat acute thromboembolism from arteriosclerosis or complications of angiography.

References

1. Adams HP, Damasio HC, Putman SF, Damasio AR (1983) Middle Cerebral artery occlusion as a cause of isolated subcortical infarction. Stroke 14:948–951
2. Taneda M, Shimada N, Tsuchiya T (1985) Transient neurological deficits due to embolic occlusion and reopening of the cerebral arteries. Stroke 16:522–524
3. Saito I, Serugawa H, Shiokawa S, Tsustsumi (1987) Middle cerebral artery occlusion: correlation of computed tomography and angiography with clinical outcome. Stroke 18:863–868
4. Bozzao L, Fantozzi LM, Bastianello S, Boassao A, Fieschi C (1989) Early collateral blood supply and late parenchymal brain damage in patients with middle cerebral artery occlusion. Stroke 20:735–740
5. Mohr JP, Gautier JC, Hier DB, Stein RW (1986) Middle cerebral artery. Stroke 1:377–450
6. Zeumer H, Hündgen R, Ferbert A, Ringelstein EB (1984) Local intra-arterial fibrinolytic therapy in inaccessible internal carotid occlusion. Neuroradiology 26:315–317
7. Del Zoppo GJ, Ferbert A, Otis S, Brückmann H, Hacke W, Zyroff J, Harker LA, Zeumer H (1988) Local intra-arterial fibrinolytic therapy in acute carotid territory stroke. Stroke 19:307–313
8. Mori E, Tabuchi M, Yoshida T, Yamadori A (1988) Intracarotid urokinase with thrombo-embolic occlusion of the middle cerebral artery. Stroke 19:802–812
9. Théron J, Courtheoux P, Casaco A, Alachkar F, Notari F, Ganem F, Maiza D (1989) Local intra-arterial fibrinolysis in carotid territory. AJNR 10:753–756
10. Siepmann G, Müller-Jensen M, Goossens H, Lachenmeyer L, Zeumer H (1991) Local intra-arterial fibrinolysis in acute middle cerebral artery occlusion. Neuroradiology 33:[Suppl]:69–71
11. Zeumer H, Freitag HJ, Grzyska U, Neunzig HP (1989) Local intra-arterial fibrinolysis in acute vertebrobasilar occlusion. Technical developments and recent results. Neuroradiology 31:336–340
12. Tsai FY, Lavin M, Matovich VB, Berberian BM, Alfieri KM. Percutaneous transluminal angioplasty adjunct to thrombolysis for acute MCA rethrombosis. AJNR (in press)
13. Bougousslavsky J, Barnett HJM, Fox AJ, et al (1986) Atherosclerotic disease of the middle cerebral artery. Stroke 17:1112–1120
14. Mandai K, Sueyoshi K, Fukunaga R, et al (1994) Acetazolamide challenge for three-dimension-time-of-flight MR angiography of the brain. AJNR 15:659–665

Local intra-arterial fibrinolysis in vertebrobasilar artery occlusion: urokinase versus recombinant tissue plasminogen activator

T. E. Mayer[1], M. Mull[2], H. Brückmann[1], A. Thron[2]

[1] Neuroradiologie, Medizinische Universität, Lübeck, Germany
[2] Neuroradiologie, Klinikum RWTH, Aachen, Germany

Abstract. From 1987 to 1994 local intra-arterial fibrinolysis was performed in 49 patients with occlusion of the vertebrobasilar system. Urokinase (13 patients) and high-dose recombinant tissue plasminogen activator (rTPA) (36 patients) was used in 25 patients semiselectively and in 24 patients with microcatheters at the thrombus side. Of all patients, 53% survived, 65% of them with good outcome. rTPA showed a better recanalisation rate than urokinase, when a microcatheter was used (81%). The superselective microcatheter procedure was superior to the proximal vertebral catheter treatment. The best results were obtained if the preceding coma lasted not longer than 3 h; of these 27 patients 63% survived, 76% of them with only minor deficits.

Key words: Fibrinolysis – Vertebrobasilar system

Correspondence to: T. E. Mayer

The natural history of acute vertebrobasilar occlusion is well known as being extremely bad [1]. Even with accompanying heparinisation and antiplatelet aggregation therapy 80–90% of the patients die [2]. Although no prospective controlled data exist, retrospective studies showed an improvement of the prognosis, up to 30% →

Fig. 1. Distribution of the level of consciousness in the urokinase and rTPA group (6 times as many comatose patients)

Fig. 2. Outcome related to catheter technique

Fig. 3. Recanalisation rate in comparison to technique and fibrinolytic agent

Fig. 4. Outcome according to fibrinolytic agent

Fig. 5. Outcome regarding recanalisation

Fig. 6. Good outcome and mortality as cumulative curve regarding time (impairment of consciousness)

Fig. 7. Outcome related to level of consciousness

Fig. 8. Relative outcome realted to time range of coma (stupor and somnolence)

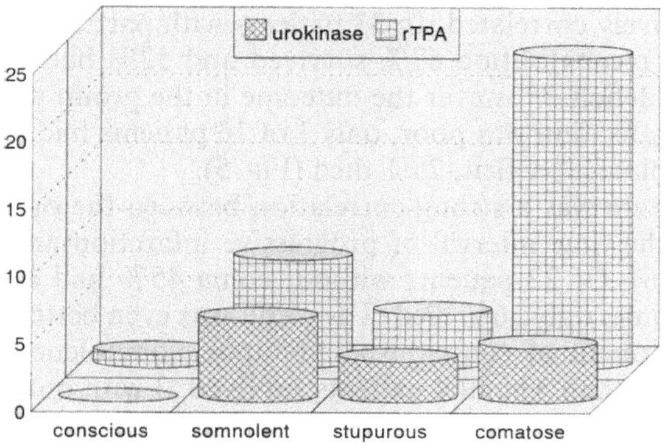

figure 1

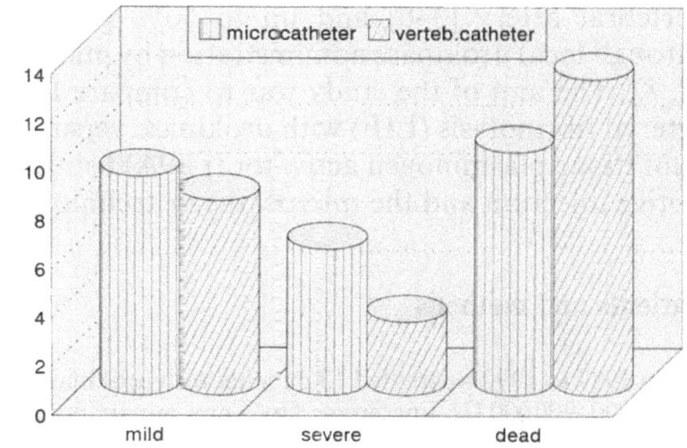

figure 2

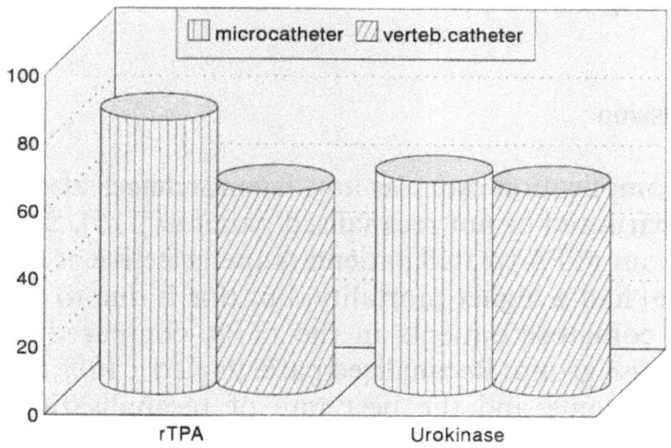

figure 3

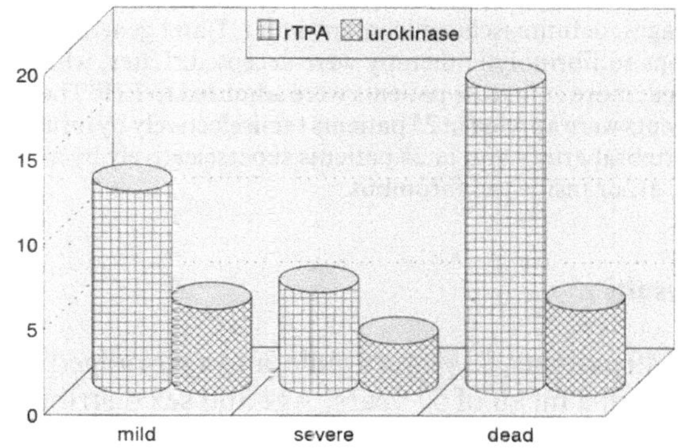

figure 4

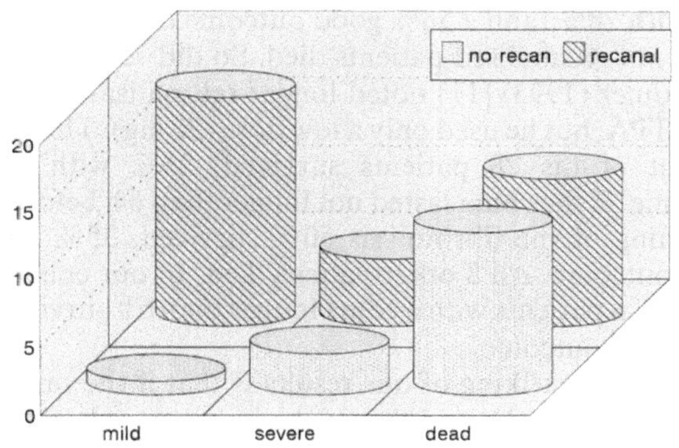

figure 5

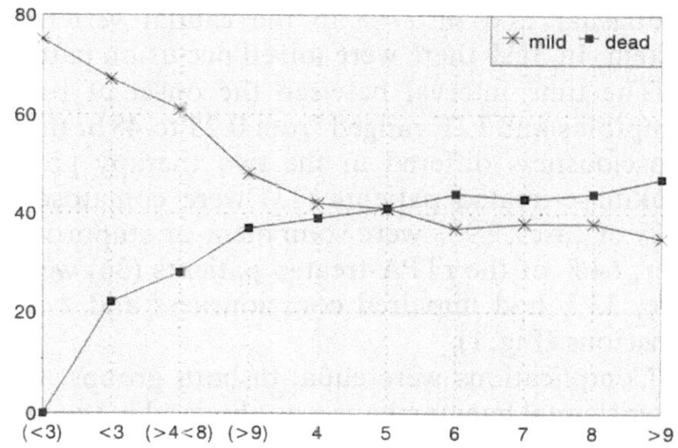

figure 6

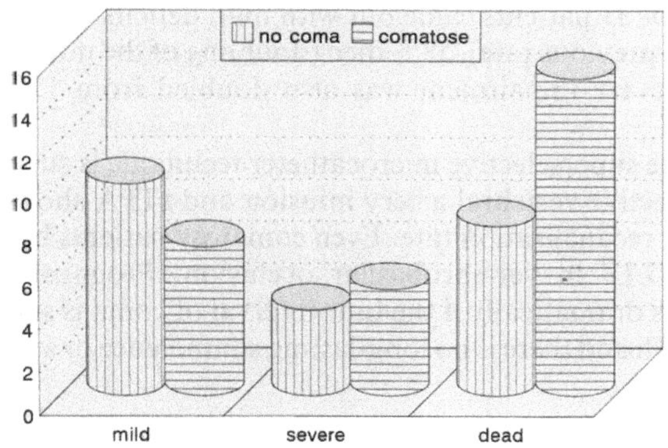

figure 7

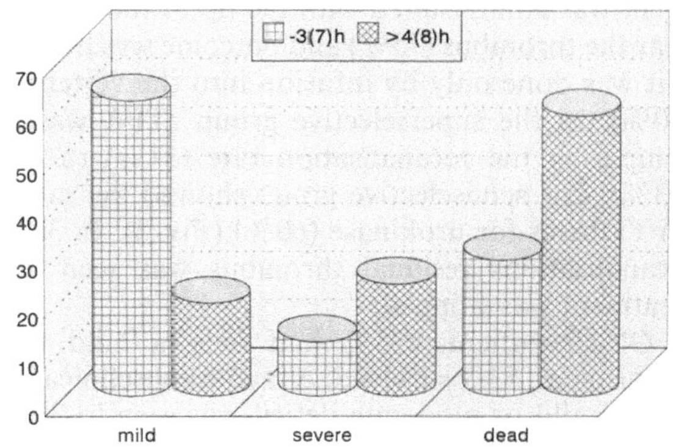

figure 8

survival, if fibrinolytic agents were infused into the vertebral artery [3–6] and up to 50% good outcome through local urokinase administration by microcatheters [7, 8]. The aim of the study was to compare local intra-arterial fibrinolysis (LIF) with urokinase versus recombinant tissue plasminogen activator (rTPA) using a semiselective injection and the microcatheter technique.

Patients and methods

From 1987 to 1990 we treated 13 patients with urokinase at dosages of 150000–900000 IU. Encouraged by a preliminary positive experience with the more thrombus-selective rTPA we have changed the therapy since August 1990 and administered rTPA to 36 patients with doses from 25 to 140 mg with a mean dose 75 mg. In the first years of the study no strict time limit existed, and only haemorrhages, definite ischaemic infarcts on CT and general contraindications to fibrinolytic therapy were accepted. Later, when rTPA was used, more comatose patients were admitted to LIF. The fibrinolytic agents were applied in 25 patients semiselectively by infusion into the vertebral artery and in 24 patients superselectively by a microcatheter at, or inside the thrombus.

Results

Of 49 patients, 73% were male, and ages ranged from 25 to 79 with a mean of 57 years. Age and sex distribution were nearly the same in both therapy groups. According to the classification of Archer and Horenstein [9], the occlusion was located in 17% at the top of the basilar artery, in 25% midbasilar and in 27% in the caudal vertebrobasilar system. In 31% there were mixed occlusion patterns.

The time interval between the onset of brain stem symptoms and LIF ranged from 0.25 to 48 h. the state of consciousness differed in the two therapy groups: the urokinase-treated patients (13) were comatose only in 31% of cases; 69% were somnolent or stuporous. However, 64% of the rTPA-treated patients (36) were comatose, 33% had impaired consciousness and 1 was fully conscious (Fig. 1).

Complications were equal in both groups. Only one parenchymal haemorrhage was observed in the rTPA and urokinase group. Haemorrhagic infarction occurred in 1 urokinase and 3 rTPA patients.

The recanalisation rate was higher if the fibrinolytic agent was administered with the tip of the microcatheter near the thrombus (75%) and outcome was better (Fig. 2) if it was done only by infusion into the vertebral artery (60%). In the superselective group rTPA was superior comparing the recanalisation rate (81%) to urokinase (63%). The semiselective group showed the same results for rTPA as for urokinase (60%) (Fig. 3). In 36% of the recanalisations residual thrombus was seen when the treatment was stopped.

Of 49 patients, 35% had only a mild remaining impairment, 53% survived. A favourable clinical outcome with a mild or moderate deficit was seen in 38% of the urokinase and 33% of the rTPA group. Severe deficit remained in 23% of the urokinase and 17% of the rTPA group. The rate of death was 38% om the urokinase and 50% in the rTPA group (Fig. 4).

Recanalisation and favourable clinical outcome are positively correlated. In 33 patients with partial or complete recanalisation 67% survived and 52% had only a mild deficit. However the outcome in the group with no recanalisation was poor, only 1 of 16 patients had a mild neurological deficit, 75% died (Fig. 5).

There was a strong correlation between the outcome and the time interval of progressive infarction and LIF (Fig. 6). Of 22 patients without coma 45% had a good outcome; only 36% died. The result was even better if the impairment of consciousness (stupor, somnolence) was shorter than 4 h; all 4 patients survived, 3 with only mild defects. Twelve of 27 comatose patients survived, 7 with a good outcome (Fig. 7). Of 5 patients who were in coma for only 2–3 h, 3 survived with only little neurological impairment (Fig. 8).

Discussion

The complication rate was low, haemorrhages also occur in heparinised or not recanalised patients [1, 5]. Summarised, our rTPA treated patients (superselective or semiselective) had a higher mortality, but this is due to 6 times more comatose patients in the rTPA compared to the urokinase group. Recanalised patients had a 50% favourable outcome and the best rate of recanalisation was obtained by high dose rTPA and placement of the microcatheter near or inside the thrombus or embolus (81%). Möbius et al. [10] reported a similar recanalisation rate with 78% (and a 56% good outcome of 18 cases). All of his not recanalised patients died. So did 75% of ours.

Zeumer (1993) [11] noted longer recanalisation times with rTPA, but he used only a low dose (20 mg). Thirty-six percent of his 28 patients survived, 25% with good outcome. If the coma lasted not longer than 6 h before the beginning of the fibrinolysis 50% survived, 35% had a good outcome. All 8 other patiens died. In our collective even 3 of 8 patients with a coma longer than 6 h survived, 1 with good outcome.

The most striking of our results is that if the onset of coma was up to 3 h and the stroke in progress lasted not longer than 7 h 61% had a good outcome, 72% (of 18 patients) survived. From the 4th h of coma and 8th h of stupor or somnolence the outcome became worse, only 19% of 31 patients came out with mild deficits (one third of the previous rate), 58% died (doubling of the mortality) and severe impairment was also doubled from 11% to 23%.

The superselective microcatheter technique is superior to selective vertebral artery infusion and rTPA showed a better recanalisation rate. Even comatose patients benefit from LIF in vertebrobasilar occlusion. Prognosis improves dramatically if the time interval of coma is shorter than 3 h and there is no long-lasting somnolence or stupor.

References

1. Kubik CS, Adams RD (1946) Occlusion of the basilar artery. A clinical and pathological study. Brain 69:73

2. Brückmann H, Ferbert A, Del Zoppo GJ, Hacke W, Zeumer H (1986) Acute vertebral-basilar thrombosis. Acta Radiol 369 [Suppl]: 38–42
3. Zeumer H, Hacke W, Kolmann HL, Poeck K (1982) Lokale Fibrinolysetherapie bei Basilaris-Thrombose. Dtsch Med Wochenschr 107: 728–731
4. Del Zoppo GJ, Ferbert A, Otis S, Brückmann H, Hacke W, Zyroff J, Harker LA, Zeumer H (1988) Local intra-arterial fibrinolytic therapy in acute carotid territory stroke. Stroke 19: 307–313
5. Hacke W, Zeumer H, Ferbert A, Brückmann H, Del Zoppo GJ (1988) Intraarterial fibrinolytic therapy improves outcome in patients with acute vertebrobasilar occlusive disease. Stroke 19: 1216–1222
6. Matsumoto K, Satoh K (1991) Topical intraarterial urokinase infusion for acute stroke. In: Hacke W, Del Zoppo GJ, Mori E (eds) Thrombolytic therapy in acute ischemic stroke. Springer, Berlin Heidelberg New York, pp 207–212
7. Zeumer H, Freitag HJ, Grzyska U, Neunzig HP (1989) Local intraarterial fibrinolysis in acute vertebrobasilar occlusion. Neuroradiology 31: 336–340
8. Pfeiffer G, Thayssen G, Arlt A, Siepmann G, Zeumer H, Kunze K (1991) Vertebrobasilar occlusion: outcome with and without local intraarterial fibrinolysis. In: Hacke W, Del Zoppo GJ, Mori E (eds) Thrombolytic therapy in acute ischemic stroke. Springer, Berlin Heidelberg New York, pp 216–220
9. Archer CR, Horenstein S (1977) Basilar artery occlusion. Clinical and radiological correlation. Stroke 8: 383–390
10. Möbius E, Berg-Dammer E, Kühne D, Kunitsch G, Nahser HC (1989) Lokale Fibrinolysetherapie bei Basilaris-Thrombose. Dtsch Med Wochenschr 107: 728–731
11. Zeumer H, Freitag HJ, Zanella F, Thie A, Arning C (1993) Local intra-arterial fibrinolytic therapy in patients with stroke: urokinase versus recombinant tissue plasminogen activator (rTPA). Neuroradiology 35: 159–162

Percutaneous transluminal angioplasty for ostial stenosis of the vertebral artery

Y. Kaku[1], Y. Yonekawa[2], T. Andoh[1], N. Sakai[1], H. Yamada[2]

[1] Department of Neurosurgery, Gifu University, Tsukasa-machi 40, Gifu 500, Japan
[2] Department of Neurosurgery, Zürich University, Zürich, Switzerland

Abstract. We report our experience of percutaneous transluminal angioplasty (PTA) for symptomatic aterosclerotic stenosis of the origin of the vertebral artery (VAO stenosis). Seventeen cases of haemodynamically significant VAO stenosis without evidence of distal embolism were treated by PTA. Fifteen lesions (88%) were successfully dilasted, with improvement in symptoms. One intimal dissection occured during PTA, which required surgical vascular reconstruction. Radiographic follow-up studies demonstrated two cases of restenosis (13.3%). One was consequently treated by surgical vascular reconstruction, and the other remained asymptomatic. In patients with haemodynamically significant VAO stenosis, these stenotic lesions can be treated by PTA techniques with low morbidity.

Key words: Vertebral artery, ostial stenosis – percutanous transluminal angioplasty, distal embolism

Percutaneous transluminal angioplasty (PTA) is now applied to selected cases with supra-aortic arterial stenoses. This technique appears to be effective for the treatment of haemodynamically significant atherosclerotic lesions. Stenosis at the origin of the vertebral artery (VAO stenosis) is frequently smooth, and it rarely has an ulcerated plaque. Angioplasty of this type of lesion can be safely performed without cerebral protection. In contrast, VAO stenosis with an obvious ulcerative plaque involves a considerable risk of embolization. We report our experience with PTA in 17 cases of haemodynamically significant atherosclerotic VAO stenosis. Four patients who had VAO stenosis with evidence of distal embolism and were consequently treated by surgical vascular reconstruction are also reported.

Patients and methods

We treated 21 patients with VAO stenoses since 1990; there were 19 men and 2 women, ranging in age from 32 years to 80 years (mean age 61.4). Seventeen patients with haemodynamically significant VAO stenosis (> 70%, bilaterally) presented clinically with symptoms of vertebrobasilar insufficiency, including subjective dizzy feelings of a vascular type, ataxia, diplopia, and drop attack. Four patients presented with embolic stroke in the vertebro-basilar system: 2 with cerebellar infarction, 1 with brain stem infarction, and 1 with occipital lobe infarction.

PTA was performed in 17 patients with haemodynamically significant VAO stenoses, while 4 patients who had VAO stenosis with evidence of distal emobilsm were treated by surgical vascular reconstruction.

PTA was attempted on the dominant vertebral artery for haemodynamically significant atherosclerotic stenosis. Patients were maintained on an oral antiplatelet (160 mg aspirin or 200 mg ticropidine per day) for at least 1 week before the procedure. PTA was performed from a transfemoral approach under local anaesthesia. A 5-F tapered diagnostic catheter with a 0.035-in. angled guidewire was advanced through the stenotic segment of the vertrebral artery. An exchange guidewire (length 300 cm, diameter 0.035 in.) was then introduced into the distal segment of the vertebral

Correspondence to: Y. Kaku

artery. The 5-F diagnostic catheter was immediately removed and then exchanged for a 5-F balloon dilatation catheter. The balloon used for angioplasty of VAO stenoses was 4–5 mm in diameter and 2 cm in length. The balloon was then inflated with a pressure of 5–8 atm for 30–50 s. One to three inflations were performed until the stenotic lesion was successfully dilated. After the procedure, patients were closely observed for 24 h with systemic heparinisation (1000 IU/h). Follow-up angiography was performed 3 months after angioplasty.

Results

PTA was successfully performed, in 15 out of 17 patients with angiographical improvement (< 30% residual stenosis). In all patients with angiographical improvement there was improvement in symptoms without further episodes of vertebrobasilar insufficiency. Intimal dissection occurred during PTA in 1 case, requiring surgical vascular reconstruction. Radiographic follow-up studies demonstrated 2 cases of restenosis (13.3%); 1 was subsequently treated with surgical vascular reconstruction and the other remained asymptomatic. In the group treated by surgery, all vascular reconstructions performed had good results.

Discussion

PTA has become a well-established technique for treating atherosclerotic stenoses in supra-aortic arteries. This technique appears to be effective for the treatment of haemodynamically significant stenotic lesions. Stenosis at the origin of the vertebral artery is frequently smooth, and it rarely has an ulcerated plaque. This site has been recognised as an infrequent donor source for distal embolism, in contrast to occlusive disease of the internal carotid artery origin, which is generally accepted as a frequent potential source of distal embolism. Angioplasty of VAO stenosis may be safely performed without cerebral protection.

Selection of patients with VAO stenosis for angioplasty remains controversial. For patients with haemodynamically significant stenotic lesions (> 70% stenosis) of both vertebral arteries, PTA may be a viable alternative way of improving blood flow in the posterior circulation. Among our 21 patients, 4 (19%) with high-grade or near-occlusion VAO stenosis demonstrated distal embolism from the VAO stenosis. In consideration of the relatively higher occurrence of distal embolism from VAO stenosis, severe unilateral stenosis or near-occlusion of the vertebral origin should be considered a source of distal embolism. Accordingly, patients with this type of stenosis may also be candidates for PTA to reduce the risk of distal embolism.

In conclusion, in patients with haemodynamically significant VAO stenosis, these stenotic lesions can be treated by PTA techniques, with low morbidity.

References

1. Fisher CM, Gore I, Okabe N, et al (1965) Atherosclerosis of the carotid and vertebral arteries: extracranial and intracranial. J Neurpathol Exp Neurol 24:455–476
2. Higashida RT, Tsai FY, Halbach VV, et al (1993) Transluminal angioplasty for atherosclerotic disease of the vertebral and basilar arteries. J Neurosurg 78:912–918
3. Caplan LR, Amarenco P, Rosengart A, et al (1992) Embolism from vertebral artery origin occlusive disease. Neurology 42:1505–1512
4. Motarjeme A, Keifer JW, Zuska AJ (1982) Percutaneous transluminal angioplasty of the brachiocephalic arteries. AJR 138:457–462
5. Courtheoux P, Tournade A, Théron J, et al (1985) Transcutaneous angioplasty of vertebral artery atheromatous ostial stricture. Neuroradiology 27:259–264
6. Cartlidge NEF, Whisnant JP, Elveback LR (1978) Carotid and vertebrobasilar transient cerebral ischemic attacks. A community study, Rochester, Minnesota. Mayo Clin Proc 52:117–120
7. Théron J, Courtheoux P, Henriet JP (1984) Angioplasty of supraaortic arteries. J Neuroradiol 11:187–200

Thrombolytic treatment of acute vertebrobasilar artery occlusion

Fong Y. Tsai, Randall Higashida, Violet Matovich, Melissa Gurley, Karen Garby

UMKC-Truman Medical Center, 2301 Holmes St. Kansas City, MO 64108, USA

Abstract. Acute occlusion of the vertebrobasilar artery often presents as progressive stroke, which can lead to coma and brain death. We present our experience with thrombolybie treatment in 29 patients.

Key words: Vertebro-basilar artery thrombosis – urokinase – thrombolysis

Acute occlusion of the vertebrobasilar artery frequently presents as progressive stroke, which can lead to coma and brain death [1–5]. Heparinization may enhance spontaneous autolysis of small thrombi, but rapid clinical deterioration requires more aggressive recanalization if fatal sequelae are to be avoided. We describe our experience with thrombolytic treatment in 29 patients.

Correspondence to: F. Y. Tsai

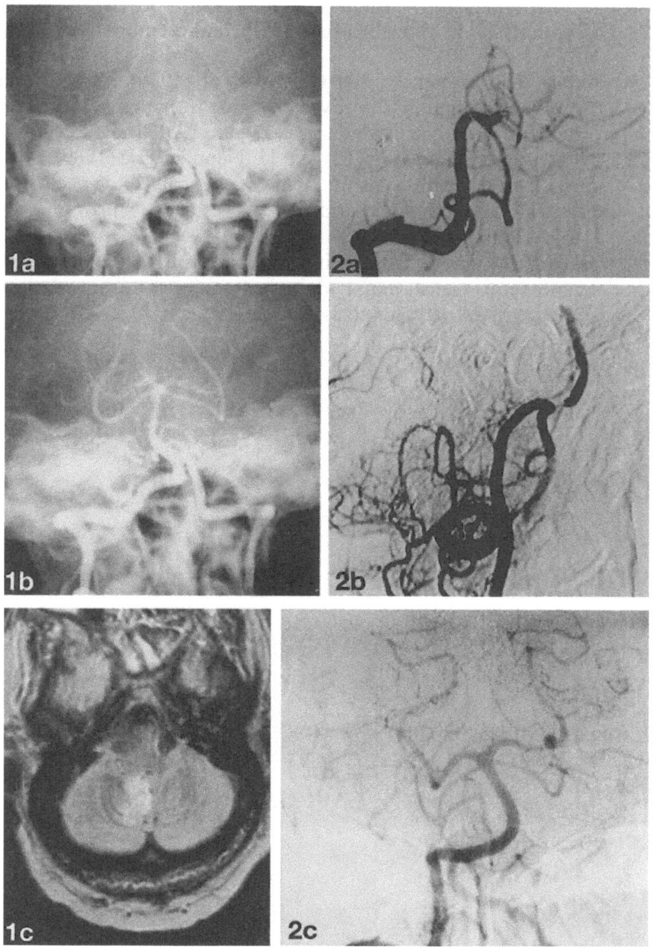

Fig. 1. **a** Vertebral angiography showed thrombus at the proximal basilar artery, with occlusion. **b** After thrombolysis, the basilar artery was patent. **c** MRI showed an sympotomatic infarct in the vermis

Fig. 2. **a** Vertebral angiography showed occlusion of the basilar artery distal to a severe stenosis. **b** After partial thrombolysis, the basilar artery was partially open. **c** Six months after PTA and thrombolysis, follow-up angiography showed a normal basilar artery

Methods

Thrombolysis was performed through a Tracker 18 catheter, advanced to the occluded segment of the vertebral and/or basilar artery utilizing a coaxial technique through a 5-F catheter. Following the initial bolus dose of 250000 IU, intermittent injections of 80000 IU urokinase were given every 15 min. All patients were given 3000 U of heparin intravenously during thrombolysis and 1000 U every hour. A continous heparin drip was maintained after thrombolysis, and oral therapy continued for 3 months. Angioplasty, in selected patients, was performed using a Stealth catheter with a balloon size of 2.5 mm × 1.5 cm. Nitroglycerin was given intraarterially prior to the balloon inflation.

Results

Over the past 8 years, we have treated 29 patients (17 men and 12 woman) with acute vertebrobasilar occlusion.

They ranged in age from 35 to 72 years, averaging 55 years. Five patients died of brain stem and cerebellar infarcts. We were unable to advance the catheter to the basilar artery in 2 patients. Two other patients developed reocclusion, and 1 died 3 weeks later of a brain stem infarct, despite successful recanalization. Twenty-four patients survived after thrombolysis. One patient had severe deficits, 5 had moderate deficits and 18 patients had mild residual symptoms. No hemorrhagic complications were encountered. Despite treatment, approximately 60% had significant MRI findings of residual infarct (Fig. 1), but one-third were asymptomatic. The sites of occlusion varied: there was occlusion in the distal vertebral and proximal basilar artery in 12 patients, in the proximal basilar artery in 7 patients, in the mid-basilar artery in 3 patients, and in the distal basilar artery in 7 patients. Eight patients had significant bilateral vertebral artery stenosis. Three patients had chronic occluded right vertebral arteries, and 1 had chronic left vertebral artery occlusion. Five patients had basilar artery stenosis and 3 had proximal vertebral artery stenosis.

Discussion

We need to rely upon the clinical picture to identify the site of acute occlusion, but initial symptoms and signs may be very subtle [1–5]. Additionally, it may not be possible to distinguish acute from chronic occlusion on angiographic features. Clinical deterioration may progress rapidly, or take hours or even days from the initial onset of symptoms. The speed of deterioration depends upon many variables, including site of occlusion, collaterals, size of thrombus and extension of the embolus. The patient may not be comatose early on with proximal basilar artery occlusion, as opposed to distal basilar occlusion, if there are good collaterals from carotid circulation to the posterior cerebral arteries.

In the investigation of vertebrobasilar stroke, diagnostic angiography must include selective bilateral carotid and vertebral injections to look for contralateral or bilateral vertebral artery occlusion [1–8]. The deaths which occured in our study were due to various causes. In those patients with bilateral vertebral artery occlusion, there may be failure to advance the Tracker catheter to the basilar artery. We failed on two occasions for this reason. These patients may have had severe stenosis or chronically occluded vertebral segments with propagation of the embolus, resulting in occlusion of the entire basilar artery. Another patient died 3 weeks after a successful recanalization, in which thrombolysis was begun about 7 h after the onset of acute progressive deterioration. Two other patients died after experiencing reocclusion of the basilar artery due to proximal severe stenosis. Although percutaneous transluminal angioplasty (PTA) carries some potential risk of arterial rupture, it may not be as high as the risk of reocclusion of the basilar artery. One survivor with severe stenosis in the proximal basilar artery received PTA after thrombolysis to avoid reocclusion (Fig. 2) [9].

References

1. Archer CR, Horenstein S (1977) Basilar artery occlusion: clinical and radiological correlation. Stroke 8:383–387
2. Caplan LR, Pessin MS, Mohr JP (1992) Vertebrobasilar occlusive disease. In: Barnett HJM, Mohr JP, Stein BM, Yatsu FM (eds) Stroke: pathophysiology, diagnosis and management 2nd ed. Churchill Livingstone, New York, pp 443–515
3. Caplan LR (1983) Bilateral distal vertebral artery occlusion. Neurology 33:552–558
4. Bogousslavsky J, Gales PC, Fox AJ, Barnett HJM (1986) Bilateral occlusion of the vertebral artery. Neurology 36:1309–1315
5. Tsai FY, Teal J, Hieshima G, et al (1982) CT in acute posterior fossa infarcts. AJNR 3:149
6. Zeumer H, Hacke W, Ringelstein ER (1983) Local intra-arterial thrombolysis in vertebro-basilar thrombo-embolic diesease. AJNR 4:401–404
7. Hacke W, Zeumer H, Ferbert A, et al (1988) Intra-arterial thrombolytic therapy improves outcome in patients with acute vertebro-basilar occlusive disease. Stroke 19:1216–1222
8. Zeumer H, Freitag HJ, Grzyska U, Neunzig HP (1989) Local intra-arterial fibrinolysis in acute vertebrobasilar occlusion: technical developments and recent results. Neuroradiology 31:336–340
9. Tsai FY, Lavin M, Metovich V, Berberian B, Alfieri K (1994) Percutaneous transluminal angioplasty adjunct to thrombolysis for acute MCA rethrombosis. AJNR (in press)

Percutaneous transluminal angioplasty for stenosis at the origin of the vertebral artery using snare catheters

K. Kazekawa[1], T. Kawano[1], Y. Kaneko[1], S. Yoshimura[2], M. Takamiya[3]

[1] Department of Neurosurgery, Fukuoka Tokushukai Medical Centre, Kasuga, Fukuoka, Japan
[2] Department of Neurosurgery, National Cardiovascular Centre, Suita, Osaka, Japan
[3] Department of Radiology, National Cardiovascular Centre, Suita, Osaka, Japan

Abstract. We report a technique for holding a guiding catheter during percutaneous transluminal angioplasty (PTA) for stenosis at the origin of the vertebral artery. A loop snare, introduced via the brachial artery, is used to fix the guiding catheter in the proximal subclavian artery. Then, through this guiding catheter, the PTA balloon is introduced to the stenotic site.

Key words: Intraventional instrumentation – Percutaneous transluminal angioplasty – Vertebral artery – loop snare catheter

In 24 patients, PTA of stenoses at the origin of the vertebral artery has been performed mostly using the femoral approach. However, in patients with severe atherosclerosis, introduction of the guiding catheter into the right subclavian artery was difficult and, even if successfully inserted, it easily dropped into the aortic arch during the procedure. We have devised a new technique to overcome these problems.

Case Report

Case 1

A 56-year-old man with vertebrobasilar insufficiency had severe stenosis of the origin of the right vertebral artery and a hypoplastic left vertebral artery. Initially, we were unable to introduce the 8-F

Correspondence to: K. Kazekawa

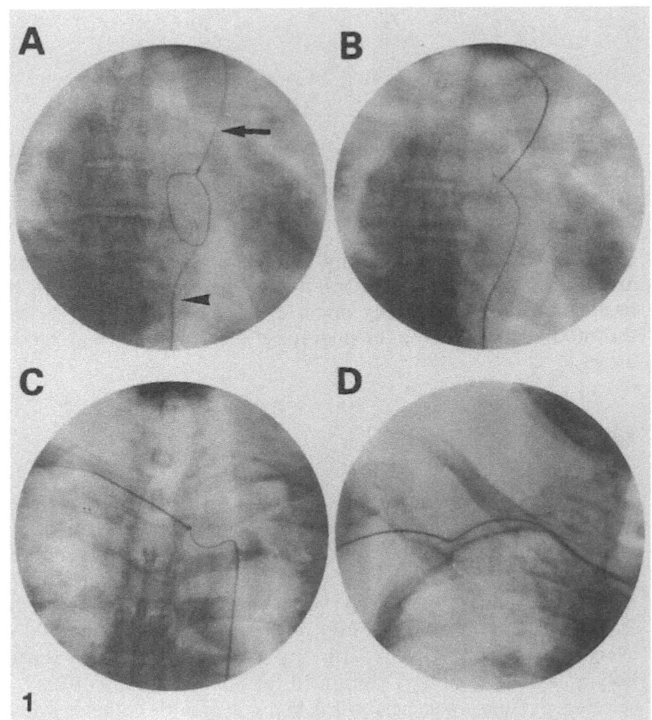

Fig. 1 A–D. Case 1. Advancing guiding catheter into the right subclavian artery. **A** A right-angled snare is introduced via the right brachial artery (*arrow*) and a 0.035 guidewire, through an 8-F guiding catheter via the femoral artery (*arrow head*). **B** The snare grasps the guide wire. **C** The snare is withdrawn into the right subclavian artery. **D** The guiding catheter enters the subclavian artery, following the guide wire

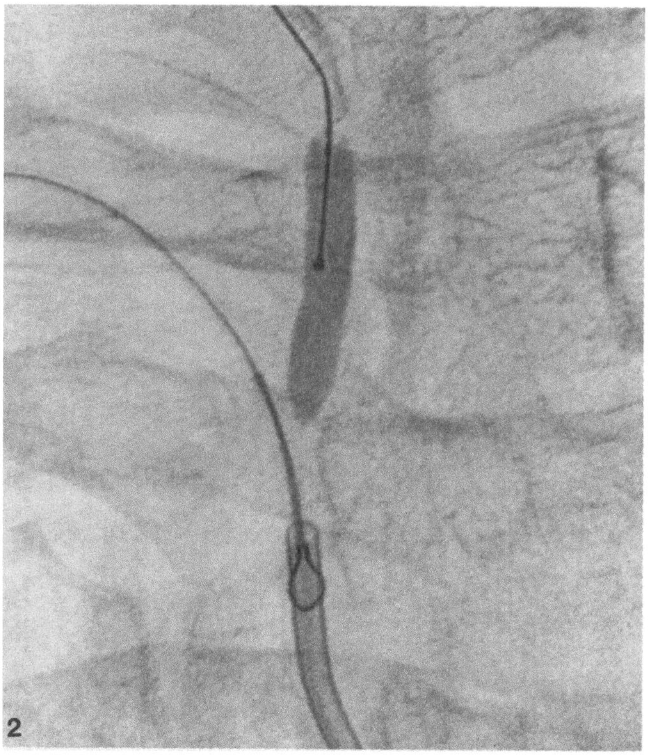

Fig. 2. A 4-mm-diameter balloon was fully inflated through the guiding catheter folded by the snare

guiding catheter into the right subclavian artery via the femoral artery, due to tortuosity of the innominate artery. Therefore, we inserted a snare catheter into the right brachial artery and advanced it into the thoracic aorta, where the 0.035 guidewire could be grasped. The snare was then gently withdrawn into the right subclavian artery, to advance the guiding catheter into the innominate artery (Fig. 1). After this procedure, PTA was successfully achieved using a 5-mm-diameter balloon through the guiding catheter via the femoral artery.

Case 2

A 76-year-old man with vertebrobasilar insufficiency had severe stenosis of the origin of the right vertebral artery and occlusion of the left. A 4-mm-diameter PTCA balloon could not be introduced, because the guiding catheter in the right subclavian artery dropped into the aorta during the procedure. A snare was therefore inserted into the right brachial artery to hold the 8-F guiding catheter at the proximal right subclavian artery (Fig. 2). Following this procedure, PTA was successfully performed via the femoral approach.

Case 3

A 70-year-old man with vertebrobasilar insufficiency was shown to have severe stenosis at the origin of the right vertebral artery and occlusion of the left. The femoral approach was not possible because of atherosclerosis. A right-angled snare was inserted into the right brachial artery and an 8-F guiding catheter was inserted into the left brachial artery. The snare was advanced into the aortic arch to hold the guiding catheter The snare was then withdrawn into the innominate artery and fixed the guiding catheter (Fig. 3). Following this procedure, PTA was performed successfully using a 4-mm-diameter balloon via the left brachial artery.

Discussion

The technique described here is a modification of the snare chatheter technique used to make a transductal arteriovenous catheter loop in the method of Porstmann et al. [1]. We used this technique for three patients and all were successfully treated. The technique is not very difficult, so that we can perform the described procedure within 1 h. With this technique, the guiding catheter is placed stably, and catheterisation and replacement of the PTA balloon are performed as usual. The technique can be used in patients with severe atherosclerosis of the femoral arteries. In case 3, PTA using the right brachial approach seemed to be dangerous, because the subclavian-vertebral artery angle was too acute to allow the balloon to be advanced. In such cases, our technique makes it possible to access the vertebral artery from the contralateral brachial artery. The snare described here is soft enough not to damage the vessel wall and has been used effictively to retrieve foreign bodies [2–4]. Our novel technique may provide access to lesions in the vertebrobasilar territory, which cannot be treated by conventional techniques.

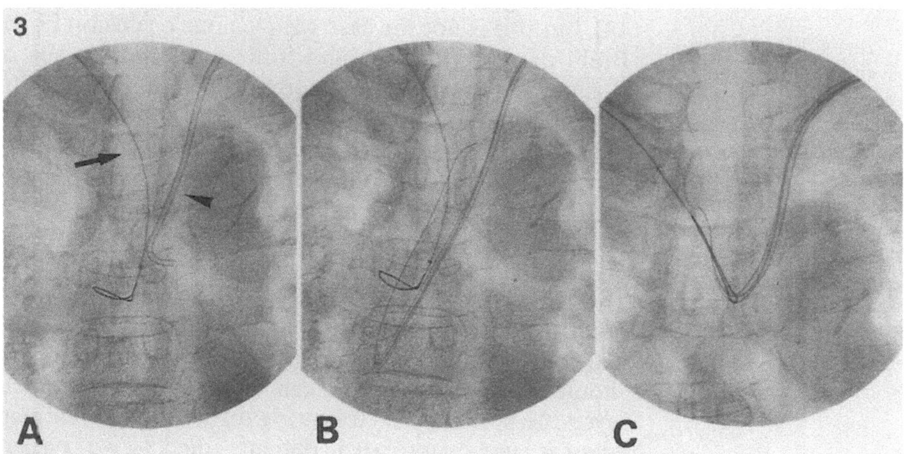

Fig. 3A–C. A snare has been introduced via the right brachial artery (*arrow*) and a guiding catheter via the left brachial artery (*arrow head*). **B** Through the guiding catheter a 0.035 guidewire was inserted into the snare. **C** The snare grasped the guiding catheter

References

1. Porstmann W, Wierny L, Warnke H, Gerstberger G, Romaniuk PA (1971) Catheter closure of patent ductus arteriosus. 62 cases treated without thoracotomy. Radiol Clin North Am 9:203–218
2. Yedlicka JW Jr, Carlson JE, Hunter DW, Castañeda-Zuñiga WR, Amplatz K (1991) Nitinol gooseneck snare for removal of foreign bodies: experimental study and clinical evaluation. Radiology 178:691–693
3. Sanchez RB, Robert AC, Valji K, Lengle L, Bookstein JJ (1992) Wallstent misplaced during transjugular placement of an intrahepatic portosystemic shunt: retrieval with a loop snare. AJR 159:129–130
4. Malden ES, Darcy MD, Picus D, et al (1992) Transvenous retrieval of misplaced stainless steel Greenfiled filters. J Vasc Interv Radiol 3:703–708

Thrombolytic treatment for acute dural sinus thrombosis

Fong Y. Tsai, Ai-Ming Wang, Violet B. Matovich, M. Lavin, B. Berberian, W. Yuh

UMKC-Truman Medical Center, 2301 Holmes St. Kansas City, MO 64108, USA

Abstract. We have treated 29 patients with acute dural sinus and/or deep venous thrombosis, While 18 of 20 survivors received intravascular thrombolysis, all 9 of the patients in whom urokinase was not administered died.

Key words: Dural sinus thrombosis – Thrombolysis – Urokinase – Venous infarction

Acute dural sinus occlusion may lead to severe venous congestion, hemorrhage and infarction, with potentially fatal consequences if diagnosis and treatment are not timely. Although early diagnosis is essential, reports in the imaging literature have not clearly described the patterns of venous occlusive disease [1–6]. Our purpose is to report our experience with 29 patients with acute dural sinus and/ or venous thrombosis, to outline a management strategy and document patient response.

Materials and methods

In analyzing these 29 patients, who presented from January 1989 to May 1993, we separated them into categories of treatment, i.e. with or without thrombolysis, and reviewed the results in these two therapeutic groups. Dural sinus venography was performed via the percutaneous transfemoral vein approach, utilizing a 5-F angiographic catheter as a guide. The catheter was advanced to the jugular bulb and a no. 18 Tracker catheter (preferably with multiple side holes) was then advanced into the dural sinus coaxially through it. We prefer to perform transverse sinus venography and thrombolysis from the contralateral transverse sinus through the torcular herophili. Thrombolysis was performed by bolus injection of 250000 IU urokinase directly to the clot, followed by 80000 IU every 15 min until thrombolysis was achieved or 1000000 IU were infused (Fig. 1) [7]. Intradural sinus pressure was measured before, during and after the completion of thrombolysis.

Correspondence to: F. Y. Tsai

Results

Nine of the 29 patients died from either massive hemorrhage or edema. None of those who died received direct thrombolysis, but only anticoagulants and other supportive treatment. These 9 consisted of 7 females and 2 males, aged from 9 months to 61 years with a mean age of 38 years. Of the 20 patients who survived, all but 2 received urokinase. This group consisted of 9 males and 11 females, ranging in age from 6 days to 44 years, with a mean age of 26 years. No predisposing factors were identified in 10 patients, but of the remaining 17, 2 were hypercoagulable, 3 were post-partum, 2 were on oral contraceptives, 3 were IV drug abusers, 1 had posterior fassa surgery 3 days previously, 2 were dehydrated infants, 2 had recent trauma and 2 were alcoholics.

Discussion

Although thrombolysis has been used extensively to treat acute arterial occlusion, thrombolytic treatment of acute dural sinus thrombosis is just beginning [8–12]. Thrombolysis is not suitable therapy for patients with edema or hemorrhage associated with acute arterial occlusion [13, 14], but this is not the case with venous occlusion [7–12]. Brain parenchymal changes from acute dural sinus occlusion are the result of increasing sinus pressure and venous congestion. The stages progress with the severity of clinical and imaging manifestations. Thus, thrombolytic treatment for acute dural sinus thrombosis is to release the occlusion and prevent venous congestion.

Thrombolytic treatment should be initiated as soon as possible to relieve venous congestion.

The five stages seen in venous occlusive disease occur because of varying degrees of venous congestion, and even if there is cerebral edema or hemorrhage, thrombolytics should not be withheld. Even with massive venous infarcts, no patients died following thrombolytic treatment, whereas most untreated patients died. Two patients

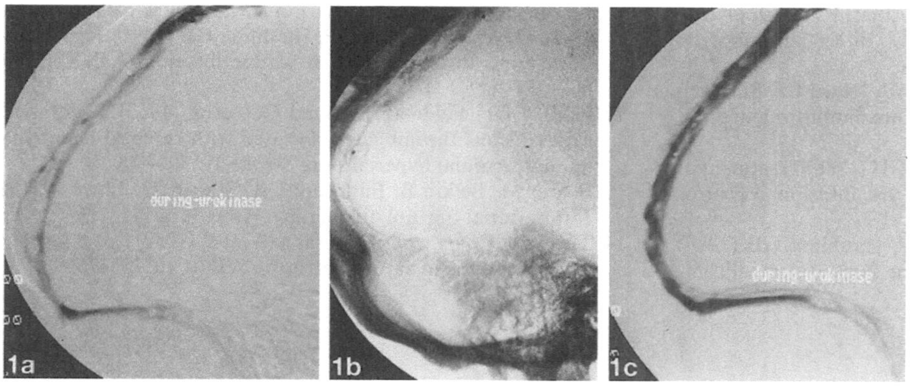

Fig. 1. a Dural sinography shows thrombosis of the sagittal sinus with an extensive filling defect. **b** Lateral view of skull shows infusion catheter with radiopaque markers indicating the extent of the side holes. **c** After thrombolysis, the sagittal sinus is open

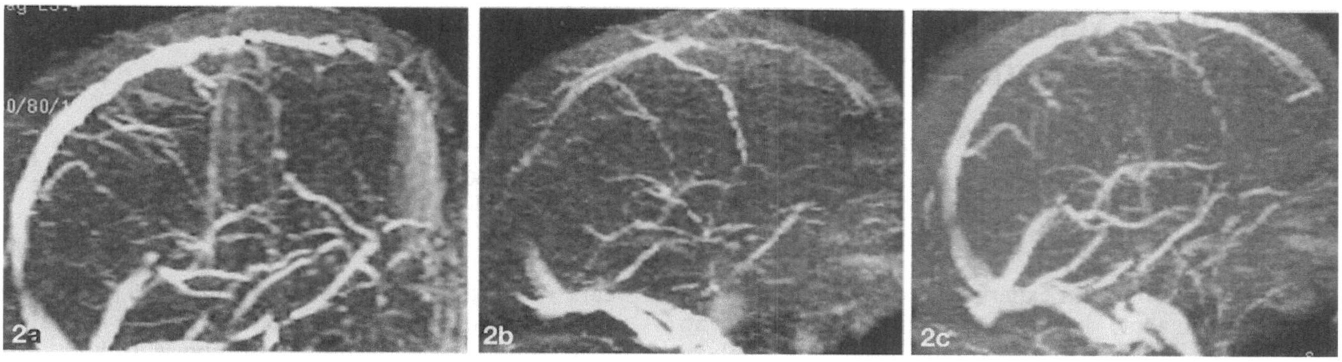

Fig. 2. a 2D time-of-flight MR venography shows partial thrombosis of the frontal sagittal sinus. **b** Follow-up MR venography after a 4-day trial of heparinization: extensive thrombosis of sagittal sinus, with clinical deterioration. **c** Repeat MR venography after thrombolysis: the sagittal sinus is open

received anticoagulants without thrombolysis and survived. However, the neurological deficits suffered by these patients were much worse than in patients who received even delayed thrombolysis. One patient had bilaterial blindness due to bilateral occipital lobe infarcts from sagittal sinus thrombosis and one a massive hemorrhage in the right parietal lobe. The other 7 untreated patients all died. Those patients who have no parenchymal changes may be treated initially with anticoagulation. Recently, 6 additional stage I patients had complete clinical recovery, although 2 had some residual thrombosis on follow-up imaging studies. None of these patients required thrombolytic treatment. However, several of our stage II patients did require thrombolysis because after a few days of anticoagulant therapy they deteriorated clinically to the point of converting from partial to complete superior sagittal thrombosis (Fig. 2). Although parenchymal changes in stage III can be reversed with thrombolytic treatment, heparinization can not stop further deterioration with clinical and imaging changes. Stage IV disease, however, is associated with true infarction. Improvement is possible with appropriate therapy, but some changes may be irreversible. Venous pressures high enough to reach stage V result in generalized disruption of the blood-brain barrier and inadequate cellular perfusion; stage V means significant, irreversible infarction and is inevitably fatal. We believe that once parenchymal changes are seen on imaging examinations or the patient shows clinical deterioration, thrombolytic treatment is essential to avoid permanent brain tissue damage and clinical dysfunction. Previous reports state that it might take several hours, even days, to disperse the thrombosis because retrograde injection through the ipsilaterial sinus is similar to generalized infusion, in which urokinase is washed down with the venous blood flow to the heart [8–11]. Our technique is easier and allows us to measure intrasinus pressure proximal to the thrombosis.

References

1. Gates PC, Barnett HJM (1986) Venous disease in cortical venus and sinuses. In: Barnet HJM, Stein BM, Mohr JP, Yatsu FM (eds) Stroke, 2nd edn. Churchill Livingstone, New York, pp 731–762
2. Zilkha A, Diaz AS (1989) Computed tomography in the diagnosis of superior sagittal sinus thrombosis. J Comput Assist Tomogr 4:124–126
3. Brant-Zawadzki M, Chang GY, McCarty GE (1982) Computed tomography in dural sinus thrombosis. Arch Neurol 39:446–447
4. McMurdo SK Jr, Brant-Zawadzki M, Bradley WG Jr, Chang GV, Berg BO (1986) Dural sinus thrombosis: study using intermediate field strength MR imaging. Radiology 161:83–86
5. Snyder TC, Sachdev HS (1986) MR imaging of cerebral dural sinus thrombosis. J Comput Assist Tomogr 10:889–891
6. Sze G, Simmons B, Krol G, Walker R, Zimmerman RD, Deck MD (1988) Dural sinus thrombosis: verification with spin-echo techniques. AJNR 9:679–686

7. Tsai FY, Higashida RT, Matovich VB, Alfieri KL (1992) Acute thrombosis of intracranial dural sinus: direct thrombolytic treatment. AJNR 13:1137–1141
8. Halbach VV, Higashida RT, Hieshima GB, Dowd CF, Barnwell SL (1989) Venography and venous pressure monitoring in dural sinus meningimas. AJNR 10:1209–1213
9. Scott JA, Pascuzzi RM, Hall PV, Becker GH (1988) Treatment of dural sinus thrombosis with local urokinase infusion. J Neurosurg 68:284–287
10. Higashida RT, Helmer E, Halbach VV, Hieshima GB (1989) Direct thrombolytic therapy for superior sagittal sinus thrombosis. AJNR 10:S4–S6
11. Smith TP, Higashida RT, Barnwell SL, Halbach VV, Dowd CF, Fraser KW, Teitelbaum GP, Hieshima GB (1994) Treatment of dural sinus thrombosis by urokinase infusion. AJNR 15:801–807
12. Hanley DF, Feldman E, Borel CO, et al (1988) Treatment of sagittal sinus thrombosis associated with cerebral hemorrhage and intracranial hypertension. Stroke 19:903–909
13. Belkin M, Belkin B, Bucknam CA, Straub JJ, Lowe R (1986) Intra-arterial fibrinolytic therapy. Arch Surg 121:769–773
14. Théron J, Courtheoux P, Casasco A, et al (1989) Local intraarterial fibrinolysis in carotid territory. AJNR 10:753–765

Acute dural venous sinus thrombosis in children: endovascular thrombolytic treatment

A. M. Wang[1], F. Y. Tsai[2], A. N. Shetty[1], M. Goetting[3], I. Gebara[3]

[1] Department of Diagnostic Radiology, and [3] Pediatrics, William Beaumont Hospital, 3601 West 13 Mile Road, Royal Oak, MI 48073, USA
[2] Department of Radiology, University of Missouri-Kansas City, School of Medicine, Missouri, USA

Abstract. We report our experience in seven children with symptomatic acute dural venous sinus thrombosis, who underwent percutaneous endovascular thrombolytic treatment with urokinase. Brain MRI and venous MR angiography were performed in each patient before and after treatment to plan and to assess the safety and efficacy of this treatment. The method we used seems to provide a safe and effective treatment to dissolve blood clots and to recanalize the thrombosed venous drainage in the brain with encouragging clinical outcome.

Key words: Cerebrovascular disease – Acute dural venous thrombosis – Percutaneous endovascular thrombolysis – Urokinase

In the early literature, the incidence of dural venous sinus thrombosis (DSVT) in children was found to be low [1]. Recently, because of the advancement of new diagnostic neuroimaging techniques (CT and MRI), much higher incidences have been reported [2–4]. In childhood, acute DVST is usually found in children less than 5 years of age [5]. In neonates, compression and distortion of the dural sinuses with molding during birth may be the cause. Infection from sepsis or as an extension of osteomyelitis, otitis media or mastoiditis, as well as severe dehydration or hypercoagulable state, are the common causes of acute DVST in children. The clinical presentations are variable and nonspecific. The traditional treatments are supportive treatment, treatment of the underlying disease, control of increased intracranial pressure, and anticoagulation [5].

Recently, the use of urokinase has been reported, with encouraging preliminary results [6]. Over a period of 1.5 years (November 1991 through June 1993), we have treated seven children with symptomatic acute DVST with or without cerebral venous thrombosis (CVT), using urokinase injected directly into the thrombosed dural sinus.

Correspondence to: A. M. Wang

Patients and methods

Seven patients (six boys, one girl), ranging in age from 2 weeks to 18 years, presented with high index of clinical suspicion of acute DVST, in which the diagnosis was confirmed by MRI, magnetic resonance angiography (MRA) and dural sinus venography (DSV). Each patient had brain MRI and MRA prior to and 1 week after the percutaneous endovascular thrombolytic treatment (PETT) with urokinase. The brain MRI and venous MRA were performed using a 1.5 T unit. The intracranial venous MRA was performed using the

Fig. 1 a–f. A 14-day-old boy presenting with seizures. Sagittal (**a**) and oblique coronal **b**) venous MRA shows no venous flow in the straight sinus (SS), deep cerebral venons system, right transverse sinus (TS) and sigmoid sinus, duplicated posterior superior sagittal sinus (SSS) on the right, with soft tissue swelling over the parietal region and a promiment emissary vein (*white arrow*) as collateral drainage. *DSV:* A Tracker-18 catheter (**c** *thick arrow*) was advanced through the right TS to the anterior SSS. Venography (DSV) shows lack of blood flow through the right duplicated posterior the right lateral sinus (LS) and the right internal jugular vein (IJV). The anterior SSS (*arrow*), left duplicated SSS (*white arrow*), left LS (*long white arrow*) and left IJV (*thick white arrow*) are patent. The Tracker-18 catheter was then withdrawn to the right duplicated posterior SSS and right LS, and a total of 150,000 IU of urokinase was injected into these thrombosed sinuses. DSV (**d**) shows recanalization of the right duplicated SSS (*white arrow*), right LS (*short white arrow*) and right IJV (*thick white arrow*). One week after treatment. Sagittal (**e**) and oblique coronal (**f**) venous MRA shows resulution of the soft tissue swelling and re-establishment of the blood flow in the thrombosed dural sinuses and deep cerebral veins

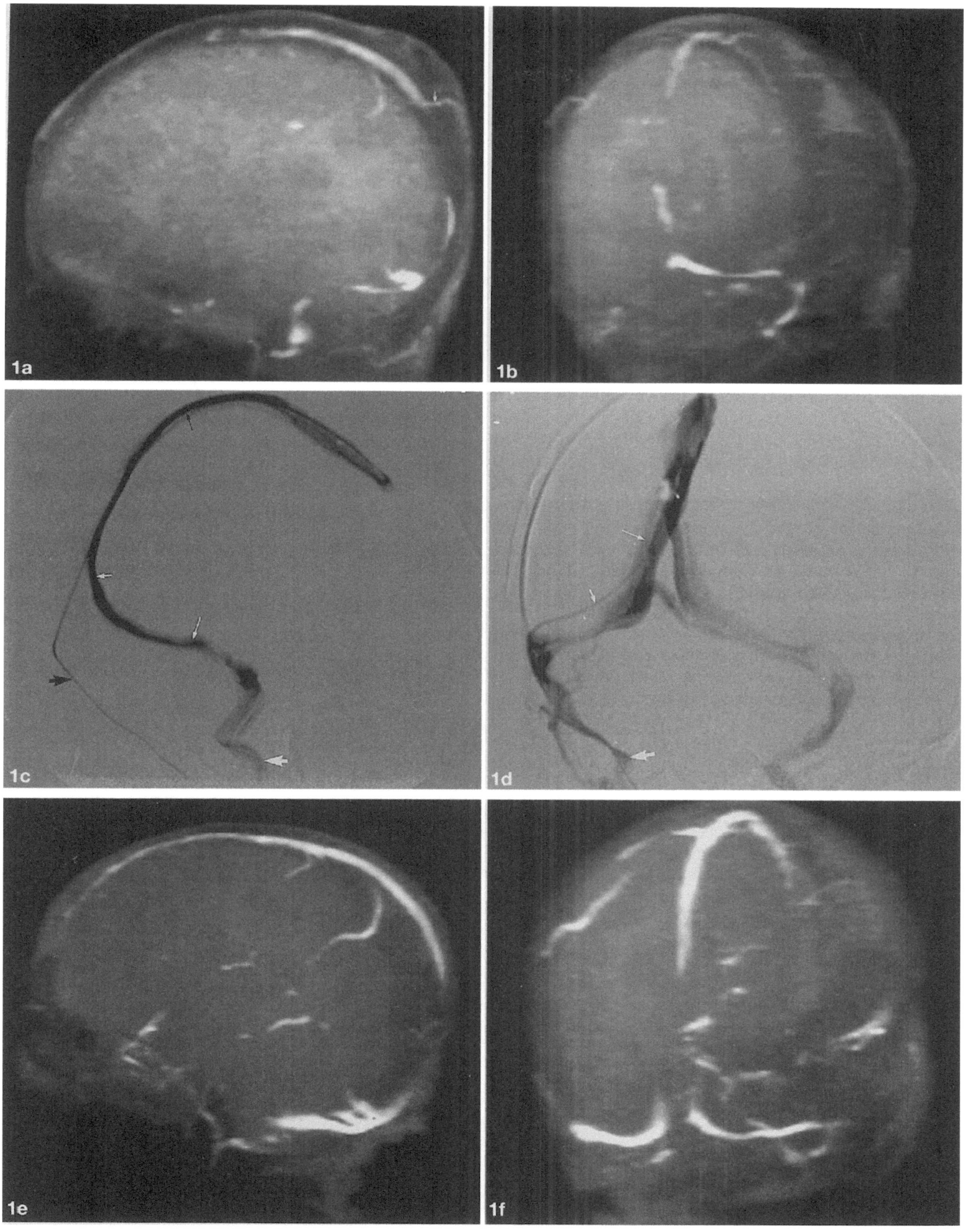
1a
1b
1c
1d
1e
1f

2D sequential time-of-flight (TOF) technique in the oblique sagittal and transverse plans. Clinical status was also recorded. DSV was performed via the percutaneous transfemoral vein ($n = 5$) or transjugular vein approach ($n = 2$), utilizing a coaxial angiographic 5-F catheter system in which a Tracker-18 catheter was placed retrogradely into the dural sinus. After the confirmation of the DVST, the Tracker catheter was then repositioned to the thrombosed dural sinuses. Thrombolysis was performed by a bolus injection of 50,000 IU urokinase every 10–15 min, until thrombolysis and recanalization were evident on DSV (Fig. 1). The total dose of urokinase injected for each patient ranged from 100,000 to 1,525,000 IU.

Results

Contributing factors included mastoiditis ($n = 3$), diarrhea ($n = 3$), and premature birth with right subclavian vein catheterization ($n = 1$). The clinical features are lethargy ($n = 4$), seizure ($n = 3$), headache ($n = 2$) and esotropia ($n = 2$). Clinically, six patients recovered completely; that one patient did not show any improvement was due to coexsisting basilar artery occlusion. MRI findings before the treatment were scalp soft tissue swelling ($n = 4$), brain edema ($n = 6$), brainstem infarct ($n = 1$), and identification of the blood clots ($n = 7$). Follow-up MRI study 1 week after the treatment showed complete resolution of these changes, except for the brainstem infarct. Pretreatment venous MRA showed occlusion of the superior sagittal sinus ($n = 5$), torcular Herophili ($n = 5$), lateral sinus [right ($n = 4$), left ($n = 1$), bilateral ($n = 2$)], straight sinus ($n = 3$), internal jugular vein ($n = 2$), and jugular bulb ($n = 2$). Post-treatment venous MRA showed complete recanalization of all the thrombosed dural sinuses and cerebral veins, except in one case where there was partial recanalization of the occluded jugular bulb and ipsilateral sigmoid sinus.

Discussion

The diffculty of early diagnosis of acute DVST in childhood is a serious clinical problem which entails a high mortality and morbidity rate without treatment [5]. MRI may show scalp soft tissue swelling, brain edema, brain infarcts and hemorrhage and may identify the blood clots as a lack of signal void (acute) or high signal intensity (subacute) in the dural sinuses and/or in the cerebral venous system [2–5]. 2D sequential TOF venous MRA is a rapid and reliable noninvasive imaging technique which can identify the normal and thrombosed dural sinus as well as the large deep cerebral venous system. The T1 shortening effect of extracellular methemoglobin from subacute blood clots or hemorrhage may result in hyperintensity mimicking the patency of venous flow in a TOF gradient-echo imaging. However, in our experience, 2D TOF imaging together with maximum-intensity projection using ray-tracing algorithm venous MRA showed extracellular methemoglobin thrombus to be significantly less intense than the normal venous flow. In addition, T1-weighted MRI also helped us to differentiate the high-signal thrombosed blood clots from the normal venous flow. Phase-contrast MRA, if available, will add confidence to differentiation of a thrombosed dural sinus from normal venous flow [7].

Urokinase is a direct-acting activator of plasminogen. The reasons that we chose urokinase as the thrombolytic agent in our study are its short half-life (13–20 min), rapid onset of action, low allergic reaction, and least clinically significant bleeding among the thrombolytic agents [8].

Although the number of patients is small (seven patients), the results are encouraging. From our study, PETT with urokinase seems to be a safe, rapid and effective treatment to dissolve blood clots and recanalize the venous drainage in the brain, with good clinical outcome in children with symptomatic acute DSVT.

References

1. Shlers H, Courville CB (1936) Thrombosis of internal cerebral veins in infancy and childhood: review of the literature and report of five cases. J Pediatr 8:600–623
2. Hulcelle PJ, Dooms GC, Mathurin P, Cornelis G (1989) MRI assessment of unsuspected dural sinus thrombosis. Neuroradiology 31:217–221
3. Virapongse C, Cazenave C, Quisling R, Sarwar M, Hunter S (1987) The empty delta sign: frequency and significance in 76 cases of dural sinus thrombosis. Radiology 162:779–785
4. Yuh WTC, Simonson T, Wang AM, et al (1994) MRI of intracranial venous thrombosis. AJNR 15:309–316
5. Muller SM, Golden GS, Swaiman KF, et al (1982) Vascular diseases of the brain and spinal cord. In: Swaiman KF, Wright FS (eds) The practice of pediatric neurology, vol 2. Mosby, St. Louis, pp 765–822
6. Tsai FY, Higashida RT, Matovich V, Alfieri K (1992) Acute thrombosis of the intracranial dural sinus: direct thrombolytic treatment. AJNR 13:1137–1141
7. Tsuruda JS, Shimakawa A, Pelc NJ, Saloner D (1991) Dural sinus occlusion: evaluation with phase-sensitive gradient-echo MR imaging. AJNR 12:481–488
8. Bell WR, Sarahara AA (1989) Review of thrombolytic therapy and thrombolytic disease. Physicians and Scientists, Glenview, Illinois

Densitometry of cerebral circulation in patients with vasospasm during percutaneous transluminal angioplasty

T. Shibuya, H. Kushi, Y. Katayama, T. Tsubokawa

Department of Neurological Surgery, Nihon University School of Medicine, 30-1 Ohyaguchi-Kamimachi Itabashi-Ku, Tokyo, Japan

Abstract. Recently, percutaneous transluminal angioplasty (PTA) has been recognized as a useful therapy for symptomatic vasospasm following subarachnoid haemorrhage. However, some patients have not had a favourable response PTA. In the present study, we attempted to characterise the haemodynamics of such patients by employing densitometric analysis of digital subtraction angiography (DSA). Ten patients underwent PTA because of severe symptomatic vasospasm. The time-density curve (TDC) for each patient was obtained during the PTA procedure by densitometric analysis. Vasospasm was found to be associated with a delayed peak time of the TDC; this was normalized after PTA and neurological improvement was also seen. In contrast, the peak time of TDC remained delayed in three patients who did not show neurological improvement even though the affected vessels were successfully dilated. Delayed TDC that persists after PTA is due to an elevated cerebrovasular resistance in the peripheral microcirculation. The densitometric analysis provides valuable information for choosing suitable therapeutic approaches during PTA.

Key words: Angioplasty – Time-density curve – Cerebral blood flow – Digital subtraction angiography – Vasospasm

The haemodynamics of cerebral circulation in patients with vasospasm following subarachnoid haemorrhage is not yet completely understood. During the last decade, the incidence of permanent neurological deficits caused by vasospasm has fallen markedly owing to the availability of percutanous transluminal angioplasty (PTA).

Nevertheless, there is a group of patients do not respond favourably to PTA. In the present study, we attempted to characterise haemodynamics of such patients by means of densitometric analysis of digital subtraction angiography (DSA).

Materials and methods

A total of ten patients with severe symptomatic vasospasm caused by subarachnoid haemorrhage were examined (Table 1). They underwent PTA with a balloon catheter when their neurological symptoms progressed in spite of the induced hypertension and hypercolaemic therapy. The densitometric analysis was carried out with DSA during the PTA procedures. The region of interest was set as a 32×32 matrix on the lateral view, at a peripheral branch of the middle cerebral artery, avoiding contamination with major cortical veins (Fig. 1). Time-density curves (TDC) before and after PTA were compared. The outcome was evaluated 6 months after the onset of subarachnoid haemorrhage.

Results

Spasm was revealed in the supraclinoid portion of 14 internal carotid arteries and the proximal portion of 14 middle cerebral arteries (Table 1). All of these lesions were

Table 1. Clinical summary of ten patients treated by PTA

Case	Age	Site of aneurysm	Interval from SAH to PTA (days)	Interval from NS to PTA (hours)	Vessels treated	TDC analysis: Delay to peak	TDC analysis: Revovery	Outcome
1	47	MCA	9	10	both IC, M1	Yes	Yes	GR
2	46	Acomm, Pcomm	14	12	both IC, M1	Yes	Yes	GR
3	36	Acomm	12	9	IC, M1	Yes	No	D
4	51	BAPcomm	7	48	IC, M1	Yes	No	D
5	42		6	6	IC, M1	Yes	Yes	GR
6	52	MCA	10	24	both IC, M1	Yes	No	D
7	46	Both Pcomm	7	12	RIC, M1	Yes	Yes	GR
8	59	Acomm	10	4	IC, M1	Yes	Yes	GR
9	38	Acomm	10	24	both IC, M1	Yes	No	MD
10	48	MCA	10	4	RIC, M1	Yes	Yes	GR

SAH, subarachnoid haemorrhage; PTA, percutaneous transluminal angioplasty; NS, neurological signs; TDC, time-density curve; Pcomm, posterior communicating; Acom, anterior communicating; BA, basilar bifurcation; MCA, middle cerebral artery; IC, internal carotid artery; GR, good recovery; D, dead; MD, moderate disability

Correspondence to: T. Shibuya

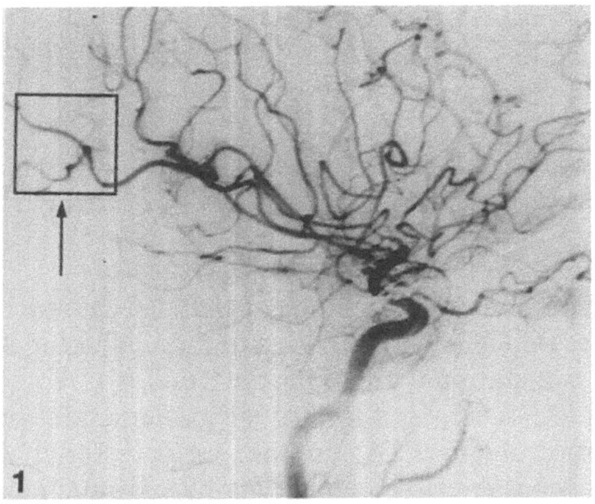

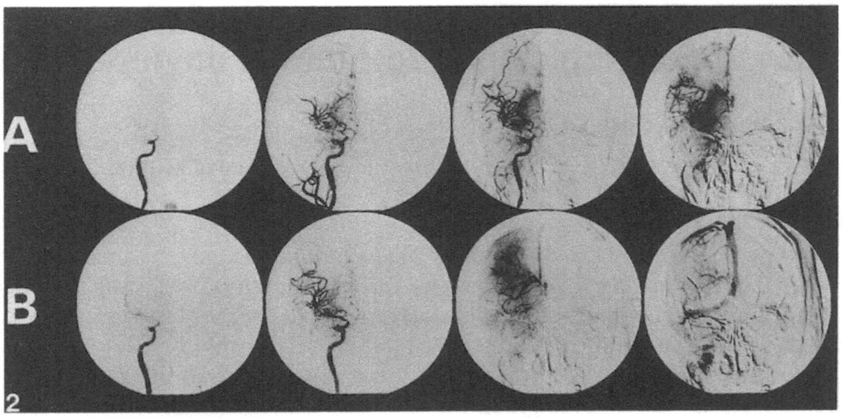

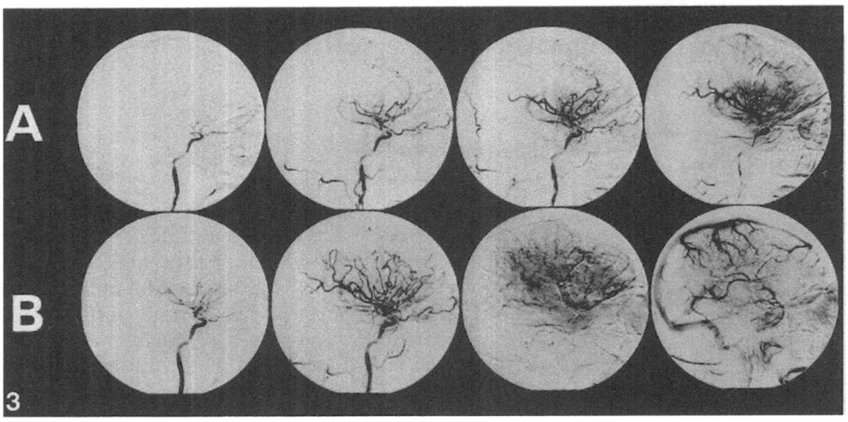

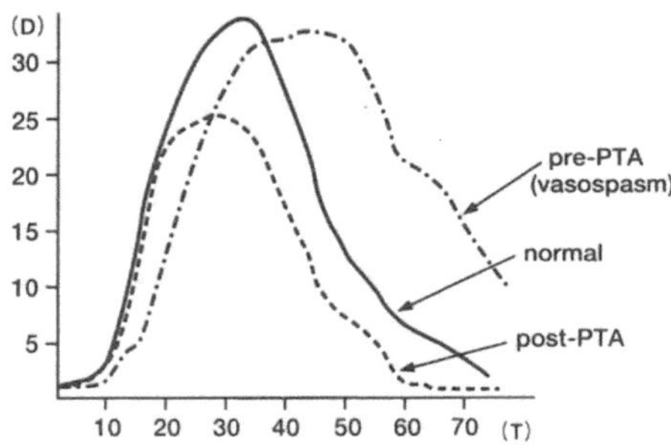

4

Fig. 1. Case 7. Right internal carotid angiogram, lateral view. The square area (*arrow*) indicates the region of interest on the middle cerebral artery perfusion area, avoiding contamination with major cortical veins

Fig. 2 A. B. Case 7. Right internal carotid angiogram, anteroposterior view. **A** Diffuse, severe vasospasm of the supraclinoid segment of the right internal carotid artery and proximal middle cerebral artery before PTA. **B** After PTA, demonstrating normal luminal diameters

Fig. 3 A, B. Case 7. Right internal carotid angiogram, laterial view. **A** Before PTA, demonstrating diffuse severe vasospasm and delay in circulation. **B** After PTA, in which the diameter of the internal carotid and middle cerebral arteries was normalised. Cerebral circulation also improved

Fig. 4. Case 7. Time-density curve revealed delay of peak time before PTA and was normal after PTA

classified as severe (diameter of stenotic region <50%) and diffuse (length of stenotic region >20 mm) (Fig. 2). Out of these lesions, 27 (96.4%) were successfully dilated by PTA (Fig. 3). However, only seven of the ten patients (70%) demonstrated neurological improvements. Vasospasm was found to be associated with delayed peaking of TDC, which became normal after, PTA, together with neurological improvement (Fig. 4). In contrast, peaking of the TDC remained delayed in three patients whose neurological symptoms did not improve even though the affected vessels were successfully dilated.

Discussion

There is no efficient medical treatment for severe symptomatic vasospam following subarachnoid haemorrhage. Undoubtedly, PTA is useful in such patients [1–3] unless the brain tissue is irreversibly damaged [4, 5]. The effect of PTA is naturally attributable to the dilatation of affected vessels, which can easily be assessed by visual inspection of the DSA [6–8]. However, the cerebral blood flow is not only dependent on the diameter of affected vessels, but also on cerebrovascular resistance. An unchanged peak time of the TDC after PTA appears to reflect an elevated cerebrovascular resistance in the peripheral circulation. Thus, persistent neurological symptoms after PTA may be attributable to unimproved cerebral blood flow owing to the elevated cerebrovascular resistance. Densitometric analysis of DSA is useful for detecting such a condition during PTA procedures.

The elevation of peripheral cerebrovascular resistance may be caused by disturbances in microcirculation, as the consequence of prolonged hypoperfusion in the territory of affected vessels. To improve microcirculation, urokinase and nicardipine can be used, together with a superselective papaverine infusion [3]. Densitometric analysis of DSA provides valuable information for choosing such a therapy during the PTA procedure.

Densitometric analysis of DSA suggests that neurological symptoms that persist after PTA are due to an elevated cerebrovascular resistance in the peripheral circulation. This technique is useful for choosing therapeutic approaches during the PTA procedure.

References

1. Livingston K, Hopkins LN (1993) Intraarterial papaverine as an adjunct to transluminal angioplasty for vasospasm induced by subarachnoid hemorrhage. AJNR 14:346–347
2. le Roux PD, Newell DW, Eskridge J, Mayberg MR, Winn HR (1994) Severe symptomatic vasospasm: the role of immediate postoperative angioplasty. J Neurosurg 80:224–229
3. Kaku Y, Yonekawa Y, Tsukahara T, Kazekawa K (1994) Superselective intra-arterial infusion of papaverine for the treatment of cerebral vasospasm after subarachnoid hemorrhage. J Neurosurg 77:842–847
4. Yonas H, Sekhar L, Johnson DW, Gur D (1989) Determination of irreversible ischemia by xenon-enhanced computed tomographic monitoring of cerebral blood flow in patients with symptomatic vasospasm. Neurosurgery 24:368–372
5. Grosset DG, Straiton J, Trevou M du, Bullock R (1992) Prediction of symptomatic vasospasm after subarachnoid haemorrhage by rapidly increasing transcranial Doppler velocity and cerebral blood flow changes. Stroke 23:674–679
6. Fischer CM, Kistler JP, Davis JM (1980) Relation of cerebral vasospasm to subarachnoid hemorrhage, visualized by computerized tomographic scanning. Neurosurgery 6:1–9
7. Hirata Y, Nonaka N, Matsukado Y, Takahashi M (1987) Clinical application of dynamic digital subtraction angiography in cerebrovascular ischemic diseases. Kumamoto Med J 40:103–117
8. Touho H, Karasawa J, Tazawa T, Yamada K, Kobayashi K (1988) Intra-arterial digital subtraction angiography for evaluation of cerebral circulation, part 1. Jpn J Stroke 10:79–84

Intervention: fistulae

Transvenous embolisation of dural arteriovenous fistulae with coils

H. C. Nahser[1], D. Kühne[1], H. Henkes[1], F. Mosler[1], E. Berg-Dammer[2]

[1] Department of Neuroradiology, Alfried-Krupp-Krankenhaus, Essen, Germany
[2] Department of Neurology, Alfried-Krupp-Krankenhaus, Essen, Germany

Abstract. In 32 of 69 patients with a dural fistula at the cavernous sinus, transvenous embolisation was used when glaucoma and loss of vision could not be controlled by transarterial embolisation, or in 16 where there was cortical drainage of the fistula. Exact closure of the fistulous points in the cavernous sinus was performed using platinum microcoils. These resulted in primary or secondary clinical and radioanatomical cure as documented by follow-up angiography in all but 4 patients, who had persistent symptoms, or their ocular signs recurred. No additional cortical drainage developed. In a second operation, the cavernous sinus and the origin of the ophthalmic vein were occluded totally with coils. In 16 fistulae at the transverse/sigmoid sinus, transvenous coil embolisation was used when cortical drainage or a intolerable bruit persisted after arterial embolisation. A definitive occlusion was achieved in all but one case, as documented by angiography 3 months later. There were no major complications, but all the patients complained of headache, and/ or vomiting and vertigo within the first 2–3 weeks.

Key words: Cavernous sinus – Transverse sinus – Dural arteriovenous fistula – Coil occlusion

Neuroradiological interventional treatment of dural arteriovenous fistulae consists mainly of embolisation with liquids or particles via the transarterial approach. A definite occlusion was not always achieved, when there was an arterial supply by branches of the vertebral or internal carotid artery [1]. Here we focus on cases of dural fistulae of the cavernous and transverse sinus treated by transvenous coil occlusion, and discuss whether this technique can be applied with an acceptable risk and whether long-term results are acceptable.

Patients and methods

In 32 of 69 patients with a dural fistula at the cavernous sinus, transvenous embolisation was used when glaucoma and loss of vision could not be controlled by transarterial embolisation with polyvinyl alcohol particles via branches of the external carotid artery in 16 cases, when there was cortical drainage of the fistula. Closure of the fistulous points in the cavernous sinus was first performed. The technique was as follows: at first direct arterial embolisation of external carotid feeders was chosen to reduce the flow of the fistula. Then a guiding catheter was placed in the jugular bulb. From this point an approach to the cavernous sinus was possible via the ipsi- or contralateral inferior petrous sinus, even if the sinus was not visible in the standard angiogram or if it was not participating in the drainage of the fistula. After exact localisation of the fistulous compartment, only this compartment of the cavernous sinus was occluded with coils of variable size. This resulted in primary or secondary clinical and radicanatomical cure as documented by control angiography in all but 4 patients, who had persistent symptoms, or whose ocular signs recurred. No additional cortical drainage developed. In a second operation, the cavernous sinus and the origin of the ophthalmic vein were occluded totally with coils. In these cases too, the symptoms resolved.

In 16 of 65 cases with fistulae at the transverse/sigmoid sinus, transvenous coil embolisation was used. The main indication was cortical drainage which had led to haemorrhage or to raised intracranial pressure. In 10 cases the transvenous approach to the fistula was via the ipsilateral sigmoid sinus, and in 6 from the contralateral side. In 5 of these where there was a thrombotic occlusion of the adjacent sinus system, 2 cases in the medial transverse sinus, 2 in the caudal sigmoid sinus and 2 occluded both caudally and medially. These thrombosed parts of the sinus were passed with the Tracker catheter with the exception of one additional case, later treated by open surgery. A definite occlusion was achieved in all cases treated with platinum coils, as documented by angiographic control 3 months later. There were no major complications, but all the patients complained of headache, vomiting and vertigo within the first 2–3 weeks.

Discussion

Transvenous coil occlusion used in cases of cavernous sinus and transverse sinus dural fistulae led to a high rate of effective closure of the fistulae. This leads to amelioration or complete resolvement of symptoms in these patients. There was negligable morbidity and no mortality. As in the series of Gobin et al. [2] a thrombosed or occluded sinus can be passed through with a microcatheter with no further risk of vessel laceration. In conclusion, definitive occlusion of dural fistulae in the cavernous or transverse/sigmoid sinuses which cannot be closed by transarterial embolisation is possible via the transvenous approach.

References

1. Lasjaunias PL, Rodesch G (1993) Lesion types, hemodynamics and clinical spectrum. In: Awad IA, Barrow DL (eds) Dural arteriovenous malformations. AANS, Park Ridge, Ill
2. Gobin YP, Houdart E, Rogopoulus A, Casasco A (1992) Percutaneous transvenous embolisation through the thrombosed sinus in transverse sinus dural fistula. AJNR 14:1102–1105

Correspondence to: H. C. Nahser, Department of Neuroradiology, Alfried-Krupp-Krankenhaus, Alfried-Krupp-Strasse 21, D-45117 Essen, Germany

Transvenous embolisation for cavernous dural arteriovenous shunts: case selection and methods of embolisation

A. Takahashi[1], M. Ezura[1], Y. Fujii[1], T. Yoshimoto[2]

[1] Division of Intravascular Neurosurgery, Department of Neurosurgery, Kohnan Hospital, Sendai, Japan
[2] Department of Neurosurgery, Tohoku University of Medicine, Sendai, Japan

Abstract. To evaluate the efficacy of transvenous embolisation for cavernous dural arteriovenous shunts (CdAVS) as a primary treatment modality, angiographic classification based on the drainage system and embolisation methods were analysed. From May 1987 to March 1994, of 76 cases admitted we treated 53 cases (7 men, 46 women aged 38–85 years, average 64.3 years; bilateral lesions in 9) of CdAVS by transvenous embolisation. Based on the venous drainage pattern and shunting architecture, the appropriate approach and method of embolisation were selected. Sixty transvenous embolisation procedures (via the superior ophthalmic vein in 22, the inferior betrosal sinus in 36, both in 2) were performed. Immediately after embolisation, we achieved complete radioanatomical cure in 33 cases (62.3%). Complete cure rate at follow-up (average follow-up 8.9 months) was 94.3%. Complications included transient cavernous sinus syndrome in 8, redirection of venous flow in 2, posterior ischaemic optic neuropathy in 1, and cerebral infarction in 1. Transvenous embolisation for CdAVS would offer satisfactory therapeutic efficacy when applied considering venous drainage pattern and shunting architecture.

Key words: Dura mater – Arteriovenous shunts – Embolisation – Vein – Coils

Clinical features of cavernous dural arteriovenous shunts (CdAVS) are mainly related to venous drainage [1]. Because of this, and the abundant dural arterial network, we were forced to develop the method of transvenous embolisation [2]. We present our experiences of treating CdAVS using transvenous embolisation as primary treatment, during the past 7 years.

Materials and methods

We treated 53 cases of CdAVS from 76 cases admitted. In these 53 cases, transvenous embolisation was used as primary treatment. There were 7 men and 46 women, aged between 38 and 85 years (average age 64.3). AV shunts involved the left cavernous sinus in 25 cases, the right in 9 and both cavernous sinuses in 9 (17.0%). Accordingly, 62 CdAVS were embolised.

We classified them into three types, based on the pattern of venous drainage on angiography. Type I referred to patients whose venous drainage was directed only anteriorly. Type II referred to those whose venous drainage was directed only posteriorly. Type III referred to those whose venous drainage was directed not only anteriorly but also posteriorly. Anterior venous drainage consists of superior and inferior ophthalmic veins. Posterior venous drainage consists of superior and inferior petrosal sinuses. Shunting architecture could be classified into two groups. One type was "diffuse" AV shunts and another was "localized". Based on these angiographic classifications, the symptoms and signs were analysed and embolisation methods were selected.

If the lesion was type II or III, we tried to catheterise the cavernous sinus through the inferior petrosal sinus (IPS). This approach was designated as the posterior approach. If the lesion was type I, we catheterised the sinus through the superior ophthalmic vein (SOV). This was designated as the anterior approach. However, for this group, it is worth trying to catheterise the sinus through the IPS.

For the anterior approach, Doppler ultrasound flowmetry was used to detect the exit point of the SOV. A small skin incision was made to expose the junction between the angular vein and the SOV. Then the SOV was carefully dissected and the direction of venous outflow was detected by Doppler. Direct catheterisation using a 3F polyethylene catheter, or Tracker catheter, was made. Special care was taken to preserve the continuity of the SOV during and after the embolisation.

Correspondence to: A. Takahashi, Division of Intravascular Neurosurgery, Department of Neurosurgery, Kohnan Hospital, 4-20-1, Nagamachi-Minami, Taihaku-ku, Sendai 982, Japan

Results

Type I lesions were found in 17 cases (32%), type II in 9 (17%), type III in 27 (51%). Cortical venous drainage was seen in 35 cases (66%) (type I, 7; type II, 7; type III, 21), but not in 18 (34%) (type I, 10; type II, 2; type III, 6). As regards clinical features, one patient with cortical venous drainage showed intracerebral haemorrhage. The presentation on admission is shown in Table 1. Table 1 also shows the relationship between venous drainage type and clinical presentation. Chemosis and exophthalmos were closely related to type I lesions, while diplopia and tinnitus were related to type II lesions.

Sixty procedures were carried out (Table 2). Ipsilateral approach to the lesion was used in 48 procedures (80%), while contralateral approach was necessary in 12 procedures (20%). Posterior approach was used in 36 procedures (60%), while anterior approach was necessary in 22 procedures (36.6%). To complete the procedure, it was necessary to use both anterior and posterior approach in 2 procedures. Of 21 procedures for type I lesions, anterior approach was used in 18 procedures (85.7%), while it was possible to enter the cavernous sinus through angiographically occluded IPS in 3 procedures (14.3%). Of 9 procedures for type II lesions, all procedures were done through posterior approach. Of 30 procedures for type III lesions, posterior approach was used in 24 procedures (80%), while anterior approach was utilised in 4 procedures (13.3%) and anterior, together with posterior, approach was necessary in 2 procedures (6.7%).

Table 1. Clinical presentation and relationship to type of venous drainage

	Total (53 cases) (%)	Type I (17 cases) (%)	Type II (9 cases) (%)	Type III (27 cases) (%)
Diplopia	44 (83.0)	12 (70.6)	9 (100.0)	23 (85.2)
Blephaloptosis	13 (24.5)	2 (11.8)	2 (22.2)	9 (33.3)
Tinnitus	25 (47.2)	7 (41.2)	6 (66.7)	12 (44.4)
Ophthalmia	27 (50.9)	10 (58.8)	3 (33.3)	14 (51.9)
Chemosis	40 (75.5)	17 (100.0)	3 (33.3)	20 (74.1)
Exophthalmos	28 (52.8)	15 (88.2)	1 (11.1)	12 (44.4)
Decreased visual acuity	12 (22.6)	3 (17.6)	1 (11.1)	8 (29.6)
Increased intra-ocular pressure	7 (13.2)	4 (23.5)	0 (0.0)	3 (11.1)

Table 2. Route of venous approach

Approach	Ipsilateral (%)	Contra-lateral (%)	Total (%)
Unilateral IPS	24	9	33 (55.0)
Bilateral IPS	2	–	2 (3.3)
MS + IPS	0	1	1 (1.7)
SOV + IPS	2	0	2 (3.3)
FV to SOV	2	0	2 (3.3)
Direct SOV	18	2	20 (33.3)
Total	48 (80.0	12 (20.0)	

IPS, Inferior petrosal sinus; MS, marginal sinus; SOV, superior ophthalmic vein; FV, facial vein

Angiographically complete cure was obtained in 33 cases (62.3%) immediately after the embolisation. Follow-up angiography between 1 and 35 months later (average 8.9 months later) revealed complete cure in 50 cases (94.3%). Angiographic and clinical follow-up showed no recurrence, except for one patient, who experienced tinnitus due to a new dAVS formation at a distant sinus. Complications were as follows: transient cavernous sinus syndrome involving trigeminal and/or oculomotor, abducens nerves was observed in 8 cases. This was considered to be due to compression of these nerves by embolic materials and was resolved within several months in all instances. Visual disturbance due to redirection of shunt flow into the SOV was seen in 2 cases. Immediate re-embolisation was done in 1 case, but partial impairment in unilateral visual acuity remained. Posterior ischaemic optic neuropathy and cerebral infarction due to accessory transarterial embolisation, were each seen in 1 case. Two cases showed new lesions involving the inferior petrosal sinus, one symptomatic and another nonsymptomatic.

Discussion

For the treatment of CdAVS, we had embolised the lesions by transarterial embolisation using oestrogen [3]. However, transarterial embolisation had limitations because of abundant collaterial dural networks. Then, transvenous embolisation had been developed [2, 4–7]. The experiences of the past 7 years have convinced us that transvenous embolisation is the first-choice treatment for this clinical entity.

Clinical features were analysed with regard to the venous drainage pattern. Except for the symptoms due to the AVs itself (tinnitus), clinical presentations were related to the venous drainage pattern. Ocular disturbances, including chemosis, exophthalmos, decreased visual acuity and increased intraocular pressure, were mainly related to type I (anterior drainage) lesions. The fact that chemosis, exophthalmos and decreased visual acuity were associated with some cases of type II (posterior drainage lesions), may be related to the change of the venous drainage pattern. In these cases, the venous drainage pattern was changed from type III or type I into type II because of the progressive outflow obstruction, due to the high venous flow. The incidence of cavernous sinus syndromes such as diplopia and blephaloptosis was higher in type II (posterior drainage). Tinnitus was also associated in higher incidence with type II lesions. Cases with type III venous drainage showed the characteristics of both type I and type II. Cortical venous reflux is one of the most reliable indicators of possible brain symptoms such as intracranial haemorrhage and venous infarction. The incidence of intracranial haemorrhage of CdAVS is lower than in lesions involving other major sinuses. However, we found cortical venous drainge in 66% of cases. If the lesion has this venous drainage, aggressive treatment should be considered to prevent future brain symptoms.

Analysis of venous drainage patterns was also essential to select the approach of transvenous embolisation. Although it was possible to enter the affected cavernous sinus in 14.3% of type I lesions by posterior approach, it was easier to use anterior approach for this type. All cases of type II were embolised successfully using posterior approach. In type III lesions, 80% were successfully treated by posterior approach, while anterior approach was necessary in 13.3% and simultaneous anterior and posterior approach was used in 6.7%. The anterior approach using direct exposure of the SOV may require certain experience. However, this is an easier, and more instant method than an anterior approach through a facial vein. Although transfemoral transfacial vein approach is considered a more elegant method, lengthy manipulation around the junction of the angular vein and the SOV may cause mechanically induced spasms, which may require emergent obliteration of the AV shunt because of acute deterioration of optic nerve function.

Complications of the transvenous approach were classified into three types: perforation of venous structures, over-embolisation, and redirection of venous outflow. Perforation of venous structures has been reported in the literature, as the most serious complication [8]. We have never encountered this complication; however, it should be prevented by using small and flexible catheters and guide wires with careful manipulation. Over-embolisation may cause a cavernous sinus syndrome. To prevent this complication, selective venous pouch embolisation for localized AV shunts is recommended. For diffuse AV shunts, it is necessary to use whole cavernous sinus packing or venous outflow occlusion. In this situation, the distal part of the cavernous sinus or venous outflow tends to be embolised loosely. This may cause over-embolisation of the rest of the sinus. Therefore, it is recommended to pack the distal compartment as tightly as possible. Redirection of venous outflow was observed when AV shunts could not be obliterated completely [6]. In such a situation the remaining shunt flow was redirected into another available venous pathway. This complication would be symptomatic when the venous outflow is redirected into the SOV (especially into the central retinal vein) or into the cortical vein. Therefore, critical analysis of venous drainage patterns before the embolisation is essential. When it occurs emergency re-embolisation using a transvenous and/or transarterial approach should be followed. We have observed the appearance of new dural AV shunts involving remote sinuses in two cases. Both cases involved the ipsilateral inferior petrosal sinus which was chateterised at the time of embolisation. A similar case was reported by Yamashita et al. [9]. The relationship between transvenous embolisation and newly developed dAVS is not clear. Carful observation of the long-term follow-up is needed.

References

1. Lasjaunias P, Chiu M, Terbrugge K, Tolia A, Hurth M, Berenstein A (1986) Neurological manifestations of intracranial dural arteriovenous malformations. J Neurosurg 64:724–730
2. Takahashi A, Yoshimoto T, Kawakami K, Sugawara T, Suzuki J (1989) Transvenous copper wire insertion for dural arteriovenous malformations of cavernous sinus. J Neurosurg 70:751–754
3. Suzuki J, Komatsu S (1981) New liquid embolisation method using estrogen for dural arteriovenous malformation and meningiomas. Surg Neurol 16:438–442
4. Peterson EW, Valberg J, Whittingham DS (1969) Electrically induced thrombosis of the cavernous sinus in the treatment of carotid-cavernous fistula (abstract). In: Drake CG, Duvoisin R (eds) Proceedings of the Fourth International Congress Series, vol 193. Excerpta Medica, Amsterdam, p 105
5. Teng MMH, Guo WY, Huang CI, Wu CC, Chang T (1988) Occlusion of arteriovenous malformation of the cavernous sinus via the superior ophthalmic vein. AJNR 9:539–546
6. Halbach VV, Higashida RT, Hieshima GB, Hardin CW, Pribram H (1989) Transvenous embolization of dural fistulas involving the cavernous sinus. AJNR 10:377–383
7. Komiyama M, Morikawa K, Fu Y, Yagura H, Yasui T, Baba M (1990) Indirect carotid-cavernous sinus fistula: transvenous embolization from the external jugular vein using a superior ophthalmic vein approach. A case report. Surg Neurol 33:57–63
8. Halbach VV, Higashida RT, Hieshima GB, Hardin CW, Yang PJ (1988) Transvenous embolization of direct carotid cavernous fistulas. AJNR 9:741–747
9. Yamashita K, Taki W, Nakahara I, Nishi S, Sadato A, Kikuchi H (1993) Development of sigmoid dural arteriovenous fistulas after transvenous embolization of cavernous dural arteriovenous fistulas. AJNR 14:1106–1108

In vitro evaluation of mechanically detachable coils

M. P. Marks, C. C. Tsai, H. Chee

Department of Radiology, Stanford University Medical Center, Stanford, CA 94305, USA

Abstract. This study was designed to evaluate the physical characteristics of mechanically detachable coils constructed of platinum, tantalum, and nitinol. Four physical characteristics of the coils were assessed: pliability of stiffness, shape memory, friction generated by introduction through a microcatheter, and stability following placement. Although we demonstrated that stiffer metals (tantalum > platinum > nitinol) exert greater frictional forces within the catheter and a greater resistive force during bending, we also demonstrated that they are more stable following placement.

Correspondence to: M. P. Marks

Key words: Interventional instrumentation, coils – Interventional neuroradiology, models – Aneurysm, therapeutic blockade – Arteries, therapeutic blockade

Platinum coils have been widely used to treat vascular lesions of the central nervous system, such as aneurysms, arteriovenous fistulae and arteriovenous malformations [1–4]. Various implantable devices have been used to treat these lesions. We report in vitro studies of coil materials.

Materials and methods

Mechanically detachable coils [5] were constructed with simple helical (4 mm × 10 cm and 8 mm × 30 cm) and pretzel shapes (4 mm × 5 cm), from three metals using 0.003″ and 0.004″ wire. Coils were assessed for frictional resistance in an 0.018″ microcatheter set in a fixed figure-of-eight position and frictional forces were measured with pushing and pulling. Stiffness or pliability was measured using a bending-stiffness tester. Stability following deployment was assessed in a pulsatile flow system utilizing a 1-cm glass aneurysm model.

Results

Frictional resistance at deployment was found to be greatest for tungsten, intermediate for platinum, and least for nitinol. These differences were statistically significant ($P<0.05$) in both 0.003″ and 0.004″ sizes. Frictional forces were less dependent on coil length, but depended instead on the complex 3D coil shape and the diameter of the turns in the shape. The 5-cm pretzel coil consistently created more frictional force than the 10-cm or 30-cm simple helical coils ($P<0.0002$). Despite being shorter, the 4-mm simple helical coil exerted more frictional force than the 8-mm coil ($P<0.05$). Pliability testing showed that tungsten generated a far greater resistance to bending when compared to platinum, which was itself greater than nitinol ($P<0.01$). Stiffer metals (tungsten and platinum) had a far greater rise in resistive force, particularly at greater deflection angles, when compared to a softer metal (nitinol). Assessments of coil stability in a pulsatile system showed that larger coils constructed of larger diameter wire (0.004″) were generally more stable. The softer metal (nitinol) was far less stable than platinum or tungsten.

Discussion

Our data suggest that a family of coils composed of different metals is indicated for various intravascular needs.

References

1. Guglielmi G, Viñuela F, Duckwiler G, et al (1992) Endovascular treatment of posterior circulation aneurysms by electrothrombosis using electrically detachable coils. J Neurosurg 77:515–524
2. Cascasco AE, Aymard A, Gobin P, et al (1993) Selective endovascular treatment of 71 intracranial aneurysms with platinum coils. J Neurosurg 79:3–10
3. Guglielmi G, Viñuela F, Briganti F, Duckwiler G (1992) Carotid-cavernous fistula caused by a ruptured intracavernous aneurysm: endovascular treatment by electrothrombosis with detachable coils. Neurosurgery 31:591–597
4. Smith MD, Russell EJ, Levy R, Crowell RM (1990) Transcatheter obliteration of a cerebellar arteriovenous fistula with platinum coils. AJNR 11:1199–1202
5. Marks MP, Chee H, Liddell RP, et al (1994) A mechanically detachable coil for the treatment of aneurysms and occlusion of blood vessels. AJNR 15:821–827

Clinical use of mechanically detachable coils for interventional neuroradiology

T. Terada[1], Y. Kinoshita[1], M. Tsuura[1], H. Yokote[1], K. Nakai[1], K. Itakura[1], S. Hayashi[2], J. Minamikawa[3], T. Kuriyama[4]

[1] Wakayama Medical College, Iban-cho 27, Wakayama city, 640 Japan
[2] Kokuritsu Minami Wakayama Hospital, Wakayama, Japan
[3] Kishiwada Municipal Hospital, Osaka, Japan
[4] Wakayama Red Cross Hospital, Wakayama, Japan

Abstract. We report our clinical experience of mechanically detachable coils (MDC) for neurointerventional radiology. We embolised nine patients with various cerebrovascular diseases using 84 MDC: three had intracranial aneurysms, five dural arteriovenous fistulae, and one a cerebral arteriovenous malformation. All were successfully embolised by MDC except one, in whom premature coil detachment occurred and the residual coil was retrieved by the snare technique. The advantage of MDC is the accurate and compact coil positioning compared with conventional microcoils. However, special care must be taken to avoid premature coil detachment and coil stretch, both possible complications of MDC.

Key words: Cerebrovascular disease – Embolisation – Interventional neuroradiology – Microcoil

Correspondence to: T. Terada

Recently, various types of microcoil have been used for interventional neuroradiological procedures [1–3]. Newly developed mechanical detachable coils (MDC) have several advantages over conventional microcoils. We used MDCs for neurointerventional cases, and the efficacy is discussed.

Materials and methods

Embolisation was performed with MDC in nine patients with various types of cerebrovascular disease. Three had cerebral aneurysms (1 giant posterior inferior cerebellar artery (PICA) aneurysm); 1 internal carotid cavernous giant aneurysm; 1 vertebral artery dissecting aneurysm); five had dural arteriovenous malformations (3 cavernous sinus; 1 transverse-sigmoid sinus; 1 cavernous-marginal sinus) and one had a cerebral arteriovenous malformation (AVM).

A Tracker 18 two-tip marker catheter was navigated into the lesions where coil embolisation was to be performed, under fluoroscopic control. A total of 84 MDC variously sized from 2 mm to 8 mm

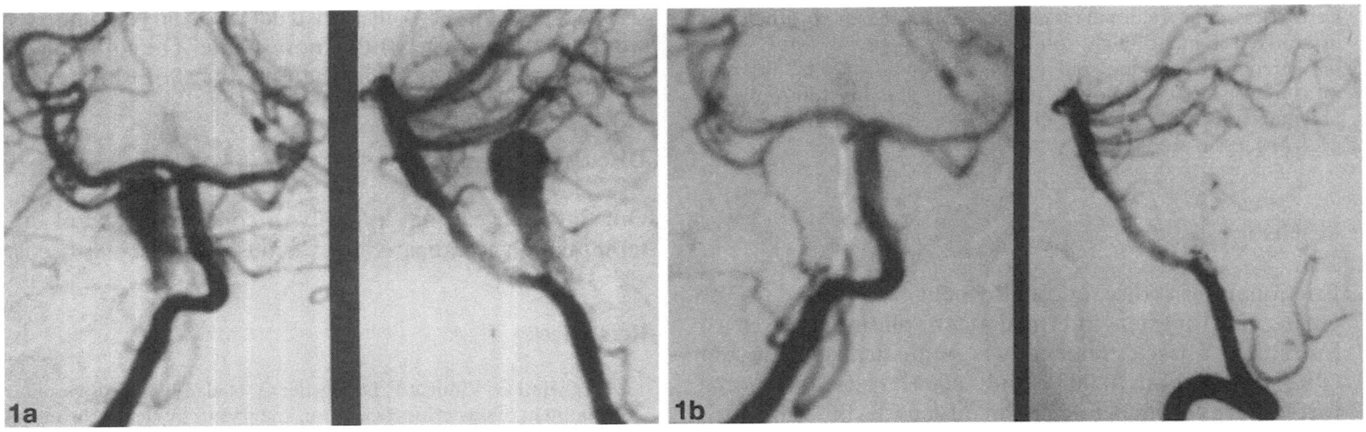

Fig. 1a, b. Case 1. Right PICA giant aneurysm. a Right vertebral angiogram before embolisation: *left*, anteroposterior, *right*, lateral; a partially thrombosed giant aneurysm is demonstrated. b After embolisation. The aneurysm has been embolised completely using MDC

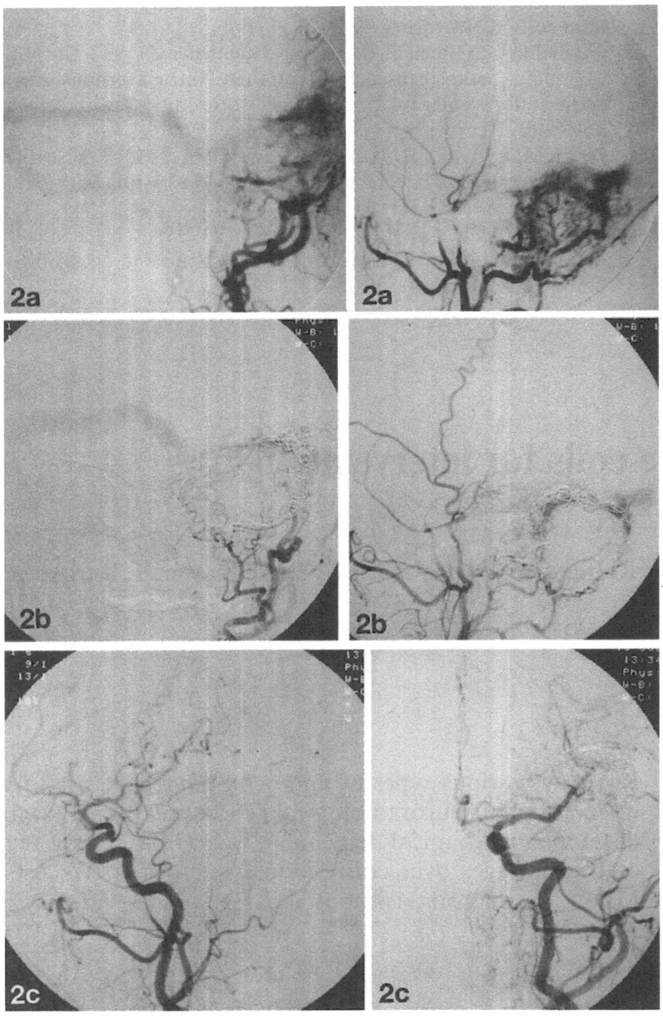

Fig. 2a–c. Case 2. a Left external carotid angiogram: *left*, anterioposterior; *right*, lateral. A dural AVM at the transverse-sigmoid sinus is demonstrated. Main feeding arteries are from occipital artery. The left internal jugular vein is occluded. b The left transverse-sigmoid sinus has been embolised using microcoils, although the AVF is still patent. c Left common carotid angiogram after MDC embolisation. The dural AVM has almost totally diappeared, although a small, faint fistula is opacified in the capillary phase

diameter were used as embolic materials. Detachable balloons were used with MDC in two cases of aneurysm to obliterate the parent artery.

Results

All the lesions were completely embolised using 84 MDC, except one transverse-sigmoid dural arteriovenous fistula; a faint slow-flow fistula remained on a follow-up angiogram. Four MDC streched during the insertion and retrieval procedure, and although three were easily retrieved one became detached inside the catheter. A special retrieval technique was applied in this case.

Case reports

Case 1

A 59-year-old woman with a history of progressive left hemiparesis and lower cranial nerve palsy was admitted to our hospital. A partially thrombosed giant PICA aneurysm was found on angiography and MRI (Fig. 1a). A Tracker 18 two-tip marker catheter was navigated into the aneurysm lumen and the aneurysm was embolised using three 7-mm, five 6-mm and two 5-mm diameter MDCs. The vertebral artery and PICA were kept patent and the aneurysm was completely obliterated (Fig. 1b). The clinical course was uneventful and the clinical signs improved slightly after embolisation. Follow-up angiography 6 months after embolisation showed complete obliteration of the aneurysm.

Case 2

A 65-year-old woman with a transverse-sigmoid dural AVM was treated by transvenous embolisation with conventional microcoils (Fig. 2a, b). One microcoil migrated into the right cardiac ventricle during the procedure. Finally, it resulted in incomplete occlusion and a retroauricular bruit reappeared. The second transvenous embolisation was performed using MDC to prevent coil migration.

The fistula was almost totally obliterated by this procedure, although a faint slow arteriovenous shunt still remained on a 3 months follow-up angiogram (Fig. 2c).

Discussion

MDC have several advantages over conventional microcoils [2, 3]. The most remarkable advantage is their retrievability, making appropriate and tight coil positioning possible without coil migration, by repeating coil positioning. Also, embolisation by MDC is faster than that by conventional microcoils, owing to the length of the coil. The disadvantage of the MDC is the high price.

Compared with GDC, MDC have both advantages and disadvantages. The advantages of MDC over GDC are the quick detachment and the fact that there is no generation of emboli during coil detachment. The disadvantages are premature detachment and coil stretch during the procedure, although the latter complication also occurs with GDC. Premature detachment is thought to happen when MDC pass through a sharp bend. The other disadvantages of MDC are the hard connecting joint at the end of the coil and the motion of MDC when released. These are serious problems when ruptured cerebral aneurysms are being embolised.

References

1. Guglielmi Gm Viñuela F, Duckwiler G, et al (1992) Endovascular treatment of posterior circulation aneurysms by electrothrombosis using electrically detachable coils. J Neurosurg 77:515–524
2. Hodes JE, Aymard A, Gobin YP, et al (1992) Endovascular occlusion of intracranial vessels for curative treatment of unclippable aneurysms: report of 16 cases. J Neurosurg 75:694–701
3. Taki W, Nishi S, Yamashita K, et al (1992) Selection and combination of various endovascular techniques in the treatment of giant aneurysms. J Neurosurg 77:37–42

Embolisation of vascular lesions of the head and neck

M. Takahashi[1], T. Nishimura[1], T. Katoh[1], H. Isoda[1], T. Masui[1], T. Mochizuki[1], M. Kaneko[1], K. Gotoh[2]

[1] Department of Radiology, Hamamatsu University School of Medicine, 3600 Handa-cho, Hamamatsu, Japan
[2] Department of Interventional Neuroradiology, Iizuka Hospital, 3-83 Yoshio-cho, Iizuka, Japan

Abstract. We reviewed 33 patients with vascular head and neck lesions treated by embolisation using a Tracker 18 catheter or direct needle injection. The lesions involved haemangiomas, venous malformations, extracranial arteriovenous malformations (AVMs), cavernous dural AVMs and ruptured dissecting or pseudoaneurysms. The cavernous dural AVMs were treated with radiation therapy in addition. We had a satisfactory outcome in 28 (85%) patients who underwent complete embolisation. No significant complications arose. These results suggest that embolisation therapy in the head and neck is an effective, safe and, in some cases, indispensable alternative.

Key words: Haemangioma – Arteriovenous malformation (AVM) – Aneurysm – Cavernous dural AVM – Embolisation

Vascular lesions in the head and neck are often difficult to treat. We review the clinical outcome of endovascular treatments given for various vascular disorders in the head and neck, and assess these procedures for efficacy, limitations and complications.

Correspondence to: M. Takahashi

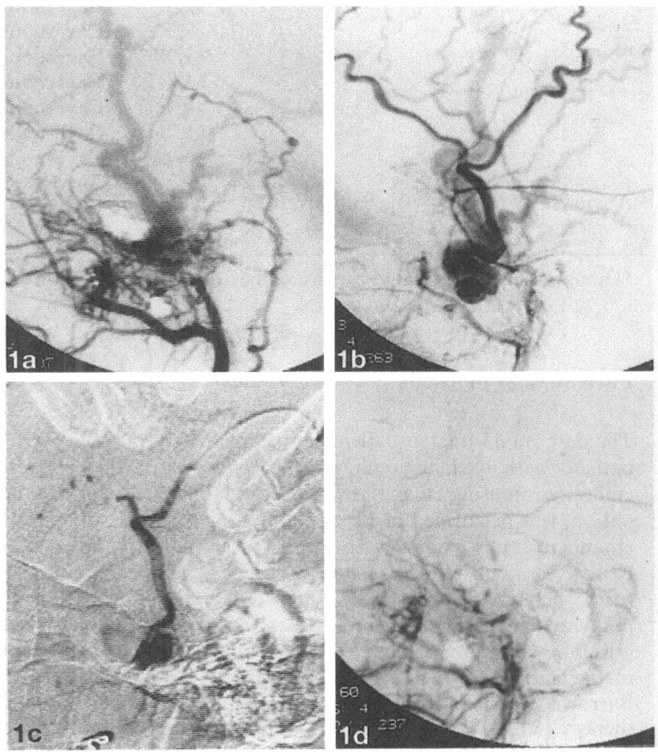

Fig. 1 a–d. Traumatic arteriovenous fistula of the scalp (patient 15). **a** Left external carotid artery. **b** Contralateral injection. **c** Embolisation using NBCA-lipiodol under flow control. **d** Left after external carotid artery embolisation

Table 1. Summary of 33 patients treated

	Preoperative or palliative	Age years/ sex	Location	Embolic material	Radiation	Outcome	Complications
Haemangioma	Preoperative	10/M	Nasal cavity	GS	–	Excellent	–
		15/F	Cheek	Eth + GS	–	Excellent	–
		28/F	Nasal cavity	GS	–	Good	–
		17/M	Nasal cavity	GS	–	Good	–
		25/M	Nasal cavity	Est + GS	–	Good	–
		68/F	Gingiva	Est + GS	–	Good	–
	Palliative	36/M	Tongue	GS	–	Excellent	–
		80/F	Floor of mouth	Eth	–	Excellent	–
		60/F	Cheek, lip, gingiva	Eth	–	Good	Transient necrosis
		13/M	Cheek, lip	GS + Eth	–	No change	–
		14/F	Cheek, lip	GS	–	No change	–
		16/F	Cheek	GS + Eth	–	No change	Submandibular adenitis
		62/M	Cheek, orbit	Est + GS	–	No change	–
Arteriovenous malformation	Preoperative	29/M	Cheek, lip	GS + coils	–	Good	–
	Palliative	22/M	Scalp	NBCA	–	Excellent	–
		14/F	Gingiva	PVA	–	Excellent	–
		50/M	Ear	Est + Eth + GS + coils	–	Good	–
Venous malformation	Palliative	65/F	Cheek[a]	Eth	–	Excellent	–
		24/F	Cheek[a]	Eth	–	Excellent	–
Cavernous dural arteriovenous malformation	Palliative	54/F	Cavernous sinus	Spongel	32.3 Gy	Good	–
		51/F	Cavernous sinus	Spongel	30.0 Gy	Excellent	–
		50/M	Cavernous sinus	Spongel	30.6 Gy	Excellent	–
		46/F	Cavernous sinus	Spongel	49.5 Gy	Good	–
		63/F	Cavernous sinus	Spongel	45.0 Gy	No change	–
		35/F	Cavernous sinus	Spongel	42.0 Gy	Excellent	–
		59/F	Cavernous sinus	Spongel	37.6 Gy	Excellent	–
		31/M	Cavernous sinus	Spongel	30.0 Gy	Excellent	–
		61/F	Cavernous sinus	Spongel	30.6 Gy	Excellent	–
		44/F	Cavernous sinus	Spongel	30.6 Gy	Excellent	Impaired vision
		61/F	Cavernous sinus	Spongel	30.6 Gy	Excellent	–
		55/M	Cavernous sinus	Spongel	30.6 Gy	Excellent	–
Aneurysm	Palliative	55/F	Left carotid artery	Coils	–	Excellent	–
		60/F	Right VA distal	Balloon	–	Excellent	–

[a]These lesions were treated by direct injection; catheterisation was used in all the rest

Patients and methods

The data on 33 treated patients are summarised in Table 1. Of 13 patients with haemangioma, superselective transcatheter arterial embolisation using ethanol, oestrogen, gelatin sponge, or a combination, was performed in 12, and direct injection sclerotherapy of ethanol in 1. In 4 patients with arteriovenous malformation (AVM), palliative embolisation was done for 3 and a preoperative measure for 1; gelatin sponge, coils, cyanoacrylate (NBCA) lipidol and polyvinyl alcohol were used as embolic agents. Direct needle injection sclerotherapy was also carried out in 2 patients with venous malformations. In 12 patients with cavernous dural AVM (D type in Barrow's classification), combined embolisation and irradiation therapy (30.0–49.5 Gy: mean 33 Gy) was performed. As an emergency measure to stop the bleeding, endovascular treatment was done on 2 patients with a ruptured pseudoaneurysm of the carotid artery or a ruptured dissecting aneurysm of the vertebral artery.

Results

Overall, 28 patients (85%) in whom adequate embolisation was performed had satisfactory results. The remaining 7 patients did not achieve a good outcome. These included 2 patients who had not received sufficient ethanol because of severe pain. Characteristics of our results were as follows: (1) Slow-flow venous malformations and haemangioma of the floor of the mouth had almost completely disappeared after direct needle injection sclerotherapy with ethanol. (2) Superselective embolisation with a Tracker 18 catheter, using ethanol or gelatin sponge in the feeders, was also effective in the patients with haemangioma. (3) A one-shot injection of NBCA for a traumatic scalp arteriovenous fistula, under flow control by digital compression on the drainers and jugular vein, brought immediate and complete disappearance of arteriovenous shunting without any complications. (4) Combined embolisation and irradiation was effective in relieving symptoms (excellent or good outcome in all but 1 patient) for up to 6 months. (5) Intravascular embolisation brought about a complete arrest of bleeding from the pseudoaneurysm of the carotid artery and was beneficial in preventing rerupture of the dissecting aneurysm of the vertebral artery. (6) Complications: ethanol-induced transient skin necrosis or submandibular adenitis was seen in 2 patients. Transient impairment of visual acuity, probably related to venous congestion, was also recognized in 3 patients with cavernous dural AVM.

Discussion

This study revealed embolisation therapy as a safe and effective treatment option for patients with vascular lesions in the head and neck. High-flow vascular malformations involve arteriovenous fistula or arteriovenous haemangioma, and low-flow vascular malformations involve capillary, cavernous and venous haemangioma [1, 2]. Complete ablation of cavernous haemangioma was obtained by means of direct injection sclerotherapy or superselective arterial injection sclerotherapy. For the high-flow type, flow control is important for appropriate embolisation. Transvenous embolisation [3] is now considered to be the best choice for cavernous dural AVM. However, a combined therapy, with mild embolisation using gelatin sponge and radiotherapy (up to 30 Gy), would also be recommended for older age groups.

References

1. Djindjian R, Merland JJ (1978) Superselective arteriography of the external carotid artery. Springer, New York Berlin Heidelberg
2. Merland JJ, Riché MC, Monteil JP (1980) Classification actuelle des malformations vasculaires. Ann Clin Plact Esthét 25:105
3. Halbach VV, Higashida RT, Hieshima GB (1989) Transvenous embolization of dural fistulas involving the cavernous sinuses. AJNR 10:379–383

Measurement of blood flow velocity by Doppler-tipped guidewires in patients with arteriovenous malformations and fistulae

G. Benndorf[1], P. Podrabsky[1], E. Wellnhofer[2], G. Biamino[1], H. P. Molsen[4], E. Fleck[2], W. Lanksch[3], R. Felix[1]

[1] Department of Radiology, Universitätsklinikum Rudolf Virchow, Berlin, Germany
[2] Department of Internal Medicine/Cardiology, Deutsches Herzzentrum, Berlin, Germany
[3] Department of Neurosurgery, Universitätsklinikum Rudolf Virchow, Berlin, Germany
[4] Institute of Neuroradiology, Klinikum Berlin-Buch, Berlin, Germany

Abstract. Intraluminal blood flow velocity measurement is a new invasive Doppler technique providing functional information during angiography or interventional procedures in dural sinuses. It can be used easily and safely without significant loss of time during the procedure. Flow velocity in dural sinuses, in our patient group, ranged between 8 and 45 cm/s in nondraining veins. In vessels draining an arteriovenous malformation (AVM) blood flow velocity was remarkably higher: up to 134 cm/s in the straight sinus. The highest velocity in dural arteriovenous fistulae (DAVF) was found in one patient to be 165 cm/s in the transverse sinus. Flow pattern was usually found to be laminar and only remarkably turbulent in proximal arterialised sinuses and direct at fistula sites. Pulsatility was evident in nonarterialised as well as in arterialised sinuses. Information about flow velocity and flow pattern of the dural sinuses is of complementary value to angiography. Ongoing studies should demonstrate the usefulness of this technique in the management of patients undergoing endovascular treatment of brain AVMs or AVF.

Key words: Blood flow velocity – Dural sinuses – Doppler guidewire – Arteriovenous malformations – Arteriovenous fistulae

The superficial location of dural sinuses beyond the skull limits satisfactory access for transcranial Doppler Sonography (TCD) in adults. Aaslid et al. [1] measured flow velocity in the straight sinus due to its deeper location in the brain. A few magnetic resonance angiography studies have also reported on flow velocity measurements in dural sinuses [2]. Increased flow velocity in patients with vascular malformations represents one of the most important risk factors for bleeding [3].

New technical developments in the intravascular field, such as the miniaturised Doppler-tipped guidewire, make it possible to reach cerebral vessels and to measure flow directly in these patients [4–7].

The purpose of this study was intraluminal measurement of blood flow in dural sinuses utilising miniaturised Doppler-tipped guidewires in patients with arteriovenous malformations (AVMs) and fistulae (AVF).

Correspondence to: G. Benndorf, Department of Radiology, Universitätsklinikum Rudolf Virchow, Augustenburger Platz 1, 13353 Berlin, Germany

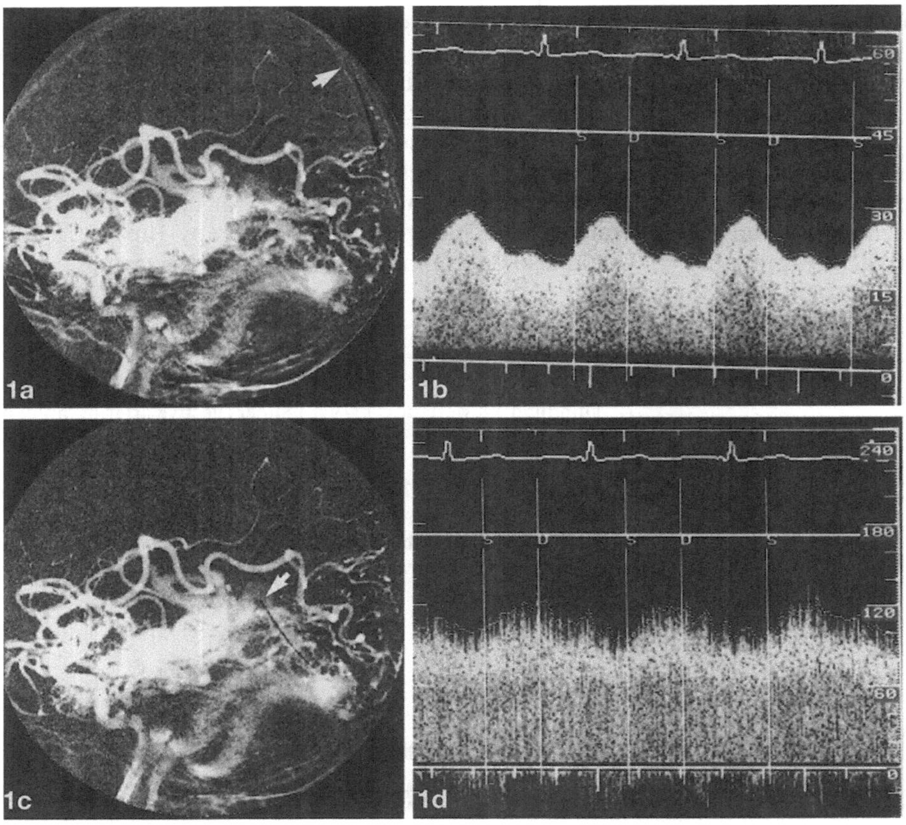

Fig. 1 a–d. A 30-year-old woman with a large arteriovenous malformation (AVM) of the left temporal lobe. **a** Road mapping of the wire position (*arrow*) in the superior sagittal sinus. **b** Velocity at this point with a Systolic peak (*MPV*) of 29 cm/s. Pulsatility index 0.3. Well-delineated outline to the curve indicating no significant turbulence. **c** Wire position (*arrow*) in the mainly draining straight sinus. **d** Velocity in this arterialised sinus is remarkably higher (122 cm/s), but pulsatility index is almost the same (0.4). Note oscillations of the outline, indicating disturbed flow

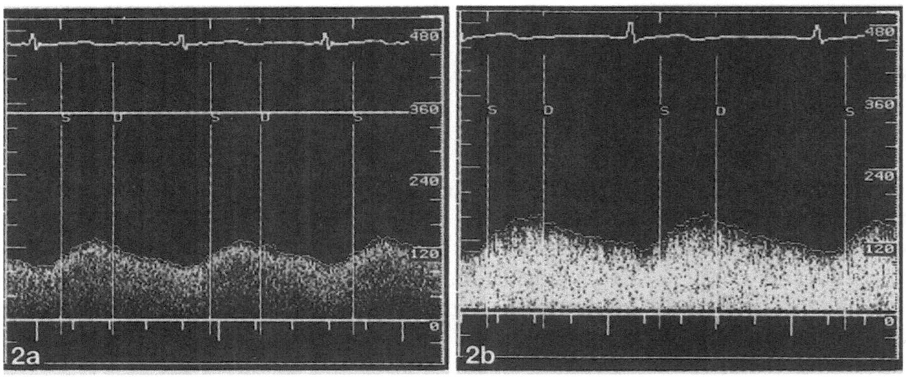

Fig. 2 a, b. High flow in patients with an AVM and a dural arteriovenous fistula (AVF). **a** A 49-year-old woman with a brain stem AVM and single draining falcine sinus. Flow velocity in this sinus with a systolic peak (*MPV*) of 134 cm/s; pulsatility index 0.5. **b** A 57-year-old man with a dural AVF of the right transverse sinus (partially thrombosed) and main venous drainage through the left transverse sinus. Flow velocity in this sinus with a systolic peak (*MPV*) of 165 cm/s: pulsatility index 0.5

Methods

Twenty-two patients (8 female, 15 male) aged between 31 and 60 with brain AVMs or dural AVF, and two patients without arteriovenous shunts were included. One had a stenosis of the superior sagittal sinus caused by a falx meningioma and one patient came for angiography after complete surgical removal of his AVM.

During diagnostic angiography or endovascular treatment the dural sinuses were catheterised in a retrograde fashion with a 5.2 F/3 F coaxial system. Measurements were performed in the superior sagittal, transverse and sigmoid sinuses and the straight sinus, monitored by road-mapping. We used a 0.018″ Doppler guidewire. Its floppy tip consists of a miniaturised transducer (12 MHz), which emits a pulsed wave with a 28° ultrasound beam. Flow velocity is calculated by fast Fourier transformation and presented in two terms: maximum peak velocity (MPV), average peak velocity (APV).

Results

Flow velocities between 11 and 165 cm/s MPV in sinuses draining an AV shunt were found. The highest flow velocity (134 cm/s, Fig. 1 a) in a dural sinus draining an AVM was measured in the straight sinus of a patient with an AVM of the brain stem. In one patient with a dural AVF, a flow velocity of 165 cm/s (Fig. 2 b) was found in the transverse sinus. Flow velocity in nonarterialised sinuses has been found to be between 11 and 42 cm/s. In one patient with a falx meningioma we found increased flow velocity of more than 80 cm/s in the area of the compressed superior sagittal sinus.

Flow pattern was usually found to be laminar (Fig. 1 b), and was disturbed only in proximal segments of

AV shunt draining sinuses (Fig. 1d). Pulsatile flow was evident in almost all sinuses (nonarterialised and arterialised by blood draining the AV shunt).

Discussion

Our first experiences show that flow parameters in venous sinuses are easy to assess with Doppler guidewires. Flow parameters can be obtained in real time during superselective angiography or interventional procedures. In adults with brain AVM, Hassler [8] performed intraoperative measurements of venous flow velocity, and recorded velocities as high as 39 cm/s. Flow velocities up to 134 cm/s in AVM-draining vessels have never been described before. We found flow velocity in the nonarterialised straight sinus had a mean of 27.6 cm/s, comparable with values reported using TCD [1]: 23.3 cm/s in 9 healthy subjects. Mattle et al. [2] found in an MR study of 10 healthy subjects and 21 patients a mean flow velocity of 33.3 cm/s in the superior sagittal sinus (compared with 27.9 cm/s in nonarterialised sinuses in our group).

A laminar pulsatile flow pattern was found in almost all our patients. Although we did not perform any statistical tests, the mean pulsatility index has not been found to be clearly lower in nondraining than in draining sinuses in patients with brain AVMs, and cannot primarily be considered as characteristic of AV shunt draining veins, as stated by other groups [9]. Significant flow disturbances in AVM-draining veins or sinuses were only found in proximal segments of these vessels, as also described by Nornes and Grip [10], who found turbulences only up to 1 cm distal from the nidus.

High degree turbulence was found in dural AVFs, in which the retrograde flow probably represents an increased vascular resistance to the antegrade flow. The reversal point of retrograde flow has never been described before and could be the major factor in the aetiology of bruits in these patients.

Although this technique is not primarily designed for measurements in large vessels such as dural sinuses, and in validation studies performed by Doucette et al. [11] was found to be accurate only in tubes up to 4.7 mm diameter, we believe that flow measurements made in dural sinuses are relatively reliable. There is no doubt that studies in healthy subjects for assessment of normal values are necessary.

References

1. Aaslid R, Newell DW, Stoos R, Sorteberg W, Lindegard KF (1991) Assessment of cerebral autoregulation dynamics from simultaneous arterial and venous transcranial Doppler in humans Stroke 22:1148–1154
2. Mattle H, Edelmann RR, Moshe AR, Atkinson DJ (1990) Flow quantification in the superior sagittal sinus using magnetic resonance. Neurology 40:813–815
3. Pasqualin A, Barone G, Cioffi F, Rosta L, Scienca R, Da Pian R (1991) The relevance of anatomic and hemodynamic factors to a classification of cerebral arteriovenous malformations. Neurosurgery 28:370–379
4. Benndorf G, Richer CS, Helden A von, Molsen HP, Biamino G, Felix R (1993) Intraluminal blood flow measurement in cerebral arteries by intravascular pulsed Doppler. Neuroradiology 35 [Suppl]:60
5. Benndorf G, Richter CS, Chammas S, Wellnhofer E, Biamino G, Felix R (1994) Intraluminal blood flow measurements in supraaortic arteries by Doppler tipped guide wire. AJR [Suppl] 162:50
6. Benndorf G, Podrabsky P, Unterberg A, Biamino G, Lanksch W, Felix R (1994) Evaluation of blood flow in dural sinuses by Doppler-tipped guide wire in patients with cerebral arteriovenous malformations and fistulas. Neuroradiology [Suppl] 36:55
7. Chaloubka JC, Viñuela F, Kimme-Smith C, Robert J, Duckwiler G (1994) Use of a Doppler guide wire for intravascular blood flow measurements: a validation study for potential neurologic endovascular applications. AJNR 15:509–517
8. Hassler W (1986) Hemodynamic aspects in angioma patients. Acta Neurochir 37 [Suppl]:1–136
9. Westra S, Curran JG, Duckweiler G, Zaninovic AC, Hall TR, Martin NA, Boechat MI, Viñuela F (1993) Pediatric intracranial vascular malformation: evaluation of treatment results with color Doppler US. Radiology 186:775–783
10. Nornes H, Grip A (1980) Hemodynamic aspects of cerebral arteriovenous malformations. J Neurosurg 53:456–464
11. Doucette JW, Corl PD, Payne HM (1990)) Validation of a Doppler guidewire for assessment of coronary flow. Circulation 82:611–621

Intervention: AVMs

Technical options for endovascular treatment of different types of arteriovenous malformation

S. Perini[1], A. Pasqualin[2], L. Rosta[1], P. Zampieri[1], F. Alessandrini[1], A. Benati[1]

[1] Department of Neuroradiology, City Hospital, Verona, Italy
[2] Department of Neurosurgery, City Hospital, Verona, Italy

Abstract. We compared two technical procedures for endovascular treatment of cerebral arteriovenous malformations (AVMs): suture thread embolisation (108 cases) and liquid glue injection (23 cases). The value of both embolic agents, the clinical and angiographic results, and complications were assessed. Embolisation with glue allows more selective occlusion of the AVM nidus and a definitive cure of the malformation; polylene suture threads completely occlude direct AV fistulae. The overall complication rate in our series was 8.5% in the glue group and 19.5% with suture thread treatment.

Key words: Arteriovenous malformations - Embolisation - Endovascular therapy

For endovascular treatment of cerebral arteriovenous malformations (AVMs), our Department uses two techniques: injection of suture threads into the feeding vessels of the malformation [1, 2] and direct injection into the nidus of a mixture of NBCA (Histo-acryl Braun) and Lipidol ultrafluid [3].

The aim of this report is to establish the value of both embolic agents, assess angiographic and clinical results, and determine the incidence of complications with the two procedures.

Materials and methods

According to technique, we evaluated two groups of patients. The first group (108 patients: mean age 28.5 years, 16 paediatric subjects) were embolised with suture threads. The AVMs were in eloquent or critical and non-critical areas in 50 and 58 cases, respectively; AVM volume was < 20 ml in 44 cases (13%) and < 20 ml in 64 cases (60%). Deep feeders were found in 43 cases (40%), 21 of which were embolised. Embolisation was a presurgical procedure in 71 patients (65%); it was followed by radiosurgery in 14 cases (13%) and performed without associated procedures in 23 patients (21%). In 13 of the last subgroup an angiographic control was performed after a follow-up period of 6 months to 4 years. The second group (23 patients: mean age 25.7 years, 2 children) were embolised with liquid glue, starting from June 1993. In all cases, the AVM site was eloquent or critical. AVM volume was > 20 ml in 4 of 23 cases, and < 20 ml in the other 19. Deep feeders were embolised in 3 of 23 cases. Radiosurgery was performed after embolisation in 16 patients, and microsurgery in 4 cases. Embolisation was the sole therapeutic procedure in 4 patients.

Correspondence to: S. Perini, Servizio di Neuroradiologia, Ospedale Maggiore, I-37126 Verona, Italy

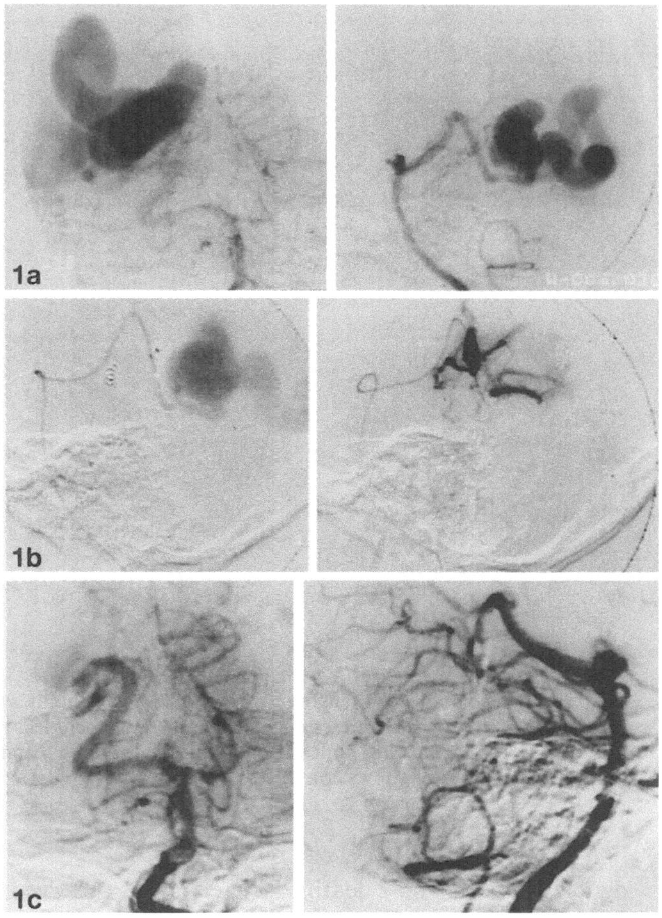

Fig. 1. a Right occipital direct AV fistula. **b** Selective embolisation with 5- to 8-cm-long polylene suture threads. **c** Obliteration of AV shunt persists after 6 months

Results

In the first group (suture threads), complete occlusion was achieved in 4 of 108 cases (3.5%) (all direct AV *fistulae* embolised with 3- to 6-cm threads). In the remaining 104 of 108 cases (96.5%), occlusion was incomplete (mean 37%, range 5–70%). Angiographic control showed complete AVM nidus recanalisation in 13 patients. In the second group (liquid glue), complete occlusion was achieved in 4 of 23 cases (17.5%). In the remaining 19 patients (82.5%) there was remarkable reduction of AVM volume (from 70% to 90%), followed by radio- or microsurgery.

Haemorrhage occurred in 5 cases (4.5%), causing a transient neurological deficit in 2 cases, a permanent

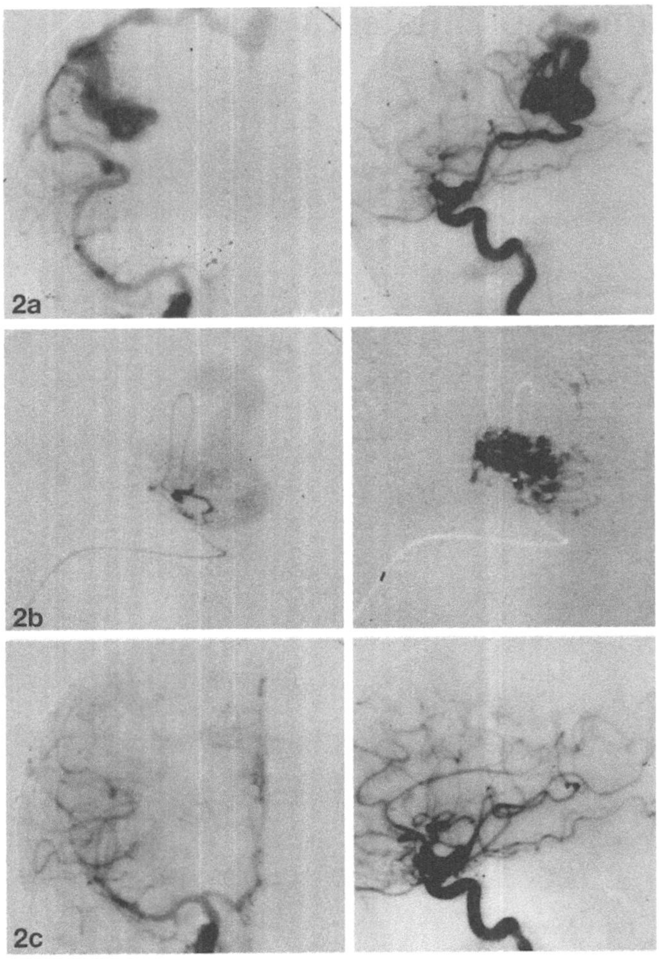

Fig. 2. a Right rolandic AVM. **b** Selective embolization of nidus with NBCA; the tip of the microcatheter completely occludes the perforating rami, allowing controlled injection of glue. **c** Angiography 8 months later shows complete cure

deficit in 1 case, and 2 deaths. Ischaemia was observed in 16 cases (15%), causing a transient or permanent deficit in 9 and 7 cases, respectively. This was probably a result of venous engorgement; it was never observed when embolisation was extended to the afferent artery. The overall complication rate in the first group was 19.5%, with a stroke rate (death + permanent deficit) of 9%. In the second group, headache was the most frequent symptom, occurring in 9 of 23 cases within a few hours of glue injection and persisting for 1–7 days.

Seizures were observed in 2 of 23 patients, 2 and 4 days after treatment. There were 2 cases (8.5%) of motor impairment. In 1, severe monoparesis (left leg with foot plegia) occurred after injection into the right anterior cerebral artery, causing reflux in the feeder. Complete recovery occurred within 10 days. In the second patient, severe left hemiparesis was observed 8 days after treatment; this was caused by a right parietal haematoma surrounding the AVM nidus, probably due to delayed venous occlusion. Eight months later, only a mild motor deficit of the left hand persisted.

Discussion

From our results, the following considerations emerge. (1) Intravascular navigation with microcatheters of variable flexibility and progressive suppleness for glue injection is safer and more distal than with flow independent microcatheters for injection of suture threads. (2) Liquid glue allows more selective occlusion of the AVM nidus, allowing permanent cure or giving scope for a range of associated treatments (radio- or microsurgery). (3) The overall complication rate in our series is 8.5% in the liquid glue group and 19.5% with the suture thread treatment (stroke rate 9%). (4) Suture threads 3–5 cm long completely occlude AV fistulae; we think that, for these high-flow shunts, threads are a safer embolic agent than glue, which in these cases must be injected pure or through a calibrated-leak balloon microcatheter. (5) Haemorrhage occurred with both procedures, probably due to venous engorgement. This complication must be carefully avoided during both procedures.

References

1. Benati A, Beltramello A, Colombari R, Maschio A, Perini S, DaPian R, Pasqualin A, Scienza R, Rosta L, Piovan E, Scarpa A, Zamboni G (1989) Preoperative embolisation of arteriovenous malformations with polylene threads: techniques with wing micro-catheter and pathologic results. AJNR 10:579–586
2. Benati A, Perini S, Pasqualin A, Pecoraro MG, Maschio A, Rostal L, Piovan E, Zampieri P (1994) Embolization of cerebral AVMs with polylene threads: technical procedure, results and complications. In: Pasqualin A, Da Pian R (eds) New trends in management of cerebro-vascular malformations. Vienna
3. Picard L, Moret J, Lepoire J (1984) Traitement endovasculaire des angiomes artério-veineux intra-cérébraux. J Neuroradiol 11:9–28

Cyanoacrylate embolisation in the management of brain arteriovenous malformations in 104 patients

T. ApSimon, M. Khangure, J. Ives, B. Stokes

Interventional Neuroradiology Unit, Department of Diagnostic Radiology, Royal Perth Hospital, Box X2213 GPO, Perth, Western Australia 6001

Abstract. Transfemoral cyanoacrylate tissue glue embolisation (TGE) has been used over a 10-year period in combination with other modalities of treatment, predominantly surgical excision (SE) and stereotactic focused radiotherapy (radiosurgery; SRS) in 104 patients. The results have been assessed in terms of the final outcome of the patient from all modalities of treatment. Outcomes were classed as successful (84%), unsucsessful (15%) and incomplete (1%). The predominant and most successful mode of therapy has been TGE combined with SE, with successful outcome in 49% of 104 patients. TGE plays a significant role in facilitating SRS and in the management of the higher grade brain arteriovenous malformations, which are hardly suited to treatment by any single modality.

Key words: Brain arteriovenous malformation – Cyanoacrylate embolisation – Surgical excision – Radiosurgery – Treatment outcomes

The purpose of this study is to report the immediate and delayed results of transfemoral cyanoacrylate tissue glue embolisation (TGE) and to assess the part it has played in patient management and final outcome.

Patients and methods

Patients. The patients form part of a larger group of patients with BAVM treated in Western Australia since late 1983. During this period, a substantial number of patient have been treated by stereotactive radiosurgery (SRS) alone, surgical excision (SE) alone, a combination of SRS and SE or by conservative management with no interference. This latter group, in whom TGE has not been performed or attempted, is not included in this report. There were 49 female and 56 male patients, aged 1–65 years.

Treatment methods. All patients have been treated primarily by TGE in the Radiology Department. Calibrated-leak balloon catheter systems [1, 2] were used exclusively from late 1983 to 1987 inclusive, using balloons and microcatheters manufactured at Royal Perth Hospital [3]. These techniques were subsequently replaced by nonballoon microcatheters, principally the Tracker microcatheter and guidewire system and, increasingly since 1990, the Magic flow-directed catheter system. Cyanoacrylate tissue glues have been combined with Pantopaque or Lipiodol ultra-fluid in varying proportions [4] and with finely divided metallic tantalum for increased radio-opacity. In 3 patients, additional intraoperative embolisation has been performed at craniotomy.

Correspondence to: T. ApSimon

Table 1. Brain AVM embolisation in 104 patients, 1983–1994

% Nidus occlusion	Patients
100	11
>90	30
60–85	38
<60	24
Nil	1

Table 2. Successful outcome: 87 patients

Facilitation of surgical excision	51
Facilitation of radiosurgery (alive and well)	23
Complete occlusion by embolisation	11
Palliation of main symptoms by embolisation (embolisation sole treatment 5)	11

Results

TGE was performed 399 times and 3 patients additionally received small-particle embolisation with either surgical silk suture or polyvinyl alcohol. Follow-up varies from 10 years to 4 months.

The percentage of nidus occlusion obtained is shown in Table 1. In one patient, the procedure was abandoned because of complications before any embolisation was achieved. To assess TGE in the context of the management of the patient as a whole, we divide the results into the following three groups.

Successful outcome (Table 2)

Facilitation of SE (patients alive and well). TGE was performed as a prelude to successful surgical removal of the malformation. Of the 51 patients in this group, 3 required a second operation to achieve total excision. There were 3 others in whom a nidus remaining after subtotal excision was treated by SRS.

Facilitation of SRS (patients alive and well). In some patients the nidus was initially too large, but following preliminary TGE a more restricted target was achieved for SRS. In the remainder of this group, the nidus was within the treatable size for SRS ab initio, but TGE was employed to reduce the risk of repeated haemorrhage while awaiting SRS. Of the 23 patients, 4 have complete occlusion on angiographic follow-up, 7 have incomplete occlusion at the 2 ½ year stage, and in 11 patients follow-up is as yet incomplete.

Table 3. Unsuccessful outcome: 16 patients

Insufficient occlusion	5
Deficit after surgical excision	2
Deficit after embolisation, preventing further treatment	2
Haemorrhage and death during embolisation	3
Haemorrhage and death after embolisation	2
Delayed haemorrhage and death (1 yr) after embolisation and radiosurgery	2

Complete occlusion by TGE (patients alive and well). Of the 11 patients showing complete occlusion at initial and early follow-up, 1 patient went on to surgical excision and 4 of the other 10 show minor degrees of recanalisation over a 1- to 3-year follow-up.

Successful palliation of main symptoms by TGE alone (patients alive and well). Palliation includes occlusion of associated intranidal or venous aneurysms, relief of disabling headache, reversal of significant neurological deficits, and improvement of dementia and dominant hemisphere dysfunction.

No patient who suffered recurrent haemorrhage after embolisation or a disabling or persisting significant neurological deficit has been included in the successful outcome category. Patients whose pretreatment deficit was unchanged or improved by TGE are included in group 1.

Unsuccessful outcome (Table 3)

Insufficient occlusion. The 5 patients are alive and well and free of recurrent haemorrhage. However, TGE failed to achieve sufficient size reduction for SRS or preoperative control for SE.

Deficit following surgical excision. Both patients were intact after embolisation, the deficits being attributable to technical difficulty in removing a massive malformation in one and inability to achieve sufficient postsurgical haemostasis in the other. Patients with minor or transitory deficit after SE are excluded.

Deficit following transfemoral embolisation, preventing further treatment. This occurred in one patient due to reflux of cyanoacrylate glue into the dominant hemisphere, reaching the middle cerebral inferior Sylvian trunk during embolisation of a temporal lobe malformation. In the other patient, the deficit was due to intracerebral and intraventricular haemorrhage occurring between planned 1st- and 2nd-stage embolisation of a choroid plexus and ventricular AVM.

Haemorrhage and death during TGE. The three fatal haemorrhages were all associated with the use of the calibrated-leak balloon catheter technique, rupturing a feeding pedicle, or the dysplastic vessels of the AVM nidus.

Haemorrhage and death after TGE. In one of these patients, the fatal intraventricular haemorrhage occurred 48 h after almost total TGE occlusion of a choroidal and temporal malformation. In the second, fatal haemorrhage arose from a dilated tortuous Huebner's artery remote from the nidus, 7 days after high-grade subtotal occlusion of a large posterior frontal AVM.

Delayed haemorrhage and death 1 year after TGE and SRS. Both patients suffered fatal haemorrhage from the nidus approximately 1 year after combined treatment.

Incomplete treatment

One patient is awaiting further staged embolisation.

Discussion

Since the early reports of cyanoacrylate tissue glue embolisation in BAVM [5, 6] over 10 years ago, numerous reports of series of treated patients have been published [7–9]. It is clear that in experienced hands, complete or high-grade subtotal occlusion of malformation nidus can be achieved [7, 9]. However, in our view it is the success or failure of embolisation in the broader context of patient clinical management that is important. That is the objective of our study.

We have approached brain AVM management as a team with our neuro- and radiosurgical colleagues. Malformations of lower Spetzler grades [10] in non-eloquent brain and accessible sites remain optimally treated by surgical excision. Many malformations in more difficult sites can be rendered amenable to safe low-morbidity surgical excision by preliminary embolisation [8, 10]. This has been our preferred objective and remains the largest single group for which embolisation is employed.

For malformations in deeper or more eloquent sites, different strategies have been employed. Malformations which have not bled and are within the size limitations for SRS have been treated by this modality alone. TGE has been combined with SRS in two main ways. For the smaller malformations with a significant risk of recurrent haemorrhage, preliminary embolisation has been employed to reduce vascularity, occlude associated arterial and intranidal aneurysms, and reduce the risk of recurrent haemorrhage pending the 2½-year delay between SRS treatment and final nidus closure [11]. Even if total nidus occlusion is achieved, we proceed to SRS to prevent delayed recanalisation and possible haemorrhage at some future date.

Secondly, we have combined SRS with TGE in larger nonsurgical malformations, attempting to occlude substantial portions of the nidus permanently with glue-cast, and to close the residual smaller remaining nidus by SRS [8]. The validity of this treatment in our hands remains questionable. In no patient with a nidus exceeding 5 cm in diameter has it produced total occlusion. Whilst only 2 of our patients treated by combined TGE and SRS have suffered recurrent haemorrhage to date, only much more prolonged follow-up will determine whether there is a sustained benefit.

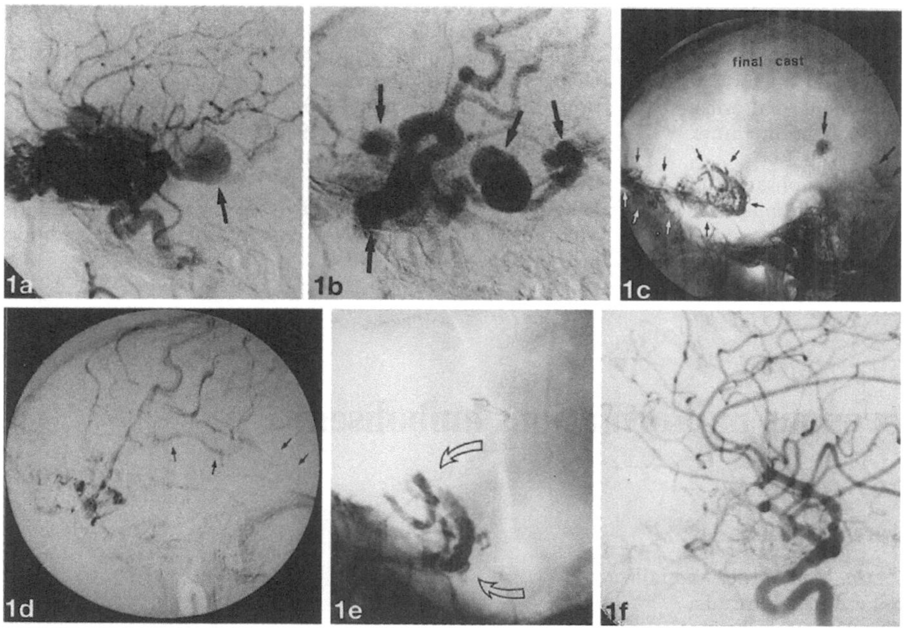

Fig. 1a–f. Spetzler grade 6 inferior frontal arteriovenous malformation (AVM) managed by extensive embolisation and partial surgical excision. Man aged 36 years, with headache, drowsiness and left hemiparesis due to inferior thalamic haemorrhage and venous pseudoaneurysm formation associated with a massive right mesial inferior frontal AVM. Malformation deemed inoperable (Spetzler grade 6) and much too large for radiosurgery. **a** Left carotid angiogram showing nidus and early filling of thalamic aneurysm arising from the vein of Rosenthal (*arrow*). **b** Venous phase. Four aneurysms on deep venous drainage (*arrow*). Note partly clotted pseudoaneurysm. **c** Final glue cast after 11 embolisations (*small arrows*). Note glue deposits in aneurysm at the posterior end of vein of Rosenthal (*single arrow*) and in straight sinus (*twin arrow*. **d** Late venous phase final postembolisation angiogram. Limited patent nidus on superior aspect of AVM with one superficial draining vein: No deep venous drainage. Note patent internal cerebral vein and straight sinus (*small arrows*). Patient underwent surgical resection of the anterior half of the embolised malformation including the small residual patent area. **e** 15-month follow-up angiogram preliminary film. Persisting cyanoacrylate glue cast in posterior and deeper parts of nidus (*arrows*). **f** Right carotid arteriogram; residual patent nidus demonstrated

Treatment of large hypervascular brain AVMs remains a major challenge. Major devascularisation has sometimes facilitated remarkable surgical feats without deficit, and total excision remains the preferred objective. Occasionally, we have combined total embolisation of the deeper portion with excision of the more accessible parts (Fig. 1). Rarely, sequential TGE, SE and finally SRS have been combined to eliminate difficult malformations. If TGE fails to achieve substantial control, then the difficulties of SE remain severe. This was significant in the first of our two major postsurgical deficits.

The percentage of occlusion achieved relates approximately to successful outcome of SE [7]. Other important factors include the timing after embolisation and the vascularity of the border zone around the nidus. We prefer that SE follow within 1 and no later than 3 weeks after TGE. An AVM nidus surrounded by a zone of small-vessel collateral hypervascularity within normal brain (the "non-sprouting angiogenesis" of Lasjunias and Berenstein [12] represents a major hazard of intra- or postoperative haemorrhage. This was the cause of our second major post-SE deficit.

The unsuccessful outcomes in 16 patients (15%) present an ongoing challenge. By better patient selection and by avoiding some high-risk patients, we can reduce the incidence of deficit and unsuccessful treatment. Thus, there must always be patients who have to be managed conservatively. With the abandonment of the calibrated-leak balloon technique, haemorrhage during TGE is now rare [13], but haemorrhage in the postembolisation period and during or following SE remains a serious complication, the principal cause of significant morbidity [7].

References

1. Kerber C (1976) Balloon catheter with a calibrated leak. A new system for superselective angiography and occlusive catheter therapy. Radiology 120:547–550
2. Debrun GM, Viñuela F, Fox AJ, Kan S (1982) Two different calibrated-leak balloons: experimental work and applications. AJNR 3:407–417
3. ApSimon HT, Khangure MS (1986) Improved technique of bucrylate embolisation in brain arterio-venous malformation. Acta Radiol 369:618–620
4. Cromwell LD, Kerber C (1979) Modification of cyanoacrylate for therapeutic embolisation. Preliminary experience. AJR 132:799–801
5. Cromwell LD, Harris AB (1980) Treatment of cerebral arteriovenous malformations. A combined neurosurgical and neuroradiological approach. J Neurosurg 52:705–708
6. Debrun G, Viñuela F, Fox AJ, Drake CG (1982) Embolisation of cerebral arteriovenous malformations with bucrylate: experience of 46 cases. J Neurosurg 56:615–627
7. Berenstein AB, Lasjuanias P, Choi IS (1992) Endovascular

treatment of arteriovenous malformations of the brain. In: Valavanis A (ed) Interventional neuroradiology. Springer, Berlin Heidelberg New York
8. Deruty R, Pelissou-Guydat I, Mottolese C et al (1993) The combined management of cerebral arteriovenous malformations. Experience with 100 cases and review of the literature. Acta Neurochir 123:101–112
9. Viñuela F (1992) Functional evaluation and embolisation of intracranial arteriovenous malformations in interventional neuroradiology. In: Viñuela F (ed) Endovascular therapy of the central nervous system. Raven Press, New York
10. Spetzler RF, Martin NA (1986) A proposed grading system for arteriovenous malformations. J Neurosurg 67:17–28
11. Yamamoto M, Jimbo M, Ide M (1993) Post-irradiation volume changes in gamma unit treated cerebral arteriovenous malformations. Surg Neurol 40:485–490
12. Berenstein A, Lasjuuanias P (1992) Surgical neuro-angiography, vol 4: Endovascular treatment of cerebral lesions. Springer, Berlin Heidelberg New York
13. Khangure MS, ApSimon HT (1989) Vessel rupture during calibrated-leak balloon AVM embolisation – some additional mechanisms. AJNR 8:970

Histopathology of arteriovenous malformations embolised with cyanoacrylate

W. Chong[1], **H. T. ApSimon**[2], **M. Khangure**[2], **V. Ojeda**[3]

[1] Department of Imaging, Monash Medical Centre, Melbourne, Australia
[2] Department of Radiology, Royal Perth Hospital, Perth, Australia
[3] Department of Pathology, Sir Charles Gairdner Hospital, Perth, Australia

Abstract. The histopathology of brain arteriovenous malformations (AVMs) embolised with cyanocrylate in 21 patients was available for study. Histotoxicity of cyanoacrylate had been implicated as the cause of angionecrosis as well as parenchymal necrosis. This study suggests that another mechanism, namely ischaemia, could explain all these changes.

Key words: Arteriovenous malformation – Cyanoacrylate – Toxicity – Embolisation

Widespread and focal necrosis of vessel walls adjacent to isobutyl-2-cyanoacrylate (IBCA) in cerebral arteriovenous malformations (AVMs) and in arteries of animals that had been embolised by IBCA has been reported [1–4]. Only Vinters et al. [1] reported embolic material in the extravascular space. A review of the histopathology of 21 AVMs that had been embolised with cyanoacrylate was performed to further assess these findings.

Materials and methods

The time between embolisation and resection ranged from 1 day to 6 years. About half the patients were embolised with IBCA and the remainder with *N*-butyl-cyanoacrylate. These were mixed with tantalum powder, iophendylate or lipiodol and in some cases also with acetic acid in proportions of 0.005 to 0.01% by volume. The specimens were fixed in formalin and routinely embedded in paraffin. Sections of 5–6 µm were obtained and stained with haemotoxylin and eosin. Some were also stained with orcein for elastic fibres and prussian blue reaction for haemosiderin. The number of sections per case available for examination varied from 1 to 12. A representative slide was chosen to determine the proportion of vessels containing embolic material and the proportion of vessels that were necrotic (widespread or focal). The presence or absence and type of vessel wall inflammation were documented. In the parenchyma (which mainly included the interstices of the AVM and in some cases a small amount of brain tissue) a search for the presence of embolic material, haemorrhage, inflammation and gliosis was carried out.

Correspondence to: W. Chong, Diagnostic Imaging, Monash Medical Centre, Locked Bag No. 29, Clayton, Victoria 3168, Australia

Results

Vessels

The proportion of vessels containing embolic material ranged from 6% to 50% per case. In 11 cases (52%), focal to widespread necrosis of vessel walls was seen in vessels that contained embolic material (Fig. 1). The time interval of these cases ranged from 2 days to 10 months, with most cases up to 1 month. In these cases, angionecrosis was also seen in non-embolised vessels. In 10 cases (48%), no angionecrosis was seen in any available section. Most were over the 1 month post-embolisation interval.

Chronic inflammation was present in the walls of vessels embolised in all 21 cases. Acute inflammation was seen in cases less than 6 weeks post-embolisation.

Foreign body reaction was seen in the lumen as well as in the intima of embolised vessels (Fig. 1). None was seen in the parenchyma or in the non-embolised vessels. The lumen of embolised vessels consisted of a meshwork-like matrix with the embolised material appearing as black particles (Fig. 1).

All embolised vessels were distended.

Parenchyma

In all cases, no embolic material was seen in the parenchyma, even in the presence of extensive parenchymal necrosis and angionecrosis. No significant recent bleeding

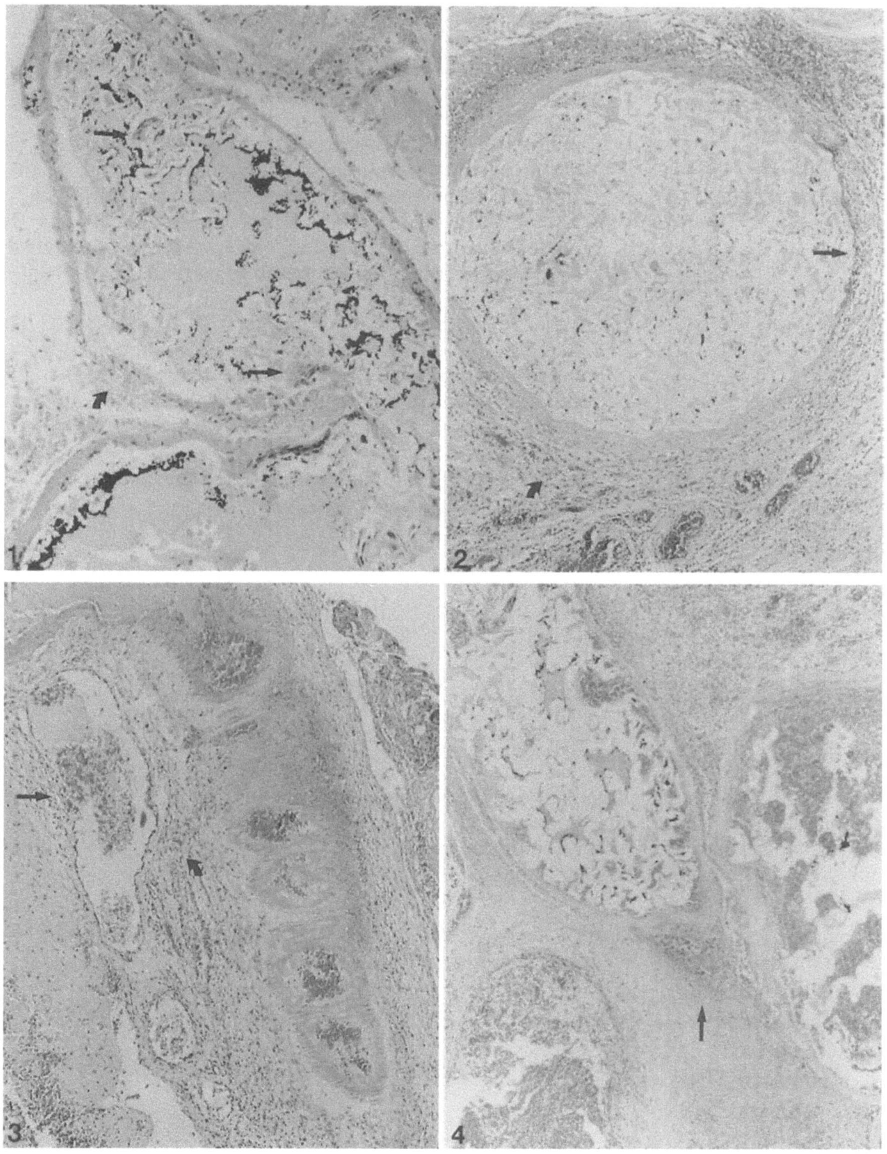

Fig. 1. Section of arteriovenous malformation (AVM) embolised 8 months before resection. Foreign body giant cells are seen in the lumen of embolised vessels (*arrow*). Focal angionecrosis is seen (*curved arrow*). H & E, orginal magnification X10

Fig. 2. Section of AVM embolised 4 weeks before resection. The vessel lumen is filled with embolic material. Focal angionecrosis (*arrow*) and parenchymal inflammation (*curved arrow*) are seen. H & E, original magnification X4

Fig. 3. Section of AVM embolised 15 days before resection. No embolic material is seen in the vessel lumen. However, angionecrosis (*arrow*) and interstitial necrosis (*curved arrow*) are seen. H & E, original magnification X4

Fig. 4. Section of AVM embolised 10 days before resection. One of the three vessels seen in this section does not contain emboli. The vessels appear intact. Focal parenchymal necrosis is seen (*arrow*). Surgical haemorrhage is present. H & E, original magnification X4

was seen apart from that assumed to be caused by the surgical procedure. Old haemorrhage was only seen in patients who had a previous bleed or surgery prior to the most recent resection producing the study material.

Mild to extensive chronic inflammation was present in the parenchyma surrounding embolised vessels in most cases (Fig. 2). However, inflammation and necrosis was also seen around non-embolised vessels (Fig. 3). Gliosis was seen in all cases. No foreign body giant cells were seen. In 5 cases, necrosis of the parenchyma was seen around embolised vessels with necrotic as well as intract walls (Fig. 4).

Other findings

There were no observable differences between the AVMs that were embolised with the two cyanoacrylates. No malignancy was seen. Those cases with the longest post-embolisation period had the largest percentage of intact vessels. Eosinophilia and cellular atypia, typical of cytotoxic reactions, were not present.

Discussion

The histotoxity of cyanoacrylate has been implicated as a cause of angionecrosis [1, 2]. Certain radicals (viz. the ethyl and methyl radicals) of the compound cause transmural necrosis when applied directly to the blood vessels but these are more toxic than IBCA [1, 2]. Tantalum is known to be inert [5] and studies have shown that the use of oily contrast media does not result in necrosis or fibroblastic scarring in lymph nodes or lungs [6]. The lack of foreign body reaction and embolic material in the parenchyma, and the presence of perivascular inflammation and necrosis involving both embolised and non-embolised vessels suggests that cyanoacrylate per se may not be the cause of angio- or parenchymal necrosis. The parenchymal inflammatory infiltrate was entirely in keeping with the response following ischaemic brain injury. Both ischaemic necrosis and gliosis are also seen de novo in non-embolised AVM [7]. In embolised AVMs they could be the result of the procedure. A possible mechanism for the angionecrosis is vessel distension in embolised vessels resulting in occlusion of the vasa vasorum, subsequent necrosis of the wall adjacent and downstream to the emboli. Occlusion of vessels supplying the AVM by emboli result in distal parenchymal necrosis. Further studies of AVMs embolised with cyanoacrylate and other agents are important to verify this theory.

References

1. Vinters HV, Lundie MJ, Kaufman JCE (1986) Long term pathological follow up of cerebral arteriovenous malformations treated by embolization with bucrylate. N Engl J Med 314:477–483
2. Vinters HV, Galil KA, Lundie MJ, Kaufman JCE (1985) The histotoxicity of cyanoacrylates. A selective review. Neuroradiology 27:279–291
3. White RI Jr, Strandberg JV, Gross GS, Barth KH (1977) Therapeutic embolization with long term occluding agents and their effects on embolized tissues. Radiology 125:677–687
4. Kish KK, Rapp SM, Wilner HI, Wolfe D, Thomas LM, Barr J (1983) Histopathologic effects of transarterial bucrylate occlusion of intracerebral arteries in mongrel dogs. AJNR 4:385–387
5. Vinters HV, Debrun G, Kaufmann JCE, Drake CG (1981) Pathology of arteriovenous malformations embolized with isobutyl-2-cyanoacrylate (bucrylate). J Neurosurg 55:819–825
6. Elliott GB, Elliott KA (1968) The variable fate of oily contrast media after lymphography compared with residues in other sites. AJR 104:851–859
7. Escourolle R (1971) Manual of basic neuropathology, 2nd ed. Saunders, Philadelphia, pp 77–79

A new mixture for embolisation of arteriovenous malformations

K. Kazekawa[1], T. Kawano[1], H. Iwata[2], J. Hamada[3], S. Yoshimura[4]

[1] Department of Neurosurgery, Fukuoka Tokushukai Medical Center, Kasuga, Fukuoka 816, Japan
[2] Department of Surgical Research, National Cardiovascular Center, Suita, Osaka, Japan
[3] Department of Neurosurgery, Kumamoto University School of Medicine, Kumamoto, Japan
[4] Department of Neurosurgery, National Cardiovascular Center, Suita, Osaka, Japan

Abstract. We report a new liquid material for embolisation of arteriovenous malformations (AVMs) using ethylene vinyl alcohol copolymer (EVAL). The liquid material is a mixture of EVAL, iopamidol and ethanol. Because of its low viscosity, it is easily handled and can be injected through any microcatheter. Histopathological study of resected AVMs verified less inflammatory reaction.

Key words: Embolisation – Arteriovenous malformations – Ethylen-vinyl-alcohol-copolymer – Ethanol

The perfect liquid embolic material has yet to be described. We have developed a new mixture which has a number of advantages.

Materials and methods

The ethylene vinyl alcohol copolymer (EVAL) and ethanol mixture

A mixture of 4 g EVAL, 60 g lopamidol 300 and 36 g of 99.9% ethanol was warmed at 80°C for 30 min. EVAL can be dissolved easily in a mixture of lopamidol and ethanol at 80°C (Table 1). After the EVAL was dissolved the mixture was sterilised at 121°C for 20 min. The new material must be warmed just before use because EVAL precipitates in the mixture of lopamidol and ethanol after several hours at room temperature.

Correspondence to: K. Kazekawa

Table 1. Composition of the new mixture

Material	Amount (g)
Ethylene vinyl alcohol copolymer	4
Iopamidol	60
Ethanol (99.9%)	36

Viscosity: 33.2 cp (37°C)

Clinical experience

We treated seven patients with the EVAL and ethanol mixture (Table 2). After embolisation procedures, three patients underwent total resection of their arteriovenous malformations (AVMs) which were histopathologically examined on routine haematoxylin and eosin staining.

Results

In the seven patients, 21 pedicles were successfully embolised with the EVAL and ethanol mixture. The symptoms of three cases with progressive neurological deficits gradually improved following embolisation. In cases 5 and 6, histopathological examination showed a few neutrophils in the vessel wall of the nidus. In case 7, the patient complained of headache during the embolisation procedure. CT findings showed a high density area around the nidus and the patient underwent emergency craniotomy.

Table 2. Summary of 7 patients embolised with EVAL and ethanol mixture

Case	Age (years) sex	Presentation	Location and size of AVM	No. of pedicles embolised	Surgical resection	Complication of embolisation
1	39, M	Progressive hemiparesis	Frontoparietal (large)	3	–	–
2	12, F	Progressive hemiparesis	Frontoparietal (large)	4	–	–
3	38, M	Progressive hemiparesis	Frontoparietal (large)	4	–	–
4	35, M	Seizure	Temporal (large)	5	–	–
5	25, F	Subarachnoid haemorrhage	Thalamus (medium)	2	+	–
6	45, M	Headache	Temporal (small)	2	+	–
7	25, M	Subarachnoid haemorrhage	Temporal (small)	2	+	Intracerebral haemorrhage

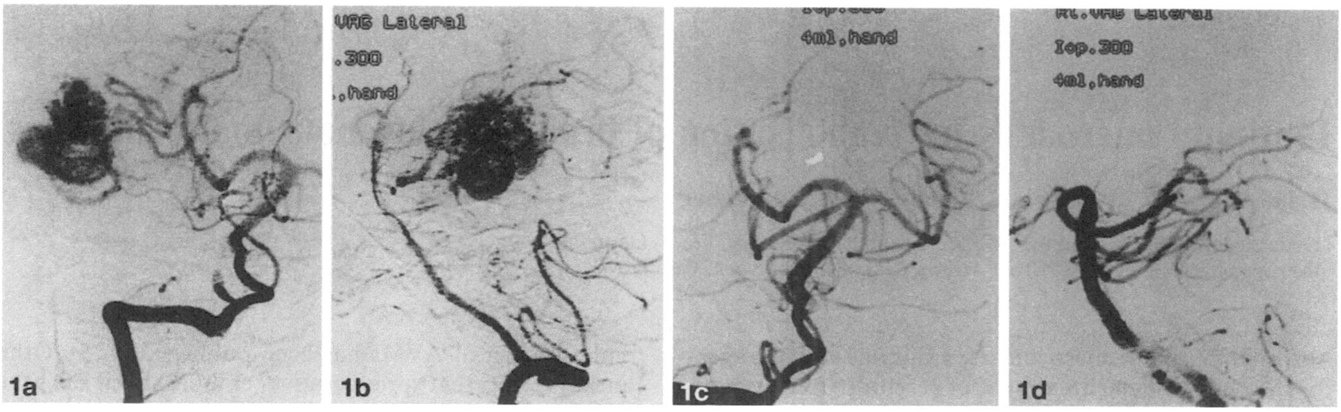

Fig. 1. Pre-embolisation carotid angiogram: anteroposterior (**A**) and lateral (**B**) views: a small arteriovenous malformation (AVM) is fed by the right posterior cerebral artery. **C, D** Postembolisation angiogram. The nidus is almost completely obliterated

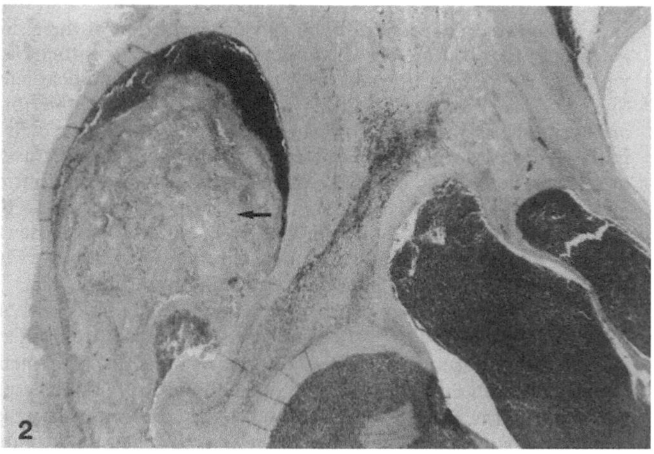

Fig. 2. Photomicrograph of AVM embolised with EVAL and ethanol mixture. There are a few neutrophils in the walls of the vessel embolised with EVAL (*arrow*)

Total resection of the nidus was successfully achieved without neurological deficit in this patient. His specimen demonstrated severe dilation and angionecrosis of embolised vessels and showed histological haemorrhage.

Illustrative case

A 45-year-old man (case 6) suffered from persistent headache. There were no neurological deficits. Angiography demonstrated an AVM in the right temporal lobe which was fed by two main feeders arising from right posterior cerebral artery (Fig. 1A, B). Embolisation of these two feeding pedicles was performed with EVAL and ethanol mixtures (Fig. 1C, D). Seven days after embolisation the AVM was totally removed without sequelae. Histopathological evaluation demonstrated that slight inflammatory reactions in the vessel wall embolised with EVAL (Fig. 2).

Discussion

Intravascular surgery has become more important recently for the treatment of AVMs [1]. Numerous embolic agents have been utilised for the embolisation of AVMs, and cyanoacrylate glues are currently considered the best liquid agents [1, 2]. However, control delivery of cyanoacrylates through microcatheters is difficult to achieve because it polymerises quickly and becomes a hard mass after polymerisation. Taki et al. [3] reported a liquid material for embolisation of AVMs using EVAL. Since this mixture is of low viscosity and not adhesive, the delivery of sufficient volume can be easily achieved. Surgical resection of AVMs after embolisation with EVAL can also be easily achieved because EVAL does not make a hard mass [2]. Histopathological study on AVMs embolised with EVAL demonstrated that a little inflammatory reaction was seen in the vessels [2–4]. However, some microcatheter systems cannot be used with the EVAL and DMSO mixture because DMSO dissolves the systems.

Intra-arterial infusion of very small volumes of anhydrous DMSO has been reported to be extremely angiotoxic [2]. Therefore we have selected ethanol as the solvent of EVAL and added iopamidol as a radiopaque agent. The mixture of EVAL, iopamidol and ehtanol has many advantages for embolisation of AVMs, as has the EVAL, metrizamide and DMSO mixture. Long-term follow-up of embolised AVMs with the new mixture is further needed to determine the usefulness in the treatment of AVMs.

References

1. Debrun G, Viñuela F, Fox AJ, Drake CG (1982) Embolisation of cerebral arteriovenous malformations with bucrylate: experience in 46 cases. J Neurosurg 56:615–627
2. Linsky ME, Sekhar LN (1993) Direct thrombosis of aneurysms (letter). J Neurosurg 78:1006–1007
3. Taki W, Yonekawa Y, Iwata H, Uno A, Yamashita K, Amemiya H (1990) A new liquid material for embolisation of arteriovenous malformations. AJNR 11:163–168
4. Fukushima T, Ohsfiro S, Tschimochi H, et al (1992) Clinicopathological evaluation of EVAL embolisation in arteriovenous malformations. Neurol Surg 209:439–444

Platinum microcoils for embolisation of brain arteriovenous malformations

H. Henkes[1], H. C. Nahser[1], D. Kühne[1], E. Berg-Dammer[2]

[1] Department of Neuroradiology, Alfried Krupp Krankenhaus, Essen, Germany
[2] Department of Neurology, Alfried Krupp Krankenhaus, Essen, Germany

Abstract. Platinum microcoils are a suitable embolic agent for the endovascular treatment of cerebral arteriovenous malformations (AVMs). Our experience with over 200 embolisations in more than 50 patients showed that coil embolisation of AVMs is a safe, effective and well-tolerated procedure. Coils are used primarily for preoperative embolisation, but are also of value to reduce the size of an AVM to a degree that allows stereotactic radiation. Since coil embolisation appears to be very safe, it is especially recommended for the rare cases of palliative AVM embolisation. Despite some disadvantages (e.g. high costs of the material, the long time required to introduce many coils, restrictions in catheter choice), platinum microcoils can replace other embolic agents in endovascular AVM treatment indicated for various different conditions.

Key words: Malformations, arteriovenous – Coil occlusion – Endovascular therapy

---

The use of particulate agents for embolisation of cerebral arteriovenous malformations (AVMs) dates back to the very beginning of endovascular treatment [1]. In 1988, Young et al. [2] proposed the use of platinum wire obtained from the distal tips of 0.014-in. or 0.013-in. guidewires. In the same year, Hilal et al. [3] introduced fibre-coated platinum coils for the endovascular treatment of arteriovenous fistulas and intracranial aneurysms. Since that time, limited experience with coil embolisation of AVMs has been published [4, 5]. Other authors feel that preoperative embolisation of brain AVMs with microcoils is of doubtful value [6].

Method

Embolisation of brain AVMs is performed by using a mono- or biplane digital subtraction unit. After systemic heparinisation, a soft 6 F guiding catheter is introduced into the corresponding internal carotid or vertebral artery via a transfemoral approach. The strategy is to achieve a centripedal or homogeneous reduction of the nidus. According to this principle, the target feeding vessel is catheterised with a Tracker-18 or, if necessary with a Tracker-10 microcatheter. Straight coils of various lengths (2, 3, 5 mm), with and without fibres are available from various companies. Embolisation of the coils is initiated in a position of the catheter tip that precludes the occlusion of nutrient vessels. To avoid excessive increases of pressure during introduction of the coils, a distance of 1 or 2 cm between the tip of the catheter and the nidus is desirable. The length of the coils is chosen to allow the most distal lodgement into the nidus, without venous passage on one hand and proximal occlusion on the other. Thus, in most cases the procedure starts with straight 2-mm coils without fibres. If these coils penetrate to the venous side, or if many coils are lodged into a vessel that is already occluded in its distal segment, larger coils are advantageous. The same applies to fistulous compartments of the nidus. Fibres attached to the coils greatly increase their thrombogenicity. The ability of the coils to penetrate the nidus may, however, be decreased. The number of coils that can be introduced via a single Tracker is apparently unrestricted, especially when there is limited tortuosity of the catheterised vessel and injection of the coils is possible. When the shunt is significantly slowed down, final occlusion of the dependent compartment of the nidus can be achieved by the injection of polyvinyl alcohol (PVA) particles. We never inject bucrylate in a coil-containing vessel. If the nidus is formed by fistulous and plexiform compartments, coil occlusion of the fistula and bucrylate embolisation of the plexus may be considered. We rarely perform proximal coil occlusion of a distally embolised feeder [4].

Correspondence to: H. Henkes, Department of Neuroradiology, Alfried Krupp Krankenhaus, Alfried Krupp Strasse 21, D-45117 Essen, Germany

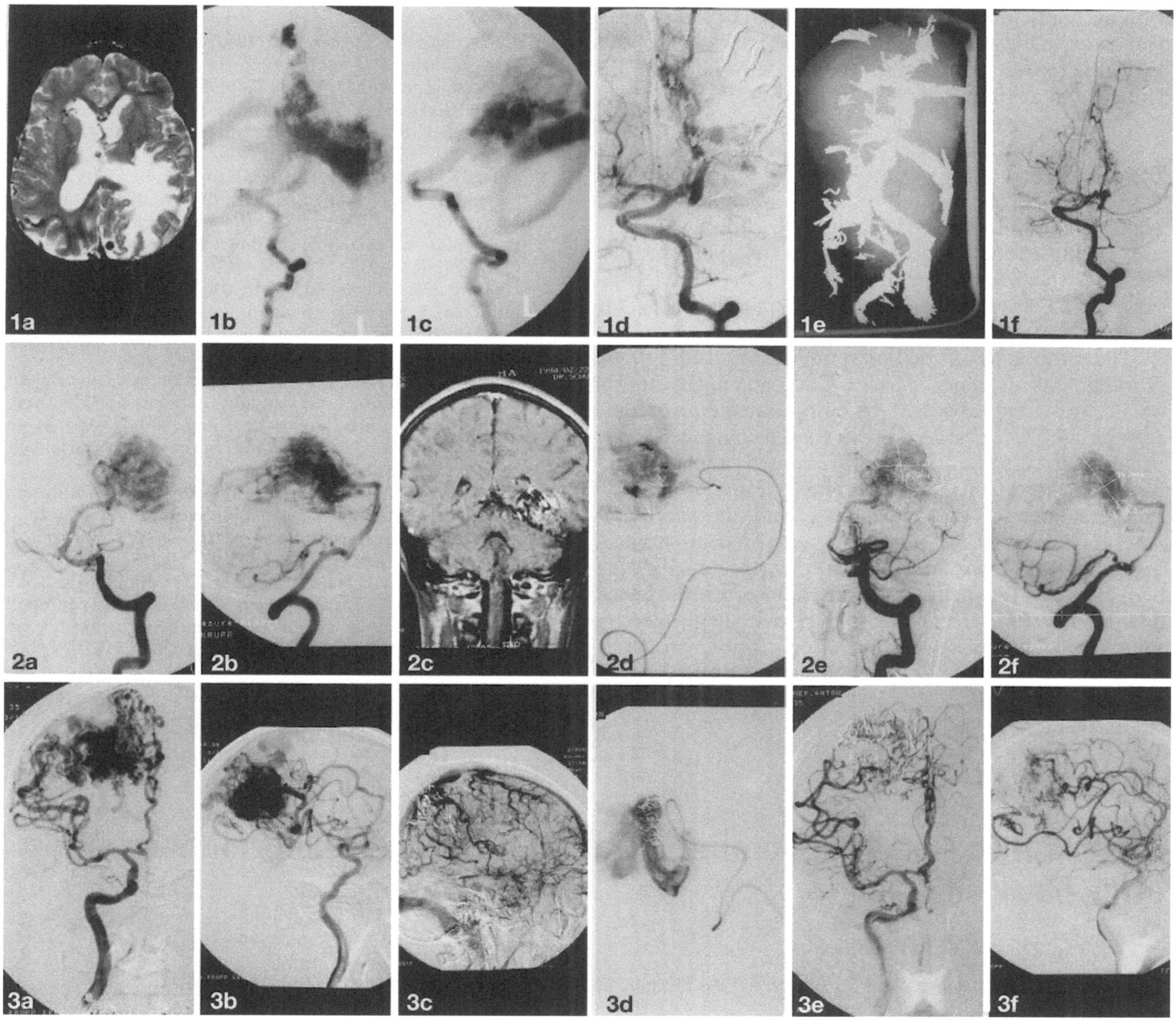

Fig. 1 a–f. Coil embolisation of a cerebral AVM prior to microneurosurgical resection of the nidus in a 2-year-old boy with a large left occipital AVM. **a** The nidus was supplied mainly be the left PCA. **b, c** In 6 sessions, 1405 coils (4925 mm) were inserted into the nidus via the left PCA and MCA. The angiogram obtained after the last embolisation demonstrated extensive devascularisation of the angioma (**d**). The nidus was resected microsurgically and the postoperative course was uneventful. **3** Radiograph of the resected nidus. **f** Postoperative angiography confirmed complete removal of the malformation

Fig. 2 a–f. Coil embolisation of a cerebral AVM prior to stereotactic radiosurgery in a 24-year-old woman. **a–c** The left temporo-occipital AVM measured 3.5×3.5×2 mm (**b, c**), and was thus too large for primary radiosurgery. It was decided to reduce the size of the nidus. **d** Via a Tracker-18 catheter, 377 microcoils (844 mm) were inserted into the nidus. **e, f** After three sessions, the nidus was significantly reduced in size. The angioma was later irradiated stereotactically

Fig. 3 a–f. Coil embolisation of a cerebral AVM as a palliative measure in a 56-year-old man. The large AVM in the right parietal lobe (**a, b**) was associated with a complete thrombosis of the internal venous system (**c**). Thus, the AVM was deemed inoperable. Fistulous (**d**) and plexiform compartments of the nidus were catheterised and occluded with platinum microcoils. With significant devascularisation of this nidus (**e, f**) the frequency of the patient's seizures was reduced and cognitive impairment less marked

Results

During the last 3 years, more than 50 AVM patients have been treated by coil embolisation of their vascular malformation in over 200 sessions. During that time, coil embolisation according to the above method has proved very safe. In no case, could clinically significant complications be related to this embolic agent. Surgical handling of coil-containing vessels and niduses was possible without difficulty in 26 patients who underwent microsurgical resection of the embolised AVM. In 4 cases of staged treatment with intervals of several months, no recanalisation and only limited recruitment of surrounding vessels was observed.

Three representative cases are shown to illustrate the clinical and angiographic results (Figs. 1–3).

Discussion

An ideal embolic agent for brain AVMs should be safe in use, readily available, easily deposited via all microcatheters, effective in permanently occluding the catheterised vessel, well tolerated and readily manipulable by the surgeon [7].

The properties of platinum microcoils fullfil these requirements in many aspects. Coils are highly radiopaque, providing excellent visibility under fluoroscopic conditions. Their positioning can be well controlled. They occlude the vessels and when fibre coated induce thrombus formation. Coils induce minimal, if any, inflammatory reactions of the vessel wall, and the platinum-irridium alloy can be cut with standard neurosurgical instruments. Drawbacks of this embolic agent include the high costs and the fact that they cannot be introduced via flow-guided catheters. Owing to their size, they are rarely suitable for complete intranidal deposition, which is essential for complete devascularisation of an AVM by endovascular means.

References

1. Luessenhop AJ, Spence WT (1960) Artificial embolization of cerebral arteries. Report of use in a case of arteriovenous malformation. JAMA 172:1153–1155
2. Yang PJ, Halbach VV, Higashida RT, Hieshima GB (1988) Platinum wire: a new transvascular embolic agent. AJNR 9:547–550
3. Hilal SK, Khandji AG, Chi TL, Stein BM, Bello JA; Silver AJ, Schumacher KJ (1988) Synthetic fiber-coated platinum coils successfully used for endovascular treatment of arteriovenous malformations, aneurysms and direct arteriovenous fistula of the CNS. AJNR 9:1030
4. Nakstad PH, Bakke SJ, Hald JK (1992) Embolization of intracranial arteriovenous malformations and fistulas with polyvinyl alcohol particles and platinum fibre coils. Neuroradiology 34:348–351
5. Nahser HC, Kühne D (1993) Strategy of endovascular treatment of mixed plexiform and fistulous intracranial arteriovenous malformations. In: Lorenz R, Klinger M, Brock M (eds) Advances in neurosurgery, vol 21. Springer, Berlin Heidelberg New York, pp 290–292
6. Berenstein A, Lasjaunias P, Choi IS (1993) Endovascular treatment of arteriovenous malformations of the brain. In: Valavanis A (ed) Interventional neuroradiology. Springer, Berlin Heidelberg New York, pp 93–110
7. Deveikis JP, Manz HJ, Luessenhop AJ, Caputhy AJ, Kobrine AL, Schellinger D, Patronas N (1994) A clinical and neuropathologic study of silk suture as an embolic agent for brain arteriovenous malformations. AJNR 15:263–271

Preoperative embolisation of cerebral arteriovenous malformations using black silk

A. P. Karapurkar, R. Ramakantan

Departments of Neurosurgery and Radiology, K.E.M. Hospital and Seth G.S. Medical College, 400012 Bombay, India

Abstract. Since 1990 patients having cerebral arteriovenous malformations (AVMs) have been advised to undergo embolisation followed by surgery if the AVM was more than 3 cm in diameter. Sixty-one patients underwent embolisation of the cerebral AVM with silk suture material: 1.8 F or 1.5 F Balt Magic MP catheters were used. There were no permanent neurological complications. Temporary complications included Todd's palsy in two patients after fits occurred immediately following the procedure. Technical complications included spasm of the cerebral artery and rupture of the catheter due to occlusion of the tip of the catheter. Fracture of the catheter due to spasm occurred in two patients.

Key words: Arteriovenous malformations, cerebral – Embolisation – Silk, black

Correspondence to: A. P. Karapurkar

Silk embolisation, like other thread techniques [1] is an effective pre-operative treatment for cerebral arteriovenous malformations (AVMs). We describe its use in 61 patients. Embolisation can also be followed by radiosurgery or linear accelerator therapy for obliteration of the nidus.

Materials and methods

Of the 106 patients seen in the Department of Neurosurgery since 1990, 61 were referred for preoperative embolisation with black silk. There were 47 male and 14 female patients: 30 AVMs were cortical, 22 were large and 9 were deep.

A Magic MP catheter with its marker cut off was negotiated into or close to the AVM nidus. Superselective angios were done. Embolisation was done with pieces of 4/O black silk. If the flow was slow or the feeding artery was small, 1.5-cm-long pieces were used. If the flow was high or the feeding artery large, 3- to 5-cm-long pieces were injected. To enable injection of the silk, the hub of the catheter was replaced by a 1-to-6 F adapter and the silk pieces introduced by a forceps.

Results

The rate of blood flow through the AVM was reduced in all cases: 5 were reduced in size from 0 to 30%. 31 from 30 to 70%, 18 from 70 to 90% and 7 by more than 90%. No AVM could be obliterated completely. Cortical arteries as well as perforators were easily embolised. The perforators included anterior choroidals, branches of the posterior medial and lateral choroidals, and the thalamoperforators and lenticulostriate arteries. Arteries of eloquent areas were embolised if the amytal test was negative. For perforators, Magic 1.5 MP catheter is used and 5/0 black silk is the embolic material.

There was no mortality. Transient neurological deficit following grand mal fits occurred in 2 patients. There were no permanent neurological deficits in any patient. Technical complications have included occlusion of the magic with proximal rupture. This has never caused any problem. Occasional spasm of the cerebral artery has occurred. On two occasions, in the same patient, the catheter could not be withdrawn and broke off on forceful withdrawal. One catheter lay in the middle cerebral trunk and the other in the posterior cerebral artery. In another patient the catheter fractured in the middle cerebral stem with its distal tip lying in the peripheral cortical branch. In both patients there was no neurological deficit immediately after the procedure nor on long-term follow-up. Both patients underwent successful embolisation and excision of the AVM. No neurological complication ensued despite the catheter having fractured in large cerebral arteries.

Of these patients 45 underwent surgical exploration. There were 5 deaths in the early post-operative period. In 40 patients the AVM was excised totally. In none of the excised or autopsied specimens was any reaction seen around the AVM. The AVM could easily be excised. The black silk suture could often be seen through the wall of the artery and could be followed into the nidus. None of the complications referred to by Deveikis et al. [2] were seen in our patients. Two patients underwent radiosurgery with complete cure on long-term follow-up. Silk meets the criteria suggested by Purdy et al. [3].

References

1. Benati A, Beltramello A, Colombari R, et al (1989) Preoperative embolization of cerebral arteriovenous malformations with polyethylene threads: techniques with wing microcatheter and pathologic results. AJNR 10:579–586
2. Deveikis JP, Manz HJ, Luessenhop AJ, et al (1994) A clinical and neuropathologic study of silk suture as an embolic agent for brain arteriovenous malformations. AJNR 15:263–271
3. Purdy PD, Samson D, Batjer HH, Risser RC (1992) Arteriovenous malformations of the brain: choosing the right embolic materials to enhance safety and ease of excision. J Neurosurg 77:217–222

Endovascular therapy of basal ganglion, thalamic, and brainstem arteriovenous malformations

M. P. Marks, A. M. Norbash, G. K. Steinberg, M. Marcellus

Department of Radiology, Stanford University Medical Center, Stanford, CA 94305, USA

Abstract. Central arteriovenous malformations (AVMs) in locations including the basal ganglia, thalamus, and brainstem are difficult to treat. These AVMs have a poor natural history and are prone to multiple hemorrhages. This study evaluated the results of endovascular treatment alone and combined with surgery and/or radiosurgery. Embolization achieved significant size reduction (mean 42.9%). In our series, 9/26 (34.6%) were thrombosed with embolization alone or embolization combined with surgery. There was a higher rate of therapeutic complications in this group than in patients with AVMs elsewhere, and endovascular therapy alone did not appear to alter the natural history of these lesions, which are prone to hemorrhage.

Key words: Arteriovenous malformations, cerebral – Brain, hemorrhage – Endovascular therapy, embolization

Correspondence to: M. P. Marks

Deep arteriovenous malformations (AVMs) are more difficult to treat than those on the surface of the brain [1–4]. We reviewed our experience of treating lesions of this type.

Methods

We treated 26 patients aged 5–67 years (mean 29.5) by 1–4 staged embolization procedures (mean 1.7), using flow-directed and guide-wire-directed catheters. They had AVMs in the basal ganglia alone (6), thalamus (5), basal ganglia and thalamus (11), or brainstem (4). Of the 26 patients, 23 (88.5%) had prior hemorrhage (1–8 episodes each), and 22 had fixed neurologic deficits (84.6%) consisting in hemiparesis, aphasia, or cranial nerve palsies deficits. Ten patients (38.5%) had previously failed radiation therapy. The AVMs varied in size from 1.5 to 9 cm (mean 4.28 cm). Of the 23/26 patients, 23 (88.5%) were embolized (secure vascular access could not be achieved in the other 3): 21 (91.3%) of these were treated with *N*-butyl cyanoacrylate, and 3 (13%) had additional therapy, utilizing a new approach involving temporary circle of Willis occlusion with proximal embolization using small polyvinyl alcohol particle spray (150 μm). Lesion diameter was measured in three orthogonal planes before treatment, and volume reduction as a result of treatment was appropriately determined.

Results

Measured volume reduction varied from zero to 100% (mean 42.9%), with 3 patients (11.5%) having complete lesion obliteration. New fixed deficits occurred in 6 patients (23%), consisting of visual field defects or worsening hemiparesis. Clinical follow-up is 1-60 months (mean 12.4). Twenty-one patients are clinically unchanged, but 5 patients (19.2%) had recurrent hemorrhages and 3 of these died.

Discussion

Endovascular therapy of basal ganglia, thalamic, and brainstem AVMs can result in a significant volume reduction, suggesting that this technique can be used on lesions in these locations as an adjunctive treatment prior to radiosurgery.

References

1. Spetzler RF, Martin N (1986) A proposed grading system for arteriovenous malformations. J Neurosurg 65:476–483
2. Heros RC, Korosue K, Diebold PM (1990) Surgical excision of cerebral arteriovenous malformations: late results. Neurosurgery 26:570–578
3. Hamilton MG, Spetzler RF (1994) The prospective application of a grading system for arteriovenous malformations. Neurosurgery 34:2–7
4. Marks MP, Lane B, Steinberg GK, Chang PJ (1990) Hemorrhage in intracerebral arteriovenous malformations: angiographic determinants. Radiology 176:807–813

Monitoring shunt flow by jugular bulb oxygen saturation during therapeutic embolisation of cerebral arteriovenous malformations

T. Hirayama[1], Y. Katayama[1], T. Tsubokawa[1], K. Himi[2]

[1] Department of Neurological Surgery, Nihon University School of Medicine, Tokyo 173, Japan
[2] Department of Radiology, Nihon University School of Medicine, Tokyo 173, Japan

Abstract. The shunt flow to perfusion flow ratio in patients with cerebral arteriovenous malformation (AVM) can be evaluated from the arterial and jugular bulb oxygen saturations (S_aO_2 and S_jO_2). We employed this technique to assess the progress of shunt obliteration during therapeutic embolisation procedures. Data from a consecutive series of 15 large supratentorial high-flow AVMs (maximum diameter >4 cm) were analysed. The S_jO_2 before embolisation was significantly higher than the S_jO_2 at the end of the embolisation. Continuous monitoring of S_jO_2 revealed a progressive decrease in association with an increase in the circulation time, as well as disappearance of early veins and evidence of steal during the embolisation procedure. This technique is useful for real-time assessment of the progress of embolisation.

Key words: Arteriovenous malformation – Embolisation – Oxygen saturation – Jugular bulb

The draining veins of cerebral arteriovenous malformations (AVMs) contain highly oxygenated blood [1], as evidenced by the intra-operative findings commonly denoted as red veins [2], since arterial blood flow directly through a shunt does not deliver oxygen to the brain tissue. We have monitored the jugular bulb oxygen saturations (S_jO_2) during preoperative embolisation procedures in a consecutive series of large AVMs to estimate the shunt flow ratio. Hypaeremic oomplications may well be reduced by staged preoperative embolisation [3], avoiding abrupt changes in the shunt flow ratio. The aim of the present study was to determine whether or not S_jO_2 sensitively reflects changes in the shunt flow ratio during embolisation procedures.

Correspondence to: T. Hirayama

Materials and methods

We treated 15 patients with large AVMs in whom the S_jO_2 was measured continuously during planned preoperative embolization. The AVMs with a maximum diameter of greater than 4 cm were included in the present study. The AVM volume was calculated as the product of the three angiographic diameters multiplied by 0.52 with correction for the magnification factor according to the methods reported by Pasqualin et al. [4]. We employed *N*-butyl-cyanoacrylate polyfilament polyethylene threads (PPTs; diameter, 300 μm; length, 5–10 mm) and/or polyvinyl alcohol particles as embolisation materials. Embolisation was performed several times, each separated by 1 week, through 1–3 feeding arteries at each session. The embolisation materials were injected via a microcatheter, usually until the mean blood pressure of the feeding artery was elevated to approximately 80 mmHg. A fibre-optic catheter system was used for continous measurement of S_jO_2. The tip of the catheter was placed in the jugular bulb. The catheter was placed on the dominant side based on the findings of CT and previous angiography. The oxygen saturation of the systemic arterial blood (S_aO_2) was monitored by pulse oximetry at the finger. The S_jO_2 in cases of AVM represents a composite of the oxygen saturation of the shunt flow ($S_{js}O_2$) and of the perfusion flow ($S_{jp}O_2$). Thus,

$$S_jO_2 \times (F_{shunt} + F_{perfusion}) = S_{js}O_2 \cdot F_{shunt} + S_{jp}O_2 \cdot F_{perfusion} \qquad (1)$$

Table 1. Jugular bulb oxygen saturation in 15 patients with large arteriovenous malformation

Stage	n	Jugular bulb oxygen saturation (%)
Pre-embolisation	15	84.1 ± 12.7
Clinical and/or angiographic steal	7	93.6 ± 4.4**
No clinical and/or angiographic steal	8	75.9 ± 11.8
Post-embolisation	15	74.2 ± 10.9***

Statistical significance: ** $P<0.002$. compared to no clinical and/or angiographic steal (unpaired t-test); $P<0.0001$, compared to pre-embolisation (paired t-test)

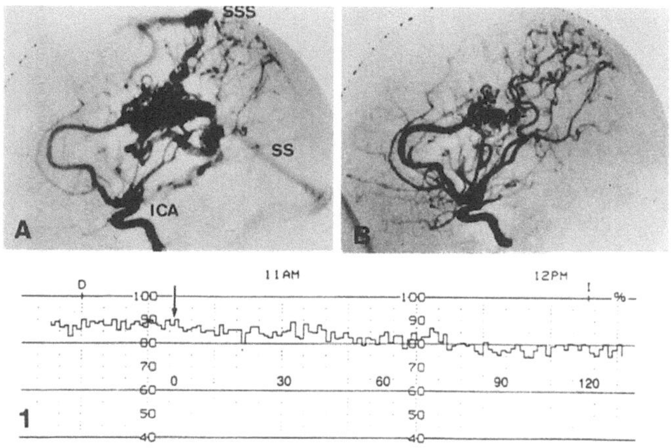

Fig. 1. Case with a moderate shunt flow; 16-year-old male. Total arteriovenous malformation volume, 12.5 cm^3. *Upper:* Angiograms before (**A**) and after (**B**) embolisation through the pericallosal artery. ICA internal carotid artery; SS, straight sinus; SSS, superior sagittal sinus. *Lower:* Chart demonstrating changes in the S_jO_2 during the embolisation procedure using polyethylene threads. The numbers of threads injected are shown on the *abscissa*

Equation 1 can be rewritten as:

$$F_{perfusion} = F_{shunt}\,(S_{js}O_2 - S_jO_2)/(S_jO_2 - S_{jp}O_2) \quad (2)$$

The shunt flow ratio can thus be expressed as:

$$F_{shunt}/(F_{perfusion} + F_{shunt}) = (S_jO_2 - S_{jp}O_2)/(S_{js}O_2 - S_{jp}O_2) \quad (3)$$

Since blood flowing directly through the shunt does not deliver oxygen to the brain tissue, the saturation of this blood flowing through the shunt can be assumed to be the same as the saturation of the systemic aterial blood (S_aO_2). Then, Eq. 3 can be re-written as:

$$F_{shunt}/(F_{tissue} + F_{shunt}) = (S_jO_2 - S_{jp}O_2/(S_aO_2 - S_{jp}O_2) \quad (4)$$

The $S_{jp}O_2$ can be assumed to be within the range of 50–75% since the brain did not seem globally ischaemic in any cases of the present study. The shunt flow ratio can therefore be evaluated from the S_aO_2 and S_jO_2 measurements.

Results

The S_jO_2 determined for withdrawn jugular bulb blood before embolisation ranged from 58 to 97% (mean ± SD = 84.1 ± 12.7%), showing a significant positive correlation with the AVM volume ($r = 0.66$, $P<0.001$). The S_jO_2 was significantly greater in patients with AVMs demonstrating clincial and/or angiographic steal (93.6 ± 4.4%) than in those with no clinical and/or angiographic steal (75.9 ± 11.8%; $P<0.002$, unpaired t-test, Table 1).

The S_jO_2 decreased following embolisation in association with an increase in the circulation time, the disappearance of early draining veins from the AVM, and evidence of steal on angiography (Fig. 1). Although the embolisation was not complete in many cases in the present study because of the large AVM volumes, the S_jO_2 determined for jugular bulb blood withdrawn at the end of the final embolisation procedure ranged from 54 to 91% (74.2 ± 10.9%, Table 1), which was significantly lower than that observed before embolisation ($P<0.0001$, paired t-test). A large decrease was generally observed when the embolisation had been performed through all major feeding arteries. When PPTs were employed, a gradual decrease in S_jO_2 was noted as the number of PPTs injected increased (Fig. 1). S_jO_2 did not return to the original level within the period of observation ranging up to 2 h, in so far as an appropriate amount of embolisation material was injected.

Discussion

We demonstrated that S_jO_2 was markedly elevated in cases with a large AVM volume. This supports the hypothesis that a high S_jO_2 in cases with AVMs reflects drainage from the shunt. The initial slow and later rapid decreases in S_jO_2 can be accounted for by an exponential decrease in shunt flow as the embolisation progressed.

Based on the values we obtained, Eq. 4 indicates that the shunt flow ratio is more than 0.5 in many cases with large AVMs. For example, an S_jO_2 of 90% indicates that the shunt flow ratio is within the range of between 0.6 and 0.8. Estimation of the shunt flow ratio in patients with AVMs from the S_jO_2 is thus relatively simple. Furthermore, data from repeated measurements are readily available in so far as the catheter resides in the jugular bulb. Continuous monitoring of S_jO_2 employing a fibreoptic catheter during the embolisation procedure provided a real-time information regarding the progress of embolisation of the AVMs.

References

1. Bauer BL, Beck B, Moessler U (1975) Investigation on volume and pressure overloading of the heart in cerebral angiomas. In: Pia HW, Gleave JRW, Grote E, Zierski J (eds) Cerebral angiomas. Springer, Berlin Heidelberg New York, pp 101–110
2. Feindel W, Yamamoto YL Hodge CP (1971) Red cerebral veins and the cerebral steal syndrome. Evidence from fluorescein angiography and microregional blood flow by radioisotopes during excision of an angioma. J Neurosurg 35:167–179
3. Spetzler RF, Martin NA, Carter LP (1987) Surgical management of large AVMs by staged embolization and operative excision. J Neurosurg 67:17–28
4. Pasqualin A, Barone G, Cioffi F (1991) The relevance of anatomic and hemodynamic factors to a classification of cerebral arteriovenous malformations. Neurosurgery 28:370–379

Spinal fistulae

Angiography of medullary and dural vascular malformations: relationship between venous drainage and outcome

L. Brunereau, Y. P. Gobin, A. L. Bailly, J. J. Merland

Department of Neuroradiology, Lariboisière Hospital, 2 rue Ambroise Paré, F-75010 Paris, France

Abstract. A series of 151 medullary and dural vascular malformations is reviewed, and two patterns of venous drainage that were observed are described: local and extensive. In this study, these patterns of venous drainage were correlated with the patient outcome, but were not related to the type of vascular malformation determined according to the current classification of spinal vascular malformations.

Key words: Angiography, spinal – Arteriovenous malformations – Spinal cord

We studied 151 consecutive cases of intra-medullary and dural vascular malformations. The purpose of this study was to analyse the relationship between the pattern of venous drainage and outcome. All patients underwent clinical examination and transfemoral angiography in the neuroradiology department of Lariboisière Hospital.

The current classification of spinal vascular malformations [1] includes intramedullary arteriovenous malformations (iAVM), perimedullary arteriovenous fistulae or malformations (pAVF), and spinal dural arteriovenous fistulae (sDAVF). Three types of perimedullary arteriovenous fistulae are described: from type 1 to type 3, arterial and venous calibre and blood flow velocity increase.

Materials and methods

We retrospectively analysed 140 spinal vascular malformations and 11 intracranial dural arteriovenous fistulae with perimedullary venous drainage (icDAVF) [2]. According to the classification of Merland, the 140 spinal vascular malformations broke down as follows: 67 iAVMs, 34 pAVFs (8 type 1, 14 type 2, 12 type 3), and 39 sDAVFs.

Analysis was clinical and angiographic. We only studied spontaneous clinical history before treatment. The clinical history was classed as sudden or progressive.

Symptoms were considered as sudden when they appeared within 24 h or less. Sudden symptoms were subarachnoid haemorrhage, medullary haematoma, or motor and sensory deficit. Symptoms were considered as progressive when they appeared over several days or several months. Progressive symptoms were motor, sensory or sphincter disturbances.

Angiographic analysis included diameter, length and blood flow velocity of dominant draining veins.

By means of angiographic analysis, two patterns of venous drainage were described, local and extensive: local venous drainage is characterised by short veins less than two vertebral bodies long, enlarged diameter, and high blood flow, and extensive venous drainage by veins longer than two vertebral bodies, normal diameter, and low blood flow.

Correspondence to: L. Brunereau

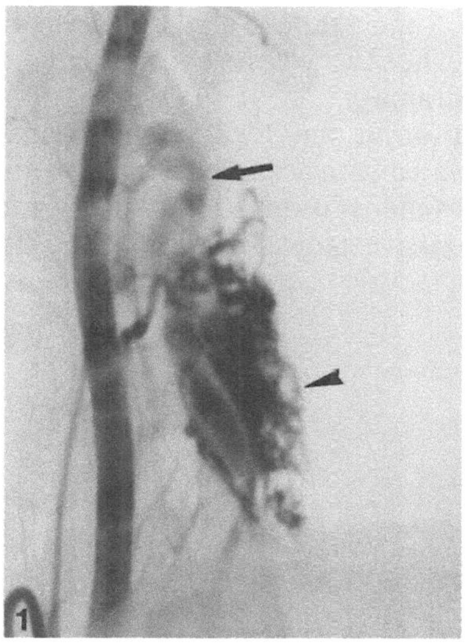

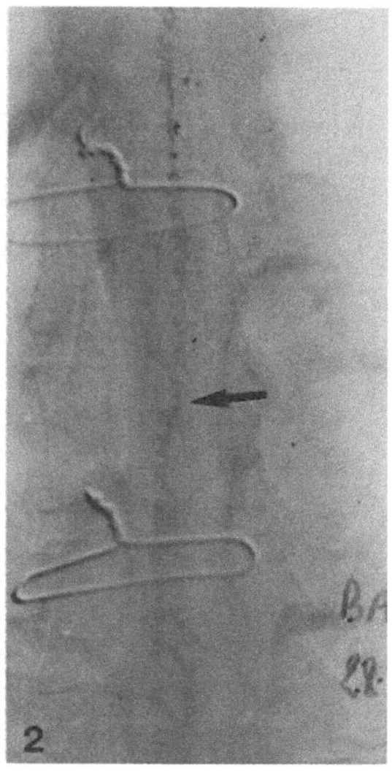

Fig. 1. Cervical intramedullary arteriovenous malformation (*arrowhead*) with typical local venous drainage (*arrow*)

Fig. 2. Perimedullary arteriovenous fistula type 1 with typical extensive venous drainage (*arrow*)

Table 1. Venous drainage and clinical course (patients)

Vascular lesion	Symptoms	Venous drainage	
		Local	Extensive
Intramedullary arterio- venous malformations	Sudden	49	12
	Progressive	0	6
Perimedullary arterio- venous fistulae	Sudden	13	1
	Progressive	5	15
Dural arteriovenous fistulae (spinal)	Sudden	1	0
	Progressive	0	38
Dural arteriovenous fistulae	Sudden	5	0
	Progressive	0	6

These patterns of venous drainage were not related to the type of vascular malformation determined according to the classification of Merland. Local and extensive venous drainage are illustrated in Figs. 1 and 2.

Results (Table 1)

In cases of iAVM, 61 malformations demonstrated a sudden clinical history. In these cases, 49 malformations demonstrated local venous drainage, and the other 12, extensive venous drainage.

In cases of pAVF, 14 had a sudden clinical history; 13 of these cases demonstrated local venous drainage and 1 demonstrated extensive venous drainage. Twenty cases had a progressive clinical history. In these cases, 15 cases demonstrated extensive venous drainage and 5 local venous drainage.

In cases of sDAVf, 38 had a progressive clinical history and extensive venous drainage. Only 1 case had a sudden history and local venous drainage.

In cases of icDAVF, 5 had a sudden clinical history and local venous drainage. The other 6 cases had a progressive history and extensive drainage.

For each type of malformation – local venous drainage was significantly correlated with a sudden clinical history ($P<0.05$); – extensive venous drainage was significantly correlated with a progressive clinical history ($P<0.05$).

Discussion

In this study, two patterns of venous drainage were demonstrated: local, characterised by short veins, large diameter, and high blood flow; and extensive, characterised by long veins, normal diameter, and low blood flow. These two patterns of venous drainage were significantly correlated with the outcome ($P<0.05$). Therefore, in each type of dural and medullary vascular malformation, analysis of the draining veins could help in the choice between conservative and more aggressive treatment.

References

1. Merland JJ, Reizine D (1987) Malformations vasculaires vertébro-médullaires. Encycl Med Chir (Paris) [Radiodiagnostic II]:31671 G10 22p
2. Guegen B, Merland JJ, Riché MC, Rey A (1987) Vascular malformations of the spinal cord: intrathecal perimedullary arteriovenous fistulas fed by medullary arteries. Neurology 37:969–979

Embolisation of the parent artery of a spinal dural arteriovenous malformation

T. Kaji[1], M. Katayama[1], H. Yokoyama[1], T. Irie[1], S. Kusano[1], S. Ishihara[2], T. Miyazawa[2], K. Shima[2]

[1] Department of Radiology, National Defense Medical College, 3-2 Namiki, Tokorozawa, Saitama, Japan, 359
[2] Department of Neurosurgery, National Defense Medical College, Saitama, Japan

Abstract. We report a spinal dural arteriovenous malformation (AVM), clinically manifest as subarachnoid haemorrhage. The patient was treated with transarterial embolisation of the left vertebral artery (the parent artery) using mechanically detachable coils, followed by occlusion of the nidus with polyvinyl alcohol particles via the collateral vessels because selective catheterisation of the feeding artery was considered difficult. In a situation such as this, embolisation of the parent artery should be considered as a therapeutic strategy, with the anticipation that collateral vessels would subsequently develop.

Key words: Arteriovenous malformation, spinal – Vertebral artery, embolisation – Interventional neuroradiology

The spinal dural arteriovenous malformation (AVM) is an unusual entity and remains a therapeutic challenge. The therapeutic goal is to embolise or remove the shunt or nidus and embolisation or ligation of the proximal feeding artery or the parent artery is ineffective due to the development of the collateral vessels. We report a spinal dural AVM in which the nidus was occluded via the collateral vessels after transarterial embolisation of the left vertebral artery (the parent artery), together with a review of the literature.

Case report

A 77-year-old man who experienced sudden headache and vomiting was shown on CT to have a subarachnoid haemorrhage. Neurological examination was normal. According to the Glasfow coma scale, the level of consciousness was E4V5M6. He had been treated for diabetes mellitus. There was no relevant history such as trauma.

MRI showed a flow void on the anterior part of the medulla oblongata. Emergency cerebral angiography was conducted with a suspicion of cerebral aneurysm. Minute vessels had grown as if to surround the left vertebral artery at the level of C1, which drained into the medullary vein through a dilated tortuous vein (Fig. 1). These findings led to a diagnosis of dural AVM arising where the vertebral artery perforated the dura mater. No vessels other than the left vertebral artery were identified as feeding arteries.

The patient was referred for transarterial embolisation for the following reasons: surgical procedures were anatomically difficult; his diabetes mellitus was not well controlled; and the probability of recurrence of haemorrhage due to rupture of the AVM was considered high. He underwent embolisation therapy 27 days after admission. Because selective catheterisation of the feeding artery was considered to be difficult to perform due to its fine vascular architecture, embolisation of the vertebral artery (the parent artery)

Correspondence to: T. Kaji

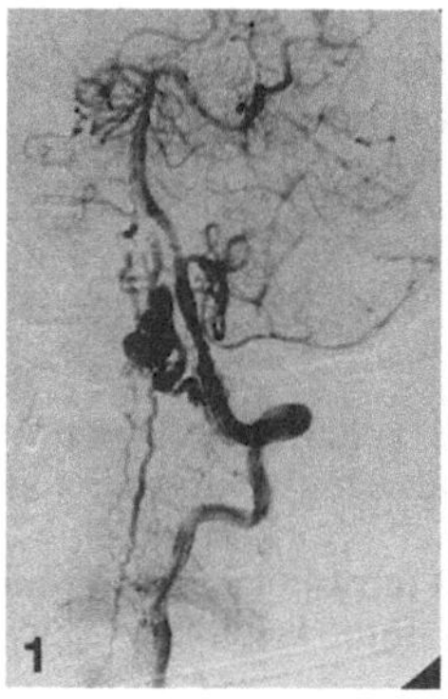

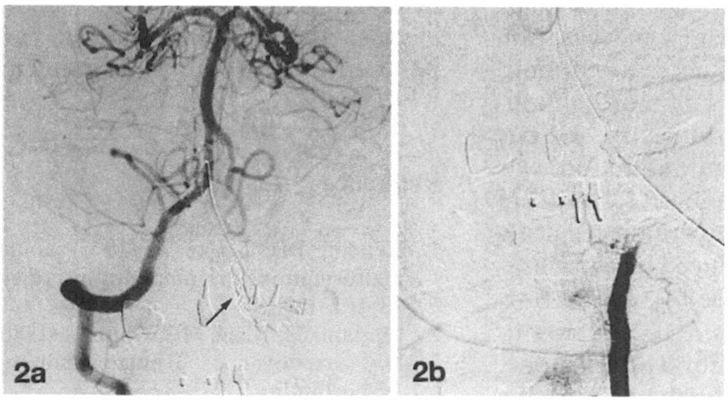

Fig. 1. Left vertebral angiography shows that minute vessels had grown as if to surround the left vertebral artery at the level of C1, which drained into the medullary veins through a dilated vein

Fig. 2a, b. Vertebral angiography after embolisation. **a** The left vertebral artery was occluded using mechanically detachable coils (*arrow*). **b** Six months later, there were no collateral vessels from the right vertebral or the posterior inferior cerebellar arteries

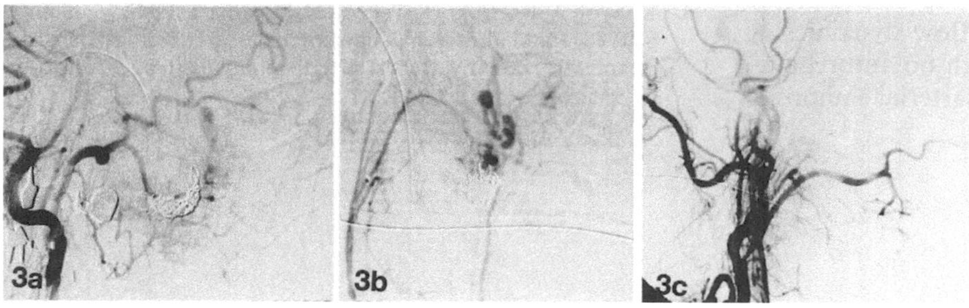

Fig 3. Left external angiography. 22 days after embolisation revealed the development of collateral vessels supplied from the occipital (**a**) and the ascending pharyngeal (**b**) arteries, which were embolised with polyvinyl alcohol particles. Another angiogram 6 months after embolisation showed no collateral vessels (**c**)

was scheduled, with the anticipation that the collateral vessels would subsequently develop. A preoperative balloon occlusion test revealed no evidence of neurological abnormalities. To fill the vertebral artery supplying the feeding artery, 21 mechanically detachable coils (MDCs) were used as emboli (Fig. 2). No complication of transarterial embolisation was encountered. Angiography immediately after embolisation showed no sign of the development of collateral vessels. Angiography 22 days after therapeutic embolisation revealed no evidence of development of a feeding artery from the vertebral or posterior inferior cerebellar arteries (Fig. 2), but it did show collateral supply from the occipital and ascending pharyngeal branches of the left external artery (Fig. 3). These were embolised with 300–700 μm of polyvinyl alcohol particles. Six months after, he was again subjected to angiography, which confirmed that the collateral arteries supplied from the occipital and ascending pharyngeal arteries had been embolised (Fig. 3). Since then, there has been no evidence that collateral vessels have developed and the patient has made a satisfactory recovery.

Discussion

Spinal AVM has been classified as single-coil (type 1), glomus (type 2), or juvenile (type 3). Since Kendall and Logue [1], followed by Merland et al. [2], reported that type 1 is in fact dilated tortuous veins which have been arterialised due to a fistula near the nerve root, it has been recognized as spinal dural AV fistula. Spinal dural AVM occurs most commonly in men in their fifties to seventies, who account for 80% or more of patients. It is associated with initial manifestations, such as leg weakness, sensory disturbance, and pain and often characterised by slow progression. Haemorrhage, as seen in our patient, is a rare clinical manifestation of spinal dural AVM.

The pathophysiology of spinal dural AVM can be explained by the following: the AV pressure gradient decreases with increasing venous pressure in the coronal venous plexus and medullary veins of the surface of the spinal cord, which results in spontaneous reduction in the intraspinal blood flow and eventual ischaemic myelopathy [3]. However, it is not known why reflux into radiculomedullary veins occurs or why an increase in venous pressure exerts a direct effect on the intrathecal blood ciruclation.

The therapeutic principle is to reduce the venous pressure by removing the AV shunt. Surgery and transarterial embolisation are acceptable options for spinal dural AVM. Surgical procedures include stripping, removal of the AV shunt, coagulation, and clipping of the draining vein. In this case, surgical procedures were thought to be difficult because the patient's diabetic condition was uncontrolled, the nidus was located within the forament magnum at the level of C1, and the draining vein ran on the anterior part of the medulla oblongata (Fig. 1).

Whether transarterial embolisation is as effective as surgery remains controversial, although some investigators advocate its effectiveness if both the nidus and the draining vein can be embolised. The following materials for embolisation are used: occlusion by balloon, particles, liquid embolic material, and microcoils. In our patient, because selective catheterisation of the feeding artery was considered difficult, the left vertebral artery (the parent artery) was embolised using MDCs. The probability of recurrence of haemorrhage is considered high when the initial clinical manifestation of AVM is haemorrhage. Therefore we first reduced the venous pressure by embolising the parent artery to prevent recurrent haemorrhage up to the time when collateral circulation developed. Then the shunt was scheduled to be embolised via the collateral artery. Embolisation of the parent artery is thought to be ineffective due to the development of collateral vessels unless the fistula is successfully closed. To our knowledge, our patient is the first reported case in which embolisation of the parent artery was considered as a necessary option.

Brain stem infarction is the most common complication of embolisation of the vertebral artery. In our patient, the probability of brain stem infarction was considered low because embolisation induced reflux from the contralateral vertebral artery. Haemorrhage resulting from changes in blood flow that are induced by embolisation had been reported in only one case [4]. Blood flow dynamics can be divided into three types: (1) blood flow to the shunt is fed from the ipsilateral vertebral artery alone, (2) it is fed from not only the ipsilateral but also the contralateral vertebral artery, and (3) it is fed from the basilar artery and both the ipsilateral and contralateral vertebral arteries. For type 3, blood flow dynamics is maintained by small dilated vessels with no autoregulation. In addition, it is thought that transarterial embolisation induces a sudden increase in blood flow in the small vessels, the so-called normal pressure breakthrough phenomenon which results in haemorrhage.

References

1. Kendall BE, Logue V (1977) Spinal epidural angiomatous malformations draining into intrathecal veins. Neuroradiology 13:181–189
2. Merland JJ, Riché MC, Chiras J (1980) Intraspinal extramedullary arteriovenous fistulae draining into medullary veins. J Neuroradiol 7:271–320
3. Aminoff MJ, Barnard RO, Logue V (1974) The pathophysiology of spinal vascular malformations. J Neurol Sci 23:255–263
4. Kondoh T, Norihiko T, Takeda N, Suyama T, Oi S, Matsumoto S (1988) Fatal intracranial haemorrhage after balloon occlusion of an extracranial vertebral arteriovenous fistula. J Neurosurg 69:945–948

A simple, practical classification of spinal vascular lesions

Y. Kikuchi[1], D. A. Rufenacht[2], B. C. Chu[1], K. Miyasaka[1]

[1] Department of Radiology, Hokkaido University School of Medicine, Kita-15 Nishi-7, Kita-ku, Sapporo, 060, Japan
[2] Department of Neuroradiology, Hospital Cantonal Universitaire de Genève, Geneva, Switzerland

Abstract. Spinal vascular lesions seen at our institution were reviewed and classified into three types: dural and extramedullary arteriovenous fistulae and intramedullary arteriovenous malformations, according to the simplified form originally proposed by Riché and Merland. Representative cases are illustrated for better understanding of these uncommon lesions.

Key words: Spinal arteriovenous malformation – Spinal arteriovenous fistula – Spinal dural arteriovenous fistula

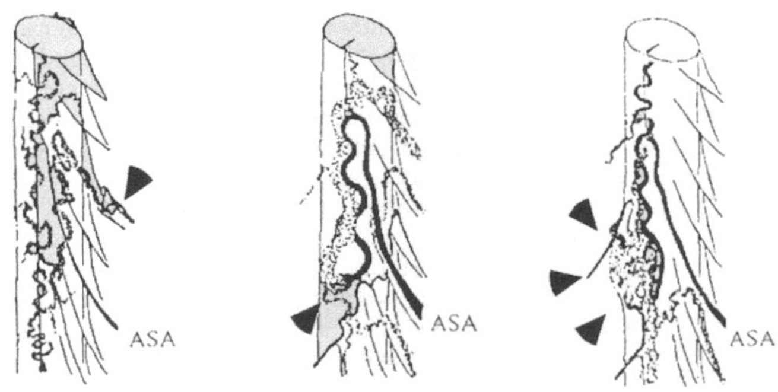

Fig. 1 a–c. Classification of spinal vascular lesions. **a** Dural and **b** extramedullary arteriovenous fistulae (AVFs). **c** Intramedullary arteriovenous malformation (AVM). *Arrowheads* point to the location of the fistula or nidus. *ASA* Anterior spinal artery

Spinal vascular lesions are relatively uncommon and this fact leads to lack of knowledge and experience. In addition, different classifications of these lesions are used by different authors, which further makes understanding of the lesions difficult. We illustrate a simple, practical classification of spinal vascular lesions with representative cases in each type for better understanding and treatment.

Materials and methods

Spinal vascular lesions seen in our institution and affiliated hospitals over the last 10 years were reviewed, and illustrative cases were chosen. Special attention was paid to the findings on selective artiography regarding the location of shunt between artery and vein. MRI and myelograms were also reviewed when available. These lesions were classified according to the simplified version of the Riché and Merland classification [1].

Correspondence to: Y. Kikuchi

Results (Fig. 1)

Spinal vasular lesions could be classified into the following three types.

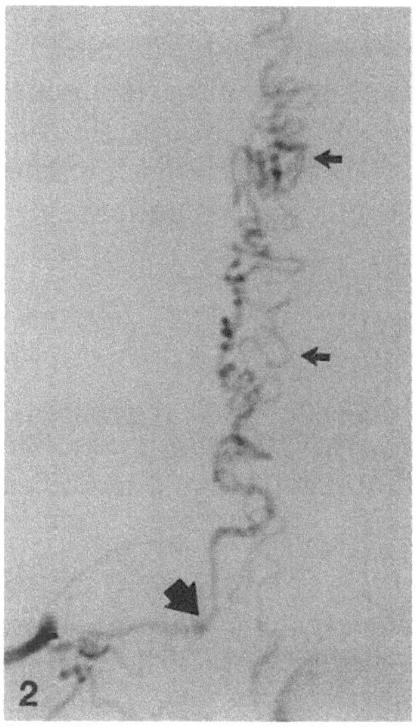

Fig. 2. Dural AVF. Angiogram shows shunt (*large arrow*) between radiculomeningeal artery and medullary vein (*small arrows*)

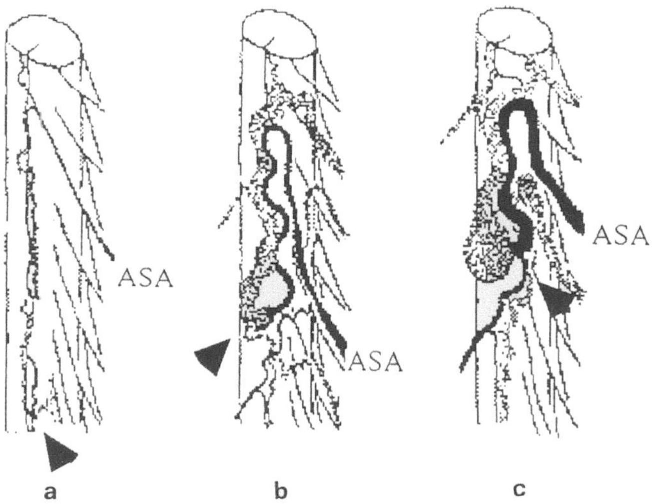

Fig. 3a–c. Extramedullary (perimedullary) AVF. These lesions can be subdivided according to the size of the vessels involved into three types: **a** type I: small (1–2 mm); **b** type II: medium (3–4 mm); **c** Type III: large (> 5 mm)

Dural arteriovenous fistula (AVF) (Fig. 2)

Dural AVFs are the most common spinal vascular lesions. They are acquired lesions, found mostly in elderly males, who classically present with a progressive myelopathy due to venous congestion. The lesion consists of an abnormal connection between a radiculomeningeal artery and radicular vein [2]. There is no contribution of the anterior or posterior spinal arteries. The preferred treatment in these fistulae is endovascular embolisation with adhesive liquid material, and not with particulate material or surgery [3].

Extramedullary (perimedullary) AVF (Figs. 3, 4)

These lesions, probably congenital, are found mostly in young patients. The lesion consists of a single, often large, abnormal connection between an anterior or posterior spinal artery and a medullary vein. These lesions are always superficial to the cord. Multiple dilated arteries and draining veins adjacent to the fistula can mimic the nidus of an arteriovenous malformation (AVM). There is nearly always a saccular dilatation of the vein at the site of the fistula. These fistulae are most frequently found at the conus medullaris. They can be further divided by the size of the vessels involved into three types: I–III. Treatment can be by endovascular embolisation or surgery.

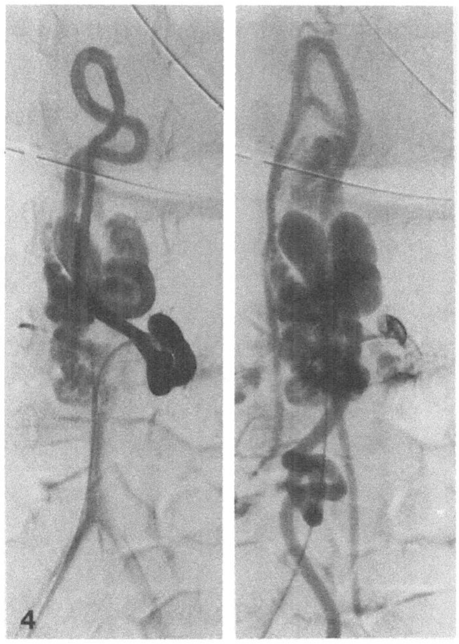

Fig. 4. Extramedullary AVF type III in a 4-year-old girl. Selective angiogram, left L2, shows clover-leaf shape venous pouch at L1/2 just beyond the point of the fistula

Intramedullary AVM (Fig. 5)

These are found in young patients who present with progressive myelopathy, or intramedullary or subarachnoid haemorrhage. In this lesion, there is a network of pathological vessels interposed between the arterial feeders and draining veins, which is located superficially or deep in the cord. The preferred method of treatment is endovascular, although in some instances surgery is feasible.

Discussion

The important point is not to make a misdiagnosis of intramedullary AVM in those cases where the lesion is in fact an extramedullary AVF. Because extramedullary AVFs can be treated by surgical or neurointerventional methods, curative results are obtained before irreversible damage develops in the spinal cord. In addition, embolisation with small particles for an extramedullarly AVF carries significant risks of deterioration of the neurological deficit, due to venous thrombosis induced by particles that pass through the shunt.

This simple classification method should direct neuroradiologists and neurosurgeons to an appropriate diagnosis of these complex spinal vascular lesions for better treatment strategy and good results for the patients.

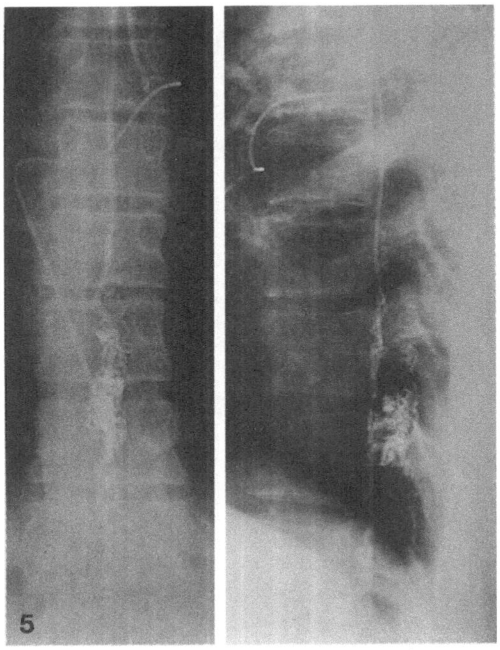

Fig. 5. Intramedullary AVM in a 22-year-old man. Frontal and lateral selective angiography shows a compact nidus at T9/10

References

1. Riche MC, Reizine D, Melki JP, Merland JJ (1985) Classification of spinal cord vascular malformations. Radiat Med 3:17–24
2. Symow LJ, Kuyama J, Kendall B (1984) Dural arteriovenous malformation of the spine: clinical features and surgical results in 55 cases. J Neurosurg 60:239–247
3. Nichols DA, Rufenacht DA, Jack CR, Forbes GS (1992) Embolization of spinal dural arteriovenous fistula with polyvinyl alcohol particles: experience in 14 patients. AJNR 13:933–940

Gamma knife

Value of embolisation therapy in gamma-knife radiosurgery for arteriovenous malformations

H. Jokura[1], A. Takahashi[2], Y. Fujii[2], N. Boku[2], T. Otsuki[3], T. Yoshimoto[3]

[1] Jiro Suzuki Memorial Clinic, Gamma House, Furukawa, Japan
[2] Division of Interventional Neurosurgery, Khonan Hospital, Sendai, Japan
[3] Department of Neurosurgery, Tohoku University School of Medicine, Sendai, Japan

Abstract. We treated 135 patients with arteriovenous malformations (AVMs) between November 1991 and December 1993 by gamma-knife radiosurgery. Intravascular embolisation using mostly oestrogen-alcohol and polyvinyl acetate was combined in 89 patients (63.7%) in an attempt to reduce the size of the AVMs before radiosurgery. Embolisation reduced the average volume of the nidus from 11.8 ml to 5.6 ml, and the number of niduses larger than 10 ml was reduced from 29 to 15. The average dose of radiation administered to the periphery of the nidus was 22.5 Gy. Complete obliteration of the nidus at 1 year and 2 years after radiosurgery, according to volume, is as follows – < 1 ml: 15/33, 21/26; 1–4 ml: 6/29, 10/18; 4–10 ml: 1/20, 3/11; > 10 ml: 0/14, 0/10. This obvious tendency for smaller AVMs to be obliterated earlier indicates that embolisation is valuable not only in making large AVMs a radiosurgically treatable size, but also in reducing the amount of rebleeding by shortening the latent period.

Key words: Radiosurgery – Arteriovenous malformation – Embolisation

It is well known that the volume of the nidus is critical in radiosurgery, and that a few years are needed to achieve complete obliteration of the nidus [1, 2]. In an attempt to widen the indications for radiosurgery and to decrease the amount of latent period bleeding, we combine embolisation with gamma-knife radiosurgery.

In this paper we discuss the value of embolisation therapy in arteriovenous malformation (AVM) radiosurgery, based on the results of our angiographic follow-up after gamma-knife radiosurgery.

Patients and methods

We treated 135 patients from November 1991 to December 1993. Ninety-three patients (68.9%) had a history of bleeding before radiosurgery. Conventional fractionated irradiation of 30 Gy in 3 weeks had been given to 8 patients at least 3 years prior to radiosurgery. Eighty-six patients (63.7%) were embolised before radiosurgery (Figs. 1, 2).

The main liquid embolisation materials we use are oestrogen-alcohol and polyvinylacetate [3]. The treatment parameters of radiosurgery are as follows – mean number of isocentres: 2.3 shots; mean marginal dose: 22.5 Gy, mean covering isodose: 59.7%; and mean maximum dose: 38.8 Gy.

All the patients, except those who refused or those with a schedule conflict, were followed by angiography at 1 year and 2 years.

Results

Embolisation decreased the average nidus volume from 11.8 to 5.6 ml in 86 cases. The number of niduses larger than 10 ml decreased from 29 to 15.

Table 1 shows the results of angiographic follow-up after gamma-knife surgery. The 1-year follow-up clearly shows that smaller AVMs tend to be effectively obliterate. At the 2-years follow-up, obliteration proceeds in every volume group and the difference between each group becomes smaller, but the correlation between volume and obliteration is still obvious. During follow-up (average 21.6 months), there was no treatment-related mortality or major morbidity.

Bleeding during the latent period happened in 8 cases (3.3% per year), 6 of which had a history of previous bleeding.

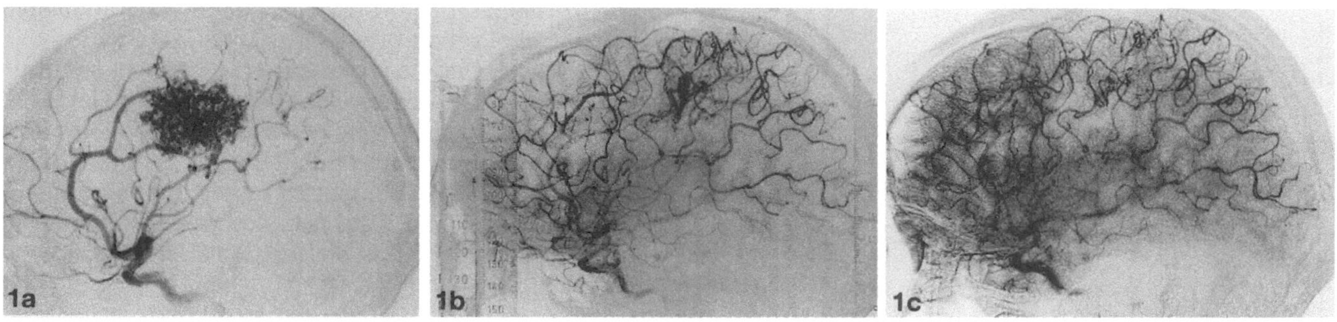

Fig. 1 a–c. Case 1. **a** Arteriovenous malformation (AVM) of 25.8 ml in motor cortex. **b** After embolisation, volume has decreased to about 3 ml. **c** Angiogram 1 year after radiosurgery shows almost complete obliteration

Correspondence to: H. Jokura, Jiro Suzuki Memorial Clinic, Gamma House 3-1-3-5, Minamimachi, Furukawa-city, Miyagi 989-61, Japan

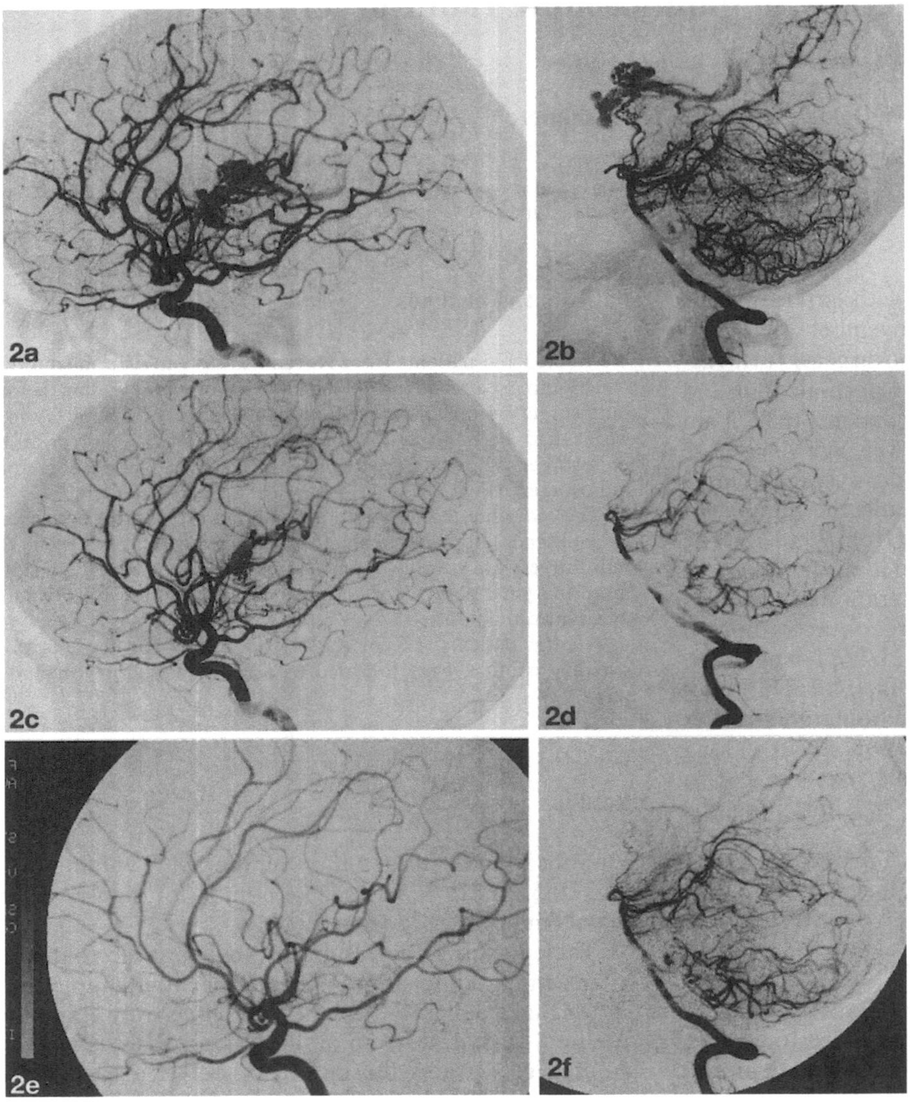

Fig. 2a–f. Case 2. **a, b** Thalamic AVM before embolisation. **c, d** At the time of gamma-knife treatment, almost complete obliteration of posterior part of nidus fed by thalamoperforating arteries. **e, f** Complete obliteration at 1 year

Table 1. Degree of obliteration related to volume of nidus

Volume of nidus (ml)	100 (%)	Obliteration (%)				Total
		> 90	50–90	< 50	0	
1. At 1 year						
< 1	21 (80.8)	3	2	0	0	26
1–4	10 (52.6)	6	2	0	0	18
4–10	3 (27.3)	4	4	0	0	11
> 10	0	3	6	1	0	10
Total	34	16	14	1	0	65
2. At 2 years						
< 1	15 (45.5)	8 (24.2)	7	2	1	33
1–4	6 (20.6)	6 (20.6)	16	1	0	29
4–10	1	3	8	4	4	20
> 10	0	1	5	5	3	14
Total	22	18	36	12	8	96

Discussion

In radiosurgery, to achieve complete obliteration of the nidus within a few years, the volume should be less than 10 ml [1, 2]. Embolisation of the nidus to decrease the volume as a pretreatment for radiosurgery is an attractive idea [4]. In our series, the target volume became about half the pre-embolisation volume.

It is said that the bleeding rate before complete obliteration is almost the same as without treatment [1, 2]. If this is true, we should make the greatest possible effort to achieve earlier complete obliteration. Our data show that small AVMs are obliterated earlier. Embolisation of AVMs even less than 10 ml may decrease the amount of bleeding by means of early obliteration after radiosurgery.

References

1. Lunsford LD, Kondziolka D, Flickinger JC, et al (1991) Stereotactic radiosurgery for arteriovenous malformation of the brain. J Neurosurg 75:512–524

2. Steiner L, Leksell L, Forster DMC (1974) Stereotactic radiosurgery in intracranial arteriovenous malformations. Acta Neurochir 21 [Suppl]: 195–209
3. Takahashi A, Yoshimoto T, Sugawara T (1991) New liquid embolization method for brain arteriovenous malformations: combined infusion of estrogen-alcohol and polyvinyl acetate. Neuroradiology 33 [Suppl]: 190–192
4. Guo WY, Wilkholm G, Lindquist C, et al (1993) Combined embolization and gamma knife radiosurgery for cerebral arteriovenous malformations. Acta Radiol 34: 600–606

Effectiveness of embolisation using oestrogen-alcohol combined with polyvinyl acetate of arteriovenous malformations before gamma-knife radiosurgery

Y. Fujii[1], **A. Takahashi**[1], **M. Ezura**[1], **H. Jokura**[2], **T. Yoshimoto**[3]

[1] Division of Intravascular Neurosurgery, Kohnan Hospital, Sendai, Japan
[2] Jiro Suzuki Memorial Clinic Gamma House, Furukawa, Japan
[3] Department of Neurosurgery, School of Medicine, Tohoku University, Sendai, Japan

Abstract. We investigated 75 cases of arteriovenous malformations treated by gamma-knife radiosurgery following embolisation, and established the effectiveness of nidus volume reduction. The volume was reduced to 54% on average by embolisation. In cases of more than 10 cm^3, the volume was reduced to 50% on average by embolisation. Although the bleeding rate after embolisation in this series was 2.7%, it is not known if embolisation reduces the bleeding rate. In this series, no recurrence was shown after embolisation using oestrogen-alcohol combined with polyvinyl acetate.

Key words: Arteriovenous malformation – Gamma knife – Embolisation – Radiosurgery

We measured nidus volume of arteriovenous malformations (AVMs) before and after embolisation prior to gamma-knife radiosurgery. The effectiveness of embolisation using oestrogen-alcohol combined with polyvinyl acetate before gamma-knife treatment of the embolisation was evaluated.

Patients and methods

The age of our 75 patients ranged from 5 to 63 years (mean 29 years). All patients were embolised using oestrogen-alcohol combined with polyvinyl acetate. Initial symptoms were bleeding in 52, seizures in 20, ischaemic symptoms in 1 and 2 patients were asymptomatic. The average period from embolisation to gamma-knife treatment was 15 months.

The nidus volume was measured by multiplication of the three dimensions on angiography by 0.5:

Volume = horizontal diameter × longitudinal diameter × vertical diameter × 0.5.

Before multiplication, each diameter was carefully corrected for magnification based on the angiography performed for the radiosurgery to remove the influence of each different magnification [1, 2].

Correspondence to: Y. Fujii, Division of Intravascular Neurosurgery, Kohnan Hospital, 4-20-1, Nagamachi Minami, Sendai, Japan

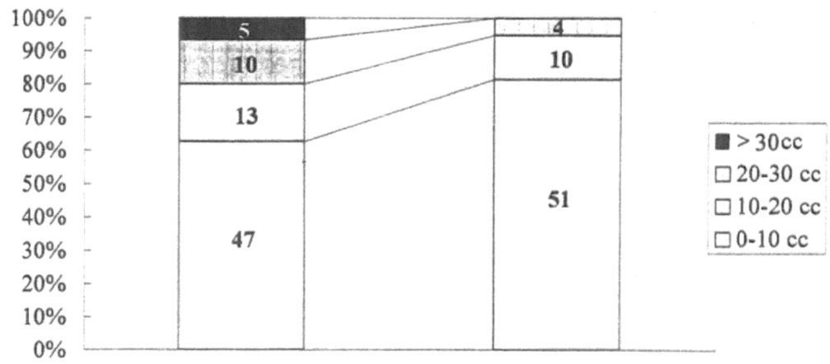

Fig. 1. Volume reduction (%) following embolisation

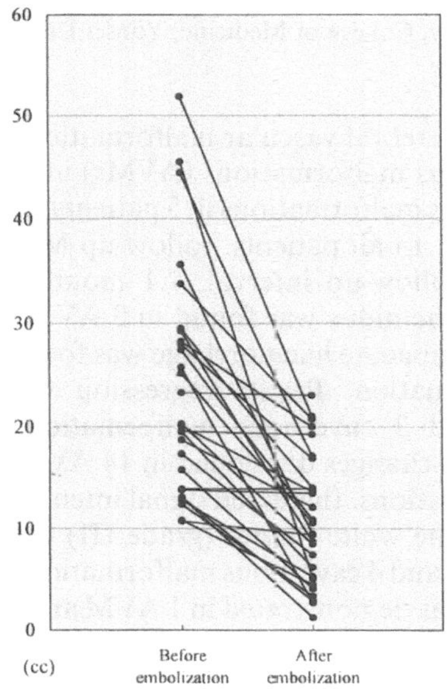

Fig. 2. Effects of embolisation on AVMs whose initial volume was more than 10 cm^3

Results

The volume of the nidus before embolisation was 0.5–51.9 cm^3 (mean 11.8 cm^3) and it decreased to 0.2–23.0 cm^3 (mean 5.7 cm^3) after embolisation. The volume was thus reduced by 54% on average by the embolisation (Fig. 1).

The nidus volume was more than 10 cm^3 (relatively difficult for radiosurgery) in 28 cases before embolisation, and 14 after embolisation. The volume was reduced to 50% on average by embolisation (Fig. 2).

The bleeding rate in this series after embolisation was 2.7% per year.

These cases had no recurrence after embolisation using oestrogen-alcohol combined with polyvinyl acetate.

Discussion

Recently, AVMs have been treated by a gamma-knife unit, and successful results have been reported by many authors. However, fewer cases of AVM treated by gamma-knife radiosurgery following embolisation have been reported.

The weak point of treatment by a gamma-knife unit is the considerable delay of evident effectiveness. It often needs 1 or 2 years to manifest itself [3]. However, the effectiveness of embolisation is immediate. For example, it may be that cases of AVM with a cerebral aneurysm, or a varix or very high flow shunt, should be treated by embolisation.

Although the bleeding rate after embolisation in this series was 2.7%, it is not known if embolisation reduces the bleeding rate.

After embolisation, the size of the nidus was stable and rather smaller than before embolisation. This result shows the usefulness of this chemical embolisation method.

References

1. Noorbehesht B, Fabricant JI, Enzmann DR (1987) Size determination of supratentorial arteriovenous malformations by MR, CT and angio. Neurosurgery 29:512–518
2. Pasqualin A, Barone G, Cioffi F, Rosta L, Scinza R, Pian RD (1987) The relevance of anatomic and hemodynamic factors to a classification of cerebral arteriovenous malformations. Neurosurgery 28:370–379
3. Yamamoto M, Jimbo M, Ide M, Lindquist C, Steiner L (1993) Postradiation volume changes in gamma unit-treated cerebral arteriovenous malformations. Surg Neurol 40:485–490

MRI demonstration of short-term treatment response after stereotactic radiosurgery for cerebral vascular malformations

Yong Kook Hong[1], **Dong Ik Kim**[1], **Sang Sub Chung**[2]

[1] Department of Diagnostic Radiology, College of Medicine, Yonsei University, Seoul, Korea
[2] Department of Neurosurgery, College of Medicine, Yonsei University, Seoul, Korea

Abstract. We treated 48 cerebral vascular malformations, including 26 arteriovenous malformations (AVMs) in 26 patients, and 22 cavernous malformations in 5 patients, by stereotactic radiosurgery. In all patients, follow-up MRI was performed (mean follow-up interval, 7.1 months). Complete regression of the nidus was found in 3 AVMs. Complete resorption of subacute haemorrhage was found in 1 cavernous malformation. Partial regression was found in 15 AVMs and 3 cavernous malformations. Radiation-induced signal changes developed in 14 AVMs and 4 cavernous malformations. Increased signal intensity of an extensive area of the white matter (grade III) was demonstrated in 4 AVMs and 4 cavernous malformations. Perifocal enhancement was demonstrated in 1 AVM and 3 cavernous malformations. There were 15 AVMs more than 2 cm in diameter, and 3 of these demonstrated grade III radiation-induced change, while 1 showed perifocal enhancement. Grade III changes were demonstrated in all 3 cavernous malformations more than 2 cm in diameter. Perifocal enhancement was demonstrated in 2 of 3 cases. The therapeutic response to radiosurgery in AVMs was favourable. However, cavernous malformations showed a relatively poor therapeutic response to radiosurgery in the short-term on follow-up MRI. Extensive radiation-induced MRI signal changes within brain parenchyma were frequently demonstrated in cavernous malformations larger than 2 cm in diameter.

Key words: Arteriovenous malformation – Cavernous angioma – Radiosurgery – Magnetic resonance imaging

Correspondence to: Yong Kook Hong, Department of Diagnostic Radiology, College of Medicine, Yonsei University, C.P.O. Box 8044, Seoul, 120-752 Korea

Radiosurgery has been used in the treatment of many intracranial diseases. One of the most reputed indications is the treatment of small, deep-seated intracerebral arteriovenous malformations (AVMs) [1–4]. There have been reports of stereotactic radiosurgery for cavernous malformations, and they showed different results [5, 6]. We reviewed follow-up magnetic resonance (MR) images after radiosurgery in cerebral vascular malformations, including AVMs and cavernous malformations, to investigate the therapeutic response of these vascular malformations and radiation-induced regional brain injury.

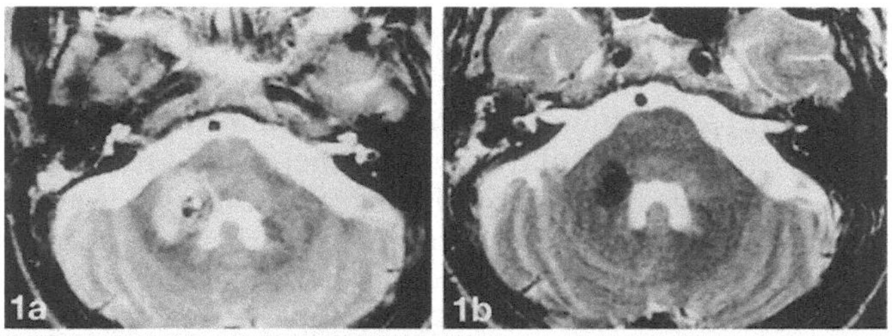

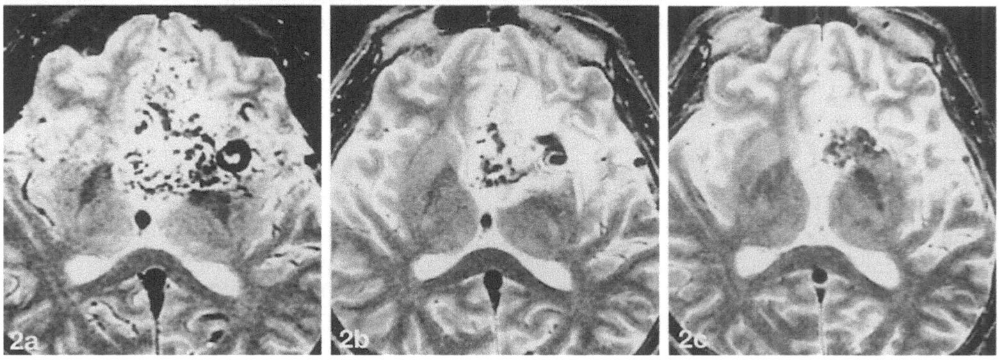

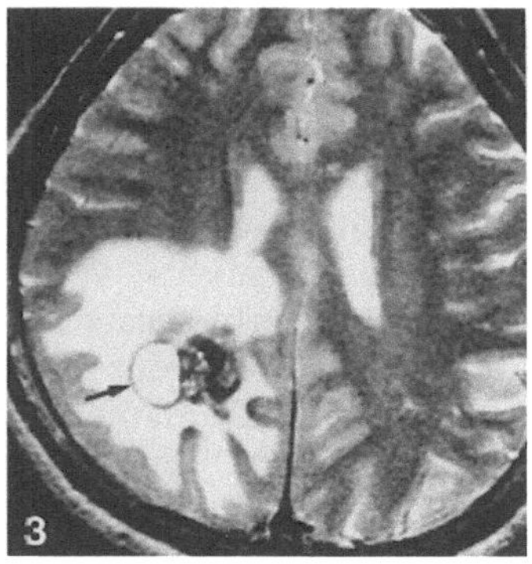

Fig. 1 a, b. Cavernous angioma in right cerebellar peduncle. **a** T2-weighted image shows high signal-intensity subacute haemorrhage before radiosurgery. **b** Six-month follow-up after radiosurgery shows resorption of subacute haemorrhage, which remains as focal haemosiderin deposit

Fig. 2 a–c. AVM in left frontal lobe. **a** T2-weighted image demonstrates huge nidus with draining veins before radiosurgery. **b** 6-month follow-up after radiosurgery demonstrates decreased size of nidus and radiation-induced perilesional high signal. **c** 12-month follow-up after radiosurgery demonstrates further decrease of nidus size and obliteration of draining veins. The extent of radiation-induced high signal is also diminished

Fig. 3. 6-month follow-up image after radiosurgery for cavernous angioma shows extensive radiation-induced high signal in the white matter and combined cystic change or rebleeding (*arrow*)

Materials and methods

We treated 48 cerebral vascular malformations, including 26 AVMs in 26 patients and 22 cavernous malformations in 5 patients with gamma-knife radiosurgery. The age of the patients ranged from 16 to 47 (mean: 27) years. The maximal doses applied to treat AVMs ranged from 30 to 50 Gy (mean: 43 Gy), with marginal doses of 15–25 Gy (mean: 23 Gy). The mean maximal diameter of the AVM nidus was 2.5 cm (range: 0.5–5.0 cm). The maximal doses for cavernous malformations were 25–50 Gy (mean: 39 Gy), with marginal doses of 13–25 Gy (mean: 20 Gy). The mean maximal diameter of cavernous malformations was 1.0 cm (range: 0.3–2.5 cm).

The follow-up MRI after gamma-knife surgery was performed with a 1.5-T imager. In all patients, T1- and T2-weighted spin-echo images, and gadolinium-enhanced T1-weighted iamges were obtained. Regular MRI follow-up was performed every 6 months after radiosurgery. Three patients were followed up three times, and two patients, twice. The remaining 26 patients were followed up once. The mean follow-up interval was 7.1 months.

On follow-up MRI, the changes in signal intensity and size of malformations were carefully assessed. Radiation-induced changes of regional parenchyma, including signal intensity change and enhancement of regional brain parenchyma, were also evaluated. The changes in the white matter were divided into three grades. Grade I was when the thickness of perifocal high signal intensity on T2-weighted image was less than 1 cm, and grade II was when the thickness of perifocal high signal intensity on T2-weighted image was between 1 and 2 cm. Grade III was when there was extensive high signal intensity along the cerebral white matter.

Results

Complete regression of the AVM nidus was found in 3 AVMs (11.5%). Two AVM nidi showed complete regression 12 months after radiosurgery, and the remaining 1 AVM nidus showed complete regression 6 months after radiosurgery. Partial regression was found in 15 AVMs (57.7%), and the size of 7 AVM nidi had shrunk by more than half. Fourteen out of 22 cavernous malformations showed subacute haemorrhage on MRI before radiosurgery. One of them showed complete resorption of subacute haemorrhage, which remained as a focal haemosiderin deposit at the 6-month follow-up (Fig. 1). Three cavernous malformations showed minimal resorption of subacute haemorrhage on the follow-up MRI. Eight cavernous malformations showed haemosiderin spots without subacute haemorrhage in MR studies before radiosurgery, and they showed no interval change after short-term follow-up MR studies after radiosurgery. Partial regression in 14 AVMs and 2 cavernous malformations were found on the 6-month follow-up MRI. Among 14 AVMs, 4 AVMs that were followed up more than twice showed progressive decrease in nidus size (Fig. 2). One AVM showed partial regression of the nidus at 18 months, and one cavernous malformation, at 12 months.

Grade I radiation-induced changes in the white matter were observed in 8 AVMs (30.8%), and grade II changes, in 2 AVMs (7.7%). Grade III radiation-induced changes were demonstrated in 3 AVMs (11.5%) and 4 cavernous malformations (18.2%). Radiation-induced cystic change or rebleeding was suspected at 6-month follow-up in 1 cavernous malformation (Fig. 3). Perifocal enhancement was demonstrated in 4 cases, including 1 of AVM and 3 of cavernous malformation. Three (20%) of 15 AVMs larger than 2 cm in diameter demonstrated grade III radiation-induced changes. One of these AVMs demonstrated perifocal enhancement. Grade III change was demonstrated in all 3 cavernous malformations larger than 2 cm in diameter, and perifocal enhancement in 2 of 3 cases.

Discussion

In gamma-knife surgery of cerebral AVMs, 73–78% of the total obliteration rate has been achieved [7–9]. The incidence of adverse radiation reactions resulting in permanent neurological deficits is only about 3%. Obliteration of the AVM nidus can take up to 2 years. Moreover, total obliteration of the nidus is obtained 5 years after irradiation has been reported [7]. In our short-term follow-up study, the obliteration rate could not be determined. However, early decrease in the size of AVM nidus was observed 6 months after radiosurgery. One small AVM nidus was totally obliterated in 6 months, and two small AVMs showed total obliteration 12 months after radiosurgery. Our study showed that the obliteration rate of small AVMs is greater than that of larger AVMs.

Weil et al. [5] reported that they treated 6 patients with cavernous malformation of the brainstem using gamma knife radiosurgery. During the 2-year follow-up period after radiosurgery, no change in the size and shape of the cavernous malformations was observed. Two of these patients suffered recurrent haemorrhage, and three developed progressive signs compatible with radiation-induced injury. Kondziolka et al. [6] reported that 4 of 24 angiographically occult vascular malformations showed a decrease in size on postradiosurgery MRI. In our study, only 1 cavernous malformation showed complete disappearance of the methaemoglobin portion. Minimally decreased size of the methaemoglobin portion was observed in 3 cavernous malformations on the short-term follow-up MRI. However, we were not sure whether this represented true regression of the lesions or only resorption of the methaemoglobin surrounding the cavernous malformation.

Evaluation of the long-term effectiveness of stereotactic radiosurgery for cerebrovascular malformations will require extended follow-up. The therapeutic response to radiosurgery in brain AVMs was favourable. However, it was controversial in cavernous malformations, because the latter showed a relatively poor response to radiosurgery in this short-term follow-up. The extensive radiation-induced MR change in the regional brain tissue was more frequently demonstrated in cavernous malformations larger than 2 cm in diameter.

References

1. Kemeny AK, Davis PS, Foster DM (1989) Results of stereotactic radiosurgery of arteriovenous malformations. Analysis of 52 cases. J Neurol Neurosurg Psychiatry 52:554–558
2. Lunsford LD, Kondziolka D, Flickinger JC, et al (1991) Stereotactic radiosurgery for arteriovenous malformations of the brain. J Neurosurg 75:517–524
3. Steiner L, Lindquist C, Adler JR, Torner JC, Steiner M (1992) Clinical outcome of radiosurgery for cerebral arteriovenous malformations. J Neurosurg 77:1–8
4. Sutcliffe JC, Foster DMC, Walton L, Dias PS, Kemenny AA (1992) Untoward clinical effects after stereotactic radiosurgery for intracranial arteriovenous malformations. Br J Neurosurg 6:177–185
5. Weil S, Tew JM, Steiner L (1990) Comparison of radiosurgery and microsurgery for treatment of cavernous malformations of brain stem (abstract). J Neurosurg 72:3365
6. Kondziolka D, Lunsfold L, Coffey RJ, et al (1990) Stereotactic radiosurgery of angiographically occult vascular malformations: Indications and preliminary experience. Neurosurgery 27:892–900
7. Yamamoto M, Jimbo M, Kobayashi M, et al (1992) Long-term results of radiosurgery for arteriovenous malformation: neurodiagnostic imaging and histological studies of angiographically confirmed nidus obliteration. Surg Neurol 37:219–230
8. Leksell L (1983) Stereotactic radiosurgery. J Neurol Neurosurg Psychiatry 46:797–803
9. Steiner L (1984) Treatment of arteriovenous malformation by radiosurgery. In: Wilson CB, Steiner BM (eds) Intracranial arteriovenous malformations. Williams & Wilkins, Baltimore, pp 295–313

Stereotactic radiosurgery for arteriovenous malformations: 1-year follow-up

K. Suzuki[1], T. Hirai[2], A. Makino[2], A. Moriki[2], M. Yoshida[2], T. Nishimura[1], M. Kaneko[1]

[1] Department of Radiology, Hamamatsu University School of Medicine, 3600 Hamda-cho, Hamamatsu, Shizuoka, 431-31 Japan
[2] Gamma Unit Center, Heisei Memorial Hospital, Fujieda, Japan

Abstract. To define treatment factors related to early obliteration of arteriovenous malformations (AVMs), we followed 71 patients treated using the gamma knife for 1 year. Abnormal signal intensity suggesting radiation-induced change was demonstrated on MRI in 11 of 42 patients examined; only 1 showed neurological deterioration. Neurological impairment observed in 5 of the 71 patients was associated with rebleeding. This result supports the importance of early AVM obliteration. Total obliteration was confirmed in 18 of 60 patients examined. Higher peripheral doses were given smaller treatment volumes using higher peripheral isodense levels in the patients with total obliteration. Early obliteration could be expected in the patients treated with effective irradiation parameters.

Key words: Radiosurgery – Arteriovenous malformations

Gamma-knife radiosurgery has proved effective in the treatment of cerebral arteriovenous malformations (AVMs). More than 80% total obliteration rate at 2 years has been reported [1]. However, obliteration is not an instantaneous result and a patient is at risk of haemorrhage during a latency period. We therefore analysed 1-year follow-up results to define factors related to early obliteration.

Patients and methods

Between November 1991 and January 1993, 71 Japanese patients with AVMs were treated using the gamma knife. The mean age at radiosurgery was 31 years (range 9–66 years). The clinical characteristics of treated patients are summarised in Table 1.

Twenty-two of the AVMs (31.0%) were located in deep cerebral structures and 10 (14.0%) were in the posterior fossa. Most (81.6%) were classified as grade II or III according to the Spetzler and Martin grading system [2].

Stereotactic angiography and computed tomography (CT) were carried out to determine the target volume. In all but 3 cases with a metallic clip, stereotactic magnetic resonance imaging (MRI) was also performed to obtain more accurate anatomical information. A newly developed stereotactic assisted software system was routinely used.

According to the size and location of the AVM, a suitable radiation dose was given to the target. The dose-volume isoeffect curve derived by Flickinger et al. [3] was used as a guideline. Table 2 lists the treatment parameters used.

Follow-up CT or MRI was scheduled at 1, 3, 6 and 12 months after treatment. Angiography was recommended 1 year after radiosurgery or earlier if CT or MRI suggested AVM obliteration.

Correspondence to: K. Suzuki

Table 1. Clinical characteristics of 71 patients with arteriovenous malformations

Characteristic	Cases (%)
Sex	
Male	40 (56.3)
Female	31 (43.7)
Clinical presentation	
Intracranial haemorrhage	52 (73.2)
Convulsion	11 (15.5)
Others	8 (11.3)
Karnofsky Performance Score	
100	38 (53.5)
90	18 (25.4)
80	3 (4.2)
70	7 (9.9)
60	5 (7.0)
Prior treatments	
Craniotomy	14 (19.7)
Embolisation	10 (14.1)
Radiosurgery	2 (2.8)
Conventional radiotherapy	1 (1.4)
None	44 (62.0)

Table 2. Parameters used in radiosurgical treatments

Parameters	Mean ± SD
Number of shots	3.2 ± 0.3
Isodose level (%) at periphery of AVM	54.0 ± 1.4
Maximum dose (Gy)	39.9 ± 1.1
Peripheral dose (Gy)	21.0 ± 0.5
Volume treated (ml)	4.2 ± 0.5

We used the criteria of total obliteration defined by Steiner et al. ("no longer filling of the nidus, normal circulation time and normalised of the afferent and efferent vessels") [1]. Partial obliteration was defined as "more than 25% decrease in AVM size on MRI or angiogram". Abnormal intensity surrounding the target on MRI images was regarded as radiation-induced change.

Statistical analyses were carried out using Student's *t*-test or Fisher's exact test.

Results

AVM obliteration

Among the 71 patients treated, AVM obliteration of 60 patients (84.5%) was assessed on angiography or MRI. Total obliteration was confirmed in 18 patients (30.0%) on the angiogram, partial obliteration in 36 patients

Table 3. Differences in treatment parameters related to obliteration of AVM

Parameters	Obliteration of AVM	
	(+) (18)	(−) (42)
Number of shots	2.6 ± 2.3	3.4 ± 2.3
Peripheral isodose level (%)	60.5 ± 16.6	51.1 ± 7.6**
Maximum dose (Gy)	40.8 ± 10.6	39.9 ± 8.1
Peripheral dose (Gy)	23.3 ± 2.7	20.2 ± 3.9*
Volume treated (ml)	2.5 ± 2.2	5.2 ± 5.2*

All values expressed as mean ± standard deviation
* $P<0.01$, ** $P<0.05$

Table 4. Differences in treatment parameters related to radiation-induced change on MRI

Parameters	Radiation-induced change	
	(+) (11)	(−) (31)
Number of shots	3.3 ± 2.6	2.9 ± 1.8
Peripheral isodose level (%)	52.3 ± 7.5	54.2 ± 13.1
Maximum dose (Gy)	40.9 ± 7.1	39.5 ± 8.1
Peripheral dose (Gy)	21.2 ± 3.5	20.9 ± 4.1
Volume treated (ml)	4.6 ± 3.5	4.5 ± 5.8

All values expressed as mean ± standard deviation

(60.0%) and no change in 6 patients (10.0%) on angiography or MRI.

Table 3 represents the differences in treatment parameters related to total obliteration. There were significant differences in the dose and isodose level at the AVM margin and treated volume.

Radiation-induced change

MRI 1 year after radiosurgery were obtained in 42 patients (59.2%). Radiation-induced change was observed in 11 patients (26.2%). Three of 11 AVMs were totally obliterated and 7 were partially obliterated. The change occurred regardless of AVM obliteration ($P=1.00$).

As shown in Table 4, there were no significant differences in treatment parameters between patients with and without radiation-induced change.

Neurological impairment

Five patients (7.0%) represented neurological deterioration within 1 year after treatment. Two of them were due to rebleeding; 2 were radiation-induced. Impairment was significantly associated with rebleeding ($P<0.05$), but not with radiation-induced change ($P=1.00$). In 3 patients (4.2%), rebleeding occurred within 1 year after treatment. All 3 patients had a previous history of intraventricular haemorrhage.

Discussion

We found significant differences in the peripheral dose, treatment volume and dose homogeneity related to early obliteration of the AVM. Neurological impairment was significantly associated with rebleeding, but not with radiation-induced change. It is important to achieve early obliteration and it was associated with some effective irradiation parameters.

References

1. Steiner L, Lindquist C, Steiner M (1992) Radiosurgery. In: Symon L, et al (eds) Advances and technical standards in neurosurgery, vol. 19. Springer, Vienna New York, pp 20–102
2. Spetzler RF, Martin NA (1986) A proposed grading system for arteriovenous malformation. J Neurosurg 65:476–483
3. Flickinger JC, Lunsford LD, Wu A, Kalend A (1992) Predicted dose-volume isoeffect curves for stereotactic radiosurgery with the ^{60}CO gamma unit. Acta Oncol 30:363–367

Long-term follow-up of arteriovenous malformations treated by the gamma-knife: CT and MRI following angiographically confirmed nidus obliteration

M. Yamamoto[1], **M. Jimbo**[1], **M. Ide**[1], **Y. Ono**[2]

[1] Departments of Neurosurgery, Tokyo Women's Medical College Dai-ni Hospital, Tokyo, Japan
[2] Department of Radiology, Tokyo Women's Medical College Dai-ni Hospital, Tokyo, Japan

Abstract. CT and MRI obtained after complete nidus obliteration had been angiographically confirmed were reviewed in nine patients who had undergone treatment with a gamma knife arteriovenous malformations (AVMs). The patients ranged in age from 9 to 54 years (mean 23 years). The period between angiographic confirmation of nidus obliteration and these most recent examinations was 18–24 months (mean 34 months). These results disclosed that radiosurgery-induced changes in a nidus may continue for several years after angiography has shown complete AVM obliteration. These late changes can be considered to involve further obliteration of the remaining or recanalising vessels, reflecting an ongoing process from coagulation necrosis to liquefaction necrosis.

Key words: Arteriovenous malformation – Radiosurgery – Computed tomography – Magnetic resonance imaging

It is clear that radiosurgical treatment can result in arteriovenous malformation (AVM) obliteration after a 1- to 3-year latency period [1–12]. In this investigation, we analysed subsequent changes in the nidus demonstrated by means of CT and MRI following angiographically confirmed nidus obliteration.

Patients and methods

Among 39 patients with AVMs treated by means of gamma-knife radiosurgery since 1978, complete nidus obliteration has thus far been angiographically demonstrated in 20 cases, between 1 and 5 years after radiosurgery. In 9 of these 20 patients, CT and MRI were performed more than 1 year after angiographic confirmation of nidus obliteration. The period between angiographic confirmation of nidus obliteration and these most recent examinations was 12–84 months (mean 33 months) and the period between gamma unit treatment and these most recent examinations was 25–96 months (mean 52 months). The patients ranged in age from 9 to 54 years (mean 24 years) at the time of radiosurgery. There were six females and three males. The AVM manifested with intracranial haemorrhage in all cases. The location of the nidus was supratentorial in eight cases and infratentorial in one. The preradiosurgical nidus volume ranged from 0.15 cm^3 to 24.15 cm^3, with a mean and median of 3.59 cm^3 and 0.68 cm^3, respectively. None of the patients had undergone either radiation for the AVMs or interventional radiology before radiosurgery. However, a cerebrospinal fluid shunt operation had been carried out in three cases and a craniotomy in two. In performing the gamma-knife treatment, the nidus was completely covered in nine cases. In one case, the nidus could not be completely covered due to its size. The selected target dose given at the periphery was 25 Gy or more in five cases, 20–25 Gy in three and less than 20 Gy in one.

Results

On CT, the obliterated nidus was isodense in seven cases and had a mixture of iso- and hypodense areas in the other two. Calcification was identified in four patients, in one of whom no calcification had been seen on CT before gamma-knife treatment. Contrast-enhanced CT demonstrated nidus enhancement in seven cases. In seven cases, serial post-obliteration follow-up CT studies were performed. In one of the seven cases, post-obliteration density changes occurred; an increase followed by a subsequent decrease was recognized between 1 and 3 years post-obliteration. In four of the seven cases, a significant time-related decrease of contrast enhancement was observed 1–3 years after angiographically confirmed nidus obliteration.

Seven patients were examined by MRI. On T1-weighted imaging, the nidus was shown to be hypointense in six cases, and had a mixture of hypo- and isointense areas in the remaining case. On T2-weighted imaging, however, nidus intensity was more varied than that on T1-weighted imaging; hyperintense in two, hypointense in two and a mixture of hyper- and hypointense areas in three. No flow signal void was demonstrated in any of these cases. Following gadolinium administration, the nidus enhanced in six cases; remarkably in five and moderately in two. In six cases, serial post-obliteration follow-up MRI was carried out. In two of the six cases, time-related intensity increases were observed on T2-weighted imaging. In two of the six cases, a time-related decrease in gadolinium enhancement was observed following angiographically confirmed nidus obliteration. In three of the six cases, significant gadolinium enhancement persisted 3 years or more after angiographic confirmation of nidus obliteration. In one of the three cases, however, a moderate decrease in gadolinium enhancement was shown between the 3rd and the 4th post-obliteration years.

Discussion

As is widely accepted, angiographically confirmed disappearance of the nidus should be the goal in all AVMs treated radiosurgically [3, 6, 7]. Therefore, the majority of

Correspondence to: M. Yamamoto, Department of Neurosurgery, Tokyo Women's Medical College Dai-ni Hospital, 2-1-10 Nishiogu, Arakawa-ku, Tokyo, Japan

patients are periodically examined by means of CT and MRI to assess the attainment of this treatment goal [7, 13, 14]. However, few CT and MRI studies of the long-term results following complete obliteration, confirmed by angiography, have been published to date. In particular, relatively little information is available on post-obliteration, time-related changes in nidus enhancement, contrast enhancement on CT, and gadolinium enhancement on MRI. In this study, post-obliteration CT and MRI findings (after angiographically confirmed nidus obliteration) were analysed in ten patients treated with a gamma knife.

Although there are a few exceptional cases, post-obliteration CT and MRI findings of the nidus can be summarised as follows:

1. The nidus is isodense on CT, except for areas of calcification.
2. Contrast-enhanced CT shows enhancement, either remarkably or moderately, within 1–2 years after angiographic confirmation of nidus obliteration. This nidus enhancement tends to disappear afterwards.
3. T1-weighted MRI reveals hypo- and/or isointensity. Although intensity varies on T2-weighted MRI, a hyperintense area tends to appear or to increase in size within the nidus with the passage of time.
4. Post-gadolinium MRI shows significant enhancement which tends to persist for several years following angiographic confirmation of nidus obliteration.

The most marked nidus changes induced by irradiation using a gamma knife are evident by the end of the 2nd radiosurgical year [11, 14]. However, these results show that radiosurgery-induced changes in the nidus may continue for several years after angiography has demonstrated complete AVM obliteration. Based on the results, as well as the autopsy findings reported elsewhere [12], these late changes can be considered to involve further obliteration of the remaining or recanalising vessels and to reflect an ongoing process from coagulation necrosis to liquefaction necrosis.

Acknowledgements. We would like to thank Bierta E. Barfod for her assistance in correcting the English manuscript. This study was supported by scholarships from the Royal Swedish Academy of Sciences, the Japanese Society for the Promotion of Science, the Japan Private School Promotion Foundation and the Dr. Itoe Okamoto International Exchange Fund.

References

1. Colombo F, Benedetti A, Pozza F, Marchetti C, Chierego G (1989) Linear accelerator radiosurgery of cerebral arteriovenous malformations. Neurosurgery 24:833–840
2. Fabrikant JI, Lyman JT, Hosobuchi Y (1984) Stereotactic heavy-ion Bragg peak radiosurgery for intra-cranial vascular disorders: method for treatment of deep arteriovenous malformations. Br J Radiol 57:479–490
3. Friedman WA, Bova FJ (1992) Linear accelerator radiosurgery for arteriovenous malformations. J Neurosurg 77:832–841
4. Jimbo M (1988) Radiotherapy for cerebral arteriovenous malformation by gamma knife. In: Takakura K (ed) Treatment of cerebral and spinal arteriovenous malformations (in Japanese). Gendai-Iryo, Tokyo, pp 117–128
5. Kjellberg RN, Hanamura T, Davis KR (1983) Bragg-peak proton-beam therapy for arteriovenous malformations of the brain. N Engl J Med 309:269–274
6. Lindquist C, Steiner L (1988) Stereotactic radiosurgical treatment of arteriovenous malformations. In: Lunsford LD (ed) Modern stereotactic neurosurgery. Nijhoff, Boston, pp 491–505
7. Lunsford LD, Kondziolka D, Flickinger JC, Bissonette DJ, Jungreis CA, Maitz AH, Horton JA, Coffey RJ (1991) Stereotactic radiosurgery for arteriovenous malformations of the brain. J Neurosurg 75:512–524
8. Steinberg GK, Fabrikant JI, Marks MP, Levy RP, Frankel KA, Phillips MH, Sher LM, Silverberg GD (1990) Stereotactic heavy-charged particle Bragg peak radiation for intracranial arteriovenous malformations. N Engl J Med 323:96–101
9. Steiner L (1984) Treatment of arteriovenous malformation by radiosurgery. In: Wilson CB, Stein BM (eds) Intracranial arteriovenous malformation by radiosurgery. Williams and Witkins, Baltimore, pp 295–313
10. Steiner L, Lindquist C, Steiner M (1989) Radiosurgery with focused gamma-beam irradiation in children. In: Edwards MSB, Hoffman HI (eds) Cerebral vascular disease in children and adolescents. Williams and Wilkins, Baltimore, pp 367–388
11. Yamamoto M, Jimbo M, Ide M, Lindquist C, Steiner L (1993) Postradiation volume changes in gamma unit-treated cerebral arteriovenous malformations. Surg Neurol 40:15–21
12. Yamamoto M, Jimbo M, Kobayashi M, Toyoda C, Ide M, Tanaka N, Lindquist C, Steiner L (1992) Long-term results of radiosurgery for arteriovenous malformation: neurodiagnostic imaging and histological studies of angiographically-confirmed nidus obliteration. Surg Neurol 37:219–230
13. Noorbehesht B, Fabrikant JI, Enzmann DR (1987) Size determination of supratentorial arteriovenous malformations by MR, CT and angio. Neuroradiology 29:512–518
14. Quisling RG, Peters KR, Friedman WA, Tart RP (1991) Persistent nidus blood flow in cerebral arteriovenous malformation after stereotactic radiosurgery: MR imaging assessment. Radiology 180:785–791

Stereotactic radiosurgery of intracranial meningiomas

Y. Kida, T. Kobayashi, T. Tanaka

Department of Neurosurgery, Komaki City Hospital, 1-20 Thobusi, Komaki City, Japan 485

Abstract. Stereotactic radiosurgery of intracranial meningiomas was attempted using gamma knife. The most frequent sites of the tumour were cavernous sinus and petroclival followed by tentorium and falx. The mean tumour diameter was 27.1 mm and the marginal tumour dose ranged from 10 to 20 Gy (mean 14.4 Gy). Serial imaging studies showed a tumour shrinkage in 13.6, 43.5 and 55.5% of tumours at 6, 12, 24 months, respectively. Only three tumours (5.8%) (all malignant) enlarged after radiosurgery. Tumours with narrow attachments, like tentorial and ventricular meningiomas, responded better than the wide-based tumours such as cavernous sinus and petroclival meningiomas. Symptomatic oedema occurred in 6 cases (11.5%) and required some treatment, with excellent (3) and poor recovery (2).

Key words: Gamma knife - Meningioma - Radiosurgery - Stereotaxy

Radiosurgery (RS) has been well accepted as one of the main treatment methods of cerebral arteriovenous malformations and acoustic neuromas. However, the role of RS in the treatment of meningiomas is controversial, because of relatively low sensitivity to irradiation, lack of evidence of efficacy as well as the risk of radiation-induced oedema.

Materials and methods

There were 52 patients (18 men and 34 women) with meningioma treated with the gamma knife since May 1991. Their ages ranged from 21 to 91 years (mean 55.3 years). The tumour diameter ranged from 11.1 to 46.1 mm with a mean of 27.1 mm. The tumours were cavernous (16), petroclival (13), tentorial (7), falcine or convexity (6), ventricular (3), sphenoid ridge (2) and other (5). After localisation with MRI and dose-planning, RS with the gamma knife was carried out. The relationship between tumour size, maximum and marginal doses for each tumour location is demonstrated in Table 1. Follow-up studies with MRI were performed every 3 months.

Results

During the follow-up period after RS (6–36 months), one patient committed suicide and one died of prolonged radiation-induced oedema. Neurologically 13 improved, 31 stationary and 8 worsened. Radiological studies demonstrated a tumour shrinkage in 13.6, 43.5, 55.5% of tumours at 6, 12 and 24 months after RS (Table 2). Central low intensity on MRI, which indicates central tumour necrosis, was found in 33.3% at 12 months and in 50.0% at 24 months. Only three tumours, all of which were malignant, enlarged even after RS. Therefore, 49 of 52 tumours (94.2%) were well controlled. As for the tumour location, falx and convexity meningiomas showed the best response, followed by ventricular and tentorial lesions. In contrast, many petroclival and cavernous meningiomas

Correspondence to: Y. Kida

Table 1. Relationship between tumour size and maximum and marginal tumour dose for each location

Location	Number	Mean size (mm)	Maximum dose (Gy)	Marginal dose (Gy) (%)
Parasellar	16	29.3	26.9	13.4 (49.8)
Tentorial	7	23.6	31.6	17.3 (54.8)
Petroclival	13	27.0	26.9	13.2 (49.0)
Falx, convexity	6	22.9	33.6	16.8 (50.0)
Ventricle	3	21.1	32.3	15.7 (48.6)
Sphenoid ridge	2	35.0	24.0	12.0 (50.0)
Others	5	30.8	29.8	14.2 (47.7)
Mean		27.1	28.8	14.4 (50.0)

Table 2. Response of 52 meningiomas to radiosurgery, assessed by MRI

	Follow-up period (months)				
	3	6	12	18	24
Major shrinkage	0	1	1	2 (1)[a]	2 (1)
Minor shrinkage	2 (1)	5 (2)	16 (7)	8 (4)	8 (7)
No change	50 (4)	37 (8)	21 (6)	14 (4)	8 (1)
Larger	0	1	1 (0)	0	0
Responders (%)	3.8	13.6	43.5	41.6	55.5
Central necrosis (%)	9.6	22.7	33.3	37.5	50.0

[a] Central low signal intensity

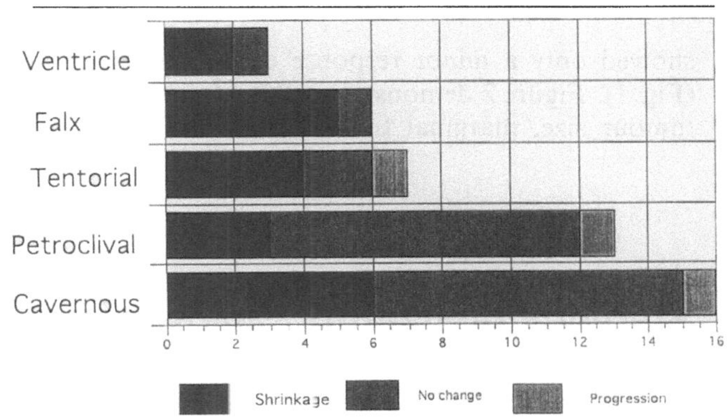

Fig. 1. Effects of radiosurgery on tumours in various locations

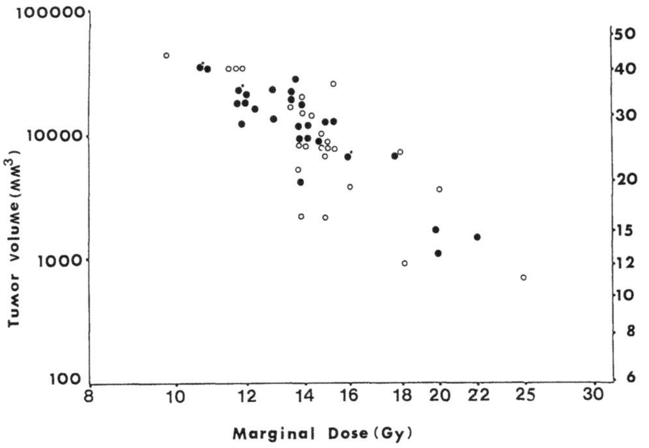

Fig. 2. Relationship between tumour size, marginal tumour dose and response. ○ tumour shrinkage, ● no change, progression

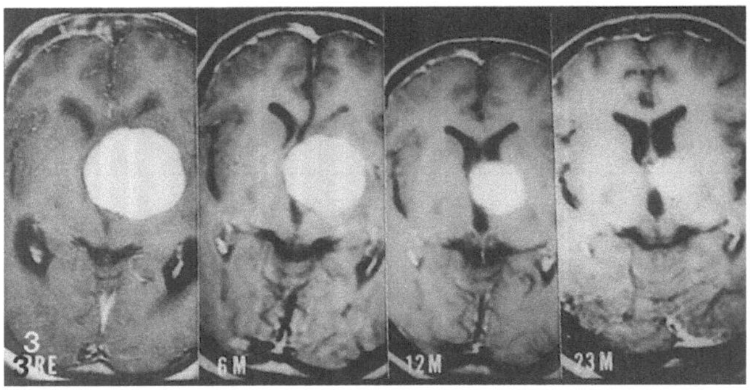

Fig. 3. Malignant meningioma of diaphragma sellae recurred even after two operative resections (*left*). This large tumour was treated with staged radiosurgery, with an interval of 4 months, using a marginal dose of 12 Gy. It showed considerable shrinkage 12 and 23 months later

showed only a minor response or no obvious changes (Fig. 1). Figure 2 demonstrates the relationship between tumour size, marginal tumour dose and the response, between which no apparent correlation was found (Fig. 2). Staged RS was tried in large tumours with an interval of 2–7 months. Even though they were treated with less than 12 Gy of marginal dose, two showed tumour shrinkage and another central necrosis (Fig. 3).

Discussion

The main strategy for the treatment of meningioma is operative resection. However, it is so often difficult to eradicate the tumour totally, especially those growing near vital structures or in the skull base. RS seems to be one of the options for these tumours [1–3]. In our study it is clear that RS can control the tumour growth except for malignant lesions [2]. Moreover, tumour shrinkage was obtained in 43.5% at 12 months and 55.5% at 24 months, which is in agreement with the report by Kondziolka et al. [3]. No correlation was verified between tumour size, the marginal dose and the response. Of interest in ventricular, tentorial, falcine and convexity meningiomas, those with narrow attachment demonstrated superior responses to the cavernous and petroclival ones, which had wide-based attachment. Therefore blood circulation in the tumour and blood vessels damage after RS may correlate with the appearance of central necrosis and shrinkage of the tumours. Radiation-induced oedema following RS is the most troublesome complication and therefore the treatment and irradiation dose must be carefully determined.

References

1. Engenhart R, Kimmig BN, Hover KH, Wowra B, Sturm V, Kaick G, Wannenmacher M (1990) Stereotactic single high dose radiation therapy of benign intracranial meningiomas. Int J Radiat Oncol Biol Phys 19:1021–1026
2. Coffey RJ, Cascino TL, Shaw EG (1993) Radiosurgical treatment of recurrent hemangiopericytomas of the meninges: preliminary results. J Neurosurg 78:903–908
3. Kondziolka D, Lunsford LD, Coffey RJ, Flickinger JC (1991) Stereotactic radiosurgery of meningiomas. J Neurosurg 74:552–559

Stereotactic gamma radiosurgery for malignant pineal tumours

Y. Mori[1], T. Kobayashi[2], Y. Kida[2], T. Tanaka[2]

[1] Department of Neurosurgery, Nagoya University School of Medicine, 65, Tsuruma-cho, Showa-ku, Nagoya, Japan
[2] Gamma Knife Center, Komaki City Hospital, Komaki City, Japan

Abstract. Seven patients with pineal tumours, including three malignant teratomas, two malignant germ cell tumours, one germinoma and one pineoblastoma were treated by radiosurgery (RS). Their mean age was 13.7 years. RS has been applied to residual pineal tumours after surgical resection, conventional irradiation, and/or chemotherapy. Those multimodality treatments were also used after RS in some cases. In five of seven cases, the tumours were stable or decreased in size with a mean follow-up time of 18.9 months after RS. Dissemination in the cerebrospinal fluid space developed in four patients, two of whom died 12 and 13 months after RS, respectively.

Correspondence to: Y. Mori

Table 1. Clinical characteristics and radiosurgical dose

Case	Age/sex (years)	Diagnosis	Prior treatments			Mean diameter (mm)	Dose (Gy) maximum/ Marginal
			Surgery	Radiation	Chemotherapy		
1	14/F	Malignant teratoma (HCG)	–	–	PE	28.3	30/15
2	12/M	Malignant teratoma (HCG, AFP)	partial (twice)	–	PE	19.8	36/18
3	15/M	Malignant teratoma (HCG, AFP)	partial (4 times)	whole spine + local	PVB PEB	34.8	22/11
4	15/M	Malignant germ cell tumour (HCG)	–	–	PE PVB	15.0	32/25.7
5	21/F	Malignant germ cell tumours (HCG, AFP)	–	–	PE	20.6	38/20.9
6	16/M	Germinoma?	–	local	PE	9.6	36/18
7	3/F	Pineoblastoma	Partial	–	–	35.3	25/12.5
Mean	13.7					23.3	31.3/17.3

PE (–B), cisplatin + etoposide + bleomycin; PVB, cisplatin + vinblastin + bleomycin; HCG, human chorionic gonadotropin; AFP, alpha-fetoprotein

Table 2. Outcome after radiosurgery (RS) and additional treatments

Case	Additional treatments			Post-RS follow-up (month)	Response	Other findings	Overall follow-up (month)	Outcome
	Surgery	Radiation	Chemotherapy					
1	Subtotal	Whole skull + radiosurgery	PE IT-MTX	31	Partial[a]	Dissemination	33	Alive
2	–	Radiosurgery (twice)	PE Ac-D MTX	20	Progression	Dissemination	32	Alive
3	–	–	–	9	Partial		86	Alive
4	–	–	PE	23	Complete	Radiation injury	26	Alive
5	–	Whole skull spine	PE + I	13	Complete	Dissemination	21	Died dissemination
6	–	–	–	24	None		32	Alive
7	–	Local	PE	12	Progression	Dissemination	14	Died tumour progression + dissemination
Mean				18.9			34.9	

PE (+ I), cisplatin + etoposide (+ ifosamide); MTX, methotrexate; IT, intrathecal
[a] Volume reduction ⩾ 50%

The other five patients are alive with a mean follow-up period of 21.4 (range 9–31) months after RS (41.8 months after diagnosis). In conclusion, RS will be one of the effective methods in the treatment of malignant pineal tumours.

Key words: Pineal body – Germ cell tumour – Pineoblastoma – Radiosurgery – Gamma knife

Pineal tumours other than germinoma and mature teratoma are not easily controlled by surgical resection, chemotherapy and/or conventional irradiation [1–8]. The role of stereotactic radiosurgery for the control of these tumours is discussed.

Patients and methods

Seven patients (4 males and 3 females) with pineal tumours, including three malignant teratomas, two malignant germ cell tumours, one germinoma, and one pineoblastoma were treated by stereotactic radiosurgery between May 1991 and June 1994 (Table 1). Their mean age was 13.7 (range 3–21) years. Radiosurgery was applied to residual pineal tumours after surgical resection, external beam radiation, and/or chemotherapy. Those multimodality treatments were also used after radiosurgery in some cases.

Results

In five of seven cases, the tumours were stable or decreased in size with a mean follow-up time of 18.9 months after the radiosurgery (Table 2). Dissemination in the cerebro-

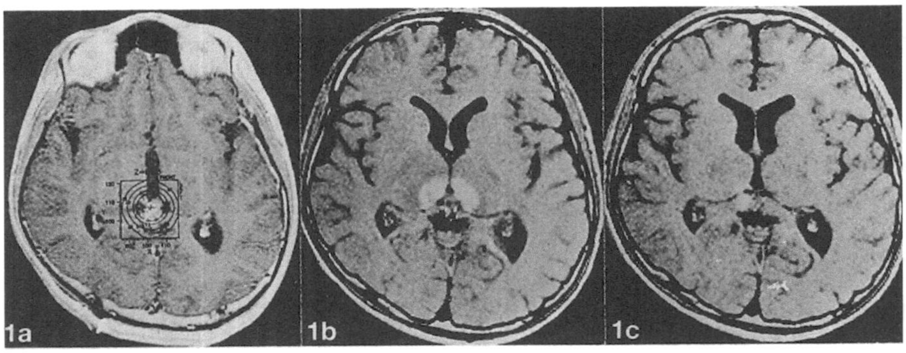

Fig. 1 a–c. Case 4. Gadolinium enhanced MRI. **a** Dose planning (32/25.7 Gy) of radiosurgery for residual pineal tumour after chemotherapy. **b** Twelve months after radiosurgery. The size of the tumour has decreased but symmetrical contrast-enhancing areas are seen in the thalamus, thought to be radiation-induced. **c** Seventeen months after radiosurgery. The pineal tumour has decreased in size. The enhancing area in the thalamus has disappeared

spinal fluid (CSF) space developed in four patients, two of whom died 12 and 13 months after radiosurgery, respectively. The other five patients are alive with a mean follow-up period of 21.4 months (range 9–31) after radiosurgery (41.8 months after diagnosis). No treatment-related clinical side-effects occurred.

A 15-year-old boy presented with headache and Parinaud's sign, and had increased serum human chorionic gonadotrophin (HCG) on admission. At first he received chemotherapy with cisplatin and etoposide and the size of the tumour decreased. Subsequently, radiosurgery with a marginal dose of 25.7 Gy was performed (Fig. 1 A). The patient is well with a normal serum HCG level 23 months after radiosurgery, and MRI showed marked regression of the pineal tumour (Fig. 1 C). MRI 12 months after radiosurgery revealed a symmetrical contrast-enhancing area in the thalamus (Fig. 1 B), which almost disappeared on later MRI (Fig. 1 C). The patient developed no additional neurological deficits and the enhancement was thought to be due to transient radiation-induced changes.

Discussion

Of the varieties of intracranial germ cell tumours, germinoma and mature teratomas are curable by conventional irradiation and surgery, respectively. In addition, successful treatment of germinoma with cisplatin-based chemotherapy has been reported [6]. However, the treatment of malignant germ cell tumours is controversial. These tumours show resistance to chemotherapy and irradiation, and recurrence or dissemination of the tumour cells in the CSF are frequent. About half of patients with malignant germ cell tumours die within 12–14 months [2, 5, 7]. Among pineal parenchymal tumours, pineoblastoma is a highly malignant, infiltrating tumour with a pronounced tendency to disseminate throughout the CSF [1, 4]. Borit et al. [1] reported that seven of eight patients with pineoblastoma died within 2 years of their first craniotomy.

In the cases presented here, local control of pineal tumours was obtained in five of seven cases. Five patients with malignant teratoma or malignant germ cell tumours survived 9–31 (mean 19.2) months after radiosurgery, or 21–86 (mean 39.6) months after diagnosis. Four of five survived longer than 2 years from diagnosis and are alive in good condition.

These patients with malignant pineal tumours who had been treated by a combination of conventional therapies and gamma radiosurgery have survived longer than previously reported cases. Stereotactic radiosurgery will be one of the effective methods in the treatment of malignant pineal tumours.

References

1. Borit A, Blackwood W, Mair WGP (1980) The separation of pineocytoma from pineoblastoma. Cancer 45:1408–1418
2. Gzirjak S, Vajda J, Pasztor E (1992) Management of pineal region tumours. Neurol Res 14:241–247
3. Edwards MSB, Hudgins RJ, Wilson CB, Levin VA, Wara WM (1988) Pineal region tumors in children. J Neurosurg 68:689–697
4. Herrick MK, Rubinstein LJ (1979) The cytological differentiating potential of pineal parenchymal neoplasms (true pinealomas). A clinicopathological study of 28 tumours. Brain 102:289–320
5. Kirkove CS, Brown AP, Symon L (1991) Successful treatment of a pineal endodermal sinus tumor. J Neurosurg 74:832–836
6. Kobayashi T, Yoshida J, Noda S, Kida Y, Teraoka M, Itoh J (1990) Combination chemotherapy with CDDP and etoposide (P-E therapy) for intracranial germ-cell tumors. Shouni No Noshinkei 15:409–416
7. Nakagawa K, Aoki Y, Akanuma A, Sakata K, Karasawa K, Terahara A, Onogi Y, Hasezawa K, Muta N, Sasaki Y (1992) Radiation therapy of intracranial germ cell tumors with radiosensitivity assessment. Radiat Oncol 10:55–61
8. Sebag-Montefiore DJ, Douek E, Kingston JE, Plowman PN (1992) Intracranial germ cell tumours. I. Experience with platinum-based chemotherapy and implications for curative chemoradiotherapy. Clin Oncol 4:345–350

Follow-up imaging studies in patients treated with radiosurgery for metastatic melanoma

C. S. Zee, Z. Petrivich, G. Luxton, L. Petrus, M. J. Apuzzo

University of Southern California School of Medicine, Department of Radiology, LAC + USC Imaging Science Center, 1744 Zonal Ave, Los Angeles, CA 90033, USA

Abstract. Our aim was to evaluate the efficacy of stereotactic radiosurgery for treatment of intracranial metastatic melanomas. A total of 13 patients with 35 intracranial metastatic melanoma lesions were treated with stereotactic radiosurgery. On imaging studies, complete remission was found in 5 of 35, partial remission in 20 of 35, stable disease in 8 of 35, and progression in 2 of 35. In addition, relapse was later seen in 3 of the 28 lesions that initially showed partial remission or stable disease. Stereotactic radiosurgery is an effective and safe therapy for brain metastatic melanomas. It can be applied as primary treatment or for a relapse in a patient previously treated by whole-brain irradiation.

Key words: Metastatic melanoma – Radiosurgery

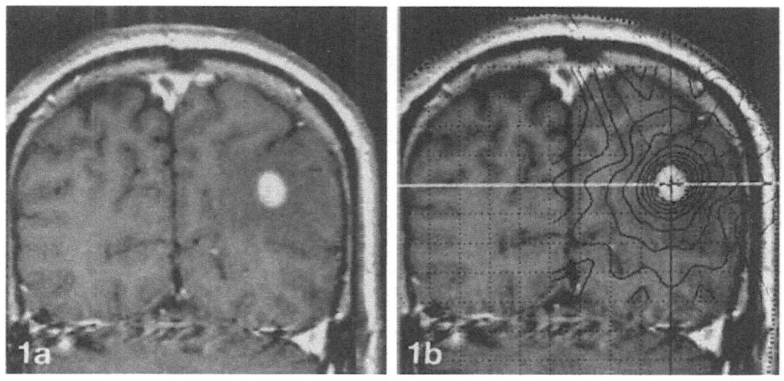

Fig. 1. Treatment plan for a left parietal metastasis. This lesion resolved entirely following treatment. **a** Contrast-enhanced coronal image shows an enhancing nodule. **b** Treatment plan with 80% isodose line at the periphery of the lesion

Management of intracranial metastatic melanoma is controversial. Types of therapy available include whole-brain radiation, fractionated radiation, stereotactic radiosurgery and immunotherapy. We attempted to evaluate the efficacy of stereotactic radiosurgery using a linear accelerator for treatment of intracranial metastatic melanoma, by performing follow-up MRI.

Methods

Between July 1991 and August 1994, 13 patients with 35 intracranial metastatic melanoma lesions were treated with radiosurgery. Their ages ranged from 30 to 85 years; there were 6 men and 7 women. The median dose of radiation used in these patients was 1800 cGy, with a range from 1250 to 2500 cGy.

A description of the preparation of the linear accelerator, patient immobilization, target localization, and treatment planning has been published previously [1, 2]. Collimators between 17.5 mm and 30 mm have been used.

Follow-up study was obtained initially within 3 months of treatment, and then at 3-month intervals for up to 2.5 years. MRI studies were performed using 1.5 T imagers. The patient was given 20 ml Gd-DTPA prior to the examination. Magnetization transfer technique, when available, was used for contrast-enhanced.

Results

A total of 35 lesions were treated in 13 patients. Complete resolution of the enhancing lesion was found in 5 lesions (Fig. 1a, b). Partial regression of the enhancing lesion was detected in 20 lesions. Stable disease with the size of enhancing lesions unchanged was seen in 8 lesions. There were lesions that increased in size despite treatment. Of the 28 lesions that initially partially regressed or were stable, 3 later showed relapse. New lesions were detected in most patients during follow-up (Fig. 2).

Of 3 patients with metastatic disease confirmed to the brain, 3 survived longer than 2 years. Overall, 5 patients died (3 of brain metastasis, 2 of disseminated disease); 4 patients are still alive; all developed additional metastatic lesions in the brain. Unfortunately, 4 patients were lost to follow-up.

Correspondence to: C. S. Zee

Discussion

Our data indicate that stereotactic radiosurgery is an effective therapy for brain metastatic melanomas. The majority of the lesions (30/35) treated with stereotactic radiosurgery showed improvement or stable disease on the follow-up MRI. Relapse was seen in only 5 of 35 lesions. However, our main problem seems to be the appearance of new lesions on the follow-up MRI. In 1 patient, a metastatic lesion was detected on the initial study (March 1993) and was treated with radiosurgery. The lesion remained stable in size for 3 months and was then surgically removed because of hemorrhage into the lesion. Subsequently, the patient developed four new lesions at different times, and each was treated with stereotactic radiosurgery. The results were favorable, with either partial remission or stable disease. However, a recent follow-up examination (August 1994) revealed six new metastatic lesions involving both the cerebral hemisphere and the cerebellum. In this case, each lesion responded favorably to radiosurgery. Prolongation of quality life span was achieved, albeit limited.

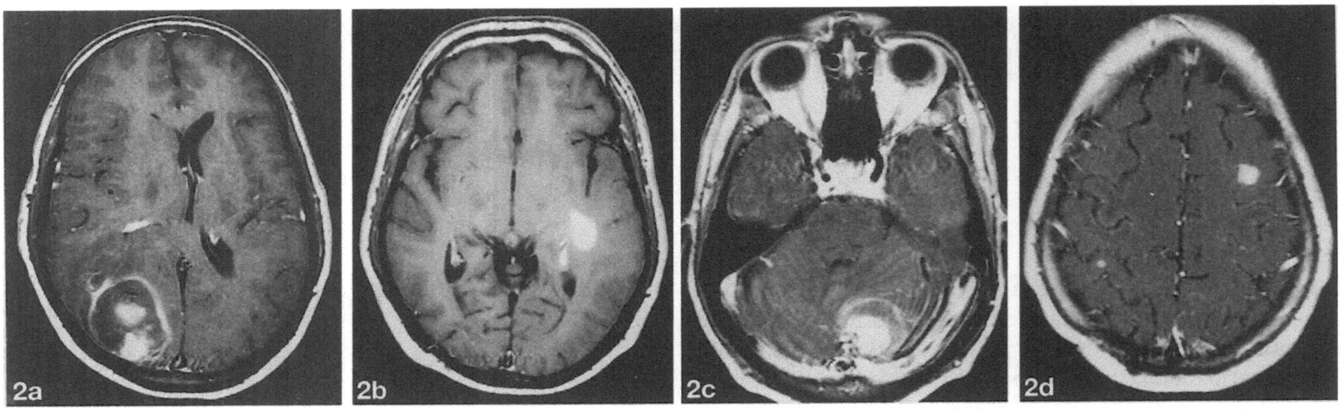

Fig. 2. "Successful" treatment of individual metastases in a patient with development of new lesions. **a** (September 1992) A contrast-enhanced axial image shows a large ring-enhancing lesion with hemorrhage. This was treated 6 months before the study and regressed 3 months after treatment. Owing to sudden enlargement secondary to hemorrhage, it was removed surgically. **b** (September 1993) A contrast-enhanced axial image shows a new metastasis in the left temporal lobe. This was treated successfully with stereotactic radiosurgery and showed marked regression. **c, d** (September 1994) Contrast-enhanced axial images show multiple new metastases

Our complications were self-limited symptoms including nausea, vomiting, and transient hemiparesis. On the initial follow-up imaging study, a transient increase in the edema surrounding the lesion was observed in some cases; these patients were all treated with corticosteroids and showed response. Both acute and delayed radiation injury to the central nervous system in patients undergoing stereotactic radiosurgery have been described by various authors [3–6].

The decision on treating patients with metastatic melanoma is extremely complicated. The goal should be improvement and maintenance of quality of life. Optimum management of intracranial metastatic melanoma remains a dilemma. Owing to the limited number of our patients and the various factors that may affect treatment, we have focused on the follow-up imaging findings on each lesion. The results seem to indicate a favorable outcome for individual lesions.

References

1. Pastyr O, Hartmann GH, Schlegel W, et al (1989) Stereotactically guided convergent beam irritation with a linear accelerator: localization-technique. Acta Neurochir 99:61–64
2. Engenhart R, Kimmig BN, Hover KH, et al (1993) Long-term follow-up for brain metastases treated by percutaneous stereotactic single high-dose irradiation. Cancer 71:1353–1361
3. Kjellberg RN (1979) Isoeffective dose parameters for brain necrosis in relation to proton radiosurgical dosimetry. In: G Szikla (ed) Stereotactic irradiation. Elsevier/North Holland, Amsterdam, pp 157–166
4. Loeffler JS, Sidon RL, Wen PY, Nedze LA, Alexander E (1990) Stereotactic radiosurgery of the brain using a standard linear accelerator: a study of early and late effects. Radiother Oncol 17:311–321
5. Hirsch A, Noren G (1988) Audiological findings at stereotactic radiosurgery in acoustic neurinomas. Arch Otolaryngol 106:244–251
6. Harris JR, Levene MB (1976) Visual complications following irradiation for pituitary adenomas and craniopharyngiomas. Radiology 120:167–171

Gamma-knife treatment for metastatic brain tumours

K. Ehara[1], N. Tamaki[1], M. Hamasaki[2], H. Yamamoto[2], S. Matsumoto[2]

[1] Department of Neurosurgery, Kobe University, Kobe, Japan
[2] Shin-Suma Hospital Gamma Knife Centre, Kobe, Japan

Abstract. We investigated the relationship between various patients' treatment protocols of gamma knife (GK) treatment, and clinical or neuroradiological outcomes in 51 patients with metastatic brain tumours. We treated 51 patients with brain metastases. Patients were divided into three groups. Group A received more than 20 Gy marginal dose; group B received less than 20 Gy marginal dose; group C patients were treated by radiosurgery combined with conventional radiotherapy. Twenty of 38 patients (74%) had improved or stable clinical conditions during follow-up. All group A cases, 60% of group B, and 77% of group C patients had satisfactory clinical outcomes. Neuroradiological control of tumour size was achieved in 29 of 38 patients (76%). No patients in group A had neuroradiological recurrences.

Key words: Radiotherapy – Metastatic brain tumour – Gamma knife – Radiosurgery

According to the recent literature, gamma knife (GK) treatment results in clinical benefits in patients with brain metastases in comparison with surgery or conventional radiotherapy [1–5]. We investigated the relationship between various patients' treatment protocols of GK treatment, and clinical or neuroradiological outcomes in 51 patients with metastatic brain tumours.

Patients and methods

Among 342 cases treated by the Gamma Knife Centre from December 1992 to August 1994, 51 cases of brain metastasis were treated. A clinical summary of these 51 patients is shown in Table 1. Their mean age is 62.5 ± 11.6 years. There were 26 males and 25 females. Multiple brain metastases were treated in 22 cases (43%). About 40% of the metastases came from lung cancer.

According to the treatment protocols, patients were divided into three groups. Group A (high dose group) received more than 20 Gy and group B (medium dose group) less than 20 Gy marginal dose. Group C (combination group) patients were treated by radiosurgery combined with conventional radiotherapy.

Among 51 cases, 38 were followed for more than 6 months.

Results

As shown in Table 1, there were differences in size in these groups. Most of group A patients had smaller tumours of less than 2.5 cm. However, group B and C patients usually had larger tumours or those very close to the critical neural structures. The distribution of the marginal dose was different in these groups. In most cases, patients in group A were treated with 20–25 Gy, and those in group B with between 15 and 20 Gy.

The clinical results are shown in Table 2. Twenty of 38 cases (74%) had improved or stable clinical conditions during follow-up. All group A cases, 60% of group B, and 77% of group C patients had satisfactory clinical conditions. Only 7 of 21 patients (33%) died because of a central nervous system lesion. One patient had intracerebral bleeding after radiosurgery that required craniotomy [6].

The neuroradiological results are shown in Table 3. Neuroradiological control of tumour size was achieved in 29 of 38 patients (76%).

In group A especially, no patients had neurological and neuroradiological recurrence.

Mean survival time did not differ in these groups, because the conditions of primary lesions were, in most cases, the most important factors for survival.

Discussion

Therapeutic endeavours for patients with metastatic brain tumours are aimed at improving the quality of life. Whatever the modality of treatment for cerebral metastasis, average survival rates of more then 12 months are rarely reported. According to the Japan Brain Tumour Registry of 1832 cases of brain metastasis from lung cancer, only 471 cases (42.7%) were totally resected. One-year survival after surgery was 31.1%, that of a combination of surgery plus radiation was 31.4%, and that of radiation alone was 23.2% [7]. Excellent results were reported for both GK and the modified linear accelerator in comparison with surgery or conventional radiotherapy [1–5]. Reported mortality and the rate of recurrence were 0% and from 3.9 to 8.7%, respectively, and were lower than those of microsurgery. The lengths of hospital stay and the risks in treatment were smaller in radiosurgery than in microsurgery. Average survival rates were compatible with those of the surgery plus radiation group. From these data, radiosurgery seems to provide the same advantages to patients as craniotomy. Small single or double tumours in particular should be treated by high-dose GK therapy. If the tumour is large, surgery or combination therapy should be considered. Even if these treatments are difficult, GK can provide patients with some benefits.

In conclusion, treatment planning of radiosurgery for brain metastasis should consider the patients' various clinical conditions. Most of the patients had some neurological (74%) and neuroradiological (76%) benefits during follow-up. High-dose single treatment had the best results, followed by those of the combination group.

Correspondence to: K. Ehara, Department of Neurosurgery, Kobe University School of Medicine, 7-5-1 Kusunoki-cho Chuo-ku, Kobe, Japan 650

Table 1. Patient characteristics and treatment protocol

	Patients	Age years	Sex (male:female)	Mean diameter (cm)	Maximum dose (Gy)	Marginal dose (Gy)	Coverage of isodose (%)
Group A	14	64.1 ± 5.1	9:5	1.96 ± 0.43	40.1 ± 5.2	21.1 ± 2.3	52.9 ± 10.7
Group B	28	62.5 ± 13.9	11:17	3.10 ± 0.79	30.3 ± 7.9	14.4 ± 2.9	48.6 ± 6.8
Group C	9	59.8 ± 11.4	6:3	2.47 ± 1,21	33.6 ± 6.5	18.1 ± 4.0	53.9 ± 6.7
Total	51	62.5 ± 11.6	26:25	2.67 ± 0.93	33.5 ± 8.1	16.9 ± 4.1	50.7 ± 8.7

Table 2. Treatment protocol and neurological outcome

	Patients	Improved or stable	Worse	Dead (CNS)	Dead (primary)	Tumour control
Group A	14	9	0	0	6	100%
Group B	28	12	3	5	5	60%
Group C	9	7	0	2	3	77%
Total	38	28	3	7	14	74%

Table 3. Treatment protocol and neuroradiological outcome

	Patients	Complete response	Partial response	No change	Progression	Tumour control
Group A	14	1	0	8	0	100%
Group B	28	0	0	13	7	65%
Group C	9	0	1	6	2	77%
Total	38	1	0	27	9	76%

References

1. Kahlström L, Karlson B, Lindquist C, Norén G, Rähn T (1991) Gamma knife surgery for cerebral metastasis. Acta Neurochir [Suppl] 52:87–89
2. Coffey RJ, Lunsford LD, Flickinger JC (1992) The role of radiosurgery in the treatment of malignant brain tumors. Neurosurg Clin North Am 3:231–244
3. Somaza S, Kondziolka D, Lunsford LD, Kirkwood J, Flickinger JC (1993) Stereotactic radiosurgery for cerebral metastatic melanoma. J Neurosurg 79:661–666
4. Kida Y, Kobayashi T, Tanaka T, Oyama H, Iwakoshi T (1993) Gammaradiosurgery of metastatic brain tumors. Neurol Surg (Tokyo) 21:991–997
5. Loeffler J, Alexander E III (1993) Radiosurgery for the treatment of intracranial metastasis. In: Loeffler J, Alexander E III, Lunsford LD (eds) Stereotactic radiosurgery. McGraw-Hill, New York, pp 197–206
6. Motozaki T, Ban S, Yamamoto T, Hamasaki M (1994) Peritumoral haemorrhage after radiosurgery for metastatic brain tumor. Neurol Surg (Tokyo) 22:789–793
7. Keiji Sano (1992) The seventh report from the Brain Tumor Registry of Japan. Neurol Med Chir 32 [Suppl]:537–547

Contrast media

New contrast media for neuroradiology

U. Speck

Contrast Media Research, Schering Laboratories, D-13342 Berlin, Germany

Abstract. Neuroradiological requirements of contrast media (CM) are defined by the specific pathologies to be diagnosed and the highest possible standard of safety. Improvements in technology have now made large-scale production of nonionic dimeric X-ray CM feasible. The first such compund is iotrolan. Since 1988 it has proved to have very good tolerance in myelography and related subarachnoid applications. Animal experiments have indicated distinctly improved vascular tolerance, including the blood-brain barrier. Clinical trials have confirmed better tolerance. Contrast in selective angiographic procedures has proved to be surprisingly good. In MRI perfusion imaging of the brain can be performed using gadolinium DTPA or new magnetites allowing rapid injection due to their superior tolerability. Ultrasound contrast media can increase the sensitivity of transcranial Doppler sonography.

Key words: Contrast media – Iotrolan – Magnetic resonance imaging – Ultrasound

Today's contrast media are used in three different imaging techniques, namely X-radiography, magnetic resonance imaging and ultrasound, each one characterised by different physics, equipment, imaging capabilities and clinical applications. Contrast media contribute to the vasualisation of the subarachnoid space to the extent that it is accessible through the cerebrospinal fluid (CSF), the lumen of the blood vessels, the blood flow, the blood-brain-barrier (BBB) and tissue perfusion.

Since the introduction of tri-iodinated urographic X-ray contrast media a large variety of iodinated products have been developed (Table 1). These belong to four different classes: the strongly hypertonic conventional ionic contrast media (e.g. diatrizoate), which in most countries is no longer used in neuroradiology, the ionic low osmolar ioxaglate, the tri-iodinated nonionic contrast media, and the hexaiodinated nonionic products.

The tri-iodinated nonionic molecules are also referred to as "monomers" because all the iodine atoms are bound to just one benzene ring. The hexaiodinated contrast media are called "dimers"; the six iodine atoms are equally distributed over two benzene rings firmly linked to each other.

Whereas the monomers, at a concentration of 300 mg iodine/ml, have twice the osmolality of blood or, for instance, CSF, the dimers are isotonic with body fluids at all usual concentrations.

Isovist contains iotrolan as the active ingredient; this belongs to the class of nonionic isotonic dimers. It was introduced in 1988 as a myelographic contrast medium. Since then production technology has improved to such an extent that its use as a general vascular agent has

Table 1. Types of water-soluble contrast medium

ionic		non-ionic	
high osmolar	low osmolar	low osmolar	isotonic
Diatrizoate (Urografin, Angiovist, Renografin etc.)	Ioxaglate (Hexabrix)	Metrizamide (Amipaque)	Iotrolan (Isovist)
Iothalamate (Conray)		Iopamidol (Iopamiro, Niopam, Solutrast)	Iodixanol (Visipaque)
Iodamide (Uromiro)		Iohexol (Omnipaque)	
Metrizoate (Isopaque)		Ioversol (Optiray)	
Ioxithalamate (Telebrix)		Iopentol (Imagopaque)	
Ioglicate (Rayvist)		Iomeprol (Iomeron)	

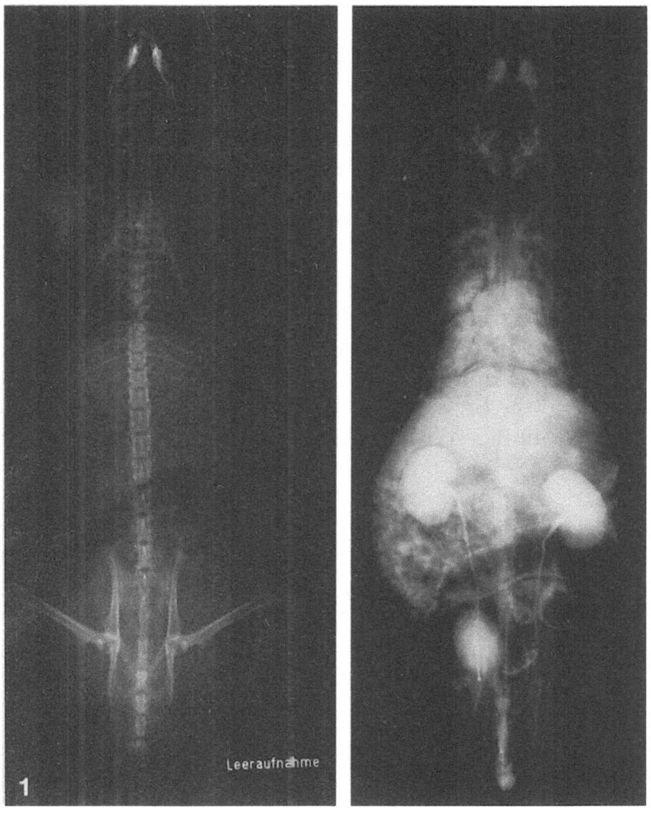

Fig. 1. a Radiography of a rat after Injection of iotrolan equivalent to 20 g iodine/kg. **b** Control rat. Note extent of abdominal space

Table 2. Other than Local (heat, pain) adverse events in double-blind randomised studies comparing iotrolan with nonionic monomers

	Iotrolan (%)	Pooled reference (%)	P-value
Total number of patients at risk	1207	1203	
Generalised heat	8.5	12.3	0.0012
Other adverse events	4.06	5.48	0.061
- severe	0.99	1.16	0.419
- mild	3.07	4.32	0.063

Table 3. Use of contrast media in MRI

Magnevist Gd DTPA
- Blood-brain barrier
- MR angiography
- Cerebral blood flow (e.g. T 2* gradient-echo)
- CSF (e.g. 2 mM Gd DTPA)
T 2-CM (e.g. Dy, Magnetites)
- Cerebral blood flow
Macromolecules
- MR angiography
- Capillary permeability

become possible. Since dimers are somewhat more viscous than monomers, a concentration of 280 mg iodine/ml was chosen for angiography and CT enhancement. This turned out to be fully satisfactory in all vascular neuroradiological applications.

The intravenous LD 50 in rats reaches 28 g iodine/kg body weight. This is equal to about 60 g contrast medium/kg and reaches 20% of the total dry weight (all organic material plus the bones) of the animals. After the injection one can hardly recognize anything but the contrast medium in the rat on a radiograph (Fig. 1). It is doubtful that we will ever find a less toxic compound considering that the space for soluble organic molecules within the organism is somewhat limited.

In animal experiments iotrolan proved to be particularly well tolerated by the BBB. Based on Evans' blue uptake in the brain as the indication for BBB disruption, iotrolan induced no more damage than saline upon prolonged injection into the internal carotid artery [1]. In clinical studies excellent visualisation of the small branches of the cerebral arteries was observed, in spite of the slightly lower iodine concentration of Isovist-280 than of the nonionic monomers (300 mg iodine/ml).

The European clinical trials comparing iotrolan with noionic monomeric contrast media for vascular use revealed a significant reduction in local side effects such as pain and heat [2]. Also, generalised heat and nausea, vomiting and cardiovascular reactions occured less frequently than with the already very well-tolerated nonionic monomers (Table 2). Less osmotically driven increases in blood volume may contribute to the cardiovascular tolerance of iotrolan.

For MRI a number of contrast media similar to gadopentetate have been introduced. In addition to the very sensitive visualisation of a variety of pathologies that are due to a nonfunctioning BBB, MR angiography can be improved by paramagnetic contrast media, and information on cerebral blood flow can be obtained by using T2-weighted gradient-echo sequences [3]. Dilute gadolinium DTPA-meglumine has been used to outline and follow CSF after subarachnoid injection in monkeys [4].

Newly developed well-tolerated magnetites may be even more suitable for perfusion imaging. Animal experiments indicate that water-soluble macromolecular gadiolinium chelates could improve the specificity of diagnosis due to capillary-leak characterisation [5] (Table 3).

Finally, ultrasound contrast media are being introduced into clinical practice. Whereas the fist products have their main application in cardiology, clinical trials indicate that newly developed media will facilitate the detection of flow in severely obstructed carotid arteries and will also substantially improve signals in transcranial Doppler ultrasound examination [6].

In conclusion, new contrast media will further contribute to the safety and performance of neuroradiology. In MRI in particular, improved visualisation of functions and greater specificity of diagnosis may be achieved.

References

1. Wilcox J, Evill CA, Sage MR (1986) Effects of intracarotid ionic and non-ionic contrast material on the blood-brain barrier in a rabbit model. Neuroradiology 28:271–274
2. Böck JC, Sander B, Hierholzer J, Haustein J, Scholz M, Radke KH, Schörner W, Lanksch W, Felix R (1992) MRI of regional cerebral blood flow in intracranial tumours: Comparison of HMPAO-SPECT with a magnetic resonance technique. Forstschr Röntgenstr 157:378–383
3. Di Chiro G, Knop RH, Girton ME, Dwyer AJ, Doppman JL, Patronas NJ, Ganzow OA, Brechbiel MW, Brooks RA (1985) MR cisternography and myelography with Gd-DTPA in monkeys. Radiology 157:373–377
4. Shames DM, Kuwatsuru R, Vexler V, Mühler A, Brasch RC (1993) Measurement of capillary permeability to macromolecules by dynamic magnetic resonance imaging: A quantitative noninvasive technique. Magn Reson Med 29:616–622
5. Bogdahn U, Becker G, Schlief R, Reddig J, Hassel W (1993) Contrast-enhanced transcranial color-coded real-time sonography. Stroke 24:676–684

EEG changes after intravenous ionic and nonionic contrast medium administration

M. Signorino[1], C. Calzolari[1], L. Provinciali[1], F. Menichelli[2], U. Salvolini[1]

[1] Istituto Malattie del Sistema Nervoso, Università di Ancona, Italy
[2] Servizio di Neuroradiologia, USL 12, Ancona, Italy

Abstract. With the aim of investigating EEG changes after the random administration of two types of contrast medium (iopamidol and methylglucamine iothalamate in balanced groups), we reviewed 40 patients suffering from lung cancer and at risk of cerebral metastases who were undergoing brain CT. The patients were assessed using a checklist prepared to investigate the side effects of the contrast media (CM), and the EEG was recorded before, during and after CM administration. The EEG signals were analysed quantitatively (computerised spectral analysis) to study the background activity in terms of power spectra. No adverse clinical side effects were observed during the study. The results of the quantitative analysis showed that administration of methylglucamine iothalamate increases fast activity power and frequency only in the frontal regions.

Key words: Contrast medium – Electroencephalographic spectral analysis – Computed tomography

In recent years, there has been a growing interest in reducing the side effects of radiographic Contrast media (CM). The neurotoxic side effects of CM vary with the method of administration and include both nonfocal events such as headaches [1], meningeal irritation [2], generalised seizures [3], attention deficits [4] and behavioural disturbances [5], and focal events such as aphasia, hemiplegia and partial epileptic attacks [6]. The occurrence of seizures in patients having intravenous CM is very low [7] but increases to 6–9% if the patient has primary or secondary brain tumours [8, 9]. The neurotoxic effects depend directly on the method of administration and are dose-dependent, subarachnoid CM having the greatest toxic effect on nervous tissue [3].

For many years, investigations of biological effects of drugs on the central vervous system (CNS) have been carried out using EEG and its computer analysis [10]. Ionic and nonionic CM have also been evaluated using EEGs during preclinical and clinical investigations. Nonionic CM show a lower level of EEG abnormalities than the ionic [11]. Furthermore, striking unilaterial EEG suppression is seen when ionic CM is used for intracarotid injection [12].

We made a direct comparison of EEG changes induced by ionic and nonionic CM given i.v. in patients at risk of neurological side effects. As far as we know, only clinical studies had hitherto been carried out on this subject [13].

Correspondence to: M. Signorino, Clinico Neuroligica, Ospedali di Torrette, I-60100 Ancona, Italy

Methods

With consent, 40 patients with lung cancer and possible brain metastases underwent CT with CM for staging. In 20 patients (12 men, 8 women, average age 67.3 years), Iopamidol (Iopamiro 300) (3 ml/kg) was adminstered. As a comparison, the other 20 (16 men, 4 women, average age 65.2 years) received infusions of methylglucamine iothalamate 3 ml/kg. Exclusion criteria were: agitation, treatment with psychotropic drugs, need for premedication and history of allergy or epilepsy.

All patients underwent quantitative and traditional EEG before, during and after CM administration. About 1 h before the CT, the patients were sent to the EEG laboratory to be prepared for the subsequent recording. First, the baseline recording was carried out, and then one of the two drugs was administered by drip infusion over 20–30 min. About 10 min after the beginning of the infustion, the second EEG recording was made. About 10 min after the infusion was finished, the third recording was made. During the next 20 min, the patients underwent CT. Brain metastases were found in 8 patients of the iopamidol group and in 5 of the methylglucamine iothalamate group.

Before and after CM administration, a checklist was completed to monitor any symptoms (sleepiness, irritability, tiredness, paraesthesia, movement difficulties, headaches) and any neurological signs (orientation, reactivity, loss of strength, sensitivity, neck rigidity, seizures).

The EEG was recorded from 16 Ag-AgCl electrodes placed according to the 10–20 system with the exception of three electrodes on the sagittal line, with linked ear-lobes as a reference during psychosensorial rest with eyes closed. Spectral analysis was carried out selecting 60 artefact-free epochs (20 for each condition) each lasting 2 s. Each epoch underwent FFT in the frequency range 0.5–28.5 Hz. The average of the 20 spectra obtained in this way was then calculated for each channel (mean spectra). The global spectrum resulting from the average of the 16 channels was then calculated. Each mean spectrum was then subdivided into 7 bands in steps of 4 Hz, considering absolute and relative power log, mean and peak frequency.

The spectral descriptor values in each group were compared with the aid of the t-test as corrected using Bonferroni's criterion for the number of bands studied.

EEG artefacts were found in 4 and 7 subjects, respectively, in the iopamidol and methylglucamine Iothalamate groups. The EEGs were excluded from further processing and analysis.

Results

There were no adverse clinical side effects in any of the patients in either group.

Methylglucamine iothalamate group

A significant power increase in the 20.5–24.5 Hz band occurred in the "during" phase compared with the baseline in Fp1 and Fp2 leads (Fig. 1). In the "after" phase, this increase was only noted in Fp1. A significant increase in

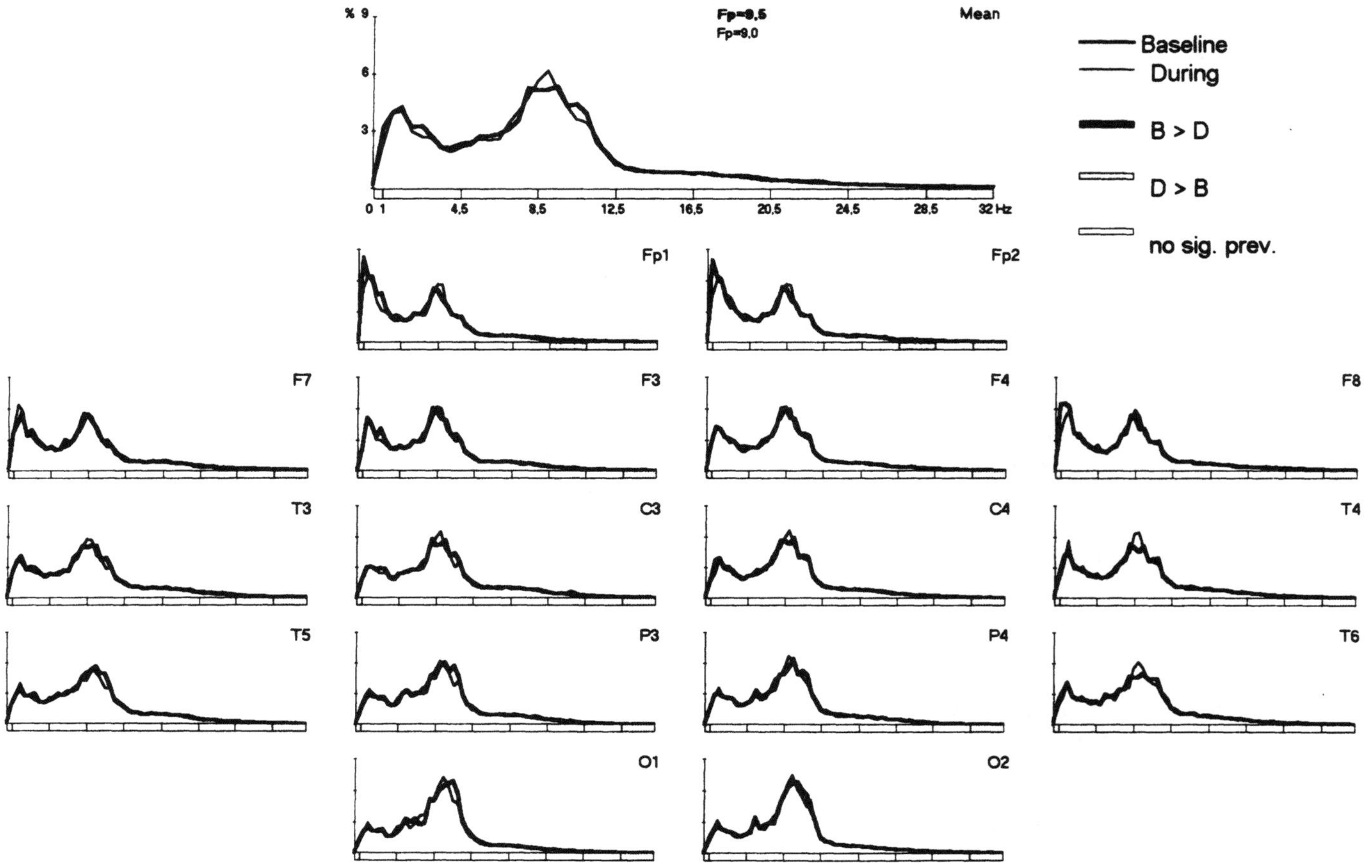

Fig. 1. Mean relative spectra obtained from EEG recordings of the methylglucamine iothalamate group: baseline (*thick lines*) and "during" (*thin lines*). The scalp leads are indicated in the top right of each Cartesian system. The abscissa shows the frequencies from 1 to 32 Hz and the ordinate shows the log RP value. At the top of each map, the "global spectrum" is plotted as the mean of the 16 regional spectra. Blank segments of the abscissa indicate no statistically significant difference; grey indicate that statistical analysis was not performed, Dark grey indicate higher power in the "during" stage

peak frequency in the 20.5- to 24,5 Hz band in Fp1 (20.9 vs 22.0 Hz, $df=12$, $t=3.31$) and in mean frequency in the 16.5–20.5 Hz band in F7 (18.2 vs 18.4 Hz, $df=12$, $t=4.71$) in the "during" phase, as compared with the baseline, was recorded. An increase in mean frequency in the 16.5–20.5 Hz band was also noted in Fp1 in the "after" as against the "during" phase (18.2 vs 18.4 Hz, $df=12$, $t=3.39$).

Iopamidol Group

No significant power, peak and mean frequency differences in the various bands were noted in any derivation when either the "during" or "after" phase was occurred with the baseline (Fig. 1).

Discussion

We used electrophysiological methods based on computerised techniques, as in a previous study dealing with intrathecal administration of nonionic CM [14].

We found no change from the background activity when iopamidol was administered, despite our previous study [14]. This may be explained by the greater neurotoxic effects of direct contact with the brain tissue after subarachnoid infusion.

A notable result is that the EEG spectral analysis shows changes only after methylglucamine iothalamate. However, these changes are slight, restricted only to the frontal derivations. This contrasts with the results of Artru et al. [12], probably because of the different methods of administration. Changes observed during and after administration of methylglucamine iothalamate concern EEG fast activity. An increase in this activity is usually seen with stimulant drugs such as D-amphetamine, caffeine and nicotine (10) and can indicate an excitatory state in the CNS, which could predispose to the appearance of excitatory side-effects such as behavioural disturbances. Furthermore, the frontal location of fast activity changes may be explained both by considering the functional activation of frontal lobes, involved in behavioural changes, and the greater occurrence of anterior metastases in our patients.

We found no significant spectral changes in the EEG slow bands. The appearance of slow potentials is generally considered "lesional" and, when it follows the administration of CM, is regarded as due to diffuse alteration of the blood-brain barrier (BBB). Thus, we can assume that the CM used in this study do not significantly alter the BBB.

The bioelectrical changes after intravenous administration of these CM are detectable even when patients do not complain of side effects; furthermore this study confirms that there may be advantages related to the use of nonionic CM.

Acknowledgements. We thank V. Durazzi, L. Ferrini, S. Cercaci, S. Acciarri and C. Castelli for their technical assistance.

References

1. Meador K, Hamilton WJ, El Gammal TAM, Demetropoulos KC, Nichols FT III (1984) Irreversible neurologic complication of metrizamide myielography. Neurology 34:817–821
2. Gelmers HJ (1979) Adverse side effects of metrizamide in myelography. Neuroradiology 18:119–123
3. Picard L, Vespignani H, Vieux-Rochat P, More CH, L'Esperance G, Montaut J, Weber M, Roland J (1979) Complications neurologiques graves des myelographies au métrizamide. J Neuroradiology 6:3–14
4. Yu YL, du Boulay GH, Paul E (1986) Influence of certain factors on the manifestations of the adverse effects of metrizamide myielography. Neuroradiology 28:339–343
5. Schmidt RC (1980) Mental disorders after myelography with metrizamide and other water-soluble contrast media. Neuroradiology 19:153–157
6. Angiari P, Crisi G, Merli GA (1984) Aphasia and right hemiplegia after cervical mielography with metrizamide. Neuroradiology 26:61–63
7. Witten DM, Hirsch FD, Hartman GW (1973) Acute reactions to urographic contrast medium. AJR 119:832
8. Lozito JC (1977) Convulsions: a complication of contrast enhancement and computerized tomography. Arch Neurol 34:649
9. Leonardi M, Lavaroni A, Biasizzo E, Fabris G, Penco T, Zappoli F (1989) High-dose contrast-enhanced computed tomography (CECT) with iopamidol in the detection of cerebral metastases. Neuroradiology 31:148–150
10. Glaze DG (1990) Drug effects. In: Daly DD and Pedley TA (eds), Current practice of clinical electroencephalography. 2nd edn. Raven Press, New York, pp 489–512
11. Corsico N, Tirone P (1987) EEG studies in the conscious unrestrained rat: a tool for a study of immediate and delayed neurotoxicity of contrast media. In: Calabrò A, Leonardi M (eds) Computer aided neuroradiology. CIC Edizioni Internazionali, Rome, pp 255–258
12. Artru AA, Stout D, Katz RA, Freund PR (1990) EEG suppression and Increased Blood-Brain Barrier permeability following intracarotid injection of Iothalamate Meglumine (Conray) in dogs. J Neurosurg Anesthesiol 2:105–113
13. McCullough M, Davies P, Richardson R (1989) A large trial of intravenous Conray 325 and Niopam 300 to assess immediate and delayed reactions. Br J Radiol 62:260–265
14. Provinciali L, Signorino M, Giovagnoli AR, Baroni M, Angeleri F, Salvolini U, Pasquini U (1988) Lumbar myelography with iopamidol: a methodological approach to the investigation of side effects. Neuroradiology 30:528–533

Iometrol: a neuropharmacological profile

A. La Noce, F. Demicheli, I. Filatori, L. Miragoli, P. Tirone

Bracco SpA, Pharmacology Department, Via E. Folli, 50, I-20134 Milan, Italy

Abstract. Iomeprol is a new nonionic monomeric contrast medium for intravascular use. This study assesses its neurological safety. First, microdialysis experiments have shown that small amounts of iomeprol can be detected in the cerebrospinal fluid (CSF) following the intravascular administration of the compound without any apparent damage to the blood-brain barrier. Secondly, no significant changes in the normal parameters of visual-evoked potentials or in the basal levels of several neurotransmitters have been observed following direct administration of iomeprol to the rat's nervous system. It is concluded that iomeprol is highly neurotolerable, possibly because of its low molecular toxicity.

Key words: Contrast media – Blood-brain barrier – Neurotoxicity

Correspondence to: A. La Noce

Mild neurological adverse effects are occasionally observed after intravascular administration of nonionic iodinated contrast media (CM). In subjects with impaired blood-brain barrier (BBB) intregrity, CM are likely to reach the nervous tissue after intravenous injection. When injected into the carotid artery, some nonionic CM have been reported to induce a disruption of the BBB [1]. Thus, regardless of the intravascular route of administration, CM can come into direct contact with nervous structures, and perhaps exert a chemotoxic action on neurological functions.

For this reason the neurological safety of iomeprol has been carfully evaluated. In the first part of the study, the passage of iomeprol through the BBB was investigated. Following intracarotid or intravenous injection in rats, the concentration of iomeprol in the CSF was measured by means of a microdialysis probe implanted into the lateral ventricle. Penetration into the brain tissue following intracisternal injection in dogs was assessed by CT. Finally, the neurological effects of administering iomeprol

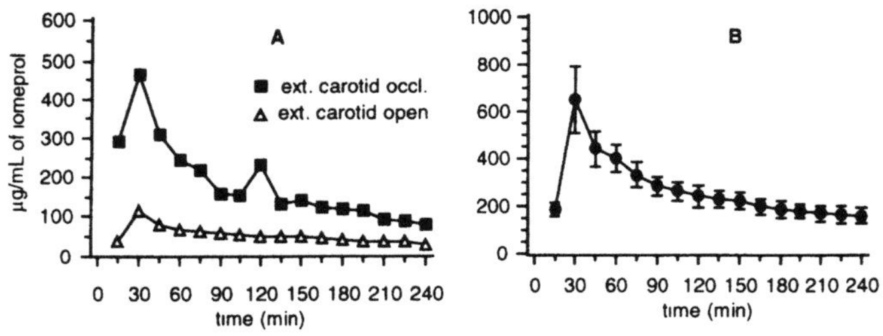

Fig. 1. Concentration of iomeprol in the cerebrospinal fluid following intracarotid (*A*; $n = 3$ for each group) or intravenous (*B*; $n = 10$) administration. *Bars* represent standard errors of the mean. The values were corrected for the "relative loss" of iomeprol through the probe, measured in vivo

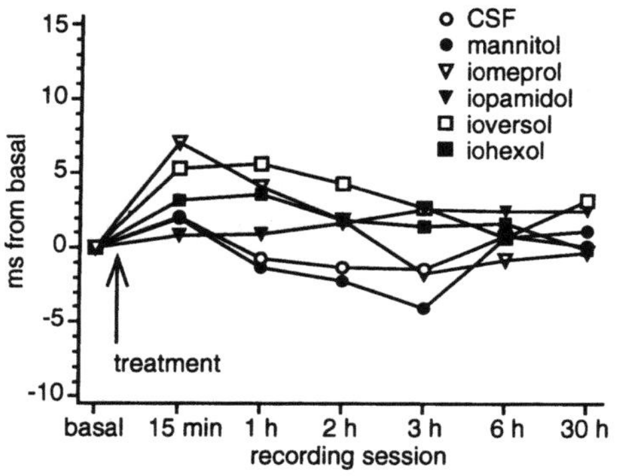

Fig. 2. Mean differences of P1 peak latency of visual evoked potentials with respect to basal mean value for the contrast media indicated

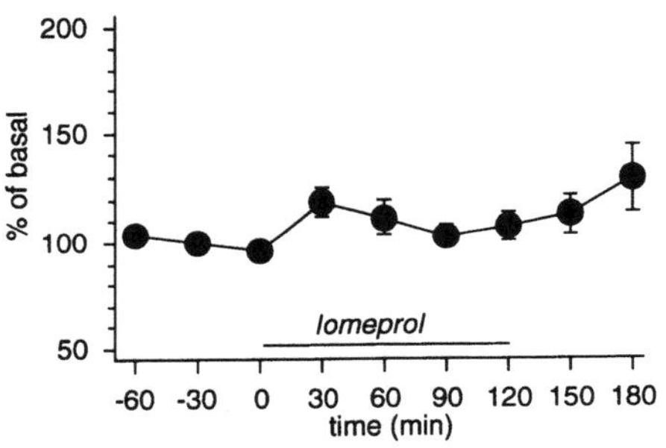

Fig. 3. Mean changes in dopamine levels following administration of iomeprol into the corpus striatum. Values are expressed as a percentage of the baseline levels. *Bars*, standard errors of the mean. The *line* indicates the period of iomeprol administration

directly to the central nervous system were investigated by recording visual-evoked potentials and by measuring the levels of a number of neurotransmitters in vivo.

In each experiment the concentration of iomeprol was 300 mg (iodine)/ml.

Methods

To study the passage of iomeprol through the BBB, a concentric microdialysis probe was inserted into the lateral ventricle of anaesthetised (sodium pentobarbital, 30 mg/kg i.p) rats. Iomeprol

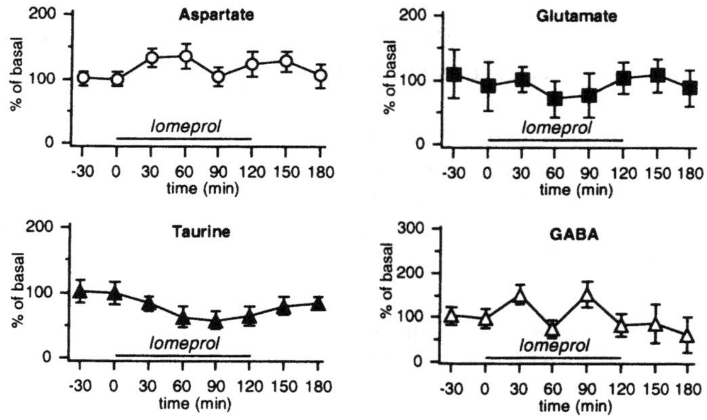

Fig. 4. Mean changes of the levels of amino acid indicated following administration of iomeprol into the hippocampus. Values are expressed a percentage of the corresponding baseline levels. *Bars*, standard errors of the mean. The *line* indicates the period of iomeprol adminstration

was injected into the common carotid artery [600 mg (iodine)/kg] with the external carotid open or occluded, or into the caudal vein [5 g (iodine)/kg]. Dialysate samples (7.5 µl) were collected at 15-min intervals for 4 h after injection. The concentration of iomeprol in the dialysate samples was measured by HPLC coupled with UV detection. In some rats damage to the BBB as results of i.c. or i.v. iomeprol adminstration was verified by injecting a 2% (w/v) solution of Evans' blue (3 ml/kg).

Brain tissue penetration was studied by serial CT performed 1–24 h after intracisternal injections to anaesthetised dogs of 50 mg (iodine)/kg of one of the following CM: iomeprol, iopamidol, or ioversol.

Pattern visual-evoked potentials (PVEP) were recorded in conscious rats with chronic implants of epidural electrodes in the cerebral cortex and with a cannula in the lateral ventricle, following intraventricular administration of 100 mg (iodine)/kg of iomeprol. Recordings were taken from 15 min to 30 h after CM administration. Iopamidol, iohexol and ioversol were used as reference compounds in different groups of rats.

The levels of dopamine in the striatum and of glutamate, aspartate, taurine and GABA in the hippocampus were measured in freely moving rats with chronic implants with a microdialysis probe in one of the above cerebral regions. A solution of iomeprol in the CSF [20 mg (iodine)/ml], isosmolal to the CSF, was adminstered locally through the probe for 60 min. All neurotransmitters were measured by HPLC coupled to electrochemical detection.

Results

The concentrations of iomeprol found in the lateral ventricle following i.c. or i.v. injection of iomeprol are illustrated in Fig. 1 A, B, respectively. The concentration peaked in the second dialysate sample, collected from 15 to 30 min after injection. It can be noted that, following intracarotid injection, the CSF concentrations of iomeprol were considerably higher when the external carotid artery was occluded. However, injection of Evans's blue to control rats that received the same dose of iomeprol, revealed no damage to the BBB.

CT in dogs gave comparable results for all CM. The CM penetrated maximally into the brain tissue surrounding the fluid spaces between the 4th and 6th hours, as indicated by the Hounsfield numbers recorded in selected brain areas. Complete recovery was not achieved within 24 h of the injection of the CM.

For PVEP recording, the most prominent result concerned the latency of the P1 peak of the response. A significant difference ($P < 0.05$) from controls was found for the P1 delay of the ioversol group, although all groups of rats treated with a CM exhibited a variable increase in P1 latency 15 min after treatment (Fig. 2).

Brain microdialysis did not reveal any significant changes in the basal levels of the analysed neurotransmitters after local administration of iomeprol, as illustrated in Figs. 3 and 4.

Discussion

We have shown that intravascularly administered iomeprol can enter the CSF of rats without there being any apparent damage to the BBB. However, only low liquoral concentrations were attained with high doses of the compound. Evans' blue injection demonstrated that no gross disrupture of the BBB occurred after intracarotid or intravenous iomeprol administration. This result is at variance with other nonionic or dimeric CM [2]. It is likely that slight, localised BBB damage was present or that only a slight passage of iomeprol at the blood CSF interface occurred. The CT study demonstrated that iomeprol, like the other CM, penetrates into the brain parenchyma when injected into the liquoral space.

These results confirm that the neurotoxicity of CM needs special attention, even when the CM is intravascular administered to patients whose BBB is apparently unimpaired.

PVEP is a sensitive indicator of the neurotoxicity of a broad range of substances in animals and humans [3]. In this study, iomeprol did not produce important modifications of the PVEP after direct administration into the CSF at high doses. A significant effect of ioversol on P1 latency was observed. This result is of particular interest, considering that the P1 peak in rats closely corresponds to the P100 peak in humans [4]. The P100 peak is the PVEP parameter most commonly considered clinically. Finally, a solution of iomeprol isosmolal to the CSF and administered directly into the brain tissue, did not change the basal levels of several neurotransmitters involved in epileptogenesis.

In conclusion, the above studies have demonstrated that iomeprol, in addition to a good systemic tolerability (5), also exhibits a high level of neurotolerability, comparable to those of myelographic CM. This can be attributed to its low molecular toxicity, as indicated by the results of measurements on neurotransmitter concentrations in which only chemotoxicity is assessed, and to its formulation possessing favourably low values for osmolality and viscosity.

References

1. Wilson AL, Evill CA, Sage MR (1991) Effects of nonionic contrast media on the blood-brain barrier. Invest Radiol 26:1091–1094
2. Wilcox J, Evill CA, Sage MR (1986) Effects of intracarotid ionic and non-ionic contrast material on the blood-brain barrier in a rabbit model. Neuroradiology 28:271–274
3. Mattson JL, Albee RR (1988) Sensory evoked potentials in neurotoxicology. Neurotoxicol Teratol 10:435–443
4. Hudrell HK, Boyes WK (1991) The comparability of rat and human visual-evoked potentials. Neurosci Biobehav Rev 15:159–164
5. Rosati G (1994) Clinical pharmacology of iomeprol. Eur J Radiol 18 [Suppl 1]:S51–S60
6. Gallotti A, Uggeri F, Favilla A, Cabrini M, De Haen C (1994) The chemistry of iomeprol and physico-chemical properties of its aqueous solutions and phamaceutical formulations. Eur J Radiol 18 [Suppl 1]:S1–S12

Ioxaglate in cerebral angiography: clinical safety, tolerability and efficacy of premedication with atropine

M. Ochi[1], A. Ogino[1], K. Hayashi[1], A. Yasunaga[2], S. Shibata[2]

[1] Department of Radiology, Nagasaki University School of Medicine, Japan
[2] Department of Neurosurgery, Nagasaki University School of Medicine, 1-7-1 Sakamoto, Nagasaki 852, Japan

Abstract. This study looked at 223 consecutive cerebral angiograms to investigate the clinical safety and tolerability of ioxaglate and the efficacy of premedication with atropine. Ioxaglate induced mild adverse reactions (nausea, vomiting and urticaria) in 3.6% of patients premedicated with atropine and in 5.4% of patients who did not receive atropine. There was no significant difference between the two groups in the incidence of adverse reactions. However, the incidence of nausea and/or vomiting (1.3%) was lower than previously reported. Ioxaglate retains anticoagulant potency, and the incidence of ioxaglate-induced reactions appears to be acceptably low. Ioxaglate is considered suitable for cerebral angiography, especially when systemic heparinisation is undesirable.

Key words: Ioxaglate - Cerebral angiography - Contrast media - Complications

In cerebral angiography, selection of the contrast medium is important for clinical safety, especially with regard to thromboembolic complications. The potential for thrombotic complications is higher with nonionic than with ionic contrast agents [1]. The contrast agent should be an anticoagulant, especially when systemic heparinisation is undesirable. Ioxaglate is an ionic dimer and retains anticoagulant potency [2]. However, with increasing anticoagulant potency, contrast agents also become more chemotoxic [3]. We evaluated the clinical safety, tolerability, and efficacy of atropine as premedication before cerebral angiography with ioxaglate.

Patients and methods

Between January 1990 and October 1993, 230 consecutive patients underwent cerebral angiography with ioxaglate for diagnosis or as a neuroinventional procedure in our institution. These included 7 patients who received steroids before examination and were then excluded from this study. We studied 223 (92 male and 131 female) patients aged 10 months to 86 years (mean 51.7 years), with body weight from 9 to 87 kg (mean 55.3 kg). The main clinical indications for cerebral angiography were known or suspected brain tumours and cerebrovascular diseases. Patients who underwent emergency cerebral angiography for evaluation of an acute subarachnoid haemorrhage were also included this study. These included 27 patients who had a history of allergy: 3 had a history of adverse reaction to contrast media, 2 had asthma, 1 had both asthma and drug allergy, 1 had both asthma and food allergy, 7 had allergies to drugs other than contrast media, 9 had food allergies, 1 had food and drug allergy, 2 had atopy and 1 had allergic rhinitis.

Correspondence to: M. Ochi

Table 1. Characteristics of the patients and volumes of contrast medium injected

	Patients premedicated with atropine (186)	Patients premedicated without atropine (37)
Number of men/women	81/105	11/26
Age (years)		
Range	0–86	7–80
Mean	51.0	55.6
Weight (kg)		
Range	9–87	23–70
Mean	55.6	53.5
Contrast medium volume (ml)		
Range	10–250	10–120
Mean	82.8	75.6

The examination procedure consisted of carotid and/or vertebral angiography with a femoral approach. Most examinations were performed on a high-definition digital subtraction angiography system, using a 5-F heparin-coated catheter. The total volumes of ioxaglate injected were 10–250 ml (mean 81.6 ml). Of 223 patients, 112 (50.2%) underwent angiography without systemic heparinisation.

Of the 223 patients, 186 received atropine, with or without diazepam and/or pentazocine, before examination. These were 81 males and 105 females, aged between 10 months and 86 years (mean 52 years). The remaining 37 patients underwent angiography without previous administration of atropine. They included 11 male and 26 female patients, aged between 7 and 80 years (mean 56). Differences between these two groups in age range, body weight and total volume of contrast medium injected were not significant (Table 1).

Subjective discomfort, such as the sensation of warmth and vascular pain induced by contrast medium injection were reported by patients at the end of the procedure. Patients under general anaesthesia or markedly sedated were excluded from this assessment of subjective events. The adverse clinical reactions, clinical safety, tolerability and image quality were assessed by the referring neurosurgeons and neuroangiographers. All patients were monitored closely in the neurosurgical department and followed for at least 24 h after the angiographic procedure.

Results

All angiograms were of good quality. Frequency and intensity of injection-induced discomfort, pain, and sensation of warmth, are summarised in Table 2. Almost half the patients felt a sensation of warmth during the contrast injection. The intensity of warmth sensation was mild to moderate. Eighteen of 170 patients (10.6%) felt mild to

Table 2. Injection-induced discomfort in 170 patients[a]

	None	Mild	Mod-erate	Severe
Pain during injection	152	16	2	0
Sensation of warmth	89	75	6	0

[a]Patients examined under general anaesthesia or markedly sedated were excluded

Table 3. Contrast medium-related adverse reactions

	Urticaria	Nausea	Vomiting
Patients premedicated with atropine	5 (2.6%)	1 (0.5%)	1 (0.5%)
Patients premedicated without atropine	2[a] (5.4%)	0	1[a] (2.7%)

[a]One patient had both urticaria and vomiting

moderate pain. None of the patients experienced severe injection-related discomfort. Adverse reactions other than discomfort are presented in Table 3. Among the 186 patients premedicated with atropine, 5 (2.6%) had urticaria, 1 (0.5%) experienced nausea, and 1 (0.5%) experienced vomiting. Among the patients not premedicated with atropine, 2 patients (5.4%) experienced urticaria, and 1 (2.7%) of these 2 also experienced vomiting. There were no significant differences between the patients who received atropine and those who did not receive atropine in the incidence of adverse reactions. None of the patients in this study experienced severe adverse reactions.

Discussion

In cerebral angiography, selection of the contrast medium is important for clinical safety, especially in thromboembolic complications. Numerous in vivo studies suggest that the potential for thrombotic complications is greater with nonionic than with ionic contrast agents [4]. A scanning electron microscopy study revealed clot formations in the catheters of patients who received nonionic low osmolar contrast media, while no coagulation process was found in the catheters of patients who received ioxaglate [5]. If nonionic contrast agents are used, anticoagulation can be achieved by systemic heparinisation. However, systemic heparinisation is undesirable in patients with acute bleeding (e.g., subarachnoid haemorrhage). The ionic low osmolar contrast medium (ioxaglate) markedly inhibited thrombus growth, whereas all nonionic low osmolar contrast media (iopamidol, ioprmide and iohexol) promoted thrombus growth [6]. This anticoagulant activity of ioxaglate is an excellent property for cerebral angiography.

However, injection-induced discomfort, nausea, vomiting, and urticaria were more common with ioxaglate than with nonionic low osmolar contrast media [7]. Although the incidence of ioxaglate-related adverse events in cerebral angiography was reported to be 27% [8], the incidence of adverse reactions in our patients (4%) seemed to be acceptably low.

In our series, there were no significant differences seen between patients reveiving atropine and those not receiving atropine in the incidence of mild adverse reactions (nausea, vomiting, and urticaria). Unfortunately, the reason for the lower incidence of mild adverse reactions in our study is still not clear. There were no serious adverse events during our study. Although the number of patients in this study was too small to assess the statistical analysis of severe adverse reactions, none of our patients experienced severe side effects.

In summary, ioxaglate induced mild adverse reactions in 4% of our patients. The incidence of nausea and/or vomiting (1.3%) appeared to be acceptably low. All of them were transient and no serious events occurred in our study. The use of ioxaglate for cerebral angiography seems to be appropriate, especially when systemic heparinisation is undesirable. Because of the small size of our study, further studies are necessary to confirm the results.

References

1. Fareed J, Walenga JM, Saravia GE, Moncada RM (1990) Thrombogenic potential of nonionic contrast media? Radiology 174:321–325
2. Kopko PM, Smith DC, Bull BS (1990) Thrombin generation in nonclottable mixture of blood and nonionic contrast agents. Radiology 174:459–461
3. Dawson P (1993) The clotting issue: etiologic factors in thromboembolism. 1. Chemistry, pharmocology, and toxicity of angiographic contrast agents. Invest Radiol 28:S25–S30
4. Piessens JH, Stammen F, Vrolix MC, Glazier JJ, Benit E, De Geest H, Willems JL (1993) Effects of an ionic versus a nonionic low osmolar contrast agent on the thrombotic complications of coronary angioplasty. Cathet Cardiovasc Diagn 28:99–105
5. Casalini E (1992) Role of low-osmolality contrast media in thromboembolic complications: scanning electron microscopy study. Radiology 183:741–744
6. Levi M, Biemond BJ, Sturk A, Heok J, ten Cate JW (1991) Variable effects of radiological contrast media on thrombus growth in a rabbit jugular vein thrombosis model. Thromb Haemost 66:218–221
7. Brismar J, Jacobsson BF, Jorulf H (1991) Miscellaneous adverse effects of low- versus high-osmolarity contrast media: a study revised. Radiology 179:19–23
8. Palmers Y, DeGreel D, Grynne BH, Smits J, Put E (1993) A double-blind study comparing safety, tolerability and efficacy of iodixanol 320 mgI/ml and ioxaglate 320 mgI/ml in cerebral arteriography. Eur J Radiol 17:203–209

Intracranial haemodynamic changes during injection of contrast medium in carotid and vertebral angiography

S. Iwasaki[1], H. Nakagawa[1], T. Taoka[1], A. Fukusumi[1], M. Nakane[1], H. Ohishi[2], H. Uchida[1], M. Takeshima[3], T. Morimoto[3], J. Sakaki[3]

[1] Department of Radiology, Nara Medical University, Nara, Japan
[2] Department of Oncoradiology, Nara Medical University, Nara, Japan
[3] Department of Neurosurgery, Nara Medical University, Nara, Japan

Abstract. The purpose of this study was to study changes in intracranial arterial pressure during contrast injection for angiography. Fifteen arteries in 13 patients undergoing angiography for chemotherapy (11 patients) and for embolization of arteriovenous malformations (AVM) (2 patients) were examined with permission. The arterial pressure was measured through a Tracker 18 catheter inserted into the basilar artery or to the top of the internal carotid artery. The contrast medium was injected at 9 ml/1.5 s via a 5.5-F catheter or a 7-F guiding catheter placed at the orifice of the vertebral or internal carotid artery. During the injection of contrast medium no peak of a shock wave was detected. Pressure elevation during the injection was 5 mm Hg (mean) in both the systolic and the diastolic pressure in the top of the internal carotid atery, and 3 mm Hg systolic and 7 mm Hg diastolic in the basilar artery. The result proved directly that in man the injection of contrast medium exerts only a minimally harmful influence on aneurysms around the circle of Willis.

Key words: Cerebral angiography – Blood pressure – Contrast medium – Aneurysm

The purpose of this study is to look at changes caused in arterial pressure in the basilar artery and the top of the internal carotid artery, by the injection of contrast medium for angiography. The study consisted of two parts:

I. Experimental: the reliability of a microcatheter in measuring pressure was studied using an experimental system.
II. Clinical: the pressure was measured in patients through a microcatheter inserted into the basilar artery and the top of the internal carotid artery during angiography.

Materials and methods

I. Experimental. Measurement of pressure through a microcatheter (Tracker 18) and the direct measurement were compared with regard to a shock wave and a portion of elevated plateau following the shock wave, using an experimental system filled with water (Fig. 1).

II. Clinical Fifteen arteries in 13 patients undergoing angiography for chemotherapy or embolisation of an arteriovenous malformation (Table 1) were examined with informed consent.

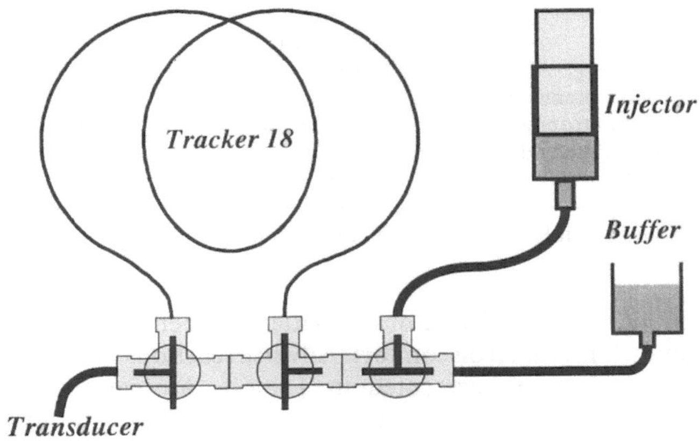

Fig. 1. Experimental system to assess the reliability of a microcatheter for measuring pressure

Table 1. Distribution of patients

Case	Age (years)	Sex	Pathology
1	21	M	Glioblastoma
2	22	F	Arteriovenous malformation
3	28	F	Glioblastoma
4	37	M	Glioblastoma
5	40	M	Glioblastoma
6	41	F	Glioblastoma
7	43	F	Glioblastoma
8	46	F	Metastasis
9	60	M	Arteriovenous malformation
10	61	M	Anaplastic astrocytoma
11	61	F	Glioblastoma
12	62	F	Astrocytoma
13	44	F	Pineal tumour

The arterial pressure was measured through a Tracker 18 catheter inserted into the basilar artery or to top of the internal carotid artery. Contrast medium was injected, 9 ml/1.5 s, via a 5.5-F catheter or a 7-F guiding catheter placed at the orifice of the vertebral of the internal carotid artery. The contrast medium was 300 mgI/dl iopamidol warmed to body temperature.

Results

Experimental

A small peak of a shock wave could be detected through the Tracker 18 catheter, but the value measured at the large peak was lower than that obtained by direct

Correspondence to: S. Iwasaki

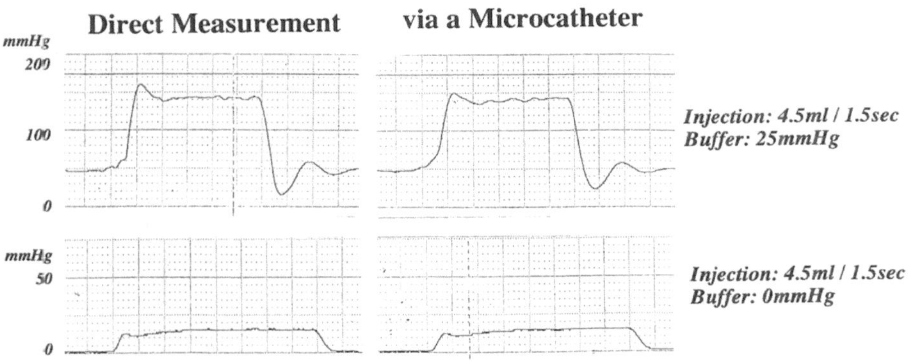

Fig. 2. Pressure tracings obtained through the experimental system

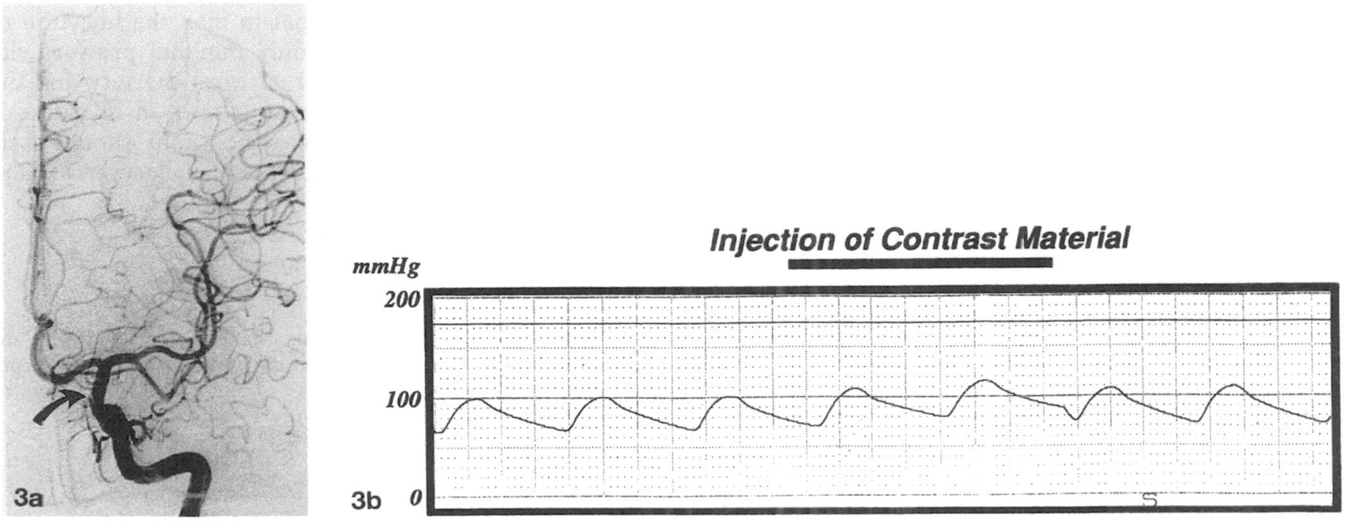

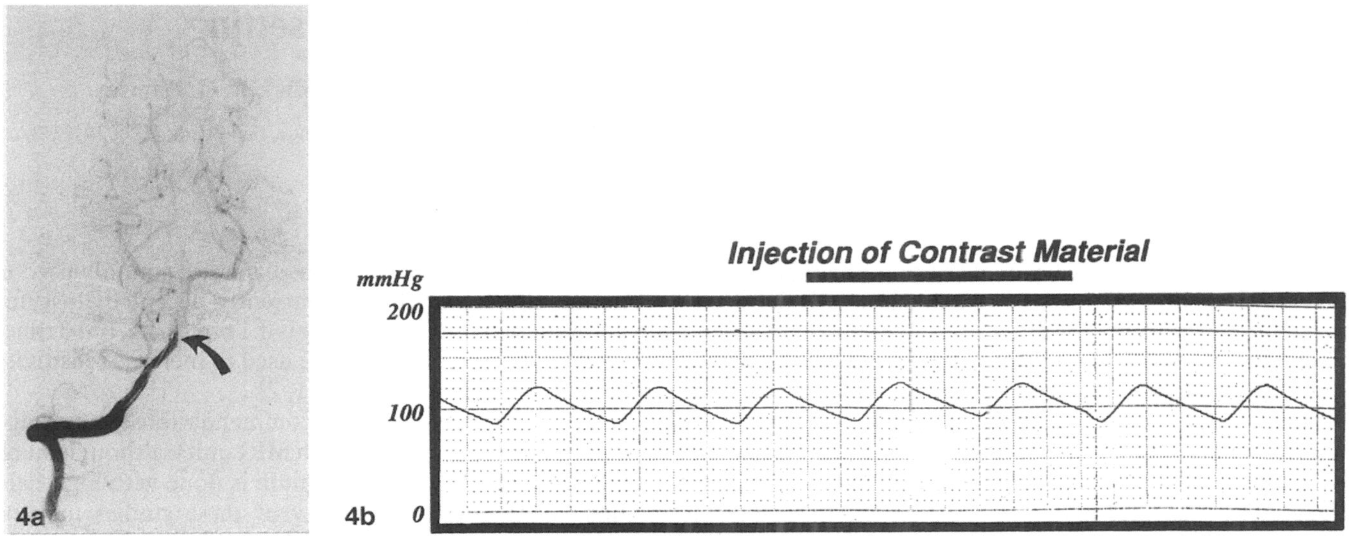

Fig. 3a, b. Case 6. **a** Left internal carotid angiogram during measurement of arterial pressure. The tip of the microcatheter is visible (*arrow*). **b** Pressure tracing obtained through the microcatheter shows 101/66 (mean mmHg; systolic/diastolic) before and 14/11 (maximum mmHg; systolic/diastolic) elevation during injection. *Bar*, injection of contrast medium (9 ml/1.5 s)

Fig. 4. a Vertebral angiogram during measurement of arterial pressure. The tip of the microcatheter is visible (*arrow*). **b** Pressure tracing obtained through the microcatheter shows 122/85 (mean mmHg; systolic/diastolic) before and 3/7 (maximum mmHg, systolic/diastolic) elevation during injection. *Bar*, injection of contrast medium (9 ml/1.5 s)

Table 2. Arterial pressure in the distal internal carotid (cases 1–12) and the basilar (case 13) artery, measured via a microcatheter

Case	Age (years)	Resting pressure (mm Hg)		Pressure elevation during injection (mm Hg)	
		systolic	diastolic	systolic	diastolic
1	21	113	86	5	2
2	22	66	59	0	0
		69	64	0	0
3	28	97	79	7	6
4	37	82	75	0	3
5	40	134	89	5	7
6	41	101	66	14	11
7	43	112	82	12	8
8	46	99	92	3	3
		95	90	3	6
9	60	103	78	5	4
10	61	87	63	6	9
11	61	113	65	4	7
12	62	117	85	5	6
mean		99	77	5	5
13	44	122	85	3	7

measurement (Fig. 2). At the plateau portion, no difference was noted between the measurement through the Tracker 18 and direct measurement (Fig. 2).

Clinical

At the top of the internal carotid artery, the systolic pressure was 99 mm Hg (mean) and the diastolic pressure was 77 mgHg (mean) (Table 2).

During the injection of contrast medium no peak of a shock wave was detected. The pressure elevation during the injection was 5 mm Hg (mean), both systolic and diastolic, in the top of the internal carotid artery, and 3 mm Hg systolic and 7 mm Hg diastolic in the basilar artery (Table 2).

Discussion

This study directly proved that in man the injection of contrast medium provokes only minimal pressure elevation at the top of the internal carotid artery and the basilar artery. This result suggests that an injection of contrast medium for cerebral angiography should exert only a minimally harmful influence on aneurysms around the circle of Willis.

Reference

1. Hilal SK (1966) Hemodynamic changes associated with the intra-arterial injection of contrast media. Am J Roentgenol 86:615–633

Field strength and gadolinium enhancement in the clinical setting

J. Prager[1], J. Rosenblum[2], D. Kim[2], G. Karczmar[2], G. Lowe[3], M. M. Tomiak[1]3, D. C. Huddle[1], R. G. Ramsey[1]

[1] Department of Radiology, Evanston Hospital/Northwestern University Medical School, 2650 Ridge Avenue, Evanston, IL 60201, USA
[2] The University of Chicago Hospitals, Chicago, Ill, USA
[3] Stanford University Hospital, Palo Alto, California

Abstract. While the efficacy of gadolinium-based contrast agents in routine MRI has been well described, there has been little exploration of differences in contrast enhancement at differing field strengths. We measured the signal intensity of the nasal mucosa and the thalamus before and after contrast medium administration. Imaging was on 0.1 T and 0.3 T units and two 1.5 T units. Enhancement was found to be greater at the high-field than of the low-field MRI, the mid-field MRI having an intermediate value. Overall, we noted less contrast enhancement at lower field strengths and feel that in appropriate clinical situations, consideration should be given to higher contrast dose, or other means of increasing contrast on infused scans, when low-field MRI units are used.

Key words: Contrast enhancement – MRI – Field strength

Correspondence to: J. Prager

Gadolinium-based contrast media are commonly used in routine clinical MRI. The currently accepted dose for gadolinium in routine imaging is 0.1 mmol/kg, but 3 times this dose, 0.3 mmol/kg, can be used to increase sensitivity for subtle enhancing lesions [1, 2].

Drug company dosage recommendations do not distinguish different field strength MRI units, although much research on the use of gadolinium is done with high field units [3, 4]. The applicability of these studies may be limited, because low- or mid-field MR units are commonly used in the clinically setting and, theoretically, the effects of paramagnetic contrast media may be quite different from those at high field strengths. The most prominent factor is longer T1 relaxation times at higher field strengths, which results in a greater proportional effect of gadolinium than at low field strengths.

This is a retrospective study examining the degree of enhancement on routine examinations. Normal structures with and without a blood-brain barrier (brain paren-

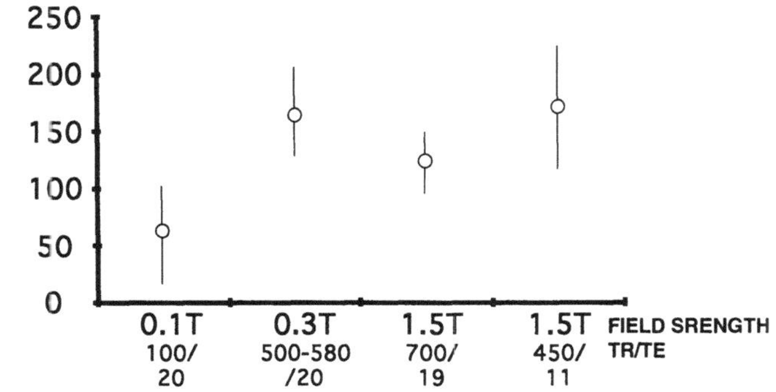

Fig. 1. Percentage enhancement versus field strength on four different MRI units. (CTR, TE in ms)

chyma and nasal mucosa, respectively) were studied with high-, mid-, and low-field MRI and quantitative gadolinium enhancement was compared.

Materials and methods

We randomly selected 33 MRI examinations of the brain with images before and after gadolinium enhancement. Of these studies, 11 were performed at 0.1 T, 6 at 0.3 T 11 on one 1.5 T imager and 6 on another. Gadolinium-DTPA was used at a dose of 0.1 mmol/kg. Images were obtained immediately after contrast medium administration.

T1-weighted axial images were performed before and after infusion using TR/TE 450/11 ms on one 1.5 T unit, TR/TE 700/19 ms on the other TR/TE 520–580/20 ms on the 0.3 unit, and PS3D 100/20 ms on the 0.1 T unit, parameters used routinely in the clinical setting. The 700/19-ms sequence on the second 1.5 T unit was originally selected to optimize the number of slices and the signal-to-noise ratio.

Signal intensity was measured in the thalamus and nasal mucosa, before and after injection using circular regions of interest placed in areas of homogenous signal intensity. The average value of several samples taken within each region of interest was used in calculations; three studies were not included because reliable values could not be obtained.

Enhancement (E) was defined as the change in contrast in a specific tissue following administration of gadolinium using the formula $E = -[M_{Gd}/M)/(T_{Gd}/T)] \times 100$, where M_{Gd}, M = average signal intensity of nasal mucosa with and without gadolinium; and T_{Gd}, T = average signal intensity of thalamus with and without gadolinium.

This formula takes into account tissue contrast before and after gadolinium administration. This is preferable to simple assessment of contrast following infusion (lesion conspicuity), which only takes the end-point of a process into consideration.

Results

Enhancement ranged from 20% to 102% (mean 65.3%) on the low-field magnet and from 103 and 225% (mean 161%) on a high-field unit. This has statistical significance ($P < 0.01$ by the two-tailed t-test). Enhancement ranged from 129% to 206% (mean 158%) on the 0.3 unit. The high-field unit that used heavier T1 weighting had a mean enhancement value of 184%, while the 1.5 T unit that used relatively less T1 weighting had a mean enhancement value of 135% (Fig. 1).

Discussion

A new technique for quantifying contrast enhancement is described, which uses nasal mucosa as a model for tissue with intense enhancement. The nasal mucosa covering the inferior turbinate consists of a thick membrane with a dense venous plexus and large vascular spaces. The thalamus is a homogeneous, easily measured structure and can be used to assess background enhancement in areas of the brain with an intact blood-brain barrier.

Enhancement of tissue without a blood-tissue barrier at 1.5 T was more than twice that at 0.1 T in this study. As expected, at 1.5 T a decrease in T1 weighting (TR 700 ms) resulted in lower mean enhancement values than at TR 450 ms. The degree of T1 weighting is critical when the mid-field units and the high-field units are compared. The mid-field unit had greater average enhancement values than the high-field unit with less T1 weighting, but lower average values than the high-field unit with greater T1 weighting.

Even with the same dose of gadolinium (0.1 mmol/kg), there are significant differences in enhancement at low-, mid-, and high-field units. This suggests that in the appropriate clinical setting it may be advisable to be more liberal with high-dose gadolinium administration or to use additional means of increasing contrast enhancement, such as magnetization transfer [5, 6].

References

1. Yuh WTC, Engelken JD, Muhonen MG, et al (1992) Experience with high-dose gadolinium MR imaging in the evaluation of brain metastases 13:335–345
2. Mathews VP, King JC, Elster AD, Hamilton CA (1944) Cerebral infarction: effects of dose and magnetization transfer saturation at gadolinium-enhanced MR imaging. Radiology 190:547–552
3. Hudgins PA; Elster AD, Runge VM, Kashanian FK, Goldstein HA (1993) The efficacy and safety of gadopentetate dimeghimine in the evaluation of patients with suspected tumor of the extracranial head and neck. J Magn Reson Imaging 3:345–349
4. Elster AD, Rieser GD (1989) Gadolinium-DTPA-enhanced cranial MR imaging in children: initial clinical experience and recommendations for as use. AJNR 10:1027–1030
5. Tomiak MM, Rosenblum JD, Prager JM, Metz CE (1994) Magnetization transfer: a potential method to determine the age of multiple sclerosis lesions. AJNR 15:1569–1574
6. Prager JM, Rosenblum JD, Huddle DC, Diamond CK, Metz CE (1994) The magnetization transfer effect in cerebral infarction. AJNR 15:1497–1500

Study of gadoteridol comparing single, double and triple doses

Y. Korogi[1], M. Takahashi[1], K. Yamaguchi[2], T. Maehara[3]

[1] Department of Radiology, Kumamoto University, Kumamoto, Japan
[2] Department of Radiology, Yamagata University, Yamagata, Japan
[3] Department of Radiology, Kanto Teishin Hospital, Tokyo, Japan

Abstract. We studied 144 patients with a high suspicion of brain metastases with MRI after an initial injection of 0.1 mmol/kg gadoteridol followed by additional injection of 0.2 or 0.3 mmol/kg gadoteridol. Both lesion detection and lesion contrast increased significantly with an additional dose. The triple was more effective than the double dose. No significant adverse effects were noted. There appear to be advantages to the use of higher doses of gadoteridol in patients with suspected brain metastases.

Key words: Brain neoplasms, magnetic resonance imaging – Magnetic resonance imaging, contrast enhancement – Contrast media, paramagnetic

Gadoteridol, a nonionic, low-osmolality contrast agent, has been developed recently and tested at higher doses. Several studies suggest that gadoteridol can be administered safely at doses up to 0.3 mmol/kg and that increased lesion contrast, delineation, and detection can be attained with such doses [1–4]. The purpose of this study was to evaluate the value of double and triple doses of gadoteridol compared with a single dose in screening for brain metastases.

Materials and methods

We studied 144 cancer patients referred for investigation of possible brain metastases. MRI was performed with both medium-field and high-field strength imagers. T1-weighted images and T2-weighted images were obtained before contrast medium injection, followed by additional injection with serial T1-weighted images. A dose of 0.1 mmol/kg gadoteridol was injected i.v. with imaging, followed by additional injection of 0.1 mmol/kg (/group I, total dosage of 0.2 mmol/kg; 74 patients), or 0.2 mmol/kg (group II, total dosage of 0.3 mmol/kg: 70 patients) with imaging after 15 min. There were 55 men and 19 women with a mean age of 61 years in group I, and 43 men and 27 women with a mean age of 60 years in group II. Image analysis was performed blindly. In the quantitative analysis, contrast ratio was defined as SI (lesion) – SI (normal brain parenchyma adjacent to the lesion) : SI (normal brain parenchyma), where SI is the signal intensity measured. Additional diagnostic information was also evaluated qualitatively.

Results

Four cases in group I and one case in group II were excluded from image analysis. Most patients, i.e. 64 of 70 cases in group I and 58 of 60 in group II, showed presumed metastatic lesions on MRI. In group I, more metastases were seen in 23 of 64 cases (35.9%) after the double dose. In group II, the number of metastases seen was higher after the triple dose in 28 of 58 cases (48.3%). In no case were fewer metastases visualized after the double or triple dose. The total number of lesions detected was improved by 121% and 144% (means) after the double and triple doses, respectively, compared with the single dose (Fig. 1). There was a significant increase in the total number of lesions between the initial and additional doses in both groups. In group II only, new lesions were demonstrated with triple doses in two cases not seen to have any lesions on single dose administration (Fig. 2). After the additional dose there was improved visualisation and definition of lesion borders as additional information. The mean lesion contrast ratios were 0.53 and 0.92 after single and double doses, respectively, and 0.47 and 0.99 after single and triple doses, repectively. The percentage increase in the contrast ratio between the initial and high doses was 173% for group I and 211% for group II ($P<0.01$, t-test).

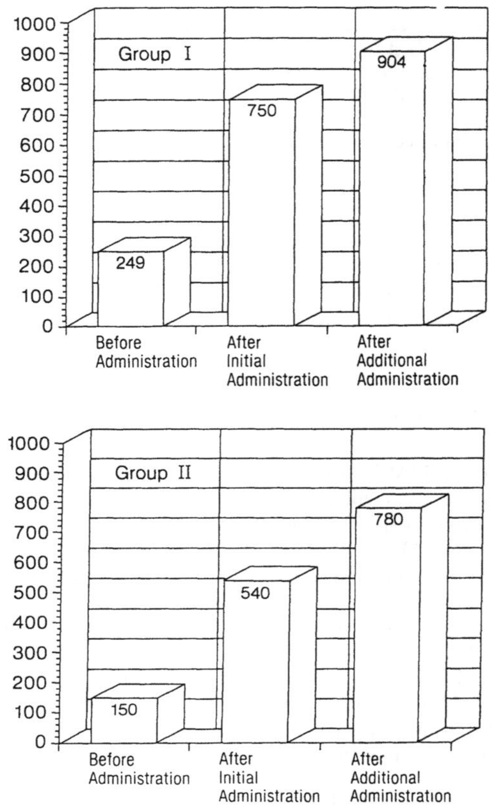

Fig. 1. Total number of lesions identified

Correspondence to: Y. Korogi, Department of Radiology, Kumamoto University School of Medicine 1-1-1, Honjo, Kumamoto City, 860 Japan

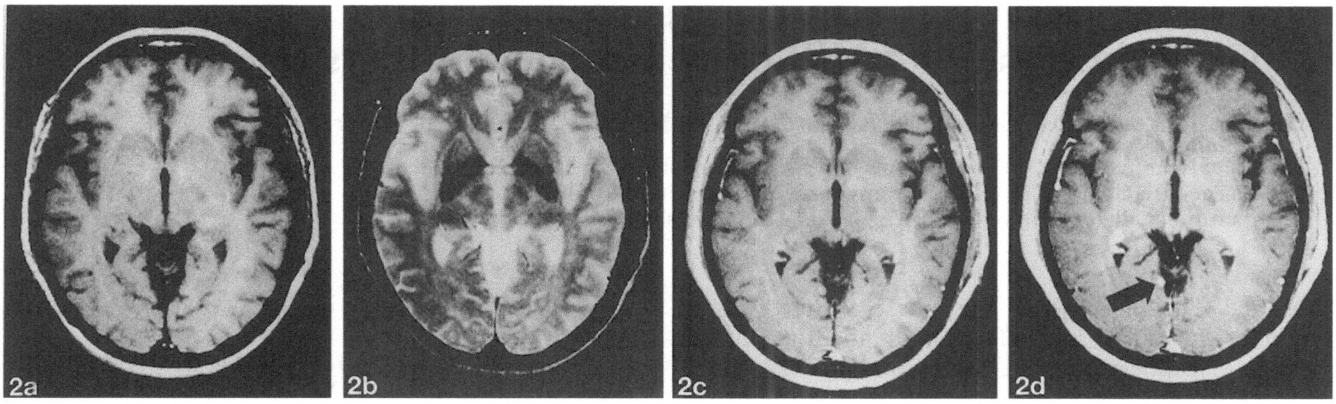

Fig. 2a–d. A 51-year-old woman with lung cancer. **a** Axial T1-weighted (600/15) and **b** T2-weighted (2300/90) images. **c** T1-weighted (600/15) initial-dose and **d** high-dose (0.3 mmol/kg) studies. A small metastasis could be identified only on the high-dose study (*arrow*). In retrospect, there was faint contrast enhancement on the initial-dose study. This lesion was thought to be a solitary metastasis from lung cancer, since no other lesions were demonstrated

Adverse reactions were observed in 2 (2.8%) and 1 (1.4%) cases in groups I and II, respectively. All adverse reactions were mild and required no treatment.

Discussion

Recent studies have shown that central nervous system (CNS) lesions imaged with higher doses of gadolinium exhibit greater enhancement [1–5]. Our results in 144 patients with a clinical suspicion of brain metastases have demonstrated that high-dose (cumulative doses of 0.2 and 0.3 mmol/kg) gadoteridol-enhanced MRI examinations have advantages over 0.1 mmol/kg examinations in detection of early and/or small metastases. After the additional dose, there was a marked qualitative improvement in lesion conspicuity and detection. Quantitative image analysis demonstrated a significant increase in the mean lesion contrast between the initial-dose and high-dose studies. Although both double and triple doses were effective, the study with the triple dose detected more lesions than that with the double dose. Lesion contrast was also significantly higher with the triple dose. All in all, the triple dose may be more appropriate for the detection of suspected brain metastases. The additional information gained by high-dose examinations may lead to improved management of patients with malignancy.

References

1. Runge VM, Kirsch JE, Burke VJ, et al (1992) High-dose gadoteridol in MR imaging of intracranial neoplasms. JMRI 2:9–18
2. Yuh WTC, Engelken JD, Muhonen MG, et al (1992) Experience with high-dose gadolinium MR imaging in the evaluation of brain metastases. AJNR 13:335–345
3. Yuh WTC, Fisher DJ, et al (1992) Review of the use of high-dose gadoteridol in the magnetic resonance evaluation of central nervous system tumors. Invest Radiol 27 (Suppl 1]:39–44
4. Yuh WTC, Fisher DJ, Engelken JD, et al (1991) MR evaluation of CNS tumors. Dose comparison study with gadopentate dimeglumine and gadoteridol. Radiology 180:485–491
5. Haustein J, Laniado M, Niendorf H, et al (1993) Triple-dose versus standard-dose gadopentate dimeglumine: a randomized study in 199 patients. Radiology 186:855–860

Injection of gadoversetamide, a new gadolinium chelate: ultra-high dose usage for MRI of the central nervous system

M. Kuhn[1], H. Youssef[1], R. Grossman[2], K. Maravilla[3], G. Hammer[1], L. Meis[1], J. Underwood[1]

[1] Division of Neuroradiology, Southern Illinois University School of Medicine, Springfield, Ill, USA
[2] Department of Radiology, University of Pennsylvania Philadelphia, Pa., USA
[3] Department of Radiology, University of Washington, Seattle, Wash., USA

Abstract. The objective of this phase II study was to evaluate the safety and effectiveness and the optimal dosage of gadoversetamide. Eighty-one patients underwent two complete MRI examinations of the head or spine between 1 and 5 days apart. Each received two different randomized intravenous doses of gadoversetamide, either 0.1, 0.3 or 0.5 mmol/kg. Identical imaging parameters and injection rates were maintained. Baseline and follow-up hematologic and blood and urine chemistry tests were obtained. Vital signs were obtained at predetermined intervals. Seventy-three patients completed the study, for a total of 146 injections. No clincally significant or life-threatening adverse effects were noted, nor were clinically significant changes in vital signs or laboratory values attributable to the contrast agent observed. Gadoversetamide is a new non-ionic gadolinium chelate which, based on these preliminary studies, appears to be safe and effective over a wide range of doses for MRI of the head and spine

Key words: Gadoversetamide – Magnetic resonance imaging – Brain – Spine

This article reports the initial phase II experimental results with high dose (0.3 mmol/kg) as well as ultra high dose (0.5 mmol/kg) injection of gadoversetamide (*N,N′,N″*-bis-(*N*-2-methoxyethyl)carbamoylmethyl)diethylenetriamine-*N,N′,N″*-triacetato)-gadolinium(III), a new nonionic, low osmolar MRI contrast medium similar in its physicochemical characteristics to gadodiamide and gadoteridol [1–7].

Methods and materials

This randomized prospective multicenter, multidose, double-blind study was conducted at six sites. A total of 81 male and female patients (18 years old or older) with suspected central nervous system (CNS) pathology were enrolled, and informed consent was obtained from each. Patients were randomized to receive two unique IV doses of gadoversetamide. The three possible pairs of doses were: 0.1 mmol/kg and 0.3 mmol/kg; 0.1 mmol/kg and 0.5 mmol/kg; and 0.3 mmol/kg and 0.5 mmol/kg. A minimum of 24 h between the two doses was used to allow for adequate washout of gadoversetamide before the second dose. Both doses were administered within a 7-day period, and the patients did not undergo any intervention that would have altered the pathologic process or structural abnormalities between dosing sessions.

All patients were closely observed and monitored for the occurrence of adverse events for 2 h after administration of gadoversetamide and again at 24 h after the injection. Vital signs were obtained immediately before, immediately after, and approximately 1 h and 2 h after IV injection of gadoversetamide for each dose. Analyses of blood and urine samples were performed as a prestudy screen 24 h before each dose, and repeated 24 h after administration of gadoversetamide.

Commercially available MR imagers with field strengths ≥ 0.5 T were used. In each patient both T1- and T2-weighted spin-echo (SE) images were obtained prior to gadoversetamide administration at each session. Post-injection T1-weighted SE images were obtained on each patient within 1 h after gadoversetamide administration with the same imaging parameters as the unenhanced T1-weighted SE images (i.e., same TR and TE, same imaging plane and same slice thickness.)

In each patient, the unenhanced T1- and T2-weighted images were compared with the enhanced images (T1-weighted only) by a single unblinded reader at each study site. The investigator evaluated the following information: whether or not the imaging session was diagnostic; the presence or absence of disease; and added diagnostic information with contrast enhancement. To determine the optimal enhancing dose of gadoversetamide, the principal investigator blindly selected the better diagnostic images obtained from the individual contrast dose comparisons of gadoversetamide using only the form attached in the case report form.

Results

Of the 81 patients enrolled a total of 73 were evaluable (50 brains and 23 spines), giving a total number of 146 injections. In this preliminary data, no serious or life-threatening adverse reactions were reported or observed in the 81 patients participating at the 6 trial centers in this study. Examination of the post-injection vital signs, physical examination, hematology, serum chemistry, and urinalysis compared with the pre-injection data revealed no clinically significant changes that were clearly attributable to the admimistration of gadoversetemide. Grades for heat, cold, and pain were analyzed at the site of injection to see whether they were significantly different from zero. No complaints of heat, cold, or pain at the injection site were reported. A total of 9 patients experienced adverse reactions that were drug related, consisting in: mild rash, metallic taste, mild palpitations, dizziness, headache, chest pressure and whole-body pruritus. Except for the pruritus, which was successfully treated with diphenhydramine hydrochloride, these reactions resolved without intervention.

Correspondence to: M. Kuhn, Southern Illinois University School of Medicine, Department of Radology, 800 East Carpenter Street, Springfield, IL 62769, USA

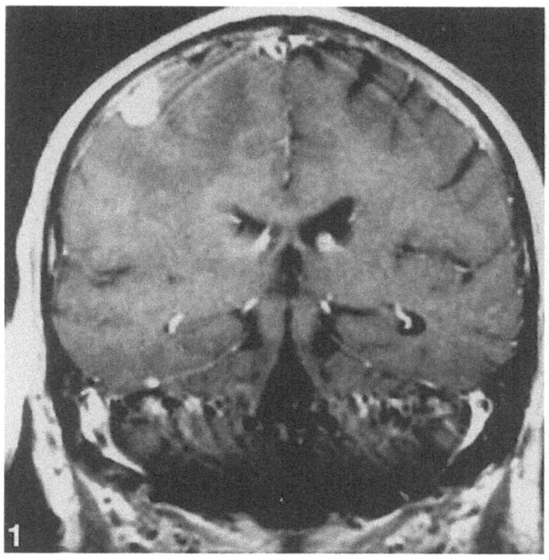

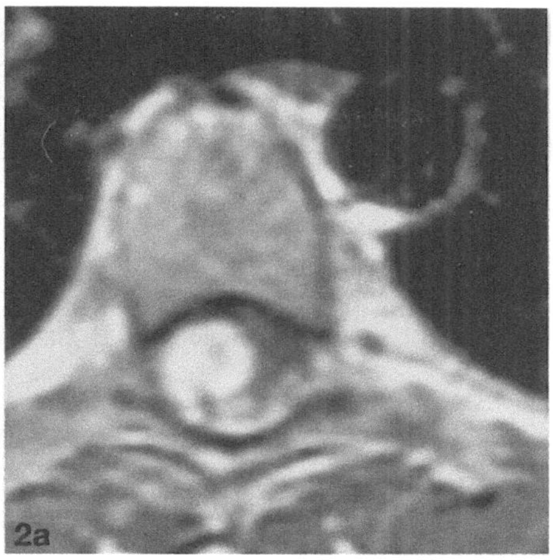

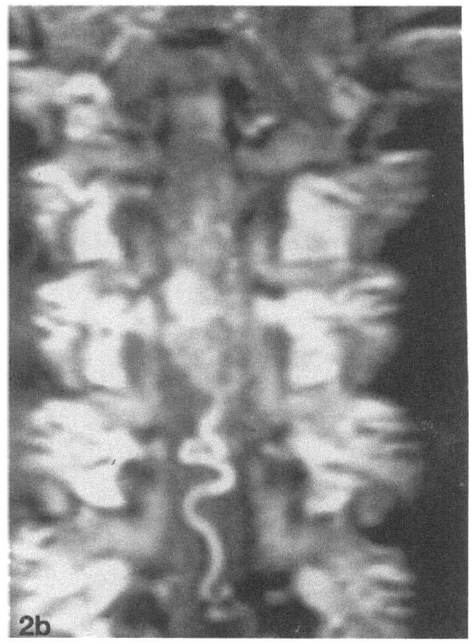

Fig. 1. An 83-year-old woman with a history of carcinoma of the colon. With gadoversetamide administration three metastatic lesions were seen, including this one in the right posterior frontal lobe

Fig. 2a, b. A 28-year-old woman with a past history of hemorrhagic myelitis. Contrast-enhanced images demonstrate a spinal arteriovenous malformation. (**a**) An intensely enhancing, enlarged vessel is well demonstrated on the coronal image (**b**)

Discussion

Gadoversetamide is a new nonionic gadolinium chelate contrast agent, which is reported to demonstrate extracellular fluid space distribution and elimination by glomerular filtration. As this study remains blind, the efficacy of ultra-high-dose (0.5 mmol/kg) gadoversetamide cannot be fully assessed at this time. However, in phase I trials and in this preliminary phase II study, results on the safety of gadoversetamide demonstrate no serious or life-threatening adverse reactions; whether reported or observed, that were attributable to gadoversetamide. No clinically significant changes in blood analysis, urinalysis, physical examination, or vital signs have been reported or observed.

Figures 1 and 2 represent images recorded with gadoversetamide and demonstrating pathology within the central nervous system.

Gadoversetamide appears to be safe at a wide range of doses for MRI examination of the head and spine.

References

1. Vogl TJ, Mack MG, Juergens M, et al (1994) MR diagnosis of head and neck tumors: Comparison of contrast enhancement with triple-dose gadodiamide and standard-dose gadopentetate dimeglumine in the same patients. AJR 163:425–432
2. Sze G, Brant-Zawadski M, Haughton VM, et al (1991) Multicenter study of gadodiamide injection as a contrast agent in MR imaging of the brain and spine. Radiology 181:693–699
3. Wagoner MV, O'Toole M, Quay SC (1990) Nonionic magnetic resonance imaging contrast agents. Clinical trial experience of safety, tolerance, and efficacy of gadodiamide injection. Invest Radiol 25:S39–S41
4. Greco A, McNamara MT, Lanthiez P, Quay SC, Michelozzi G (1990) Gadodiamide injection: nonionic gadolinium chelate for MR imaging of the brain and spine – phase II–III clinical trial. Radiology 176:451–456
5. Yuh TC, Engelken JD, Muhonen MG, Mayr NA, Fisher DJ, Ehrhardt JC (1992) Experience with high-dose gadolinium MR imaging on the evaluation of brain metastases. AJNR 13:335–345
6. Yuh TC, Fisher DJ, Engelken JD, et al (1991) MR evaluation of CNS tumors: dose comparison study with gadopentetate dimeglumine and gadoteridol. Radiology 180:485–491
7. Runge VM, Kirsch JE, Thomas GS (1991) High dose applications of gadolinium chelates in magnetic resonance imaging. Magn Reson Med 22:358–363

Phase III multicenter evaluation of high-dose gadoteridol in neurologic pathology: comparison of 0.1 mmol/kg gadopentetate dimeglumine and 0.3 mmol/kg gadoteridol in patients with lesions of the central nervous system

H. Youssef, M. Kuhn, G. Hammer, L. Meis, T. Burk, T. Pencek

Division of Neuroradiology, Southern Illinois University School of Medicine, 800 E. Carpenter Street, Springfield, IL 62769, USA

Abstract. In this phase III multicenter study, 164 patients with suspected intracranial or spinal pathology underwent magnetic resonance imaging (MRI) to evaluate the safety of gadoteridol as a neurological MR contrast agent and to compare the efficacy of 0.1 mmol/kg of gadopentetate dimeglumine and 0.3 mmol/kg of gadoteridol. One serious adverse event was reported, which resolved spontaneously without residual effects. No other clinically significant changes were noted in laboratory values, vital signs, or physical examination. Comparison of gadopentetate dimeglumine and gadoteridol scans demonstrated visualization of 194 versus 285 brain lesions, respectively ($P = 0.0001$) and 70 versus 77 spine lesions ($P = 0.0625$). A potential change in patient management occurred in 10 patients (7.6%). Data from this study indicate that gadoteridol at a dose of 0.3 mmol/kg yields increased lesion detection and diagnostic information compared with 0.1 mmol/kg of gadopentetate dimeglumine in MRI of intracranial and spinal lesions.

Key words: Gadopentetate dimeglumine – Gadoteridol – Magnetic resonance imaging

Doses up to 0.3 mmol/kg of gadoteridol have been studied, without reports of serious adverse event or laboratory variation [1–14]. On the basis of these data, our study was designed to investigate whether high concentration gadoteridol (0.3 mmol/kg) has a significant influence in the evaluation of pathology within the central nervous system (CNS) when compared with the standard dose examination with gadopentetate dimeglumine (0.1 mmol/kg).

Methods and materials

This phase III open-label study was conducted at 22 sites. We enrolled 164 patients with suspected CNS pathology and from 18 to 85 years of age; their mean age was 49 years. Each patient enrolled was to have had a 0.1 mmol/kg gadopentetate dimeglumine MRI examination not less than 24 h but not more than 7 days, before the 0.3 mmol/kg gadoteridol MRI examination. A single dose of gadoteridol (0.3 mmol/kg) was administered to each patient. Imaging was performed any time up to 1 h after injection of gadoteridol. Each patient was monitored for clinical reactions. Serum chemistry and hematologic analysis and urinalysis were performed.

Correspondence to: M. Kuhn

Results

Safety

A total of 26 adverse events were reported in 16 of the 164 (105%) patients who received gadoteridol. Of these 26 events 25 (96%) were rated by the investigators as mild or moderate in intensity and non-serious in nature. One event (seizure) was considered serious by the investigator. No treatment was given and the event resolved spontaneously.

Of the patients who received gadoteridol, 10 patients (6%) had differences between the results of the physical examination performed before dosing and the examination at the 24 h post-dose evaluation. Vital signs demonstrated no overall age- or sex-related trends that were of clinical significance.

Applying the established laboratory guidelines, we recorded 32 post-dose changes in a total of 25 patients. None of these laboratory changes were considered by the investigator to be clinically significant.

Efficacy

One hundred-and-thirty-one patients (100 brain, 31 spine) with pathology were analyzed for efficacy.

In comparing pre- and post-dose gadoteridol images, the investigator determined that the post-dose images provided additional diagnostic information (improved visualization, definition of lesion borders and number of lesions) for 79 of 100 patients (79%) with brain pathology (Fig. 1) and 21 of 31 patients (68%) with spine pathology. This diagnostic information would have led to a change in MR diagnosis in 12 of 79 patients with brain pathology (15%) and 2 of 21 (10%) with pathology involving the spine. A change in the management/therapy in these patients would have occurred in 13 of 79 patients (16%) with brain pathology and 4 of 21 patients (19%) with spine pathology.

In comparing post-dose gadoteridol images with all pre- and post-dose gadopentetate dimeglumine images for additional information, the investigators determined those post-dose gadoteridol images that provided additional diagnostic information for 55 of 100 patients (55%; 95% CI: 45%, 65%; $P = 0.3150$) with brain pathology and 18 of 31 patients (58%; 95% CI: 41%, 75%; $P = 0.3630$) with pathology involving the spine. This additional diagnostic information would have led to a change in MR diagnosis in 10 of 55 patients (18%) with pathology of the

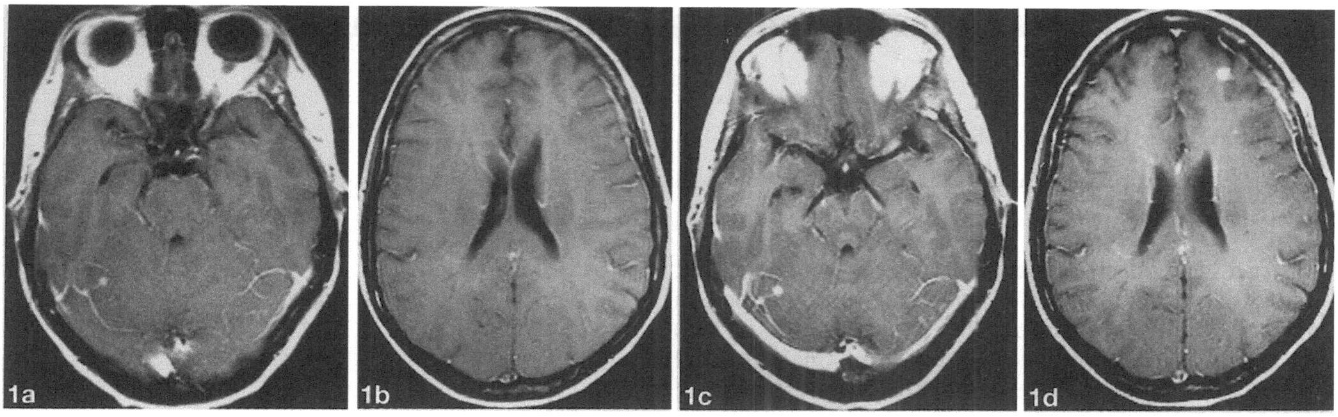

Fig. 1a–d. A 44-year-old woman with cerebral metastases (**a, b**). Images gadopentetate dimeglumine (0.1 mmol/kg) demonstrate a lesion in the right cerebellar hemisphere. After gadoteridol (0.3 mmol/kg) two further lesions are seen with greater clarity (**c, d**). The cerebellar metastasis enhances more with the triple dose. Courtesy of Dr. M. Brant-Zawadski

brain and 2 of 18 patients (11%) with spine pathology. A change in the management/therapy in these patients would have occurred in 7 of 55 patients (13%) with brain pathology and 3 of 18 patients (17%) with pathology of the spine. A statistically significant (sign test, $P = 0.0001$) difference between gadoteridol and gadopentetate dimeglumine was observed in the number of lesions visualized on post-dose brain scans (285 versus 194, respectively).

Discussion

One serious adverse event (seizure) was reported, which resolved spontanously without residual effects. No other serious or life-threatening changes were noted in laboratory values, vital signs, or physical examination. A statistically significant difference between gadoteridol and gadopentetate dimeglumine, favoring gadoteridol, was observed in the number of lesions visible on contrast-enhanced brain images (285 versus 194, respectively). An example of this is shown in Fig. 1. The difference between the number of lesions seen on the gadoteridol and gadopentetate dimeglumine images in patients with spinal pathology also approached statistical significance (77 versus 70 respectively). A potential change in patient management occurred in 10 patients (7.6%).

Our data indicate that gadoteridol at a dose of 0.3 mmol/kg also provides better detection of lesions and more diagnostic information in MRI of intracranial and spinal pathologies than the standard-dose examination with gadopentetate dimeglumine, 0.1 mmol/kg.

References

1. Brant-Zawadski M, Berry I, Osaki L, et al (1986) Gd-DTPA in clinical MR of the brain. I. Intra-axial lesions. AJNR 7:781–788
2. Berry I, Brant-Zwadski M, Osaki L, et al (1986) Gd-DTPA in clinical MR of the brain. II. Extra-axial lesions and normal structures. AJNR 7:789–794
3. Carr DH, Brown J, Bydder GM, et al (1984) Gadolinium-DTPA as a contrast agent in MRI: initial clinical experience in 20 patients. AJR 143:215–224
4. Healy ME, Hesselink JR, Press GA, Middleton MS (1987) Increased detection of intracranial metastases with intravenous Gd-DTPA. Radiology 165:619–624
5. Dillon WP, Norman D, Newton TH, Bolla K, Mark A (1989) Intradural spinal cord lesions: Gd-DTPA-enhanced MR imaging. Radiology 170:229–237
6. Felix R, Schorner W, Laniado M, et al (1985) Brain tumors: MR imaging with gadolinium-DTPA. Radiology 156:681–688
7. Hesselink JR, Healy ME, Press GA, Brahme FJ (1988) Benefits of Gd-DTPA for MR imaging of intracranial abnormalities. J Comput Assist Tomogr 12:266–274
8. Russell EJ, Geremia GK, Johnson CE, et al (1987) Multiple cerebral metastases: detectability with Gd-DTPA-enhanced MR imaging. Radiology 165:609–617
9. Breger MK, Papke RA, Pojunas KW, Haughton VM, Williams AL, Daniels DL (1987) Benign extra-axial tumors: contrast enhancement with Gd-DTPA. Radiology 163:427–429
10. Sze G, Abramson A, Krol G, et al (1988) Gadolinium-DTPA in the evaluation intradural extramedullary spinal disease. AJR 150:911–921
11. Sze G, Krol G, Zimmerman RD, Deck MDF (1988) Intramedullary disease of the spine: diagnosis using gadolinium-DTPA-enhanced MR imaging. AJR 151:1193–1204
12. Runge VM, Gelblum DY, Pacetti ML, Carolan F, Heard G (1990) Gd-HPDO3A in clinical MR imaging of the brain. Radiology 177:393–400
13. Runge VM, Kaufman DM, Woo ML, Adelman LS, Jacobson S (1989) Experimental trials with Gd(DO3A – a nonionic magnetic resonance contrast agent. Nucl Med Biol 16:561–567
14. Yuh WTC, Fisher DJ, Engelken JD, et al (1991) MR evaluation of CNS tumors: dose comparison study with gadopentetate dimeglumine and gadoteridol. Radiology 180:485–491

Effects of Gd-DTPA on dynamic MRI employing gradient-echo pulse sequences

T. Fukuhara, S. Tsuchida, T. Kageyama

Department of Neurological Surgery, Fukuyama Municipal Hospital, 5-23-1 Zaou-cho, Fukuyama, Hiroshima, 721 Japan

Abstract. The effects of Gd-DTPA on gradient-echo MR images a few minutes after injection were analysed in normal subjects. A transient loss in signal intensity was seen only after a double-dose injection on sequential images. From these, three parameters were established: time to bottom (TB), gap of TB compared with the straight sinus (Gap) and ratio of reduction value compared with the straight sinus (RRV). By analogy with dynamic CT, TB may reflect cerebral blood flow, RRV may reflect cerebral blood volume and Gap may show the local changes in cerebral blood flow.

Key words: Flash - Gd-DTPA - Gradient-echo - Magnetic resonance imaging

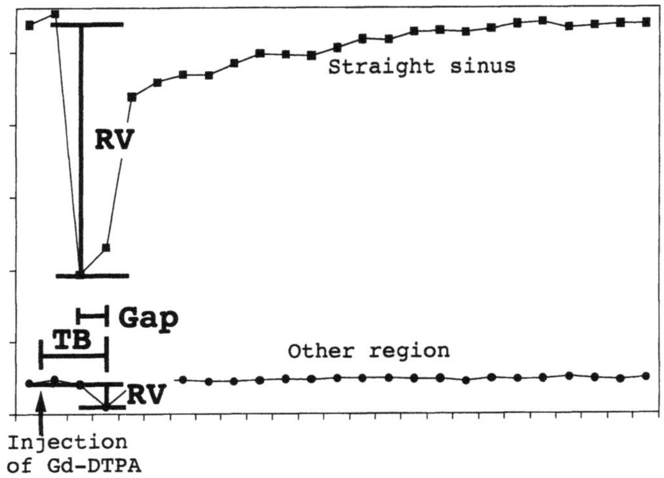

Fig. 1. Time-signal intensity (*SI*) curve of the double-dose group on FLASH images. Reduction in SI was observed 21–31 s after injection. No reduction was seen in the single-dose group. *ACA*, anterior cerebral artery

Although gradient-echo pulse sequences have been used in performance of clinical MRI [1], the effects of Gd-DTPA a few minutes after injection have not been fully analysed. We examined these effects in relation to the cerebral circulation.

Materials and methods

MR images were obtained with a 1.0-T whole-body imaging system. MR images of 25 healthy subjects were examined. Performed pulse sequences were as follows: a T1-weighted image (spin-echo (SE) sequence, TR/TE = 550/15) and a FLASH image (gradient-echo sequence, TR/TE = 33/18, flip angle = 30°). After the first FLASH image had been obtained a compact bolus of Gd-DTPA was injected through an intravenous line placed in the antecubital fossa of the right arm. The subjects were classified into two groups according to the amount of Gd-DTPA injected: 0.1 mmol/kg (single-dose group, $n = 13$) or 0.2 mmol/kg (double-dose group, $n = 12$). At 10 s after the injection, the enhanced FLASH images were obtained successively at a level that included the basal ganglia (total 262 s for 24 FLASH images). The T1-weighted image was then repeated to obtain the contrast-enhanced image. Signal intensity (SI) was taken from several regions of interest (ROI): the anterior cerebral artery (ACA) territory, putamen, internal capsule, thalamus of the right hemisphere and the straight sinus. The enhancement was compared between the final FLASH image and the enhanced T1-weighted SE image at the same level. Statistical comparisons were made using ANOVA.

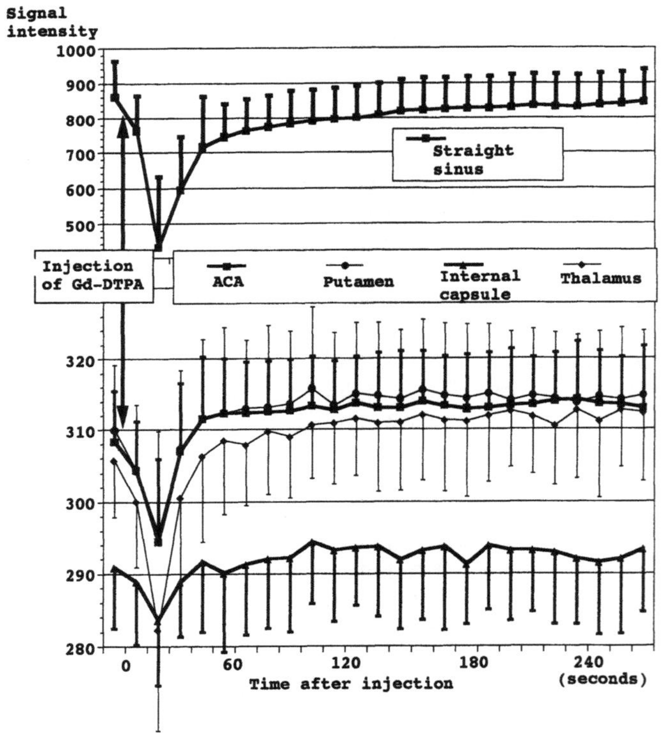

Fig. 2. Parameters obtained from the time-SI curve. *TB*, time to bottom; *Gap*, gap of TB of each region compared with the straight sinus; *RV*, reduction value: difference in SI before injection and at bottom

Results

Comparisons of contrast enhancement between T1-weighted SE and FLASH images appear in Table 1. Contrast enhancement was greater on T1-weighted SE images only in the double-dose group. Figure 1 shows the

Correspondence to: T. Fukuhara

Table 1. Changes in signal intensity (mean ± standard deviation) before and after contrast enhancement

Region of interest	Single-dose						Double-dose					
	FLASH		*F* value	Spin-echo		*F* value	FLASH		*F* value	Spin-echo		*F* value
	before	after		before	after		before	after		before	after	
Anterior cerebral artery	300.0 ±10.7	306.3 ±11.8	15.6*	576.0 ±28.4	603.8 ±24.0	5.2	312.8 ±4.5	317.5 ±5.5	23.9***	570.3 ±22.4	593.8 ±23.5	148.6****
Putamen	316.3 ±6.1	320.5 ±8.8	5.5	627.2 ±27.4	657.2 ±21.7	7.2*	307.8 ±10.0	312.3 ±9.1	5.2	611.7 ±20.4	639.5 ±22.6	36.5***
Internal capsule	297.5 ±6.7	299.2 ±6.7	0.7	572.5 ±19.7	585.8 ±26.1	2.7	290.2 ±9.7	291.8 ±9.9	1.7	544.0 ±20.7	555.5 ±24.6	33.8***
Thalamus	307.5 ±8.5	316.5 ±7.8	12.9*	575.2 ±37.3	622.7 ±15.3	15.2*	303.3 ±10.1	313.2 ±8.7	18.7**	570.3 ±20.2	603.5 ±19.2	59.9****

*$P<0.05$; **$P<0.01$; ***$P<0.005$; ****$P<0.001$

sequential SE change of the double-dose group on FLASH image in each ROI. The SI reduction was seen 21–31 s after the injection in all ROI in the double-dose group; this reduction was not seen in the single-dose group. This reduction was small in the internal capsule and large in the straight sinus. The reduction of each ROI was compared with that of the straight sinus (Fig. 2). Time to bottom (TB), gap of TB of each ROI compared with the straight sinus (Gap) and the ratio of reduction value between each ROI and the straight sinus (RRV) were established. The reduction of SI was judged absent if the reduction value was less than 5. Among 12 subjects in the double-dose group, the TB of the straight sinus was 21–31 s in 9 subjects, 10–20 in 2 subjects and 32–42 in 1 subject. The TB of the ACA, putamen and thalamus was 21–31 s in 9 subjects and 10–20 in 3 subjects. In the internal capsule, TB was absent in 2 subjects, 21–31 s in 6 subjects, 10–20 in 2 subjects and 32–42 in 1 subject. The degree of Gap was divided into three classes: TB shorter than the straight sinus (fast Gap), longer TB (slow Gap) and no Gap. In the ACA, putamen and thalamus, 10 subjects had no Gap and 2 had a fast Gap. In the internal capsule, 9 had no Gap and 1 had a slow Gap. The degree of RRV was divided into five groups; less than 10, 10–20, 20–30, 30–40 and more than 40. In the ACA, 8 had RRV of 20–30 and 4 had 30–40. In the putamen, 7 subjects had RRV of 20–30, 2 had 10–20, 2 had 30–40 and 1 had RRV more than 40. In the internal capsule, 5 had RRV more than 40, 2 had 20–30, 2 had 30–40 and 1 had 10–20 (2 subjects did not have RRV because of a lack of TB). In the thalamus, 5 had RRV of 20–30, 5 had 10–20, 1 had RRV less than 10 and 1 had RRV more than 40.

Discussion

Although the diagnostic results of postcontrast SE and FLASH images have been reported to be equivalent with respect to contrast enhancement [1], gradient-echo images are more sensitive to local magnet field inhomogeneity [2]. This high sensitivity is reported to cause transient SI loss when Gd-DTPA passes through the cerebrovascular system in high concentrations [3]. Some groups have tried to assess cerebral circulation with the FLASH sequence [3, 4]; our work establishes the basic data needed to evaluate cerebral circulation. We analysed three parameters from sequential changes of SI. The concept of these parameters was derived from the functional image of dynamic (FID) CT [5].

According to the theory of FID-CT, TB may reflect cerebral blood flow and RRV may reflect cerebral blood volume. Gap, obtained by comparison with the TB of the straight sinus, may reflect the local difference in cerebral blood flow. These data must now be compared with data from patients affected by pathologic conditions or with other measurements of cerebral blood flow taken simultaneously.

References

1. Schörner W, Sander B, Henkes H, Heim T, Lanksch W, Felix R (1990) Multiple slice FLASH imaging: an improvement pulse sequence for contrast enhanced MR brain studies. Neuroradiology 32:474–480
2. Winkler ML, Ortendahl DA, Hylton NM, Crooks LE, Carlson JW, Kaufman L (1988) Characteristics of partial flip angle and gradient reversal MR imaging. Radiology 166:17–26
3. Edelman RR, Mattle HP, Atkinson DJ, Hill T, Finn JP, Mayman C, Ronthal M, Hoogewoud HM, Kleefield J (1990) Cerebral blood flow: assessment with dynamic contrast-enhanced T2*-weighted MR imaging at 1.5 T. Radiology 176:211–220
4. Houkin K, Kamiyama H, Iwasaki Y, Abe H (1992) Evaluation of cerebral blood circulation using fast magnetic resonance imaging (Turbo-FLASH). Neurol Surg 20:1155–1160
5. Nagata K, Asano T (1989) Early detection of cerebral ischaemia by means of FID-CT (functional image of dynamic CT). Prog CT 11:541–555

Early and delayed MRI of the cranium and lumbosacral spine following augmented dose (0.3 mmol/kg) gadolinium dimeglumine adminstration in clinically normal, asymptomatic subjects

J. R. Jinkins[1], G. T. Gee[1], C. Bazan III[1], R. A. Rauch[1], L. Xiong[1], F. K. Kashanian[2]

[1] The University of Texas Health Science Center San Antonio, TX 78240-7800, USA
[2] Berlex Imaging, Wayne, NJ 07470-7358, USA

Abstract. The purpose of this study was to determine the normal enhancement patterns seen during cranial and lumbosacral MRI at 1.5 T utilizing and augmented dose (0.3 mmol/kg) of intravenous gadopentetate dimeglumine. Several intracranial and intraspinal tissues were seen to enhance in a series of clinically normal, asymptomatic volunteer subjects. These normally enhancing structures included the spinal nerve roots, the petrous segments of the seventh cranial nerve, the leptomeninges, the facet joints, and the intervertebral discs. Recognition of this normal enhancement pattern associated with an expanded gadopentetate dimeglumine dosage is important, since such enhancement after a standard gadolinium contrast medium dosage (0.1 mmol/kg) is generally thought to signify the presence of pathology. In addition, this normal enhancement pattern suggests that use of an expanded contrast dosage in the lumbosacral spine could actually reduce the conspicuity of lesions, by obscuring true pathologic enhancement. Thus, the use of an augmented contrast medium dose may be contraindicated for lumbosacral spine studies in most clinical settings.

Key words: Spine – Magnetic resonance imaging – Cranium – Contrast media, paramagnetic

Correspondence to: J. R. Jinkins, Director of Neuroradiology, The University of Texas Health, Science Center, 7703 F Curl Drive, San Antonio, TX 78240-7800, USA

There is a widespread impression that larger doses of MRI contrast media confer great diagnostic benefit. We set out to explore the effects of triple-dose contrast enhancement of the normal head and spine.

Materials and methods

We carried out a prospective MRI study of 12 volunteer subjects (median age: 25 years), all of whom were clinically normal on neurologic examination. Conventional spin echo T1-weighted (600/20) axial and sagittal MRI of the cranium and lumbosacral spine was performed on each subject a total of three times: prior to contrast medium injection, immediately after administration of 0.3 mmol/kg gadopentetate dimeglumine i.v., and after a delay of 30–60 min. The MR images were then read by an observer blinded to the relationship of contrast administration to the imaging process.

Results

Enhancement of the horizontal and vertical segments and ganglion of the seventh cranial nerve within the temporal bone was observed bilaterally in all 12 volunteers on both immediate and delayed contrast-enhanced images. Sixty-

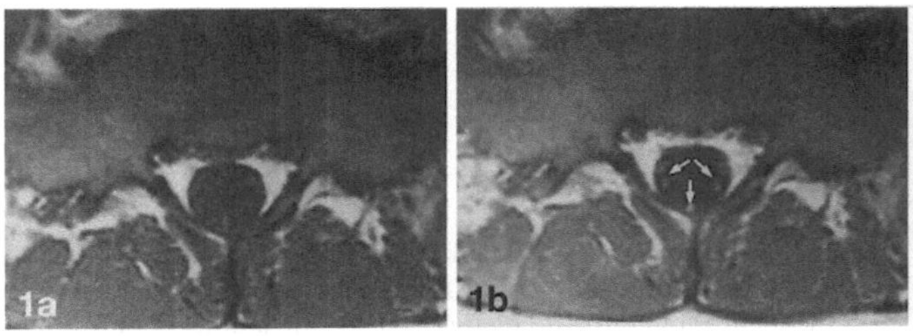

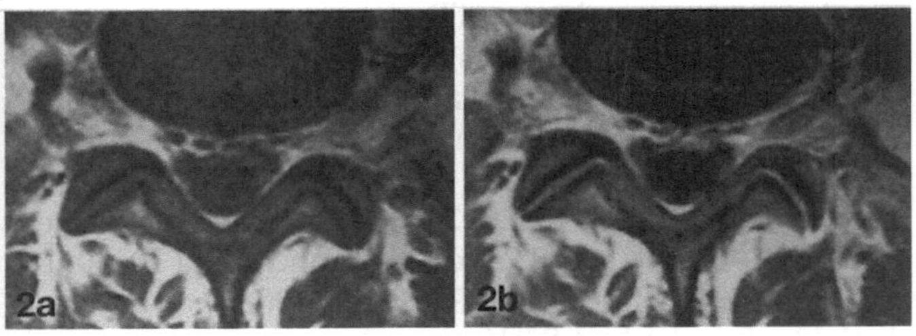

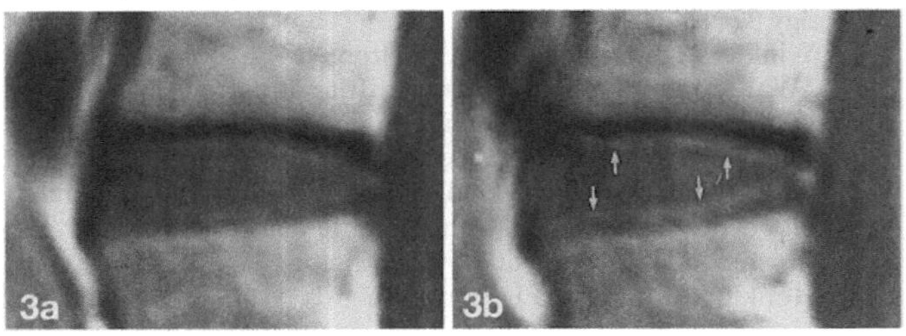

Fig. 1 a, b. Normal lumbosacral nerve root enhancement. **a** Axial T1-weighted (600/20) spin-echo image demonstrates no abnormality. **b** Following administration of 0.3 mmol/kg Gd-DTPA i.v. there is universal nerve root enhancement (*arrows*)

Fig. 2 a, b. Normal lumbosacral face joint enhancement. **a** Axial T1-weighted (600/20) spin echo image at L4-5 demonstrates no abnormality. **b** By 40–60 min after 0.3 mmol/kg Gd-DTPA i.v. there is marked bilateral enhancement of the tissues of the facet joints

Fig. 3 a, b. Normal intervertebral disc enhancement. **a** Sagittal T1-weighted (600/20) spin-echo image through the L4-5 intervertebral disc shows no abnormality. The T2-weighted image also showed normal configuration and intensity. **b** By 40–60 min after 0.3 mmol/kg Gd-DTPA i.v. there is linear intervertebral disc enhancement (*arrows*) paralleling the vertebral endplates, probably reflecting a normal diffusion pattern typical of the nutritional physiology of this tissue

four percent of the subjects demonstrated normal diffuse enhancement of the intrathecal spinal nerve roots in the lumbosacral region on early contrast-enhanced MRI; this frequency rose to 91% on the delayed examination. Other normal postcontrast findings included peripheral intervertebral disc enhancement paralleling the vertebral endplates on the delayed postenhancement images and diffuse facet joint enhancement on both early and delayed studies.

Discussion

In conclusion, 0.3 mmol/kg Gd-DTPA seems to be too large a dose for routine investigation of suspected lumbosacral nerve root, leptomeningeal, intervertebral disc, and face joint disease [1]. The same is true when evaluation of the ganglion and horizontal-vertical segments of the seventh cranial nerve is to be carried out by contrast-enhanced MRI [2]. However, the cisternal and intracanalicular segments of the seventh cranial nerve and the cisternal segments of the remaining cranial nerves, the spinal cord (conus medullaris), and the cerebrum, cerebellum and brainstem visually show no enhancement on either early or delayed imaging at a dose of 0.3 mmol/kg Gd-DTPA i.v. in clinically normal, asymptomatic subjects. Thus, the use of an augmented contrast medium dose in the search for lesions in these latter locations may thus improve conspicuity without the obscuration of lesions by enhancement of normal structures [3, 4].

References

1. Jinkins JR (1993) MR of enhancing nerve roots in the unoperated lumbosacral spine. AJNR 14:193–202
2. Gebarski SS, Telian SA, Niparko JK (1992) Enhancement along the normal facial nerve in the facial canal: MR imaging and antomic correlation. Radiology 183:391–394
3. Haustein J, Laniado M, Niendorf H-P, et al (1993) Triple-dose versus standard-dose gadopentetate dimeglumine: a randomized study in 199 patients. Radiology 186:855–860
4. Yuh WTC, Fisher DJ, Mayr-Yuh NA, et al (1992) Review of the use of high-dose gadoteridol in the magnetic resonance evaluation of central nervous system tumors. Invest Radiol 27:S39–S44

CT technique

Assessment of carotid artery stenosis with spiral CT angiography

J. Link, J. Brossmann, U. Stock, P. Marquart, M. Heller

Department of Radiology, Christian-Albrechts-University of Kiel, Arnold-Heller-Strasse 9, D-24105 Kiel, Germany

Abstract. Spiral CT angiography was performed in 16 patients with 26 internal carotid artery stenoses using both maximum-intensity projection (MIP) and surface-shaded display (3D). The degree of stenosis was determined according to the technique of the NASCET study by measuring maximal stenosis in relation to the postbulbar internal carotid artery. The degree of stenosis in each case was classified as total occlusion (100%), severe (70–99%), moderate (30–69%) or mild (0–29%). There was a significant correlation between the 3D and the MIP techniques in all categories of stenosis. Compared with digital subtraction angiography (DSA), both spiral CT angiography showed a good correlation in the moderate and severe stenosis and occluded groups. In the group with mild stenosis, correlation between either spiral CT angiography technique and DSA was poor.

Key words: Maximum-intensity projection – Surface-shaded display – Carotid artery stenosis

Spiral CT angiography, which can be postprocessed using the maximum-intensity projection (MIP) [1–3] and surface-shaded display (3D) techniques [4, 5] is a new modality for assessment of carotid artery stenosis. This study was performed to evaluate the accuracy of the MIP and 3D techniques compared with digital subtraction angiography (DSA), in determining the degree of carotid artery stenosis.

Materials and methods

In 16 patients (10 men, 6 women aged 50–75 years, mean 61 years), 26 carotid artery stenoses were studied with the 3D and MIP techniques and the results then compared with those of DSA. Spiral CT angiography was performed as follows: data acquisition time 32 s; slice thickness 2 mm; table speed 2 mm/s; range 6.4 cm. With a flow of 3 ml/s (start delay, 12 s), 100 ml contrast medium was injected into the antecubital vein. The degree of stenosis was determined according to the NASCET study of measuring maximal stenosis in relation to the postbulbar internal carotid artery [6, 7]. The degree of narrowing was classified as: total occlusion (100%), severe (70–99%), moderate (30–69%) and mild (0–29%) stenosis. The Spearman rank test was used to compare the different modalities.

Results

The 26 stenoses included 6 mild, 3 moderate, 11 severe and 6 absolute stenoses (occlusions). In 77% of stenoses (20 of 26), the classification determined by the 3D and MIP techniques, was the same ($r=0.89$; $P=0.0001$). The correlation between the MIP and 3D techniques in the different subgroups was as follows: mild stenosis ($r=0.81$; $P=0.686$), moderate stenosis ($r=0.1$; $P=0.3173$), severe stenosis ($r=0.77$; $P=0.154$), occlusion ($r=1$; $P=0.253$). The comparison of DSA and MIP showed overall agreement in 81% (21 of 26) ($r=0.89$; $P=0.0001$). The correlation in the different groups of stenosis was as follows: mild stenosis ($r=0.54$; $P=0.2248$); moderate stenosis ($r=1$; $P=0.3173$); severe stenosis ($r=0.88$; $P=0.0057$), occlusion ($r=1$; $P=0.253$). DSA and the 3D technique agreed in 73% (19 of 26) ($r=0.86$; $P=0.0001$): mild stenosis ($r=0.53$; $P=0.2372$), moderate stenosis ($r=1$; $P=0.3173$), severe stenosis ($r=0.69$; $P=0.289$), occlusion ($r=1$; $P=0.0253$).

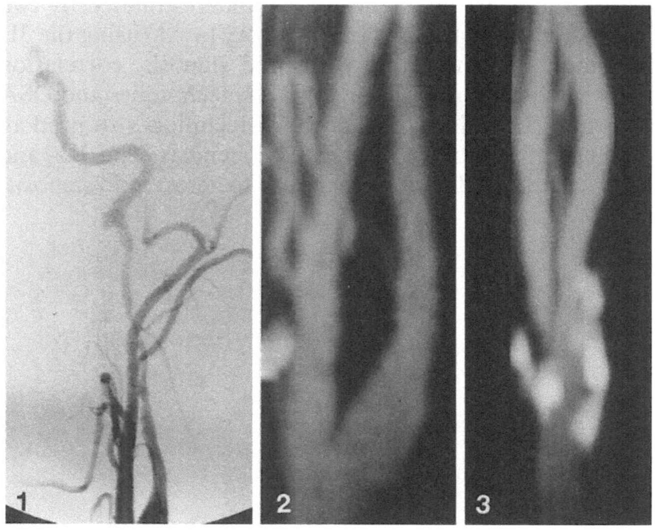

Fig. 1. Dissection of internal carotid artery, with severe stenosis and poststenotic aneurysm, on digital subtraction angiography

Fig. 2. Dissection of internal carotid artery with severe stenosis, shown by maximum-intensity projection

Fig. 3. Severe stenosis of internal and external carotid artery with calcified plaque shown by MIP

Discussion

The overall agreement of spiral CT angiography using the 3D and MIP techniques for the assessment of carotid artery stenosis was good (77%). Compared with DSA, correlation with MIP (81%) was superior to that with the 3D technique (73%) for all 26 stenoses. Both spiral CT angiography techniques showed a good correlation with DSA in detecting moderate stenosis (100%) and occlusion (100%). In the group with severe stenosis, correlation between MIP and DSA (91%) (10 of 11) (Figs. 1, 2) was

Correspondence to: J. Link

better than the correlation between the 3D technique and DSA (73%) (8/11). The correlation between MIP and 3D techniques in the group with severe stenosis was only 73%, owing to the good differentiation of calcified plaques and contrast medium with MIP (Fig. 3). In the 3D technique there may be difficulties in differentiating between calcification and contrast medium. In the remaining 3 of the 11 cases, the degree of stenosis was underestimated by two categories ($n = 2$) and by one category ($n = 1$) using the 3D technique. In the group with mild stenosis, correlation between both spiral CT angiography techniques and DSA was only 33%. However, both CT techniques showed an agreement of 67% in mild carotid stenosis. The 3D- and MIP technique do not make it easy to detect mild stenosis.

References

1. Castillo M (1993) Diagnosis of disease of the common carotid artery bifurcation. AJR 161:395–398
2. Marks MP, Napel S, Jordan JE, Enzmann DR (1993) Diagnosis of carotid artery disease: preliminary experience with maximum-intensity-projection spiral CT angiography. AJR 160:1267–1271
3. Napel SA, Marks MP, Rubin GD, Dake MD, McDonnell CH, Song SM, Enzmann DR, Brooke Jeffrey R (1992) CT angiography with spiral CT and maximum intensity projection. Radiology 185:607–610
4. Dillon EH, van Leeuwen MS, Fernandez MA, Eikelboom BC, Mali WPTM (1993) CT angiography: application to the evaluation of carotid artery stenosis. Radiology 189:211–219
5. Schwartz RB, Jones KM, Chernoff DM, Mukherji SK, Khorasani R, Tice HM, Kikins R, Hooton SM, Stieg PE, Polak JF (1992) Common carotid artery bifurcation: evaluation with spiral CT. Radiology 185:513–519
6. North American Symptomatic Carotid Endarterectomy Trial Collaborators (1991) Benefical effect of carotid endarterectomy in symptomatic patients with high-grade carotid stenosis. N Engl J Med 325:445–453
7. Fox AJ (1993) How to measure carotid stenosis. Radiology 186:316–318

Clinical application of three-dimensional CT angiography to cerebrovascular disease

M. Ueda[1], S. Okawara[2]

[1] Department of Neurosurgery, Tomakomai Neurosurgical Hospital, 1-12-20 Koyo-cho, Tomakomai 953, Japan
[2] Department of Neurosurgery, Okawara Neurosurgical Hospital, Muroran, Japan

Abstract. Three-dimensional CT angiography (3D-CTA) was used in the investigation of 47 patients with cerebrovascular disease (CVD), and compared with conventional angiography. With the exception of 4 patients with stenosis of the internal carotid artery C4 portion, 16 occlusive lesions were visualized on 3D-CTA as clearly as on conventional angiography. In 16 patients with non-ruptured cerebral aneurysm, 3D-CTPA revealed all the aneurysms demonstrated by conventional angiography. No complications arising from the procedure were encountered. Although this technique requires further development and clinical evalution, 3D-CTA is a valuable tool in the investigation of patients with CVD.

Key words: Cerebrovascular disease – Spiral computed tomography – Three-dimensional CT angiography

3D-CTA is a new angiographical method with minimal risk to patients [1–4]. We evaluated the usefulness of 3D-CTA in the diagnosis of patients with CVD and postoperative evaluation. We compared 3D-CT images with images obtained from conventional angiography.

Correspondence to: M. Ueda

Patients and methods

We studied 31 patients with occlusive CVD and 16 with non-ruptured cerebral aneurysm.

In this procedure, spiral CT was performed in the usual way with the patient in the supine position. A scout view of the head and upper cervical spine was obtained. A no. 20 or larger intravenous infusion line was placed and connected to an injector. An intravenous infusion of non-ionic iodinated contrast solution was continued at a rate of 2 ml/s for 50 s. Volume mode scanning was begun 25 s after the start of the infusion of contrast medium. The CT table was withdrawn at a velocity of 1.5 mm/s while scanning was performed (120 kV, 150 mA, 50 s continuous exposure). This resulted in a 3D volume acquisition of approximately 75 mm. 3D reconstruction was performed using the shaded-surface rendering method with a lower threshold of about 150 HU and reconstruction time of 5 min. The total examination time of 3D-CTA was about 20–30 min. The evaluation of 3D-CTA was as follows: (1) 1 mm original axial image (window: 300, level: 35, window: 1500, level: 150); (2) 3D image reconstructed by the shaded-surface rendering method; (3) multiplanar reconstruction (MPR) image.

Conventional angiography was performed with an intra-arterial digital subtraction angiography (IA-DSA) system.

Results

Of the 26 patients with occlusive CVD, 10 did not demonstrate intracranial vascular pathology on either 3D-CTA or IA-DSA. Sixteen patients demonstrated oc-

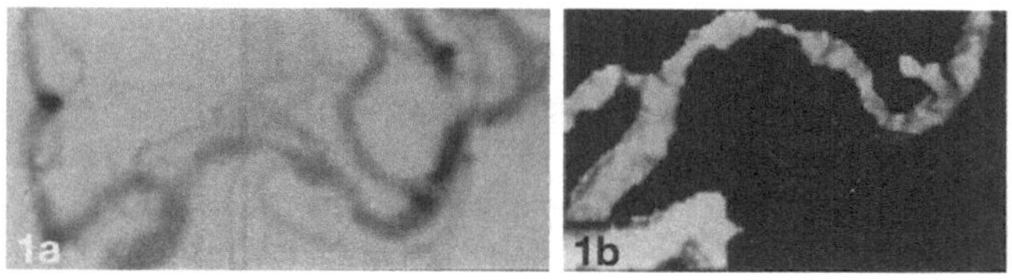

Fig. 1 a, b. Case 13. **a** Left carotid angiogram shows severe stenosis of the middle cerebral artery sphenoidal segment. **b** 3D-CTA also shows this stenosis

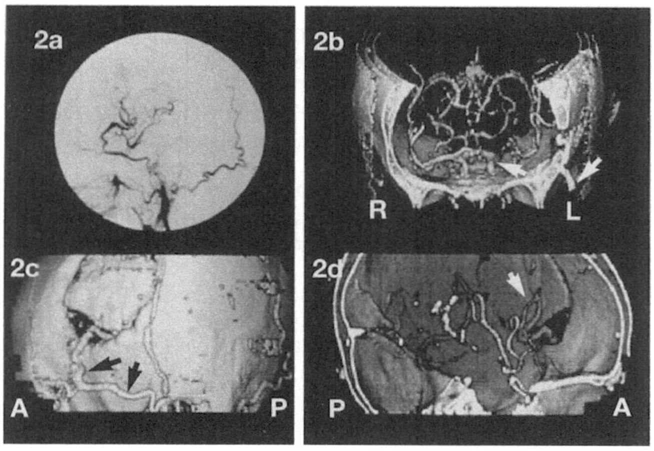

Fig. 2 a–d. Case 18. **a** Left carotid angiogram shows the patency of superficial temporal middle cerebral artery bypass. **b–d** On 3D-CTA, the left superficial temporal artery (*arrowhead*) is seen to connect with a branch of the middle cerebral artery through the cranial window (*arrow*); left intracranial carotid artery (*curved arrow*) is not seen

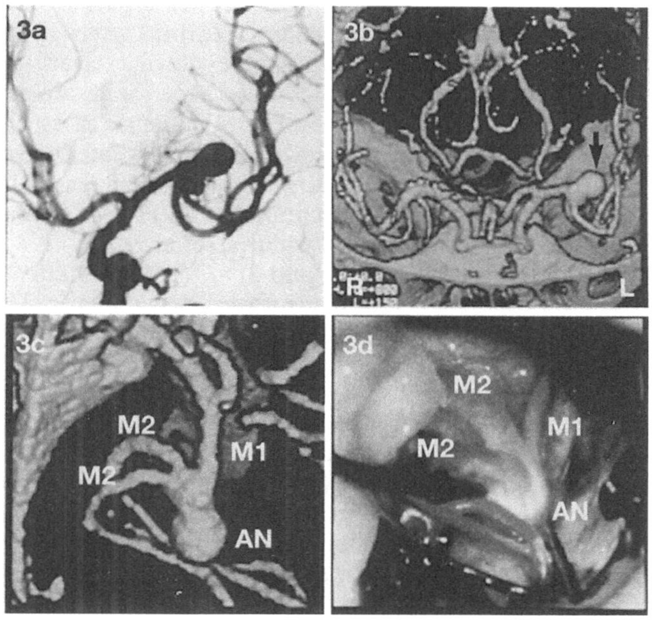

Fig. 3 a–d. Case 32. **a** Left carotid angiogram shows an unruptured aneurysm of the middle cerebral artery, also seen on 3D-CTA (**b**; *arrow*). **c** Operative view of 3D-CTA. **d** Intraoperative photograph. *AN*, aneurysm; *M1*, sphenoidal, *M2*, insular segments of middle cerebral artery

Table 1. IA-DSA and 3D-CTA findings in 16 patients with unruptured cerebral aneurysms

Patient	Age (years)/sex	DSA		3D-CTA	
		Aneurysm on site	Size (mm)	Original image	3D image
22	55 F	L ICA	3	Non-diagnostic	Diagnostic
23	57 F	R ICA	5	Diagnostic	Diagnostic
24	76 F	L ICA	10	Diagnostic	Diagnostic
25	53 M	L ICA	30	Diagnostic	Diagnostic
26	68 F	L ICA	8	Diagnostic	Diagnostic
27	58 M	L MCA	8	Diagnostic	Diagnostic
28	41 F	R MCA	6	Diagnostic	Diagnostic
29	50 M	L MCA	5	Suggestive	Diagnostic
30	52 F	R MCA	4	Non-diagnostic	Diagnostic
		R MCA	6	Diagnostic	Diagnostic
31	59 F	R MCA	7	Diagnostic	Diagnostic
		L MCA	4	Non-diagnostic	Diagnostic
32	57 M	L MCA	12	Diagnostic	Diagnostic
33	48 F	R MCA	7	Diagnostic	Diagnostic
34	43 F	R MCA	6	Diagnostic	Diagnostic
35	64 M	AcomA	4	Suggestive	Diagnostic
36	62 F	BA	4	Diagnostic	Diagnostic
37	54 M	BA	6	Diagnostic	Diagnostic

L, left; *R*, right; *ICA*, internal carotid artery; *MCA*, middle cerebral artery; *AcomA*, anterior communicating artery; *BA*, basilar artery

clusive lesions on IA-DSA (cases 1–16). Apart from 4 patients with stenosis of the internal carotid artery in the C4 portion, all occlusive lesions were shown as clearly by 3D-CTA as by IA-DSA. 3D-CTA was superior in showing calcification of the arterial wall. In 4 patients (cases 17–20), 3D-CTA revealed patency of the bypass after extracranial-intracranial bypass surgery. In 1 patient (case 21), 3D-CTA revealed the disappearance of the carotid stenotic lesion 3 days after carotid endarterectomy.

The findings of IA-DSA and 3D-CTA in 16 patients with non-ruptured cerebral aneurysm, are summarised in Table 1. 3D-CTA revealed all aneurysms demonstrated by IA-DSA. All aneurysms were clearly visualised on 3D-CTA. 3D-reconstructed views from different angles were helpful in determining the direction of the aneurysm, its shape, the size of neck, and its relationship with parent arteries and adjacent bony structures. 3D views from above and below were especially useful in providing information that was not available from conventional angiograms. Operative views were also helpful in planning and performing surgery.

Although our experience with 3D-CTA was limited, we did not encounter any complications.

Discussion

The advantages and disadvantages of 3D-CTA are listed as follows: advantages: short scanning time; 3D-capacity; possibility of screening examination and surgical planning; disadvantages: radiation exposure; use of contrast medium; no demonstration of small vascular lesions; impossibility of distinguishing arteries from venous and bony structures; limited field of view.

References

1. Aoki S, Sasaki Y, Machida T, Ohkubo T, Minami M, Sasaki Y (1992) Cerebral aneurysms: detection and delineation using 3D-CT angiography. AJNR 13:1115–1120
2. Gholkar A, Isherwood I (1988) Three-dimensional computed tomographic reformations of intracranial vascular lesions. Br J Radiol 61:258–261
3. Harbaugh RE, Schlusselberg DS, Jeffery R, Hayden S, Cromwell LD, Pluta D (1992) Three-dimensional computerized tomography angiography in the diagnosis of cerebrovascular disease. J Neurosurg 76:408–414
4. Schwartz RB, Jones KM, Chernoff DM, Mukherji SK, Khorasani R, Tice HM, Kikinis R, Hooton SM, Stieg RE, Polak JF (1992) Common carotid artery bifucation: evaluation with spiral CT. Radiology 185:513–519

Spiral CT angiography of brain aneurysms and arterovenous malformations

R. Tadmor, M. Faivel, A. Eyal

Department of Radiology-Neuroradiology, Tel Aviv University, Sheba Medical Center, Tel-Hashomer 52621, Israel

Abstract. The new Elscint CT system, using dual-slice spiral acquisition with continuous bed motion, collects in 30 s, twice the data and double the area length of spiral CT system. It allows overlapping thin axial slices, thus improving 3D reconstruction, 2D reformations, and maximum intensity projection (MIP) for spiral CT angiography. Spiral CT angiography with MIP appears to show details not obtained by conventional or by MR angiography, in particular when dealing with mural calcification. Excellent demonstration and delineation of normal blood vessels arteriovenous malformations and aneurysms were acquired. It seems that a reduction of contrast medium volume will not degrade the image quality. Limitations in MIP reconstruction are encountered when bone is close to the vascular lesion.

Key words: Spiral CT angiography – Brain arteriovenous malformations – Brain aneurysms

Correspondence to: R. Tadmor

The spiral CT scanner is a recent achievement of CT technology. It allows for fast volumetric data acquisition, while continuous table transport and X-ray tube rotation are taking place. If combined with a dynamic intravenous contrast injection, imaging of the blood vessels is obtained. By using special imaging processing and maximum intensity projection (MIP) spiral CT angiography is achieved [1–3].

Since the duration of one spiral scan at present amounts to 32 s, it is possible to perform an entire study with a single breath-hold. This feature is highly advantageous for chest and abdominal evaluation, as well as for neck and head studies.

The Elscint Twin CT is a new system, which using dual-slice spiral acquisition with continuous bed motion collects twice the data in 30 s. Therefore it doubles the length of the area scanned.

This new CT system also enables thinner volumetric imaging with excellent 2D reformation and 3D reconstruction, as well as MIP for spiral CT angiography.

We report on our experience of evaluating the accuracy and detail demonstration using dual-slice spiral CT angiography in cases of aneurysms and arterovenous malformations (AVMs).

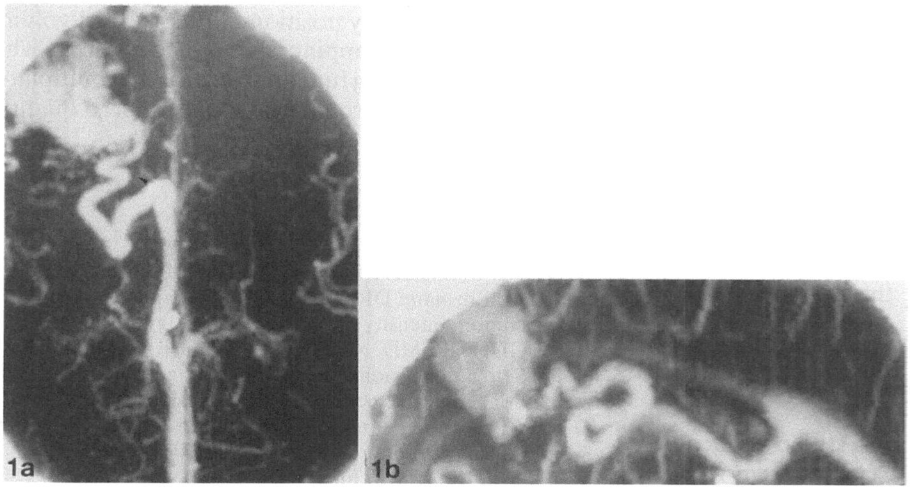

Fig. 1 a, b. Spiral CT angiography of right frontal arteriovenous malformation (AVM). **a** Axial view of late arterial early venous phase. **b** Lateral view; note nidus of AVM with small zones of calcification and a large, tortuous, deeply draining vein

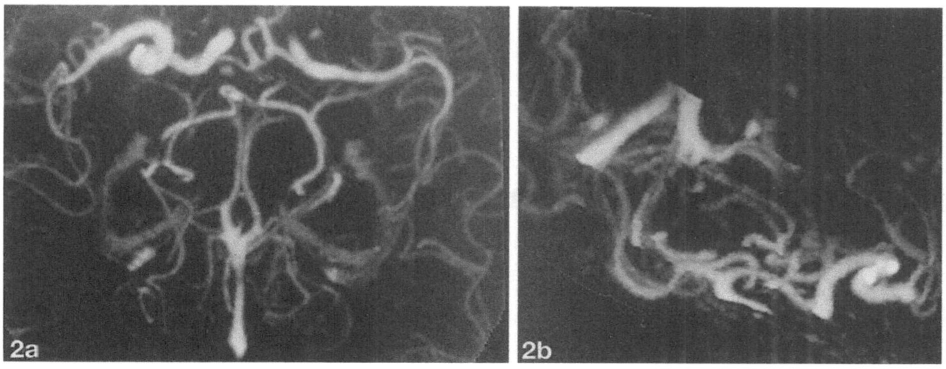

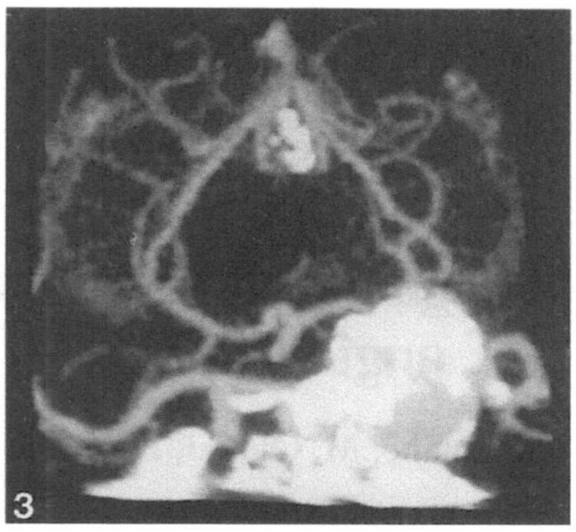

Fig. 2 a, b. Spiral CT angiography. Calcification in a loop of the middle cerebral artery (not an aneurysm!) **a** Axial view. **b** Oblique rotation and unfolding of the loop

Fig. 3. Spiral CT angiography of a giant carotid artery aneurysm with large areas of surface calcification. Slight rotation of a coronal view

Materials and methods

All scans for this study were performed with an Elscint CT twin, dual-slice spiral CT scanner (Elscint, Haifa, Israel), which allows scanning of two slices at the same time. This system is equipped with twin beams and two closely packed solid state detector arrays mounted on an advanced slip ring gantry, enabling the performance of double-helix spiral scans.

In this dual-slice system the table moves at twice the speed of a conventional scanner for the same slice thickness (pitch = 2), while maintaining full coverage and image quality.

Scans described in this work were performed with dual 1.0 mm slices at 2 mm/s table speed and reconstructed at both 1.3 mm and 2.0 mm ("fused") effective thicknesses. Carotid arteries and neck areas were scanned mainly in the dual 2.5 mm, 5.0 mm/s helix mode and reconstructed as both 3.2 mm and 5.0 mm ("fused") effective slices.

An injector was used, programmed to deliver 40–80 ml contrast medium (60% concentration) at rates of 2.5–3.0 ml/s. Helical scanning was initiated 20–25 s after the start of the injection. For visualisation of the late venous phase a repeat scan was performed without contrast injection.

All image processing functions, 2D reformation, 3D reconstruction and MIP for spiral CT angiography were available on the scanner operator console, as well as on the independent diagnostic console connected to the main system through a local area network (Ethernet) for image transfers.

Results

Among the patients submitted to the twin-spiral CT studies, more than 30 patients had AVMs, aneurysms or other vascular problems.

Generally, superb visualisation of the circle of Willis and more peripheral blood vessels was obtained. All AVMs were clearly shown, including early arterial and late venous phases (Fig. 1). Intracranial calcification adjacent to the wall of an arterial loop was detected, thus differentiating it from a small calcified middle cerebral artery aneurysm and an arteriogram was avoided (Fig. 2). Large surface calcification and a giant carotid aneurysm were demonstrated by the spiral CT angiography (Fig. 3). In a 4-year-old child the aneurysm was well shown using only 40 ml contrast medium. Limitations in MIP reconstruction are present when bone is close to the high-density vascular lesion.

Discussion

The MIP function is another 3D volume presentation technique, in which projections of a selected volume are shown in such a way that only the pixels with the highest value CT numbers are displayed for any line of sight. This technique is particularly suitable for viewing contrast-enhanced blood vessels in a scanned volume, and producing images comparable to conventional angiography. Real-time manipulation of the projection adds to the 3D "feeling" and enables selection of the best view for presenting a particular pathology or anatomical detail. The MIP function enables the removal of bone and other-high-density tissue that may obstruct the vascular structures in the projection images.

Using helix scans for head and neck studies is beneficial, especially when imaging the vascular system with fast contrast medium injections, since time is a very important factor in obtaining optimal enhancement [1–4]. The volume acquisition of helical scans enables reconstruction of slices at any position in the scanned volume, including highly overlapping slices. These slices, when used in image processing functions such as 3D multiplanar reformatting or MIP, produce images of superb quality.

References

1. Napel SA, Marks MP, Rubin GD, Dake MD, McDonnel CH, Song SM, Enzmann DR (1992) CT angiography with spiral CT and maximum intensity projection. Radiology 185:607–610
2. Rubin GD, Dake MD, Napel SA, McDonnell CH, Jeffery RB Jr (1993) Three-dimensional spiral CT angiography of the abdomen: initial clinical experience. Radiology 186:147–152
3. Dillon EH, Van-Leeuwen MS, Fernandez MA, Mali WP (1993) Spiral CT angiography. AJR 160:1273–1278
4. Marks MP, Napel SA, Jordan JE, Enzmann DR (1993) Diagnosis of carotid artery disease: preliminary experience with MIP spiral CT angiography. AJR 160:1267–1271

Diagnosis of unruptured intracranial aneurysms with three-dimensional CT angiography

S. Tanabe, M. Ohtaki, K. Hashi

Department of Neurosurgery, Sapporo Medical University, School of Medicine, South-1, West-16, Chuo-ku, Sapporo, 060 Japan

Abstract. The usefulness of three-dimensional CT angiography (3D-CTA) for the diagnosis of unruptured cerebral aneurysms was compared with that of MR angiography (MRA) and digital subtraction angiography (DSA).

Thirty-three patients in whom unruptured cerebral aneurysms were suspected on the basis of CT, MRI, or MRA investigations were included in this study. CT was performed with a bolus injection of non-ionic contrast medium. The presence of 41 cerebral aneurysms was confirmed by 3D-CTA in 24 of the 33 cases. In the remaining 9 cases, no aneurysm was shown by 3D-CTA. 3D-CTA revealed more detailed features of aneurysms and the vessels involved than did MRA and DSA. It revealed even small aneurysms with a diameter of 1 mm, and it gave more useful information about surgical approaches to large aneurysms. We conclude that 3D-CTA is an effective contribution to the screening for and diagnosis of cerebral aneurysms.

Key words: Spiral computed tomography – three-dimensional computed tomography angiography unruptured – Cerebral aneurysm unruptured – Diagnosis – surgical simulation image

Correspondence to: S. Tanabe

Three-dimensional CT angiography (3D-CTA) is a new, minimally invasive technique for the diagnosis of cerebral aneurysms. The purpose of this study was to compare the diagnostic value of 3D-CTA for unruptured cerebral aneurysms with that of MRA and DSA, by reference to operative findings.

Table 1. Location of 41 unruptured aneurysms shown by 3D-CTA in 24 patients

	Single aneurysm		Multiple aneurysms	
Patients	15		9	
Aneurysms	15		26	
Artery				
Anterior cerebral:	4		5	
Anterior communicating		3		4
Distal anterior cerebral		1		1
Middle cerebral	4		3	
Internal carotid:	4		12	
Cavernous portion		1		3
Carotid-ophthalmic				1
Posterior communicating		3		2
Anterior choroidal				3
Terminal internal carotid				3
Basilar	2		5	
Vertebral	1		1	

Table 2. Unruptured single aneurysms shown by 3D-CTA

Case	Age (years)/Sex	Artery with aneurysm	Size (mm)	Diagnostic utility
1	36 M	Anterior communicating	12	3D-CTA> DSA
2	64 M	Middle cerebral	20	3D-CTA > DSA, MRA
3	44 M	Middle cerebral	3	3D-CTA = DSA > MRA
4	67 F	Posteior communicating	6	3D-CTA = DSA, MRA
5	64 M	Posterior communicating	7	3D-CTA < DSA
6	34 M	Posterior inferior cerebellar	8	3D-CTA = DSA > MRA
7	45 F	Posterior communicating	5	3D-CTA < DSA
8	71 F	Basilar	8	3D-CTA + DSA > MRA
9	51 M	Middle cerebral (thrombosed)	27	3D-CTA[a] > DSA, MRA
10	64 F	Intracavernous carotid	3	3D-CTA < DSA, MRA
11	82 F	Basilar (fusiform)		3D-CTA[a] > MRA
12	64 M	Anterior cerebral (A1–A2)	2	3D-CTA > DSA, MRA
13	51 F	Distal anterior cerebral	5	3D-CTA = DSA > MRA
14	51 F	Middle cerebral	6	3D-CTA = DSA > MRA
15	49 M	Anterior cerebral (A1–A2)	2	3D-CTA > DSA, MRA

[a] Using maximum-intensity projection

Table 3. Unruptured multiple aneurysms shown by 3D-CTA

Case	Age (years)/Sex	Artery with aneurysms	Size (mm)	Diagnostic utility
16	56 M	Basilar	9	3D-CTA + DSA, MRA
		Posterior communicating	7	3D-CTA = DSA > MRA
		Terminal internal carotid	12	3D-CTA + DSA > MRA
17	72 F	Middle cerebral	2	3D-CTA > DSA, MRA
		Anterior communicating	14	3D-CTA > DSA, MRA
18	66 F	Basilar	10	3D-CTA = DSA
		Anterior cerebral (A1–A2)	6	3D-CTA = DSA
		Intracavernous carotid	13	3D-CTA = DSA
19	53 F	Anterior communicating	14	3D-CTA > DSA
		Distal anterior cerebral	2	3D-CTA = DSA
		Middle cerebral	5	3D-CTA + DSA
20	52 M	Middle cerebral	6	3D-CTA = DSA > MRA
		Anterior choroidal	1.5	3D-CTA > DSA, MRA
21	60 F	Posterior communicating	6	3D-CTA > DSA
		Cavernous carotid	5	3D-CTA > DSA
		Terminal internal carotid	6	3D-CTA > DSA
22	59 M	Posterior inferior cerebellar	5	3D-CTA = DSA
		Carotid-ophthalmic	3.5	3D-CTA > DSA
		Terminal internal carotid	6	3D-CTA > DSA
		Bilateral anterior choroidal	1	3D-CTA > DSA
		Anterior cerebral (A1)	–	3D-CTA < DSA
23	80 M	Basilar	10	3D-CTA = MRA
		Anterior communicating	2.5	3D-CTA > MRA
		Intracavernous carotid	2.5	3D-CTA > MRA
24	51 F	Basilar	9	3D-CTA > MRA
		Basilar (posterior cerebral)	13	3D-CTA > MRA

Patients and methods

3D-CTA was performed in 33 patients in whom unruptured cerebral aneurysms suspected on CT, MRI, or MRA. 3D-CTA images were obtained with 120 kV, 210 mA, slice thickness 2–3 mm, image interval 1 mm, and table increment 1–3 mm/s. 3D image reconstruction was performed through surface-rendering and maximum-intensity projection (MIP) processing.

Results and discussion

The presence of 41 unruptured cerebral aneurysms was confirmed by 3D-CTA in 24 of the 33 patients in whom aneurysms were suspected after previous investigations with CT, MRI or MRA. In the remaining 9 patients 3D-CTA revealed no evidence of aneurysms.

The locations of the 41 aneurysms that were confirmed by 3D-CTA were as follows (Table 1): 7 aneurysms on the anterior communicating artery (AcomA), 2 on the distal

Table 4. Comparison of diagnostic utility for unruptured aneurysms

Diameter of aneurysm (mm)	Diagnostic utility	Number of aneurysms
1–5	CTA > MRA	8/9
	CTA < MRA	1/9 (intracavernous carotid)
	CTA > DSA	8/15
	CTA = DSA	5/15
	CTA < DSA	2/15 (posterior cxommunicating, intracavernous carotid)
6–11	CTA > MRA	6/9
	CTA = MRA	3/9
	CTA > DSA	3/13
	CTA < DSA	1/13 (posterior communicating)
12–27	CTA > MRA	6/6
	CTA > DSA	5/7
	CTA + DSA	2/7

anterior cerebral artery (ACA), 7 on the middle cerebral artery (MCA), 5 on the internal carotid (IC)/posterior cerebral (PC) arterio (IC-PC), 4 on the cavernous IC, 1 carotid-ophthalmic, 3 on the IC anterior choroidal artery (Ach), 3 on the terminal IC, 7 on the basilar artery (BA), and 2 on the vertebral artery (VA). Nine patients out of the 24 had multiple aneurysms. The locations of the suspected aneurysms that were not confirmed by 3D-CTA were on the ACA in 2 cases, the MCA in 3, the IC/OC in 2, the BA in 1, and the superior cerebellar artery in 1.

The size of the aneurysms delineated by 3D-CTA ranged from 1 to 27 mm; there were 1 giant and 8 large aneurysms (Tables 2, 3).

The usefulness of 3D-CTA in the diagnosis and operation was evaluated in comparison with MRA and DSA (Table 4). 3D-CTA was superior to MRA and DSA for showing small aneurysms with a diameter of less than 5 mm, which were located on the cavernous IC, carotid IC-ophthalmic and IC-anterior choroidal artery. For medium-sized aneurysms, there was no difference in diagnostic accuracy between 3D-CTA and DSA. With regard to large aneurysms with a diameter of over 12 mm, 3D-CTA tended to be more useful than MRA and DSA, particularly for planning an operation, because there was less difficulty in operative simulation. DSA, on the other hand, was superior for only 3 of the 16 IC aneurysms when the aneurysm shadow was overlapped on the bony structures. The accuracy of aneurysm images on 3D-CTA was confirmed by observation during the operation.

3D-CTA was capable of delineating aneurysms with diameters of over 1 mm, and also giant aneurysms, which MRA failed to reveal. For the operation, the three-dimensional image of 3D-CTA provided useful information about the shape and anatomical relationship with the parent artery and bony structure around the aneurysm in particular.

The aneurysms located in the vicinity of the cavernous sinus could be visualized by 3-D image reconstruction by elevating the threshold level to 250 HU. In addition, MIP image was able to show calcification of an arterial wall, which was useful when clips were applied to aneurysms.

The detectability of intracranial aneurysms using helical CT compared with conventional cerebral angiography

Y. Ogura[1], K. Katada[2], H. Sano[3], Y. Kato[3], T. Kanno[3], M. Nomura[1], G. Takeshita[1], S. Koga[1]

[1] Department of Radiology, School of Medicine, Fujita Health University, Fujita, Japan
[2] Department of Neurosurgery, School of Medicine, Fujita Health University, Fujita, Japan
[3] School of Health Science, Fujita Health University, Fujita, Japan

Abstract. Helical CT (HCT) was applied to the diagnosis of cerebral aneurysms. The diagnostic accuracy of HCT, including the detectability of aneurysms, was compared with that of conventional cerebral angiography in 62 aneurysms of 43 patients. The scanning parameters were 135 kV, 260 mA and 1 mm slice thickness. The couch top was moved at 1 to 1.2 mm/s during the scanning of 30 s. In a prospective study, the detection rates using HCT and angiography were 91.9% and 93.5%. Retrospectively, the detection rates with HCT and with angiography were 95.4% and 98.4%. HCT was also effective in illustrating the detailed contours of aneurysms and calcifications and thrombosed parts of aneurysms. Three-dimensional CT (3D-CT) images were helpful in diagnosing complicated vascular anomalies. Our results indicate that HCT was an effective diagnostic modality to supplement cerebral angiography.

Key words: Helical computed tomography – Cerebral aneurysm – Cerebral angiography – Three-dimensional computed tomography

Correspondence to: Y. Ogura

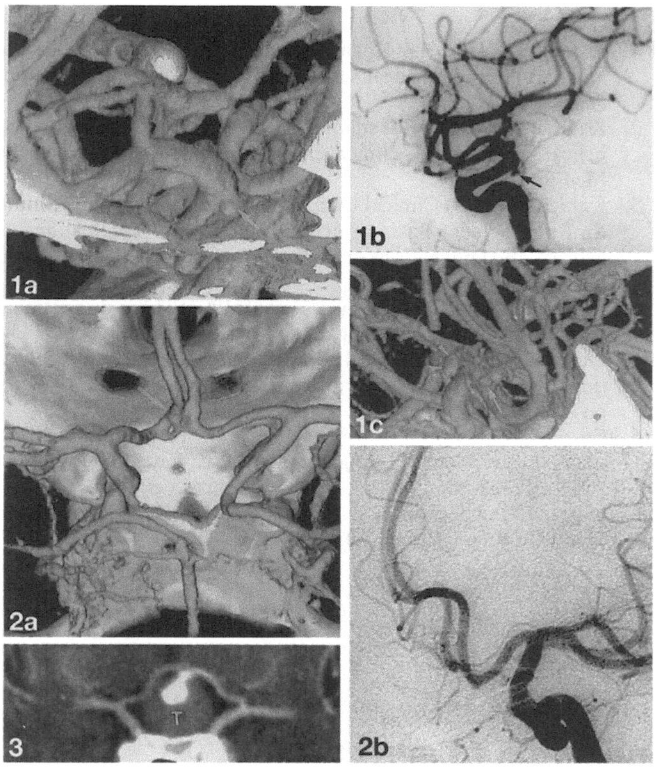

Fig. 1 a–c. A 46-year-old woman with multiple aneurysms. **a** 3D-CT, left lateral view shows an aneurysm (*arrow*) on the internal carotid artery, 1.5×2.0 mm in diameter. **b** Internal carotid angiogram, left lateral view. The aneurysm (*arrow*) is delineated as is the anterior choroidal artery. **c** 3D-CT, right lateral view, shows a 4×3.2 mm aneurysm at posterior cerebral artery (*arrowheads*) and another, 2.1 mm, at the middle cerebral artery bifurcation (*arrow*)

Fig. 2 a, b. A 67-year-old woman with suspected subarachnoid haemorrhage. Routine CT showed marked hydrocephalus. The patient was referred for HCT. **a** 3D-CT from above delineates small fenestration of distal A1 portion. A small blister-like aneurysm (*arrow*) is seen distal to the fenestration. **b** Left internal carotid angiogram. Neither fenestration nor aneurysm can be identified

Fig. 3. A 59-year-old man with an aneurysm at the anterior communicating artery. MPR coronal section. Unenhancing thrombosed portions (*T*) of aneurysm are clearly shown. Note demonstration of lenticulostriate arteries

We used helical CT (HCT) in the investigation of intracranial aneurysms; the diagnostic accuracy of 3D-CT angiography and multiplanar reconstruction (MPR) was compared with that of cerebral angiography.

Methods and materials

We studied 13 patients who underwent HCT and cerebral angiography for the diagnosis of cerebral aneurysm. The scanning parameters were: 135 kV, 260 mA, slice thickness 1 mm, couch top speed 1–1.2 mm/s. The scanning time for one rotation was 1 s, and the total scanning time was 30 s. Nonionic contrast medium (300 mgl/ml), 80–100 ml, was injected simultaneously during scanning. Using the reconstruction programme of 180° opposite beam interpolation algorighm, 60–70 axial images with 0.5 mm pitch were generated from the raw data. For postprocessing, 3D-CT images with volume-rendering technique and MPR images were obtained using a workstation. The accuracy of HCT in the diagnosis of cerebral aneurysm was evaluated prospectively and retrospectively in terms of detectability, and was compared with that of cerebral angiography. In addition to the detection of aneurysms, the detectability of abnormalities associated with aneurysms – calcification, mural thrombus, and vascular anomalies – was also evaluated.

Results

On cerebral angiograms, 58 aneurysms were diagnosed prospectively in 43 patients (Fig. 1) while in 1 patient no aneurysm was detected. In a retrospective observation of the angiograms, 61 aneurysms were detected. On HCT, 57 cerebral aneurysms were detected prospectively while 59 were detected on retrospective review. In 1 case, a blister-like aneurysm associated with small fenestration at the distal A1 portion was detected only by HCT and could not be detected even after retrospective observation of the angiogram (Fig. 2). Another three angiographically equivocal aneurysms were readily diagnosed by HCT, which were confirmed at surgery. Three aneurysms that were false-negative in prospective analysis of HCT also could not be detected by retrospective review. These consisted of two carotid-ophthalmic aneurysms and one cavernous carotid aneurysm, whose maximum diameter was 6×3 mm. Another two false-negative aneurysms, one incidental aneurysm associated with parasellar meningioma and one peripheral aneurysm on the distal anterior cerebral artery were detected on retrospective review.

A total of 62 aneurysms were detected in 43 patients. The detection rates of the aneurysms on prospective assessment by HCT and angiography were 91.9% and 93.5% respectively. Also, the detection rates of aneurysms by HCT and angiography on retrospective observation were 95.2% and 98.4% respectively.

As for associated abnormalities, calcification (in 2 cases), and mural thrombus (also in 2) of aneurysms were detected on MPR images of HCT (Fig. 3). Angiograms failed to show these findings. Anomalous arterial fenestrations were observed in three cases on 3D-CT images, which could not be assessed by cerebral angiograms.

Discussion

The possibility of rapid data acquisition and superior data continuity in the axial direction permits HCT to provide excellent three-dimensional visualisation of vascular structures. In this study, we evaluated the accuracy of HCT in the diagnosis of cerebral aneurysms in comparison with cerebral angiography. Our results indicated that the detectability of cerebral aneurysm using HCT was almost comparable to that of angiography. It also showed that the detection rate with HCT differs greatly according to the location of the aneurysm. In our series, all the aneurysms located above the anterior clinoid process could be seen retrospectively, while three of the infraclinoid aneurysms could not be detected by HCT.

HCT has definite advantages over cerebral angiography in multi-directional display of the circle of Willis, including base-view representation. This is particularly effective in diagnosing aneurysms of anterior comminication artery complex in which HCT showed superior diagnostic accuracy over cerebral angiography. The presented cases illustrated that some aneurysms and associated abnormalities could only be diagnosed by HCT, which indicated that HCT can supplement angiography. Another advantage of HCT over angiography is the delineation of the detailed contours of aneurysms. The shape and position of the aneurysmal neck and bleb, as well as the relation to parent arteries, are well appreciated by 3D-CT images.

The current limitations of HCT in the diagnosis of cerebral aneurysms are in the detection of small infraclinoid aneurysms and the delineation of narrow perforating arteries next to the aneurysm.

References

1. Katada K, Anno H, Koga S, et al (1990) Three-dimensional angiography with helical scanning CT. Radiology 177 [Suppl]: 364
2. Katada K, Anno H, Tsujioka K, et al (1991) Application of helical scanning CT – clinical experience with 174 cases. Toshiba Med Rev 38:7–17
3. Katada K (1993) Clinical usefulness of helical scan. In: Kimura K, Koga S (eds) Basic principles and clinical applications of helical scan; applications of continuous-rotation CT. Iryoukagakusya, Tokyo, pp 141–152
4. Katada K, Takeshita G, Ogura Y, et al (1993) Three-dimensional vascular imaging using helical scan. In: Kimura K, Koga S (eds) Basic principles and clinical applications of helical scan: applications of continuous-rotation CT. Iryoukagakusya, Tokyo, pp 170–182
5. Castillo M (1993) Diagnosis of disease of the common carotid artery bifurcation: CT angiography vs catheter angiography. AJR 161:395–398
6. Dillon EH, Leerwen MS, Fernandez A, Mali WPTM (1993) Spiral CT angiography. AJR 160:1273–1278

Three-dimensional CT angiography: application to detection of intracranial aneurysms

S. Imakita[1], N. Yamada[1], M. Takamiya[1], N. Hashimoto[2], Y. Kuriyama[3], T. Yamaguchi[3]

[1] Department of Radiology, National Cardiovascular Centre, Osaka, 5-7-1 Fuijishirodai, 565 Japan
[2] Department of Neurosurgery, National Cardiovascular Centre, Osaka, Japan
[3] Department of Neurology, National Cardiovascular Centre, Osaka, Japan

Abstract. We examined 20 patients with 26 intracranial aneurysms by three-dimensional CT angiography (3D-CTA) using helical scanning. Nine middle cerebral artery aneurysms, 4 basilar artery aneurysms, and 1 vertebral artery aneurysm were all clearly shown. In the demonstration of these aneurysms, 3D-CTA was equal or superior to conventional angiography. Three carotid-ophthalmic aneurysms and 1 cavernous carotid aneurysm were shown on 3D-CTA. The 3D-CTA was inferior to the conventional angiography in the demonstration of these 4 aneurysms. Six of 8 posterior communicating artery aneurysms were shown, but 2 could not be seen on 3D-CTA. In the demonstration of these aneurysms, 3D-CTA was equal or superior to the conventional angiography in 3 cases and inferior in 5. The longitudinal prolongation of intracranial vasculature could be reduced on 3D-CTA using 1 mm thick helical scanning. 3D-CTA is useful for detecting intracranial aneurysms.

Key words: Three-dimensional computed tomography angiography – Intracranial aneurysm – Helical scanning

Correspondence to: S. Imakita

There have been several reports of the clinical usefulness of high-resolution CT and three-dimensional CT angiography (3D-CTA) using rapid-sequence scanning in the diagnosis of intracranial aneurysms [1, 2]. However, the resolution of these CT studies is not always sufficient for the detection of small lesions. The purpose of this paper is to evaluate the reliability of 3D-CTA using helical scanning in showing vascular structures, and to determine its usefulness in detecting intracranial aneurysm.

Patients and methods

We studied 20 patients (12 women and 8 men, ranging in age from 50 to 69 years) with intracranial aneurysms (Table 1).

We carried out 3D-CTA using helical scanning. The procedure for 3D-CTA is summarised in Table 2.

Results

Of the 26 aneurysms 24 (92.3%) were shown on 3D-CTA, but 2 (7.7%) could not be seen. All of 9 middle cerebral artery aneurysms, 4 basilar artery aneurysms, and 1 vertebral artery aneurysm were shown on 3D-CTA. In demonstrating the orientation of these aneurysms and

Table 1. Summary of patients and aneurysms

Case no.	Age, sex	Site of aneurysm (An)	Detection of An
1	54, M	L-MCA (bifur)	CT = AG
2	52, M	R-MCA (bifur)	CT > AG
3	65, M	L-MCA (bifur)	CT > AG
4	69, M	L-MCA (bifur)	CT > AG
5	55, M	R-MCA (M1)	CT = AG
		R-MCA (bifur)	CT > AG
6	63, M	R-MCA (M2–3)	CT = AG
		L-MCA (M2)	CT > AG
7	65, M	L-MCA (bifur)	CT > AG
		BA top	CT = AG
8	64, M	BA top	CT = AG
9	59, F	BA top	CT = AG
10	59, F	BA top	CT = AG
11	65, M	R-IC-PC	CT = AG
12	62, M	L-IC-PC	CT < AG
13	64, F	R-IC-PC	CT = AG
14	64, F	R-IC-PC	CT > AG
15	50, F	R-IC-PC	CT < AG
		L-IC-PC	CT < AG
16	61, F	R-IC-PC	CT < AG
		L-IC-PC	CT < AG
17	65, F	L-IC (cavern)	CT < AG
18	51, F	R-IC-ophth	CT < AG
19	58, F	R-IC-ophth	CT < AG
		L-IC-ophth	CT < AG
20	66. F	R-VA	CT = AG

* Invisible on 3D-CTA; MCA, middle cerebral artery; BA, basilar artery; IC, internal carotid artery; PC, posterior communicating artery; VA vertebral artery; bifur, bifurcation; cavern, cavernous sinus; ophth, ophthalmic; CT, 3D-CTA; AG, conventional angiography

Table 2. Summary of the procedure for 3D-CT angiography

CT scanner:	X force, X vigor (Toshiba, Japan)
3D reconstruction system:	X link 50, X tension (Toshiba, Japan)
Scan time:	1.5 s/rotation (X force), 1 s/rotation (X vigour) Total scan time 50–100 s Scan delay time 40–75 s (after the start of injection)
Slice thickness:	1 mm or 2 mm
Table speed:	1 mm/rotation or 2 mm/rotation
Image reconstruction:	0.5 mm or 1 mm pitch, 360° interpolation
3D reconstruction method:	surface rendering, volume rendering
Matrix size:	512×512
Contrast medium:	Iohexol 350 injection via antecubital vein total volume 1.2–1.5 ml/body weight kg biphasic injection rate 1) 1.0–1.5 ml/s for 30 s 2) 0.7–1.0 ml/s

their relationship to the surrounding structure, 3D-CTA was equal or superior to conventional angiography (Fig. 1). Three carotid-ophthalmic aneurysms and 1 aneurysm of the cavernous carotid were shown on 3D-CTA. In the discrimination of these aneurysms from the surrounding structures, 3D-CTA was inferior to conventional angiography (Fig. 2). Six of 8 posterior communicating artery aneurysms (75%) were shown but 2 (25%) could not be dentified on 3D-CTA. In the discrimination of these aneurysms from the surrounding structures, 3D-CTA was equal or superior to conventional angiography in 3 of the 8 (37.5%) and inferior in 5 (62.5%). The artefactual longitudinal elongation of the intracranial vessels could be reduced on 3D-CTA using 1 mm thick instead of 2 mm thick scanning (Fig. 2).

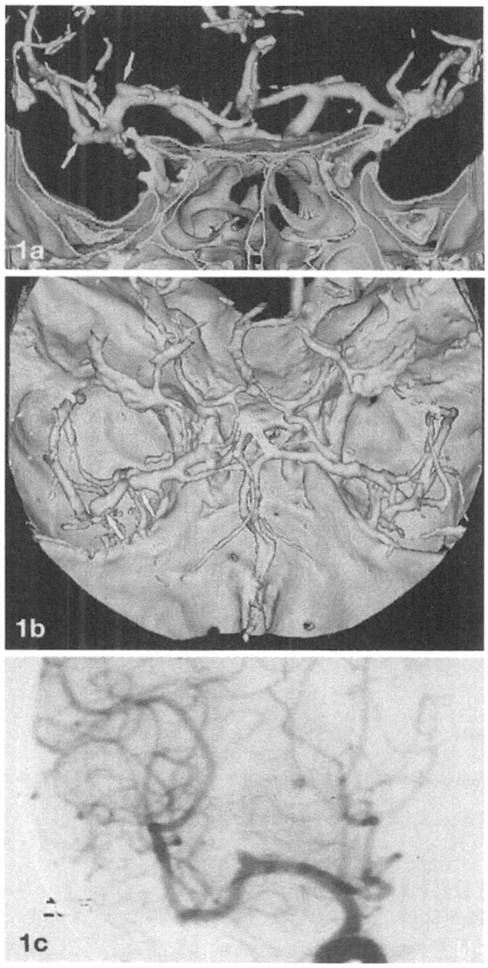

Fig. 1 a–c. Two right middle cerebral artery aneurysms (M_1 segment, bifurcation). **a, b** 3D-CTA **c** conventional angiography. The two aneurysms (*arrows*) are clearly discriminated from the surrounding structures on 3D-CTA

Discussion

Aneurysms can easily be observed from any direction on 3D-CTA. Therefore, they can be discriminated clearly from the surrounding vessels. However, aneurysms adjacent to the bone and the cavernous sinus cannot be clearly identified owing to the limitation of the threshold of CT numbers. Therefore, 3D-CTA is often inferior to conventional angiography in depicting aneurysms of the cavernous carotid, carotid-ophthalmic aneurysms, and some

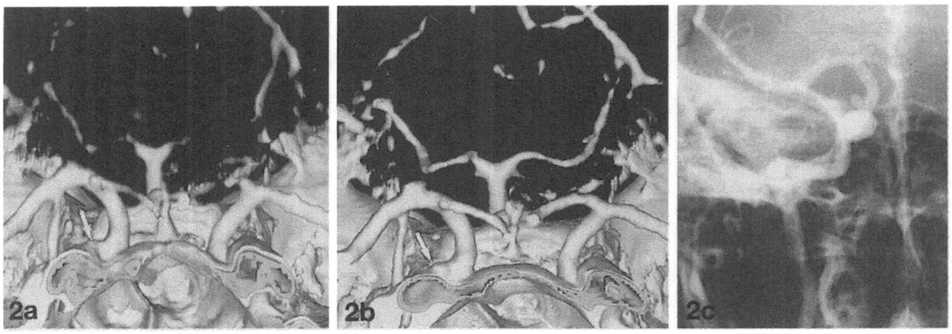

Fig. 2a–c. Case 18. Right carotid-ophthalmic aneurysm. **a, b** 3D-CTA using 2- and 1 mm thick helical scanning. **c** conventional angiography. The aneurysm (*arrow*) cannot be clearly separated from the adjacent bone. The artefactial elongation of the M_1 segment (increase in M_1 diameter) is reduced using 1 mm thick helical scanning

small posterior communicating aneurysms. Furthermore, because of the difficulty of showing the fine posterior communicating artery, small aneurysms at its origin cannot be clearly differentiated from infudibular widening on 3D-CTA.

References

1. Schmid UD, Steiger HJ, Huber P (1987) Accuracy of high-resolution computed tomography in direct diagnosis of cerebral aneurysms. Neuroradiology 29:152–159
2. Harbaugh RE, Schlusselberg DS, Jeffery R, Hayden S, Cromwell LD, Pluta D (1992) Three-dimensional computed tomography angiography in the diagnosis of cerebrovascular disease. J Neurosurg 76:408–414

Efficacy of 3D-CT angiography in surgical simulation of intracranial aneurysms

S. Nagasawa, J. Deguchi, H. Tanaka, M. Arai, T. Ohta

Department of Neurosurgery, Osaka Medical College, 2-7 Daigaku-cho, Takatsuki, 569, Osaka, Japan

Abstract. The efficacy of three-dimensional CT angiography (3D-CTA) in diagnosis and surgical planning was investigated in 38 patients with 48 intracranial aneurysms. Conformation of the diagnosis was possible in all aneurysms more than 2 mm in diameter by 3D-CTA, except those on the infraclinoid segment of the internal carotid artery. 3D-CTA showed configuartion of aneurysms and the neighbouring arterial and bony structures well. It was especially useful for: (1) multiple aneurysms, in which 3D-CTA gave good information on the accessibility of both far and near aneurysms on a single approach line; (2) giant aneurysms: the relations between the neck and parent artery were easily established by 3D-CTA images at arbitrary angles; (3) aneurysms near the skull base; and (4) aneurysms in the infraclinoid segment: the original axial images for 3D-CTA gave excellent information on structures in the extradural space.

Key words: Intracranial aneurysm – Computed tomography, Three-dimensional reconstruction – Angiography – Cerebrovascular disease

Correspondence to: S. Nagasawa

Three-dimensional CT angiography (3D-CTA) is known to give reliable information on the cerebro vascular system as well as the neighbouring bony structures of the skull base [1, 2]. This specific feature is useful not only for diagnosis of intracranial aneurysms but also for establishing surgical strategy.

Materials and methods

We investigated 28 surgically treated patients by 3D-CTA. We verified 48 intracranial aneurysms by conventional angiography. These were on the carotid artery in 25, the anterior cerebral artery in 1, the middle cerebral artery in 4 and the vertebrobasilar system in 18 cases, and ranged between 1 mm and 30 mm in diameter. Nonionic iodinated contrast medium, a total of 2 ml/kg, was infused intravenously at a rate of 1.5–2.5 ml/s. Helical scanning was begun 30–40 s after initiation of the infusion, 1–2 mm pitch for 1.5 s/cycle to produce 20–33 cycles. Images of 3D-CTA at various angles including the expected surgical approaches were created using a work Station. The views obtained in the surgical fields were compared to images of 3D-CTA, conventional digital subtraction angiography, MRI and MRA. Original axial images were also used for aneurysms in the clinoid segment of the internal carotid artery [3].

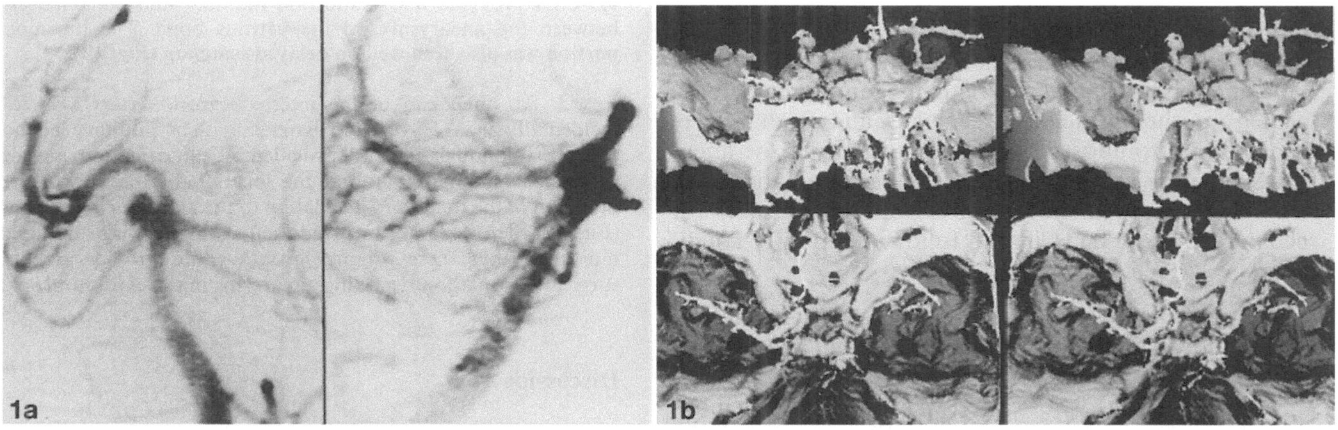

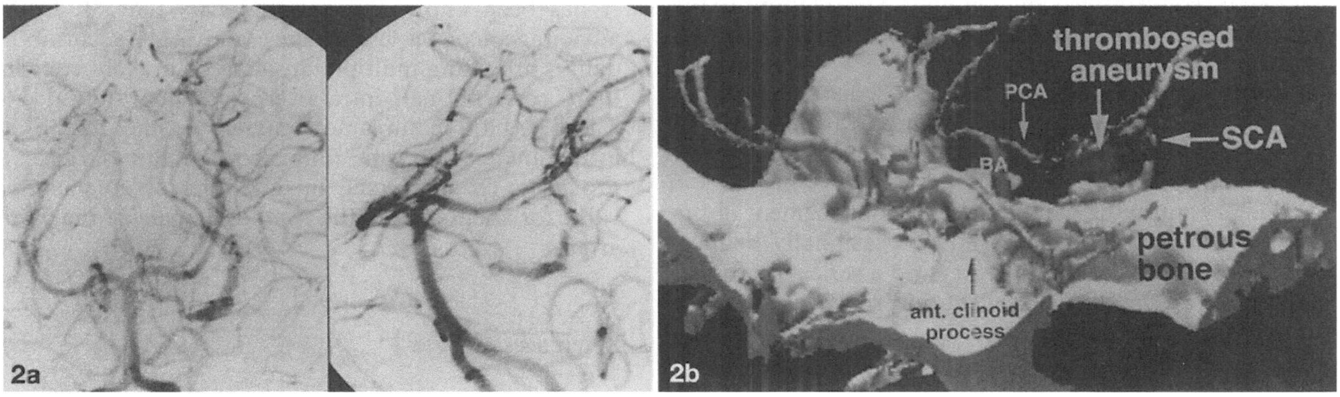

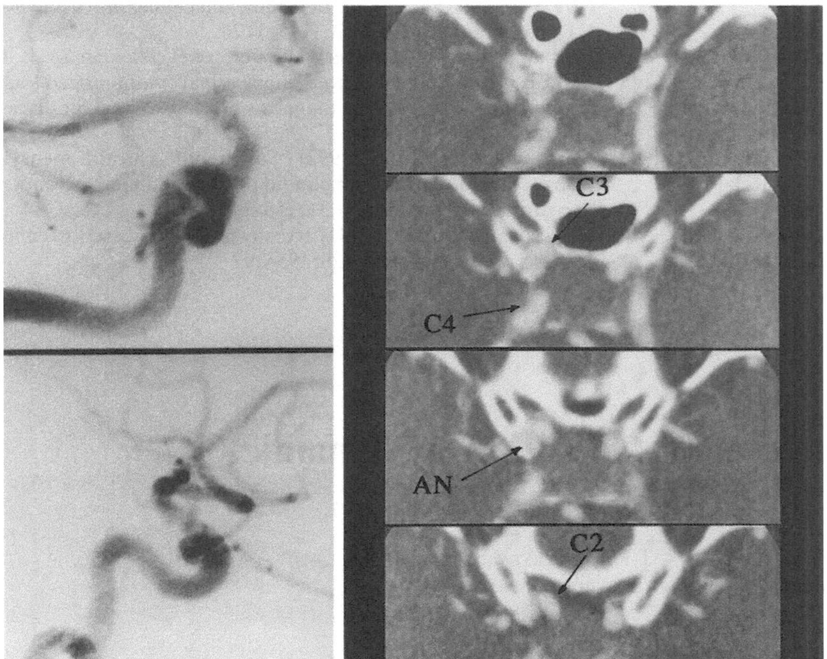

Fig. 1 a, b. Case 1. **a** Anteroposterior *left* and lateral *right* projections of left vertebral angiogram demonstrating an aneurysm at the origin of the right superior cerebellar artery. **b** Stereoscopy of 3D-CTA, showing the aneurysm and the bony spur lateral to the posterior clinoid process, viewed from the right anterolateral direction similar to the surgical approach (*top*) and from above (*bottom*)

Fig. 2. a Vertebral angiogram demonstrating a fusiform aneurysm of the left superior cerebellar artery in anteroposterior (*left*) and left anterior oblique (*right*) projections. **b** 3D-CTA showing the relationship between the aneurysm and neighbouring bony structures of the skull base and between the parent artery and two compartments of circulating blood and thrombus in the dome of the aneurysm. *BA*, basilar artery; *PCA*, posterior cerebral artery; *SCA*, superior cerebellar artery

Fig. 3. a Right internal carotid angiogram in anteroposterior (*top*) and lateral (*bottom*) projections demonstrating an aneurysm originating from the right internal carotid artery near the origin of the ophthalmic artery and projecting superolaterally. **b** Original axial images of 3D-CTA near the clinoid process with the lower slice displayed in upper row. The aneurysm (*AN*) originated at the posterolateral surface of the C3 portion of the internal carotid artery (*ICA*), extended upwards and eroded the tip of the anterior clinoid process. C_2, C_3, C_4, segments of ICA

Results

3D-CTA demonstrated all the aneurysms except for 1 of the 4 aneurysms that were less than 3 mm in diameter, 2 located in the infraclinoid segment and 2 that were completely thrombosed. The configuration of the aneurysms as well as the neighbouring arterial and bony structures were well shown and 3D-CTA was useful for recognising aneurysms in the following specific conditions:

1. Multiple aneurysms located on a single approach line; 3D-CTA provided good information about the accessibility of both far and near aneurysms.
2. Giant aneuryms whose neck was not clearly demonstrated by conventional angiography. The relations to the parent artery were easily established by obtaining images at arbitrary angles.
3. Aneurysms located near the skull base. Anatomical relations with bony structures such as the clinoid processes, jugular tubercle or petrous ridge were clearly delineated by 3D-CTA.
4. Aneurysms in the clinoid or cavernous segment of the carotid artery; although 3D-CTA occasionally demonstrated only some of these aneurysms, a series of original axial images provided excellent information on those located in the extradural space.

Illustrative case reports

Case 1. A 48-year-old man presented with a ruptured basilar artery superior cerebellar artery aneurysm on the right (Fig. 1a). 3D-CTA showed the aneurysm and a neighbouring bony spur lateral to the posterior clinoid process, which appeared to block the line of sight to the aneurysmal neck (Fig. 1b). At surgery, the spur was found on the approach line and removed for successful clipping of the neck [4].

Case 2. A 22-year-old man had a large ruptured aneurysm with partial thrombosis on the left superior cerebellar artery (Fig. 2a). 3D-CTA provided information on the neck and the relationship between the aneurysm and the petrous bone. The thrombosed portion was also seen well on delayed scanning (Fig. 2b).

Case 3. An aneurysm of the internal carotid artery was found incidentally in a 56-year-old woman with a pituitary adenoma (Fig. 3a). Although 3D-CTA provided little information, a series of original axial images showed the location of the neck and the direction of the dome and its relation to the anterior clinoid process (Fig. 3b). These data concurred well with the surgical findings, indicating that these original images could provide important surgical information regarding aneurysms in the extradural space.

Discussion

It has been known for several years that 3D-CTA is advantageous as a less invasive and more accurate modality, providing multiple projections in a shorter time, than conventional intra-arterial angiography [1, 2]. These specific features not only ensure the diagnosis of intracranial aneurysms, but also simulate surgical approaches. Original axial images were of great surgical value for aneurysms in the clinoid segment of the carotid artery.

References

1. Aoki S, Sasaki Y, Machida T, Ohkubo T, Minami M, Sasaki Y (1992) Cerebral aneurysms: detection and delineation using 3-D-CT angiography. AJNR 13:1115–1120
2. Harbaugh RE, Schlusselberg DS, Jeffery R, Hayden S, Cromwell LD, Pluta D (1992) Three-dimensional computerized tomography angiography in the diagnosis of cerebrovascular disease. J Neurosurg 76:408–414
3. Korosue K, Heros RC (1992) "Subclinoid" carotid aneurysm with erosion of the anterior clinoid process and fatal intraoperative rupture. Neurosurgery 31:356–360
4. Nagasawa S, Ohta T (1994) Exostosis of the posterior clinoid process. Acta Neurochir 126:195–197

Quantitative measurement of cerebral blood flow by dynamic CT

R. Takehara[1], D. Naka[1], Y. Naka[1], N. Tsuji[1], H. Imai[1], T. Kido[1], T. Terada[2], K. Nambu[3]

[1] Department of Neurological Surgery, Wakayama Rosai Hospital, 43T-Koya, Wakayama 640, Japan
[2] Department of Neurological Surgery, Wakayama Medical College, Wakayama, Japan
[3] Toshiba Nasu Works, Tochigi, Japan

Abstract. We propose a new "BOX-MTT method" to measure the regional cerebral blood flow (rCBF) quantitatively using a fourth-generation CT scanner. In this method, the time-density curve (TDC) of the region of interest (ROI) on the brain tissue is assumed to be proportional to convolution of the TDC of the artery feeding the ROI and the modulation transfer function (MTF). Although the transit pattern of the blood through the brain tissue is not well known, we hypothesise that the MTF is box-shaped and have named this model the BOX-MTT model. The rCBF and regional cerebral blood volume rCBV were measured by our method in eight patients with various neurological diseases. Our model fitted the original TDC well, and rCBV and rCBF values in various parts of the normal hemispheres were similar to

Correspondence to: T. Takehara

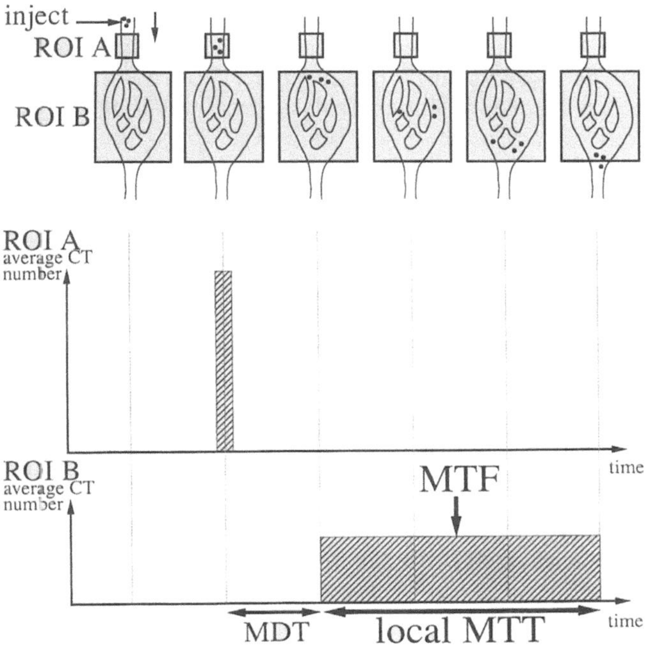

Fig. 1. Diagram of the "BOX-MTT model". Hypothesising that the local mean transit time (*MTT*) in the region of interest (*ROI*) is constant and that the mean delay time between an arterial ROI and a tissue ROI (*MDT*) is negligible, the modulation transfer function (*MTF*) is given a box shape

those measured by PET or SPECT. By applying deconvolution analysis, we found that the MTF in the brain tissue was approximately box-shaped. Our method offers quantitative rCBF values by fitting TDCs directly to the BOX-MTT model.

Key words: Cerebral blood flow – Cerebral blood volume – Dynamic computed tomography

---

It is possible to calculate regional cerebral blood flow (rCBF) by measuring the transit time in brain tissue and artery. We propose a new "BOX-MTT analysis method" for measuring rCBF quantitatively with a fourth-generation CT scanner. In this method, the original time-density curves (TDCs) are fitted directly without gamma fitting, and the transfer function in the region is regarded as box-shaped. Our method is presented in this paper.

Methods

Theory

CBF can be calculated from cerebral blood volume (CBV) and mean transit time (MTT) according to the formula:

$$\mathrm{CBF} = \mathrm{CBV}/\mathrm{MTT} \tag{1}$$

Because CBV and MTT cannot be extracted directly from the data of dynamic CT, we have developed the "BOX-MTT analysis method" to calculate them from TDC.

Principles of "BOX-MTT analysis"

In this method, the TDC of a region of interest (ROI) placed on brain tissue (Ci) is presumed to be proportional to convolution of the input function and modulation transfer function (MTF), where the input function is the TDC of the artery (Ca) feeding the ROI:

$$\mathrm{Ci} = \mathrm{K}(\mathrm{Ca} \cdot \mathrm{MTF}) \tag{2}$$

K is a constant. For the average increase in CT number in the ROI at t s after the injection of contrast medium [$\mathrm{Ci}(t)$],

$$\mathrm{Ci}(t) = \mathrm{K} \int_0^{\infty} \mathrm{Ca}(t - s)\, \mathrm{MTF}(s)\, ds \tag{3}$$

where $\mathrm{Ca}(t)$ is the average arterial CT number increment at t s after the injection.

We hypothesise that the MTF is box-shaped (not an exponential function), and call this the "BOX-MTT model". If a box-shaped MTF is proposed,

$$\mathrm{MTF}(t) = \begin{cases} \dfrac{1}{m} & (0 \le t \le m) \\ 0 & (\text{otherwise}) \end{cases} \tag{4}$$

where m is the "local MTT". In this model, we defined "local MTT" as the mean time for the contrast medium to pass through the ROI. This definition is different from the usual MTT, explained as the centre of gravity of the TDC in the ROI.

The BOX-MTT model is given by hypothesising that the local MTT in the ROI is constant and that the mean delay time between an arterial ROI and a ROI placed on brain tissue (MDT) is negligible (Fig. 1).

Applying the $\mathrm{MTF}(t)$ (Eq. 4) to Eq. 3 is equivalent to

$$\mathrm{Ci}(t) = \mathrm{K} \int_{-m}^{0} \mathrm{Ca}(t + s)\, ds \tag{5}$$

Both m and K can be calculated by fitting model 5 to the measured curves $\mathrm{Ci}(t)$ and $\mathrm{Ca}(t)$ using the least-squares method:

$$\text{local MTT} = m \tag{6}$$

$\mathrm{Ci}(t)$ can also be described as follows:

$$\mathrm{Ci}(t) = \frac{\mathrm{CBV}(-\mathrm{bHtc})}{1 - \mathrm{Htc}} \frac{1}{m} \int_{-m}^{0} \mathrm{Ca}(t + s)\, ds \quad (\mathrm{b} = 0.69) \tag{7}$$

where Htc is the haematocrit in the peripheral artery, and b is a constant relating peripheral haematocrit to tissue haematocrit. CBV is derived from Eqs. 5 and 7:

$$\mathrm{CBV} = \frac{(1 - \mathrm{Htc})m\mathrm{K}}{1 - \mathrm{bHtC}} \tag{8}$$

CBF is calculated from Eqs. 1, 6 and 8.

Input function

In the brain, it is impossible to obtain arterial TDC (Ca) directly, because there is no artery that has a sufficiently large cross-section to place the ROI in it. Since the area under the curve (AUC) following a single contrast medium bolus should be the same for all arteries and veins in the brain, where almost all contrast medium stays within the vascular system, AUC in the superior sagittal sinus ($\mathrm{AUC_{SSS}}$) is used to amplify the TDC for the ROI which was set to surround the middle cerebral artery ($\mathrm{C_{MCA}}$):

$$\mathrm{C_{MCA}} = \mathrm{ACa} \tag{9}$$

$$\mathrm{A} = \mathrm{AUC_{MCA}}/\mathrm{AUC_{SSS}} \tag{10}$$

When this method is applied to obtain an input function, Eq. 8 should be corrected based on Eq. 9:

$$\mathrm{CBV} = \mathrm{A}\,\frac{(1 - \mathrm{Htc})m\mathrm{K}}{1 - \mathrm{bHtc}} \tag{11}$$

Cases

We examined eight patients with neurological diseases.

A 40-ml bolus of iodinated contrast medium was administered via the antecubital vein at the rate of 8 ml/s using a mechanical injector. The CT images were scanned with 5 mm slice thickness and with a scan duration of 1 s. In 2 cases, a series of 20 scans was initiated 3 s after the start of the injection with 7 s interscan delay. For the other 6 cases, a series of 24 scans without interscan delay was started 6 s after the injection.

The ROI were set on an MCA branch, the superior sagittal sinus (SSS), putamen, thalamus, MCA territory and white matter in the frontal lobe to obtain the TDCs. The average CT number of the pixels within the ROI was determined for each scan and plotted against time.

The BOX-MTT analysis was performed for each ROI to calculate the rCBV, local MTT and rCBF. Direct calculation of MTF was also performed by deconvoluting the formula Ci = K(Ca · MTF) (deconvolution analysis), to prove the hypothesis that the MTF in the ROI is box-shaped.

Results

Our model fitted the original TDC well, and a box-shaped MTF was obtained from each ROI.

The rCBV and rCBF values of 8 cases were calculated in various parts of the normal hemispheres. The rCBV values (mean ± SD%) were 2.7 ± 0.91 in the putamen, 2.2 ± 0.74 in the thalamus, 3.5 ± 1.33 in the MCA territory, 2.9 ± 0.83 in the MCA territory except major vessels, and 2.1 ± 0.99 in the frontal white matter. The rCBF values were 73 ± 17 (mean ± SD ml flow/100 ml brain tissue/min) in the putamen, 50 ± 22 in the thalamus, 78 ± 38 in the MCA territory, 52 ± 15 in the MCA territory except major vessels, and 23 ± 15 in the frontal white matter.

Discussion

We speculated the wash-out pattern of blood from the tissue is box-shaped rather than exponential [1–3]. By applying deconvolution analysis, we found that the wash-out pattern in the brain tissue was approximately box-shaped. Out method fits raw data to the BOX-MTT model and provides direct calculation of MTT without gamma fitting. Therefore, it is not necessary to use unstable factors (e.g., MTT, lung circulation, and recirculation of contrast medium) derived from gamma fitting.

Both rCBF and rCBV values were similar to those measured by PET or SPECT. The CBF value in the thalamus was lower than reported values in our series. As the thalamus is supplied by the vertebrobasilar system, there might be a slight difference in the arrival time of contrast medium between the carotid and vertebral systems, which might result in rCBF changes.

Out method offers new quantitative rCBF measurements using a fourth-generation CT scanner.

References

1. Gobbel GT, Cann CE, Fike JR (1991) Measurement of regional cerebral blood flow using ultrafast computed tomography. Stroke 22:768–771
2. Gobbel GT, Cann CE, Iwamoto HS, Fike JR (1991) Measurement of regional cerebral blood flow using ultrafast computed tomography: experimental validation. Stroke 22:772–779
3. Gobbel GT, Cann CE, Fike JR (1993) Comparison of xenon-enhanced CT with ultrafast CT for measurement of regional cerebral blood flow. AJNR 14:543–550

3D-CT reconstructions and rapid prototyping models in craniospinal diseases: preliminary clinical experience

L. Valvassori[1], N. Colombo[1], S. Sforza[2], V. Branca[1], E. Boccardi[1], S. Taggi[2], S. Villa[2], F. Tovazzi[2], M. Sberna[1], G. Scialfa[1]

[1] Neuroradiology Department, Ospedale Niguarda Ca'Granda, Milano, Italy
[2] Mirus Lob Project/ACR Foundation, Milan, Italy

Abstract. The evolution of computer science and its application to medical imaging has led to a great interest in post-elaboration of CT data. Head and neck and neuroradiology are certainly some of the best fields of application of this new technique. Based on CT image acquisition of osseous tissues in different pathologies, a new method is being tested, which includes the possibility of producing solid models from 3D offline reconstructions, by a rapid prototyping technique.

Correspondence to: L. Valvassori

Key words: Computed tomography, technology – Computed tomography, three-dimensional – Treatment planning

In the last few years post-processing techniques for treatment of CT data have been greatly changing and becoming quicker and cheaper [1]. Sometimes it seems as if technological evolution has overtaken real clinical necessities but in 3D reconstructions have become a currently used imaging modality in many institutions and, thanks to advances in computer science, they are no longer limited to CT data and bone tissue diseases [2].

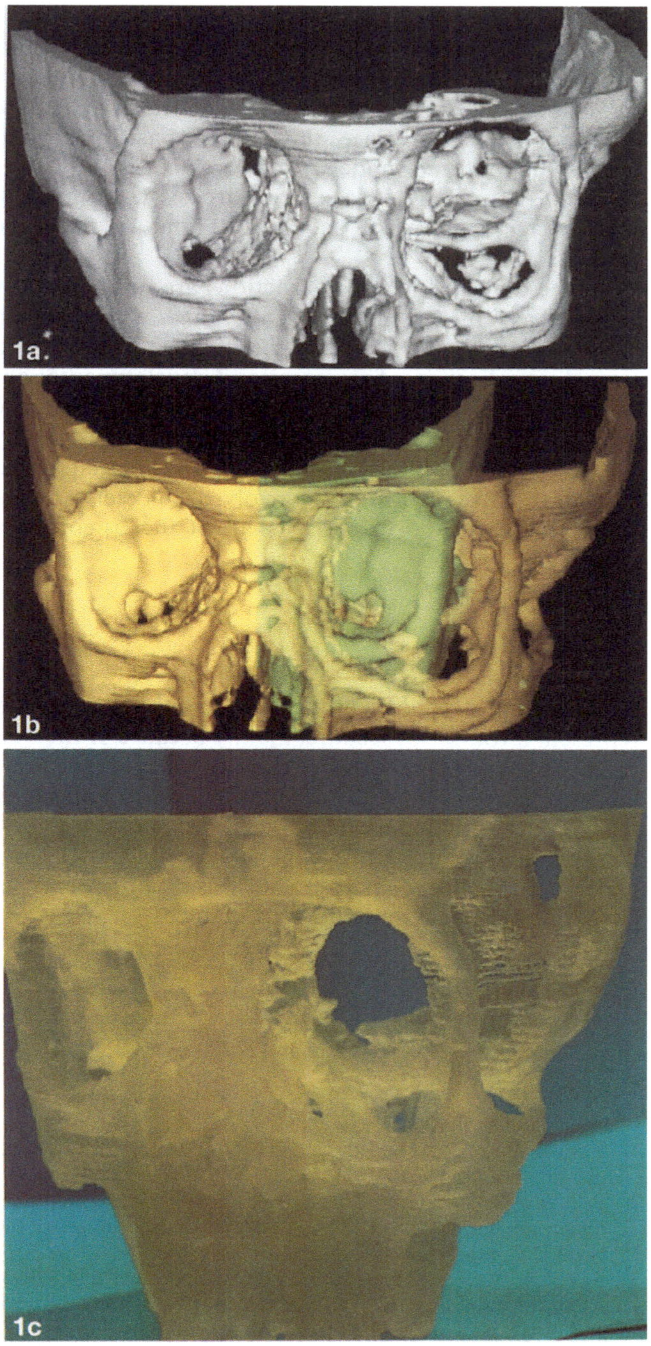

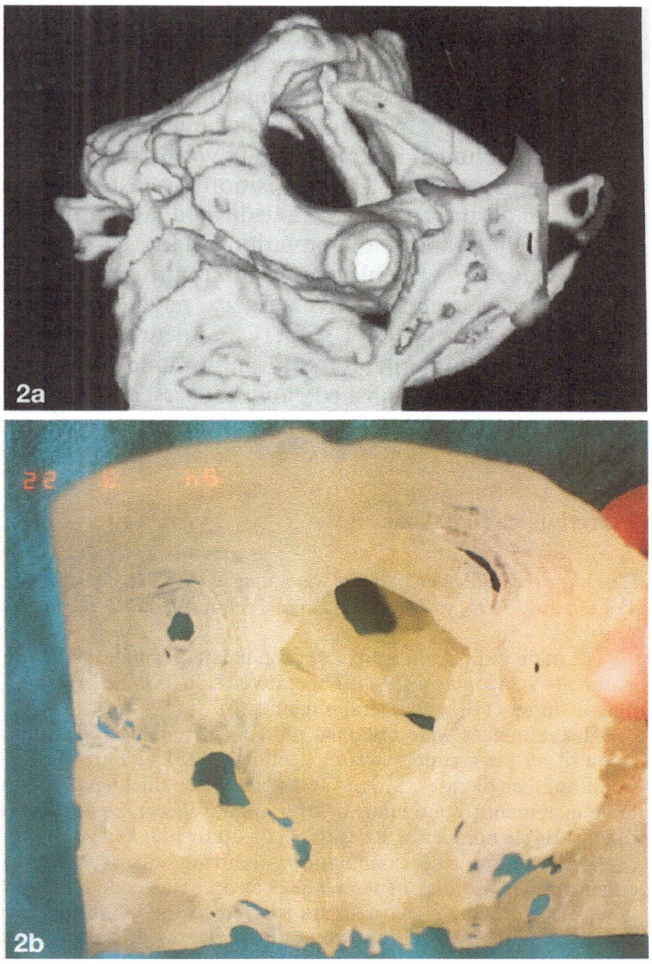

Fig. 1. a Offline 3D reconstruction in a 14-year-old patient suffering from von Recklinghausen's disease. A complex malformation of the left orbital cavity is present, with dysplasia of the greater wing of the sphenoid **b** Video surgical simulation, for reconstruction of the left orbit, obtained by mirroring the right orbit on the left. Solid model obtained by stereolithography

Fig. 2. Solid model obtained by stereolithography. Congenital malformation of the craniocervical junction in a young patient, consisting of aplasia of the right arch of C1 with rotation and upward dislocation of C2. Offline 3D reconstruction. View from above showing the great deformity of the spinal canal. Corresponding solid model

Current applications still concern mostly malformative and traumatic alterations but, whereas years ago only rough images, which took a long time to be reconstructed, were available, today new tools, strictly connected to hardware and software technology, are at our disposal. We are therefore able to achieve different post-processing modalities in almost realtime. With regard to CT, cranio-spinal diseases best satisfy the need for a complete preoperative assessment of patients, given the complexity of the anatomical regions and the difficulty of surgery [3, 4].

Together with "conventional" 3D images, two additonal tools are being tested in our hospital: video surgical simulation and solid models production.

In 1991, a new project was started consisting of a laboratory dedicated to offline image elaboration, reconstruction and visualization of potentially any digitally acquired image.

So far, 3D reconstructions have been obtained with the Siemens Somatom DRH (taking over 1 h) and with the then new, and much faster, Siemens HiQ, using the software implemented on the scanners. Such a procedure had some obvious drawbacks. The time required to process the images meant that no new patients were acquired. The software itself also had clear limits in terms of obtaining different views, eliminating artefacts, making cuts in different planes, and performing measures. As a result, little clinical interest was shown by physicians in this imaging modality. The acquisition of a faster scanner, but above all the creation of a dedicated laboratory, has dramatically changed the situation. Many co-operative studies have been established in different branches, such as plastic and reconstructive surgery, maxillofacial surgery, dental surgery, ENT surgery and neurosurgery.

The aim of this paper is to show how model production is technically accomplished, and to present the initial application of such a method to clinics.

Materials and methods

One hundred and seven patients were imaged by CT from September 1992 to July 1994, with specific clinical requests for 3D reconstructions.

The main indications were: craniospinal malformations (30) and trauma (45), neoplasms (9), preoperative evaluation before cranioplastic surgery (10) and dental implants (6).

All the images were obtained on a Siemens HiQ CT scanner. Acquisition programmes were as follows: 125 kV, 140 mAs (in a small number of cases, 375 mAs), 1–2 mm slice thickness, 1–2 mm table increments (contiguous or overlapping slices), 2 s acquisition time, variable number of slices (from 25 up to 100) and zooming.

At the end of the examination, archiving was accomplished either on the hard disk of the scanner or on a magnetic removable tape, on which data sets were transferred to the laboratoy. This was because the two stations are not yet integrated in a local area network.

We developed ad hoc programs for reading and writing Siemens Somatom, ACR-NEMA and DICOM file format.

First of all we performed data analysis to find out a good structure of interest segmentation. Then we chose a suitable threshold to compute the best isosurface fitting the structure bounds.

We used this geometry to obtain both good anatomical 3D images by rendering and a suitable input for CATIA, a CAD system. Once the isosurface was a CATIA structure, we obtained output for stereolithography systems by writing an appropriate triangular mesh in an STL ASCII file format.

Using different external services, we tested some rapid prototyping (RP) technologies. Generally, stereolithography was preferred because it was both cheaper and faster than others.

We have a research agreement with an Italian stereolithographic service, so that the time needed for each model is about 1 week and the maximum cost for a complex model is $ 1200, with an average cost for each of $ 600.

Results

All the images and models obtained were judged as satisfactory by both neuroradiologists and surgeons. From a technical point of view, it is important to acquire very good images, since this is the basis for good reconstructions and models: 1 or 2 mm slices, no movement by the patient, sedation or narcosis when needed, low dosage, and rapid acquisition time to minimize artifacts.

Three-dimensional reconstructions are now generally accepted as a further image modality, highly beneficial in specific pathologies, where it is critical to have a good spatial visualization of fractures and developmental abnormalities, as well as evaluation of asymmetry, before the surgical treatment. Surgical simulation may be greatly helped by the possibility of handling a solid anatomical copy of the osseous structures involved, so determining a correct surgical approach and plan of the osteotomies (Figs. 1, 2).

Discussion

At this time it is difficult to imagine that this could represent a routine procedure, mainly because of the cost in money and time. For particular clinical requests, however, such as the study of complex malformations of the craniocervical junction or of the face, in which a good therapeutical result greatly depends upon a correct and precise preoperative assessment, this methodology is likely to have many more benefits than costs.

Acknowledgement. This research is supported by the ACR Foundation

References

1. Fishman EK, Magid D, Ney DK, et al (1991) Three-dimensional imaging. Radiology 181:321–337
2. Pellizzari C, Chen G, Spelbring D, et al (1989) Accurate three-dimensional registration of CT, PET and/or MR images of the brain. J Comput Assist Tomogr 13:20
3. Ray CE, Maffee MF, Friedman M, Tahmoressi CN (1993) Applications of three-dimensional CT imaging in head and neck pathology. Radiol Clin North Am 31:181–194
4. Zonneveld F, Lobregt S, Meuten J van der (1989) Three-dimensional imaging in craniofacial surgery. World J Surg 13:328–342

CT-based stereotactically guided microsurgical resection of small lesions in "eloquent" brain areas

D. Van Roost[1], C. Cedzich[1], L. Solymosi[2]

[1] Neurochirurgische Universitätsklinik, Bonn, Germany
[2] Neuroradiologie, Radiologische Universitatsklinik, Bonn, Germany

Abstract. CT-based stereotactic guiding was used for microsurgical resections of 22 small lesions located deep in functionally important brain areas, and supported in 12 cases by intraoperative functional cortical mapping. The latter consisted of direct cortical recording of somatosensory evoked potentials and their phase reversal over the central sulcus. Stereotactic guiding allowed for small, well-centred craniotomies and was found to be very reliable for transfer of a preoperatively planned transsulcal approach into the operation field. In only one case did intraoperative brain swelling cause a surface shift and a morphological disagreement between planning and initial operative findings. In this case the ambiguity was overcome by the simultaneous use of functional mapping. Otherwise, CT morphology alone proved to be reliable for the identification of the rolandic structures near the vertex, while it was of little use for the identification of motor and sensory structures near the sylvian fissure.

Key words: Stereotaxis - Computed tomography - Evoked potentials - Functional mapping

In functionally critical brain areas, even very small lesions become symptomatic and are easily detected by modern digital imaging techniques. However, the concern of causing no new deficit may then jeopardize the surgical consequences, which would not be debated if another brain area was involved. This study examines the feasibility of resecting lesions from functionally important brain areas with the aid of CT-based stereotactic guiding, and with the facility of cortical mapping by evoked potentials.

Patients and methods

In a 3-year period, we operated on 22 patients with small lesions. The exact localization of these lesions was prerolandic and rolandic in 14 patients, postcentral in 4 patients, and 1 patient each had a lesion within the superior temporal gyrus, the optic radiation, the cerebral peduncle and the internal capsula. The histological diagnosis was metastasis in 8 cases, cavernous angioma in 6, glioblastoma in 5, and astrocytoma, tuberculoma and granuloma in 1 case each. The size of lesions ranged between 5 and 28 mm with a mean value of 17 mm and a standard deviation of 8 mm.

A Riechert-Mundinger stereotactic frame was used for guiding, which was based on CT morphology and enhanced by i.v. contrast medium. The frame was mounted close to or below the skull base and artefact-free fixation pins and head posts were used. In 20 cases the stereotactic frame was left on the head for navigation during the microsurgical procedure, while in 2 cases the stereotactic placement of a guiding catheter preceded the microsurgical procedure.

Additionally to stereotactic guiding, somatosensory evoked potentials (SEP) were recorded for the intraoperative localization of the central sulcus in 12 patients. After stimulation of the median nerve at the wrist, SEP were recorded from the cortex directly by means of strip or grid electrodes, placed over the suspected central sulcus. A typical potential with N20/P20 peaks was available from the primary sensory cortex and its phase reversal, i.e. a typical P20/N20, was recorded from the primary motor cortex. The exact stimulation and recording parameters are listed in Table 1.

Table 1. Stimulation and recording methods

SEP	
Stimulation	Bipolar
Intensity	20 mA
Frequency	5.3 Hz
Duration	300 µs
Recording	Strip/grid electrode
Filter	30 Hz–3 kHZ
Repetition	50–250
Sensitivity	10–20 µV/div

Results

The cortex surface was inconspicuous in 21 patients, i.e. the lesion was not detectable at the brain surface, either by inspection or by palpation. A tumorous infiltration was observed in only 1 patient; in another patient with a subcortical cavernous angioma the cortex was faintly stained. The distance from the cortex surface to the tumour border was 16 mm on average, with a standard deviation of 7 mm, with the exception of the lesion of the cerebral peduncle, which was located at a depth of 78 mm from the frontal cortex. The CT-based stereotactic guiding allowed an uncomplicated, quick and accurate localization in all patients, and surgical removal of the lesion through a small, well-centred craniotomy. The approach to the lesions around the central sulcus could, as a rule, be planned at the CT desk with such detail that afterwords, in the operating theatre, the guiding cannula pointed to the right sulcus to be entered. However, in 1 case the stereotactic guidance did not mark the sulcus aimed at on the CT, but an adjacent gyrus, due to brain swelling with a shift at the surface. Anti-oedematous measures corrected the morphological disagreement between planning and initial operative findings. In this case, and in 11 other cases, the SEP phase reversal method was used intraopera-

Correspondence to: D. Van Roost, Neurochirurgische Universitätsklinik, Sigmund-Freud-Strasse 25, D-53127 Bonn, Germany

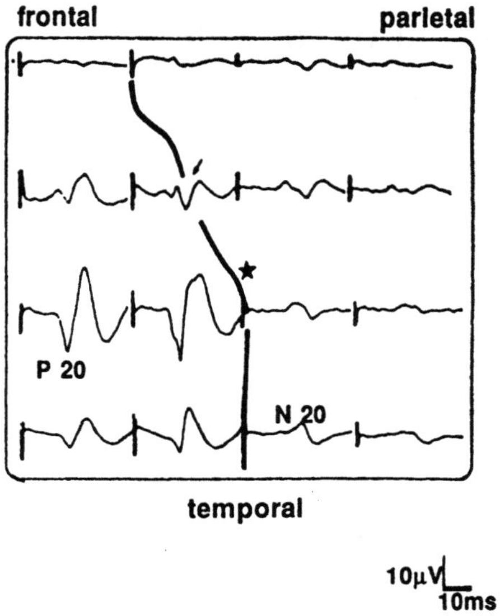

Fig. 1. Potentials recorded from the cortex after median-nerve stimulation. A typical P20 is obtained over the precentral gyrus and a typical N20 over the postcentral gyrus. The *star* indicates the course of the central sulcus. The *arrow* indicated an intermediate potential form which can sometimes be recorded directly over the central sulcus

tively as a functional method for the localization of the central sulcus and of the postcentral and the precentral gyri. In all these cases we obtained a typical phase reversal (Fig. 1). In 9 of the 12 patients SEP phase reversal corroborated the sulcal and gyral approach in the central region, which turned out to be well-definable on a CT-morphological base near the vertex. In the other 3 patients the SEP phase reversal intraoperatively distinguished motor and sensory brain areas near the sylvian fissure, where CT morphology proved to be of little use. Postoperatively 3 patients showed an improvement in their deficits, 5 had no deficit, 6 an unchanged neurological deficit, 5 a temporary new motor deficit and only 3 patients demonstrated a permanent new deficit.

Discussion

With the above-described combination of CT-based stereotactic guiding and the intraoperative SEP phase reversal method for the microsurgical resection of small lesions deep in functionally important brain areas, we obtained good functional results, as demonstrated by the morbidity rate of 13.6%. With CT-based stereotactic guiding a perfectly centred, small craniotomy for a transcerebral or trans-sulcal approach is possible. The possibility of preoperative planning led us to prefer the stereotactic method over an intraoperative ultrasonic localization.

The intraoperative use of functional cortical mapping makes it possible to correct for an eventual disagreement between preoperative imaging and the operation field, whereas image-based preoperative cortical mapping would be subjected to the same mechanisms that led to the disagreement and thus could not correct for it. The method has already been discribed in the 1950s [1] and was used in the 1970s during epilepsy surgery [2–5], and later also during tumour surgery [6–13]. The success rate of phase reversal has been reported in the literature to be between 91.4% [9] and 93.8% [12].

The combination of two already well-known methods seems to be of great help for surgery of small lesions within functional, critical brain areas.

References

1. Woolsey CN, Erickson TC (1950) Study of the postcentral gyrus of man by evoked potential technique. Trans Am Neurol Assoc 75:50–52
2. Goldring S (1978) A method for surgical management of focal epilepsy, especially as it related to children. J Neurosurg 49:344–356
3. Goldring S, Gregorie EM (1984) Surgical management of epilepsy using epidural recordings to localize the seizure focus. J Neurosurg 60:457–466
4. Gregorie EM, Goldring S (1984) Localization of function in the excision of lesions from the sensorimotor cortex. J Neurosurg 61:1047–1054
5. Ojemann GA (1979) Brain organization for language from perspective of electrical stimulation mapping. Behav Brain Sci 6:189–220
6. Black P, Ronner SF (1987) Cortical mapping for defining the limits of tumor resection. Neurosurgery 20:914–919
7. Cedzich C, Taniguchi M, Schramm J (1991) Die exakte Bestimmung des Sulcus centralis mittels SEP-Phasenumkehr. Z EEG-EMG 21:96
8. Firsching R, Klug N, Börner U, Sanker P (1992) Lesions of sensorimotor evoked potentials and ultrasound guided surgery. Acta Neurochir 118:87–90
9. King RB, Schell GR (1987) Cortical localization and monitoring during cerebral operations. J Neurosurg 67:210–219
10. Lueders H, Lesser RP, Hahn J (1983) Cortical somatosensory evoked potentials in response to hand stimulation. J Neurosurg 58:885–894
11. Nuwer M (1991) Localization of motor cortex with median nerve SEPs. In: Schramm J, Moller A (eds) Intraoperative neurophysiologic monitoring, Springer, Berlin Heidelberg New York, pp 35–41
12. Wood CC, Spencer DD, Allison T, McCarthy BR, Williamson PD, Goff WR (1988) Localization of human sensorimotor cortex during surgery by cortical surface recording of somatosensory evoked potentials. J Neurosurg 68:99–111
13. Woolsey CN, Erickson TC, Gilson WE (1979) Localization in somatic sensory and motor areas of human cerebral cortex as determined by direct recording of evoked potentials and electrical stimulation. J Neurosurg 51:476–506

Development and early trials of real-time CT fluoroscopy

K. Katada[1], H. Anno[1], Y. Ogura[2], G. Takeshita[2], S. Koga[2], K. Nonomura[3], H. Sano[3], T. Kanno[3], S. Sata[4], Y. Shibata[4]

[1] Fujita Health Iniversity, School of Health Sciences, Toyoake, Japan
[2] Department of Radiology, Fujita Health University, Toyoake, Japan
[3] Department of Neurosurgery, Fujita Health University, Toyoake, Japan
[4] CT Engineering Department, Nasu works, Toshiba Corporation, Ohtawara, Japan

Abstract. A CT fluoroscopy system that permits real-time monitoring of CT images was developed. In phantom studies the images were displayed at a rate of 6 per s, with a delay time of 0.67 s. Early clinical trials in aspiration of intracranial haematoma and brain tumour biopsy indicated that CT fluoroscopy is useful for CT-guided intervention on the central nervous system.

Key words: CT fluoroscopy – CT-guided intervention – Stereotactic surgery – Real-time reconstruction

In the last 45 years CT-guided intervention has become a modality of choice for selected neurosurgical diseases [1–3]. However, the time interval required for image reconstruction resulted in inaccuracy in CT-guided procedures. The purpose of this study is to develop a CT fluoroscopy (CTF) system that can provide real-time reconstruction of CT images, and to apply CTF to neurosurgical interventions.

Methods and subjects

A prototype CT scanner with third-generation geometry equipped with s slip-ring and solid-state detector system was used. CTF was conducted by continuing 1-s scan up to 50 s, with the parameters of 120 kV and 50 mA (50 mAs). The CT images were consequently reconstructed by continously acquiring raw data with a 256×256 matrix, using a newly developed array processor and reconstruction algorithm (Fig. 1). Reconstructed images were displayed on the monitor and were recorded on a videocassette recorder. Experimental and volunteer studies were performed, and the results were evaluated in terms of temporal resolution and image quality. A total of 14 clinical cases underwent CTF, 5 involved diseases of the central nervous system. These consisted of stereotactic punctures and aspirations of intracerebral haematomas (3), ventricular tapping for the drainage of intraventricular haematoma accompanying moyamoya disease (1), and a biopsy of thalamic glioma (1).

Results

Phantom studies revealed that the CTF system achieved the temporal resolution of 6 images per s, with a delay time of 0.67 s. CTF of the volunteer successfully visualised real-time reconstruction of the hand-in-motion with sufficient image quality. Clinical trials of CTF in monitoring puncture and aspiration were successful in 4 cases. In spite of image deterioration due to metallic artefacts from the stereotactic frame or puncture needle, the process of needle puncture and placement, and also the processes of irrigation and aspiration, were monitored by CTF (Fig. 2, 3). In a case of thalamic glioma, biopsy was not successful due to deterioration of the patient's condition. There were no complications attributable to CTF.

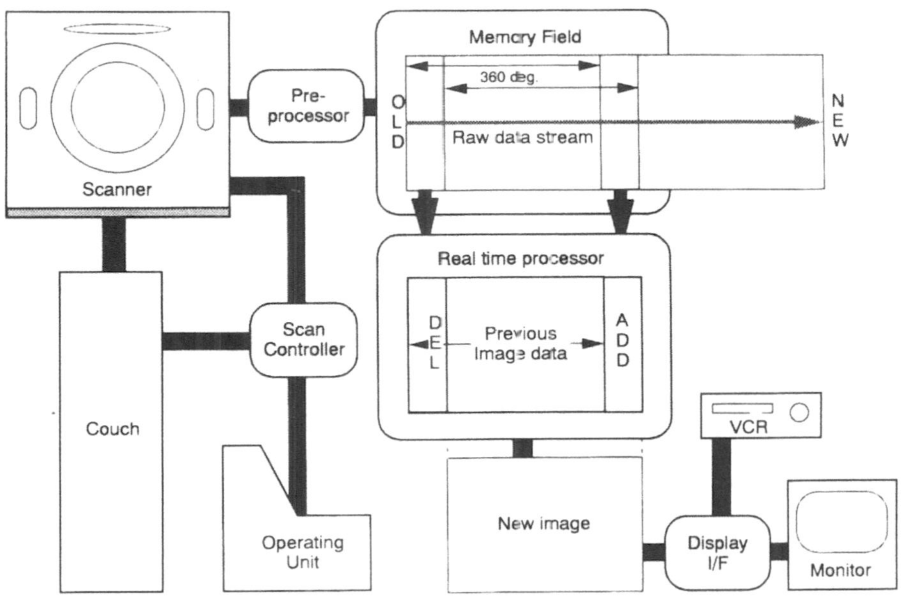

Fig. 1. Block diagram of CT fluoroscopic system

Correspondence to: K. Katada

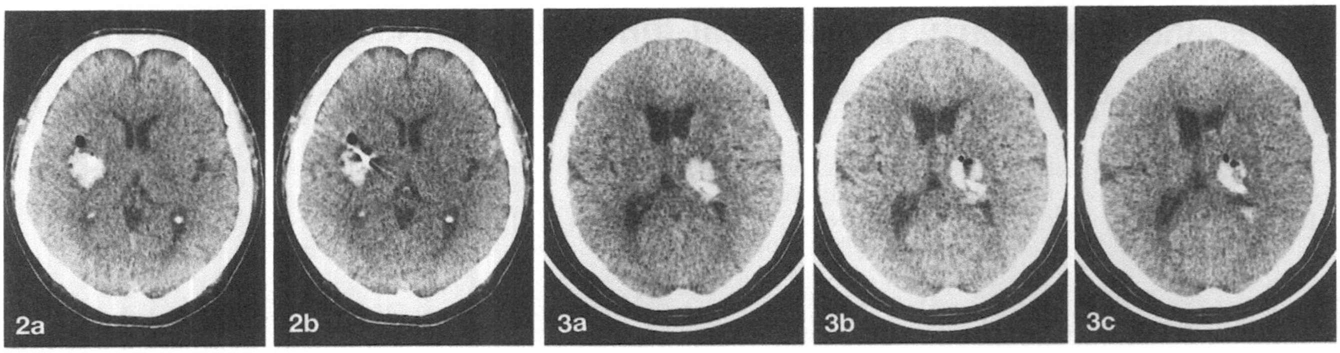

Fig. 2. CT fluoroscopy-guided puncture of intracerebral haematoma in a 60-year-old man with hypertensive putaminal haemorrhage. CT fluoroscopic images **a** before and **b** after insertion of drainage tube in real-time

Fig. 3 a–c. A 52-year-old woman with hypertensive thalamic haemorrhage. CT fluoroscopy showed the process of haematoma irrigation and aspiration in real-time. **a** Before **b** after irrigation. Normal saline solution is seen at the centre of the haematoma, with air bubbles. **c** After aspiration. The normal saline solution has disappeared, together with part of the haematoma. Note the fluid level in ipsilateral lateral ventricle, indicating communication between haematoma cavity and ventricle

Discussion

Attempts to utilise CT for the guidance of biopsy originated in 1976 [4]. Shortly after the initial trial, its application to central nervous system lesions started [1–3]. One of the limitations of these conventional CT-guided interventions was the interruption of the procedure because of the time interval required for image processing. In order to improve on this situation, the real-time CT system was developed [5] and was applied to clinical cases. Our initial clinical trial showed that CTF had definite advantages over conventional procedures in several respects. Real-time monitoring of puncture, tube positioning, irrigation, aspiration and biopsy improved the accuracy and success rate of these procedures. It also contributes to improved safety of the procedure by reducing the number of punctures and by allowing earlier detection of any complications earlier.

The current CTF system has various limitations and disadvantages: the scan angle is basically limited to an axial direction, and metallic artifacts from stereotactic frames and puncture needles sometimes degrade the quality of the fluoroscopic images. The major disadvantage of CTF will be the use of ionic radiation. Although the X-ray dose used in CTF is approximately one-tenth used in conventional CT (50 mAs), it is 10 times that needed for conventional fluoroscopy. Further reductions of dosage are anticipated with improvement of the system.

References

1. Gleason CA, Wise BL, Feinstein B (1978) Stereo tactic localization (with computed tomographic scanning), biopsy and radiofrequency treatment of deep brain lesions. Neurosurgery 2:217–222
2. Moran CJ, Naidich TP, Gado MH, Marchosky JA (1979) Central nervous lesions biopsied or treated by CT-guided needle placement. Radiology 131:681–686
3. Matsumoto K, Hondo H (1984) CT-guided stereotaxic evacuation of hypertensive intracerebral hematomas. J Neurosurg 61:440–448
4. Haaga JR, Alfidi RJ (1976) Precise biopsy localization by computed tomography. Radiology 118:603
5. Katada K, Anno H, Koga S, et al (1993) Initial trial with CT fluoroscopy (abstract). Radiology 190:662

Nuclear medicine

Quantitative mean transit-time distribution pattern of brain tissue using nondiffusible tracers

P. Lindner, O. Nickel

Department of Radiology and Nuclear Medicine, Municipal Hospital, Weinberg 1, D-31134 Hildesheim, Germany

Abstract. Positron emission tomography (PET) measurements have shown that the mean transit time (MTT) of cerebral tissue, or the ratio of cerebral blood volume to cerebral blood flow (CBV/CBF), is a very good parameter for characterising cerebral perfusion and function. The MTT takes into account the effects of vasodilation, for instance in ischaemia. The aim of this paper is to demonstrate the possibility of calculating quantitative MTT values of brain tissue with the use of a firstpass of nondiffusible tracers. Functional images of the local MTT distribution can be generated. Application and results in patients with unilateral carotid stenosis or acute infarcts are reported. Additionally, an investigation of the brain-heart relationship is possible, by combining a first-pass dynamic brainstudy with a steady-state blood pool examination of the heart to calculate the ejection fraction. The application of the method to fast CT scanners is reported.

Key words: Cerebral blood flow – Mean transit time – Dynamic computed tomography – Functional images – Carotid stenosis

Positron emission tomography – the gold standard for cerebral blood (CBF) measurement – has shown [1] that the function and metabolism of the brain depend on the oxygen extraction rate and the ratio of cerebral blood volume to cerebral blood flow (BBV/CBF). This ratio is a tissue mean transit time (MTT). These results showed that CBF and CBV can vary simultaneously, for instance when there is vasodilatation in ischaemic areas. Tissue MTTs of nondiffusible tracers (blood is also, in normal cases, a nondiffusible liquid) are well suited to quantitative characterisation of the behaviour of brain tissue perfusion.

Materials and methods

In fact, there is a theory on MTTs that is as valuable for diffusible as for nondiffusible tracers. In the theory of Meier and Zierler [2], the MTT is the ratio of the distribution volume (V) of the tracer in the volume of measurement to the blood flow (f-blood together with tracer) through the volume of measurement.

$$\text{MTT} = V/f = \text{CBV/CBF}$$

In the case of diffusible tracers (xenon, etc.), the distribution volume is the whole brain tissue, including the volume of the vessels. In the case of nondiffusible tracers (technetium pertechnetate or X-ray contrast media), the distribution volume is the volume of blood (together with nondiffusible tracer) only.

In consequence, Meier and Zierler developed the famous "height over area" formula for CBF:

CBF	=	height/area × lambda × 100
CBF/CBV	=	1/MTT = height/area
CBV	=	lambda × 100
Height	=	Amount of tracer in the volume of measurement ("peak of time-tracer curve")
Area	=	Area of externally measured time-tracer curve
lambda	=	Partition coefficient; the ratio of distribution volume to weight of distribution volume

The lambda value is 1 ml/g for diffusible tracers and approximately 0.05 ml/g for nondiffusible tracers.

When nondiffusible tracers (such as radionuclide or contrast media) are given by injection into the cubital vein, approximations are necessary to take account of the problems of bolus dispersion and recirculation during the firstpass of the tracer. We have shown the following, the approximations to be valid [3, 4].

$$\text{Height} = \frac{1}{(t_m - t_0)} \int_{t_0}^{t_m} Q(t)\,dt \times C_k$$

$$\text{Area} = \int_{t_0}^{t_m} (Q(t) - U(t))\,dt$$

were: t_0 = beginning, t_m = maximumtime of, t_g = end of first pass $Q(t)$; $U(t)$ = recirculation correction; Ck = 2,3 dispersion correction factor.

Consequently:

MTT = area/height, and calculation of the MTT is possible by measurement of height and area from timetracer curves.

Using these approximations, CBF values from normal volunteers, and patients were established, and a computer programme was developed which allows us to calculate functional images of the mean transit times of regional distribution of tissue.

Clinical investigations, results and discussion

With the use of a gamma/camera, a fast CT scanner with rotating detection system, or a digital subtraction angiography (DSA) apparatus, the following investigations have been made. For the radionuclide studies, a bolus injection of 18–20 mCi technetium pertechnetate in 2 ml saline is rapidly injected and immediately followed by a flush of 20 ml saline. A serial scintigram of three frames/s is generated over a detection time of 1 min. X-ray studies by fast CT scanners, or by DSA techniques are made with a bolus injection of 30–40 ml contrast-medium, also followed by a flush of 20 ml saline.

Correspondence to: P. Lindner

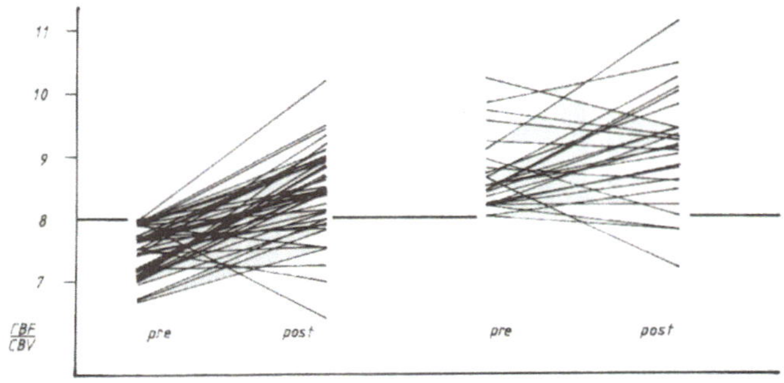

Fig. 1. Ratio of cerebral blood flow to cerebral blood volume (CBF/CBV) before and after carotid surgery

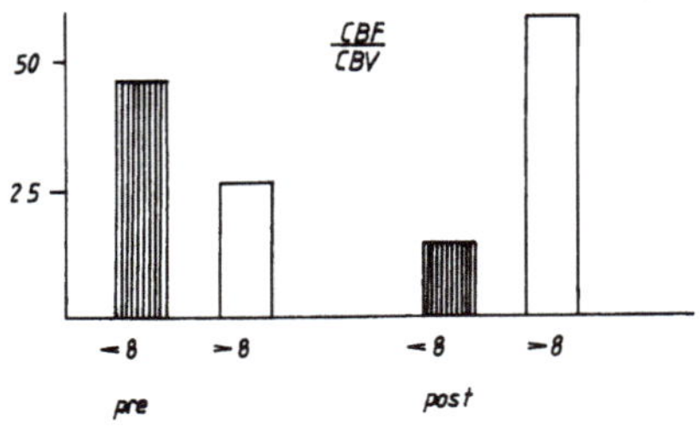

Fig. 2. Success of carotid surgery. CBF/CBV values greater than 8 correspond to normal or short MTT values, and CBF/CBV values smaller than 8, to increased MTT values (more than 7.5 s)

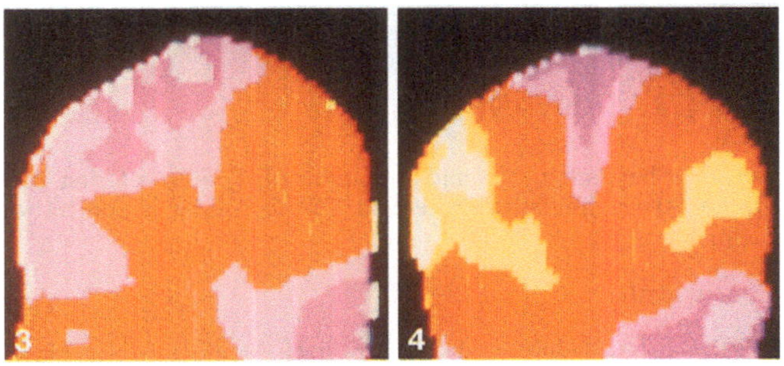

Fig. 3. Patient with high-grade carotid stenosis on left side with reduced CBF in left hemisphere

Fig. 4. Same patient as in Fig. 3, after surgery. Normal, high CBF distribution in both hemispheres

A DSA is made with three frames/s over a detection time of about 40 s.

A computer program computes quantitative blood flow values over selected regions of interest (both hemispheres) and generates parametric images, which show the of regional distribution of tissue MTTS.

Patients with proven carotid stenosis

Investigations and results from 37 patients with angiographically proven carotid stenosis before and after carotid surgery (10 days after surgery) are shown in Figs. 1 and 2.

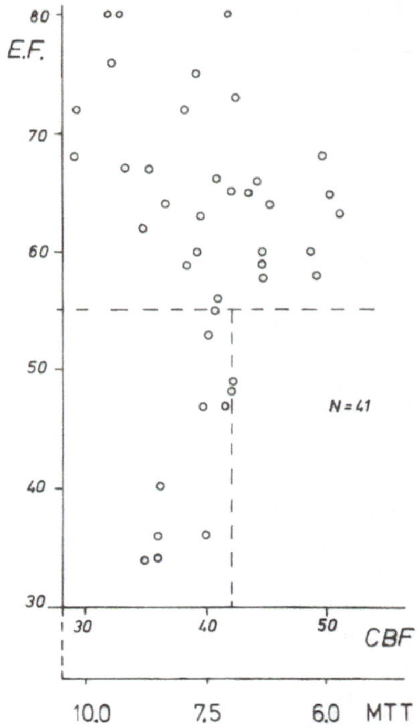

Fig. 5. Results of combined investigation of CBF (first-pass study) and ejection fraction of the heart (MUGA study)

Functional images (MTT distribution) from patient before and after carotid surgery (left side) are shown in Figs. 3 and 4.

Discussion. The haemodynamic relevance of stenosis for cerebral tissue blood flow can be quantitatively evaluated. The capacity of collaterals and function of the circulus arteriosus Willisi can be estimated. Decrease of CBF in both hemispheres can be calculated. Follow-up of carotid stenosis is possible. Increased MTT values before surgery decrease to normal MTT values after surgery in 90% of patients.

Brain-heart relationship

The method allows nearly simultaneous measurement of CBF and the ejection fraction (EF) of the heart.

After a bolus first-pass study for evaluation of MTT, the investigation of heart function is possible with the same injection, by means of a MUGA heart study in the steady state. The EF is calculated.

The results in 42 patients are shown in Fig. 5.

Discussion. Simultaneous registration of CBF and EF can help to decide whether a decreased heart function (EF less than 50%) is accompanied by an increased MRR or not. Normally, an EF of less than 50% also causes a decreased CBF (less than 40–42 ml/min per 100 g). A normal CBF (more than 42 ml/min per 100 g) is mostly associated with a normal EF (EF more than 50%). In patients with decreased CBF (less than 40 ml/min per 100 g) and normal EF (more than 50%), vascular reasons for the decrease of CBF, for instance carotid stenosis, are assumed. Combined investigation of CBF and EF (brain-heart relationship) can help to select high-risk patients for surgery. The influence of drugs on the brain-heart relationship can be investigated.

We also applied this method on a fast CT scanner. After a bolus injection of 30 ml contrast medium into the aortic arch, the dynamic sequence of 3 images/s was established and a digital-subtraction CT sequence was performed. In this way we obtained similar data to those yielded by the nuclear medicine technique and were able to apply region-of-interest techniques. Preliminary results are reported.

The application of nondiffusible tracers (during time of first pass) is more sensitive to changes of blood flow and blood volume than the use of diffusible tracers such as xenon, because the distribution volume of the nondiffusible tracer is the blood volume itself. The accuracy of the method is 5–10% for the nuclear medicine technique. The sensitivity seems to be very high. The method is in expensive and quick (acquisition time 1 min) and gives reliable results.

References

1. Gibbs J, Wise R, Leenders K, Jones T (1983) The relationship of regional cerebral blood flow, blood volume and oxygen metabolism in patients with carotid occlusion: evaluation of perfusion reserve. J Cereb Blood Flow Metab 3 (Suppl 1]:S590–S591
2. Meier P, Zierler KL (1954) On the theory of the indicator-dilution method for measurement of blood flow and volume. J Appl Physiol 6:731–743
3. Lindner P, Wolf F, Schad N (1980) Assessment of regional blood flow by intravenous injection of 99 mm technetium pertechnetate. Eur J Nucl Med 5:229–235
4. Lindner P (1983) Quantitative, noninvasive cerebral blood flow measurements with nondiffusible tracers using a heart-rate-dependent recirculation correction: application in carotid surgery. Eur J Nucl Med

Cerebral blood flow studies with xenon CT and PET before and after acetazolamide

B. Haubitz[1], T. Koch[1], H. E. Heissler[2], W. Burchert[3], E. Rickels[2], K. Holl[4], H. Becker[1]

[1] Department of Neuroradiology, Medical School, Hanover, Germany
[2] Department of Neurosurgery, Medical School, Hanover, Germany
[3] Department of Nuclear Medicine, Medical School, Hanover, Germany
[4] Neurosurgical Department, Landesnervenklinik, Linz, Austria

Abstract. Stable xenon computed tomography and positron emission tomography were used to measure cerebral blood flow in the same 22 patients suffering from cerebrovascular diseases. Using a special regression analysis [model equation $y = ax$; least median square approximation (LMS)] of hemisphere blood flow and the blood flow in the area of the middle cerebral artery, a correlation of cerebral blood flow values could be determined. These findings indicate the reliability of both cerebral blood flow measurement methods for investigation of clinical problems.

Key words: Stable xenon computed tomography – Positron emission tomography – Cerebral blood flow

---

Different methods have been used for the measurement of cerebral blood flow and cerebral reserve capacity. Stable xenon computed tomography (CT) and positron emission tomography (PET) measurements of cerebral blood flow are both based on the Kety-Schmidt equation [1]. Nevertheless, there are no studies using both methods for the measurement of local cerebral blood flow in the same patients.

Correspondence to: B. Haubitz, Abteilung Neuroradiologie, Medizinische Hochschule, D-30625 Hannover, Germany

Patients and methods

A comparative study was performed in the same patients, using stable xenon CT and PET. Flow maps were generated before and after i.v. injection of 1 g acetazolamide [2] 10 min after baseline images. We studied 22 patients (16 men/6 women) suffering from cerebrovascular disease (2 unilateral carotid stenose, 6 bilateral carotid stenoses, 8 combinations of carotid occlusion and stenosis, 2 unilateral carotid occlusions, 1 bilateral carotid occlusion, and 3 stenoses of the middle cerebral artery). A xenon blood flow system was used, with an inhalation time of 4.5 min and a 33% xenon/67% O_2 mixture. Two baseline images and six enhanced images with a slice thickness of 1 cm were generated. For PET (axial solution 5 mm (full width half mean), field of view 10.8 × 45 cm, a bolus injection of 3.7 GBq (^{15}O) H_2O, 10 ml in 8–10 s was used. The PET slice was reconstructed according to the direction of the corresponding slice of the stable xenon CT investigation.

Results

Figure 1 gives an example of corresponding flow maps generated with stable xenon CT and PET. Using the model equation y = ax and the least median square approxi-

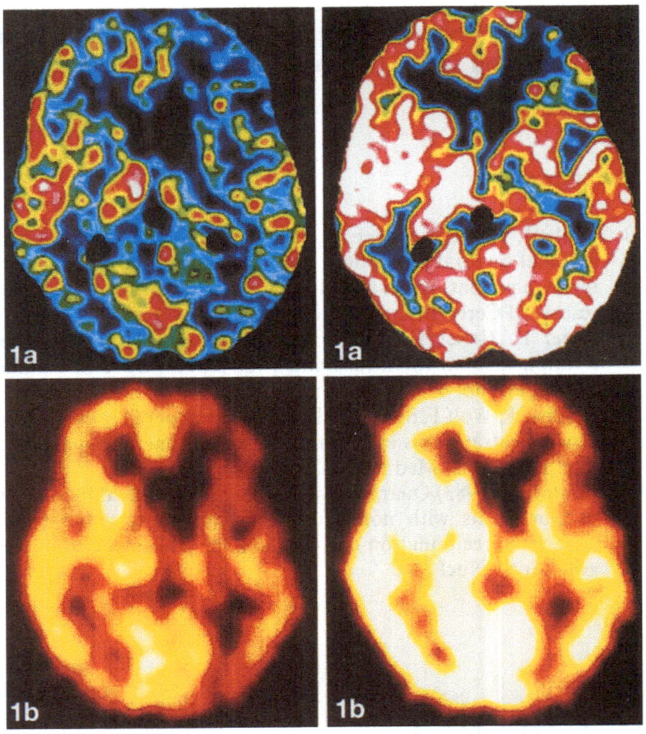

Fig. 1 a, b. A 58-year-old man suffering from bilateral carotid stenosis (more severe on the left side). **a** Stable xenon computed tomography: *left,* baseline value; *right,* stimulated image. **b** Positron emission tomography before (*left*) and after (*right*) stimulation with 1 g acetazolamide

mation (LMS) [3], a good correlation of cerebral blood flow values measured with the two methods could be demonstrated, in baseline studies of the hemisphere values and of the values in the middle cerebral artery area (Fig. 2). A similar correlation could be shown in blood flow values after stimulation. The statistical procedure identifies outlier values, which were differently included in the calculation, leading to a robust regression.

Discussion

This optimal statistical comparison of two methods for cerbral blood flow measurement demonstrates the reliability of stable xenon CT and of PET analyses.

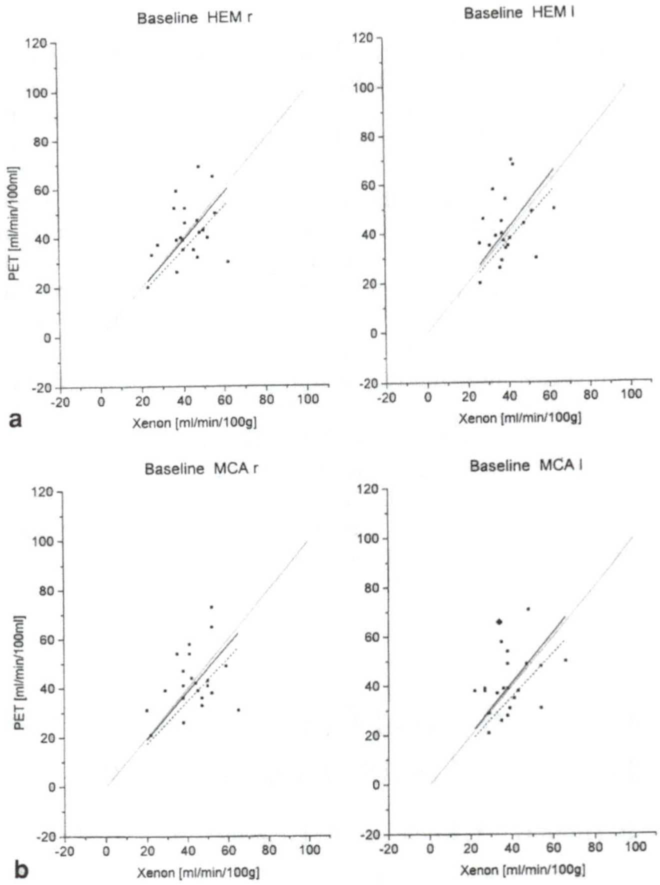

Fig. 2 a, b. Regression analysis. **a** Baseline hemisphere blood flow, **b** baseline blood flow in the area of the middle cerebral artery. *Ordinate, PET* (ml/min, per 100 ml); *abscissa,* stable xenon CT (ml/100 g brain tissue per min); ***quadrate points,*** individual pairs of measured cerebral blood flow values; ***rhomb points,*** classified as outliers; ***thin solid line,*** ideal line $y = x$; thick solid line, standard regression (least square); *dotted line,* robust regression (least median square)

References

1. Kety SS, Schmidt CF (1948) The nitrous oxide method for the quantitative determination of cerebral blood flow in man: theory, procedure and normal values. J Clin Invest 27:478–483
2. Vorstrup S, Henriksen L, Paulson OB (1984) Effect of acetazolamide on cerebral blood flow and cerebral metabolic rate for oxygen. J Clin Invest 74:1634–1639
3. Dallal GE, Rousseeuw PJ (1992) LMSMVE: A programme for least median of squares regression and robust distances. Comput Biol Med 25:384–391

^{99m}Tc-HMPAO single-photon emission tomography in the standing position in cerebral infarction

N. Tsuda, K. Negoro, M. Morimatsu

Department of Neurology, Yamaguchi University School of Medicine, Yamaguchi, Japan

Abstract. Consecutive ^{99m}Tc-HMPAO studies were performed before and after standing, to the cerebral flow perfusion of the cerebral infarction and normal control. In normal subjects, standing stress decreased the blood flow of the superior frontal, the parietal and the inferior frontal lobes significantly. Standing stress did not decrease the blood flow of the superior frontal lobe and temporal lobe in lacunar infarct patients. The blood flow between standing and supine positions changed significantly around the cerebral infarct in a patient with middle cerebral artery occlusion.

Key words: Sing-photon emission tomography - Cerebral infarction - Standing stress

Materials and methods

We studied five patients with cerebral infarcts (4 cases of lacunar infarction, 1 of middle cerebral artery (MCA) occlusion) and six normal controls, using ^{99m}Tc-HMPAO single-photon emission tomography (SPECT). After inserting a needle into the vein, the patient lay on a bed in a quiet room for 15 min. Then the patient was instructed to move from the supine to the standing position in about 5 min. The patient was injected with 288 MBq of ^{99m}Tc-HMPAO in a bolus. The patient remained standing for 5 min after the injection, and first SPECT scan then started. After that, the patient was injected with another 432 MBq of ^{99m}Tc-HMPAO in a bolus, while the patient remained on the SPECT bed. The second SPECT scan then started. The investigation was carried out using a rotatory digital gamma camera. After reconstruction, the tomographic images in the first step were subtracted from the images in the second step to obtain those during standing. Regions of interest (ROI) were drawn on the cerebellar hemispheres, cortical regions (superior frontal, temporal, inferior frontal, parietal and occipital), and basal ganglia bilaterally. The RI count index was expressed as a ratio of activity in each ROI to mean counting rate over cerebellar region. Then the percentage activity change of each ROI during standing was calculated as follows: 100(Rxs/Rcs)/(Rxr/Rcr), where Rxs/Rcs and Rxr/Rcr are the relative activity ratio of each ROI count (Rx) to the cerebellum (Rc) at standing (s) and at rest (r).

Results

Normal control

The ratios between standing and supine positions changed significantly in the superior frontal, the parietal and the inferior frontal lobes (Fig. 1).

Cerebral infarcts

Lacunar infarcts. Standing stress did not decrease the blood flow of the superior frontal lobe and temporal lobe in patients with lacunar infarcts (Fig. 2).

MCA occlusion. The blood flow between standing and supine positions changes significantly around the cerebral infarct.

Discussion

In normal subjects, the blood flow of the superior frontal, the parietal and the inferior frontal lobes decreased after standing. The local cerebral blood flow in the brain stem revealed a tendency to increase in the hypotensive state in rats [1]. The results suggest that the blood flows preferentially to the vertebrobasilar artery rather than to the carotid artery when the cerebral blood flow decreases in

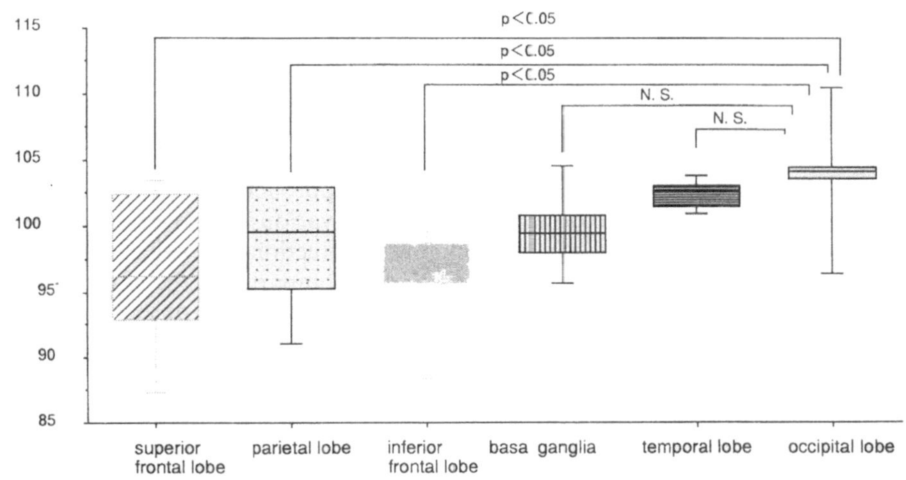

Fig. 1. The ratios in standing and supine positions changed significantly in the superior frontal, parietal and inferior frontal lobes in normal controls

Correspondence to: N. Tsuda

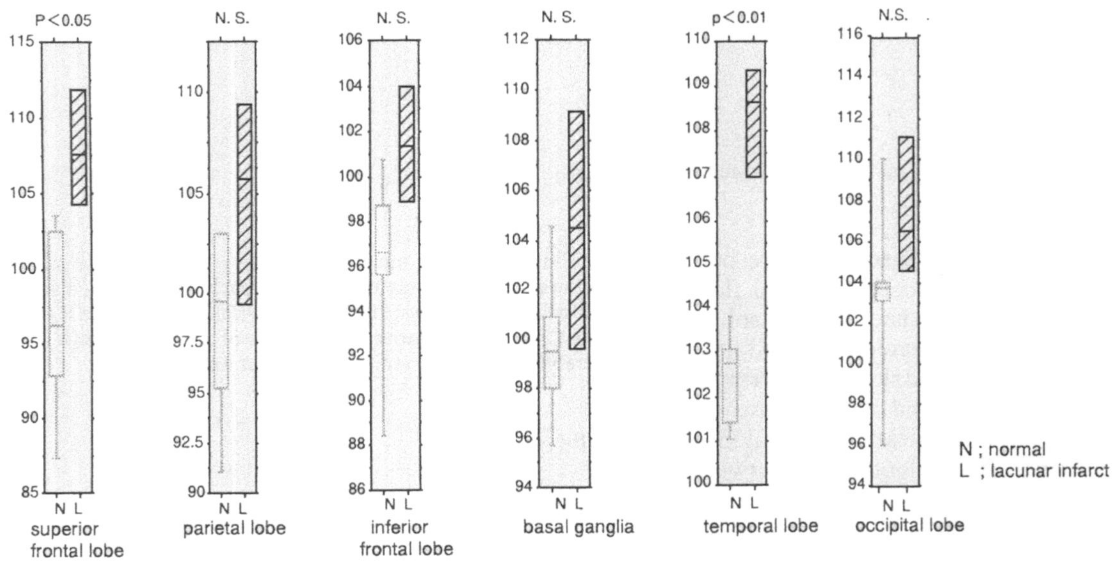

Fig. 2. Standing stress did not decrease the blood flow to the superior frontal and temporal lobes in patients with lacunar infarcts

the standing position. On the other hand, standing stress did not decrease the blood flow of the superior frontal lobe or the temporal lobe in patients with lacunar infarcts. The reason is unknown, but dysfunction of the vertebrobasilar artery may occur in patients with lacunar infarcts. Standing SPECT suggests postural cerebral hypoperfusion, possibly related to silent cerebral ischaemia, as in Hayashida et al. [2, 3].

References

1. Niwa K, Shinohara Y, Takizawa S, Takagi S (1993) Regional differences in autoregulation of cerebral blood flow. Study using hypotensive rats by exsanguination in the awake state. Jpn J Stroke 303–309
2. Hayashida K, Hirose Y, Kaminaga T, Ishida Y, Imakita S, Takamiya M, Yokota I, Nishimura T (1993) Detection of postural cerebral hypoperfusion with technetium-99m-HMPAO brain SPECT in patients with cerebrovascular disease. J Nucl Med 34:1931–1935
3. Hayashida K, Nishimura T, Uehara T, Kaminaga T, Hirose Y (1992) Raise up 99mTc-HMPAO brain SPECT for detecting the change in cerebral perfusion pressure. Nippon Acta Radiol 52:1036–1038

An error in cerebral blood flow measured by ^{123}I-IMP single-photon emission tomography and a microsphere model

S. Ohta[1], Y. Kumon[1], S. Sakaki[1], K. Murase[2], S. Tanada[2], K. Hamamoto[2]

[1] Department of Neuroradiological Surgery, Ehime University School of Medicine, Shigenobu-cho, Onsen-gun, Ehime, 791-02, Japan
[2] Department of Radiology, Ehime University School of Medicine, Shigenobu-cho, Onsen-gun, Ehime, 791-02, Japan

Abstract. We studied errors arising from back flow from brain to blood and blood-borne radioactivity of ^{123}I-iodamphetamine (^{123}I-IMP), both of which are neglected in the microsphere model. We used an analytical approach to compare cerebral blood flow (F), calculated at various-study times by microsphere analysis, and the unidirectional clearance from blood to brain (K_1) using two-compartment analysis, including parameters representing these assumptions explicitly. The values of back flow (k_2) and initial distribution volume (V_0) were very small, and did not seem to influence the estimation of F in the microsphere model. However, regression analysis between each F and K_1 revealed that F at 5 min was overrestimated because blood-borne radioactivity was neglected, while F at 53 min was underrestimated owing to the effect of k_2. The highest correlation of F with K_1 was observed at 13 min. We should be aware of regional overestimation on earlier images due to the blood-borne radioactivity, and underestimation on later images due to the back flow when analysing cerebral blood flow by ^{123}I-IMP single photon emission tomography (SPECT) and the microsphere model.

Correspondence to: S. Ohta

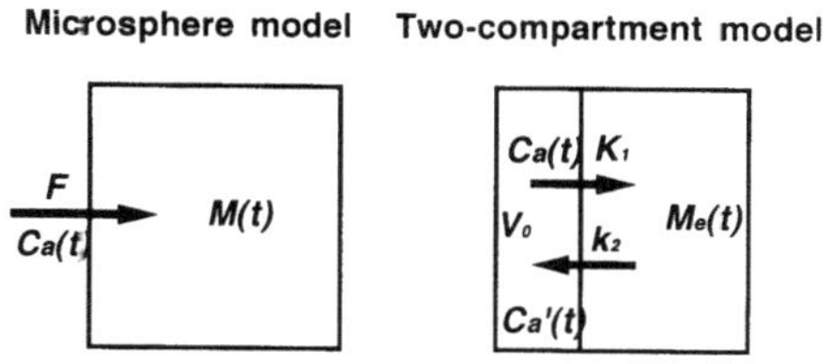

Fig. 1. Diagrams of microsphere model and two-compartment model

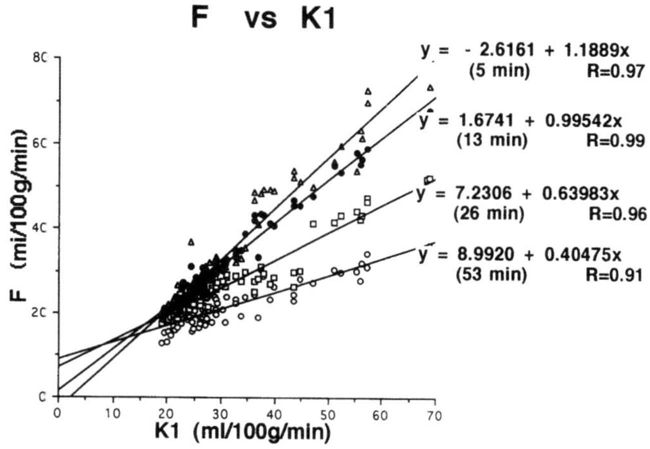

Fig. 2. Relationship between F at various study times in the microsphere model and K_1 in the two-compartment model, calculated using whole SPECT data. The highest correlation of F with K_1 was observed after 13 min

Key words: ^{123}I-Iodoamphetamine (^{123}I-IMP) – Single photon emission tomography – Cerebral blood flow – Microsphere model

---

Cerebral blood flow (CBF) measurement by SPECT using ^{123}I-iodoamphetamine (^{123}I-IMP) and the microsphere model requires the assumption that back flow of ^{123}I-IMP from brain to blood (k_2) and blood-borne radioactivity are negligible 1]. We examined the validity of these assumptions by comparing F (CBF) using microsphere analysis with unidirectional clearance (K_1) from blood to brain by two-compartment analysis, including parameters representing these assumptions explicitly.

Model configuration (Fig. 1)

Microsphere model. When delivery and entrance of the tracer to the brain depends only on blood flow and the tracer is trapped in the brain for a long time, whole brain tissue has only one compartment, which is characterised by the microsphere model;

$$\frac{dM(t)}{dt} = FCa(t)$$

where $M(t)$ is the total radioactivity of the brain measured by SPECT and $Ca(t)$ the radioactivity of the lipophilic

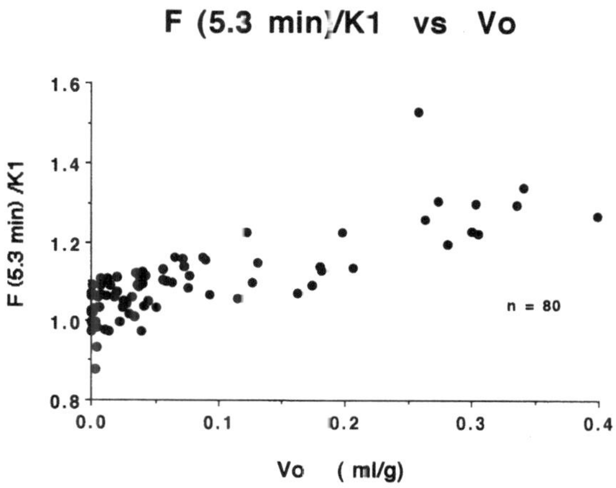

Fig. 3. Relationship between the ratio of F to K_1 and V_0 after 5.3 min. Overestimation of F increased as V_0 increased

^{123}I-IMP in the arterial blood, which can pass the blood-brain barrier.

Two-compartment model. When a barrier is assumed to exist between the vascular components and the brain parenchyma, the two compartment model, including three parameters, is characterised as follows:

$$\frac{dMe(t)}{dt} = K_1Ca(t) - k_2Me(t)$$

$$M(t) = Me(t) + V_0\{Ca(t)' + Ca(t)\}$$

where $M(t)$ is the total radioactivity in the brain measurable by SPECT, $Me(t)$ the radioactivity in the extravascular space, and $Ca(t)$ and $Ca(t)'$ the lipophilic and hydrophilic tracers in the arterial blood, respectively. K_1 is the initial clearance from blood to brain parenchyma related to blood flow, k_2 the back flow from brain to blood, and V_0 the initial distrubution volume occupied by the lipophilic and hydrophilic tracers not extracted and passing through the vascular space.

Method

We performed dynamic ^{123}I-IMP SPECT studies in eight patients. We injected 6 mCi ^{123}I-IMP intravenously and 20 dynamic scans with frame durations of 160 s were obtained. Arterial radioactivities extracted and not extracted by octanol were used as $Ca(t)$ and $Ca(t)'$, respectively. We calculated F using data obtained after 5, 13, 26 and 53 min according to the microsphere model. K_1, k_2 and V_0 were calculated using whole dynamic data and the two-compartment model by the time-weighted integration method [2].

Results

The values of K_1, k_2 and V_0, calculated using whole SPECT data according to the two-compartment model, were 0.25 ± 0.08 (mean ± SD ml g^{-1} min^{-1}), 0.0083 ± 0.0037 (min^{-1}) and 0.029 ± 0.025 (ml g^{-1}). However, regression analysis revealed that F after 5 min was overestimated compared with K_1, while F after 53 min was underestimated, and the highest correlation of F with K_1 was observed

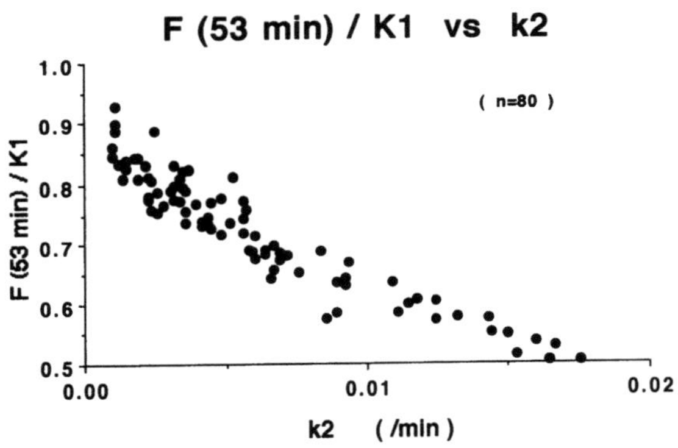

Fig. 4. Relationship between the ratio of F to K_1 and k_2 after 53 min. Underestimation of F increased as k_2 increased

after 13 min (Fig. 2). Figure 3 shows that overestimation of regional F after 5.3 min increased more than K_1 when the regional V_0 was larger. Figure 4 shows that the underestimation of regional F after 53 min became more pronounced as the regional k_2 increased.

Discussion

The values of back flow (k_2 and V_0) seemed to be small enough to be negligible in the estimation of F based on the microsphere model. However, the values of F in the microsphere model varied with the measuring time of SPECT. The estimation of F in the early and late periods was sensitive to blood-borne radioactivity and back flow of the tracer from brain to blood. It is concluded that we should be aware of overestimation caused by blood-borne radioactivity in the earlier images of ^{123}I-IMP SPECT, and of underestimation, caused by back flow of ^{123}I-IMP from brain to blood in the later images as seen in the microsphere model.

References

1. Kuhl DE, Barrio JR, Huang SC (1982) Quantifying local cerebral blood flow by N-isopropyl-p-[^{123}I] iodoamphetamine (IMP) tomography. J Nucl Med 23:196–203
2. Ohta S, Meyer E, Thompson CJ, Gledde A (1992) Oxygen consumption of the living human brain, measured after a single inhalation of positron-emitting oxygen. J Cereb Blood Flow Metab 12:179–192

Discrepancies in regional cerebral blood flow measured by ^{133}Xe single photon emission tomography and stable Xe CT methods

M. Matusuda[1], H. Lee[1], K. Kuribayashi[1], J. Handa[1], H. Ohnishi[2], K. Masuda[2]

[1] Department of Neurosurgery, Shiga University of Medical Science, Seta, Ohtsu, Shiga 520-21, Japan
[2] Radiology Service, Shiga University of Medical Science, Seta Ohtsu, Shiga 520-21, Japan

Abstract. Single photon (Xe SPECT) and stable xenon-enhanced computed tomography (Xe CT) were performed in 50 patients with chronic cerebrovascular disease. The regional cerebral blood flow (rCBF) values at the level 5 cm above the orbitomeatal line on the normal side were compared and correlated between the two methods. Xe SPECT recorded significantly higher values in the anterior cerebral artery territory than Xe Ct, without correlation. In the middle cerebral artery territory, Xe CT showed significantly higher values than Xe SPECT, with good correlation. Basal ganglia showed higher values in Xe CT than in Xe SPECT, with some correlation. Closely approximate values were measured in the posterior cerebral artery territory, without correlation. Both methods gave closely approximate and well-correlated values in hemispheric CBF. The discrepancies of rCBF values between the two methods are discussed.

Key words: Single photon emission tomography – Computed tomography – Xenon inhalation – Regional cerebral blood flow

Correspondence to: M. Matusuda

Stable xenon-enhanced computed tomography (Xe CT) and single photon emission computed tomography with ^{133}xenon inhalation (Xe SPECT) are now widely used as a means of regional cerebral blood flow (rCBF) measurement. We determined the correlation of rCBF values measured by Xe SPECT and Xe CT in the same patients.

Methods

We studied 50 patients, neurologically stable in the chronic stage of a unilateral hemisphere lesion due to a cerebral infarct or subarachnoid haemorrhage, by Xe SPECT and Xe CT with an interval of 2–5 days. There were 27 men and 23 women, average age 53.9 ± 15.9 years (range 20–83 years).

Xe SPECT was performed using 4 NaI scintillation cameras rotating around the subject's head. Data acquisition started 60 s before ^{133}Xe inhalation. The patient inhaled ^{133}Xe gas (650 MBq/l in air) for 80 s. Data acquisition continued for a further 180 s in the washout phase. The rCBF values were calculated according to the method described by Kanno and Lassen [1] and Celsis et al. [2]. No correction for attenuation was made and the slice thickness was 12 mm. The Xe CT study was performed as follows: After two baseline scans, the patient started to inhale a mixture of gas (30% Xe, 30–50% O_2 and air) and underwent scans every 30 s for a 5-min inhalation period. The slice thickness was 8 mm.

Table 1. Regional cerebral blood flow[a] measured by Xe SPECT and Xe CT in the same patients[b]

	Territory				
	Anterior cerebral	Middle cerebral	Posterior cerebral	Basal ganglia	Cerebral hemisphere
Xe SPECT	45.5 ± 9.8	42.6 ± 9.8	42.5 ± 8.6	46.7 ± 10.0	42.7 ± 8.8
Xe CT	41.9 ± 11.2*	46.9 ± 11.6***	41.9 ± 10.2	52.1 ± 14.7**	44.3 ± 9.5

[a] mean ± SD ml/100 g per min
[b] $n = 50$ (except for HS, $n = 32$)
* $P < 0.05$; ** $P < 0.005$; *** $P < 0.001$

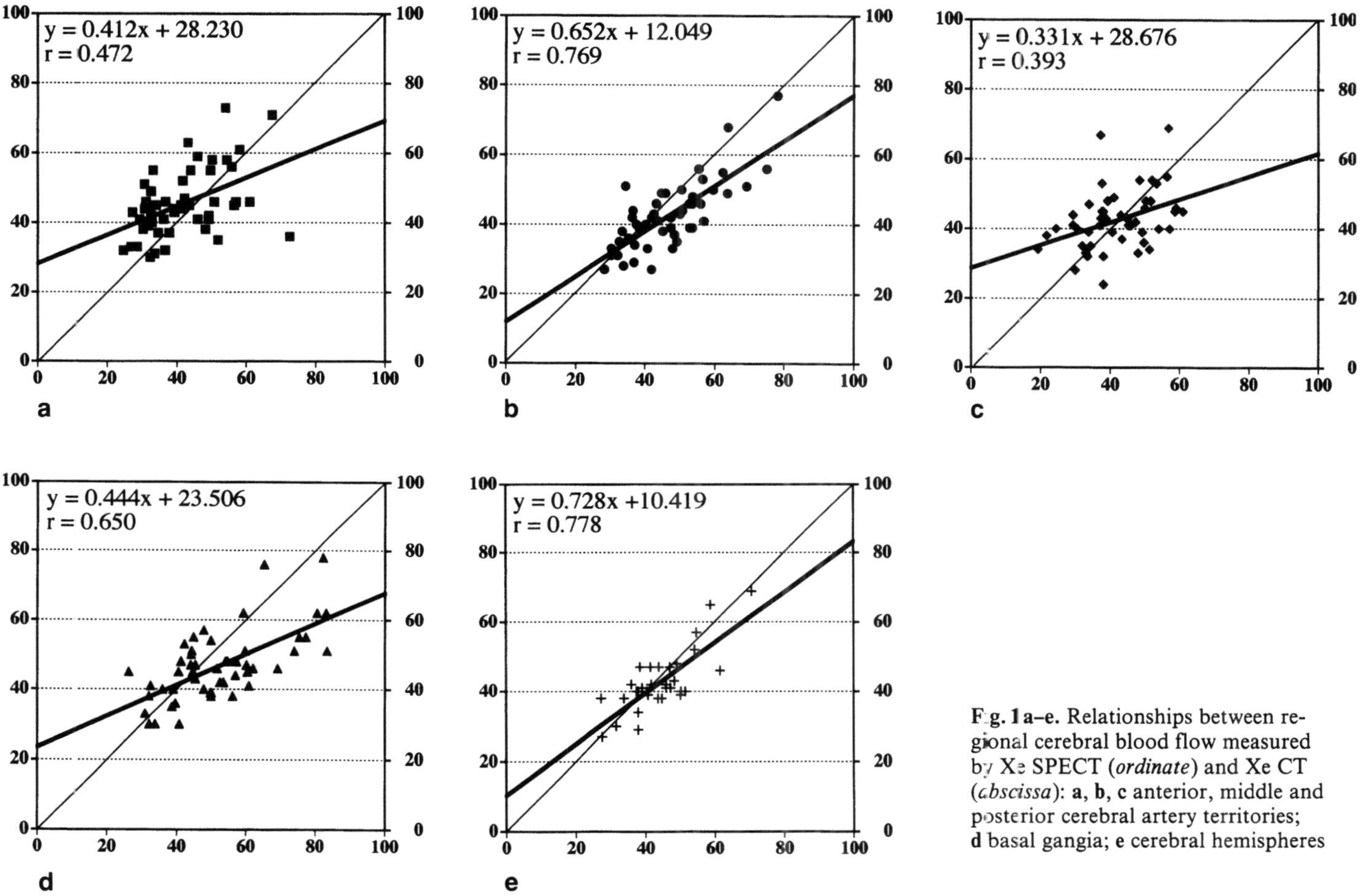

Fig. 1 a–e. Relationships between regional cerebral blood flow measured by Xe SPECT (*ordinate*) and Xe CT (*abscissa*): **a**, **b**, **c** anterior, middle and posterior cerebral artery territories; **d** basal gangia; **e** cerebral hemispheres

Regions of interest (ROI) were drawn at 5 cm above the orbitomeatal line, according to the vacular territories of the anterior cerebral artery (ACA), the middle cerebral artery (MCA) and the posterior cerebral artery (PCA), and the anatomical boundary of the basal ganglia (BG) and the cerebral hemisphere (HS). The rCBF in the HS was not measured in the first 18 patients. The rCBF values were compared and correlated between Xe SPECT and Xe CT in the corresponding ROIs on the intact side. A paired *t*-test was used for statistical analysis. A *P* value of < 0.05 was considered significant. Correlation was tested with linear regression analysis.

Results

The mean systemic blood pressure was not different between Xe SPECT and Xe CT: 94.9 ± 11.1 and 94.8 ± 18.9 mmHg, respectively. The rCBF values are shown in Table 1, and the relationship between the corresponding values in Fig. 1. In the ACA, Xe SPECT yielded a significantly higher value than Xe CT (8.6%), and no correlation was found between the values given by the different methods. In the MCA and the BG, Xe CT recorded 10.1% and 11.6%, respectively, significantly higher value than Xe SPECT. There was good correlation for the MCA, and fairly good for the BG. Closely approximate values were obtained by either method in the

PCA and the HS. Good correlation was obtained for the HS, but not for the PCA.

Discussion

The rCBF in the ACA measured significantly higher (8.6%) by Xe SPECT than by XE CT, and there was no correlation between the results of the different methods. In 8 cases, Xe SPECT gave more than 40% higher values than Xe CT. Hyperfrontal distribution [3], which had been reported in the two-dimensional ^{133}Xe method and later regarded as an artefact due to gamma rays scattering from the nasopharyngeal airway [4], was still observed by our SPECT study [5]. Correlation between the two methods was good in the MCA, although Xe CT yielded a significantly 10.1% higher value than Xe SPECT. This difference between the values cannot be explained. In the BG, the rCBF measured by Xe SPECT was 11.6% significantly lower than by Xe CT. The lower rCBF by Xe SPECT could be attributable to attenuation of radioactivity from deep structures before reaching the detectors. Only HS showed well-correlated, closely similar values between the two methods. Since quantification by Xe SPECT is reported to be valid for ROI 3 cm or larger in diameter and composed predominantly of grey matter [6], the larger the ROI are, the more reliable the rCBF values. Good correlation is reported between the two-dimensional ^{133}Xe method and Xe CT in the global CBF [7].

Although we measured rCBF on the apparently normal side, the values obtained are not necessarily those that would be found in a normal brain. Some discrepancies in the rCBF values is inevitable between the two methods, since the corresponding ROI cannot be the same. In our preliminary study, discrepancies in the rCBF between the two methods were larger when ischaemic lesions were included in the ROI. It is said that owing to Compton scatter, true rCBF cannot be measured by Xe SPECT in ischaemic lesions [8]. We should be aware of these discrepancies between and characteristics of the method used.

References

1. Kanno I, Lassen NA (1979) Two methods for calculating regional cerebral blood flow from emission computed tomography of inert gas concentrations. J Comput Assist Tomogr 3:71–76
2. Celsis P, Goldman T, Henriksen L, Lassen NA (1981) A method for calculating regional cerebral blood flow from emission computed tomography of inert gas concentrations. J Comput Assist Tomogr 5:641–645
3. Ingvar DH (1975) Patterns of brain activity revealed by measurements of regional cerebral blood flow. In: Ingvar DH, Lassen NA (eds) Brain work. The coupling of function, metabolism and blood flow in the brain. Munksgaard, Copenhagen, pp 397–413
4. Devous MD Sr, Stokely EM, Chehabi HH, Bonte FJ (1986) Normal distribution of regional cerebral blood flow measured by dynamic single-photon emission tomography. J Cereb Blood Flow Metab 6:95–104
5. Matsuda M, Lee H, Shiino A, Handa J (1992) A few comments on the evaluation of rCBF by means of ^{133}Xe SPECT (in Japanese with English abstract). CI Kenkyu 14:465–473
6. Rezai K, Kirchner PT, Armstrong C, Ehrhard JC, Heistad D (1988) Validation studies for brain blood flow assessment by radioxenon tomography. J Nucl Med 29:348–355
7. Stringer WA, Marion DW, Bouma GJ, Muizelaar JP, Braun IF, Fatouros PP, Marmarou A (1992) Correlation of xenon-133 and stable xenon-enhanced computed tomographic cerebral blood flow measurements in patients with severe head injury. In: Yonas H (ed) Cerebral blood flow measurement with stable xenon-enhanced computed tomography. Raven Press, New York, pp 233–237
8. Holm S, Vorstrup S, Lassen NA, Paulson OB (1985) Physical factors affecting calculated cerebral blood flow values in hypoperfused areas in single-photon emission computed tomography. In: Hartmann HS (ed) Cerebral blood flow and metabolism measurement. Springer, Berlin Heidelberg New York, pp 234–237

MIX
Papier aus verantwortungsvollen Quellen
Paper from responsible sources
FSC® C105338

If you have any concerns about our products,
you can contact us on
ProductSafety@springernature.com

In case Publisher is established outside the EU,
the EU authorized representative is:
Springer Nature Customer Service Center GmbH
Europaplatz 3, 69115 Heidelberg, Germany

Printed by Libri Plureos GmbH
in Hamburg, Germany